Depression in Medical Illness

Depression in Medical Illness

Edited by:

Arthur J. Barsky, MD
Vice Chair for Academic Affairs
Department of Psychiatry
Brigham and Women's Hospital
Professor of Psychiatry
Harvard Medical School
Boston, Massachusetts

David A. Silbersweig, MD
Chairman, Department of Psychiatry
Co-Director, Institute for the Neurosciences
Brigham and Women's Hospital
Stanley Cobb Professor of Psychiatry
Harvard Medical School Academic Dean (Partners HealthCare)
Harvard Medical School
Boston, Massachusetts

Associate Editor:

Robert J. Boland, MD
Vice Chair for Education
Department of Psychiatry
Brigham and Women's Hospital
Associate Professor of Psychiatry
Harvard Medical School
Boston, Massachusetts

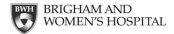

New York   Chicago   San Francisco   Athens   London   Madrid   Mexico City
Milan   New Delhi   Singapore   Sydney   Toronto

Depression in Medical Illness

1 2 3 4 5 6 7 8 9 DSS 21 20 19 18 17 16

ISBN 978-0-07-181908-4
MHID 0-07-181908-8

This book was set in Myriad Pro by Aptara, Inc.
The editors were Andrew Moyer and Christie Naglieri.
The production supervisor was Catherine Saggese.
Project Management was provided by Amit Kashyap, Aptara, Inc.
RR Donnelley was printer and binder.

This book is printed on acid-free paper.

Library of Congress Cataloging-in-Publication Data

Names: Barsky, Arthur J., editor. | Silbersweig, David A., editor.
Title: Depression in medical illness / edited by Arthur J. Barsky,
David A. Silbersweig.
Description: New York : McGraw-Hill Education, [2016]. | Includes
   bibliographical references.
Identifiers: LCCN 2016005101| ISBN 9780071819084 (hardcover : alk. paper) |
   ISBN 0071819088 (hardcover : alk. paper)
Subjects: | MESH: Depressive Disorder–diagnosis | Behavioral Medicine
Classification: LCC RC537 | NLM WM 171.5 | DDC 616.85/270651–dc23 LC record
available at http://lccn.loc.gov/2016005101

"To our patients"

CONTENTS

CONTRIBUTORS

Elizabeth Alfson, MD
Department of Psychiatry
Atrius Health
Peabody, Massachusetts

Stanley Ashley, MD
Frank Sawyer Professor of Surgery
Harvard Medical School
Brigham and Women's Hospital
Boston, Massachusetts

Geena Athappilly, MD
Clinical Director of Women's Mental Health
Brigham and Women's Hospital
Instructor in Psychiatry
Harvard Medical School
Boston, Massachusetts

Orit Avni Barron, MD
Women's Mental Health Psychiatrist
Brigham and Women's hospital
Instructor in Psychiatry
Harvard Medical School
Boston, Massachusetts

Gaston Baslet, MD
Division of Neuropsychiatry
Department of Psychiatry
Brigham and Women's Hospital
Assistant Professor of Psychiatry
Harvard Medical School
Boston, Massachusetts

Emily Benedetto, MSW, LCSW
Program Manager
Primary Care Behavioral Health Integration
Cambridge Health Alliance
Somerville, Massachusetts

Jhilam Biswas, MD
Forensic Psychiatrist
Bridgewater State Hospital
Bridgewater, Massachusetts

Robert Boland, MD
Vice Chair for Education
Department of Psychiatry
Brigham and Women's Hospital
Associate Professor of Psychiatry
Harvard Medical School
Boston, Massachusetts

Ilana Braun, MD
Chief, Division of Psychosocial Oncology
Dana Farber Cancer Institute Department of Psychiatry
Brigham and Women's Hospital
Assistant Professor of Psychiatry
Harvard Medical School
Boston, Massachusetts

Melissa Bui, MD
Clinical Fellow in Psychiatry
Brigham and Women's Hospital
Instructor in Psychiatry
Harvard Medical School
Boston, Massachusetts

James Cartreine, PhD
Research and Clinical Psychologist
Brigham and Women's Hospital
Instructor in Psychiatry
Harvard Medical School
Boston, Massachusetts

Daniela Carusi, MD, MSc
Department of Obstetrics and Gynecology
Brigham and Women's Hospital
Assistant Professor of Obstetrics and Gynecology
Harvard Medical School
Boston, Massachusetts

Hongtu Chen, PhD
Department of Psychiatry
Brigham and Women's Hospital
Assistant Professor of Psychology
Harvard Medical School
Boston, Massachusetts

Kirk Daffner, MD
Chief, Division of Cognitive and Behavioral Neurology
Director, Center for Brain/Mind Medicine
Brigham and Women's Hospital
J. David and Virginia Wimberly Professor of Neurology
Harvard Medical School
Boston, Massachusetts

David DeMaso, MD
Psychiatrist-in-Chief and Chairman of Psychiatry,
    Boston Children's Hospital
George P. Gardner & Olga E. Monks Professor of Child Psychiatry &
    Professor of Pediatrics Harvard Medical School
Boston, Massachusetts

Vivian Ecker, MD
Psychiatrist, Counseling and Mental Health Services
Harvard University
Instructor in Psychiatry
Harvard Medical School
Boston, Massachusetts

Mark Eldaief, MD, MMSc
Division of Cognitive and Behavioral Neurology
Departments of Neurology and Psychiatry
Brigham and Woman's Hospital
Center for Brain Science
Harvard University
Assistant Professor of Neurology
Harvard Medical School
Boston, Massachusetts

Jane Epstein, MD
Department of Psychiatry
Boston VA Healthcare System
Assistant Professor of Psychiatry
Harvard Medical School
Boston, Massachusetts

Jane Erb, MD
Medical Director, Brigham Depression Center
Department of Psychiatry
Brigham and Women's Hospital
Assistant Professor of Psychiatry
Harvard Medical School
Boston, Massachusetts

John Fromson, MD
Chief of Psychiatry, Brigham and Women's Faulkner Hospital
Vice Chair for Community Psychiatry
Brigham and Women's Hospital
Associate Professor of Psychiatry
Harvard Medical School
Boston, Massachusetts

Michael Gaziano, MD
Chief, Division of Aging
Department of Medicine
Brigham and Women's Hospital
Professor of Medicine
Harvard Medical School
Boston, Massachusetts

David Gitlin, MD
Vice Chair for Clinical Programs
Chief, Division of Medical Psychiatry
Brigham and Women's/Faulkner Hospitals
Assistant Professor of Psychiatry
Harvard Medical School
Boston, Massachusetts

Hilary Goldberg, MD, MPH
Division of Pulmonary Medicine
Brigham and Women's Hospital
Assistant Professor
Harvard Medical School
Boston, Massachusetts

John Grimaldi, MD
Consulting Psychiatrist, Infectious Diseases Unit
Department of Psychiatry
Brigham and Women's Hospital
Instructor in Psychiatry
Harvard Medical School
Boston, Massachusetts

Florina Haimovici, MD
Director of Reproductive Endocrinology and Infertility Psychiatry
Department of Psychiatry
Brigham and Women's Faulkner Hospital
Assistant Professor of Psychiatry
Harvard Medical School
Boston, Massachusetts

Jessica Harder, MD
Division of Neuropsychiatry
Department of Psychiatry
Brigham and Women's Hospital
Instructor in Psychiatry
Harvard Medical School
Boston, Massachusetts

Howard Hartley
Division of Cardiology
Department of Medicine
Brigham and Women's Hospital
Associate Professor of Medicine
Harvard Medical School
Boston, Massachusetts

Robert Jamison, PhD
Pain Management Center
Brigham and Women's Hospital
Professor, Departments of Anesthesia and Psychiatry
Harvard Medical School
Boston, Massachusetts

Hadine Joffe, MD, MSc
Vice Chair for Psychiatric Research
Director, Division of Women's Mental Health
Brigham and Women's Hospital
Director of Psycho-Oncology Research, Dana Farber Cancer Institute
Associate Professor of Psychiatry
Harvard Medical School
Boston, Massachusetts

Inder Kalra, MD
Attending Psychiatrist
Albert Einstein Healthcare Network
Philadelphia, Pennsylvania

Jeffrey Katz, MD, MSc
Director, Orthopedic and Arthritis Center for Outcomes Research
Brigham and Women's Hospital
Professor of Medicine and Orthopedic Surgery
Harvard Medical School
Boston, Massachusetts

Matthew Kim, MD
Clinical Director, Division of Endocrinology, Diabetes and
  Hypertension
Brigham and Women's Hospital
Instructor in Medicine
Harvard Medical School
Boston, Massachusetts

Meghan Kolodziej, MD
Instructor in Psychiatry
Brigham and Women's Hospital
Harvard Medical School
Boston, Massachusetts

Joshua Korzenik, MD
Director of Crohn's and Colitis Center
Department of Medicine
Brigham and Women's Hospital
Assistant Professor of Medicine
Harvard Medical School
Boston, Massachusetts

David Kroll, MD
Associate Psychiatrist
Department of Psychiatry
Brigham and Women's Hospital
Instructor in Psychiatry
Harvard Medical School
Boston, Massachusetts

Katy LaLone, MD
Assistant Professor of Psychiatry
Case Western Reserve University
MetroHealth Medical Center
Cleveland, Ohio

Joshua Leo, MD, MPH
Psychiatric Consultation Service
Beth Israel Deaconess Medical Center
Instructor in Psychiatry
Harvard Medical School
Boston, Massachusetts

Susan Mackie, MD
Department of Medicine
Brigham and Women's Hospital
Instructor in Medicine
Harvard Medical School
Boston, Massachusetts

Eleni Maneta, MD
Assistant in Psychiatry
Boston Children's Hospital
Instructor in Psychiatry
Harvard Medical School
Boston, Massachusetts

Lindsay Merrill, MD
Playa Vista Mental Health Psychiatric and Counseling Services
Los Angeles, California

Fremonta Meyer, MD
Department of psychosocial Oncology and Palliative Care
Dana Farber Cancer Institute
Brigham and Women's Hospital
Assistant Professor of Psychiatry
Harvard Medical School
Boston, Massachusetts

Laura Miller, MD
Medical Director of Women's Mental Health
Edward Hines Jr. VA Hospital
Professor of Psychiatry,
Loyola University Stritch School of Medicine,
Maywood, Illinois

Pamela Mirsky, MD
Medical Director, Consultation–Liaison Psychiatry
Banner University Medical Center Tucson
Assistant Professor of Psychiatry
University of Arizona College of Medicine
Tucson, Arizona

Leena Mittal, MD
Director of the Reproductive Psychiatry Consultation Service
Brigham and Women's Hospital
Instructor in Psychiatry
Harvard Medical School
Boston, Massachusetts

Laura Morrissey, MSW, LICSW
Clinical Social Worker
Center for Brain/Mind Medicine, Department of Psychiatry
Brigham and Women's Hospital
Boston, Massachusetts

Michael Mufson, MD
Department of Psychiatry
Brigham and Women's Hospital
Assistant Professor of Psychiatry
Harvard Medical School
Boston, Massachusetts

Olivia Okereke, MD, SM
Departments of Psychiatry and Medicine
Brigham and Women's Hospital
Associate Professor of Psychiatry
Harvard Medical School
Boston, Massachusetts

Megan Oser, PhD
Director, Psychology and CBT/Behavioral Medicine
Department of Psychiatry
Instructor in Psychiatry
Harvard Medical School
Boston, Massachusetts

Jaya Padmanabhan, MD
Department of Psychiatry
Beth Israel Deaconess Medical Center
Instructor in Psychiatry
Harvard Medical School
Boston, Massachusetts

Eliza Park, MD, FAPM
Assistant Professor of Psychiatry
Lineberger Comprehensive Cancer Center
University of North Carolina at Chapel Hill
Chapel Hill, North Carolina

David Perez, MD
Assistant in Neurology and Psychiatry
Massachusetts General Hospital
Instructor in Neurology
Harvard Medical School
Boston, Massachusetts

John Peteet, MD
Department of Psychosocial Oncology and Palliative Care
Dana Farber Cancer Institute Department of Psychiatry
Brigham and Women's Hospital
Associate Professor of Psychiatry
Harvard Medical School
Boston, Massachusetts

Stuart Pollack, MD
Medical Director, Advanced Primary Care Associates,
   South Huntington
Brigham and Women's Hospital
Instructor in Medicine
Harvard Medical School
Boston, Massachusetts

Shreya Raj, MD
Division of Neuropsychiatry
Department of Psychiatry
Brigham and Women's Hospital
Instructor in Psychiatry
Harvard Medical School
Boston, Massachusetts

Audra Robertson Meadows, MD
Department of Obstetrics and Gynecology
Brigham and Women's Hospital
Instructor in Obstetrics and Gynecology
Harvard Medical School
Boston, Massachusetts

Arturo Saavedra, MD, PhD, MBA
Vice Chairman for Clinical Affairs
Department of Dermatology
Massachusetts General Hospital
Associate Professor of Dermatology
Harvard Medical School
Boston, Massachusetts

Laura Safar, MD
Director, Division of Neuropsychiatry
Department of Psychiatry
Brigham and Women's Hospital
Instructor in Psychiatry
Harvard Medical School
Boston, Massachusetts

Paul Sax, MD
Clinical Director, Division of Infectious Diseases,
    Department of Medicine
Brigham and Women's Hospital
Professor of Medicine
Harvard Medical School
Boston, Massachusetts

Naomi Schmelzer, MD, MPH
Director, Emergency and Psychiatry Services
Department of Psychiatry Brigham and Women's Faulkner Hospital
Harvard Medical School
Boston, Massachusetts

Sejal Shah, MD
Assistant Director, Division of Medical Psychiatry
Department of Psychiatry
Brigham and Women's Hospital
Instructor in Psychiatry
Harvard Medical School
Boston, Massachusetts

Samata Sharma, MD, MPH
Division of Consultation Liaison Psychiatry
VA Boston Healthcare System
Instructor in Psychiatry
Harvard Medical School
Boston, Massachusetts

David Silbersweig, MD
Chairman, Department of Psychiatry
Co-Director, Institute for the Neurosciences
Brigham and Women's Hospital
Stanley Cobb Professor of Psychiatry
Harvard Medical School Academic Dean (Partners HealthCare)
Harvard Medical School
Boston, Massachusetts

Arielle Stanford, MD
Medical Director, Clinical Science at Alkermes
Boston, Massachusetts

Emily Stern, MD
Director, Functional and Molecular Neuroimaging
Director, Functional Neuroimaging Laboratory
Departments of Radiology and Psychiatry
Brigham and Women's Hospital
Associate Professor of Radiology
Harvard Medical School
Boston, Massachusetts

John Sullivan, MD
Division of Neuropsychiatry
Department of Psychiatry
Brigham and Women's Hospital
Instructor in Psychiatry
Harvard Medical School
Boston, Massachusetts

Charles Surber, MD
Instructor in Psychiatry
University of Michigan Health System
Ann Arbor, Michigan

Joji Suzuki, MD
Director, Division of Addiction Psychiatry
Brigham and Women's Hospital
Instructor in Psychiatry
Harvard Medical School
Boston, Massachusetts

Ajay Wasan
Vice Chair for Pain Medicine
Department of Anesthesia
University of Pittsburgh School of Medicine
Pittsburgh, Pennsylvania

John Winkelman, MD, PhD
Chief, Sleep Disorders Clinical Research Program
Massachusetts General Hospital
Associate Professor of Psychiatry
Harvard Medical School
Boston, Massachusetts

David Wolfe, MD, MPH
Director of Research, BWH Depression Center
Brigham and Women's Hospital
Instructor in Psychiatry
Harvard Medical School
Boston, Massachusetts

Rachel Yung, MD
Department of Medical Oncology
Dana Farber Cancer Institute
Instructor in Medicine
Harvard Medical School
Boston, Massachusetts

PREFACE

As our knowledge expands and our understanding evolves, we have come to appreciate a confluence between what were previously thought to be independent entities: depression and major medical illness. The associations between depression and medical illness are more intimate and more extensive than previously appreciated. We are beginning to see how the disease processes that overtake the body also affect the brain, and conversely how brain disorders like depression can affect medical illnesses. Depression influences the occurrence, presentation, course, and outcome of many medical illnesses, and conversely, comorbid medical illnesses can affect the onset, presentation, course, and outcome of depression. We owe this enhanced understanding to recent advances in scientific methods, to more precise clinical observation, and to greater diagnostic precision.

Thus the time is ripe for a text based on the premise that depression and medical illness are inextricably bound together and must be viewed through a single lens in order to truly understand them, diagnose them, and treat them. The organization and content of this text are based on this premise. Throughout, we emphasize not simply a critical distillation and balanced summary of the available empirical evidence, but equally important, an active synthesis, formulation, and analysis of that evidence. All of the chapters are authored by the members of our Department of Psychiatry at the Brigham and Women's Hospital, including several who were on our faculty at the time but have since moved to other institutions. In the chapters devoted to specific medical disorders, psychiatrists with particular expertise in those areas have been joined by other eminent Brigham medical specialists or subspecialists. Thus we aim to make these chapters valuable not just for psychiatrists and other mental health professionals, but also for a wide range of medical specialists as well.

The relationships between depression and medical illness are complex; each is in itself multifactorial, and furthermore their interrelationships are bidirectional. Medical illness may cause depression via direct pathophysiological action in the brain, and depression may also result from the psychological and emotional response to the stress, physical suffering, and disability imposed by the medical illness. Depression may also be caused by the medications used to treat the medical illness. Conversely, depression may lead to or exacerbate a co-occurring medical illness, via biological and/or behavioral mechanisms. In addition, antidepressant pharmacotherapy and somatic treatments for depression have systemic effects and can thereby exacerbate medical illness. Finally, both depression and medical illness may co-occur because they can both result from the same underlying pathophysiological process, for example, inflammation, or from the same neurobehavioral risk factors, such as alcoholism.

The book is organized in five sections. The first two chapters provide a conceptual and intellectual framework for understanding depressive illness. In chapter 1, we clarify the use of the term depression, since it can refer both categorically to a diagnosable disorder as well as dimensionally to symptoms (affective, cognitive, behavioral, and somatic) that exist along a spectrum of severity. Particular attention is given here and throughout the text to the clinical, epidemiological, and neurobiological overlap of depression and anxiety. Chapter 2 goes on to address the neurobiology of depression, considering systems-level, cellular, molecular, genetic, and epigenetic factors, including what we know about the neurocircuitry and neurochemistry of the disorder, as well as the findings emerging from structural and functional neuroimaging.

In Section 2, Chapters 3 and 4 discuss the general principles of depression diagnosis and treatment. Here and throughout the book, we emphasize the importance of diagnostic precision, screening, early intervention, measurement-based care, the individualization of treatment, and collaborative care. The discussion of diagnosis attends to boundary issues (e.g., with anxiety), the clinical interview, screening and the use of rating scales, the assessment of suicide, and special cross cultural and ethnic considerations in diagnosis. Chapter 4 begins with a general approach to the patient and goes on to discuss specific considerations imposed on depression treatment by the concurrent presence of medical illness. Pharmacotherapies and the most recent somatic therapies are discussed, along with the psychotherapies for which there is evidence of efficacy in the medically ill.

The chapters in Section 3 carefully, comprehensively, and critically assess what we know about depression when it is comorbid with the full range of major medical disorders, including sleep disorders and substance use disorders. The focus is on those particular aspects of depression that are specific and unique when it occurs in medically ill patients. Each chapter follows the same format: epidemiology; pathophysiology; clinical presentation; course and natural history; assessment and differential diagnosis; and treatment. When there is insufficient empirical evidence, we discuss the limits of what is known and suggest guidelines for proceeding, given the current state of our knowledge. We pay particular attention to the phenomenology of the medical illness and of depression, the course of untreated and treated depression when co-occurring with the medical illness, the impact of depression on the course of the medical illness, and of the effect of medical illness on the course of the depression. These chapters focus on the aspects of depression assessment and treatment that are unique to the particular medical illness being considered: What is the pathophysiology of the relationship? How treatment-responsive or treatment-refractory is depression when it is associated with this particular medical illness? What are the depressive side effects of medications used to treat these medical conditions? What are the effects of antidepressants on the medical illness?

Section 4 is devoted to special patient populations and the importance of the settings in which care is delivered. Here we address issues specific to the medically ill child who is depressed and the elderly medical patient who is depressed. The final chapters in this section discuss particular issues that arise in the settings in which the depression care is delivered, including the care of the surgical patient, collaborative care in ambulatory medical practices, the emergency department, and the depressed medical inpatient.

The book concludes with a glimpse into the future. We are moving toward greater understanding of the final common pathways mediating depressive symptoms and medical illnesses, and toward a more complete understanding of the relevant neurophysiological and pathophysiological processes. We look forward to the development of multimodal biomarkers that will lead to targeted therapies and more precise and individualized treatment planning. We will also witness a more seamless integration of depression care into general medical care, greater diagnostic precision, and earlier identification and intervention. We are entering a truly promising era in the understanding and the care of medically ill patients who are depressed.

Arthur Barsky, MD
David Silbersweig, MD
Boston, Massachusetts

SECTION I

Basic Concepts

CHAPTER 1

The Relationships Between Depression and Medical Illness

Melissa Bui, MD
Michael Mufson, MD
David Gitlin, MD

INTRODUCTION

Medicine has a long and complex past that mirrors the course of human history. Indeed, the major historical milestones of medicine cannot be understood outside of cultural context. A current of reductionist thought flows throughout the history of medicine, and has been pivotal in identifying and defining disease, and directing treatment into specialized, highly developed fields. However, this may have led to the creation of artificial boundaries around assessment and management, resulting in fractured, and at times, sub-optimal patient care. A more contemporary approach has reconceptualized the patient within a larger clinical and practical context. This transition demonstrates the value of an interdisciplinary approach, in which the patient, rather than the illness is the focus of treatment rather than the identified illness. There is also a transition toward a greater mechanistic understanding of illnesses. These developments have resulted in a greater appreciation of the overlap between physical and mental health, two areas which have at times occupied opposite poles of medical practice due to dualistic thinking, but which undeniably influence one another and can never be fully disentangled.

This textbook focuses its lens at this interface, examining the relationship between medical disorders and the most ubiquitous mental illness, depression. The associations between medical illness and depressive illness now appear to be more extensive and more intimate than previously appreciated. These associations may be considered coincidental, causal, or the result of a common underlying pathological process. The implications of these associations are shifting clinical practice in a new and more unified direction.

In this chapter, we will review differential diagnosis of depressive disorders within medically ill populations, including brief considerations of screening and treatment of depression in medical settings and an approach for stratification and treatment that can be implemented in both inpatient and outpatient settings. This discussion is followed by a closer examination of the relationship between depression and medical illness, reviewing diseases and treatments known to cause depression and examining depression as a final common pathway for both emotional and physiological disturbances. Finally, we review the synergistic effects of depression and medical illness, ranging from diminished functional status and decreased quality of life to increased rates of suicide and other forms of physical mortality. Although treatment is not a specific focus of this chapter and is covered in great depth later in this textbook, this chapter reiterates key themes of early intervention and collaborative care, as such principles of treatment can be implemented in the medical setting and are critical to optimizing outcomes.

In order to best appreciate the current understanding of depression in medically ill patients, it is helpful to begin with an historical perspective. This review reflects the natural evolution of man's approach to "madness." Early pioneers in the field produced rich descriptions of psychopathology, whereas later generations would propose causal mechanisms and modes of treatment.

HISTORICAL CONTEXT

Historical accounts of what constitutes a depressive disorder are long and varied. Yet as Stanley Jackson noted in his history of Melancholia and Depression, descriptions of depression date back over two millennia, yet have a remarkable consistency. Jackson describes the wide variety of terms for depression over the years, including feeling down, blue, unhappy, feeling dispirited, discouraged, disappointed, dejected, despondent, melancholy, sad, depressed, and despairing. For Jackson, depression is at the heart of being human.[1]

The term melancholia dates back to the humoral theory during Greek and Roman times When Aristotle identified a "melancholic temperament" that he related to overproduction of "black bile".[2] This early observation of the mind-body interaction in depression permeates our conceptualization of depression.

In the mid-nineteenth century, Griesenger described "stadium melancholicum" as the initial period of the disease and one that could "precede insanity," which we would now term psychotic depression[3] and various forms of major depression; he may have been the first to posit a hereditary predisposition for depression.[3] At the same time, Falret identified the concept of "circular insanity" or bipolar disorder, and also noted that it was "very hereditary".[4] In the 1880s, Emil Kraepelin delineated "manic depressive insanity" as a new nosologic entity, distinguishing it from dementia praecox and Bleuler schizophrenia and suggesting that all were part of the same spectrum: "the classification of states by definite fundamental disorders is the experience that all morbid forms brought together here as a clinical entity, not only pass over the one into the other without recognizable boundaries, but they may even replace each other in one and the same case".[5–8] In the mid-twentieth century, Karl Leonhard continued the Kraepelinian tradition and also introduced the concept of unipolar versus bipolar depression, that is, pure melancholia and pure depression.[9] He identified five "pure depressions" subtypes, including agitated, hypochondriacal, self-tortured, suspicious and apathetic, again illustrating the diverse phenotypes of depressive disorder. Leonhard also looked toward genetics and heredity as the etiology of these disorders.[10]

In the 1970s, Akiskal and McKinney elucidated a unified hypothesis of depressive disorder[11] that included interactions with medical illness. They introduced a stress diathesis model in which the interactions between genetics, neurobiological development, and interpersonal factors all impact the diencephalic centers of reinforcement and conceptualized depression as a "psychobiological final common pathway" based on genetic vulnerability,[11] while emphasizing that physiologic stressors, *including medical illness*, could all be directly related to the emergence of depression. They also suggested acute and chronic stress, *including chronic disease*, could lead to depression.

In 1997, advances in our understanding of molecular neuroscience led Duman et al. to emphasize that depression is a heterogeneous illness that can result from the dysregulation of several neurotransmitters or metabolic systems.[12] They emphasized the need for a broader understanding of the biologic basis of depression including the role of growth factors, genetic predispositions related to monoamine enzymes, receptors and proteins and noted risk factors for depression including medical illnesses. They too emphasized a stress diathesis model that includes both responses to stress and genetic vulnerability, a model that is very germane to our focus on depression in medical illness.

Today it is postulated by Kendler et al.[13] that major depression is a "prototypical multifactorial disorder" influenced by many factors including predisposing genetics, exposure to disturbed family environment, childhood sexual abuse, premature parental loss, predisposing personality traits, early-onset anxiety or conduct disorder, exposure to traumatic events and major adversities, low social support, substance misuse, prior history of major depression, low self-esteem and recent stressful life events. It has also been proposed by Parker[14] that "neurobiological processes lead to an obligatory depressed mood component alone or via recruitment of other neurobiological processes determining the dimensional expression of, for example, anxiety, irritability, hostility, fatigue, with such features… joining depression to define in part, mood state parameters." This diverges from a unitarian paradigm for depression toward an emphasis on subtypes that could eventually be defined by neuroimaging, and ultimately result in more specific treatment models. Chapter 2 focuses upon the brain circuit abnormalities that have been identified and are transforming the understanding of depression in medical illness.

Finally, though the theories of causality of depression have adopted a more integrative neurobiological model, the history of how to treat depression is also filled with competing models that reflect the historical paradigms of the day. During the psychoanalytic era, the guiding paradigm was Freud's "Mourning and Melancholia"[15] emphasizing the concept of loss in the affective state of grief and mourning in which the emotional world becomes "poor and empty" and distinguishing this from melancholia (depression) wherein it is the ego itself that is lost and becomes worthless. The grief stricken patient complains of the loss of a loved one whereas the melancholic focuses on his own inadequacies.

In the early 1950s, Bibring expanded this by focusing on the decrease in self-esteem seen in melancholic depression in contrast to grief. An "ego psychologist," Bibring describes the role of lost self-esteem in depression, particularly helplessness of the ego, another consideration in individuals with medical illness.[16] Aaron Beck then introduced the concept that early emotional deprivation leading to change in cognitive perceptions underlies depression and described the triad of hopeless, helpless, and worthless feelings that drive negative cognitive patterns and thoughts. Beck introduced cognitive-behavioral therapy as an evidence-based treatment modality for depression.[17]

DIAGNOSTIC CONSIDERATIONS

■ CHALLENGES IN THE DIAGNOSIS OF DEPRESSION

The current nosology and classificatory schema for the diagnosis of depressive disorders can be found in the DSM-5, which aims to "capture the heterogeneity of depressive disorders by classifying them along two dimensions: severity and chronicity.[18]" **Table 1-1** presents the DSM diagnostic criteria for various depressive disorders.

Historically, medicine has progressed through the development of objective, reproducible tests and measures of physiological and anatomical abnormality. However, psychiatry has remained dependent on phenomenological description and clinical judgment for diagnosis.[19] While patients or their healthcare providers may recognize the emergence of mood changes or physical symptoms, such as fatigue, psychomotor retardation, anorexia, and insomnia, the specific diagnosis of such disorders entails many challenges. Unlike some other fields of medicine, there are currently no biomarkers or imaging findings to conclusively support or refute the diagnosis of depressive disorder. Thus, healthcare providers frequently rely on screening tools to diagnose and track depressive symptoms over time. However, these diagnostic tools are not a substitute for seasoned clinical assessment using a structured approach.[20] Also confounding the reliability of psychiatric diagnosis is the issue of dynamic fluctuation. A patient's clinical presentation may change over brief periods of time in response to both biological and environmental factors. Without the aid of definitive biomarkers or other objective measures, clinicians are challenged with distinguishing "normal" dysphoria from pathological symptoms. This issue becomes especially problematic in the diagnostic assessment of patients who do not meet full criteria for DSM-5 disorders. In this context, there is a move from categorical toward dimensional approaches to the spectrum of mental illness.

■ DIFFERENTIAL DIAGNOSIS
Major Depressive Disorder

Major depressive disorder (MDD) has been increasingly well characterized. The illness almost always includes either persistent

TABLE 1-1 Summary of DSM-5 Diagnostic Criteria for Depressive Disorders

Diagnosis	Diagnostic Criteria
Major depressive episode	Five or more of the following symptoms for at least 2 weeks (must include either depressed mood or anhedonia) 1. Depressed or irritable mood 2. Anhedonia: Decreased interest or pleasure in most activities 3. Poor appetite or overeating 4. Insomnia or hypersomnia 5. Psychomotor agitation or retardation 6. Fatigue or loss of energy 7. Feelings of guilt or worthlessness 8. Poor concentration or difficulty making decisions 9. Suicidality: Thoughts of death or suicide, or has suicide plan
Persistent depressive disorder (dysthymia)	Three or more of the following symptoms for at least 2 years (must include depressed mood) 1. Depressed or irritable mood 2. Poor appetite or overeating 3. Insomnia or hypersomnia 4. Fatigue or loss of energy 5. Low self-esteem 6. Poor concentration or difficulty making decisions 7. Feelings of hopelessness
Adjustment disorder with depressed mood	1. The development of emotional or behavioral symptoms occurring within 3 months of an identifiable stressor or stressors. 2. Symptoms are characterized by marked distress that is out of proportion to stressor severity and results in significant distress or impairment in major functional domains (e.g., social, occupational, family). 3. The clinical picture does not meet the criteria for another mental disorder and does not reflect an exacerbation of a pre-existing mental disorder. 4. The symptoms do not represent normal bereavement. 5. Symptoms resolve within a 6-month period after the stressor(s) have ended. 6. Depressed mood, tearfulness, or feelings of hopelessness are predominant.
Depression secondary to a general medical condition	1. A persistent period of depressed mood or anhedonia. 2. The disturbance is the direct pathophysiological consequence of another medical condition. 3. The disturbance is not better explained by another mental disorder. 4. The disturbance does not occur exclusively during a period of delirium. 5. The disturbance causes significant distress or impairment in major functional domains (e.g., social, occupational, family).
Depressed phase of bipolar disorder	At least one episode of mania or hypomania, usually alternating with major depressive episodes as defined above

Data from American Psychiatric Association: Diagnostic and statistical manual of mental disorders: DSM-5, 5th edition. Arlington, VA: American Psychiatric Association; 2013.

depressed mood and/or loss of interest in all usual pleasurable areas. Common psychological features include feelings of guilt and worthlessness, impairment in decision making, low motivation, hopelessness, and suicidal ideation or behavior. In addition, MDD typically includes various physical derangements, often referred to as neurovegetative symptoms. These may include appetite disturbance (anorexia or hyperphagia), sleep impairment (insomnia or hypersomnia), psychomotor disturbance (agitation or retardation), fatigue, and concentration problems.

Most medical providers are reasonably adept at recognizing MDD, although the neurovegetative symptoms may lead providers to focus exclusively on the physical symptoms and thus miss the diagnosis. However, other depressive illnesses are less well known to medical providers. They may confuse or obscure the diagnosis but are important to recognize for optimal management and outcome. While MDD is the most commonly diagnosed and treated depressive disorder, practitioners must also be able to recognize and treat depressive entities not meeting full criteria for MDD, including persistent depressive disorder (dysthymia), minor depression, adjustment disorder with depressed mood, and secondary mood disorder due to a general medical condition. Providers also need to recognize that depressive symptoms can occur in the context of other serious psychiatric illnesses, such as schizophrenia, bipolar disorder, and posttraumatic stress disorder.

Persistent Depressive Disorder (Dysthymia)

Persistent depressive disorder is the second most common depressive disorder likely to be encountered by medical professionals.[21] It is estimated that 9.1% of the U.S. population meet criteria for current depression, and greater than one-third of them have persistent depressive disorder.[22] While MDD has been extensively studied and has a solid evidence base to guide treatment, there are fewer data to guide treatment of persistent depressive disorder. This difference can be attributed in part to the early classification of dysthymic symptoms as "chronic depression" or "depressive personality disorder," conditions which were characterological in nature and believed to respond only to psychotherapy.[23] However, numerous studies have established the effectiveness of antidepressant medications as well as cognitive and behavioral therapeutic interventions in the treatment of persistent depressive disorder.[21,24-26]

Depression with Anxious Features

Anxiety symptoms frequently co-occur along with depressive symptoms,[27] with rates of significant anxiety symptoms in the 40% to 60% range. Similarly, anxiety and depressive disorders have been demonstrated to have high rates of comorbidity in the same range,[28] and depressive illness has been shown to have increased comorbidity with most subtypes of anxiety disorders. Thus, the rate of comorbidity for posttraumatic stress disorder and depression is quite high, approaching 40%.[29] Since serious traumatic events are associated with depression, this helps to explain the strong correlation between these two illnesses. Panic disorder has also been noted to be highly comorbid with depressive illness, with a nearly sevenfold increase compared to patients without panic disorder.[30]

This frequent co-occurrence has led many researchers to study whether a depressive subtype, often called anxious depression, may best account for this syndrome rather than separate but comorbid anxiety and depressive disorders. Studies suggest that those patients with marked anxious features may have more severe mood disorders,[31] and that their course and outcomes are often worse, than patients without an anxiety component, including an increased risk of suicide.[32] Clinicians should evaluate any patient presenting with depressive illness for comorbid anxiety, and treatment approaches that include consideration of anxiety are more likely to be successful.

In the setting of comorbid medical illness, the co-occurrence of anxiety and depression may be particularly devastating to patients. Anxious symptoms may contribute to poor sleep, diminished appetite, and psychomotor acceleration, all of which may interfere with treatment and recovery from the medical condition. Anxiety may also affect the patient's ability to make difficult treatment decisions, and to tolerate unpleasant tests and procedures; for instance, anxiety often interferes with the ability of intubated patients to wean from their ventilators. Finally, as with depression, anxiety may have a direct, deleterious effect on medical conditions. For example, it has been demonstrated that PTSD is a significantly independent risk factor for coronary artery disease.[33]

Adjustment Disorder with Depressed Mood

Individuals may have some symptoms of depressive illness, particularly depressed mood, in response to an acute stressful event, and the diagnosis and/or development of a medical illness is a particularly stressful experience for many individuals. This response may include marked and persistent distress which appears out of proportion to the seriousness of the event, and may result in impairment of function in a variety of areas, including social, interpersonal, and occupational. In most cases, however, the symptoms do not rise to the level of major depression disorder, and is more accurately diagnosed as an adjustment disorder with primarily depressed mood.

Adjustment disorder with depressed mood is self-limited, almost always resolving within 6 months. It also has favorable outcomes when targeted with either psychotherapeutic interventions such as cognitive behavioral therapy, although at times may require a brief course of pharmacotherapy and close clinical monitoring.[34] However, practitioners frequently prefer to take a "watchful waiting" approach to such patients, as it is possible that their depressive symptoms may improve independently of specific, targeted treatment. While this conservative approach may be appropriate for certain cases, providers should have a structured plan for regular observation, with a low threshold to initiate treatment if the patient's symptoms worsen, or there is no concomitant mood reactivity or improvement as the patient's primary condition improves.

Complicated Grief and Bereavement

Grief is a common experience in elderly populations, due to the increased frequency of losses that occur later in life. By some estimates, over 70% of elderly individuals experience serious personal loss over a 2-year period.[35] Grief is typically associated with many depressive features. These may include sadness, decrease in pleasure, and interest in usual activities, social isolation, insomnia, and difficulty concentrating in occupational and interpersonal settings.

Although grief is a normative reaction to serious loss and is typically self-limited, some people may experience a more severe response. Such a response, which may occur in nearly 10% of bereaved older adults[36] is known as complicated grief or persistent complex bereavement disorder. The grief is both persistent and prolonged, lasting a year or more. Unrelenting yearning for the lost person, continued sadness and sorrow related to the loss, and excessive preoccupation with that person or the circumstances of the loss may be overwhelming. There may also be a tendency to avoid people and places associated with the loss.

Medical illness itself also may be experienced by many individuals as loss, and serious losses are associated with worsening of physical health, decline in function, and increase in mortality.[37] The loss of physical health and integrity may have many of the qualities of grief associated with interpersonal loss, as well as the feelings of loss of personal capacity, independence, and omnipotence over one's world. Since both interpersonal losses and physical illnesses are more likely in older individuals, complicated grief may be a more significant condition in this population. However, it may be difficult to distinguish typical grief in response to the onset or progression of illness from a more complicated grief reaction. When the course of the grief over the illness is prolonged and progressive, it is appropriate to address the issue with the patient and to consider treatment. Cognitive therapy has been suggested to be effective in the management of complicated grief.[38]

Secondary Mood Disorder Due to a Medical Condition

In patients for whom the primary medical illness does not simply precipitate depression, but is thought to be its pathophysiologic cause, clinicians should consider a diagnosis of secondary mood disorder due to a general medical condition.[39] In these cases, the depressive syndrome can be etiologically related to the patient's medical condition either by history, physical examination, or laboratory findings. The diagnosis requires that the patient's mood symptoms are not better accounted for by another mental disorder and do not occur exclusively in the course of delirium or dementia. Examples of medical illnesses that cause depressive syndromes range from hypothyroidism to pancreatic cancer to cerebrovascular lesions. Although pharmacotherapy can ameliorate certain mood or neurovegetative symptoms, complete remission of the depressive symptoms may not occur without effective treatment of the underlying medical condition. For example, depressive symptoms in Cushing disease may be resistant to antidepressant treatment but respond to steroid suppression.[40]

Depression and Comorbid Schizophrenia or Bipolar Disorder

It is not uncommon for patients diagnosed with one psychiatric condition to carry other comorbid psychiatric diagnoses, making both the diagnosis and treatment of these patients more difficult. Depression that co-occurs with schizophrenia or bipolar disorder raises particular challenges. The patient with schizophrenia may appear flat or withdrawn at baseline, making it difficult to detect a superimposed depression. However, screening tools such as the PANSS-D (Positive and Negative Syndrome Scale—Depression subscale) or the CDSS (Calgary Depression Scale for Schizophrenia) are helpful in differentiating underlying negative symptoms of schizophrenia from symptoms of a depressive disorder.[41–43]

Patients with bipolar disorder typically demonstrate classic symptoms of depression when in the depressed phase. A careful psychiatric history must be taken to assess for past manic or hypomanic episodes, for example, by using the Mood Disorder Questionnaire (MDQ).[44] Careful consideration is required before starting bipolar patients on antidepressant medications, as such medications have the potential to induce a manic or mixed state or may lead to rapid cycling of depressive or manic episodes.

■ DEPRESSION IN PATIENTS WITH MEDICAL ILLNESS
Recognition of Depression

Patients with serious medical illnesses may exhibit a spectrum of depressive symptoms without meeting formal criteria for a depressive disorder. These symptoms include grief, sadness, demoralization, and loss of interest. They may seem appropriate for patients who are newly challenged with their own mortality (**Box 1-1**). Healthcare providers not uncommonly dismiss these feelings as a "natural" response, and therefore assume that treatment is not indicated.[45] They may be reluctant to diagnose or treat patients not meeting full DSM-5 criteria for depression, and may favor a "wait and see" approach rather than exploring potential treatment options with the patient. However, subsyndromal depressive symptoms in medically ill patients may be exceptionally responsive to treatment and, in addition, treatment of depressive states may also improve medical outcomes.[46]

BOX 1-1
CLINICAL VIGNETTE 1: CHALLENGES IN DIAGNOSIS: THE PATIENT RECENTLY DIAGNOSED WITH ILLNESS

Case: A 46-year-old female is referred for evaluation of depression. Her history is significant for diagnosis of breast cancer 4 months earlier, resulting in radical mastectomy and radiotherapy. Her psychiatric history is notable for a prior episode of moderate depression following the birth of her second child, which responded well to antidepressant medication. She has not required any medication for over 10 years. She reports that she was doing well prior to her diagnosis and treatment but has had depressed mood, anergia, poor sleep and appetite for about 2 months. She notes that her husband has been distant throughout her illness, not helping very much with their two children. She has been unable to return to work as a real estate lawyer. She describes recurrent feelings of hopelessness regarding her own potential mortality as well as guilt about her role as mother and wife.

Challenge: The clinical challenge in this case is whether or not to initiate antidepressant medication given that the patient's sadness seems fitting of her new cancer diagnosis as an identifiable cause for her depression. The question then arises, where is the line between appropriate negative affect and pathologic symptomatology?

Resolution: The emotional impact of the diagnosis of a new medical illness, as well as the stress associated with the acceptance and management of that illness, can strongly influence the development of a depressive illness. In addition, the illness itself can directly bring about a depressive disorder. What is critical in the evaluation and management of the depressive illness is recognition of important neurovegetative symptoms, as well as a prior personal or family history of a mood disorder. In this patient, her symptoms meet the criteria for a major depressive disorder, and her past history of depression increases the likelihood of a serious relapse. Antidepressant medication is strongly indicated and should be initiated immediately. This treatment may occur in tandem with psychotherapy, the combination of which may ultimately have the most effective outcome.

BOX 1-2
CLINICAL VIGNETTE 2

Case: A 57-year-old male with history of type II diabetes, hypertension, COPD, and arthritis returns to his primary care physician seeking evaluation of multiple complaints. He notes worsening arthritis pain in his knees and shoulders and is having difficulty sleeping through the night. He is now experiencing daily fatigue. He no longer enjoys hobbies such repairing his antique car, and rarely leaves his house except to go to his many doctors' appointments. His primary care physician is concerned that the patient's physical complaints may have a psychological component, and is considering referring the patient to a therapist even though the patient has never reported feeling depressed.

Challenge: This highlights a common scenario in primary care treatment of depression in patients with medical illness. The patient has multiple medical problems and frequently reports nonspecific complaints, including a number of neurovegetative symptoms. This presentation may not prompt his primary care doctor to consider treatment of depression because the patient has never endorsed feeling depressed.

Resolution: DSM-5 criteria for depression do not require depressed mood to make the diagnosis of depression, and this patient's loss of interest may be sufficient to make the diagnosis.[39] Patients with underlying depressive disorders may not be forthcoming about depressive or suicidal feelings unless explicitly questioned by their healthcare providers.[47] Therefore the PHQ-9 or other validated depression questionnaire should be a standard measure of depression screening in any outpatient medical practice. If the screening suggests high risk for depression, PCP initiation of an antidepressant or referral to a psychiatrist/therapist should be considered.

Medically ill patients may also experience any of the classically described DSM-5 depressive disorders (Table 1-1). Most clinicians are familiar with the clinical picture of MDD, however, it may be harder to recognize symptoms of persistent depressive disorder, depression secondary to a general medical condition, or the depressed phase of bipolar disorder. Depressive disorders are also present across a wide range of psychiatric illness, and while certain patients will have an established diagnosis (i.e., bipolar disorder or schizophrenia), others may be newly diagnosed, or may have gone unrecognized for decades. Conversely, clinicians may be too quick to ascribe a patient's depressive symptoms to a preexisting mental illness, such as schizophrenia without considering the time course of depressive symptomatology. This may result in failure to consider potential benefits of additional treatment.

Differentiation from Medical Illness

One of the most common challenges to appropriately diagnosing depressive disorders in patients who are medically ill is determining which diagnostic criteria to use (**Box 1-2**). The symptoms of MDD include neurovegetative symptoms, such as low energy, fatigue, insomnia or hypersomnia, poor concentration, impaired sexual function, decreased appetite, and psychomotor slowing. However, these symptoms should not be counted toward a depressive diagnosis if in the clinician's judgment they are "due to a general medical condition." It is often unclear whether these neurovegetative symptoms can be used to diagnose depression in patients with cancer, congestive heart failure, chronic pain, or other conditions that are frequently complicated by disturbances of sleep or concentration or debilitating fatigue.

Koenig et al. found that using an inclusive approach (i.e., counting depressive symptoms toward the diagnosis of depression regardless of whether the clinician judges that the symptoms are due to medical or psychological causes) provided the highest sensitivity, though at the cost of poor specificity and an overall inflated rate of depression.[48] This approach provides the most liberal diagnostic strategy and is the least likely to miss patients with serious depressive disorders. Two alternatives include the exclusive and substitutive approaches. The exclusive approach eliminates from consideration certain symptoms likely to be caused by medical illness (fatigue, weight loss, poor concentration). The substitute approach replaces these symptoms with more affective ones, such as tearfulness, irritability, or social withdrawal.[45] These two approaches have the potential to more narrowly define depressive disorders within medically ill populations. However, due to the lack of consensus regarding which symptoms to exclude or substitute, there are limited data for the validity of such specific approaches. Koenig proposes an "etiologic approach," in which clinical judgment is used to decide whether to attribute each of the neurovegetative symptoms to depression or to the comorbid medical condition. This strategy yields "middle-range prevalence rates for major and minor depressions that are associated with relatively high impairment and intermediate persistence of depressive symptoms when compared with other diagnostic schemes."[48]

Screening for Depression in Medical Settings

It is estimated that 30% to 50% of patients who are medically ill have comorbid depressive disorders, so systematic screening is imperative.[47,49] Over 50% of patients with depressive disorders receive treatment exclusively from their primary care physicians, making this clinical interface a critical point for identification and treatment of individuals with depression.[50] The need for effective and systematic screening for depression in primary care and inpatient medical settings cannot be underscored strongly enough. The World Health Organization lists depression as the leading cause of disability as measured by years lived with disability, and by the year 2020 depression is projected to become the second leading contributor to global burden of disease.[51] Certain patient groups are at especially high risk for developing depressive disorders and therefore merit additional screening, such as those with chronic pain or other chronic or high mortality conditions.

Several evidence-based screening tools are frequently used in both medical and psychiatric settings to identify and track depressive symptoms over time. These include the Beck Depression Inventory (BDI) and the Patient Health Questionnaire (PHQ-9).[52,53] The PHQ-9 has the added advantage that it specifically asks patients about DSM-5 criteria for depression, and thus satisfies the etiologic approach to depression screening. An approach for screening high-risk patients for depression using the PHQ-9, and stratifying individuals with a positive score (≥10) into two treatment groups using additional risk factors for screening is presented in **Figure 1-1**. Patients who screen positive for safety concerns or bipolar risk factors should be referred to psychiatry for further assessment and management, whereas patients without additional risk factors who are in agreement with outpatient treatment may begin antidepressant therapy within the primary care setting.

By emphasizing regular screening, early intervention, and collaborative care across services and clinical disciplines, medical and mental health providers can work to bridge the gaps that separate patients from the treatment they require, and in so doing connect patients with the resources that will best serve their needs and give them the greatest chance of recovery.

The Importance of Treatment of Depression in Medical Illness

Treatment of depression does not simply have implications for the patient's mood and general quality of life, but can also improve patients' participation in their medical care, and significantly affect measures such as functional status, clinical outcomes, and even life expectancy. These far-reaching consequences have a significant impact not only on patient well-being but also on healthcare costs, making early treatment of depression not only a quality of life issue, but also an economic one.

Patients with comorbid depressive and medical disorders are particularly challenging to treat. Depressed patients are more likely than nondepressed controls to forget or miss their medications,[54,55] less likely to adhere to healthcare regimens such as diet, exercise or glucose self-monitoring,[56] and more likely to miss appointments or wait an inappropriately long time before seeking treatment.[57] These treatment-interfering behavioral issues in patients with depression likely explain part of the increased medical morbidity and mortality.

Depressed patients tend to be high utilizers of healthcare services, and frequently present with vague or medically unexplained symptoms, which may prompt their physicians to order excessive or unnecessary laboratory tests, imaging studies, or medication trials, all of which increase healthcare costs.[58] Treatment of depression by mental health providers accounts for only about 10% of the increase in medical costs among this patient population.[46]

Patients with comorbid depression and medical illness are more disabled than patients with either depression or medical illness alone.[46] And medical patients with depression suffer in multiple domains of well-being and functioning when compared to individuals with chronic medical conditions without depression.[59] Areas of impairment among medical patients with depression include worse physical functioning, poorer social functioning, and increased bodily pain. Patients with depression are also more likely to experience greater subjective distress related to their medical conditions, typically reporting two to three times more medical symptoms.[60]

Recent studies of life expectancy among individuals with serious mental illness estimates that those with MDD have a life expectancy between 7.2 and 10.6 years shorter than average.[61] This increase in mortality is not solely due to suicide, but is largely attributable to deaths from "natural" causes such as cardiovascular disease.[62] For example, there is a well-established association between depression and increased cardiac mortality, with increased cardiovascular and all-cause mortality in patients with post-MI depression, as well as in patients with comorbid depression and congestive heart failure.[63-65] There is also increased mortality among patients with comorbid depression and diabetes, with an estimated 54% greater mortality among individuals with diabetes and at least mild depression.[66] Conversely, treatment of depression can improve the course of medical illness. For example, patients with co-morbid Parkinson disease and depression demonstrated significant improvement in cognitive and executive function with successful treatment of depression.[67] Further discussion of the impact of depression on cardiovascular and endocrine health is explored in chapters 7 and 14, respectively.

Patients with depression and medical illnesses experience functional impairment that is more severe than that seen in individuals with either depression or medical illness. However, effective treatment of depression is accompanied by concomitant improvements in functional impairment and disability.[68] In addition, costs improve across every sphere of medical care, including clinic costs, laboratory fees, and expenses related to medications.[69]

Increasingly, collaborative and integrated care models have been established to recognize and manage depressive illness in the primary care setting. Development of primary care-based depression management teams, with multidisciplinary providers, including psychiatry, psychology, nursing, and social work, can aid the primary care provider in treating depression effectively in this setting. As a treatment delivery model, collaborative and integrated care not only improves medical and mental health outcomes, but does so in a cost-effective manner that persists over several years.[70] In an era of managed care,

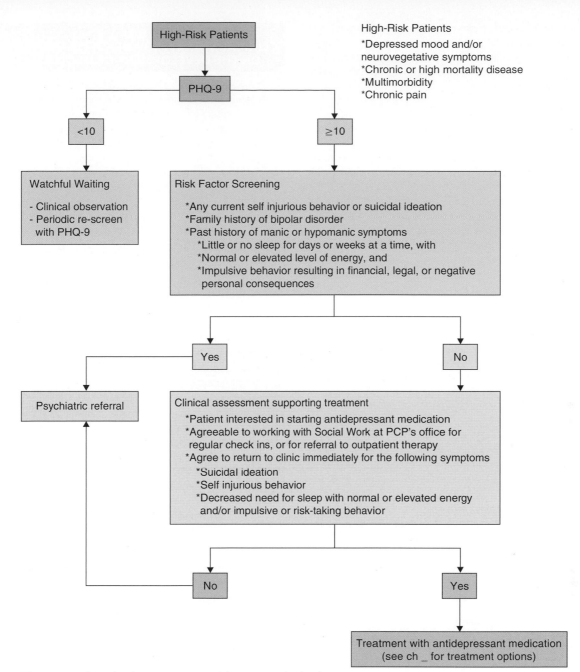

Figure 1-1 *Algorithm for management of depression in high-risk patients.*

these potential cost-savings will likely establish collaborative care as a cornerstone of the management of this patient population.

■ RELATIONSHIPS: COINCIDENCE, CAUSE, OR COMMON UNDERLYING MECHANISM

Chronic illness tends to be multifactorial, a complex interplay between genetic predisposition and environmental insult. This complexity is readily apparent among patients with cancer or diabetes, however even among diseases with a single etiologic cause such as sickle cell anemia, there is a wide variety of clinical presentations for which these patients seek medical care, ranging from asymptomatic anemia to acute pain syndrome or stroke.[71] Mental illness is similarly complex, balancing the influence of biology and environment with the individual's personal coping skills and defense mechanisms. While a single episode of depression may have a clear etiologic cause, the depressive condition far more often represents a final common pathway with multiple contributing factors.

The relationship between depression and medical illness can be conceptualized in several different ways. These two conditions may be unrelated to each other, in which case the relationship is coincidental. There may be a causal relationship between depression and medical condition. The causal relationship may be bidirectional. On one hand, the medical condition may cause or contribute to depression, either through the disease process, through its pharmacotherapy, or by causing a nonspecific, depressive response to the stress of being ill. Conversely, on the other hand, depression can cause or contribute to medical illness through its pathophysiology, through antidepressant medication, or through depressive behaviors. Finally, both the depressive and the medical illness may result from a common underlying mechanism (e.g., stress, alcoholism, or inflammation).

Coincidence

Depression and medical illness may occur in the same individual without any etiological association. They co-occur on a statistical basis alone: Since depression is common, the probability that it will co-occur with a common medical illness is substantial. However, even if the two conditions are unrelated etiologically, once present, they may then interact with each other and can result in the clinical relationships described below.

Depression Causing Medical Illness

There are three ways in which depression can cause or exacerbate medical illness. First, the pathophysiological changes that underlie or accompany depression can themselves lead to medical disorder. Thus depression is associated with HPA axis dysfunction and with inflammation, both of which have pathogenic effects. Second, the medications used to treat depression may contribute to medical illnesses. For example, selective serotonin reuptake inhibitors are associated with an increased risk of bleeding and weight gain, and some newer generation neuroleptics, given adjunctively to treat depression, are associated with the development of a metabolic syndrome and diabetes. Third, depression is accompanied by a range of unhealthy behaviors that can cause or exacerbate medical illnesses. For example, depressed individuals are less likely to adhere to their medication regimen and to exercise, and are more likely to drink alcohol (in some cases as self-medication) and smoke cigarettes. These behaviors constitute serious risk factors for a range of serious medical illness, such as cirrhosis and lung cancer.

Medical Illness Causing Depression

Medical illness may cause or exacerbate depression via pathophysiological mechanisms, as a side effect of the medical treatment, or through stress and related nonspecific effects of becoming sick. Examples of medical pathophysiology contributing to depression include the endocrine changes associated with thyroid disease and Cushing syndrome. Medical or neurologic illness may also affect the brain circuits and chemistry that underlie mood and its regulation, leading to depression. Examples of this include Parkinson disease, and strokes or other lesions in the left frontal cortex.[72,73] Medications prescribed for medical conditions, such as propranolol or interferon, may themselves contribute to depression.[74] Likewise, radiation therapy of the brain may lead to depression. In addition, the generic stress of a serious or disabling medical illness can provoke a psychological depressive reaction (**Box 1-3**).

Common Underlying Mechanisms

In some instances, the relationship between depression and medical illness is characterized as the common result of a single, underlying pathologic process. For example, stress may contribute not only to the development of depression, but also to the development and penetrance of medical disorders. Investigation is focusing on the ways in which stress is mediated, and its impact on the brain and other organ systems. Work has focused on the hypothalamic–pituitary and thyroid axes, the role of cytokines and inflammation, and the interplay between these two modulators of neurohumoral function. Chronic or repeated exposure to high levels of stress hormones precipitates both depressive behavior and chronic disease.[75] There appears to be a pathophysiologic relationship between catecholamines and cytokines, mediated by the sympathetic nervous system and cortisol, that are released in response to a cascade of hormonal precursors within the HPA axis.[75] Cortisol is known to cause insulin resistance, and other HPA axis precursors can contribute to subcutaneous fat redistribution, which has been known to promote insulin resistance. Chronically elevated levels of these stress hormones have been shown to increase the likelihood of medical conditions such as diabetes and vascular disease.[75]

■ BIOMARKERS OF DEPRESSION

The recognition of the above relationships between depression and medical illness, and of the need for a more biological taxonomy

Case: A 62-year-old female is brought to the emergency room complaining of acute chest pain and shortness of breath. Her history is negative for cardiac or pulmonary disease. Social history is notable for husband hospitalized the previous day with serious injuries after fall from roof. Psychiatric history includes Panic disorder, although patient denies any episodes × 3 years. EKG is notable for mild ST elevation but negative cardiac enzymes. She is admitted to hospital. Echocardiogram notable for apical hypokinesis. Cardiac catheterization is negative. Patient is diagnosed with Takotsubo cardiomyopathy. She is noted to be tearful and dysphoric, and psychiatric consultation is requested.

Challenge: One example of the relationship between mental distress and medical illness is the example of Takotsubo, or stress cardiomyopathy, a reversible disturbance of cardiac contractility which occurs directly in response to emotional distress, mostly in postmenopausal women.[76] Electrocardiography demonstrates ST-elevation and T-wave inversions but cardiac enzymes may only be minimally elevated and cardiac catheterization shows unobstructed coronary arteries. Definitive diagnosis of Takotsubo is usually made by ventriculogram or echocardiography, showing apical ballooning (i.e., hypokinesis of the cardiac apex) and a decreased ejection fraction (EF). There is no single confirmed cause of Takotsubo cardiomyopathy, however, evidence suggests that significantly elevated plasma catecholamine levels are instrumental in the pathophysiology of this disease.[77] The reversibility of this condition is likely a reflection of the acute, brief nature of exposure to the catecholamine surge, whereas chronic or repeated exposure to high levels of stress hormones has been shown to have negative effects on both depressive and chronic disease entities.[75]

Resolution: While patients with Takotsubo cardiomyopathy may initially present with significant impairment (EF 15–25%) it is a reversible condition and usually shows a complete recovery in 4 to 6 weeks. Therapy focused on psychosocial stressors, including Cognitive Behavioral Therapy, can help diminish risk of subsequent cardiac events.

and understanding of depression, has fueled a search for potential biomarkers (**Table 1-2**). In particular, the association between depressive illness and neurohumoral and inflammatory function has provided avenues for investigation in this area. However, the heterogeneity of depressive illness as well as the impact of medical illnesses on HPA function and inflammation complicates this search in terms of specificity.

Nevertheless, certain relationships are worth noting. The best studied of these is the dexamethasone suppression test (DST). Research has demonstrated that patients with major depression are more likely to show an impairment of DST suppression.[78] This phenomenon is even more significant in patients with more severe, melancholic depressive disorders and psychotic depression, and may be predictive of suicide risk.[79–81] These patients with more severe forms of depression, including suicidal patients, have a blunted prolactin response to a D-fenfluramine challenge test, which is associated with hypercortisolemia and reduced serotonergic activity.[82,83]

The pituitary–thyroid axis has also been studied for its neuroendocrine role in depression. This relates in part to the long-standing observation of depressive symptoms in patients with hypothyroidism. Several researchers demonstrated a blunted response of thyrotropin-stimulating hormone (TSH) to exogenous

TABLE 1-2 Potential Biologic Markers for Depression

Neuroendocrine tests
Dexamethasone suppression test
Prolactin response to D-fenfluramine
Thyrotropin-releasing hormone stimulation test
Inflammatory markers
Interleukin-6
C-reactive protein
Tumor necrosis factor-α
Interleukin-1a
CNS growth factors
Brain-derived neurotrophic factor
Glial-cell derived neurotrophic factor
Insulin-like growth factor
Neurotrophin-3
Nerve growth factor
Fibroblast growth factor-2

thyrotropin-releasing hormone (TSH). However, much like the other neuroendocrine tests, poor sensitivity and specificity make it inadequate for use as a biologic marker.[84]

More recently, researchers have explored the possibility that depression may have an inflammatory component. Inflammation plays a critical role in the etiology of many medical disorders, including Crohn disease, celiac disease, asthma, and rheumatoid arthritis. In addition, several other chronic illnesses are believed to have an inflammatory component, such as atherosclerotic cardiovascular disease and diabetes. Recent studies have suggested that depression, similar to cardiovascular disease, may also have an inflammatory component, as demonstrated by increases in inflammatory markers.[85] Serum levels of both interleukin-6 (IL-6) and tumor necrosis factor-α (TNF-α), which are pro-inflammatory cytokines, are elevated in MDD.[86] Compared to patients with treatment resistant depression, treatment responders have lower levels of IL-6.[87] Other inflammatory markers have been shown to be associated with depression, including IL-1 and C-reactive protein.[88]

Finally, there is increasing evidence of a relationship between stress and brain tropism, in which growth factors may be inhibited in the setting of chronic stress such as depression. It is known that antidepressant treatment enhances growth factor production and resultant neuroplasticity.[89] The best studied of the CNS growth factors is brain-derived neurotrophic factor (BDNF). Multiple studies and meta-analyses have demonstrated that BDNF is decreased in major depression, and that this response is reversed with antidepressant therapy.[89] Other growth factors potentially affected by depressive illness include glial cell–derived neurotrophic factor, insulin-like growth factor, neurotrophin-3, nerve growth factor, and fibroblast growth factor-2.[89] Genetic, epigenetic, and imaging biomarkers are discussed in Chapter 2.

SUMMARY

Our understanding of the relationship between depression and medical illness is in transition; what began as independent threads are now being re-conceptualized as parts of a single fabric. The manner in which these conditions are diagnosed and treated must increasingly take into account the different permutations of the interrelationships described above. As the mechanisms underlying these interrelationships are elucidated, biomarkers can be validated, and the conceptualization of depression as a medical illness will increasingly be recognized, with benefits to patients and to society at large.

REFERENCES

1. Jackson SW. *Melancholia and Depression*. New Haven: Yale University Press;1986:1–4.

2. Jackson SW *Melancholia and Depression*. New Haven: Yale University Press;1986:5–7.

3. Griesenger W. *Mental Pathology and Therapeutics*. Robertson CL, Rutherford J, trans-eds. London: New Sydenham Society; 1867.

4. Falret JP. Memoire sur la folie circulaire, forme de maladie mentale caracterisee par la reproduction successive et reguliere de l'etat manique,de l'etat mealncoliique, e d'un intervale lucide plus ou moins prolong. *Bulletin de l'Academie de Medicine*. 1854;19:382–415.

5. Kraepelin E. *Manic Depressive Insanity and Paranoia*. Mary Barclay R, Robertson GM, trans-eds. Edinburgh: E & S Livingstone; 1921.

6. Kraepelin E. *Manic Depressive Insanity and Paranoia*. Mary Barclay R, Robertson GM, trans-eds. Edinburgh: E & S Livingstone; 1921:1–10.

7. Kraepelin E. *Manic Depressive Insanity and Paranoia*. Mary Barclay R, Robertson GM, trans-eds. Edinburgh: E & S Livingstone; 1921:70–74.

8. Kraepelin E. *Manic Depressive Insanity and Paranoia*. Mary Barclay R, Robertson GM, trans-eds. Edinburgh: E & S Livingstone; 1921:167–184.

9. Leonhard K. *Classification of Endogenous Psychosis and their Differential Etiology*. New York, NY: Springer-Verlag-Wien; 1999.

10. Leonhard K. *Classification of Endogenous Psychosis and their Differential Etiology*. New York, NY: Springer-Verlag-Wien; 1999: 250–329.

11. Akiskal H., McKinney W. Overview of recent research in depression. *Arch Gen Psychiatry*. 1975;32(3):285–305.

12. Duman R, Heninger G, Nestler EJ. A molecular and cellular theory of depression. *Arch Gen Psychiatry*. 199754:597–606.

13. Kendler K, Gardner C, Prescott C. Toward a comprehensive developmental model for major depression. *Amer J Psychiatry*. 2002;59(7):1133–1145.

14. Parker G. Classifying depression: Should paradigms lost be regained? *Amer J Psychiatry*. 2000;157:1195–1203.

15. Freud S. Mourning and melancholia. *The Standard Edition of the Complete Psychological Works of Sigmund Freud Volume XIV*. (1914–1916):237–258.

16. Bibring E. The mechanism of depression. In: Greenacre P, ed. *Affective Disorders*. NY: IUP; 1953:13–48.

17. Beck A. *Depression: Clinical, Experimental and Theoretical Aspects*. NY: Harper and Row; 1967.

18. Klein D. Classification of depressive disorders in DSM V: proposal for a two-dimension system. *J Abnormal Psychol*. 2008;117(3):552–560.

19. Kendler KS, Zachar P, Craver C. What kinds of things are psychiatric disorders? *Psychol Med*. 2011;41(6):1143–1150.

20. Koenig HG, Pappas P, Holsinger T, Bachar JR. Assessing diagnostic approaches to depression in medically ill older adults: how reliably can mental health professionals make judgments about the cause of symptoms? *J Am Geriatr Soc*. 1995;43(5):472–478.

21. Barrett JE, Williams JW Jr, Oxman TE, et al. Treatment of dysthymia and minor depression in primary care: a randomized trial in patients aged 18 to 59 years. *J Fam Pract*. 2001;50(5):405–412.

22. Centers for Disease Control and Prevention (CDC). Current depression among adults—United States, 2006 and 2008. *MMWR*

Morb Mortal Wkly Rep. 2010;59(38):1229–1235. Available at http://www.cdc.gov/mmwr/preview/mmwrhtml/mm5938a2.htm

23. Howland RH, Thase ME. Biological studies of dysthymia. *Biol Psychiatry.* 1991;30(3):283–304.

24. Markowitz JC. Psychotherapy for dysthymic disorder. *Psychiatr Clin North Am.* 1996;19(1):133–149.

25. Williams JW Jr, Barrett J, Oxman T, et al. Treatment of dysthymia and minor depression in primary care: A randomized controlled trial in older adults. *JAMA.* 2000;284(12):1519–1526.

26. Ravindran AV, Anisman H, Merali Z, et al. Treatment of primary dysthymia with group cognitive therapy and pharmacotherapy: clinical symptoms and functional impairments. *Am J Psychiatry.* 1999;156(10):1608–1617.

27. Regier DA, Burke JD, Burke KC. Comorbidity of affective and anxiety symptoms in the NIMH epidemiologic catchment area program. In: Maser JD, Cloninger CR, eds. *Comorbidity of Mood and Anxiety Disorders.* American Psychiatric Association; 113–122:1990.

28. Zimmerman M, McDermut W, Mattia JI. Frequency of anxiety disorders in psychiatric outpatients with major depressive disorder. *Am J Psychiatry.* 2000;157(8):1337–1340.

29. Breslau N, Davis GC, Andreski P, et al. Traumatic events and post traumatic stress disorder in an urban population of young adults. *Arch Gen Psychiatry.* 1991;48(3):216–222.

30. Kessler RC, Stang PE, Wittchen HU, et al. Lifetime panic-depression comorbidity in the National Comorbidity Survey. *Archives of Gen Psychiatry.* 1998;55(9):801–808.

31. Fava M, Rush AJ, Alpert JE, et al. What clinical and symptom features and comorbid disorders characterize outpaitents with anxious major depressive disorder. *Can J Psychiatry.* 2006;51(13):823–835.

32. Fawcett J. Predictors of early suicide: identification and appropriate intervention. *J Clin Psychiatry.* 1988;49(10 suppl):7–8.

33. Edmondson D, Kronish IM, Shaffer JA, et al. Posttraumatic stress disorder and the risk of coronary heart disease: A meta-analytic review. *Am Heart J.* 2012;166(5):806–814.

34. Hameed U, Schwartz T, Malhotra K, West R, Bertone F. Antidepressant treatment in the primary care office: Outcomes for adjustment disorder versus major depression. *Ann Clin Psychiatry.* 2004;17(2):77–81.

35. Williams BR, Sawyer Baker P, Allman RM, et al. Bereavement among African American and white older adults. *J Aging and Health.* 2007;19(2):313–333.

36. Kersting A, Brahler E, Glaesmer J, et al. Prevalence of complicated grief in a representative population-based sample. *J Affective Disorders.* 2011;131:339–343.

37. Shear MK, Ghesquiere A, Glickman K. Bereavement and complicated grief. *Curr Psychiatry Rep.* 2013;15:406.

38. Jacobsen JC, Zhang B, Block SD, et al. Distinguishing symptoms of grief and depression in a cohort of advanced cancer patients. *Death Studies.* 2010:34(3):257–273.

39. DSM-5 American Psychiatric Association. *Diagnostic and Statistical Manual of Mental Disorders.* 5th ed. Washington, DC: American Psychiatric Association; 2013.

40. Sonino N, Fava GA. Psychiatric disorders associated with Cushing's syndrome. Epidemiology, pathophysiology and treatment. *CNS Drugs.* 2001;15(5):361–373.

41. El Yazaji M, Battas O, Agoub M, et al. Validity of the depressive dimension extracted from principal component analysis of the PANSS in drug-free patients with schizophrenia. *Schizophr Res.* 2002;56(1–2):121–127.

42. Kim SW, Kim SJ, Yoon BH, et al. Diagnostic validity of assessment scales for depression in patients with schizophrenia. *Psychiatry Research.* 2006;144(1):57–63.

43. Lako IM, Bruggeman R, Knegtering H, et al. A systematic review of instruments to measure depressive symptoms in patients with schizophrenia. *J Affect Disord.* 2012;140(1):38–47.

44. Hirschfeld RM, Williams JB, Spitzer RL, et al. Development and validation of a screening instrument for bipolar spectrum disorder: the Mood Disorder Questionnaire. *Am J Psychiatry.* 2000; 157:1873–1875.

45. Endicott J. Measurement of depression in patients with cancer. *Cancer.* 1984;53(10 Suppl):2243–2249.

46. Katon W. Epidemiology and treatment of depression in patients with chronic medical illness. *Dialogues Clin Neurosci.* 2011;13(1):7–23.

47. Goldman LS, Nielsen NH, Champion HC. Awareness, diagnosis, and treatment of depression. *J Gen Intern Med.* 1999;14(9):569–580.

48. Koenig HG, George LK, Peterson BL, Pieper CF. Depression in medically ill hospitalized older adults: prevalence, characteristics, and course of symptoms according to six diagnostic schemes. *Am J Psychiatry.* 1997;154(10):1376–1383.

49. Robinson RG, Rama Krishnan KR. *Depression and the Medically ill. Neuropsychopharmacology: The Fifth Generation of Progress.* In: Davis KL, Charney D, Coyle JT, Nemeroff C, eds. Chapter 81. American College of Neuropsychopharmacology; 2002.

50. Kerr LK, Kerr LD. Screening tools for depression in primary care: The effects of culture, gender, and somatic symptoms on the detection of depression. *West J Med.* 2001;175(5):349–352.

51. Reddy MS. Depression: The disorder and the burden. *Indian J Psychol Med.* 2010;32(1):1–2.

52. Beck AT, Steer RA. Internal consistencies of the original and revised beck depression inventory. *J Clin Psychol.* 1984;40(6):1365–1367.

53. Kroenke K, Spitzer RL, Williams JB. The PHQ-9: validity of a brief depression severity measure. *J Gen Intern Med.* 2001;16(9):606–613.

54. Gehi A, Haas D, Pipkin S, Whooley MA. Depression and medication adherence in outpatients with coronary heart disease: findings from the Heart and Soul Study. *Arch Intern Med.* 2005;165:2508–2513.

55. DiMatteo MR, Lepper HS, Croghan TW. Depression is a risk factor for noncompliance with medical treatment: meta-analysis of the effects of anxiety and depression on patient adherence. *Arch Intern Med.* 2000;160(14):2101–2107.

56. Gonzalez JS, Safren SA, Cagliero E, et al. Depression, self-care, and medication adherence in type 2 diabetes. Relationships across the full range of symptom severity. *Diabetes Care.* 2007;30(9):2222–2227.

57. Ciechanowski P, Russo J, Katon W, et al. Influence of patient attachment style on self-care and outcomes in diabetes. *Psychosom Med.* 2004;66:720–728.

58. Simon GE, VonKorff M, Barlow W. Health care costs of primary care patients with recognized depression. *Arch Gen Psychiatry.* 1995;52(10):850–856.

59. Wells KB, Stewart A, Hays RD, et al. The functioning and well-being of depressed patients: results from the Medical Outcomes Study. *J Am Med Assoc.* 1989;262:914–919.

60. Katon W, Sullivan M, Walker E. Medical symptoms without identified pathology: relationship to psychiatric disorders, childhood

and adult trauma, and personality traits. *Ann Intern med.* 2001; 134(9 Pt 2):917–925.

61. Chang CK, Hayes RD, Perera G, et al. Life expectancy at birth for people with serious mental illness and other major disorders from a secondary mental health care case register in London. *PLoS ONE.* 2011;6(5):e19590.

62. Newcomer JW, Hennekens CH. Severe mental illness and risk of cardiovascular disease. *JAMA.* 2007;298(15):1794–1796.

63. Van der Kooy K, van Hout H, Marwijk H, Marten H, Stehouwer C, Beekman A. Depression and the risk for cardiovascular diseases: systematic review and metaanalysis. *Int J Geriatr Psychiatry.* 2007;22:613–626.

64. van Melle JP, de Jonge P, Spijkerman TA, et al. Prognostic association of depression following myocardial infarction with mortality and cardiovascular events: a meta-analysis. *Psychosom Med.* 2004;66(6):814–822.

65. Junger J, Schellberg D, Muller-Tasch T, et al. Depression increasingly predicts mortality in the course of congestive heart failure. *Eur J Heart Fail.* 2005;7(2):261–267.

66. Zhang X, Norris SL, Gregg EW, Cheng YJ, Beckles G, Kahn HS. Depressive symptoms and mortality among persons with and without diabetes. *Am J Epidemiol.* 2005;161(7):652–660.

67. Dobkin RD, Troster AI, Rubino JT, et al. Neuropsychological outcomes after psychosocial intervention for depression in Parkinson's disease. *J Neuropsychiatry Clin Neurosci.* 2014;26:57–63.

68. Simon GE, Von Korff M, Lin E. Clinical and functional outcomes of depression treatment in patients with and without chronic medical illness. *Psychol Med.* 2005;35(2):271–279.

69. Katon W, Unutzer J, Fan MY, et al. Cost-effectiveness and net benefit of enhanced treatment of depression for older adults with diabetes and depression. *Diabetes Care.* 2006;29: 265–270.

70. Katon WJ, Russo JE, Von Korff M, Lin EH, Ludman E, Cichanowski PS. Long-term effects on medical costs of improving depression outcomes in patients with depression and diabetes. *Diabetes Care.* 2008;31:1155–1159.

71. Barabási AL, Gulbahce N, Loscalzo J. Network medicine: a network-based approach to human disease. *Nat Rev Genet.* 2011;12(1):56–68.

72. Patton S. Long-term medical conditions and major depression in a Canadian population study at waves 1 and 2. *J Affect Disord.* 2001;63:35–41.

73. Aben I, Verhey F, Strik J, Lousberg R, Lodder J, Honig A. A comparative study into the one year cumulative incidence of depression after stroke and myocardial infarction. *J Neurol Neurosurg Psychiatry.* 2003;74:581–585.

74. Capuron L, Neurauter G, Musselman DL, et al. Interferon-alpha–induced changes in tryptophan metabolism: Relationship to depression and paroxetine treatment. *Biol Psychiatry.* 2003;54: 906–914.

75. Champaneri S, Wand GS, Malhotra SS, Casagrande SS, Golden SH. Biological basis of depression in adults with diabetes. *Curr Diab Rep.* 2010;10:396–405.

76. Nef HM, Möllmann H, Akashi YJ, Hamm CW. Mechanisms of stress (Takotsubo) cardiomyopathy. *Nat Rev Cardiol.* 2010;7(4): 187–193.

77. Szardien S, Möllmann H, Willmer M, Akashi YJ, Hamm CW, Nef HM. Mechanisms of stress (takotsubo) cardiomyopathy. *Heart Fail Clin.* 2013;9(2):197–205.

78. Rubin RT. Psychoendocrinology of major depression. *Eur Arch Psychiatry Neurol Sci.* 1989;238:259–267.

79. Gold PW, Chrousos GP. Organization of the Stress System and its dysregulation in melancholic and atypical depression. *Mol Psychiatry.* 2002;7:254–275.

80. Rush AJ, Giles DE, Schlesser MA, et al. The dexamethasone suppression test in patients with mood disorders. *J Clin Psychiatry.* 1996;10:471–485.

81. Coryell W, Schlesser MA. The dexamethasone suppression test and suicide prediction. *Am J Psych.* 2001;158:748–753.

82. Cleare AJ, Murray RM, O'Keane V. Reduced prolactin and cortisol responses to D-fenfluramine in depressed compared to healthy matched control subjects. *Neuropsychopharmacology.* 1996;14:349–354.

83. Lee BH, Kim YK. Potential peripheral biologic predictors of suicidal behavior in major depressive disorder. *Prog Neuropsychopharmacol Biol Psychiatry.* 2011;35:842–847.

84. Arana GW, Zarzar MN, Baker E. The effect of diagnostic methodology on the sensitivity of the TRH stimulation test for depression. *Biol Psychiatry.* 1990;733–737.

85. Raison CL, Miller AH. Is Depression an inflammatory disorder? *Curr Psychiatry Rep.* 2011;13:467–475.

86. Dowlati Y, Herrmann N, Swardfager W, et al. A meta-analysis of cytokines in major depression. *Biol Psychiatry.* 2010;67:446–457.

87. Maes M, Bosmans E, De Jongh R, et al. Increased IL-6 and IL-1 receptor antagonist concentrations in major depression and treatment resistant depression. *Cytokine.* 1997;9:853–858.

88. Howren MB, Lamkin DM, Suls J. Associations of depression with C-reactive protein, IL-1, and IL-6: a meta-analysis. *Psychosom Med.* 2009;71:171–186.

89. Schmidt HD, Shelton RC, Duman RS. Functional biomarkers of depression: Diagnosis, treatment, and pathophysiology. *Neuropsychopharmacology.* 2011;36:2375–2394.

CHAPTER 2

The Neurobiology of Depression: An Integrated Systems-Level, Cellular–Molecular and Genetic Overview

David Perez, MD

Mark Eldaief, MD

Jane Epstein, MD

David Silbersweig, MD

Emily Stern, MD

INTRODUCTION

Depression is a highly prevalent and disabling mental illness characterized primarily by abnormalities of mood, cognition and behavior. Individuals with major depression frequently experience anhedonia, depressed mood, negative self-referential thinking, impaired concentration, suicidal ideation, abnormal psychomotor activity, and variable changes in appetite and sleep. Major depression is among the most studied idiopathic psychiatric conditions, with an increasingly well-understood neurobiology. These insights are a pre-requisite to the development of more targeted therapeutic strategies, and can be helpful in understanding this disorder in the context of medical illness.

In this chapter, an overview of the neurocircuits frequently implicated in mood disorders is first detailed to allow for a systems-level conceptualization of brain-behavior relationships in depression.[1] This is followed by a discussion of *in vivo* human structural, neurochemical and functional neuroimaging findings and postmortem brain abnormalities in depressed subjects. Neuroendocrine, inflammatory, neurotransmitter, cellular–molecular and genetic–epigenetic disturbances associated with depression are also summarized to provide a comprehensive multi-level understanding of this illness. The frequently encountered clinical and neurobiological intersection of depression and anxiety is discussed in **Box 2-1**. It should also be noted that the neural circuits discussed in this chapter are the same distributed brain regions frequently implicated in mood related symptoms as a consequence of medical and neurological conditions discussed elsewhere in this book. Throughout the chapter, the term "depression" will be used synonymously with major depressive disorder, unless otherwise specified, though it is relevant to highlight that a dimensional, symptom-oriented approach is increasingly being taken across traditional diagnostic boundaries.

OVERVIEW OF NEUROCIRCUITS OF PARTICULAR RELEVANCE TO MOOD DISORDERS

■ PREFRONTAL–STRIATAL–THALAMO-CORTICAL CIRCUITS

The human prefrontal cortex, anterior to the primary motor cortex, plays critical roles in many of the complex affective, cognitive, and behavioral functions (and dysfunctions) important in the neurobiology of mood disorders. From a structural perspective, the prefrontal cortex is organized into five distinct prefrontal–subcortical circuits. Cortically, these five distinct circuits include: (1) primary motor/premotor/supplementary motor; (2) oculomotor; (3) dorsolateral prefrontal cortex (dlPFC); (4) anterior cingulate cortex (ACC); (5) orbitofrontal cortex (OFC).[2] Each of these regions has distinct, parallel connections to the caudate-putamen (striatum), which in-turn projects to the globus pallidus and specific thalamic nuclei. Afferent connections from discrete thalamic nuclei project back to the same prefrontal cortical region. While these cortical–subcortical–cortical circuits have distinct motor–cognitive–affective–behavioral functions, the subcortical components of each of these circuits are implicated in the automaticity of these distinct functions.

Of particular importance for psychiatry are the three nonmotor prefrontal–subcortical circuits originating from the ACC, OFC, and dlPFC (**Fig. 2-1**).[3] The ACC, a paralimbic cortical structure, and its subcortical connections are implicated in motivated behavior, conflict monitoring, cognitive control, and affective regulation. Regions

BOX 2-1
THE INTERSECTION OF DEPRESSION AND ANXIETY

Depression is frequently comorbid with anxiety which includes generalized anxiety disorder, social phobia, posttraumatic stress disorder, and panic disorder among other disorders.[185,186] From a dimensional perspective, this overlap may be referred to as an anxious depression. High trait anxiety and neuroticism have been shown to be risk factors for the development of depression,[187] and depressed individuals show enhanced fear learning.[188] From a systems-level perspective, neuroimaging research studies have started investigating brain–behavior relationships in individuals with anxious depression compared to nonanxious depressed individuals. For example, during an emotional conflict identification task that involved categorizing emotionally valenced faces while ignoring overlaid emotional words, depressed patients with and without comorbid generalized anxiety disorder similarly demonstrated impaired ventral anterior cingulate and amygdala activations and connectivity on functional magnetic resonance imaging (fMRI); depressed only individuals, however, showed additional recruitment of lateral prefrontal regions that positively associated with task performance.[189] Resting-state functional connectivity analyses in a cohort of individuals with late-life anxious depression compared to nonanxious depressed subjects showed increased coupling of posterior Default Mode Network (DMN) regions and decreased coupling of anterior DMN in anxious depressed subjects.[190] Structural analyses in a large group of patients with nonanxious depression, mixed anxiety disorders, and anxious depression demonstrated similar rostral anterior cingulate cortex gray matter volume reductions across all patient groups compared to healthy subjects.[191] Electrophysiology studies including electroencephalography (EEG) have also been used to study brain differences in depressed individuals with and without anxiety[192]; for example, a quantitative EEG study showed right-lateralized hemispheric activation differences in patients with anxious depression compared to depressed subjects.[193] From a neuroendocrine perspective, subjects with anxious depression exhibited attenuated adrenocorticotropic hormone (ACTH) and cortisol secretion following CRH challenge compared to mixed depressed-bipolar disorder and healthy subject cohorts.[194] Anxious depressed individuals have also demonstrated impaired cortisol suppression following dexamethasone challenge.[195] Early-stage genetic investigations implicate some convergent and interrelated neurochemical and cellular–molecular pathways in the neurobiology of depression and anxious depression. For example, less robust antidepressant treatment response has been associated with anxious depressed individuals carrying the short allele of the serotonin-transporter–linked promotor region (5-HTTLPR)[196] Genes that regulate the CRH system and BDNF have also been linked to antidepressant treatment response in anxious depressed individuals.[197,198] In summary, depression and anxiety symptoms are frequently clinically interrelated and early neurobiological investigations suggest neurocircuit, cellular–molecular and genetic level relationships that warrant further research inquiry.

of the ACC located subgenually and rostral to the genu of the corpus callosum have been implicated in emotion regulation, while more dorsal regions are involved in cognitive functions and behavioral expression of emotional states.[4,5] An important cognitive function of the dorsal ACC is the ability to engage in aspects of *cognitive control*—the ability to pursue and regulate goal-oriented behavior. ACC–subcortical connections include the nucleus accumbens/ventromedial caudate, ventral globus pallidus, and ventral aspects of the magnocellular mediodorsal and ventral anterior thalamic nuclei. Deficit syndromes linked to the ACC–subcortical circuits include the

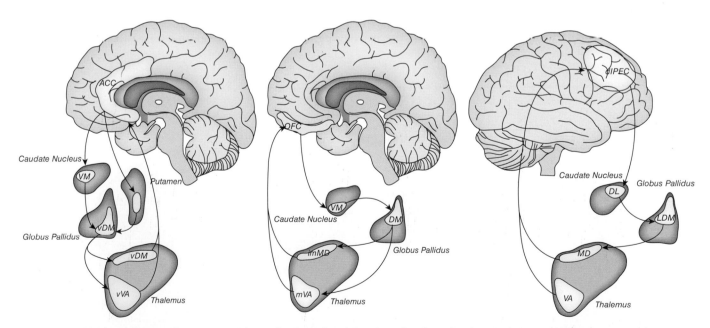

Figure 2-1 *Graphic depiction of anterior cingulate, orbitofrontal and dorsolateral prefrontal–subcortical circuits. ACC, anterior cingulate cortex; OFC, orbitofrontal cortex; dlPFC, dorsolateral prefrontal cortex; VM, ventromedial; vDM, ventral portion of dorsomedial thalamic nucleus; vVA, ventral portion of ventral anterior thalamic nucleus; DM, dorsomedial; imDM, inferomedial portion of mediodorsal thalamic nucleus; mVA, medial portion of ventral anterior thalamic nucleus; DL, dorsolateral; LDM, lateral dorsomedial; MD, mediodorsal; VA, ventral anterior. (Adapted with permission from Perez DL, Catenaccio E, Epstein J: Confusion, hyperactive delirium, and secondary mania in right hemispheric strokes: A focused review of neuroanatomical correlates,* J Neurol Neurophysiol *2011; Special Issue 1.)*

spectrum of amotivational syndromes (apathy, abulia, akinetic mutism), and cognitive impairments, including poor response inhibition, error detection and goal-directed behavior.

The OFC–subcortical circuit is implicated in socially appropriate and empathic behavior, reward-based decision making, mental flexibility, response inhibition, and emotion regulation. Similar to the regional functional specificity described for the ACC, the OFC has functional specificity along its anterior–posterior and medial–lateral axes. The medial OFC has been primarily linked to behavioral responses in the context of viscerosomatic processing, while more lateral regions mediate more external, sensory evaluations.[6] The posterior OFC is particularly important for emotion regulation. The OFC–subcortical connections include the ventromedial caudate, mediodorsal aspects of the globus pallidus interna, and the medial ventral anterior and inferomedial aspects of the magnocellular mediodorsal thalamus. OFC dysfunction, depicted in the classic personality change experienced by Phineas Gage following injury of his left medial prefrontal cortex by a metal rod in a construction accident,[7] is associated with impulsivity, disinhibition, socially inappropriate behavior, and mental inflexibility.

The dlPFC–subcortical circuit is principally involved in attentional and higher-order cognitive executive functions. Executive functions include the ability to shift sets, organization, planning, cognitive control, and working memory. Shifting sets is related to mental flexibility and consists of the ability to move between different concepts or motor plans, or the ability to shift between different aspects of the same or related concept. Working memory is the on-line maintenance and manipulation of information. The dlPFC–subcortical circuit consists of the dorsolateral head of the caudate, lateral mediodorsal globus pallidus interna, and the parvocellular aspects of the mediodorsal and ventral anterior thalamic nuclei. Dysfunction in this circuit has been linked to environmental dependence syndromes (including utilization and imitation behavior), poor organization and planning, mental inflexibility, and working memory deficits.

From a general perspective, these affective, cognitive and behavioral prefrontal–subcortical connections are closed circuits; the subcortical components are thought to be nonoverlapping across the distinct circuits in the healthy brain. Interactions across the circuits are critical for integrated brain function and occur at the cortico-cortical level (**Fig. 2-2**).[8] Reciprocal connections exist between the dlPFC–ACC and between the ACC–OFC. Given these connectivity patterns, the anterior aspects of the dorsal ACC are theorized as an integrative zone for cognitive-emotional processing.

■ FRONTO-AMYGDALAR CIRCUITS

In addition to cortical–basal ganglia–thalamic circuits, fronto-amygdalar connections are important in the neurobiology of mood. The amygdala, an almond-shaped structure in the medial aspect of the temporal lobe anterior to the hippocampus, is a critical brain region for emotional processing and affectively driven memories, fear-based behaviors, arousal, and salience determinations.[9] Bilateral amygdala lesions, as seen in the Kluver Bucy syndrome, result in loss of appropriate behavioral responses to potential threats and indiscriminate consummatory behaviors. The amygdala is composed of discrete nuclei (**Fig. 2-3**). The lateral and basal nuclei are the main sites receiving afferents from sensory cortices, heteromodal association cortices, the hippocampal–entorhinal cortex, and regulatory prefrontal regions. The central nucleus is the principal output nucleus and has efferent connections with the hypothalamus, periaqueductal gray and brainstem monoamine neurotransmitter systems among other regions. A major amygdala outflow tract is the bed nucleus of the stria terminalis. The efferent connectivity pattern of the amygdala enables activation of the fight-or-flight response in response to motivationally salient stimuli. Amygdala outflow is regulated, in part, by the prefrontal cortex. Medial prefrontal cortices, including the ACC and OFC, have reciprocal connections with the amygdala and are important in the inhibitory regulation of amygdalar function. Disruption of prefrontal efferents projecting to the amygdala result in unregulated amygdalar activity (impaired top-down inhibition) and subsequent heightened affective symptoms and emotional responses. The amygdala also interacts with the prefrontal–subcortical circuits through its connections with the mediodorsal nucleus of the thalamus.

■ CIRCUITS INVOLVING THE HIPPOCAMPAL FORMATION

Posterior to the amygdala in the medial temporal lobe lies the hippocampus and related entorhinal cortex and parahippocampus. The hippocampus is a critical node in the cortical–hippocampal system for declarative forms of memory, including episodic (biographical) and semantic (factual) subtypes.[10] Damage to this region, as seen in Alzheimer disease, results in deficits in the encoding of new information. The hippocampus, parahippocampus, and neocortical association areas comprise three critical components of this circuit. Cortical regions, including the ventromedial prefrontal cortex, anterior and posterior cingulate, dlPFC, posterior parietal and temporal cortices send afferent projections to the parahippocampus, providing cognitive, affective, motor and/or perceptual information. The

Cortico-Limbic Connectivity

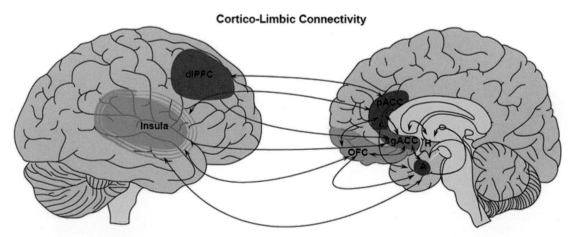

Figure 2-2 *Graphic depiction of frontolimbic neurocircuitry. Reciprocal connections are outlined among the perigenual anterior cingulate cortex (pACC), subgenual ACC (sgACC), orbitofrontal cortex (OFC), dorsolateral prefrontal cortex (dlPFC), insula, amygdala (A), and hypothalamus (H). Adapted with permission from Perez DL, Barsky AJ, Daffner K, et al. Motor and somatosensory conversion disorder: a functional unawareness syndrome? J Neuropsychiatry Clin Neurosci. 2012 Spring;24(2):141–151.*

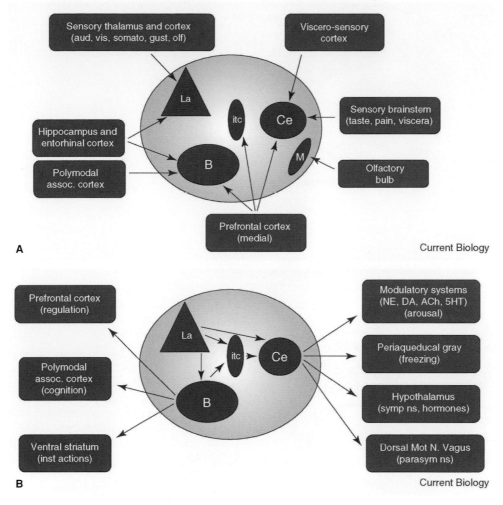

Figure 2-3 *A and B: Panel A:* inputs into specific amygdala nuclei. *Panel B:* outputs from the amygdala. B, basal nucleus; Ce, central nucleus; ict, intercalated cells; La, lateral nucleus; M, medial nucleus; aud, auditory; vis, visual; somato, somatosensory; gust, gustatory; olf, olfactory; assoc, association; NE, norepinephrine, DA, dopamine, Ach, acetylcholine; 5-HT, serotonin; parasym ns, parasympathetic nervous system; symp ns, sympathetic nervous system; inst, instinctual. (Reproduced with permission from LeDoux J. The amygdala. Curr Biol. 2007;17(20):R868–R874.)

parahippocampus in this capacity serves as a convergent site for cortical information, and subsequently projects to the hippocampus, where individual elements of memory are linked together across cognitive–affective–perceptual–behavioral domains. Reciprocal connections between the hippocampus—parahippocampus, and between the parahippocampus and neocortical regions allows for the cortical storage of this bound information. Additional regions in the declarative memory circuit include the fornix, mammillary bodies, and anterior nuclei of the thalamus (**Fig. 2-4**). As with amygdalar circuits, convergence of the prefrontal–subcortical circuits and the cortical–hippocampal system occurs at the level of the anterior thalamus. Of note, the precuneus has been implicated in retrieval of episodic memory,[11] while the inferior lateral temporal lobes are more strongly associated with semantic memory. Implicit forms of memory, such as procedural memory, involve motor-related cortical–subcortical pathways and the cerebellum.

■ **INSULAR CIRCUITS**

In addition to classic frontolimbic regions, the insula has emerged as an important region for viscerosomatic and emotional processes.[12,13] The insula sits on the inner banks of the lateral sulcus, and its posterior aspect receives viscerosomatic afferents from the thalamus. The posterior insula provides an interoceptive representation of the physiological condition of the body. The mid-insula is considered an integrative zone, in which emotional/motivational information from

ACC, OFC, and amygdalar afferents influences sensory processing. The integration of visceral-somatic, affective, and motivational information converges onto the anterior insula (right > left) which, together with the ACC, has been implicated in emotional awareness.[13] Interestingly, the insula and ACC share large spindle-shaped neurons, termed von Economo neurons, linked to social–emotional cognition.[14]

■ **THE DEFAULT MODE NETWORK**

Disturbances in intra and inter network connectivity of the default mode network (DMN) have also been theorized to play a role in the pathobiology of mood disorders (**Fig. 2-5**).[15] This widely distributed network comprises core regions that include ventral and dorsal medial prefrontal cortex, posterior cingulate cortex/precuneus, inferior parietal lobule, lateral temporal cortex, and the hippocampus. These regions co-activate when individuals are allowed to think in an unrestricted fashion, and co-deactivate when subjects engage in a broad array of cognitively demanding tasks. In addition, functional connectivity MRI analyses have revealed that low-frequency oscillations in the fMRI blood-oxygen-level-dependent (BOLD) signal are robustly correlated among these regions, further underscoring the notion that they form a coherent network (see below). DMN regions overlap with those postulated to serve a role in certain social and emotional functions in healthy individuals. For example, the dorsal medial prefrontal cortex appears to be important to self-referential processing and taking the mental perspective of others.

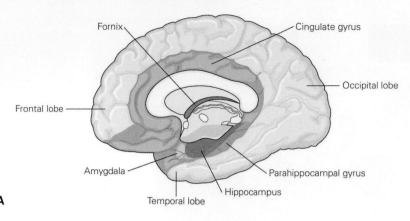

A

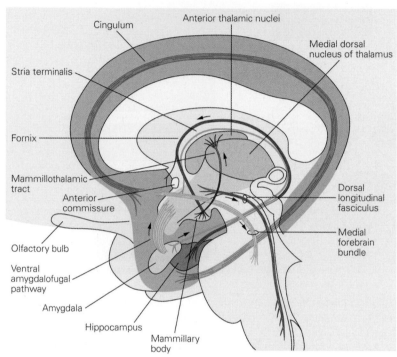

B

Figure 2-4 *The limbic system and related deep-lying structures.* **A:** *Medial brain view showing prefrontal paralimbic cortices and medial temporal lobe structures, including the amygdala and the hippocampus. (Adapted with permission from Damasio AR, Van Hoesen GW. The limbic system and the localisation of herpes simplex encephalitis.* J Neurol Neurosurg Psychiatry. *1985;48(4):297–301.)* **B:** *Interconnections of the deep-lying structures included in the limbic system. The* arrows *indicate the predominant direction of neural activity in each tract, although these tracts are typically bidirectional. (Adapted with permission from Nieuwenhuys R, Voogd J, van Huijzen C. The Human Central Nervous System: A Synopsis and Atlas. 4th ed. Berlin: Springer Verlag; 2008.)*

NEUROIMAGING ABNORMALITIES ASSOCIATED WITH DEPRESSION

Modern neuroimaging methodologies have allowed the *in vivo* examination of brain structure and function. Importantly, these techniques have shed light on important factors contributing to the range of brain disorders, including depression. Brain abnormalities in depressed patients delineated via structural and functional neuroimaging techniques are discussed below,[16] preceded by brief descriptions of the relevant imaging technologies. Postmortem brain abnormalities are also reviewed to contextualize and validate the neuroimaging findings. These abnormalities are interpreted in the context of the neuroanatomy outlined above.

■ STRUCTURAL NEUROIMAGING TECHNIQUES AND FINDINGS

Structural imaging techniques employed in studies of depression include computed tomography (CT), magnetic resonance imaging (MRI), and diffusion tensor imaging (DTI). Brain CT was first made readily available in the 1970s, and this technique uses ionizing radiation to distinguish bodily tissues based on density related differences in radiation attenuation. While particularly beneficial for acute hemorrhage detection, CT scans have limited spatial resolution, and limited ability to delineate subtle soft tissue differences.

MRI scans have significant advantages over CT in spatial resolution, and rely on the physical properties of hydrogen protons in the context of statically and dynamically applied magnetic fields to visualize and differentiate brain tissues (**Fig. 2-6**). The appearance of the brain on MRI is dependent on acquisition parameters, such as echo time (TE) and the time repetition (TR). Commonly acquired MRI sequences include T1, T2 and Fluid Attenuated Inversion Recovery (FLAIR). On T1 sequences, the white matter appears white, and gray matter structures such as the cerebral cortex and brainstem nuclei appear gray. T2 sequences display an inverse pattern of gray-white differentiation. FLAIR-based sequences use an inversion recovery pulse sequence to block cerebrospinal fluid signal and aid detection of periventricular abnormalities. FLAIR/T2 sequences are predominantly used to detect parenchymal abnormalities, while the T1 sequence provides greater anatomic visualization (and regional atrophy characterization). Quantified structural neuroimaging research in psychiatry generally utilizes high-resolution MRI scans. *Manual volumetry* is a technique that combines manual tracing of regions of interest (ROIs) with calculations that estimate cross-sectional volumes. Although readily available, this technique is highly operator dependent and time consuming. *Voxel-based morphometry* (VBM) is an automated technique that deconstructs T1-weighted images into discrete voxels of either gray or white matter. Thereafter, voxel-wise statistical parametric

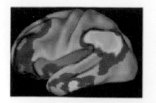
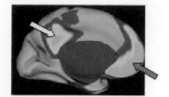
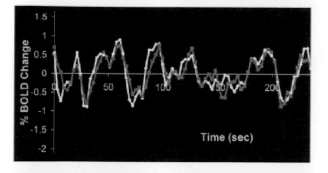
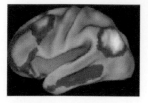
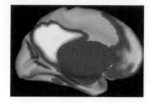

Figure 2-5 *Default mode network (DMN). Performance of a wide variety of tasks leads to decreased activity in broadly distributed regions including dorsal medial prefrontal cortex and posterior cingulate cortex/ precuneus referred to as the DMN (top row). This distributed network can be appreciated by capturing low frequency oscillations in the blood oxygen level dependent (BOLD) signal (middle row). The same regions that deactivate with task increase in activity when subjects allow their mind to freely wander and self-reflect (bottom row). (Reproduced with permission from Raichle ME. Two views of brain function. Trends Cogn Sci. 2010;14(4):180–190.)*

mapping (SPM) techniques are applied across cohorts to detect group differences.[17] Automated techniques have also been developed to specifically measure *cortical gray matter thickness*.[18,19] In addition to comparative volumetric differences, variations in the gyral morphometry may also be studied using statistical techniques.

Structural studies in depression have principally identified frontolimbic and prefrontal–subcortical circuit abnormalities (**Fig. 2-7**). Early MRI studies in depression using manual tracing techniques identified decreased frontal lobe volumes and increased subcortical and periventricular white matter lesions.[20,21] Lesion studies in patients with post-stroke depression (a secondary depression syndrome) suggested a particular association between depressed mood and left anterior frontal lesions.[22]

Hippocampal volume changes have been extensively studied in depression. Compared to healthy subjects, depressed patients exhibited hippocampal volume reductions,[23] and these structural changes have also been described in individuals in the midst of their first depressive episode.[24,25] While not all volumetric studies have cross-sectionally identified hippocampal atrophy in patients with depression, a strong association between total time depressed and hippocampal volume reductions has been reported[26]; a meta-analysis examining clinical predictors of hippocampal volume loss confirmed this finding.[27] In a 3-year longitudinal VBM study, chronically depressed patients exhibited progressive decline in hippocampal volume, with less hippocampal atrophy in remitted patients.[28]

A volumetric tracing study of hippocampal differences in nondepressed individuals with a first-degree relative with major depressive disorder compared to healthy subjects without a family history of depression, identified smaller bilateral hippocampal volumes in patients with a family history of depression and previously reported early-life adversity (abuse).[29] This suggested that hippocampal atrophy may represent a neural mechanism underlying vulnerability to the development of depression.

Amygdalar abnormalities in depression may display a dynamic pattern of volumetric change. Compared to both healthy subjects and patients with recurrent depression, patients in their first depressive episode exhibited enlarged amygdala volumes in an MRI study using volumetric tracing techniques.[30] Parallel amygdala volume increases and hippocampal volume decreases were described in a cohort of women with recent-onset depression.[31] With progressive illness duration, a longitudinal prospective study identified progressive left amygdala gray matter density reductions.[28]

In addition to medial temporal lobe abnormalities, prefrontal–subcortical structural changes have been extensively characterized in depression. Volumetric reductions in the left subgenual ACC were described in young and middle-aged women with depression compared to healthy women using manualized tracing methods,[32] however, this finding has not consistently been replicated.[33,34] Sex differences and illness duration may potentially account for some of this heterogeneity. Depressed men compared to depressed women demonstrated smaller left subgenual ACC volumes,[35] and patients with three or more episodes of untreated depression were more likely to exhibit subgenual ACC volumetric reductions compared to individuals with shorter illness durations.[36] Structural changes have also been reported in other regions of the ACC including gray matter volume reductions in the rostral ACC (using VBM), and an inverse correlation between rostral ACC volume and circulating salivary cortisol levels.[37] The OFC, like the ACC, exhibits volumetric reductions[38] and possible sex differences[39] in depression. In a large cohort of 226 depressed and 144 nondepressed elderly individuals, depressed subjects exhibited smaller OFC volumes using semi-automated tracing methods,[40] and OFC cortical thickness reductions have also been characterized.[41] Of note, late-life (geriatric) depression may have distinct pathophysiology mechanisms compared to idiopathic depression which are discussed below.[42] Caudate-putamen components of the prefrontal–cortical circuits display volumetric reductions in patients with depression.[43,44] Meta-analyses confirmed extensive prefrontal, limbic, and subcortical volumetric reductions in the rostral/pregenual ACC, dlPFC, dorsomedial PFC, OFC, insula, striatum, globus pallidus, thalamus, and hippocampus.[45–47] In addition to these regional abnormalities, enlarged pituitary and adrenal glands have been described in depression.[48,49] Other regions implicated in cognitive-affective processing, such as the cerebellum, have been less well studied and require further investigation.[50]

DTI uses T2-weighted scans and relies on the detection and quantification of the random movement of water. DTI is based on the principal that diffusion within the brain is limited by physical barriers, and the direction-dependent displacement of water molecules (i.e., axonal) is called anisotropy.[51] The anisotropic fraction quantifies white matter microstructural integrity, and decreased fractional anisotropy (FA) is associated with loss of tissue organization (including axonal degeneration, disruption and partial breakdown of cytoarchitecture, or demyelination).

While DTI imaging has been under-utilized in depression research to date, several studies have characterized prefrontal and striatal white matter abnormalities.[52,53] In a meta-analysis of 231 patients with depression and 261 healthy subjects, decreased FA was observed in the bilateral frontal, right fusiform and right occipital white matter in depressed subjects. The fiber tracts implicated in these regions included interhemispheric fibers from the genu and

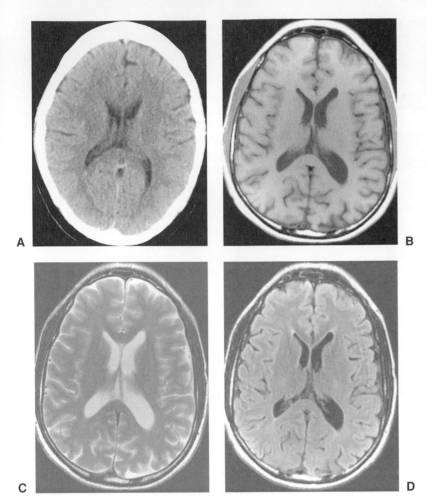

Figure 2-6 *Brain computed tomography (CT) and magnetic resonance imaging (MRI) scans.* **A:** *Axial non-contrast head CT.* **B:** *T1 MRI sequence.* **C:** *T2 MRI sequence.* **D:** *Fluid attenuated inversion recovery (FLAIR) sequence.*

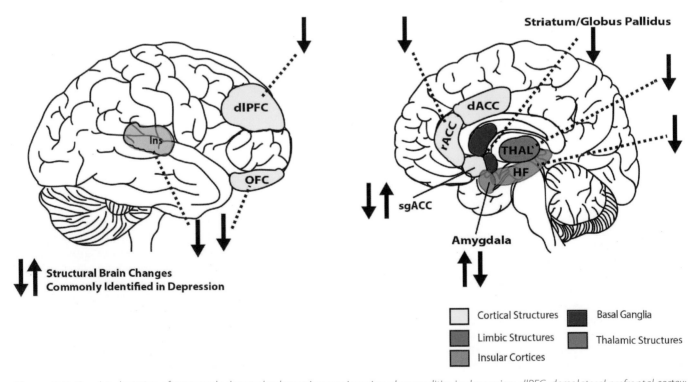

Figure 2-7 *Graphic depiction of commonly detected volumetric neuroimaging abnormalities in depression. dlPFC, dorsolateral prefrontal cortex; Ins, insula; OFC, orbitofrontal cortex; ACC, anterior cingulate cortex, d, dorsal; r, rostral; sg, subgenual; THAL, thalamus; HF, hippocampal formation. (Used with permission from David Vago PhD.)*

body of the corpus callosum, right inferior longitudinal fasciculus, and right inferior fronto-occipital fasciculus. Disruption of dlPFC-related white matter tracts have also been reported,[54] including decreased FA in mediodorsal thalamus to dlPFC pathways.[55]

Postmortem studies of depressed patients compared to matched controls revealed frontolimbic cellular abnormalities consistent with in vivo structural MRI findings. Patients with familial forms of depression exhibited reduced glial cell counts in the subgenual ACC.[56] A similar glial cell density and neuronal size reduction in the dorsal (supracallosal) ACC was found in mixed familial and nonfamilial depressed patients compared to schizophrenia, bipolar disorder, and nonpsychiatric controls.[57] In addition to glial abnormalities, layer VI pyramidal neurons in the ACC showed decreased dendritic arborization in depressed patients who died of suicide compared to controls.[58] In a specific postmortem analysis of the left prefrontal cortex, depressed subjects compared to psychiatrically healthy subjects exhibited rostral OFC reductions in cortical thickness, neuronal size, and neuronal and glial densities.[59] In addition, glial density was reduced in the caudal OFC and neuronal size and glial cell counts were reduced in the dlPFC. These glial and neuronal dlPFC abnormalities have also been replicated.[60] Left hemisphere lateralized total glial and oligodendrocyte density reductions in the amygdala have also been characterized,[61,62] as have hippocampal neuronal cell count abnormalities, particularly in the dentate gyrus.[63]

■ MAGNETIC RESONANCE SPECTROSCOPY AND FINDINGS

Magnetic resonance spectroscopy (MRS) is an MR technique that measures the average amount of distinct metabolites in a given region of brain tissue. MRS detects and quantifies molecular signals based on their magnetic resonance properties. This technique takes into account the effect of the local chemical environment on particular nuclei. Commonly detected metabolites include: N-acetyl aspartate (NAA)—a marker of neuronal integrity; choline (Cho)—an indicator of cell membrane synthesis; creatine (Cr)—a marker of cellular energy metabolism. In addition, glutamate-related metabolites (including glutamate and glutamine) can be quantified separately or as a composite (termed Glx). Gamma-amino butyric acid (GABA).[64] concentrations can also be measured.

MRS has detected abnormal glutamate, GABA and choline concentrations in depression. Decreased Glx (glutamate/glutamine) concentrations were noted in the dorsomedial/dorsal anterolateral and ventromedial prefrontal cortices in patients with depression compared to healthy controls.[65] GABA levels were also reduced in the dorsomedial/dorsal anterolateral prefrontal cortex. Studies have similarly characterized decreased ACC, amygdala, and hippocampal Glx in depression.[64] A meta-analysis of glutamate MRS abnormalities in depression found a consistent decrease in Glx and glutamate concentrations in the ACC.[66] Apart from excitatory and inhibitory neurotransmitter abnormalities, depression has been associated with basal ganglia Cho/Cr increases.[67] This finding suggests possible glial dysfunction or increased membrane turnover in depression.

■ FUNCTIONAL NEUROIMAGING TECHNIQUES AND FINDINGS

Single proton emission computed tomography (SPECT), positron emission tomography (PET), and functional MRI (fMRI) have been used to study primary and secondary depressive syndromes. SPECT detects gamma rays and measures regional cerebral blood flow (rCBF), an indirect measure of neuronal activity. Commonly injected tracers include 99mTc-hexamethyl-propylene-amine-oxime (99mTc-HMPAO) and 99mTc-ethyl cysteinate dimer (99mTc-ECD). These lipophilic tracers cross the cell membrane and remain intracellular following conversion to hydrophilic compounds. Their incorporation is proportional to rCBF in the first few minutes after injection, and subsequent blood flow modifications do not alter initial tracer distribution.[68] SPECT tracers have longer half-lives and are less expensive to manufacture than those used in PET. The limitations of SPECT include exposure to ionizing radiation and relatively limited spatial resolution, although technical advancements, including coregistration of rCBF images onto MRI scans rather than CT images have improved spatial resolution.

Brain PET imaging detects paired gamma rays emitted at 180 degrees from a given brain region and has improved spatial resolution compared to SPECT. There are several radionuclides commonly used including: carbon-11, nitrogen-13, oxygen-15, and fluorine-18. Fluorine-18 has the longest half-life and fluorodeoxyglucose (18F-FDG), an analog of glucose labeled with fluorine-18, is commonly used as a marker of regional brain metabolic activity. PET can also utilize antibody-radionuclide compounds to determine the distribution of particular brain molecules, and ligand-radionuclide compounds can measure the distribution of neurotransmitter receptors. These techniques have aided researchers in elucidating the in vivo neurochemistry of depression.

BOLD fMRI is a noninvasive, nonradiation-based neuroimaging technique that relies on the inherent magnetic properties of hemoglobin to provide a proxy for neuronal activity. Oxy- (diamagnetic) and de-oxy (paramagnetic) hemoglobin have distinct magnetic properties. Regional brain activity is associated with local vasodilation and increases in oxygenated venous blood concentration. Increases in oxy-hemoglobin due to elevated neural demands for oxygen and parallel compensatory increases in blood flow that exceed local metabolic requirements lead to elevated BOLD signal.[69] While BOLD fMRI relies on venous blood flow, other methods such as arterial spin labeling (ASL) provide an arterial phase measure of cerebral blood flow with the potential for improved spatial and temporal resolution (currently ASL has diminished signal-to-noise compared to BOLD signal). fMRI provides high spatial resolution brain images, but has relatively poor temporal resolution given its reliance on the hemodynamic response (peaks at 5–6 seconds). fMRI is also highly sensitive to head movements and cardiorespiratory artifacts, and individuals with certain metallic implants are unable to participate in MRI-based imaging. The MRI environment is also loud and confining, and individuals with claustrophobia are typically not studied.

fMRI uses a broad array of paradigm and nonparadigm experimental designs and analysis techniques to probe structure–function relationships in depression. The two most widely used paradigm types include task-based and resting-state neuroimaging studies. Task-based studies serve as a "brain-stress test" to probe the functional integrity of a given circuit or set of circuits through task performances. Examples of this include working memory tasks to probe dlPFC function and the display of affectively valenced words or faces to characterize frontolimbic emotional processing. These functional neuroimaging methods compare task-of-interest activation patterns in patient populations of interest (i.e. depression) compared to those in healthy subjects (or other relevant control cohorts such as nondepressed patients exposed to early life trauma if the depressed patient group also experienced early life trauma) to identify regional differential task-related brain activations. In resting-state neuroimaging studies, no task or induction is employed. Rather, subjects are instructed to allow their mind to freely wander while low-frequency oscillations in BOLD signal are measured.[70] This approach allows for functional connectivity analyses that probe coherent activation patterns within and across neural networks. While such analyses can also be performed with task-based imaging with great utility, their use in the resting state allows for particular investigation of the DMN, a collection of functionally coupled regions that activate during naturalistic "mind wandering" (and self-referential processing) and deactivate during many cognitive and affective tasks.

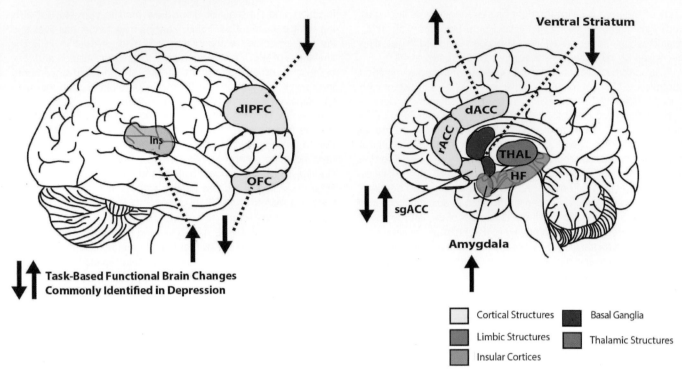

Figure 2-8 *Graphic depiction of commonly detected functional neuroimaging abnormalities in depression. dlPFC, dorsolateral prefrontal cortex; Ins, insula; OFC, orbitofrontal cortex; ACC, anterior cingulate cortex, d, dorsal; r, rostral; sg, subgenual; THAL, thalamus; HF, hippocampal formation. (Used with permission from David Vago PhD.)*

Functional neuroimaging studies in depression using SPECT, PET and fMRI demonstrate abnormal prefrontal cortex, basal ganglia, and medial temporal lobe activations (**Fig. 2-8**). One of the earliest functional brain imaging studies in depression was performed in 1985 using 18F-FDG PET and identified lower glucose metabolic rates in the left frontal cortex and bilateral caudate regions.[71] This left frontal hypoactivation was replicated and refined to the left anterior-medial prefrontal cortex by other early investigations in depression using PET and SPECT.[72,73] From a dimensional symptom perspective, early studies also linked decreased left dlPFC and striatum activations to psychomotor slowing in depression.[74,75]

Increased basal and stimuli-driven amygdala activity has been extensively characterized in depression.[76] Depressed patients with a family history of depression demonstrated increased left amygdala activation in an early PET imaging study, and this pattern of amygdalar hyperactivation was also observed in remitted subjects with a family history of depression.[77] This suggested that enhanced amygdalar activity potentially represented a trait neural biomarker for depressive illness. Subsequent fMRI studies using negative valenced emotional faces and linguistic stimuli delineated both initial elevated amygdala activity and prolonged activation (failed habituation) in patients with depression.[78,79] A number of studies have specifically linked enhanced amygdala activity to the negative attentional bias of information processing in depression. Selective increased amygdala activity to sad facial expressions (compared to happy) was demonstrated in both acutely depressed and remitted patients.[80] Importantly, enhanced amygdala activity to negatively valenced stimuli normalized following selective serotonin reuptake inhibitor (SSRI) treatment.[80,81] In addition to an association with the negative attentional bias of depression, increased amygdalar metabolic activity positively correlated with plasma cortisol levels.[82] This suggested a possible link between elevated amygdalar activity and increased hypothalamic–pituitary–adrenal (HPA) axis function.

Prefrontal cortex dysfunction also plays important roles in depression neurobiology. The subgenual ACC has been implicated in the modulation of negative mood states.[83] Several neuroimaging studies characterized elevated baseline subgenual activation in depression,[84–87] while other investigations have described reduced subgenual activations.[88] The induction of a sad mood state in healthy subjects increased BOLD activity in the subgenual cingulate on fMRI.[89,90] Treatment response to SSRIs, subgenual ACC deep brain stimulation (DBS) and anterior cingulotomy has been linked to pretreatment elevated subgenual ACC activity.[84,86,91] Mayberg et al. have suggested that depression can be potentially defined phenomenologically as "the tendency to enter into, and inability to disengage from, a negative mood state."[92] A key disturbance in depression may not be the experience of a dysphoric mood state itself, but rather the inability to shift out of a negative mood state as if "stuck in a rut." Subgenual ACC dysfunction is theorized to play a critical role in the inability to effectively modulate a negative mood state. Apart from the subgenual ACC, increased pregenual ACC activity has also been demonstrated in depressed subjects.[93,94]

In addition to the ACC, the OFC and dlPFC have exhibited dysfunction in depression. Consistent with OFC lesions linked to increased depression risk, depression severity inversely correlated with medial and posterior-lateral OFC activity in neuroimaging studies.[95,96] PET neuroimaging after induction of sadness with autobiographical memory scripts revealed prominent deactivations in the medial OFC of acute and remitted depressed patients compared to rest conditions and healthy subjects.[97] Given the efferent connections from the OFC to the amygdala, impaired OFC activations may disinhibit amygdalar output (including heighted activity in the bed nucleus of the stria terminalis) in depression. Meanwhile, the dlPFC may potentially exhibit a lateralized dysfunctional activation pattern in depression. While not consistently identified, depressed patients have demonstrated left dlPFC hypoactivity and right dlPFC hyperactivity[98]; left dlPFC hypoactivity was linked to negative emotional judgments, while right dlPFC hyperactivity was associated with attentional deficits. Modulation of the left dlPFC by repetitive transcranial magnetic stimulation (TMS) has been used to treat

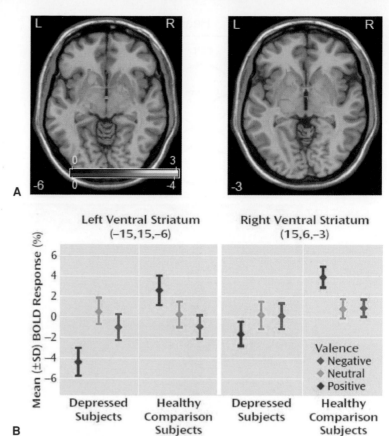

Figure 2-9 *Axial brain images (**A**) and graphs (**B**) showing significant decreased bilateral ventral striatal activations to positive stimuli in depressed versus healthy subjects. Decreased activation was particularly associated with anhedonia, or the inability to experience interest and pleasure. (Reproduced with permission from Epstein J, Pan H, Kocsis JH, et al. Lack of ventral striatal response to positive stimuli in depressed versus normal subjects. Am J Psychiatry. 2006;163(10):1784–1790.)*

depression, and the degree of intrinsic anti-correlated functional connectivity between the targeted dlPFC site and the subgenual ACC may be linked to therapeutic efficacy.[99] Such hemispheric-specific findings raise interesting questions about the importance of laterality in the study of depression circuitry, particularly in light of the fact, described above, that post-stroke depression tends to occur with left prefrontal lesions.

From a symptom-based perspective, decreased ventral striatum/nucleus accumbens activation has been linked to anhedonia. This is relevant in light of this region's role in motivation, reward and reinforcement learning. Depressed patients exposed to positively valenced words in an emotional word fMRI study demonstrated significantly less bilateral ventral striatum activation to positive stimuli compared to healthy subjects; this study also observed a positive correlation between anhedonia and diminished ventral striatum activation (**Fig. 2-9**).[100] This same cohort of patients in a task-based functional connectivity analysis demonstrated increased functional coupling between emotional processing regions (including the ventral striatum) and regions involved in linguistic, sensorimotor and self-referential (DMN) processing (**Fig. 2-10**).[101] The lack of segregation of emotional processing from cognitive and sensorimotor functions potentially represented a systems-level neural substrate for a core phenomenon of depression: the interconnection of affective disturbance with perception, cognition and behavior. Hypoactivation of the ventral striatum/nucleus accumbens in patients with depression has been replicated using affectively valenced autobiographical prompts and a facial viewing task,[102] as well as a monetary incentive reward processing task.[103] Similar to previously discussed amygdala temporal activation abnormalities, the nucleus accumbens exhibited reduced duration of BOLD activation (enhanced habituation) during a cognitive, positive-emotion appraisal task.[104]

Meta-analyses of emotionally valenced task-based functional neuroimaging studies are particularly useful in delineating neuronal dysfunction patterns in depression. An fMRI meta-analysis of negative versus positive stimuli identified increased amygdala, dorsal ACC and insula activity in depressed patients (along with increased superior and middle temporal, and precentral gyri). For positive versus negative stimuli, depressed patients exhibited reduced right striatum and cerebellar uvula activations.[105] In a meta-analysis limited to facial emotion processing studies in depression, negatively valenced facial processing increased amygdala, insula, subgenual ACC, middle cingulate, parahippocampal gyrus and caudate-putamen activations; decreased activation to negatively valenced stimuli was noted in the OFC.[106] In contrast, positively valenced facial processing showed decreased putamen, amygdala, insula, and parahippocampus activations. Facial processing functional connectivity analyses suggest enhanced amygdala–subgenual ACC connectivity, and reduced coupling between the amygdala and regulatory regions, including the dorsal ACC, dlPFC, hippocampus, parahippocampus and insula.

■ ABNORMALITIES IN RESTING-STATE NETWORKS IN DEPRESSION

Increasing interest in resting-state fMRI studies has led to the elucidation of functional connectivity abnormalities in depression. Several studies have reported altered functional connectivity within the DMN, as well as among specific cortico-limbic structures in depressed subjects when compared to match healthy controls. For example, Greicius et al.[107] employed Independent Component Analysis (ICA) to demonstrate that DMN functional connectivity was significantly increased in the subgenual anterior cingulate cortex (sgACC), medial thalamus and OFC in depressed patients, and that increased sgACC connectivity correlated with the duration of depressive episodes. Other groups have used seed-based approaches to show increased functional connectivity within a cortico-limbic circuit anchored at the sgACC and including the insula and ventromedial/orbitofrontal cortex.[108,109] Also, Sheline et al. identified a "dorsal nexus" in the dorsomedial prefrontal cortex which exhibited increased functional connectivity with the DMN,

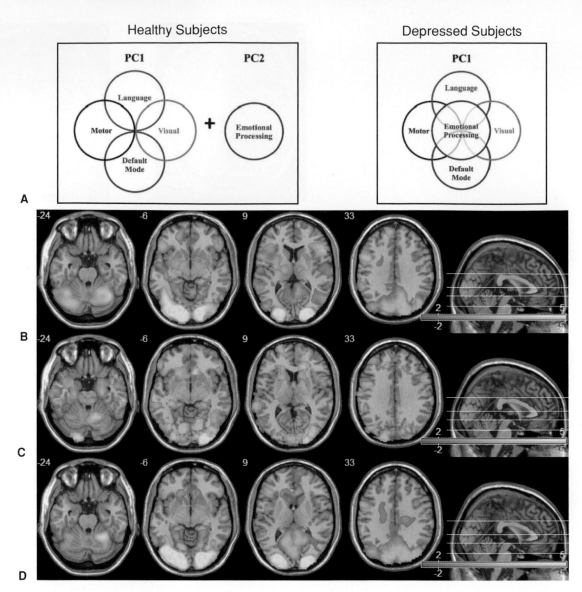

Figure 2-10 *A: Schematic depiction of network connectivity patterns in healthy controls and depressed subjects viewing positive words in a functional magnetic resonance imaging principal component analysis. **B and C:** Principle components 1 and 2 for healthy subjects demonstrating functional connectivity segregation of sensory–linguistic–motor processing regions from emotion processing circuits. **D:** Principle component 1 for depressed subjects demonstrating coherent functional connectivity between sensory–linguistic–motor processing regions and emotion processing circuits. (Reproduced with permission from Epstein J, Perez DL, Ervin K, et al. Failure to segregate emotional processing from cognitive and sensorimotor processing in major depression.* Psychiatry Res. *2011;193(3):144–150.)*

with an affective network, and with a cognitive control network in depressed subjects.[110] It should be noted that whereas functional connectivity abnormalities in the DMN and other cortico-limbic structures have been consistently reported in depression, the directionality of these abnormalities is somewhat inconsistent between studies. Employing graph theoretical metrics, resting-state fMRI data have demonstrated abnormal network metrics in depression, including increased regional homogeneity, increased nodal centrality and connectivity degree, and decreased small-worldness.[111,112] There is also evidence to suggest that successful depression treatment normalizes aberrant connectivity patterns in depression. Placebo controlled studies in healthy subjects and depressed patients have demonstrated rectification of connectivity anomalies seen in depression following the administration of selective serotonin reuptake inhibitors and ketamine.[113–115] As stated earlier, the therapeutic efficacy of TMS is correlated with the extent to which it targets dlPFC regions that are functionally correlated with the sgACC; targeting dlPFC regions that are the most functionally anti-correlated with the

sgACC yield the greatest therapeutic gain.[99] Liston et al. showed that following a 5-week treatment course of TMS to the dlPFC, correlations within the DMN decreased and better approximated correlations observed in matched healthy controls.[116] Interestingly, in that study anti-correlations between the dlPFC stimulation site (a node of the central executive network) increased following a course of TMS, suggesting that inter-network modulation may also play a role in the therapeutic effects of this modality.

■ NEUROIMAGING BIOMARKERS OF TREATMENT RESPONSE AND SUICIDALITY

While neuroimaging studies have made significant progress in delineating neurocircuit abnormalities in depression, a particularly promising convergence between clinical care and psychiatric neuroimaging in depression is the development of neurocircuit biomarkers for treatment response prediction. Early work by Mayberg et al. using FDG-PET reported that baseline hypermetabolism of the rostral ACC predicted treatment response to a mixed-group of antidepressants;

similarly, poor treatment response was predicted by rostral ACC hypometabolism.[117] Structural and functional MRI studies have subsequently demonstrated that treatment response to fluoxetine was predicted by increased gray matter in the pregenual and subgenual ACC, OFC, dlPFC, caudate nucleus and right lateralized temporoparietal regions; greater pregenual ACC activation also predicted faster symptom relief following antidepressant treatment.[118] Rostral ACC hyperactivity, as measured by electroencehalography (EEG) (increased theta), also predicted nortriptyline treatment response.[119] In addition to an association between treatment response and ACC structure–function, larger pretreatment hippocampal volumes have also been associated with improved outcomes.[120] For example, fluoxetine response was predicted by higher baseline right hippocampal volumes in a study comparing female responders to nonresponders[121]; similarly, response to a naturalistically prescribed range of antidepressants was predicted by larger pretreatment bilateral hippocampal body/tail volumes.[122] While predictors of nonpharmacologic treatment response have received less attention, cognitive behavioral therapy efficacy was predicted by low subgenual ACC and high amygdala activity during performance of a fMRI emotional word paradigm,[123] and metabolic activity in the right anterior insula has been identified as a potential treatment selective biomarker to help differentiate CBT and SSRI drug responders.[124]

In addition to biomarkers of treatment response, identifying individuals at-risk for suicidality is a difficult clinical challenge that may be aided by the future use of neuroimaging biomarkers. Studies comparing depressed individuals with and without a history of suicide have frequently, although not exclusively,[125] found reduced prefrontal activity in patients with prior suicide attempts.[126] An fMRI study of remitted depressed patients demonstrated decreased left lateral OFC activation in individuals with prior suicide attempts during high-risk decisions in a gambling task.[127] Volumetric tracings revealed decreased bilateral OFC and increased right amygdala volumes in depressed suicidal patients compared to control groups.[128] Bilateral rostral ACC and caudate, and left dorsal ACC and dlPFC, volumetric reductions have also been reported in depressed patients at high risk for suicide using VBM and cortical thickness analyses.[129,130] Subcortical white matter disruptions using DTI have been observed in depressed patients with prior suicidality.[131] Overall, these studies suggest further decreases in regulatory prefrontal activity in depressed patients at risk for suicide.

■ LATE-LIFE (GERIATRIC) DEPRESSION

Late-life depression (LLD), also known as geriatric depression, is a heterogeneous syndrome encompassing age-related changes in neurological, immune, and endocrine systems.[42,132–134] The "vascular depression" hypothesis suggests that cerebrovascular disease predisposes or perpetuates depressive symptoms in older individuals.[132–134] Clinically, vascular depression is characterized by cognitive (executive) deficits, slowed processing speed/psychomotor retardation, lack of insight, and disability out of proportion to depressive symptoms. Radiographically, cerebrovascular T2/FLAIR white matter hyperintensities from diabetes, hyperlipidemia, cardiac disease, and hypertension have been linked to this condition. Some studies have localized white matter lesions to the prefrontal cortex and temporal lobe, including disturbances in particular fiber tracts (e.g., cingulum bundle, uncinate fasciculus and superior longitudinal fasciculus.[135] LLD with prominent dysexecutive symptoms has been associated with decreased frontoparietal function, poor antidepressant response, and higher relapse rates.[136,137] Mechanistically, frontolimbic disconnection, immune dysregulation (altered neural function in areas mediating cognitive and affective processes in the context of inflammatory states,[138] and cerebrovascular hypoperfusion have been theorized to play synergistic roles in the pathophysiology of LLD.

OVERVIEW OF CELLULAR AND MOLECULAR BIOLOGICAL ABERRATIONS IN DEPRESSION

■ ABNORMALITIES IN MONOAMINERGIC NEUROTRANSMISSION

The neuromodulatory monoamine neurotransmitter systems (serotonin, norepinephrine, dopamine) have long been considered to be critical to the pathogenesis of depression. The "monoamine hypothesis" posits that depression is caused by relative deficiencies in monoamine neurotransmission. This hypothesis was borne out of observations that medications that increase the availability of monoamines in the synaptic cleft (e.g., by inhibiting monoamine reuptake or by preventing their enzymatic degradation) have antidepressant properties, while those that decrease this availability are depressogenic (**Fig. 2-11**). Monoaminergic neurotransmitter systems originate in the brainstem and send widespread projections across the cortical mantle as well as to subcortical gray matter structures. In addition, more recent evidence has emphasized the importance of the downstream intracellular effects of monoamine neurotransmission, particularly those acting upon second messenger systems and upon gene transcription and protein translation.

Serotonin

Central serotonin (5-hydroxytryptamine: 5-HT) plays important roles in cognition, emotion, impulse control, circadian and sleep–wake cycle regulation, and pain modulation among other functions.[139] Disinhibition, inappropriate social behavior, and apathy in frontotemporal dementia have been linked to a serotonergic deficit,[140] and these symptoms may be partially treated with pro-serotonergic medications. Serotonergic neurons are located in the midline brainstem raphe nuclei, including the dorsal raphe nucleus, which provides inputs to the upper brainstem, cerebral hemispheres and basal ganglia (including the substantia nigra and the ventral tegmental area [VTA]) (**Fig. 2-12A–B**). Serotonin is synthesized from L-tryptophan by tryptophan hydroxylase to produce 5-hydroxytryptophan, which is converted by L-amino acid decarboxylase to serotonin. Serotonin is stored in presynaptic vessels, and after its release into the synaptic cleft may be activated through presynaptic serotonin transporter proteins (SERT) or monoamine oxidase A–medlated metabolism. The major therapeutic action of the most widely prescribed class of antidepressants, the serotonin reuptake inhibitors, is mediated by SERT binding.

There are currently 14 different serotonin receptors, with many of these postulated to have roles in mood regulation. These are broadly classified into "5-HT" receptors numbered 1 to 7, with 5-HT1 and 5-HT2 receptors each having several different receptor subtypes. With the exception of 5-HT3 (which is an ion gated ligand channel), serotonin receptors are exclusively G-protein coupled.[141] 5-HT1 can be either pre or postsynaptic, whereas other receptor cell types are characterized by being postsynaptic. 5-HT1A and 5-HT1B receptors can act as presynaptic autoreceptors on serotonergic cells to modulate the release of serotonin, particularly in response to feedback inhibition.[142] The anxiolytic buspirone is thought to act as a selective partial agonist at the 5-HT1A receptor.[143] In contrast, the 5-HT1B receptor (as well as the 5-HT1D receptor) is frequently the target of antimigraine drugs.[141] 5-HT2 receptors typically mediate excitatory postsynaptic responses and have less binding affinity for serotonin than 5-HT1 receptors.[143] Many "typical" and "atypical" anti-psychotics bind to 5-HT2a receptors as well to 5-HT6 and 5-HT7 receptors.

Several studies have supported the importance of serotonin transmission in mood regulation, and a detailed review can be found in Lopez-Munoz and Alamo.[144] Tryptophan depletion induces a relapse of depressive symptoms in depressed subjects but not in healthy controls.[142] Much of the *in vivo* work on serotonergic transmission has utilized PET imaging to study radio-labeled ligand

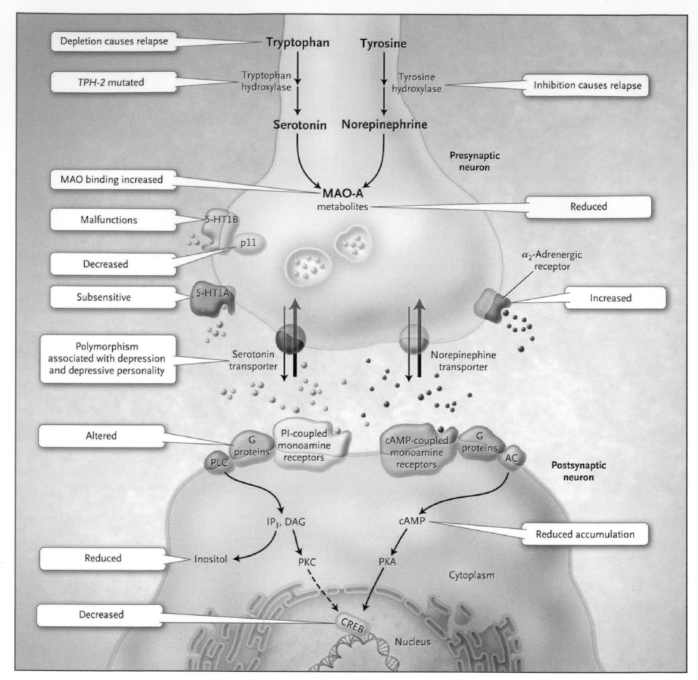

Figure 2-11 *Depiction of the monoamine-deficiency hypothesis at the synaptic level. Monoaminergic neurotransmission is mediated by serotonin or norepinephrine released from presynaptic neurons. Serotonin is synthesized from tryptophan by tryptophan hydroxylase (TPH); norepinephrine is synthesized from tyrosine, catalyzed by tyrosine hydroxylase. Monoamine transmitters are stored in presynaptic vesicles and released into the synaptic cleft. Cessation of the synaptic action of the neurotransmitters occurs through both reuptake transporters as well as feedback control of release through presynaptic 5-HT1A and 5-HT1B regulatory autoreceptors for serotonin and alpha2-noradrenergic receptors for norepinephrine. Monoamine oxidase A (MAO-A) catabolizes monoamines presynaptically. Protein p11 interacts with 5-HT1B receptors and increases their function. Postsynactically, both serotonin and norepinephrine bind to G-protein-coupled receptors: cyclic AMP (cAMP)-coupled receptors activate adenylate cyclase (AC) to generate cAMP, while phosphatidylinositol (PI)-coupled receptors activate phospholipase C (PLC). PLC generates inositol triphosphate (IP₃) and diacylglycerol (DAG). cAMP activates protein kinase A (PKA), while IP₃ and DAG activate protein kinase C (PKC). These two protein kinases affect the cAMP response element–binding-protein (CREB). Findings that support the monoamine-deficiency hypothesis include a relapse of depression with inhibition of tyrosine hydroxylase or depletion of dietary tryptophan, an increased frequency of mutations affecting the brain-specific form of TPH-2, increased specific ligand binding to MAO-A, subsensitive 5-HT1A receptors, 5-HT1B receptor malfunction, decreased p11 levels, polymorphisms in the serotonin-reuptake transporter associated with depression, an inadequate G-protein response to neurotransmitters, and reduced levels of cAMP, inositol and CREB in postmortem brain. (Reproduced with permission from Belmaker RH, Agam G. Major depressive disorder. N Engl J Med. 2008;358(1):55–68.)*

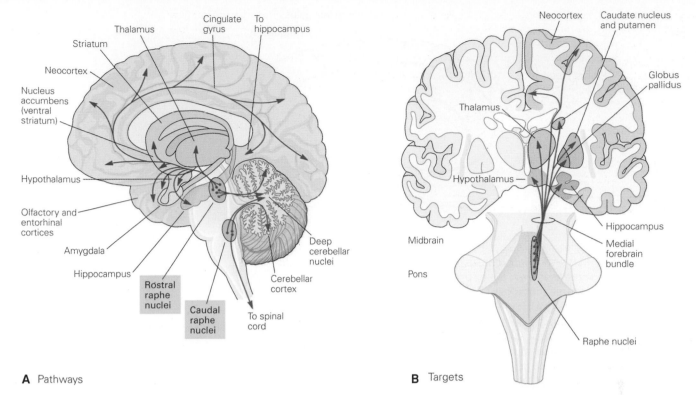

A Pathways

B Targets

Figure 2-12 *The major serotonergic brain systems arise from the raphe nuclei of the brainstem. Serotonin is synthesized in the raphe nuclei, and these neurons project throughout the neuroaxis. The serotonergic projections are the most massive and diffuse of the monoaminergic systems.* ***A:*** *Sagittal view of the raphe nuclei and its afferent connections.* ***B:*** *Coronal view of the serotonergic neurons of the raphe nuclei. (Adapted with permission from Heimer L. The Human Brain and Spinal Cord. 2nd ed. Berlin: Springer-Verlag; 1995.)*

binding.[145] However, while this technique offers significant promise in linking neuronal dysfunction patterns with serotonergic abnormalities, specific reproducible patterns have yet to be well elucidated. For example, both reduced[146] and increased.[147] 5-HT1A receptor binding has been described in limbic and paralimbic brain regions in depressed patients. Abnormalities of the serotonin 2A receptor and serotonin transporter, with variable directionality, have also been characterized.

Dopaminergic neurotransmission has been linked to motivation, the ability to experience pleasure, concentration, and psychomotor speed among other functions.[148,149] The majority of dopaminergic neurons are located in the substantia nigra pars compacta, VTA and the arcuate nucleus of the hypothalamus (**Fig. 2-13**). The nigrostriatal pathway, implicated in motor planning, motor execution and higher-order cognitive functions, consists of dopaminergic projections from the substantia nigra pars compacta in the midbrain to the dorsal striatum. Mesolimbic and mesocortical pathways originate from the VTA, and are important in the pathophysiology of idiopathic psychiatric and neuropsychiatric conditions. The mesocortical pathway mainly projects to prefrontal (particularly the ACC) and temporal (including the entorhinal region) cortices, and mediates attentional and executive functions including working memory. Dopaminergic projections from the VTA to the ventral striatum (including the nucleus accumbens), amygdala, bed nucleus of the stria terminalis, hippocampus and septum comprise the mesolimbic pathways, and serve important roles in reward processing, motivation, and hedonic experiences. Dopamine is synthesized in presynaptic neurons from tyrosine and phenylalanine via, in part, the activity of the rate-limiting enzyme tyrosine hydroxylase. Dopamine receptors are G-protein–coupled receptors divided into two broad groups: D_1 and D_2 families. D_1 receptors activate adenylate cyclase second messenger systems, while the binding of D_2 receptors lowers adenylate cyclase activity. Once released into the synaptic cleft, dopamine may be inactivated through presynaptic dopamine transporter (DAT) reuptake or is enzymatically metabolized via monoamine oxidase (A and B) and catechol-o-methyl transferase (COMT). Using probes for the dopaminergic system with PET, unmedicated depressed subjects with prominent motor retardation demonstrated significantly higher D_2 receptor binding (lower dopamine) in the bilateral putamen compared to healthy controls,[150] while depressed patients taking selective serotonin reuptake inhibitors demonstrated reduced dorsal caudate-putamen D_2 binding.[151] It remains unclear the extent to which these divergent findings are explained by medication effects and other confounds.

The locus ceruleus–norepinephrine system has been implicated in attention, stress response, pain modulation, synaptic plasticity, and arousal among other functions.[152,153] The locus ceruleus is a cluster of neurons containing norepinephrine located in the upper dorsolateral pons (**Fig. 14A–B**). These neurons have extensive afferent projections to the neocortex, hippocampus, cerebellum and thalamus. Norepinephrine, like dopamine, is synthesized from tyrosine. Dopamine is converted to norepinephrine within synaptic vessels by dopamine B-hydroxylase. Inactivation may occur either through reuptake by selective norepinephrine transporters (NET) or monoamine oxidase A and COMT-mediated metabolism. Like other monoamines, norepinephrine acts via G-protein–coupled receptors; alpha1 and beta receptors are primarily located postsynaptically and exert excitatory actions; alpha2 receptors are located both pre and postsynaptically and typically exert inhibitory effects. From a neurocircuit perspective, the ACC, OFC, central nucleus of the amygdala and paraventricular nucleus of the hypothalamus project to the locus ceruleus, providing links between the stress response and norepinephrine release. Interactions between stress and attentional networks may also be linked through norepinephrine function.

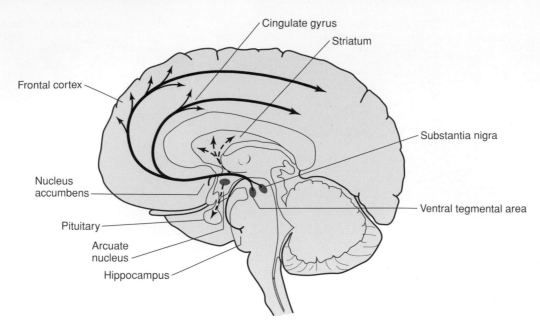

Figure 2-13 *The three major dopaminergic projections in the central nervous system. (1) The mesostriatal (or nigrostriatal) pathway: the substantia nigra pars compacta (SNc) projects to the dorsal striatum* (upward dashed arrows); *this is the pathway that degenerates in Parkinson disease. (2) The ventral tegmental area (VTA) projects to the ventral striatum (nucleus accumbens), olfactory bulb, amygdala, hippocampus, orbital and medial prefrontal cortex and cingulate gyrus* (solid arrows). *The terms "mesoaccumbens" and "mesocortical" are sometimes used to describe components of the VTA projection. (3) The arcuate nucleus of the hypothalamus projects via the tuberoinfundibular pathway in the hypothalamus, from which dopamine is delivered to the anterior pituitary* (downward dashed arrow). *(Reproduced with permission from Nestler E, Hyman S, Malenka R.* Molecular Psychopharmacology: A Foundation For Clinical Neuroscience. *2nd ed. New York: McGraw-Hill Education; 2009.)*

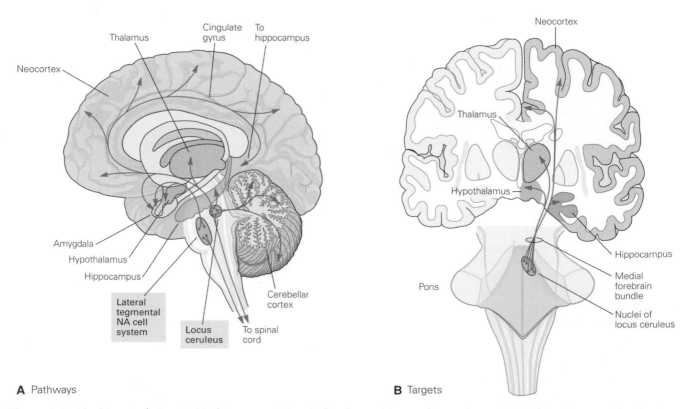

A Pathways

B Targets

Figure 2-14 *The locus ceruleus–norepinephrine system is involved in the modulation of arousal, attention, and stress among other functions.* ***A:*** *Sagittal view of afferent norepinephrine projections from the locus ceruleus and the lateral tegmental cell system.* ***B:*** *Coronal view of the major afferent projections from the locus ceruleus. (Adapted with permission from Heimer L.* The Human Brain and Spinal Cord. *2nd ed. Berlin, Springer-Verlag; 1995.)*

■ THE ROLE OF SECOND MESSENGER SYSTEMS AND SIGNAL TRANSDUCTION IN DEPRESSION

One major criticism of the monoamine hypothesis is that medications which increase the synaptic availability of monoamines do not immediately induce antidepressant effects. This suggests that their antidepressant properties are mediated by the downstream effects of monaminergic binding or by altering brain plasticity (see next section). As such, increased interest has been devoted to intracellular signaling cascades in the pathogenesis of the disorder. Specifically, many monoaminergic receptors are G-protein coupled, with receptor binding initiating the release of second messenger molecules, such as cyclic adenosine monophosphate (cyclic AMP), cyclic GMP, diacylglycerol, and inositol triphosphate.

The cyclic AMP second messenger system has been implicated in the pathophysiology of depression.[154] Cyclic AMP activates protein kinase A, which in turn phosphorylates the transcription factor CREB (cyclic-AMP-response-element-binding protein). Once phosphorylated, CREB promotes the transcription of several genes thought to be involved in the antidepressant response.[155] In addition, one of the phosphodiesterases, PDE4, might mediate the antidepressant effects of cyclic AMP, and levels of PDE4 are decreased in the brains of unmedicated depressed patients.[156]

The intracellular calcium–binding protein p11 increases 5-HT1B receptor signaling.[157] p11 is also overexpressed in rodent brains after antidepressant interventions and decreased in animal models of depression.[158] Moreover, p11 is upregulated in patients successfully treated with SSRIs and downregulated in the postmortem brains of depressed individuals.[157]

Finally, the Akt-GSK3 (glycogen synthase kinase-3) signaling pathway may also contribute to the pathogenesis of both unipolar and bipolar depression. Akt and GSK-3 are serine threonine kinases which are involved in glycogen synthesis, and Akt/GSK-3 signaling is modulated by dopamine and serotonin receptor binding.[159] Activated levels of GSK-3 are higher in the postmortem brains of unipolar- and bipolar-depressed patients.[160] Interestingly, lithium is a potent inhibitor of GSK-3, and this may explain its antidepressant and its antimanic effects.[161]

■ ALTERATIONS IN NEUROPLASTICITY IN DEPRESSION

Depression is increasingly being perceived as a disorder of neuroplasticity. As mentioned above, numerous studies have shown decreases in neuronal and dendritic density, as well as synaptic number and synaptic strength in depression, particularly in limbic regions, such as the hippocampus. This is concordant with the observations of decreased hippocampal volume noted earlier. In fact, many antidepressants enhance hippocampal neurogenesis, an important source of neural stem cells in the adult brain.

A critical mediator of neuroplasticity is brain-derived neurotrophic factor (BDNF). BDNF promotes neuronal growth in development and affects dendritic complexity and dendritic spine density.[160] BDNF expression is increased in patients successfully treated with SSRIs and is decreased in postmortem examination of depressed patients who have committed suicide.[162] Carriers of a BDNF gene polymorphism (Val66Met) have reduced hippocampal volumes on neuroimaging studies.[163]

Another critical role for BDNF is that of promoting synaptic plasticity. Synaptic plasticity refers to the possibility of changing the relative strength of a given synaptic connection (e.g., through increased postsynaptic receptor expression or through synaptogenesis). Synaptic plasticity is critical to learning and memory. Important examples of synaptic plasticity come in the phenomena of long-term potentiation (LTP) and long-term depression (LTD), which are often dependent on glutaminergic transmission through NMDA and AMPA receptors.

It was recently discovered that ketamine, an ionotropic NMDA receptor antagonist, induces rapid antidepressant effects (observed hours after administration and lasting up to 2 weeks). This discovery has sparked interest in the role of glutamate neurotransmission and synaptic plasticity in depression. Ketamine is thought to induce a variety of downstream signaling cascades after binding to the NMDA receptor, including activation of the mammalian target of rapamycin (mTor) pathway (which is itself stimulated by BDNF) and inhibition of the GSK-3 pathway.[160,164]

■ ALTERATIONS IN NEUROHORMONAL AND INFLAMMATORY MOLECULES IN DEPRESSION

It has long been recognized that environmental stress, especially when chronic and/or severe, has psychological ramifications which predispose to the depressive phenotype.[165] In recent decades, the molecular biological mechanisms through which stress induces a mood disorder have received greater attention, and have been explored in both human and animal models. For instance, in rodents chronic stress impairs dendritic arborization and induces atrophy of limbic and paralimbic cortical pyramidal neurons.[160] In humans, the volumetric decreases in the hippocampus mentioned earlier have also been linked to chronic stress exposure. A significant reason for these morphological changes is the fact that stress has been consistently shown to decrease the expression of BDNF. Moreover, there appears to be a rich interplay between BDNF expression and neurohormonal and neuroinflammatory signaling.

With respect to neurohormonal signaling, stress is a potent activator of the HPA axis, and there is ample evidence that the HPA axis is hyperactive in depression (**Fig. 2-15**). The HPA axis exists as a homeostatic neuroendocrine circuit which, in addition to several other functions, serves to respond to environmental and endogenous stress through the secretion of glucocorticoids, such as cortisol. Corticotropin-releasing hormone (CRH) is released by the paraventricular nucleus of the hypothalamus and stimulates cells of the anterior pituitary to release adrenocorticotropic hormone (ACTH, or corticotropin), which in turn stimulates adrenal corticotropin receptors to secrete glucocorticoids such as cortisol. Excessive secretion of CRH and ACTH is regulated by a negative feedback loop in which cortisol stimulates glucocorticoid receptors (GR) in the hypothalamus and anterior pituitary, causing them to decrease their secretion of CRH and ACTH, respectively.

In rodents, administration of excess levels of glucocorticoids can produce hippocampal subregion atrophy.[157] Compared to matched healthy controls, depressed patients have elevated levels of CRH in their cerebrospinal fluid, increased expression of CRH mRNA in limbic brain regions, increased CSF, urine and plasma cortisol levels and augmented cortisol secretion in response to ACTH challenges.[142,166,167] In addition, adult humans with a history of childhood trauma have increased CRH levels. Unfortunately, clinical trials with CRH receptor antagonists have thus far proved unsuccessful in treating depression.[142]

Critically, depressed patients also demonstrate an inability to downregulate CRH and ACTH secretion through stimulation of GR receptors with cortisol. This has led to the dexamethasone suppression and the dexamethasone-CRH tests.[167] Following the administration of the synthetic glucocorticoid dexamethasone, as many as 50% of depressed patients fail to suppress cortisol production, suggesting impairment at the level of the GR receptor. Indeed, there is growing data to support GR dysfunction in depression,[167] though lack of specificity limits clinical utility of the dexamethasone test.

The HPA axis is intimately regulated by inflammatory cytokines, and Pace and Miller have suggested that GR dysfunction is mediated by enhanced inflammatory signaling.[166] Depressed patients have increased levels of interleukins 1 and 6 (IL-1 and IL-6) and tumor

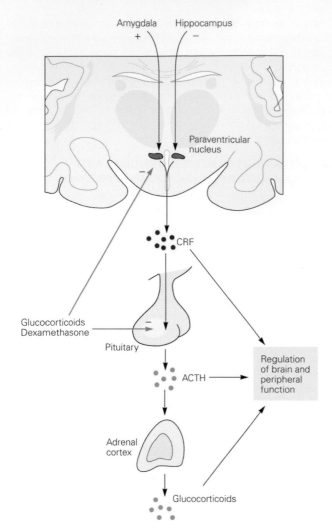

Figure 2-15 *The hypothalamic–pituitary–adrenal axis. Neurons in the paraventricular nucleus of the hypothalamus synthesize and release corticotropin-releasing factor (CRF), the key regulatory hormone in this cascade. CRF secretion follows a circadian pattern, and the effects of stress are superimposed on this circadian pattern. Excitatory fibers from the amygdala convey information about stress and activate CRF secretion and biosynthesis; inhibitory fibers descend from the hippocampus. CRF enters the hypophyseal portal system and stimulates the corticotropic cells of the anterior pituitary. These cells synthesize and release adrenocorticotropic hormone (ACTH), which enters the systemic circulation and ultimately stimulates the adrenal cortex to release glucocorticoids. In humans the major glucocorticoid is cortisol. Both cortisol and synthetic glucocorticoids such as dexamethasone act at the level of the pituitary and hypothalamus to inhibit further release of ACTH and CRF, respectively. (Adapted with permission from Nestler EJ, Hyman SE, Malenka RJ. Molecular Psychopharmacology: A Foundation For Clinical Neuroscience. 2nd ed. New York: McGraw-Hill Education; 2009.)*

necrosis factor (TNF)-α. Moreover, in response to stress induction in an experimental setting (e.g., through performing mental arithmetic or through forced public speaking), depressed patients mount a higher inflammatory response than matched healthy controls.[166] Finally, a pathogenic role for inflammatory signaling is evidenced by clinical observations. Patients treated with interferon-α (INF-α) (e.g., for hepatitis) often experience profound depression as a side effect. Also, inflammatory upregulation is considered a mechanism explaining the significant comorbidity between depression and cardiovascular disease.[168]

GENETIC AND EPIGENETIC FACTORS

While the heritability of depression based on twin studies is estimated to be between 40% and 50%,[169] the genetics of depression have thus far proven difficult to elucidate fully. Depression is a multi-genetic condition that does not adhere to simple Mendelian genetics, and genetic mechanisms implicated in depression suggest complex gene–environment interactions; an individual's genetic make-up may lead to increased susceptibility for the development of depression in the context of adverse environmental (psychosocial) influences. Approaches to the study of genetic influences in depression include association studies of candidate genes, genetic linkage studies of pedigrees with a strong family history of depression, and genome-wide association studies.

Association studies in depression have focused on monoaminergic candidate genes.[169] An intriguing interaction between polymorphisms in the promoter region of the serotonin transporter (5-HTT) gene and depression, as well as, an association between 5-HTT promoter region polymorphisms and depression related neural circuit activation patterns have emerged. The promoter activity of the 5-HTT gene is modified by sequence elements proximal to the 5′ regulatory region, termed the 5-HTT gene-linked polymorphic region (5-HTTLPR). The short "s" allele of the 5-HTTLPR is associated with lower transcription output of 5-HTT mRNA compared to the long "l" allele. A prospective-longitudinal study demonstrated that individuals with one or two copies of the short allele exhibited more depressive symptoms and suicidality following the experience of stressful life events in their early 20s compared to individuals homozygous for the long allele.[170] While the effect size may be modest, an association between the 5-HTTLPR short allele and increased depression risk following stress (particularly childhood maltreatment) has been replicated in meta-analyses.[171] Subsequent genetic-neuroimaging studies have characterized increased amygdala, ACC, and pulvinar activity in response to stress-based emotional probes in individuals carrying the short allele genotype.[172,173] Decreased rostral ACC–amygdala functional connectivity in these subjects has also been reported.[174] Short allele carriers exhibited decreased gray matter volumes in the prefrontal cortex (including the ACC and dlPFC), amygdala and hippocampus.[175,176] The regions exhibiting functional and structural associations with the short allele of the 5-HTTLPR overlap with brain regions implicated in depression neurobiology.

Genome-wide association studies in depression have largely failed to identify robust, reproducible findings.[177,178] A meta-analysis of 9,230 cases of depression and 9,519 healthy controls failed to show any single-nucleotide polymorphisms linked to depression. This suggests that genome-wide association studies have been underpowered to date, and that the genetics of depression likely includes a multiplicity of genetic polymorphisms (each with relatively small effect sizes) with complex gene–environment interactions.

Studies of epigenetic mechanisms in depression, while in their infancy, appear to hold great promise in elucidating the mechanisms by which environmental factors may affect phenotypic expression. Epigenetics is the study of heritable changes in gene activity caused by factors other than changes in the underlying nucleotide sequence. While the genomic sequence defines the potential genetic repertoire of a given individual, the epigenome delineates which genes in the repertoire are actually expressed (along with the degree of gene expression).[179] DNA methylation is one of several possible epigenetic modifications that influence gene expression. In a pioneering animal study probing the impact of early life experiences on subsequent epigenetic programming, rat pups who experienced high rates of licking and grooming behaviors (positive environmental influences) exhibited decreased methylation at the glucocorticoid receptor transcription factor binding site.[180] A postmortem study of human brains examining epigenetic glucocorticoid receptor regulation revealed increased methylation in the neuron-specific glucocorticoid receptor and decreased glucocorticoid receptor mRNA in suicide victims with a history of childhood abuse compared with nonabused suicide victims and non-suicide controls.[181] A study of highly traumatized individuals identified a possible association between increased demethylation of the FK506-binding protein 5 gene (an important regulator of the stress hormone system) in individuals with prior childhood trauma and increased risk of developing stress-related psychiatric disorders.[182] As an additional example of potential epigenetic influence, elevated antenatal maternal anxiety levels were associated with decreased OFC, dlPFC, ventrolateral PFC and medial temporal lobe gray matter in 6- to 9-year-old offspring.[183] A similar study observed a link between high maternal anxiety during pregnancy and elevated, flattened day-time cortisol profiles in adolescent offspring; this HPA axis disturbance was associated with depressive symptoms in female adolescents.[184]

THE INTERSECTION OF IDIOPATHIC DEPRESSION AND SECONDARY DEPRESSION IN MEDICAL AND NEUROLOGICAL CONDITIONS

Depression in traditional psychiatric disorders, termed primary or idiopathic depression, shares clinical and neurobiological features with depression originating in the context of medical or neurological conditions, referred to as secondary depression. In addition, while depression may at times emerge as consequence of the psycho-social stress experienced by an individual in the context of a new medical or neurological condition, medical and neurological disorders may also disrupt the same brain circuits implicated in idiopathic depression. As discussed elsewhere in this book, toxic metabolic disturbances, infectious disease, autoimmune and inflammatory disorders, cardiovascular disease, endocrinopathies, and neurological disorders such as cerebrovascular disease, demyelinating disease, dementia, and epilepsy among many other conditions have been associated with depression. The brain–behavior relationships discussed in this chapter are thus highly relevant to the pathobiology of depression in medical illness.

THE NEUROBIOLOGY OF DEPRESSION: A SYNTHESIS

Depression is a complex neuropsychiatric disorder associated with a high degree of morbidity. The neurobiological underpinnings of depression remain elusive, but efforts to better understand the genetic, molecular, synaptic and systems-level brain mechanisms giving rise to the depressive phenotype have led to promising avenues of investigation. A fundamental challenge in depression research is to develop a biological model which conceptually integrates dysfunction across the molecular and systems levels. One possible impediment to this is the fact that depression has heretofore been conceptualized as a single disease. It may well be that certain features of the depressive phenotype are referable to specific molecular and circuit aberrations. For example, as mentioned earlier in this chapter, the symptom of anhedonia may be mostly rooted in dysfunction of the dopaminergically mediated VTA to ventral striatum reward circuit. A symptom-specific, multi-level clinical and translational research approach will likely lead to future advancements in the neurobiological understanding of depression, which will subsequently aid the development of novel therapeutics and the identification of biomarkers guiding treatment selection and prognosis.

REFERENCES

1. Perez DL, Ortiz-Terán L, Silbersweig DA. Neuroimaging in psychiatry: The clinical-radiographic correlate. In: Fogel BS, Greenberg DB, eds. *Psychiatric Care Of The Medical Patient*. Oxford University Press; 2015.

2. Alexander GE, DeLong MR, Strick PL. Parallel organization of functionally segregated circuits linking basal ganglia and cortex. *Annu Rev Neurosci*. 1986;9:357–381.

3. Cummings JL. Frontal-subcortical circuits and human behavior. *Arch Neurol*. 1993;50:873–880.

4. Devinsky O, Morrell MJ, Vogt BA. Contributions of anterior cingulate cortex to behaviour. *Brain*. 1995;118(Pt 1):279–306.

5. Etkin A, Egner T, Kalisch R. Emotional processing in anterior cingulate and medial prefrontal cortex. *Trends Cogn Sci*. 2011;15:85–93.

6. Ongur D, Price JL. The organization of networks within the orbital and medial prefrontal cortex of rats, monkeys and humans. *Cereb Cortex*. 2000;10:206–219.

7. Damasio H, Grabowski T, Frank R, Galaburda AM, Damasio AR. The return of Phineas Gage: clues about the brain from the skull of a famous patient. *Science*. 1994;264:1102–1105.

8. Perez DL, Barsky AJ, Daffner K, Silbersweig DA. Motor and somatosensory conversion disorder: a functional unawareness syndrome? *J Neuropsychiatry Clin Neurosci*. 2012;24:141–151.

9. LeDoux J. The amygdala. *Curr Biol*. 2007;17:R868–R874.

10. Eichenbaum H. A cortical-hippocampal system for declarative memory. *Nat Rev Neurosci*. 2000;1:41–50.

11. Cavanna AE, Trimble MR. The precuneus: a review of its functional anatomy and behavioural correlates. *Brain*. 2006;129:564–583.

12. Craig AD. How do you feel? Interoception: the sense of the physiological condition of the body. *Nat Rev Neurosci*. 2002;3:655–666.

13. Craig AD. How do you feel–now? The anterior insula and human awareness. *Nat Rev Neurosci*. 2009;10:59–70.

14. Allman JM, Tetreault NA, Hakeem AY, et al. The von Economo neurons in the frontoinsular and anterior cingulate cortex. *Ann N Y Acad Sci*. 2011;1225:59–71.

15. Raichle ME. Two views of brain function. *Trends Cogn Sci*. 2010;14:180–190.

16. Perez DL, Murray ED, Price BH. Depression and psychosis in neurological practice. In: Daroff RB, Jankovic J, Mazziotta JC, Pomeroy SL, eds. *Neurology in Clinical Practice*. 7th ed. Philadelphia: Elsevier; 2015.

17. Ashburner J, Friston KJ. Voxel-based morphometry—the methods. *Neuroimage*. 2000;11:805–821.

18. Fischl B, Dale AM. Measuring the thickness of the human cerebral cortex from magnetic resonance images. *Proc Natl Acad Sci U S A*. 2000;97:11050–11055.

19. Chung MK, Robbins S, Evans AC. Unified statistical approach to cortical thickness analysis. *Inf Process Med Imaging*. 2005;19:627–638.

20. Coffey CE, Wilkinson WE, Weiner RD, et al. Quantitative cerebral anatomy in depression. A controlled magnetic resonance imaging study. *Arch Gen Psychiatry*. 1993;50:7–16.

21. Soares JC, Mann JJ. The anatomy of mood disorders–review of structural neuroimaging studies. *Biol Psychiatry*. 1997;41:86–106.

22. Robinson RG. Neuropsychiatric consequences of stroke. *Annu Rev Med*. 1997;48:217–229.

23. Bremner JD, Narayan M, Anderson ER, Staib LH, Miller HL, Charney DS. Hippocampal volume reduction in major depression. *Am J Psychiatry*. 2000;157:115–118.

24. Frodl T, Meisenzahl EM, Zetzsche T, et al. Hippocampal changes in patients with a first episode of major depression. *Am J Psychiatry*. 2002;159:1112–1118.

25. Zou K, Deng W, Li T, et al. Changes of brain morphometry in first-episode, drug-naive, non-late-life adult patients with major depression: an optimized voxel-based morphometry study. *Biol Psychiatry*. 2010;67:186–188.

26. Sheline YI, Sanghavi M, Mintun MA, Gado MH. Depression duration but not age predicts hippocampal volume loss in medically healthy women with recurrent major depression. *J Neurosci*. 1999;19:5034–5043.

27. McKinnon MC, Yucel K, Nazarov A, MacQueen GM. A meta-analysis examining clinical predictors of hippocampal volume in patients with major depressive disorder. *J Psychiatry Neurosci*. 2009;34:41–54.

28. Frodl TS, Koutsouleris N, Bottlender R, et al. Depression-related variation in brain morphology over 3 years: effects of stress? *Arch Gen Psychiatry*. 2008;65:1156–1165.

29. Carballedo A, Lisiecka D, Fagan A, et al. Early life adversity is associated with brain changes in subjects at family risk for depression. *World J Biol Psychiatry*. 2012;13:569–578.

30. Frodl T, Meisenzahl EM, Zetzsche T, et al. Larger amygdala volumes in first depressive episode as compared to recurrent major depression and healthy control subjects. *Biol Psychiatry*. 2003;53:338–344.

31. Lange C, Irle E. Enlarged amygdala volume and reduced hippocampal volume in young women with major depression. *Psychol Med*. 2004;34:1059–1064.

32. Botteron KN, Raichle ME, Drevets WC, Heath AC, Todd RD. Volumetric reduction in left subgenual prefrontal cortex in early onset depression. *Biol Psychiatry*. 2002;51:342–344.

33. Brambilla P, Nicoletti MA, Harenski K, et al. Anatomical MRI study of subgenual prefrontal cortex in bipolar and unipolar subjects. *Neuropsychopharmacology*. 2002;27:792–799.

34. Pizzagalli DA, Oakes TR, Fox AS, et al. Functional but not structural subgenual prefrontal cortex abnormalities in melancholia. *Mol Psychiatry*. 2004;9:325, 93–405.

35. Hastings RS, Parsey RV, Oquendo MA, Arango V, Mann JJ. Volumetric analysis of the prefrontal cortex, amygdala, and hippocampus in major depression. *Neuropsychopharmacology*. 2004;29:952–959.

36. Yucel K, McKinnon MC, Chahal R, et al. Anterior cingulate volumes in never-treated patients with major depressive disorder. *Neuropsychopharmacology*. 2008;33:3157–3163.

37. Treadway MT, Grant MM, Ding Z, Hollon SD, Gore JC, Shelton RC. Early adverse events, HPA activity and rostral anterior cingulate volume in MDD. *PLoS One*. 2009;4:e4887.

38. Bremner JD, Vythilingam M, Vermetten E, et al. Reduced volume of orbitofrontal cortex in major depression. *Biol Psychiatry*. 2002;51:273–279.

39. Lacerda AL, Keshavan MS, Hardan AY, et al. Anatomic evaluation of the orbitofrontal cortex in major depressive disorder. *Biol Psychiatry*. 2004;55:353–358.

40. Taylor WD, Macfall JR, Payne ME, et al. Orbitofrontal cortex volume in late life depression: influence of hyperintense lesions and genetic polymorphisms. *Psychol Med*. 2007;37:1763–1773.

41. van Eijndhoven P, van Wingen G, Katzenbauer M, et al. Paralimbic cortical thickness in first-episode depression: Evidence for trait-related differences in mood regulation. *Am J Psychiatry* 2013; 170:1477–1486.

42. Taylor WD, Aizenstein HJ, Alexopoulos GS. The vascular depression hypothesis: mechanisms linking vascular disease with depression. *Mol Psychiatry* .2013;18:963–974.

43. Krishnan KR, McDonald WM, Escalona PR, et al. Magnetic resonance imaging of the caudate nuclei in depression. Preliminary observations. *Arch Gen Psychiatry*. 1992;49:553–557.

44. Parashos IA, Tupler LA, Blitchington T, Krishnan KR. Magnetic-resonance morphometry in patients with major depression. *Psychiatry Res*. 1998;84:7–15.

45. Bora E, Fornito A, Pantelis C, Yucel M. Gray matter abnormalities in Major Depressive Disorder: a meta-analysis of voxel based morphometry studies. *J Affect Disord*. 2012;138:9–18.

46. Bora E, Harrison BJ, Davey CG, Yucel M, Pantelis C. Meta-analysis of volumetric abnormalities in cortico-striatal-pallidal-thalamic circuits in major depressive disorder. *Psychol Med*. 2012;42: 671–681.

47. Kempton MJ, Salvador Z, Munafo MR, et al. Structural neuroimaging studies in major depressive disorder. Meta-analysis and comparison with bipolar disorder. *Arch Gen Psychiatry*. 2011; 68:675–690.

48. Krishnan KR, Doraiswamy PM, Lurie SN, et al. Pituitary size in depression. *J Clin Endocrinol Metab*. 1991;72:256–259.

49. Rubin RT, Phillips JJ, Sadow TF, McCracken JT. Adrenal gland volume in major depression. Increase during the depressive episode and decrease with successful treatment. *Arch Gen Psychiatry*. 1995;52:213–218.

50. Shah SA, Doraiswamy PM, Husain MM, et al. Posterior fossa abnormalities in major depression: a controlled magnetic resonance imaging study. *Acta Psychiatr Scand*. 1992;85:474–479.

51. Beaulieu C. The basis of anisotropic water diffusion in the nervous system—a technical review. *NMR Biomed*. 2002;15:435–455.

52. Li L, Ma N, Li Z, et al. Prefrontal white matter abnormalities in young adult with major depressive disorder: a diffusion tensor imaging study. *Brain Res*. 2007;1168:124–128.

53. Kieseppa T, Eerola M, Mantyla R, et al. Major depressive disorder and white matter abnormalities: a diffusion tensor imaging study with tract-based spatial statistics. *J Affect Disord*. 120:240–244.

54. Blood AJ, Iosifescu DV, Makris N, et al. Microstructural abnormalities in subcortical reward circuitry of subjects with major depressive disorder. *PLoS One*. 2010;5:e13945.

55. Osoba A, Hanggi J, Li M, et al. Disease severity is correlated to tract specific changes of fractional anisotropy in MD and CM thalamus—a DTI study in major depressive disorder. *J Affect Disord*. 2013;149:116–128.

56. Ongur D, Drevets WC, Price JL. Glial reduction in the subgenual prefrontal cortex in mood disorders. *Proc Natl Acad Sci U S A*. 1998;95:13290–13295.

57. Cotter D, Mackay D, Landau S, Kerwin R, Everall I. Reduced glial cell density and neuronal size in the anterior cingulate cortex in major depressive disorder. *Arch Gen Psychiatry*. 2001;58:545–553.

58. Hercher C, Canetti L, Turecki G, Mechawar N. Anterior cingulate pyramidal neurons display altered dendritic branching in depressed suicides. *J Psychiatr Res*. 2010;44:286–293.

59. Rajkowska G, Miguel-Hidalgo JJ, Wei J, et al. Morphometric evidence for neuronal and glial prefrontal cell pathology in major depression. *Biol Psychiatry*. 1999;45:1085–1098.

60. Cotter D, Mackay D, Chana G, Beasley C, Landau S, Everall IP. Reduced neuronal size and glial cell density in area 9 of the dorsolateral prefrontal cortex in subjects with major depressive disorder. *Cereb Cortex*. 2002;12:386–394.

61. Bowley MP, Drevets WC, Ongur D, Price JL. Low glial numbers in the amygdala in major depressive disorder. *Biol Psychiatry*. 2002;52:404–412.

62. Hamidi M, Drevets WC, Price JL. Glial reduction in amygdala in major depressive disorder is due to oligodendrocytes. *Biol Psychiatry*. 2004;55:563–569.

63. Boldrini M, Santiago AN, Hen R, et al. Hippocampal granule neuron number and dentate gyrus volume in antidepressant-treated and untreated major depression. *Neuropsychopharmacology*. 2013;38:1068–1077.

64. Yuksel C, Ongur D. Magnetic resonance spectroscopy studies of glutamate-related abnormalities in mood disorders. *Biol Psychiatry*. 2010;68:785–794.

65. Hasler G, van der Veen JW, Tumonis T, Meyers N, Shen J, Drevets WC. Reduced prefrontal glutamate/glutamine and gamma-aminobutyric acid levels in major depression determined using proton magnetic resonance spectroscopy. *Arch Gen Psychiatry*. 2007;64:193–200.

66. Luykx JJ, Laban KG, van den Heuvel MP, et al. Region and state specific glutamate downregulation in major depressive disorder: a meta-analysis of (1)H-MRS findings. *Neurosci Biobehav Rev*. 2012;36:198–205.

67. Yildiz-Yesiloglu A, Ankerst DP. Review of 1H magnetic resonance spectroscopy findings in major depressive disorder: a meta-analysis. *Psychiatry Res*. 2006;147:1–25.

68. Farid K, Caillat-Vigneron N, Sibon I. Is brain SPECT useful in degenerative dementia diagnosis? *J Comput Assist Tomogr*. 35:1–3.

69. Logothetis NK, Pauls J, Augath M, Trinath T, Oeltermann A. Neurophysiological investigation of the basis of the fMRI signal. *Nature*. 2001;412:150–157.

70. Zhang D, Raichle ME. Disease and the brain's dark energy. *Nat Rev Neurol*. 2010;6:15–28.

71. Baxter LR Jr., Phelps ME, Mazziotta JC, et al. Cerebral metabolic rates for glucose in mood disorders. Studies with positron emission tomography and fluorodeoxyglucose F 18. *Arch Gen Psychiatry*. 1985;42:441–447.

72. Dolan RJ, Bench CJ, Brown RG, Scott LC, Friston KJ, Frackowiak RS. Regional cerebral blood flow abnormalities in depressed patients with cognitive impairment. *J Neurol Neurosurg Psychiatry*. 1992;55:768–773.

73. Thomas P, Vaiva G, Samaille E, et al. Cerebral blood flow in major depression and dysthymia. *J Affect Disord*. 1993;29:235–242.

74. Bench CJ, Friston KJ, Brown RG, Frackowiak RS, Dolan RJ. Regional cerebral blood flow in depression measured by positron emission tomography: the relationship with clinical dimensions. *Psychol Med*. 1993;23:579–590.

75. Hickie I, Ward P, Scott E, et al. Neo-striatal rCBF correlates of psychomotor slowing in patients with major depression. *Psychiatry Res*. 1999;92:75–81.

76. Drevets WC. Neuroimaging abnormalities in the amygdala in mood disorders. *Ann N Y Acad Sci*. 2003;985:420–444.

77. Drevets WC, Videen TO, Price JL, Preskorn SH, Carmichael ST, Raichle ME. A functional anatomical study of unipolar depression. *J Neurosci*. 1992;12:3628–3641.

78. Sheline YI, Barch DM, Donnelly JM, Ollinger JM, Snyder AZ, Mintun MA. Increased amygdala response to masked emotional faces in depressed subjects resolves with antidepressant treatment: an fMRI study. *Biol Psychiatry*. 2001;50:651–658.

79. Siegle GJ, Steinhauer SR, Thase ME, Stenger VA, Carter CS. Can't shake that feeling: event-related fMRI assessment of sustained amygdala activity in response to emotional information in depressed individuals. *Biol Psychiatry*. 2002;51:693–707.

80. Victor TA, Furey ML, Fromm SJ, Ohman A, Drevets WC. Relationship between amygdala responses to masked faces and mood state and treatment in major depressive disorder. *Arch Gen Psychiatry*. 2010;67:1128–1138.

81. Arnone D, McKie S, Elliott R, et al. Increased amygdala responses to sad but not fearful faces in major depression: relation to mood state and pharmacological treatment. *Am J Psychiatry*. 2012;169:841–50.

82. Drevets WC, Price JL, Bardgett ME, Reich T, Todd RD, Raichle ME. Glucose metabolism in the amygdala in depression: relationship to diagnostic subtype and plasma cortisol levels. *Pharmacol Biochem Behav*. 2002;71:431–447.

83. Hamani C, Mayberg H, Stone S, Laxton A, Haber S, Lozano AM. The subcallosal cingulate gyrus in the context of major depression. *Biol Psychiatry*. 2011;69:301–318.

84. Dougherty DD, Weiss AP, Cosgrove GR, et al. Cerebral metabolic correlates as potential predictors of response to anterior cingulotomy for treatment of major depression. *J Neurosurg*. 2003;99:1010–1017.

85. Konarski JZ, Kennedy SH, Segal ZV, et al. Predictors of nonresponse to cognitive behavioural therapy or venlafaxine using glucose metabolism in major depressive disorder. *J Psychiatry Neurosci*. 2009;34:175–180.

86. Mayberg HS, Lozano AM, Voon V, et al. Deep brain stimulation for treatment-resistant depression. *Neuron*. 2005;45:651–660.

87. Gotlib IH, Sivers H, Gabrieli JD, et al. Subgenual anterior cingulate activation to valenced emotional stimuli in major depression. *Neuroreport*. 2005;16:1731–1734.

88. Drevets WC, Price JL, Simpson JR Jr., et al. Subgenual prefrontal cortex abnormalities in mood disorders. *Nature*. 1997;386:824–827.

89. Liotti M, Mayberg HS, Brannan SK, McGinnis S, Jerabek P, Fox PT. Differential limbic–cortical correlates of sadness and anxiety in healthy subjects: implications for affective disorders. *Biol Psychiatry*. 2000;48:30–42.

90. Mayberg HS, Liotti M, Brannan SK, et al. Reciprocal limbic-cortical function and negative mood: converging PET findings in depression and normal sadness. *Am J Psychiatry*. 1999;156:675–682.

91. Mayberg HS, Brannan SK, Tekell JL, et al. Regional metabolic effects of fluoxetine in major depression: serial changes and relationship to clinical response. *Biol Psychiatry*. 2000;48:830–843.

92. Holtzheimer PE, Mayberg HS. Stuck in a rut: rethinking depression and its treatment. *Trends Neurosci*. 2011;34:1–9.

93. Kennedy SH, Evans KR, Kruger S, et al. Changes in regional brain glucose metabolism measured with positron emission tomography after paroxetine treatment of major depression. *Am J Psychiatry*. 2001;158:899–905.

94. Sacher J, Neumann J, Funfstuck T, Soliman A, Villringer A, Schroeter ML. Mapping the depressed brain: a meta-analysis of structural and functional alterations in major depressive disorder. *J Affect Disord*. 2012;140:142–148.

95. Drevets WC. Orbitofrontal cortex function and structure in depression. *Ann N Y Acad Sci*. 2007;1121:499–527.

96. Price JL, Drevets WC. Neurocircuitry of mood disorders. *Neuropsychopharmacology*. 2010;35:192–216.

97. Liotti M, Mayberg HS, McGinnis S, Brannan SL, Jerabek P. Unmasking disease-specific cerebral blood flow abnormalities: mood challenge in patients with remitted unipolar depression. *Am J Psychiatry*. 2002;159:1830–1840.

98. Grimm S, Beck J, Schuepbach D, et al. Imbalance between left and right dorsolateral prefrontal cortex in major depression is linked to negative emotional judgment: an fMRI study in severe major depressive disorder. *Biol Psychiatry*. 2008;63:369–376.

99. Fox MD, Buckner RL, White MP, Greicius MD, Pascual-Leone A. Efficacy of transcranial magnetic stimulation targets for depression is related to intrinsic functional connectivity with the subgenual cingulate. *Biol Psychiatry*. 2012;72:595–603.

100. Epstein J, Pan H, Kocsis JH, et al. Lack of ventral striatal response to positive stimuli in depressed versus normal subjects. *Am J Psychiatry*. 2006;163:1784–1790.

101. Epstein J, Perez DL, Ervin K, et al. Failure to segregate emotional processing from cognitive and sensorimotor processing in major depression. *Psychiatry Res*. 2011;193:144–150.

102. Keedwell PA, Andrew C, Williams SC, Brammer MJ, Phillips ML. The neural correlates of anhedonia in major depressive disorder. *Biol Psychiatry*. 2005;58:843–853.

103. Pizzagalli DA, Holmes AJ, Dillon DG, et al. Reduced caudate and nucleus accumbens response to rewards in unmedicated individuals with major depressive disorder. *Am J Psychiatry*. 2009;166:702–710.

104. Heller AS, Johnstone T, Shackman AJ, et al. Reduced capacity to sustain positive emotion in major depression reflects diminished maintenance of fronto-striatal brain activation. *Proc Natl Acad Sci U S A*. 2009;106:22445–22450.

105. Hamilton JP, Etkin A, Furman DJ, Lemus MG, Johnson RF, Gotlib IH. Functional neuroimaging of major depressive disorder: a meta-analysis and new integration of base line activation and neural response data. *Am J Psychiatry*. 2012;169:693–703.

106. Stuhrmann A, Suslow T, Dannlowski U. Facial emotion processing in major depression: a systematic review of neuroimaging findings. *Biol Mood Anxiety Disord*. 2011;1:10.

107. Greicius MD, Flores BH, Menon V, et al. Resting-state functional connectivity in major depression: abnormally increased contributions from subgenual cingulate cortex and thalamus. *Biol Psychiatry*. 2007;62:429–437.

108. Avery JA, Drevets WC, Moseman SE, Bodurka J, Barcalow JC, Simmons WK. Major depressive disorder is associated with abnormal interoceptive activity and functional connectivity in the insula. *Biol Psychiatry*. 2014;76:258–266.

109. Connolly CG, Wu J, Ho TC, et al. Resting-state functional connectivity of subgenual anterior cingulate cortex in depressed adolescents. *Biol Psychiatry* 2013;74:898–907.

110. Sheline YI, Price JL, Yan Z, Mintun MA. Resting-state functional MRI in depression unmasks increased connectivity between networks via the dorsal nexus. *Proc Natl Acad Sci U S A*. 2010;107:11020–11025.

111. Jin C, Gao C, Chen C, et al. A preliminary study of the dysregulation of the resting networks in first-episode medication-naive adolescent depression. *Neurosci Lett*. 2011;503:105–109.

112. Wu QZ, Li DM, Kuang WH, et al. Abnormal regional spontaneous neural activity in treatment-refractory depression revealed by resting-state fMRI. *Hum Brain Mapp*. 2011;32:1290–1299.

113. McCabe C, Mishor Z. Antidepressant medications reduce subcortical-cortical resting-state functional connectivity in healthy volunteers. *Neuroimage*. 2011;57:1317–1323.

114. Posner J, Hellerstein DJ, Gat I, et al. Antidepressants normalize the default mode network in patients with dysthymia. *JAMA Psychiatry*. 2013;70:373–382.

115. Scheidegger M, Walter M, Lehmann M, et al. Ketamine decreases resting state functional network connectivity in healthy subjects: implications for antidepressant drug action. *PLoS One*. 2012; 7:e44799.

116. Liston C, Chen AC, Zebley BD, et al. Default mode network mechanisms of transcranial magnetic stimulation in depression. *Biol Psychiatry* 2014;76:517–526.

117. Mayberg HS, Brannan SK, Mahurin RK, et al. Cingulate function in depression: a potential predictor of treatment response. *Neuroreport*. 1997;8:1057–1061.

118. Chen CH, Ridler K, Suckling J, et al. Brain imaging correlates of depressive symptom severity and predictors of symptom improvement after antidepressant treatment. *Biol Psychiatry*. 2007; 62:407–414.

119. Pizzagalli D, Pascual-Marqui RD, Nitschke JB, et al. Anterior cingulate activity as a predictor of degree of treatment response in major depression: evidence from brain electrical tomography analysis. *Am J Psychiatry*. 2001;158:405–415.

120. MacQueen GM. Magnetic resonance imaging and prediction of outcome in patients with major depressive disorder. *J Psychiatry Neurosci*. 2009;34:343–349.

121. Vakili K, Pillay SS, Lafer B, et al. Hippocampal volume in primary unipolar major depression: a magnetic resonance imaging study. *Biol Psychiatry*. 2000;47:1087–1090.

122. MacQueen GM, Yucel K, Taylor VH, Macdonald K, Joffe R. Posterior hippocampal volumes are associated with remission rates in patients with major depressive disorder. *Biol Psychiatry*. 2008;64:880–883.

123. Siegle GJ, Carter CS, Thase ME. Use of FMRI to predict recovery from unipolar depression with cognitive behavior therapy. *Am J Psychiatry*. 2006;163:735–738.

124. McGrath CL, Kelley ME, Holtzheimer PE, et al. Toward a neuroimaging treatment selection biomarker for major depressive disorder. *JAMA psychiatry*. 2013;70:821–829.

125. Jollant F, Lawrence NS, Giampietro V, et al. Orbitofrontal cortex response to angry faces in men with histories of suicide attempts. *Am J Psychiatry*. 2008;165:740–748.

126. Desmyter S, van Heeringen C, Audenaert K. Structural and functional neuroimaging studies of the suicidal brain. *Prog Neuropsychopharmacol Biol Psychiatry*. 35:796–808.

127. Jollant F, Lawrence NS, Olie E, et al. Decreased activation of lateral orbitofrontal cortex during risky choices under uncertainty is associated with disadvantageous decision-making and suicidal behavior. *Neuroimage*. 2010;51:1275–1281.

128. Monkul ES, Hatch JP, Nicoletti MA, et al. Fronto-limbic brain structures in suicidal and non-suicidal female patients with major depressive disorder. *Mol Psychiatry*. 2007;12:360–366.

129. Wagner G, Schultz CC, Koch K, Schachtzabel C, Sauer H, Schlosser RG. Prefrontal cortical thickness in depressed patients with high-risk for suicidal behavior. *J Psychiatr Res*. 46:1449–1455.

130. Wagner G, Koch K, Schachtzabel C, Schultz CC, Sauer H, Schlosser RG. Structural brain alterations in patients with major depressive disorder and high risk for suicide: evidence for a distinct neurobiological entity? *Neuroimage*. 54:1607–1614.

131. Jia Z, Huang X, Wu Q, et al. High-field magnetic resonance imaging of suicidality in patients with major depressive disorder. *Am J Psychiatry*. 2010;167:1381–1390.

132. Alexopoulos GS. Depression in the elderly. *Lancet*. 2005;365: 1961–1970.

133. Alexopoulos GS, Meyers BS, Young RC, Campbell S, Silbersweig D, Charlson M. 'Vascular depression' hypothesis. *Arch Gen Psychiatry*. 1997;54:915–922.

134. Alexopoulos GS, Meyers BS, Young RC, Kakuma T, Silbersweig D, Charlson M. Clinically defined vascular depression. *Am J Psychiatry*. 1997;154:562–565.

135. Sheline YI, Price JL, Vaishnavi SN, et al. Regional white matter hyperintensity burden in automated segmentation distinguishes late-life depressed subjects from comparison subjects matched for vascular risk factors. *Am J Psychiatry*. 2008;165:524–532.

136. Alexopoulos GS, Meyers BS, Young RC, et al. Executive dysfunction and long-term outcomes of geriatric depression. *Arch Gen Psychiatry*. 2000;57:285–290.

137. Kalayam B, Alexopoulos GS. Prefrontal dysfunction and treatment response in geriatric depression. *Arch Gen Psychiatry*. 1999;56:713–718.

138. Harrison NA, Brydon L, Walker C, Gray MA, Steptoe A, Critchley HD. Inflammation causes mood changes through alterations in subgenual cingulate activity and mesolimbic connectivity. *Biol Psychiatry*. 2009;66:407–414.

139. Benarroch EE. Serotonergic modulation of basal ganglia circuits: complexity and therapeutic opportunities. *Neurology*. 2009; 73:880–886.

140. Huey ED, Putnam KT, Grafman J. A systematic review of neurotransmitter deficits and treatments in frontotemporal dementia. *Neurology*. 2006;66:17–22.

141. Wang C, Jiang Y, Ma J, et al. Structural basis for molecular recognition at serotonin receptors. *Science*. 2013;340:610–614.

142. Belmaker RH, Agam G. Major depressive disorder. *N Engl J Med*. 2008;358:55–68.

143. Meltzer HY, Roth BL. Lorcaserin and pimavanserin: emerging selectivity of serotonin receptor subtype-targeted drugs. *J Clin Invest*. 2013;123:4986–4991.

144. Lopez-Munoz F, Alamo C. Monoaminergic neurotransmission: the history of the discovery of antidepressants from 1950s until today. *Curr Pharm Des*. 2009;15:1563–1586.

145. Savitz JB, Drevets WC. Neuroreceptor imaging in depression. *Neurobiol Dis*. 2013;52:49–65.

146. Drevets WC, Thase ME, Moses-Kolko EL, et al. Serotonin-1A receptor imaging in recurrent depression: replication and literature review. *Nucl Med Biol*. 2007;34:865–877.

147. Parsey RV, Ogden RT, Miller JM, et al. Higher serotonin 1A binding in a second major depression cohort: modeling and reference region considerations. *Biol Psychiatry*. 2010;68:170–178.

148. Dunlop BW, Nemeroff CB. The role of dopamine in the pathophysiology of depression. *Arch Gen Psychiatry*. 2007;64: 327–337.

149. Cools R. Role of dopamine in the motivational and cognitive control of behavior. *Neuroscientist*. 2008;14:381–395.

150. Meyer JH, McNeely HE, Sagrati S, et al. Elevated putamen D(2) receptor binding potential in major depression with motor retardation: an [11C]raclopride positron emission tomography study. *Am J Psychiatry*. 2006;163:1594–1602.

151. Montgomery AJ, Stokes P, Kitamura Y, Grasby PM. Extrastriatal D2 and striatal D2 receptors in depressive illness: pilot PET studies using [11C]FLB 457 and [11C]raclopride. *J Affect Disord*. 2007;101:113–122.

152. Benarroch EE. The locus ceruleus norepinephrine system: functional organization and potential clinical significance. *Neurology*. 2009;73:1699–1704.

153. Sara SJ. The locus coeruleus and noradrenergic modulation of cognition. *Nat Rev Neurosci*. 2009;10:211–223.

154. Carlezon WA Jr., Duman RS, Nestler EJ. The many faces of CREB. *Trends Neurosci*. 2005;28:436–445.

155. Niciu MJ, Ionescu DF, Mathews DC, Richards EM, Zarate CA Jr. Second messenger/signal transduction pathways in major mood disorders: moving from membrane to mechanism of action, part I: major depressive disorder. *CNS Spectr*. 2013;18:231–241.

156. Fujita M, Hines CS, Zoghbi SS, et al. Downregulation of brain phosphodiesterase type IV measured with 11C-(R)-rolipram positron emission tomography in major depressive disorder. *Biol Psychiatry*. 2012;72:548–554.

157. Krishnan V, Nestler EJ. The molecular neurobiology of depression. *Nature*. 2008;455:894–902.

158. Svenningsson P, Chergui K, Rachleff I, et al. Alterations in 5-HT1B receptor function by p11 in depression-like states. *Science*. 2006; 311:77–80.

159. Beaulieu JM. A role for Akt and glycogen synthase kinase-3 as integrators of dopamine and serotonin neurotransmission in mental health. *J Psychiatry Neurosci*. 2012;37:7–16.

160. Duman RS, Aghajanian GK. Synaptic dysfunction in depression: potential therapeutic targets. *Science*. 2012;338:68–72.

161. Okamoto H, Voleti B, Banasr M, et al. Wnt2 expression and signaling is increased by different classes of antidepressant treatments. *Biol Psychiatry*. 2010;68:521–527.

162. Karege F, Vaudan G, Schwald M, Perroud N, La Harpe R. Neurotrophin levels in postmortem brains of suicide victims and the effects of antemortem diagnosis and psychotropic drugs. *Brain Res Mol Brain Res*. 2005;136:29–37.

163. Szeszko PR, Lipsky R, Mentschel C, et al. Brain-derived neurotrophic factor val66met polymorphism and volume of the hippocampal formation. *Mol Psychiatry*. 2005;10:631–636.

164. Kavalali ET, Monteggia LM. Synaptic mechanisms underlying rapid antidepressant action of ketamine. *Am J Psychiatry*. 2012;169:1150–1156.

165. McEwen BS, Morrison JH. The brain on stress: vulnerability and plasticity of the prefrontal cortex over the life course. *Neuron*. 2013;79:16–29.

166. Pace TW, Miller AH. Cytokines and glucocorticoid receptor signaling. Relevance to major depression. *Ann N Y Acad Sci*. 2009;1179:86–105.

167. Pariante CM, Miller AH. Glucocorticoid receptors in major depression: relevance to pathophysiology and treatment. *Biol Psychiatry*. 2001;49:391–404.

168. Gleason OC, Pierce AM, Walker AE, Warnock JK. The two-way relationship between medical illness and late-life depression. *Psychiatr Clin North Am*. 2013;36:533–544.

169. Levinson DF. The genetics of depression: a review. *Biol Psychiatry*. 2006;60:84–92.

170. Caspi A, Sugden K, Moffitt TE, et al. Influence of life stress on depression: moderation by a polymorphism in the 5-HTT gene. *Science*. 2003;301:386–389.

171. Karg K, Burmeister M, Shedden K, Sen S. The serotonin transporter promoter variant (5-HTTLPR), stress, and depression meta-analysis revisited: evidence of genetic moderation. *Arch Gen Psychiatry*. 2011;68:444–454.

172. Hariri AR, Mattay VS, Tessitore A, et al. Serotonin transporter genetic variation and the response of the human amygdala. *Science*. 2002;297:400–403.

173. Drabant EM, Ramel W, Edge MD, et al. Neural mechanisms underlying 5-HTTLPR-related sensitivity to acute stress. *Am J Psychiatry*. 2012;169:397–405.

174. Pezawas L, Meyer-Lindenberg A, Drabant EM, et al. 5-HTTLPR polymorphism impacts human cingulate-amygdala interactions: a genetic susceptibility mechanism for depression. *Nat Neurosci*. 2005;8:828–834.

175. Frodl T, Koutsouleris N, Bottlender R, et al. Reduced gray matter brain volumes are associated with variants of the serotonin transporter gene in major depression. *Mol Psychiatry*. 2008;13:1093–1101.

176. Selvaraj S, Godlewska BR, Norbury R, et al. Decreased regional gray matter volume in S' allele carriers of the 5-HTTLPR triallelic polymorphism. *Mol Psychiatry*. 2011;16:471, 2–3.

177. Lewis CM, Ng MY, Butler AW, et al. Genome-wide association study of major recurrent depression in the U.K. population. *Am J Psychiatry*. 2010;167:949–957.

178. Wray NR, Pergadia ML, Blackwood DH, et al. Genome-wide association study of major depressive disorder: new results, meta-analysis, and lessons learned. *Mol Psychiatry*. 2012;17:36–48.

179. Booij L, Wang D, Levesque ML, Tremblay RE, Szyf M. Looking beyond the DNA sequence: the relevance of DNA methylation processes for the stress-diathesis model of depression. *Philos Trans R Soc Lond B Biol Sci*. 2013;368:20120251.

180. Weaver IC, Cervoni N, Champagne FA, et al. Epigenetic programming by maternal behavior. *Nat Neurosci*. 2004;7:847–854.

181. McGowan PO, Sasaki A, D'Alessio AC, et al. Epigenetic regulation of the glucocorticoid receptor in human brain associates with childhood abuse. *Nat Neurosci*. 2009;12:342–348.

182. Klengel T, Mehta D, Anacker C, et al. Allele-specific FKBP5 DNA demethylation mediates gene-childhood trauma interactions. *Nat Neurosci*. 2013;16:33–41.

183. Buss C, Davis EP, Muftuler LT, Head K, Sandman CA. High pregnancy anxiety during mid-gestation is associated with decreased gray matter density in 6-9-year-old children. *Psychoneuroendocrinology*. 2010;35:141–153.

184. Van den Bergh BR, Van Calster B, Smits T, Van Huffel S, Lagae L. Antenatal maternal anxiety is related to HPA-axis dysregulation and self-reported depressive symptoms in adolescence: a prospective study on the fetal origins of depressed mood. *Neuropsychopharmacology*. 2008;33:536–545.

185. Fava M, Rankin MA, Wright EC, et al. Anxiety disorders in major depression. *Compr Psychiatry*. 2000;41:97–102.

186. Ionescu DF, Niciu MJ, Mathews DC, Richards EM, Zarate CA Jr. Neurobiology of anxious depression: a review. *Depress Anxiety*. 2013;30:374–385.

187. Sandi C, Richter-Levin G. From high anxiety trait to depression: a neurocognitive hypothesis. *Trends Neurosci*. 2009;32:312–320.

188. Nissen C, Holz J, Blechert J, et al. Learning as a model for neural plasticity in major depression. *Biol Psychiatry*. 2010;68:544–552.

189. Etkin A, Schatzberg AF. Common abnormalities and disorder-specific compensation during implicit regulation of emotional processing in generalized anxiety and major depressive disorders. *Am J Psychiatry*. 2011;168:968–978.

190. Andreescu C, Wu M, Butters MA, Figurski J, Reynolds CF 3rd, Aizenstein HJ. The default mode network in late-life anxious depression. *Am J Geriatr Psychiatry*. 2011;19:980–983.

191. van Tol MJ, van der Wee NJ, van den Heuvel OA, et al. Regional brain volume in depression and anxiety disorders. *Arch Gen Psychiatry* 2010;67:1002–1011.

192. Manna CB, Tenke CE, Gates NA, et al. EEG hemispheric asymmetries during cognitive tasks in depressed patients with high versus low trait anxiety. *Clin EEG Neurosci*. 2010;41:196–202.

193. Bruder GE, Fong R, Tenke CE, et al. Regional brain asymmetries in major depression with or without an anxiety disorder: a quantitative electroencephalographic study. *Biol Psychiatry*. 1997;41:939–948.

194. Meller WH, Kathol RG, Samuelson SD, et al. CRH challenge test in anxious depression. *Biol Psychiatry*. 1995;37:376–382.

195. Rao ML, Vartzopoulos D, Fels K. Thyroid function in anxious and depressed patients. *Pharmacopsychiatry*. 1989;22:66–70.

196. Baffa A, Hohoff C, Baune BT, et al. Norepinephrine and serotonin transporter genes: impact on treatment response in depression. *Neuropsychobiology*. 2010;62:121–31.

197. Binder EB, Owens MJ, Liu W, et al. Association of polymorphisms in genes regulating the corticotropin-releasing factor system with antidepressant treatment response. *Arch Gen Psychiatry*. 2010;67:369–379.

198. Domschke K, Lawford B, Laje G, et al. Brain-derived neurotrophic factor (BDNF) gene: no major impact on antidepressant treatment response. *Int J Neuropsychopharmacol*. 2010;13:93–101.

SECTION II

Assessment and Treatment of Depression in Medically Ill Patients

CHAPTER 3

Assessment of Depression in Patients with Medical Illnesses

David Wolfe, MD, MPH
Jane Erb, MD
Jhilam Biswas, MD

INTRODUCTION

Like most medical complaints, a depressed mood in and of itself represents a symptom, and not a diagnosis. Indeed, depression is a relatively nonspecific complaint, that could reflect anything from the most debilitating psychiatric illness to a normal response to stress or loss (**Fig. 3-1**). The differential diagnosis for depression among psychiatric disorders alone is broad, requiring a thorough history, examination, and often laboratory tests to discern the underlying etiology (or at least exclude potential confounders). The assessment of mood disorders in the medically ill poses yet several additional challenges, especially since many core, neurovegetative symptoms of depression – such as fatigue, anergia, insomnia, anorexia, weight loss, and pain – often result directly from medical illnesses, themselves. Among patients with severe medical disease, assessment can be confounded by "sickness behavior," a state of decreased motivation resulting from systemic inflammation, and characterized by malaise, anorexia, insomnia, fatigue, as well as fever.[1] Similarly, delirium, especially the hypoactive subtype, can present with prominent mood symptoms, making patients appear dysphoric. Adding to the complexity in assessment, many commonly used treatments, such as steroids or interferon-α, can also lower mood as a side effect. Proper diagnosis remains critical, as the recommended treatment approaches do vary widely, depending on the etiology.

In this chapter, we review approaches for screening and diagnosing depression in the medically ill. We begin in what is likely familiar territory: the common, primary psychiatric diagnoses that present with a low mood, and their implications for medical patients. We then discuss approaches to the clinical interview, available screening tools, the potentially confounding role of delirium in this population, and the assessment of suicidal risk. Finally, we review cultural and ethnic considerations that inform the assessment of depression.

WHEN IS DEPRESSION A DISORDER?

Along with anxiety, a low mood represents a common, typical response to stressors in life. As is the case with bereavement, a certain degree of depression is considered normal, even adaptive, and does not rise to clinical attention. This phenomenon is of special relevance for individuals with medical illness, all of whom face some degree of stress, loss, or burden. Physical suffering, functional limitations, hospitalizations, frequent medical appointments, social isolation, concern about the future, reliance on caregivers, and the financial burdens are just a few examples of illness-related stress. Feeling at least somewhat discouraged is to be expected in these situations, so how do we know when depression requires clinical intervention? The DSM addresses this issue primarily by requiring the presence of "significant distress or impairment in social, occupational, or other important areas of functioning" as diagnostic criteria for a mood disorder.[2] That said, even the authors concede that normal grief and illness can coexist and that clinical judgment is ultimately required. For depression arising from a stressor (social or health-related), that crosses the line into clinical significance, the diagnosis of adjustment disorder with depressed mood represents the first point beyond uncomplicated grief or normal coping. According to the DSM 5, adjustment disorders are pervasive in general medical hospitals, with a prevalence of up to 50% among inpatients. The key feature of an adjustment disorder is the presence of a stressor bearing a clear relationship to a depression that appears to be out of proportion to the situation and/or results in functional impairment. The typical

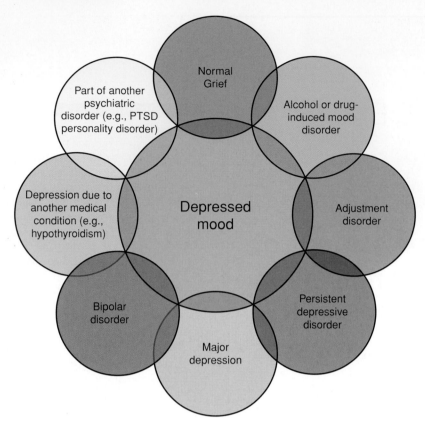

Figure 3-1 *The symptom of depression has several possible causes.*

course of adjustment disorder with depressed mood is contrasted with that of major depression in **Figure 3-2**. Adjustment disorder with depressed mood is often seen when medically ill patients receive new diagnoses, have a recurrence or worsening of their illness, or require new types of treatment, such as supplemental oxygen or chemotherapy. Notably, an exacerbation of an underlying, pre-existing mental illness, even in the context of stress, does not constitute an adjustment disorder, underscoring the importance of careful history taking in making the diagnosis.

DIAGNOSES THAT INCLUDE DEPRESSION

The diagnosis of adjustment disorder is insufficient for depression that causes severe impairment, or that arises without a clear relationship to stressors, expanding the diagnostic possibilities considerably (**Fig. 3-3**). The first task is to exclude direct medical causes for a depressed mood and ensure their adequate treatment. (In DSM 5, the formal diagnosis "mood disorder due to a general medical condition" was changed to "due to *another* medical condition, reflecting

the notion that primary depressive disorders are medical.) Examples of mood disorder due to the pathophysiology of another medical condition are found throughout this book, and can arise from a variety of diseases. The initial evaluation of depressed mood includes the exclusion of drug- or alcohol-induced mood disorders as well as of common medical illnesses causing low energy and fatigue, such as anemia and thyroid dysfunction. Taking a relatively prevalent example, hypothyroidism can present with prominent complaints of depressed or irritable mood, apathy, anergia, anhedonia, and amotivation. While clinical hypothyroidism is found in less than 4% of patients with depression, subclinical hypothyroidism is present in up to 40% of patients, and can be important to recognize.[3] The diagnosis of depression due to another medical condition also encompasses any drug-related side effects that produce a low mood. Common examples of drugs that can induce depression include isoniazid, prednisone, and interferon.

Once adjustment and substance-use disorders and medical causes are excluded, the key entity to consider in the differential

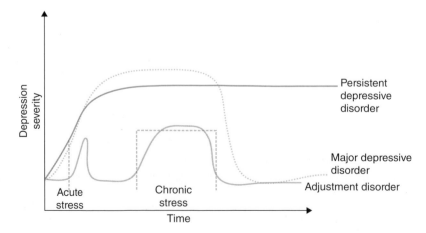

Figure 3-2 *Adjustment disorders always occur following a stressor and may be chronic. Major depression in its episodic and chronic forms can arise with or without a precipitant, and are generally marked by more severe mood symptoms.*

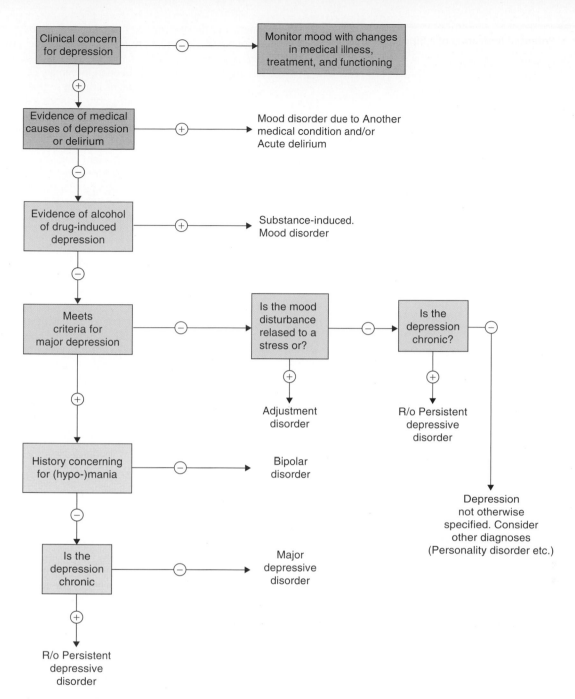

Figure 3-3 *A diagnostic pathway for assessing depression in the medically ill.*

diagnosis is major depressive disorder (MDD). MDD is marked by at least 2 weeks of depressed mood, occurring most days, causing significant distress, and accompanied by at least four other symptoms. Four of the nine diagnostic criteria (weight change, dyssomnia, psychomotor retardation or agitation, and fatigue) are also common in acute and chronic medical disease, which complicate the diagnostic process in the medically ill. In this case, greater reliance on the cognitive and affective symptoms (decreased pleasure in activities, feelings of worthlessness or guilt, helplessness, hopelessness, decreased concentration, and suicidal thoughts) may be required to make the diagnosis. Importantly, major depression may arise in the context of one or more stressors, at first resembling adjustment. Alternatively, it may arise either without a clear precipitant or coincide with the onset of a life stressor. While adjustment disorders generally respond well to supportive psychotherapy, major depres-

sion typically requires medication or a combination of treatment modalities, including cognitive behavioral therapy. In severe cases of major depression, psychotic features (typically mood-congruent, negative delusions, and auditory hallucinations) can arise, prompting treatment with antipsychotics as well as antidepressants.

Although major depression is typically believed to be episodic, marked by interspersed periods of normal mood (or euthymia), more chronic forms do exist. For clinically significant depression lasting 2 years or longer, clinicians should consider the diagnosis of persistent depressive disorder (a consolidation of the former diagnoses of dysthymia and chronic major depression, thus superseding the prior distinguishing criteria of symptom severity). These patients typically report depression beginning as early adults, if not during childhood, and have some chronic degree of mood disturbance with fluctuating severity. Earlier onset of persistent depressive

TABLE 3-1 Potential Indicators of a Bipolar Diathesis

Family history of bipolar disorder
Early onset of first depression (>age 25)
Multiple prior episodes of depression
Shorter depressive episodes
Psychosis or pathological guilt
Mood lability
Psychomotor slowing, leaden paralysis, hypersomnia, hyperphagia

Data from Mitchell PB, Goodwin GM, Johnson GF, et al. Diagnostic guidelines for bipolar depression: a probabilistic approach. Bipolar Disord. 2008;10(1 Pt 2):144–152.

disorder is associated with comorbid personality and substance-use disorders.

Evaluating a patient in the midst of a major depressive episode, regardless of duration, is important to determine whether a bipolar diathesis exists. Individuals with an underlying bipolar diathesis, or full disorder, are at risk for developing mania from antidepressants, and may face a worsened course of their mood disorder without an appropriate mood stabilizing agent.[4,5] It is therefore important to screen for a history of mania or hypomania, as well as to identify individuals at risk for developing the disorder but who have yet to manifest manic symptoms (**Table 3-1**). Unfortunately, the depressive phase of bipolar disorder is generally clinically indistinguishable from that of (unipolar) major depression. While inquiring about a past history of mania or hypomania is a necessary first step, even structured diagnostic interviews fail to identify past manic or hypomanic episodes in a significant number of patients with bipolar depression.[6] Patients with active major depression may have difficulty recalling any history of (hypo-)mania fully, so collateral information from family or friends is often useful.

Beyond these primary mood disorders, many psychiatric illnesses can present with some symptoms of depression, such as posttraumatic stress disorder, substance-use disorders, anxiety disorders, personality disorders, or eating disorders. It is always important to keep in mind that multiple diagnoses can coexist, and that a depressive disorder alone may not fully explain the clinical picture. In cases where the diagnosis is unclear, a systematic approach to excluding contributing factors, such as outlined in **Table 3-2**, can be useful.

CLINICAL INTERVIEWS IN PATIENTS WITH MEDICAL ILLNESS

The psychiatric interview of individuals with active medical illness can present various challenges, depending on the environment and nature of the referral. Certainly for patients in medical inpatient or emergency department settings, small spaces, limited privacy, noisy surroundings, interruptions, and unpredictable time constraints can all affect the quality of the interview. The same may be true for outpatient clinicians embedded in primary care offices or other specialty clinics, where mental health may not be the primary focus of the practice. In these venues, consultations may be unexpected, arising with little to no warning to the patient or provider, and require a flexible, yet efficient approach. Since the timeframe for assessment and management can be relatively short compared to customary intakes in an outpatient psychiatry clinic, it is ideal to establish rapport quickly and address the "critical" issues, such as safety, early. In this sense, operating under the assumption that the interview could be interrupted at any moment can help the clinician focus on the most important elements of the history and examination, before the patient must leave to obtain a laboratory test, or vacate the examination room.

For initial encounters, it is important to keep in mind that many patients seen in general medical settings (or who are referred from these settings), may never have seen a psychiatrist or mental health provider before. They might not have sought out psychiatric care of their own accord, and in some cases may be entirely unaware of the reasons for the referral. This situation may be especially true of medical inpatients, individuals noted to be depressed on routine screenings, and patients seeking psychiatric "clearance" for surgeries or other procedures. Many patients therefore harbor some anxiety about the psychiatric interview and how the findings will be used. Some may have misconceptions or embarrassment about mental illness, or even present with hostility toward the psychiatric provider for thinking they need mental health services. Since a comfortable and productive rapport is so important, a few strategies for managing these issues are reviewed here.

Asking patients if they are aware of the reasons for the referral – and clarifying any inaccuracies – builds the alliance from the outset. This process also gives the clinician some sense of the patient's insight into their illness, mood, and social interactions. For patients reluctant to entertain a depression diagnosis, it can also be helpful to provide some education about the impact of depression on medical disorders and the benefits of addressing both simultaneously. For patients with chronic depression, especially in the context of health or other social stressors, they may not necessarily view their low mood and related functional impairment as abnormal, or in need of treatment. Indeed, they may have gotten the message from family, friends, and even medical providers, that being depressed is "normal," appropriate, or expectable given their situation. In these cases, it often helps to portray the initial interview more as an evaluation to see "what could be done to be helpful," whether it is improving sleep, energy level, or motivation, as opposed to making a diagnosis.

For patients who have never seen a psychiatric clinician in the past, and did not seek out the evaluation on their own, anxiety about the nature of the interview is common. Patients often worry

TABLE 3-2 Comprehensive Depression Evaluation

Checklist for confounding and contributing factors		
Medical	**Psychiatric**	**Basics**
Sleep disorder (e.g., restless legs, periodic leg movements, sleep apnea)	Bipolar risk	Diet
	Psychotic symptoms	Exercise
Thyroid disorder	Alcohol and substance use (consider urine tox screen)	Engaging in pleasurable activities including socially
B12 or folate deficiency		Sense of purpose
Cognitive disorder (e.g., dementia)	Trauma history	Stable/safe living situation (e.g., domestic violence)
Delirium	Obsessive compulsive disorder	Adequate light (e.g., getting outside routinely)
	Eating disorder	

that they will be "analyzed" or somehow "tricked" into discussing things that are private. This concern may be shaped by the experience – positive or negative – of their family or friends who had previously sought mental health care. Individuals being screened for surgery or employment may be especially guarded about revealing depression symptoms or other signs of mental illness. It is not uncommon for patients to ask for some reassurance during the end of the interview; "So I'm not crazy, right?"

One helpful approach is to begin the history by inquiring about more comfortable, familiar information for the patient: their medical illness. Most patients have had more experience discussing their physical complaints. For many, discussing their pulmonary disease or diabetes is familiar and well-travelled territory, while seldom if ever have they broached the related emotional issues. Conveying or reflecting back some basic knowledge about the medical disease in an empathic manner not only serves to build the alliance, it conveys that the clinician intends to recognize and address the medical as well as psychiatric issues in the patient's care. This approach allays fears that the clinician does not understand the medical illness, or that psychiatric treatment will hinder their medical care.

In addition to increasing the comfort level of the interview, starting with the medical history also gives a sense of the time course and relative severity of the illness, important for determining the chronological relationship to mood symptoms. Transitioning to more "psychiatric" questions is then accomplished by asking how the medical illness, now well reviewed, has affected them. For instance, one might ask, "How have your spirits been holding up with all of this going on?" or "Has all this affected your activities or mood?" From there, more specific inquiries can proceed to assess hopelessness, helplessness, and self-blaming thoughts. Again, early knowledge of the patient's medical illness helps contextualize these cognitive features of depression; for example, is the illness terminal, or does the self-blame arise from a perceived burden of family? Exploring negative cognitions can also be useful in determining the nature of nonspecific symptoms, such as fatigue, common to both depression and many systemic illnesses. Given the potential time constraints mentioned above, it is also prudent to screen for suicidal thoughts as early as appropriate in the interview, ensuring an adequate opportunity to address any acute safety concerns.

In concert with the history typically reviewed during a psychiatric interview, special consideration should be given to the longitudinal course of the patient's functional impairment, social context, and health care resources. Social isolation and financial difficulties often grow as medical illness progresses, for instance, compounding the level of depression. For illnesses with a relapsing and remitting course, inquiring in more detail about possible past episodes of mood symptoms – whether formally diagnosed or not – may be helpful in formulating the current disorder. Eliciting a family history of medical as well as psychiatric illnesses similarly provides a basis not only for the patient's genetic risk but, for diagnoses that run in families, it also identifies any preconceived notions the patient may have about their illness, based on their relatives' experiences.

DEPRESSION SCREENING

Given the time constraints of many medical encounters, there is great value in employing screening tools for detecting possible cases of depression and integrating them into the clinical workflow. Although many validated tools exist, the most common remains the Patient Health Questionnaire (PHQ-9). This nine-item self-report screening instrument rates the presence or absence, and the frequency, of cognitive and physical symptoms of depression as well as suicidal thoughts. The PHQ-9 is well validated in several outpatient medical settings, though the evidence for its use in medical inpatients remains mixed.[7–11] It has also been validated in several languages, including Chinese, Thai, Spanish, French, Swahili, and British sign language.[12–17] PHQ-9 scores range from 0 to 27, with a score over 20 indicative of severe depression. A score of 10 is generally recommended as the threshold for major depression, with a sensitivity and specificity of approximately 88% for both using this cutoff.[18] A more recent meta-analysis of the validation studies, however, showed similar pooled sensitivity and specificity for scores between 8 and 11.[19,20]

A two-item version of this tool, the PHQ-2, also exists and inquires solely about depressed mood and anhedonia in the previous 2 weeks. The PHQ-2 is ideally used as the initial screen. Among primary care and obstetrics-gynecology clinic patients, the PHQ-2 score of 3 or more has a sensitivity of 83% and a specificity of 92% for detecting major depression.[21] A positive score on the PHQ-2 should prompt the administration of the full (PHQ-9) scale. It is important to note that the PHQ-9 (and PHQ-2), cannot differentiate the causes of depression, such as bipolar disorder, adjustment disorder, bereavement, or mood disorders due to substances or a general medical condition. For all of the utility of screening instruments, however, it is important to use clinical judgment and not rely solely on a score to define next steps. A positive screening score always requires further diagnostic clarification; it is critical to review responses with the patient to ensure correct interpretation and avoid misdiagnosis.

DEPRESSION RATING SCALES

Although scores on screening instruments such as the PHQ-9 correlate with depression severity and can demonstrate changes, they typically lack the precision to track specific symptoms over time. For monitoring severity and response to treatment interventions, more detailed scales covering additional symptoms and their severity, not just frequency, are required. Numerous scales exist, with the Hamilton depression rating scale (HDRS) and Montgomery-Asberg Depression Scale (MADRS) remaining the most common, serving as the primary outcomes in efficacy trials of antidepressant medications.[22,23] Both of these scales require administration by a trained individual, and involve ranking the severity of depressive symptoms, such as sleep disturbance, negative thoughts, and suicidal ideation, on Likert-type scales.

The score of the HDRS is summed from 17 items (4 additional items can be recorded but do not add to the score), with a "normal" range below 8, and a "severe" range generally considered to be 24 and above.[24] Contemporary clinical trials of medication efficacy in major depression typically require a relatively high HDRS score of 22 or higher for inclusion. On the MADRS, scores can range from 0 to 60, with a value below 7 generally considered normal, and severe depression defined at about 30 and above.[25] Scores of 30 or above on the MADRS are typical for inclusion in antidepressant studies. The HDRS and MADRS are generally speaking comparable in terms of validity and sensitivity to change, though the MADRS is seven items shorter and usually quicker to administer.[26] Although these scales are used more often in research settings, their clinical value lies in identifying individuals who are most likely to respond to antidepressants (i.e., resembled the subjects in the efficacy trials). Theoretically, this "screening for severity" may reduce unnecessary antidepressant treatment (and related side effects) in mild cases. With repeated measurement, the HDRS and MADRS can also more formally assesses change over time and treatment response (or failure), and provide guidance into which specific symptoms require additional monitoring or intervention. While remission of depression is defined as a score below a cut off (e.g., 7 for the HDRS), treatment response is typically defined as a 50% reduction in the total baseline score.

Self-report depression questionnaires do not require staff time or training, and therefore have clear advantages in routine clinical practice. As with all such instruments, however, there is a risk of patient's under- or over-reporting their symptoms in the absence of careful review and clarification of the responses. Among self-report measures, the most common is the Beck Depression Inventory, a 21-item questionnaire assessing for the negative cognitions as well as neurovegetative symptoms typical of depression.[27] In routine psychiatric practice, BDI scores useful for tracking treatment response, though, symptoms arising from medical illness (such as fatigue) can lead to misleading elevations of somatic sub-scores and as a consequence exaggerate depression severity.[28] The 16-item Quick Inventory of Depressive Symptomatology (QIDS), is also available in a self-report format that has gained acceptance following its use in the pivotal STAR*D trial.[29] The QIDS is well correlated with the HDRS, and has comparable sensitivity to change.[30] The Hospital Anxiety and Depression Scale (HADS) assesses both mood states, and was designed with medical patients in mind, though it may be confounded by the somatic symptoms of medical illnesses. With a sensitivity of approximately 0.8 to detect depression (at a cutoff score above 8), it appears to be a reasonable screening tool, though its utility in diagnosing and tracking cases of depression is relatively low.[31,32]

ASSESSING SUICIDE RISK

Suicide and related attempts arguably represent the most patent and tragic sequelae of depression. Among individuals suffering from life-threatening medical diseases, the prevalence of clinically significant suicidal ideation has been reported at approximately 7%, though this number approaches 25% when comorbid with MDD.[33] Regardless of the underlying diagnosis, detecting and stratifying suicide risk remain critical, as prompt intervention can indeed be life-saving. All patients reporting depression (or screening positive), should be directly asked about suicidal thoughts, plans, and behaviors. Individuals thought to be at significant risk for suicide are typically sent directly to an emergency department, where they can be safely evaluated by a psychiatrist and, if necessary, admitted to a psychiatric inpatient unit.

For many clinicians, inquiring about suicide can be anxiety-provoking, either due to a (false) belief that such a discussion increases the risk, or to uncertainty over how to manage a patient who appears unsafe. A study using simulated patients with depressive disorders, determined that suicide was explored by primary care physicians in only 36% of visits.[34] Clinicians in academic settings and those with personal histories of depression were more likely to inquire, while gender, medical specialty (family practice vs. internal medicine), and confidence in treating depression were not associated with the likelihood of asking about suicide. Simulated patients who reported symptoms of an MDD, as opposed to an adjustment disorder with depressed mood, were more likely to have been questioned about suicide, as were patients specifically requesting antidepressant medication. The authors speculated that the fear of insufficient experience in managing suicidal patients may have influenced clinicians' reluctance to inquire about suicide. Having a clear system for eliciting and addressing suicidal ideation, improves the comfort level for clinicians as well as patients.

The clinician can begin by asking whether the patient has ever wished he or she were dead. If endorsed, then questions about specific thoughts of suicide should follow, including whether the individual has thought about a method, begun making plans or preparations, gathered materials for the suicide such as pills, begun putting his/her affairs in order, and whether he or she intends to act on his/her thoughts. Generally speaking, the further along the patient is on this path from suicidal thought to behavior, the more concerning. Understanding what has prevented the individual from following through, can be helpful in stratifying risk as well. In the absence of active suicidal thoughts, inquiry about past ideation and past behaviors is important, as this history suggests an elevated longitudinal risk for future suicide.

For those seeking a more structured assessment, the Columbia Suicide Severity Rating Scale (C-SSRS)[35] is a validated screening tool. It is used throughout the world and in a variety of settings, including

primary care, medical homes and behavioral health organizations as well as by clergy, hospices, schools, prisons, and the military. The C-SSRS has excellent specificity and sensitivity, has been validated for both adult and pediatric populations, and is available in many languages. Although administering the scale requires training, specific mental health or other clinical training is not required. When patients screen positive for suicide risk, the scale administrator is prompted to alert a trained clinician who can more thoroughly assess the patient. What makes this tool particularly useful is that it differentiates among the wide range of suicidal ideation and related behaviors, allowing for some quantification of risk. More recently, a self-rated, computer-automated version, the eC-SSRS, is being evaluated for use in clinical trials.[36]

It is important to assess suicide risk in the routine care not only of patients with known psychiatric illness or history, but also of patients with serious physical illness. Medical illness is an independent risk factor for suicide, though the relationship between the two is complex and nuanced. Additional risk factors for suicide include being single, unemployed, and male. Having access to a firearm and a comorbid alcohol or substance abuse disorder also raise the risk for attempted and completed suicide.

Although cancer and HIV are historically associated with an increased risk for suicide, particularly in the period of time immediately following diagnosis, not all medical illnesses appear to increase this risk. In a large, longitudinal study of patients diagnosed with Parkinson's disease, the suicide rate was actually 10 times lower than that observed in the general population. Furthermore, the social profile of those who committed suicide with Parkinson's disease was the same as that of the general population except that, unlike others, being married conferred a greater suicide risk than not being married.[37] Similarly, individuals with chronic pulmonary disease were found to be more likely to commit suicide if married.[38] Authors in both studies postulated that worries about becoming dependent and burdening the spouse may have been contributing to this behavior. Therefore, the usual consideration that individuals who are single are at higher risk of suicide is not necessarily true in those with all medical illnesses.

Timing of the diagnosis of the comorbid illness is also a consideration. The risk of suicide appears to be highest soon after the diagnosis of a major medical illness is made and diminishes over time in association with initiating treatment for the medical illness. Age also appears to be a factor as younger individuals diagnosed with a major physical illness are more likely to take their lives than medically ill elderly individuals. A study that explored suicides in people aged over 65 found that individuals suffering from three or more illnesses had a threefold increase in their risk of suicide.[39]

Further study of physical illness as a risk factor for suicide is needed. However, this research is difficult because there are no standardized or uniform definitions of chronic or terminal illness, physical impairment or disability, and pain. Furthermore, identifying a good control group is challenging as those dying of "natural causes" are inevitably afflicted with physical illness. Most studies use motor vehicle accident victims as the comparison group but a subset of them are misclassified because they are actually suicides. Nevertheless, the presence of physical illness has not received the emphasis it deserves in suicide assessment and prevention strategies. A study by Demos, a UK-based think tank, challenges the notion that suicide is solely a mental health issue. Careful examination of data from a range of sources led to the conclusion that 10% of 4,390 cases of suicide occurred in individuals who were "experiencing some form of serious physical illness as an influencing factor."[40]

Individuals who end their lives through suicide have visited their primary care physicians (45%) or mental health clinicians (19%) in the last month of their lives.[4] Most studies do not report what was discussed in these final visits. Only a minority of the studies that do find that suicide was mentioned. And when such discussions were documented, most patients denied suicidal ideation. Smith et al. examined the quality of a suicide assessment of Veteran's Health Administration patients with a history of depression who died by suicide.[5] While most of these patients had undergone some suicide risk assessment within the past year, many did not at their final visit, particularly those seen by nonmental health clinicians. Patients were more likely to have reported suicidal thoughts at some previous point in the past year than at their final visit. This suggests that lifetime suicidal ideation may sometimes be a better predictor than current suicidal ideation, and highlights the importance of repeated, ongoing suicide assessment and monitoring of suicidal ideation and behaviors in the context of physical illness and depression. It is imperative to remember that denial of current suicidal thoughts does not necessarily preclude imminent risk.

ASSESSING DEPRESSION IN THE PRESENCE OF DELIRIUM

Delirium, an acute change in mental status marked by impairment of attention, disorganized or confused thinking, and fluctuating level of consciousness, is a common and significant complication in medically ill individuals. While delirium is primarily seen in the hospital setting, with a reported prevalence between 14% and 56%, cases can arise among outpatients as well, especially in the elderly.[41,42]

Delirium can mimic many psychiatric illnesses, with hallucinations, sleep disturbance, affective changes, additional disruptions in cognition, and significant agitation. The most common subtype of delirium, however, is hypoactive, where patients appear withdrawn, less interactive, and "quietly confused." In these cases, a blunted or flat affect frequently lends itself to misdiagnosis as depression. This topic is covered in greater detail in Chapter 22, though the main points are reviewed here.

Distinguishing hypoactive delirium from depression relies on assessing carefully for cognitive changes and determining if there are any related medical causes, such as new infections or medications. Typically patients with hypoactive delirium will not endorse a depressed mood, but may report low energy, anxiety, difficulty concentrating, and sleep disturbance. Testing for attention, such as asking the patient to recite the months of the year backward, as well as directly asking about the patient's mood are often sufficient to distinguish hypoactive delirium from depression. Notably, visual hallucinations are most common in delirium, but rare in major depression. The time course of delirium typically waxes and wanes over hours, whereas primary depression remains relatively static.

There are difficulties in cognition in some severe cases of depression, occasionally (and misleadingly) referred to as "pseudo-dementia." But these generally reflect lack of effort or apathy, as opposed to true dysfunction. Auditory hallucinations can occur in severe cases of either condition, but are more likely to occur in delirium. In some cases, especially those involving patients with a significant psychiatric history, or a prolonged and complicated hospital stay, distinguishing between the two can be difficult. Also, in relatively rare instances, delirious patients can appear quite tearful and endorse several signs of depression, including suicidal thoughts. In unclear situations, an electroencephalogram (EEG) can be useful by demonstrating the diffuse slowing classically seen in delirium, as well as by ruling out seizure activity. In a depressed individual without delirium or other neurologic disease, the EEG is expected to be normal.

Delirium and depression can coexist, but if they do, the immediate concern is to treat the underlying cause(s) of the delirium, while managing agitation, sleep disturbance, and subjective distress with antipsychotics. Adding antidepressants during this period may actually worsen confusion and is best considered after the delirium has resolved.

ASSESSING ANXIETY IN THE CONTEXT OF DEPRESSION

Anxiety, whether manifested in psychological tension or somatic symptoms, is common in depression, though it may also reflect another coexisting disorder. Indeed, a review of depression rating scales such as the HDRS reveals this overlap in symptoms, with several items capturing anxiety, such as agitation, "psychic" anxiety, "somatic" anxiety, and hypochondriasis. Interestingly, many of these features also appear on the corresponding anxiety rating scales. Carefully assessing the time course of the anxiety symptoms may help to distinguish the two diagnoses; did the anxiety symptoms pre-date the depression? Or did they solely arise on occasion from physical stress such as severe pain or dyspnea? In some instances, the anxiety may in fact be the heralding or most troubling symptom of depression, especially in those individuals who are under significant medical or social stress. Fortunately, first-line antidepressant medications often help generalized anxiety and panic symptoms, though more focused treatments may be indicated if there is evidence for a primary anxiety disorder diagnosis.

CULTURAL AND ETHNIC CONSIDERATIONS IN ASSESSING DEPRESSION

In this discussion of multicultural variance in depression among the medically ill, we will define culture as a shared belief system and sets of norms and values of a given ethnic group. Although cultural diversity is a defining feature of the American population, ethnic groups frequently have unequal access to health care resources. They are at greater risk of having undiagnosed comorbid depression, even while being treated for a medical condition. Latinos, African Americans, and Asian Americans of more traditional backgrounds rarely seek out specialized mental health treatment and most often come to primary care clinics[43] with somatic symptoms rather than explicit psychiatric concerns.

Stigma has a role in explaining why ethnic minorities may prefer to see medical providers rather than psychiatrists for mental health problems. Though research is sparse, studies show that mental illness stigma is stronger among all minority groups (including Native Americans, African Americans, Asians, Latinos and Middle Easterners) than it is among Caucasian Americans. (DHHS, 2001;[44-46] These groups tend to value a collectivistic, interdependent social network more than European cultures that tend value autonomy, independence, individuation, and future orientation more.[47-48] With ethnic patients, skilled physicians may first need to build rapport by exchange of casual conversation before beginning the business of taking a medical history or depression assessment. Primary care physicians often play a critical role in helping patients to normalize their experience of mental health problems through education and discussion about common misconceptions, ignorance, and discrimination associated with mental illness.

In many Asian cultures, one's individual successes and failures reflect on the family. For instance, in Filipino culture, an individual's mental illness is considered the family's mental illness.[49] Depression can therefore be a source of family shame and make it difficult for caregivers to reach out for help. In Latino culture, *marianismo* and *machismo* are important traditional values.[50] *Marianismo* refers to the ideal attribute in a woman to be moral, self-sacrificing and to endure suffering with dignity, while *machismo* refers to valuing men who are strong, protective, and defend their families. These cultural values make it difficult for individuals to discuss mental illness openly for fear of appearing weak or incapable.[45]

Different societies have differing psychological constructs for understanding depression. Debilitating depressive symptoms may not be seen as a disease or as symptoms of a pre-existing medical condition. Symptoms of depression may be interpreted as an emotional reaction to a life stressor rather than an illness that has medical treatments or

TABLE 3-3 Eliciting Culturally Based Understanding of Illness

Culturally Sensitive Methods in Learning Patient Concerns	Questions to Ask
Explore patient and their social network's definition of the problem	1. What brings you in today? 2. Sometimes people find different ways of describing their problem to family and friends. How would you tell them what's going on with you?
Explore cultural perception of the cause	1. Why do you think this is happening to you? 2. What might be causing your problem? 3. What do other people in your family or your friends think is happening to you?
Explore patient's stressors and supports	1. What makes your life better? 2. Who helps you when you have a problem? 3. Are there difficulties in your life that are causing you stress?
Explore patient's coping skills and help-seeking behaviors	1. What are some ways you are dealing with your problem? 2. Are there things you do to cope that are specific to your background? 3. Has anything stopped you from getting help in the past 4. Have you ever seen a traditional healer for your problem?
Explore how patient identifies with their culture and how important it is to their decisions.	1. For you, what is the most important part of your culture to you? 2. What types of interactions give you comfort? 3. Are there aspects of your culture or identity that makes things more difficult for you?
Help clarify different expectations between the physician and the patient	1. Sometimes doctors and patients miscommunicate because they come from different backgrounds or have different expectations for treatment. Have you been worried about this and is there anything we can do to take better care of you?

consequences; thus it might seem less urgent to the patient or the caregivers to get help.[51] Although this can feel less stigmatizing, it may stop people from considering available treatment options.

Understanding the patient's cultural background can help the clinician form an alliance, develop a more accurate formulation of his/her mental state, and increase adherence to treatment. Key factors in cultural history-taking include an exploration of the patient's traditions, values, beliefs, and family systems and of how racism and poverty may affect his/her behavior, as well as an appreciation of how language, speech patterns, and communication styles differ across cultural communities. At the same time, the clinician must recognize that professional values may conflict with or require accommodation to the emotional needs of patients from different cultures.[52]

The cultural formulation in Appendix I of DSM-IV was the first formal attempt to define cultural nuances in diagnosis and practice. It pointed to four culturally sensitive domains: the patient's relationship to his/her cultural identity; the meaning of the current illness and the experience of it; psychosocial supports; and daily functioning. This formulation was revised and updated in DSM-5. **Table 3-3** is an adaptation of the DSM model, describing how to elicit a culturally focused interview of a patient and formulate their understanding of their illness.

A common concern when assessing depression in patients of ethnic minority groups or special cultural backgrounds is whether the common depression screening instruments are valid. The following discussion focuses on the PHQ and CES-D, whose cultural validity has been examined.

The self-administered PRIME-MD PHQ-9 is a DSM criterion-based instrument for depression screening in primary care.[53] It has good validity and utility in ethnic minority patients. It is therefore generally considered to be a good screening tool for detecting depression in various ethnic groups. The PHQ-9 was examined in a large primary care sample that included Chinese American, Latino, African American, and non-Hispanic white patients. It had satisfactory reliability, sensitivity, and specificity.[54] The Spanish version of the PHQ-9 has demonstrated satisfactory diagnostic validity in general hospital inpatients[55] and in primary care outpatients.[56]

However, there are significant variations in the endorsement of individual PHQ items by ethnicity. Depressed Latino patients are more likely to endorse anhedonia, and depressed Chinese Americans are more likely to endorse psychomotor abnormalities and sleep problems and less likely to endorse appetite problems, compared with other ethnic groups.[54] Wong et al.[57] noticed that the optimal cutoff scores for the PHQ-9 used in Asian studies tended to be lower, which may imply that Asian patients tend to endorse fewer items overall.

The Center for Epidemiological Studies Depression Scale (CES-D) is another screening instrument has been widely used and validated in various cultural and ethnic populations.[58] The Spanish version of CES-D has demonstrated fair accuracy and validity in detecting depression.[56,59,60] The Chinese version of CES-D also showed satisfactory psychometric properties[61] and has been widely used for assessing depressive symptoms and comparisons with other ethnic groups.

There is variation in the endorsement of individual CES-D items across ethnic groups. Some researchers found that African Americans responded higher on "people are unfriendly" and "people dislike me" items than Whites, while matching on overall depressive symptoms, and suggested the CES-D would have greater validity after removal of these two interpersonal items.[62] A factor analysis of the CES-D in an older, community-dwelling African-American sample disclosed four factors (depressive/somatic, positive, interpersonal, and social well-being) that differ from the factor structure originally derived.[63] This finding was confirmed in a later study.[64] Administration of the CES-D in a Chinese sample revealed an overlap of affective and somatic factors, reflecting the experience and manifestation of depression in Chinese culture.[61]

A recent meta-analysis of the CES-D literature compared African Americans, American Indians, Asians, Whites, and Hispanics[65] and confirmed the original four-factor structure of the CES-D.[58] However, when Kim et al.[65] conducted an exploratory factor analysis without prespecifying the categories for sorting the items they found greater variability across racial/ethnic groups. Two additional factors (demoralization and distress) appeared in African Americans, one additional factor (alienation) appeared in Asians, and one additional factor (preoccupation) appeared in Whites.

The PHQ-9 and CES-D are better choices for detecting depression in ethnic minority groups. The Beck Depression Inventory (BDI) has limited predictive power and validity.[66–68]

CONCLUSION

Among the medically ill, depressed mood is a common yet non-specific symptom that requires thorough medical and psychiatric evaluation. Although discouragement alone is not typically grounds for clinical intervention, adjustment disorder is indeed prevalent in this population as medical illness brings a multitude of psychological, social, and functional stressors. Major depression can arise in the presence or absence of these stressors, and shares several symptoms with medical illnesses, complicating diagnosis. Several standardized instruments can detect depression and gauge its severity in this population, while cognitive examination and basic medical evaluation are often sufficient to exclude nonpsychiatric causes of a depressed mood. Regardless of cause, however, patients with depression require careful monitoring for suicidal thoughts, plans, and behaviors. Finally, consideration of cultural and ethnic differences can help the clinician improve screening efficacy, avoid misdiagnosis, and more closely understand the best ways to support patients through their illnesses.

REFERENCES

1. Dantzer R, O'Connor JC, Freund GG, Johnson RW, Kelley KW. From inflammation to sickness and depression: when the immune system subjugates the brain. *Nat Rev Neurosci*. 2008;9(1):46–56.

2. American Psychiatric Association. *DSM-5 Task Force. Diagnostic and Statistical Manual of Mental Disorders: DSM-5*. 5th ed. American Psychiatric Association

3. Wolkowitz OM, Rothschild AJ. Psychoneuroendocrinology: The Scientific Basis of Clinical Practice. 1st ed. Washington, DC: American Psychiatric Pub; 2003.

4. Luoma JB, Martin CE, Pearson JL. Contact with mental health and primary care providers before suicide: a review of the evidence. *Am J Psychiatry*. 2002;159(6):909–916.

5. Smith EG, Kim HM, Ganoczy D, Stano C, Pfeiffer PN, Valenstein M. Suicide risk assessment received prior to suicide death by Veterans Health Administration patients with a history of depression. *J Clin Psychiatry*. 2013;74(3):226–232.

6. Tsuang MT, Winokur G, Crowe RR. Morbidity risks of schizophrenia and affective disorders among first degree relatives of patients with schizophrenia, mania, depression and surgical conditions. *Br J Psychiatry*. 1980;137:497–504.

7. Watnick S, Wang PL, Demadura T, Ganzini L. Validation of 2 depression screening tools in dialysis patients. *Am J Kidney Dis*. 2005;46(5):919–924.

8. Fann JR, Bombardier CH, Dikmen S, et al. Validity of the Patient Health Questionnaire-9 in assessing depression following traumatic brain injury. *J Head Trauma Rehabil*. 2005;20(6):501–511.

9. Martin A, Rief W, Klaiberg A, Braehler E. Validity of the Brief Patient Health Questionnaire Mood Scale (PHQ-9) in the general population. *Gen Hosp Psychiatry*. 2006;28(1):71–77.

10. van Steenbergen-Weijenburg KM, de Vroege L, Ploeger RR, et al. Validation of the PHQ-9 as a screening instrument for depression in diabetes patients in specialized outpatient clinics. *BMC Health Serv Res*. 2010;10:235.

11. Rentsch D, Dumont P, Borgacci S, et al. Prevalence and treatment of depression in a hospital department of internal medicine. *Gen Hosp Psychiatry*. 2007;29(1):25–31.

12. Chen S, Fang Y, Chiu H, Fan H, Jin T, Conwell Y. Validation of the nine-item Patient Health Questionnaire to screen for major depression in a Chinese primary care population. *Asia-Pac Psychiatry*. 2013;5(2):61–68.

13. Lotrakul M, Sumrithe S, Saipanish R. Reliability and validity of the Thai version of the PHQ-9. *BMC psychiatry*. 2008;8:46.

14. Arthurs E, Steele RJ, Hudson M, Baron M, Thombs BD, Canadian Scleroderma Research G. Are scores on English and French versions of the PHQ-9 comparable? An assessment of differential item functioning. *PLoS One*. 2012;7(12):e52028.

15. Rogers KD, Young A, Lovell K, Campbell M, Scott PR, Kendal S. The British Sign Language versions of the Patient Health Questionnaire, the Generalized Anxiety Disorder 7-item Scale, and the Work and Social Adjustment Scale. *J Deaf Stud Deaf Educ*. 2013;18(1):110–122.

16. Omoro SA, Fann JR, Weymuller EA, Macharia IM, Yueh B. Swahili translation and validation of the Patient Health Questionnaire-9 depression scale in the Kenyan head and neck cancer patient population. *Int J Psychiatry Med*. 2006;36(3):367–381.

17. Merz EL, Malcarne VL, Roesch SC, Riley N, Sadler GR. A multigroup confirmatory factor analysis of the Patient Health Questionnaire-9 among English- and Spanish-speaking Latinas. *Cultur Divers Ethnic Minor Psychol*. 2011;17(3):309–316.

18. Kroenke K, Spitzer RL, Williams JB. The PHQ-9: validity of a brief depression severity measure. *J Gen Intern Med*. 2001;16(9):606–613.

19. Arroll B, Goodyear-Smith F, Crengle S, et al. Validation of PHQ-2 and PHQ-9 to screen for major depression in the primary care population. *Ann Fam Med*. 2010;8(4):348–353.

20. Manea L, Gilbody S, McMillan D. Optimal cut-off score for diagnosing depression with the Patient Health Questionnaire (PHQ-9): a meta-analysis. *CMAJ*. 2012;184(3):E191–E196.

21. Kroenke K, Spitzer RL, Williams JB. The Patient Health Questionnaire-2: validity of a two-item depression screener. *Med Care*. 2003;41(11):1284–1292.

22. Hamilton M. A rating scale for depression. *J Neurol Neurosurg Psychiatry*. 1960;23:56–62.

23. Montgomery SA, Asberg M. A new depression scale designed to be sensitive to change. *Br J Psychiatry*. 1979;134:382–389.

24. Zimmerman M, Martinez JH, Young D, Chelminski I, Dalrymple K. Severity classification on the Hamilton depression rating scale. *J Affect Disord*. 2013; 150:384–388.

25. Muller MJ, Himmerich H, Kienzle B, Szegedi A. Differentiating moderate and severe depression using the Montgomery-Asberg depression rating scale (MADRS). *J Affect Disord*. 2003;77(3):255–260.

26. Khan A, Khan SR, Shankles EB, Polissar NL. Relative sensitivity of the Montgomery-Asberg Depression Rating Scale, the Hamilton Depression rating scale and the Clinical Global Impressions rating scale in antidepressant clinical trials. *Int Clin Psychopharmacol*. 2002;17(6):281–285.

27. Beck AT, Ward CH, Mendelson M, Mock J, Erbaugh J. An inventory for measuring depression. *Arch Gen Psychiatry*. 1961;4:561–571.

28. Farmer A, Chubb H, Jones I, Hillier J, Smith A, Borysiewicz L. Screening for psychiatric morbidity in subjects presenting with chronic fatigue syndrome. *Br J Psychiatry*. 1996;168(3):354–358.

29. Trivedi MH, Rush AJ, Ibrahim HM, et al. The Inventory of Depressive Symptomatology, Clinician Rating (IDS-C) and Self-Report (IDS-SR), and the Quick Inventory of Depressive Symptomatology, Clinician Rating (QIDS-C) and Self-Report (QIDS-SR) in public sector patients with mood disorders: a psychometric evaluation. *Psychol Med*. 2004;34(1):73–82.

30. Rush AJ, Trivedi MH, Ibrahim HM, et al. The 16-Item Quick Inventory of Depressive Symptomatology (QIDS), clinician

rating (QIDS-C), and self-report (QIDS-SR): a psychometric evaluation in patients with chronic major depression. *Biol Psychiatry*. 2003;54(5):573–583.

31. Bjelland I, Dahl AA, Haug TT, Neckelmann D. The validity of the Hospital Anxiety and Depression Scale. An updated literature review. *J Psychosom Res*. 2002;52(2):69–77.

32. Spinhoven P, Ormel J, Sloekers PP, Kempen GI, Speckens AE, Van Hemert AM. A validation study of the Hospital Anxiety and Depression Scale (HADS) in different groups of Dutch subjects. *Psychol Med*. 1997;27(2):363–370.

33. Kishi Y, Robinson RG, Kosier JT. Suicidal ideation among patients with acute life-threatening physical illness: patients with stroke, traumatic brain injury, myocardial infarction, and spinal cord injury. *Psychosomatics*. 2001;42(5):382–390.

34. Feldman MD, Franks P, Duberstein PR, Vannoy S, Epstein R, Kravitz RL. Let's not talk about it: Suicide inquiry in primary care. *Ann Fam Med*. 2007;5:412–418.

35. Posner K, Brown GK, Stanley B, et al. The Columbia-Suicide Severity Rating Scale: initial validity and internal consistency findings from three multisite studies with adolescents and adults. *Am J Psychiatry*. 2011;168(12):1266–1277.

36. Mundt JC, Greist JH, Gelenberg AJ, Katzelnick DJ, Jefferson JW, Modell JG. Feasibility and validation of a computer-automated Columbia-Suicide Severity Rating Scale using interactive voice response technology. *J Psychiatr Res*. 2010;44(16):1224–1228.

37. Myslobodsky M, Lalonde FM, Hicks L. Are patients with Parkinson's disease suicidal? *J Geriatr Psychiatry Neurol*. 2001;14(3):120–4.

38. Quan H, Arboleda-Florez J, Fick GH, Stuart HL, Love EJ. Association between physical illness and suicide among the elderly. *Soc Psychiatry Psychiatr Epidemiol*. 2002;37(4):190–197.

39. Juurlink DN, Herrmann N, Szalai JP, Kopp A, Redelmeier DA. Medical illness and the risk of suicide in the elderly. *Arch Intern Med*. 2004;164(11):1179–1184.

40. Bazalgette L, Bradley W, Ousbey J, *The Truth About Suicide*. London, UK; 2011. http://www.demos.co.uk/files/Suicide_-_web.pdf?1314370102

41. Inouye SK. The dilemma of delirium: clinical and research controversies regarding diagnosis and evaluation of delirium in hospitalized elderly medical patients. *Am J Med*. 1994;97(3):278–288.

42. McCusker J, Cole M, Abrahamowicz M, Primeau F, Belzile E. Delirium predicts 12-month mortality. *Arch Intern Med*. 2002;162(4):457–463.

43. Hails K, Brill CD, Chang T, Yeung A, Fava M, Trinh NH. *Curr Psychiatry Rep*. 2012;14(4):336–44.

44. Yang LH, Kleinman A, Link BG, Phelan JC, Lee S, Good B. Culture and stigma: adding moral experience to stigma theory. *Soc Sci Med*. 2007;64:1524–1535.

45. Abdullah T, Brown TL. Mental illness stigma and ethnocultural beliefs, values, and norms: an integrative review. *Clin Psychol Rev*. 2011;31(6):934–948.

46. U.S. Department of Health and Human Services. *Mental health: Culture, race, and ethnicity–A supplement to Mental health: A report of the Surgeon General*. U.S. Department of Health and Human Services, Substance Abuse and Mental Health Services Administration, Center for Mental Health Services, Rockville; 2001.

47. Hughes Halbert C, Barg FK, Weathers B, et al. Differences in cultural beliefs and values among African American and European American men with prostate cancer. *Cancer Control*. 2007;14(3):277–284.

48. Mizelle ND. Counseling White Americans. In: Marini MA, Stebnicki, eds. *The Professional Counselor's Desk Reference*. New York, NY: Springer Publishing Company; 2009:247–254.

49. Sanchez F, Gaw A. Mental health care of Filipino Americans. *Psychiatr Serv*. 2007;58(6):810–815.

50. Andrés-Hyman RC, Ortiz J, Añez LM, Paris M, Davidson L. Culture and clinical practice: recommendations for working with Puerto Ricans and other Latinas(os) in the United States. *Professional Psychology: Res Practice*. 2006;37(6):694–701.

51. Karasz A,. Cultural differences in conceptual models of depression. *Soc Sci Med*. 2005;60:1625–1635

52. Saldana D.. *Cultural Competency: A Practical Guide for Mental Health Service Providers*. Austin, TX. Hogg Foundation for Mental Health, University of Texas at Austin; 2001

53. Kroenke K, Spitzer RL, Williams JB. The PHQ-9: validity of a brief depression severity measure. *J Gen Intern Med*. 2001;16(9):606–613.

54. Huang FY, Chung H, Kroenke K, Delucchi KL, Spitzer RL. Using the patient health questionnaire-9 to measure depression among racially and ethnically diverse primary care patients. *J. Gen. Intern. Med*. 2006;21(6):547–552.

55. Diez-Quevedo C, Rangil T, Sanchez-Planell L, Kroenke K, Spitzer RL. Validation and utility of the patient health questionnaire in diagnosing mental disorders in 1003 general hospital Spanish inpatients. *Psychosom Med*. 2001;63(4):679–686.

56. Reuland DS, Cherrington A, Watkins GS, Bradford DW, Blanco RA, Gaynes BN. Diagnostic accuracy of Spanish language depression-screening instruments. *Ann Fam Med*. 7:455–462.

57. Wong R, Wu R, Guo C, Lam JK, Snowden LR. Culturally sensitive depression assessment for Chinese American Immigrants: development of a comprehensive measure and a screening scale using an item response approach. *Asian Am J Psychol*. 2012; 3;230–253.

58. Radloff LS.. The CES-D Scale: A self-report depression scale for research in the general population. *App Psychol Measurement*. 1977;1:385–401.

59. Ruiz-Grosso P, Loret de Mola C, Vega-Dienstmaier JM, et al. Validation of the Spanish Center for Epidemiological Studies Depression and Zung Self-Rating Depression Scales: A Comparative Validation Study. *PLoS ONE*. 2012;7(10):e45413.

60. Roberts RE. Reliability of the CES-D scale in different ethnic contexts. *Psychiatry Res*. 1980;2:125–134.

61. Ying YW., Depressive symptomatology among Chinese Americans as Measured by the CES-D. *J Clin Psychol*. 1988;44:739–746.

62. Cole SR, Kawachi I, Maller SJ, Berkman LF. Test of item-response bias in the CES-D scale: Experience from the New Haven EPESE study. *J Clin Epidemiol*. 2000;53 285–289.

63. Long Foley K, Reed PS, Mutran EJDeVellis RF. Measurement adequacy of the CES-D among a sample of older African Americans. *Psychiatry Res*. 2002;109:61–69.

64. Williams CD, Taylor TR, Makambi K, et al. CES-D four-factor structure is confirmed, but not invariant, in a large cohort of African American women. *Psychiatry Res*. 2007;150:173–180.

65. Kim G, Decoster J, Huang CH, Chiriboga DA. Race/ethnicity and the factor structure of the Center for Epidemiologic Studies Depression Scale: a meta-analysis. *Cultur Divers Ethnic Minor Psychol.* 2011;17(4):381–396.

66. Azocar F, Areán P, Miranda J, Munoz RF. Differential item functioning in a Spanish translation of the Beck Depression Inventory. *J Clin Psychol.* 2001;57:355–365.

67. Leentjens AF, Verhey FR, Luijckx GJ, Troost J. The validity of the Beck Depression Inventory as a screening and diagnostic instrument for depression in patients with Parkinson's disease. *Mov Disord.* 2000;15:1221–1224.

68. Zheng YP, Wei LA, Goa LG, Zhang GC, Wong CG. Applicability of the Chinese Beck Depression Inventory. *Compr Psychiatry.* 1988;29(5):484-489.

CHAPTER 4

General Considerations in Treatment

Jane Erb, MD
David Kroll, MD
Arielle Stanford, MD
Megan Oser, PhD
Jhilam Biswas, MD

INTRODUCTION

Once a patient with potential depression is identified, comprehensively assessed, and the subtype of his/her depression defined (Chapter 3), the next task is to engage the patient in developing a treatment plan composed of evidence-based interventions to be implemented at the appropriate stage of their depression. Providing a choice of interventions and their respective benefits versus side effects is one way to engage the patient in planning treatment and improves adherence and outcomes.[1] The timing of the intervention is also important; for example, patients with severe depression are often unable to fully engage in cognitive behavioral therapy (CBT) and profit more from CBT if it is introduced during milder stages of illness or once recovery has begun.

Aiming for complete remission and optimal functioning improves outcomes. Patients who experience residual subthreshold symptoms demonstrate a more severe course of illness and experience a relapse or recurrence three times faster than patients who achieve a full remission.[2]

Achieving full remission and optimal functioning improves the mental health prognosis, and may also improve the course of the comorbid medical disorders. Some examples are as follows:

- Patients with depression following stroke are more likely to die from complications of their stroke.[3]
- Patients with diabetes and depression have worse glycemic control and higher rates of diabetic complications.[4]
- Patients with untreated depression are at greater risk of arrhythmia following myocardial infarction and other cardiac diseases than are those without depression (Chapter 7).

The care of patients with medical disorders and comorbid depression costs up to twice that of patients with chronic diseases who are not depressed.[5] It is important to note that only a fraction of these increased costs (about 1%) are attributable to mental health care. Indirect costs are substantial and include lost income and employer costs due to missed work. Costs go well beyond the monetary and also include poorer quality-of-life and increased suicide rates.[6,7] Effective treatment of the depression is likely to lower overall healthcare costs. For example, older adults with major depression or dysthymic disorder who are managed using an integrated depression care model (Chapter 23) are twice as likely as those with nonintegrated care to have at least a 50% reduction in depression symptoms,[8] and reduced total healthcare costs.[8]

In summary, treating depression to remission and minimizing risks for recurrence not only benefits patients and their families; it also has the potential to lower the costs of care and limit the other wider societal burdens of depression. In this chapter, we address methods for approaching and engaging the patient with medical illness and depression, the nuances of treating depression in the context of medical comorbidities, and the measurement of the patient's progress during treatment.

APPROACH TO THE PATIENT

The first step to successful treatment is in the approach to the patient, summarized by the checklist in **Box 4-1**.

■ STRIKE A BALANCE BETWEEN EMPATHY AND MOBILIZATION

It is fundamental to convey a genuine recognition and appreciation of the patient's distress, despair, helplessness, and hopelessness.

BOX 4-1
APPROACHING THE PATIENT CHECKLIST

Fully assess

The right treatment at the right time

Aim for full remission and optimal functioning

Engage while empathizing

Address stigma

Normalize yet minimize imperfect adherence

Support and educate caretakers

Minimize burnout

Seamless communication

The challenge is to empathize with the patient, assure that he or she feels heard, yet gently resist the patient's depressive tendency to dwell on the negative through redirecting the conversation. Otherwise, this risks reinforcing hopelessness and entrenchment. Aiming for a balance between genuine empathy with the patient's despair while at the same time identifying and reinforcing any signs of desire for change, feeling better, and engaging in life is critical. As well, western medicine is disease-focused and problem-oriented. While this is valuable in facilitating an understanding of the underlying cognitive, behavioral, psychologic, and neurologic processes of psychiatric illness, it also risks promoting an externalized focus and intensifying passivity in a patient who may already be depleted, negative, and often immobilized. It is, therefore, up to the clinician to find ways to limit reinforcing the patient's passivity without shaming or otherwise sending a message that could be interpreted by the patient as being blamed for his or her depression or trivializing its magnitude and impact. As discussed later in this chapter, continually promoting active engagement of the patient through self-care approaches and carefully timed evidence-based psychotherapies should be regarded as central. By implementing carefully identified interventions, and simultaneously aligning with any aspects of the patient that are hopeful and desiring change, more robust and sustainable progress can be made.

Motivational interviewing (MI) is a natural fit for patients with depression who are inclined to become disengaged, unmotivated, hopeless, helpless, and frankly overwhelmed.[9] MI is a communication style that embraces the balance between empathizing with the distress and negativity while simultaneously helping patients to relinquish any ambivalence about feeling better (usually linked to the sense of being overwhelmed), and encouraging them to participate actively in alleviating their depression.

■ ADDRESS STIGMAS

Despite the growing public awareness of depression, the stigma of mental illness remains a destructive attitude lurking in the background for many patients, including those who have reached out for help. Sometimes the patient's family or significant others unwittingly contribute to poor treatment adherence because of stigmatized or misinformed beliefs. Listening for and addressing this from the outset can keep treatment on track. Peer-led programs are a potent approach to neutralizing stigma and are increasingly available. These range from support groups to buddy programs for which formalized training programs are available.

■ FOCUS ON TREATMENT ADHERENCE

The sense of depletion and hopelessness that accompanies depression may contribute to poor treatment adherence, compromising the patient's capacity to engage actively in therapy, keep appointments, and take psychiatric and nonpsychiatric medications as prescribed. The expense of multidrug regimens and psychotherapy

are contributing factors, leading some patients to skip doses or not fill prescriptions because of cost.[10] In addition, a societal imperative for "quick fixes" can lead some patients to cease treatment when it doesn't seem to help immediately. Thus, imperfect treatment adherence has become the rule rather than the exception.[11]

From the outset, clinicians should engage in an open and honest dialogue about whether and how the medications are to be taken and tolerated. This can be facilitated by normalizing the likelihood that some doses will be missed, while nonjudgmentally emphasizing the importance of adherence and the consequences of nonadherence. Involve family members and significant others in these discussions whenever possible, with close attention to their concerns, belief systems, and understanding of the illness. Educating and supporting those closely involved with the patient improves outcomes for patients with depression.[12,13]

■ SUPPORT AND EDUCATE CARETAKERS

Caring for a relative or friend with depression can be difficult and stressful, and it is not unusual for such individuals to become depressed themselves, or to engage in maladaptive coping with excessive use of alcohol, or insufficient sleep, exercise, social engagement, or other restorative activities. This, in turn, can adversely affect the patient.[13] Caregivers, family, and friends may also not understand that the patient cannot help feeling and behaving as they are and cannot just "snap out of it." It is, therefore, important to maintain contact with caregivers, to find ways of involving them in the treatment when clinically appropriate, and to remain attuned to their own signals of distress and refer them for treatment when indicated.

■ PREVENT CLINICIAN BURNOUT

Similarly, clinicians working with depressed individuals must continually be aware of their own responses, which can range from increasing hopelessness to anger when a patient's depression is not responding to treatment. Working with patients with depression is often depleting; particularly at risk are clinicians who've yet to establish a healthy work–life balance. This risk is intensified when treating medically ill patients since the likelihood of treatment resistance and physical suffering and death is increased. Team-based care helps clinicians to tolerate this stressful work since it provides support and a sharing of clinical responsibility (Chapter 23).

■ MAINTAIN COMMUNICATION WITH ENTIRE CARE TEAM

It is essential in treating depression in the medically ill for all clinicians involved to be in close communication, given the heightened risk of adverse events, complications, and medication interactions. Ideally, treatment should be conducted in a setting where there is a common electronic medical record. But even when such continuity is available, some clinicians avoid documenting in the shared medical record due to confidentiality concerns. However, sophisticated information systems allow for heightened security. It is also important that only the most clinically relevant details are documented and process notes are never contained within the treatment record.

■ TREATING MULTICULTURAL POPULATIONS IN MEDICAL SETTINGS

Depression is a leading cause of disability among major ethnic groups in the United States and is one of the most common and underdiagnosed medical comorbidities in these groups. Research consistently has shown that non-European populations are much more likely to see primary care physicians than specialists for depression and are less likely to adhere to antidepressant therapy. The prevalence of depression in Chinese Americans seeking medical treatment is approximately 20%[14–16] and the prevalence among

Hispanics, seeking treatment in urban medical centers, is 22%.[17] Interestingly, the time spent in America as an immigrant seems to be a notable factor. Recent immigrants seem to be relatively more protected from the risk of psychiatric disorder. Having a "home" country with recent connections to family and friends seems to be a positive health advantage that diminishes over time with increasing isolation from home, low income, and other stresses related to minority status in the United States.[18] Depression recurrence and chronicity are higher among Mexican Americans, Puerto Ricans, and African Americans than in the white population, and these groups are the most likely among all ethnic populations to receive inadequate depression treatment.[19] These prolonged and recurrent depressions may be related to the lack of access to treatment. Because the most consistent care these patients receive is in the primary care or emergency setting, it is worth examining the emerging modalities of culturally sensitive depression treatment being used in primary care.

The biopsychosocial model of depression is not necessarily shared by all ethnic minorities. The notion of medicalizing the psychological reaction to chronic and intense emotional stress and loss may appear foreign to them.[20] The Engagement Interview Protocol (EIP) has been developed to help Chinese Americans to accept mental health treatment and a way to incorporate their worldviews into the psychiatric assessment.[15] This interview allows the clinician to work with the patient by understanding their illness beliefs and taking their narratives of their illness experience into account. Because the primary care visit has multiple time constraints, the EIP uses a direct line of questioning to gain data on the patient's developmental, immigration, educational and work history, current social environment, and stressors. Other goals include eliciting narratives on connections and networks within the host country, spiritual beliefs, marital status and issues with extended family members or cultural community members. Questions like "How do you like living in this country?" that are included in the EIP can bring about important disclosures about cultural- and immigration-related stressors through the patient's story telling. Other questions like "What do you call your problem?," "What do you fear most about this problem?," and "What kind of treatment do you think you should receive?" can be helpful in conceptualizing the patient's view of depression.[15]

The disclosure of a depression diagnosis should be done with sensitivity since these patients are less familiar with the biopsychosocial method and can find the diagnosis highly stigmatizing. Ask directly about what this diagnosis means to the patient and describe the illness using the patient's words, perhaps with words like stress, tension, anxiety, or feeling overwhelmed and tired. Clarify misconceptions around diagnostic labels and describe the biology of depression in terms that are accessible to the patient. Elicit the patients' worries about the diagnosis and prognosis, and provide reassurance.[21]

After the diagnosis is made, it is important to look at how clinicians initiate and follow up with standard depression care. Collaborative care centers that use Depression Care Managers (DCMs) to follow up with patients after they are diagnosed with depression are helpful in providing standard care (see Chapter 23). However, while collaborative care has improved treatment among all socioeconomic classes it has not been shown to overcome racial/ethnic barriers to accessing mental health care.[22] Incorporating cultural tailoring into the collaborative care model, as in the Blacks Receiving Interventions for Depression and Gaining Empowerment (BRIDGE) study, has been shown to be beneficial among African Americans. Cultural tailoring is a minority patient centered care that provides intense psychoeducation and supportive counseling that is culturally understandable. This study and a few others have shown that these patients react significantly more positively to their DCMs and find them more helpful and supportive. These patients were more likely to become connected to psychotherapy as well.[23,24]

Adherence to antidepressants can be a major issue in minority populations, especially if the patient's ambivalence about taking medication is not explored. Motivational interviewing has been shown to be helpful for Latino patients taking medications and has improved antidepressant adherence.[25,26] A method called Motivational Enhancement Therapy for Antidepressants (META) and other techniques like this are used to motivate the patient by empathizing with the patient's struggle, addressing concerns about pharmacotherapy, validating reasons for not taking the medications, and allowing the patient to decide about the regimen. This type of motivational therapy helps patients adhere to treatment and increases trust in the clinician, improvement in symptoms, daily functioning, and quality-of-life.[25] Although the studies done on culturally sensitive depression treatment have shown positive effects, relatively few have been done for selected ethnic populations. The emergence of collaborative care provides the impetus to study these techniques more rigorously, but there is much left to study. **Table 4-1** summarizes a selected group of new treatment modalities addressing cultural barriers in depression treatment.[15,17,23,24,26,27]

INTERVENTIONS

■ THE BASICS

Basic lifestyle measures for patients with comorbid medical illness and depression are an integral part of treatment, as they affect treatment response[28] and are often disrupted in patients who are medically ill. These include sleep, daylight exposure, nutritional needs, and physical activity.

Sleep

Insomnia and hypersomnia are extremely common in depression. Compared to the general population, patients with medical illness are more likely to suffer from a sleep disturbance,[29] experience physical symptoms, such as pain that interfere with sleep quality, and/or be taking a medication that affects sleep. Sleep problems are associated with general medical comorbidity and poorer cognitive function in the elderly[30,31] and with chronic illnesses in nongeriatric populations, including obesity,[32] hypertension,[33] cardiovascular disease,[34] hypercholesterolemia,[35] and diabetes.[36] There may be an association between abnormal sleep duration (either short sleep or long sleep) and higher mortality,[37] though this is controversial and there is little consensus on how to interpret such an association.[38] Regardless, it is clear that caring for patients with depression and comorbid medical conditions is likely to include management of sleep complaints.

Take a thorough sleep history, consider a primary sleep disorder (discussed in Chapter 18), and address contributing medical issues including medications, primary sleep disorders, and psychiatric and medical illnesses that may contribute to insomnia. Next, address factors and behaviors that contribute to poor sleep. Some of the most important modifiable factors include use of alcohol, caffeine, smoking, and noise and light pollution. Many commonly prescribed antidepressants have a deleterious effect on sleep architecture, ultimately suppressing deep, restorative, non-REM sleep and REM sleep. Easily implementable sleep hygiene interventions (**Box 4-2**) and specific behavioral therapies, such as sleep restriction, CBT, and structured relaxation training can be helpful for many patients.[39] If these measures are not affective or implementable, consider pharmacologic intervention for the sleep problem.

Benzodiazepines for Insomnia

Risk of respiratory depression associated with benzodiazepines is the first consideration, and these agents should be used sparingly in patients whose respiratory functions are already compromised by, for example, pulmonary disease, sleep apnea, or chronic opioid use.

TABLE 4-1 Selected Cultural Treatment Tools for Depression in Outpatient Medical Settings

Type of Treatment	Intervention Method	Populations Studied	Goals	Outcomes
Collaborative Depression Care Management (DCM) Programs	Multidisciplinary team follows up treatment and monitor symptoms while encouraging medication and psychotherapy adherence	Multiple ethnicities	Outreach and treatment	Reduction of disparity in treatment in less educated patients but no reduction in ethnic disparities in treatment
Collaborative Care Model with Cultural Tailoring	Multidisciplinary team, longitudinal follow-up of treatment with cultural/language sensitive methods	African Americans	Outreach and treatment	Positive treatment experience. Improvement is similar to standard patient care
Engagement Interview Protocol (IEP)	Semi-structured instrument integrating patient illness beliefs into psychiatric assessment.	Developed for a Chinese population	Accurate assessment and evaluation tool	A 1-hour tool that facilitates enrollment and adherence to treatment
Motivational Enhancement Therapy for Antidepressants (META)	Motivational interviewing focused on culturally relevant fears of treatment	Latinos	Reducing ambivalence and increasing medication adherence	Greater likelihood of staying on medication and achieving remission
Remote Simultaneous Medical Interpreting (RSMI)	Interpretation occurs as the clinician speaks with the privacy of a remote interpreter	Spanish and Chinese speaking individuals	Removes language barriers in real time	Greater likelihood of being diagnosed with depression
Culturally Focused Psychiatric Consultation Model (CFP)	Three consults with a culturally trained psychiatrist who reports to PCP	Urban Asian Americans and Latino Americans	Culture and language focused psychoeducation	Patients wanted this culturally sensitive program in PCP offices. Studies still tracking outcomes
Telepsychiatry-based Culturally Sensitive Collaborative Treatment (T-CSCT)	Culturally sensitive collaborative care via video-conferencing/ telephone	Chinese Americans	Remote specialized management by culturally competent psychiatrists	Still tracking treatment effect but demonstrated improved care accessibility

In the elderly, benzodiazepines are also associated with increased risks of cognitive decline and falls.[40]

Benzodiazepines and benzodiazepine receptor agonists have been associated with an increase in mortality,[39,41] but this association remains controversial and may not be causal. Despite these uncertainties, since a causal relationship between hypnotics and mortality has been suggested, clinicians are advised to use caution when prescribing hypnotics or other sedatives for patients who are medically ill.

Nonbenzodiazepine Hypnotics

Nonbenzodiazepine hypnotics such as zolpidem, zaleplon, and eszopiclone appear less likely to suppress respiration than benzodiazepines.[42] Nonetheless, they carry risks of altered mental status similar to those of the benzodiazepines. Zolpidem has been associated with parasomnias, and falls, and so particular caution is warranted with these agents.[43]

Sedating Antidepressants for Insomnia

Because of its sedating properties, mirtazapine is often useful in depressed patients with prominent sleep problems, provided that weight gain is not of special concern. Trazodone is often used for sleep in doses that are subtherapeutic for depression. The most common medical concern with trazodone, and with the tricyclic antidepressants, is the increased risk of falls. The risk of falling associated with trazodone and SSRIs in the elderly is similar to, and may even be higher than, with tricyclic antidepressants.[44] Trazodone-induced QTc prolongation is usually mild and clinical reports of this have appeared exclusively in the context of overdose.[45]

Antipsychotics for Insomnia

Use of antipsychotics, most importantly quetiapine, for insomnia has become commonplace for patients with and without major psychiatric illness.[46] However, these have a risk of adverse metabolic effects and movement disorders, even when used at low doses. These concerns, as well as the increased risk of sudden cardiac death in the elderly,[47] should prompt caution about their use for insomnia in depressed, medically ill patients. They should be reserved for cases in which other agents have clearly failed or other indications exist, for example, psychotic symptoms.

Antihistamines for Insomnia

Many patients try antihistamines such as diphenhydramine prior to seeking a prescription for sleep problems, as these are the key

---

BOX 4-2
BEHAVIORAL INTERVENTIONS THAT PROMOTE GOOD SLEEP HYGIENE[261]

Go to bed only when sleepy

If unable to fall asleep within 20 minutes, get out of bed and return only when sleepy

Get up at the same time every morning

No daytime napping

Reduce noise, light, and temperature in the bedroom

Use the bed only for sleep and sex; no TV, eating, reading using back-lit devices such as

e-readers, smartphones, or iPads in bed

Avoid nicotine and exercise for several hours before bedtime and caffeinated products late in day

Try relaxation exercises (e.g., progressive muscle relaxation) before bed ingredients in most over-the-counter sleep-aids. However, their anticholinergic properties increase the risk of confusion and other systemic anticholinergic effects (urinary retention, constipation, dry mouth, blurred vision, and confusion), particularly in the elderly or patients with central nervous system compromise.[48]

Melatonin and Ramelteon

Melatonin might be an ideal option for treating sleep problems because of its virtually nonexistent toxicity. Unfortunately, its hypnotic effects are limited in patients who are elderly or have a medical illness.[49] The melatonin receptor agonist ramelteon appears to be effective for insomnia across all adult age groups, and without a consistent pattern of adverse events, although data remain limited.[50] Interestingly, melatonin seems helpful in reversing sleep disruption induced by beta-blockers.[51] This class of agents is preferentially useful in treating difficulties with sleep initiation as opposed to sleep maintenance.

Light Exposure

Exposure to light, natural or artificial, is useful in treating patients with seasonal affective disorder.[52] Evidence for prescribing light exposure to patients with nonseasonal depressive disorders is mixed.[53,54] However, recommending increased exposure to light, such as a morning walk or other daytime activities that require going outside, as part of a comprehensive treatment plan carries minimal risk. It may be especially beneficial for depressed patients who have a shifted sleep/wake cycle, stay inside most of the day, or prefer a naturalistic treatment model.

If artificial light is used, it is important that the patient be guided to reputable light box distributers and the light box should be used as recommended. Typically, patients should use the light box soon after they wake up (to correlate with natural morning light exposure) and for no more than 45 minutes per day. Although guidelines have historically instructed patients to use a light box that provides a high "dose" (as measured in photopic lux) of at least 10,000 lux, more recent evidence indicates that lower doses can also be effective.[55] The cost of these devices is modest and adverse effects are unlikely. The risks are primarily those of activation, insomnia, and mania in the context of a bipolar diathesis.[56] To date there are no established ocular/vision risks though it is generally recommended that periodic eye examinations be conducted.[53]

Nutrition

Good general nutrition appears to be associated with better outcomes for depression, and obesity is strongly associated with a higher risk of depression.[57] People who consume diets high in processed and sweetened foods are at higher risk for depression compared to those on nutrient-rich diets, such as the Mediterranean diet and whole foods diets.[58–60] And among patients with depression, better nutritional intake is associated with higher global assessment of functioning (GAF) scores.[47,61] However, a causal relationship between poor general nutrition and depression is not firmly established. Potential causal mechanisms include a relationship between dietary factors and brain-derived neurotrophic factor (BDNF),[62] as well as several specific nutritional deficiencies that have independent causal associations with depression.

A comprehensive intervention for depression in patients with suboptimal nutrition might include consideration of the following specific nutritional needs:

Fish Oil

Although the evidence for the efficacy of fish oil is stronger for bipolar depression, it may also be effective as an adjunct to conventional treatment for major depression. Fish oil appears to be most helpful when it contains a ratio of eicosapentaenoic acid (EPA) to docosahexaenoic acid (DHA) that exceeds 60%.[63] Typical therapeutic doses for EPA + DHA lie in the 1,000 to 4,000 mg per day range.

Vitamin D

Vitamin D deficiency is associated with depression. However, there is insufficient evidence to support that vitamin D supplementation in patients who are deficient improves depression outcomes.[64,65] In a recently published small randomized placebo-controlled trial involving 36 individuals with severe depression and vitamin D deficiency at baseline, the group randomized to receive 50,000 units of Vitamin D3 weekly showed significantly more improvement in their depression as measured by Beck Depression Inventory.[66] Given the low risk, potential mood benefits, and other medical benefits of correcting the deficiency, supplementation should still be considered.

Folate

Individuals with folate deficiency are more likely to experience depression,[67] and hypofolatemia has been associated with treatment resistance.[68] Risks for folate deficiency are significantly higher in the context of pregnancy, alcoholism, and gastrointestinal disorders. Folate ultimately regulates the synthesis of the monoamine neurotransmitters serotonin, norepinephrine, and dopamine. Some anticonvulsant-class mood stabilizers such as lamotrigine and valproate interfere with conversion of folate to l-methylfolate, its biologically active metabolite. A link has been identified between a genetic mutation in the enzyme 5-methyltetrahydrofolate (-MTHF) reductase (which converts folate to l-methylfolate), and major depressive disorder, as well as other neuropsychiatric conditions.[69] Given the reductase mutation findings, and studies linking excessive folic acid (synthetic folate) supplementation with heightened risk for some cancers, supplementing specifically with l-methylfolate is ideal.[70] There appears to be stronger evidence for folate as adjunctive treatment for depression in women specifically.[71]

Heavy Metals

There is little evidence that supplementation with heavy metals such as selenium and chromium improves depression outcomes,[72,73] though for some patients with depression who lack access to nutritious food, attention to this problem such as enrollment in a food assistance program has a positive effect.[74]

Physical Activity and Relaxation

There is an association between depression and lower levels of physical activity,[75] but the extent to which prescribed exercise augments depression treatment remains a matter of debate.[76,77] It appears to improve depression outcomes to at least some extent,[78] in addition to its well-established benefits for other health parameters, including sleep. A formal exercise regimen must be tailored to the physical limitations resulting from the medical illness.

Relaxation training may also be beneficial, but the evidence supporting it arises primarily from interventions that combine psychotherapy with relaxation training and/or physical activity, rather than from these practices alone.[79] The relaxation response is a state of relaxed consciousness that is associated with decreases in physiologic indicators of stress, for example, heart rate and oxygen consumption. It can be induced by various spiritual, deep breathing, and attention-focusing techniques,[80] is virtually without risk, and has been associated with a positive effect on depressive and some medical symptoms.[81] However, its efficacy in the treatment of depressive disorders remains unproven.[82]

■ PSYCHOTHERAPY

Evidence-based psychotherapy is an important component of depression treatment in the medically ill patients. Many medical patients prefer psychotherapy to adding psychotropic medications to their regimen[83] Depressed patients have the tendency to engage in unhealthy behaviors and poor self-care, which may intensify the medical illness or increase the risk of additional medical problems.[84] For those with medical illness, psychotherapy for depression can also specifically target problematic health behaviors contributing to worsening medical conditions (such as withdrawing from social support, smoking, sedentary lifestyle, poor medication and treatment adherence).

Depression in the presence of medical illness is associated with more severe psychological, cognitive, and physical impairment[85] making psychotherapeutic treatment more complicated, associated with less robust benefits, and requiring adaptation. Despite the complex interactions between depression and medical illness, several forms of structured psychotherapy are effective in treating depression and associated problematic health behaviors, including nonadherence.[85,86] These include interpersonal psychotherapy, CBT, and mindfulness-based therapies.[87–90]

Interpersonal Psychotherapy

Interpersonal psychotherapy (IPT) has been adapted and studied for the treatment of depressed patients in primary care,[91] and for patients with coronary artery disease,[92] HIV,[93] and breast cancer.[87,94] IPT focuses on interpersonal stressors, changes, and difficulties,[87] since these often serve as causal or maintenance factors. Depression often follows a negative or stressful change in one's interpersonal environment, such as the death of a loved one, conflict with a significant other, a career change, the beginning or ending of a marriage or other relationship, or becoming medically ill.[95] Subsequently, depressive symptoms jeopardize interpersonal functioning, resulting in additional negative life events. For example, medical treatment related demands may lead to decreased social contact and support resulting in interpersonal deficits over time. Additionally, changes in roles may also result from medical illness, commonly seen as decreased ability to work or loss of work productivity.[87]

There are two key principles guiding IPT. First, depression is a medical illness. This first principle defines the problem to be solved and counteracts any tendency for the patient to blame him/herself. The second principle is that depressed mood is related to life events, and situational context. IPT makes the connection between mood and distressing life events that either precede or follow onset of depressive disorder.[96] In particular, IPT targets four core problem areas: grief, role disputes, role transitions, and interpersonal deficits.[87]

IPT is a time-limited psychotherapy comprised of three phases with a typical treatment course ranging between 8 and 20 sessions. The initial phase (sessions 1–3) involves assessment of depression severity, the interpersonal context in which the depression occurs, the patient's relationship history and patterns, capacity for intimacy, and current relationships (is to substantiate depression as an illness rather than a flaw or defect within the patient).[95] In diagnosing depression, the IPT therapist employs symptom severity measures, such as the Beck Depression Inventory (BDI-II; additional measure information provided toward the end of this chapter).[97] Further clarification of how the four problem areas relate to depression (grief, role disputes, role transitions, and interpersonal deficits) also occurs during the initial treatment phase.

In the second phase of treatment, the IPT therapist is explicit and transparent with the patient in describing the IPT model of depression and the case formulation.[95] The IPT therapist collaborates with the patient in a partnership while maintaining a relaxed and supportive therapeutic stance. During session, the events of the past week are reviewed. When the patient demonstrates success or skillful behavior in an interpersonal situation, the therapist acts as a cheerleader, reinforcing these pro-social skills. With negative outcomes or missed opportunities, the therapist empathizes, works with the patient to analyze what went wrong in the situation, generates new interpersonal options, and rehearses them with the patient. Common interpersonal skills targeted in IPT include asser-

tion of needs and wishes, promoting effective expression of anger, and taking social risks. Then the patient tests out these new options/skills in between sessions. Thus, over time, depressed patients develop a repertoire of new, adaptive interpersonal skills.[95]

In the final phase of treatment (last three sessions), the therapist reviews the patient's accomplishments to highlight the patient's competency and discusses that ending therapy is another role transition, encompassing both negative and positive aspects.[95]

IPT has been modified to specifically address the needs of medically ill patients. These modifications include decreasing session time to 45 minutes, phone sessions if the patient is too ill to travel, psychoeducation about both depressive and medical symptoms, and adaptations to the content within the four interpersonal problem areas.[98] For instance, within the psychoeducation component, patients are informed they have two medical illnesses and the "sick role" is adapted to include both illnesses.

IPT has been conducted with and without medication augmentation.[99–101] The combination of medication and IPT produces the best outcomes, making it optimal for prescribers to simultaneously provide IPT.[95] Although IPT is comparable to medication, it takes longer to achieve these benefits. IPT training resources can be found at www.interpersonalpsychotherapy.org; the International Society for Interpersonal Psychotherapy's website.

Cognitive Behavior Therapy

Cognitive behavior therapy (CBT) for depression has been adapted and studied for treating patients in primary-care[102] and in those with diabetes,[103,104] HIV,[105] cardiovascular disease,[106] chronic obstructive pulmonary disease,[107,108] Parkinson disease,[109] multiple sclerosis,[110,111] inflammatory bowel disease,[112,113] rheumatoid arthritis,[114] end stage renal disease,[115,116] and cancer.[117,118] Behavioral activation and cognitive restructuring are key components of CBT for depression.

Behavioral activation improves mood by fostering involvement in activities that bring patients into contact with reinforcing contingencies and by decreasing behaviors, such as avoidance, that perpetuate depression, such as avoidance.[88,89] Key behavioral targets include reducing reinforcement for depressive behaviors and increasing reinforcement for healthy/pro-social behaviors.[90] Particularly relevant to medical patients, behavioral activation generates nondepressed, approach-oriented behavior through behavioral scheduling, problem solving, and prioritizing, all of which contribute to an increasing sense of control over life.[89,119] These structured activation approaches target social support, emotional expression, and stress management.[120] For example, development of social skills, graduated exposure to social situations, and social anxiety reduction strategies increase positive social reinforcement and decrease negative affect.

At the beginning of treatment, in addition to establishing a strong therapeutic alliance, discussion is devoted to the function of depression and the treatment rationale. Weekly self-monitoring is the first step in systematically increasing nondepressive activities. Self-monitoring of daily activities and mood serves multiple functions: (1) to highlight current daily activities, (2) to identify potential activities to target, and (3) to obtain baseline measurement. The next treatment component focuses on identifying patients' values within a range of life domains. Then an activity hierarchy is constructed in which new values-based activities are rated from "easiest" to "most difficult" to accomplish. Patients then progress from the easiest activity through the hierarchy to the most difficulty. Both the therapist and patient thoughtfully consider the frequency and duration of each activity per week. The activity engagement is reviewed at the next session, and barriers or problems with engaging the activation plan are thoroughly discussed.[88]

The cognitive component of CBT focuses on identifying and challenging negatively biased thoughts that cause or maintain depression.[121] Therapists guide patients through structured learning experiences with techniques, such as psychoeducation, guided discovery using use of Socratic questioning, role playing, the downward arrow technique for uncovering core beliefs, and behavioral experiments to empirically test their maladaptive automatic depressive thoughts.[121] Cognitive restructuring is then used to challenge the validity of the patient's assumptions and to develop more realistic appraisals of daily situations. In addition, behavioral experiments are developed to test out unhelpful and/or rigidly held beliefs. These challenging strategies are applied in real time (daily, weekly) to help patients develop more realistic, alternative thoughts and beliefs that improve mood. Typically, about eight sessions are needed for patients to sufficiently learn the cognitive model and skills and a significant reduction in depression often occurs within this first stage of therapy. The next phase of therapy (sessions 9–16) focuses on modifying dysfunctional core beliefs and learning skills to prevent relapse.[121]

Although somewhat distinct, problem-solving therapy (PST) is derived from CBT and is thought of as a type of CBT. PST involves training patients to adopt adaptive problem-solving attitudes (e.g., increase positive problem orientation) and skills (e.g., increasing rational problem solving and decreasing impulsive and avoidant problem-solving).[122] PST is short-term and present-focused, ranging from 6 to 16 1-hour sessions. PST has strong empirical support for treating depression provided that the course of treatment includes training in problem-orientation and assignment of homework.[123] PST has demonstrated promise as an effective treatment for psychological distress and depression among medically ill patients,[123,124] including depressed patients with cancer,[125,126] cardiac disease,[127] and diabetes.[128,129]

PST teaches patients to address current life difficulties by appraising problems as solvable challenges,[130] breaking larger problems into smaller pieces and identifying specific steps toward positive change, similar to the process of change engendered by behavioral activation.[131] Patients are taught to identify emotions as cues for the presence of a problem and to inhibit automatic/impulsive responses to the problem(s). Instead, patients are taught to practice rational problem-solving skills (see **Table 4-2** for rational problem-solving activities).[120] The PST model identifies problem-solving skill

as the ability to define a problem, identify solutions, and verify the effectiveness of the employed solutions and that one's problem-solving repertoire mitigates how one experiences psychological distress leading to depression.

Applying the PST model to medical conditions means that medical patients can experience their medical problems as ongoing stressors and problem-solving skills can decrease the likelihood that one will experience heightened distress when facing ongoing medical stress. The PST manual and training tools and videos can be found on the IMPACT Collaborative Care for Depression website (http://impact-uw.org/tools/pst_manual.html).

Mindfulness-Based Therapy

Mindfulness-based therapies aim to teach mindfulness skills so that depressed patients can better connect to their experiences and their environment in real time. Here, mindfulness is defined as the skill of nonjudgmentally observing one's experiences, such as bodily sensations, emotions, and thoughts, in the present moment.[131] Most learning within mindfulness-based therapies is experiential and involves first learning basic mindfulness practices, such as mindful breathing, body scan, and mindful movement. Then mindfulness is applied in a more sophisticated way to emotions, thoughts, one's sense of self, and interpersonal processes.

The first two mindfulness treatments discussed here (mindfulness-based stress reduction [MBSR] and mindfulness-based cognitive therapy [MBCT]) utilize and require formal mindfulness meditation (i.e., sitting in silence and meditating). The latter two treatment programs (emotion regulation and acceptance and commitment therapy) involve mindfulness skills training but typically do not require that the patient employs sitting meditation practice. MBSR, developed by Jon Kabat-Zinn,[131] is a group treatment for psychological distress, depressive symptoms, and anxiety for patients with chronic disease. Originally developed for chronic pain, its effect on alleviating depression has subsequently been tested in patients with a range of medical conditions, such as cancer, heart failure, and rheumatoid arthritis.[90,132] A meta-analysis of six studies found that MBSR has significant but small effect sizes (Hedges $g = 0.26$) in treating depression in patients with various medical and somatic conditions[90] and may be most useful when integrated into a CBT program. However, among patients with recurrent and treatment-resistant depression but without major medical comorbidities, mindfulness appears to be more beneficial than either CBT or education alone.[133] MBCT is a form of MBSR, also delivered in a group format. It includes mindfulness skills training (i.e., sitting mindfulness meditation) as well as cognitive therapy exercises to improve awareness of depressive cognitions and the connection between depressive thinking patterns and behavior and mood. MBCT helps patients develop a different mode of mind to best work with these thoughts and feelings when depression threatens to overwhelm them.[134,135] MBCT has led to significant improvement in depressive symptoms among HIV-infected patients,[135] vascular disease,[136] cancer,[137] traumatic brain injury,[138] and for patients who have had a stroke.[139]

Other forms of mindfulness-based behavior therapies show promise for treating depression in medically ill patients. One such treatment is a mindfulness and emotion regulation intervention, adapted from MBCT[114] and MBSR. This treatment aims to improve emotion regulation and promote awareness and acceptance of the entire spectrum of emotional experience through training in mindfulness meditation.[133] It has been employed in patients with rheumatoid arthritis to improve regulation of negative affective responses to stressful life events, and to encourage positive affective engagement (e.g., social engagement). Adaptations in the medically ill include reducing duration of meditation times to 10 minutes. Aside from the mindfulness meditation component, the other treatment elements are based on CBT. These include emphasizing

---

TABLE 4-2 Rational Problem-Solving Activities

Defining the Problem
- Gather available facts about the problem
- Describe these facts in clear terms
- Differentiate between facts and assumptions
- Identify what makes this situation a problem
- Set realistic problem-solving goals

Generating Alternatives
- Make a list of alternative solutions
- Defer critical judgment of alternative solutions
- Think of general strategies, and tactics for each, when generating the potential solutions

Decision Making
- Evaluate each alternative by the likelihood that it will achieve desired goals and rate the value of the alternative in terms of personal, social, long-term, and short-term consequences
- Choose the alternative(s) which have highest ranking according to above

Implementing and Verifying the Solution
- Carry out chosen solution/plan
- Monitor outcomes of implemented solution
- Compare the actual outcomes with predicted outcomes
- Self-reinforcement if satisfactory or recycle through process again if outcome is unsatisfactory

emotional clarity, accepting and reframing of negative thoughts, cultivating positive emotions through pleasant event scheduling, and enhancing social relations.

Acceptance and commitment therapy (ACT) also relies heavily on mindfulness and acceptance, and includes other core components such as values-based behavioral change and activation.[140] ACT has a moderate evidence base for treating depression. It is empirically supported for treatment of chronic pain and has some evidence for improving psychological functioning, medical symptoms, and health behaviors among patients with diabetes, epilepsy, obesity, and irritable bowel syndrome. Both of these mindfulness-based CBTs place a primary emphasis on learning to relate differently to unwanted thoughts and feelings during times of negative affect such that the function of negative thoughts and emotions is altered.[133,140]

Common Features of Psychotherapy

All three psychotherapy types (IPT, CBT, mindfulness) are effective for depression among medically ill patients and have common treatment elements, principles, and goals. All aim to preserve effective and rewarding social relationships and interpersonal connections despite facing medical-related burdens while learning new ways of responding or relating to depressive symptoms. In addition, they are structured, short-term (i.e., ≤20 sessions), rely on multiple components, are present-focused, and are designed flexibly to accommodate the medical condition. All therapeutic modalities are directive with agendas and a path to follow, skills to learn, and continuous assessment of depressive symptom change.

It is important to note that insight-oriented therapeutic approaches and nondirective supportive psychotherapy are not recommended as a stand-alone treatment for depression among the medically ill. Research, although limited, suggests poorer outcomes with insight-oriented and nondirective supportive approaches in the medically ill.[82,103] Support, ventilation, clarification, and insight are all valuable, but do not in and of themselves appear to be effective treatments for depression in medically ill populations. Rather, they should be included as part of the evidence-based therapies described above. There is, however, one empirically informed exception: among HIV patients with depression, group supportive psychotherapy and psychoeducational groups have shown equivalent benefits as CBT.[141] Medically ill patients seeking treatment for depression should be informed about recommended evidence-based psychotherapies and offered these treatments as the first-line approach.

■ PHARMACOLOGIC INTERVENTIONS

Approaching pharmacologic interventions for the patient diagnosed with medical illness and depression involves following general guidelines for treating depression in conjunction with special consideration of the interactions among medical illness, aging, and the medications being prescribed.

General Considerations

Start by carefully establishing the depressive diagnosis and assessing the roles of concurrent medications, medical disease, and substance abuse. False-positive diagnoses of depression are common, perhaps even more common than false negatives, particularly in busy primary care practices where standardized assessments, re-assessments, and/or rating scales are not routinely used.[142] When considering pharmacologic treatments, differentiating between bipolar and unipolar depression is important (Chapter 3) as pharmacologic treatment guidelines for bipolar depression are substantially different.

Evidence-based treatment guidelines for nonbipolar depression[143–145] support starting with any of the newer antidepressant agents, namely selective serotonin reuptake inhibitors (SSRIs), serotonin-norepinephrine reuptake inhibitors (SNRIs), mirtazapine,

or bupropion. Most evidence suggests that all of these agents are roughly equal in efficacy when applied to the general population;[146] there is some evidence that SNRIs are more effective than SSRIs in inducing remission, particularly among the more severely depressed.[147] Remission is typically defined as PHQ-9 total score <5 or when the individual is close to symptom-free and back to functioning at his or her peak level.

Identify two or three agents that would likely have favorable side-effect profiles for the individual, and then present the menu of options and side effects to the patient. While many patients will ask the clinician to choose the "best" medicine for them, it is important to educate the patient that there is no perfect medication, none without potential side effects, and no significant differences in efficacy (though evidence has emerged over the last decade that patients with severe comorbid anxiety tend to have worse outcomes and also more difficulty tolerating the side effects of medications).[148] Patients educated on these fundamentals often find it easier to engage actively in making a decision on which medication to try.

Once the patient has identified a medication, it is generally most prudent to start with the lowest dose possible for at least the first few doses in order to assess the patient's sensitivity to the agent. Otherwise, one risks the patient having a negative experience with the medication and reduces odds of the patient persisting with a medication trial. As it appears, the patient is tolerating the medication, increase the dose as tolerated to the lower threshold for a therapeutic response. In the context of significant comorbid anxiety, it is especially important to start low and gradually titrate the dose as this population has a heightened sensitivity to the adverse effects of antidepressant class medications. Tracking response, side effects, and adherence to the regimen, while continually encouraging the patient to partner with the clinician and persevere with the medication, are all key factors. If a partial or no response is observed after 4 to 6 weeks at a therapeutic dose, switch or augment the medication. Generally the clinician will switch antidepressants if there is no response or if a partial response, consider augmenting with a complementary antidepressant. If the patient continues to respond inadequately, review the history to assure nothing has been overlooked, reassess for adherence, and then sequentially revise the regimen, including consideration of other somatic therapies, psychotherapies, and even of complementary and alternative agents. Once the patient has achieved a full remission or as close to full remission and optimal functioning as possible, prevent relapse with continuation therapy and depending on past history, consider whether maintenance therapy is indicated.

Complementary and Alternative Agents

Alternative medicines remain popular with patients who suffer from depressed mood and prefer to avoid prescription antidepressants. These agents can be difficult to manage due to a limited understanding of optimal dosing, pharmacologic mechanisms and safety profiles, and a tendency for the contents to vary. Nonetheless, they can be part of a psychiatric regimen for depression.

St. John wort and S-adenosyl methionine (SAMe) show a potential benefit for the treatment of mild depression,[149–151] but the evidence supporting their efficacy is still limited. St. John wort appears to be most promising for the treatment of mild depression,[150,151] while SAMe appears useful as an adjunctive therapy for patients who do not respond to SSRI monotherapy.[152]

St. John wort can induce the P450 enzyme CYP3A and thus affect the metabolism of other medications, including lowering serum levels of hormonal contraceptives and antiretroviral agents. St. John wort should also not be taken in conjunction with conventional antidepressants due to the risk of serotonin syndrome.[153] SAMe may affect sleep or precipitate mania in individuals with underlying bipolar disorder[154] and also has risk for serotonin syndrome when used in tandem with conventional antidepressants.[155]

■ SELECTING AN AGENT IN THE CONTEXT OF MEDICAL ILLNESS

General Considerations

Patients who responded well to and tolerated a particular agent during a prior depressive episode often respond well to the same agent if prescribed again. In the absence of a past positive antidepressant response, many clinicians will prescribe an antidepressant to which a first-degree relative has had a particularly favorable response, though this has not been well studied. Patients for whom adherence to a daily medication regimen is more difficult may struggle with antidepressants with short half-lives, such as paroxetine or venlafaxine, which more commonly cause a discontinuation syndrome when missed; fluoxetine might be considered for such patients because of its long (and forgiving) half-life. There are other important factors to consider in selecting an antidepressant, particularly in patients with significant medical comorbidity or on other medications. These are discussed below (**Table 4-3**).

Consider Target Symptoms

Certain agents might prove helpful not only for the depressed mood but also for other symptoms, which may or may not be part of the depression. For example, patients who complain of insomnia may be good candidates for mirtazapine, trazodone, or a tricyclic antidepressant (TCA),[156] mirtazapine may be an optimal choice for the patient who is anorexic or underweight. TCAs and SNRIs (such as duloxetine and venlafaxine) are effective for treating neuropathic pain.[157] Bupropion may benefit patients with comorbid fatigue or inattention, or who wish to quit smoking.[158] Bupropion or the SNRIs are helpful for patients with chronic diarrhea.

Consider other Medical Conditions and Side Effects

Arrhythmias

Prolongation of the QT interval has long served as proxy for risk of torsades de pointes and other potentially life-threatening ventricular arrhythmias.[159] TCAs, with the possible exception of nortriptyline, are associated with QTc prolongation,[160] and newer antidepressants may share this risk. The Food and Drug Administration advisory warns of dose-dependent QT interval prolongation with citalopram, and recommend that citalopram dosing be no more than 40 mg per day in individuals younger than 60 and no more than 20 mg per day in patients over age 60 or those taking medications that inhibit cytochrome P450 2C19.[161] Analysis of a large data registry revealed that citalopram, escitalopram, and amitriptyline were associated with lengthening of the QTc interval, while fluoxetine, sertraline, paroxetine, venlafaxine, duloxetine, mirtazapine, bupropion, and nortriptyline were not.[162] It is prudent to avoid citalopram, escitalopram, and TCAs in patients at risk of cardiac arrhythmias, in those coprescribed drugs that lengthen QTc (such as methadone); in those with congenital QTc prolongation; and in those taking medications that inhibit P450 2C19 (such as omeprazole) as these will increase citalopram serum levels (see drug interactions below).

Increased Risk of Bleeding

SSRIs and SNRIs have an increased risk of bleeding[90] that can be manifested as petechiae, gastrointestinal hemorrhage, ecchymosis, purpura, epistaxis, strokes, and postoperative bleeding.[163,164] The presumed mechanism for this bleeding diathesis is interference with the platelet secretory response and platelet aggregation. Patients taking SSRIs in the perioperative period may be at higher risk for adverse events including readmission, and death,[165] raising the question of whether or not SSRIs and SNRIs should be discontinued or withheld perioperatively. The predominant risk appears to be upper gastrointestinal bleeding in patients using NSAIDs, aspirin, or anticoagulants or who have a history of gastrointestinal bleeds; however, the risk of SSRIs/SNRIs plus antiplatelet agents has not been shown to be higher than the risk of antiplatelet agents alone.[166] Use caution in prescribing SSRIs and SNRIs in individuals with bleeding risks and consider adding a proton-pump inhibitor if there is concern.[167]

Increased Risk of Osteoporotic Fractures

Individuals with depression are inherently at higher risk for fractures due to reduced physical activity, more frequent falls, poor nutrition, and increased tobacco smoking in addition to the added risks of older age, medical comorbidity, and complex medication regimens. However, after controlling for these potentially confounding factors, SSRIs, SNRIs, and TCAs appear to increase the risk of fractures by almost twofold.[168] The risk may not be dose-related and appears to be greatest in the first year of treatment.[168] In the absence of a consensus, consider this risk in especially high-risk populations such as those with osteopenia or osteoporosis and those on chronic steroid therapy. Optimize intake of calcium and assuring adequate 25-OH vitamin D levels as well.

Weight Gain and Metabolic Risks

Include weight gain in the review of potentially significant side effects. For some illnesses such as malignancies or immune dysfunction, medication-induced weight gain is therapeutic, but for many patients with major medical conditions, weight gain aggravates their illness.

Antidepressants associated with weight gain include mirtazapine, TCAs (especially amitriptyline), and the monoamine-oxidase inhibitors (MAOIs) (particularly phenelzine).[169] SSRIs and SNRIs are associated with weight loss in the short term, though modest weight gain can occur in the long term.[170] Paroxetine in particular has been associated with longer-term risk for weight gain.[169] The mechanisms for this include the antihistaminic effects, the blockade of the post-synaptic 5HT2c receptors, and/or activation of the serotonin neural pathways that dampen the dopaminergic neurotransmission that reduces fat stores. There is no correlation between degree of therapeutic response and weight gain. The gain is not attributable to the recovery of weight lost as a result of the medical illness, and individuals without prior weight loss may gain weight with antidepressants. Avoid augmentation with antipsychotics in individuals who would be most adversely affected by weight gain or who have metabolic syndrome risks. Bupropion is associated with weight loss[171] and nefazodone is the most weight-neutral of the available conventional antidepressants. Lamotrigine, triiodothyronine, and buspirone are weight-neutral augmentation agents.

Anticholinergic Risks

Dry mouth, blurred vision, constipation, and paralytic ileus are the primary adverse effects associated with the anticholinergic properties of some psychotropics. With the possible exception of paroxetine, TCAs, particularly the tertiary agents such as amitriptyline, have the most potent anticholinergic properties. Of the TCAs, desipramine is least anticholinergic. Avoid these agents in patients with narrow-angle glaucoma and prostatic hypertrophy and be especially cautious in individuals taking other medications with such effects. Consider, too, the longer-term risks associated with xerostomia such as increased dental caries and periodontitis, both of which can exacerbate the inflammation associated with cardiovascular disease,[172] and other systemic consequences.

TABLE 4-3 Commonly Used Antidepressants

Generic Name	Trade Name(s) and Dosage Forms	Dosing	Pro's	Con's	P450
Fluoxetine (SSRI) Also blocks 5HT2c and at high doses, block NE reuptake Generic available	*Prozac* 10 mg green/green pulvule 10 mg scored green tablet 20 mg green/cream pulvule 40 mg green/orange pulvule 20 mg/5 mL solution *Prozac Weekly* 90 mg green/clear enteric coated capsule with visible white pellets *Sarafem* 10 mg purple 20 mg purple/pink capsules	10–20 mg qam up to 60 mg qd occasionally dosed higher 90 mg *Prozac Weekly* should only be used once stable on 20 mg qd	• Very effective for atypical depressions, anxiety, eating d/o's, OCD (as with all SSRIs) • Relatively safe in overdose (as with all SSRIs) • Long t1/2 good for noncompliant pt (less discontinuation effects) • Has the most data suggesting no significant teratogenic effects • *Sarafem* approved for PMDD	• May be agitating (as with all SSRIs) • May cause insomnia and/or aggravate restless legs (as with all SSRIs) • May cause akathisia (as with all SSRIs) • Sexual side effects (as with all SSRIs) • Long t1/2 may complicate transition to new drug and prolong side effects • May cause mild weight gain (as with all SSRIs) • Blood levels not helpful (as with all non-TCA agents) • Cognitive "fuzz" (as with all SSRIs) • Drug interactions	Potent 2D6 inhibitor Metabolized by 2D6
Sertraline (SSRI) Also mild DRI and Mild alpha 1 antagonist Generic available	*Zoloft* Scored tablets: 25 mg green 50 mg pale blue 100 mg pale yellow	25–50 mg qam (food increases absorption, increased nausea) up to 200 mg	• Second most data supporting use during pregnancy • drug of choice during breastfeeding due to relatively lower fluoxetine levels in breastmilk	• Discontinuation effects • Diarrhea common	Modest inhibitor 2D6, 2C Metabolized by multiple P450 enzymes
Paroxetine (SSRI) Mild anticholinergic (similar to desipramine) Weak NE reuptake inhibition at doses > 40 mg Inhibits Nitrous oxide synthetase Generic available	*Paxil* Tablets: 10 mg yellow 20 mg scored pink 30 mg blue 40 mg green 10 mg/5mL in 250 mL bottle *Paxil CR* 12.5 mg yellow 25 mg pink 37.5 mg blue	10 mg usually at hs up to 60 mg	• relatively more sedating, less activating • less diarrhea and nausea • inhibits nitrous oxide synthetase (increased rate impotence)	• Discontinuation effects, probably worst of the SSRIs—cholinergic rebound • Drug interactions • Most prone of SSRIs to trigger weight gain • More likely than other SSRIs to cause dry mouth, constipation, etc. (anticholinergic)	The most potent 2D6 inhibitor Metabolized by 2D6

(continued)

TABLE 4-3 Commonly Used Antidepressants (*continued*)

Generic Name	Trade Name(s) and Dosage Forms	Dosing	Pro's	Con's	P450
fluvoxamine (SSRI) Moderate alpha 1 antagonist Generic and CR available	*Luvox* Tablets: 25 mg white 50 mg scored yellow 100 mg scored peach	25–50 mg qhs up to 300 mg	• Though only approved for OCD, likely as effective as any SSRI for anxiety and depressive spectrum disorders • More potent than sertraline as alpha-1 blocker	• BID dosing usually necessary • Diarrhea can be a problem • Drug interactions	Potent 3A4, 1A2, 2C19 inhibitor
Citalopram (SSRI) R-enantiomer has mild antihistamine activity Generic available	*Celexa* tablets: 10 mg beige 20 mg pink scored 40 mg white scored *Oral Solution: 10 mg/5 mL*	10–20 mg qhs up to 60 mg	• Minimal drug interactions	• Discontinuation effects • QTc prolongation: avoid >40 mg (max 20 mg in elderly) and pairing with QTc conditions and other drugs which prolong	Weak 2D6 inhibition with hi doses Metabolized by 2C19
Escitalopram (SSRI)	*Lexapro* Oral solution 1 mg/mL Round, white-off white tablets: 5 mg unscored 10 mg scored 20 mg scored	5–10 mg qhs, increase to 20 mg in a week	• S-enantiomer of Celexa (industry sponsored studies suggested superior efficacy and more rapid onset of response of escitalopram compared to citalopram)	• Discontinuation effects • May be similar risk as citalopram re QTc (Castro et al 2012) though no FDA imposed limit	Very weak inhibition of 2D6 Metabolized by 2C19
Venlafaxine SRI only at low doses NRI in doses>~200 mg Generic available all forms	*Effexor* 25,37.5,50,75,100 mg peach tabs *Effexor XR* 37.5 mg grey/peach caps 75 mg peach caps 150 mg red caps	37.5 mg qam IR or XR	• Possibly more effective than SSRIs in severe depression • No drug interactions • Helpful with anxiety and at higher doses, concentration/ attention • Less weight gain than SSRIs • May be more effective than SSRIs in postmenopausal women (as with other non-SSRI antidepressants)	• Tachycardia and hypertension above 200 mg/d may occur • Discontinuation effects • IR form requires divided dosing • Sexual side effects • Nausea	No sig inhibition Metabolized by 2D6 and to a lesser degree, 3A4
Desvenlafaxine NRI > SRI Generic available	*Pristiq* 50 mg pinkish square tab 100 mg reddish brown square tab	Start 50 mg Up to 100 mg	• Evidence supports use for perimenopause in addition to depression • Serum levels not affected by 2D6 polymorphisms	• Same as with venlafaxine	No sig inhibition Minor 3A4 metabolism

Duloxetine SRI slightly > NRI but at *all* doses	*Cymbalta* 20 mg green caps 30 mg white/blue caps 60 mg green/blue	Start 20 mg BID, up to 30 mg BID (or 60 mg qd single dose)	• Possibly more effective than SSRIs in severe depression • Approved for pain • Increases NE in addition to 5HT at initial dosing (and DA at high dosing)	• Nausea, dry mouth, dizziness, constipation • Recently marketed (8/04) • Insert recommends VS monitoring though unlikely to produce clinically significant BP/P elevations • Avoid in uncontrolled acute narrow angle glaucoma • May increase transaminases; should avoid ETOH • As hydrolyzed to napthol in acid media, avoid in patients with delayed gastric emptying and do not crush, chew, or mix with liquids	Moderate inhibitor of 2D6 Metabolized by 2D6 and 1A2 Highly protein bound
Bupropion DRI, NRI Generic available for all forms	*Wellbutrin (IR)* 75 mg orange tab 100 mg red tab *Wellbutrin SR* 100 mg blue tab 150 mg purple tab *Zyban (wellbutrin sr)* 150 mg purple tab *Wellbutrin XL* 150 mg white tab 300 mg white tab	100 mg sr qam or 75 mg IR qam up to 450 mg in bid start 150, up to 300 once daily	• *Wellbutrin* approved for depression, *Zyban* approved for smoking cessation • Helpful in ADHD and restless legs • Most stimulating antidepressant • Very low risk sexual side effects • Least likely to induce rapid-cycling/mixed states • No weight gain • Very useful augmentation agent (though watch drug interactions)	• Bid or tid dosing necessary above 200 mg for IR • Contraindicated in epilepsy and eating disorders due to increased risk of seizures (although SR form probably safer) • May aggravate anxiety, particularly panic • Drug interactions	Moderate 2D6 inhibitor Metabolized by 2B6 (not D) to active metabolites
Mirtazapine 5HT2 and 5HT3 antag Antihist Alpha-2 blockade (releases breaks on 5HT and NE) Generic available	*Remeron* 15 mg yellow scored tab 30 mg orange scored tab 45 mg unscored white tab	15 mg qhs up to 60 mg	• Little nausea or diarrhea • Little agitation • May benefit sleep • Appetite stimulating (good choice for low weight elderly or medcally ill patients) • No drug interactions • May have fewer sexual side effects • No cardiotoxicity • Safe in overdose	• Can be too sedating • Weight gain • Rare cases of reversible agranulocytosis (1.1/1000)	No sig inhibition Metabolized by 2D6, 1A2

Fall Risks

Antidepressants carry an increased risk of falling, thought to be due to sedation, insomnia, nocturia, impaired postural reflexes, increased reaction time, orthostatic hypotension, cardiac rhythm or conduction disturbances, and movement disorders.[173] TCAs (least likely nortriptyline) are associated with orthostatic hypotension and heightened fall risk, ultimately mediated by alpha-1 blockade. There is growing evidence that SSRIs, in particular, are no less, and may even be more closely associated with an increased risk of falling in registry-based studies though this needs to be confirmed in randomized controlled trials.[174–176] Educate patients and their families about this risk, and underscore the importance of using night lights, exercising caution when making positional changes, and avoiding sudden movements. Dehydration and diminished cardiovascular reserve exaggerate this risk.

Hyponatremia

Antidepressant-induced syndrome of inappropriate secretion of antidiuretic hormone (SIADH) hyponatremia is especially common in older individuals, particularly in woman, and is apt to occur in the first few weeks of treatment.[177] SSRIs carry a higher risk of hyponatremia than TCAs and MAOIs.[44] Mild hyponatremia can be asymptomatic or present with weakness, fatigue, headaches, or loss of appetite that can easily be misinterpreted as worsening depression. It is critical that milder cases are recognized as side effects and not misinterpreted as worsening depression because increasing the antidepressant dose could further depress sodium levels, potentially leading to delirium, seizures, and even death.

Renal Disease

Declining renal function impacts the pharmacokinetics of drugs.[178] Uremia commonly reduces the absorption of medication through increasing gastric alkalinity, increased use of antacids, or increased vomiting. Alternatively, in the context of dehydration, increased serum concentration is likely. Hypoalbuminemia increases the free, bioavailable levels of acidic drugs whereas increased glycoproteins reduce the free fraction of alkaline drugs. Renal disease not only impacts the clearance of renally excreted drugs and also impairs hepatic cytochrome P450 oxidative pathways for the metabolism of these drugs. Drugs cleared through hydrolysis or reduction are not typically metabolized as quickly, leading to increased levels of bioactive metabolites. Adjust dosing for drugs excreted renally, such as lithium, gabapentin, pregabalin, and topiramate. Remember, serum creatinine in the elderly is a poor indicator of renal function due to the decreased contribution of muscle mass in this population.[178]

Hepatic Disease

Hepatic blood flow is generally reduced in hepatic failure, thereby increasing the clearance time for all drugs metabolized by the liver. Parenchymal disease will specifically impair oxidative pathways (Phase I) of metabolism but spare conjugative pathways such as glucuronidation (Phase II). In patients with hepatic disease such as cirrhosis use agents metabolized through Phase II mechanisms such as lorazepam, temazepam, and oxazepam. Drugs such as lithium, gabapentin, and pregabalin are safest in patients with hepatic disease given they are exclusively processed by the kidneys. All antidepressant-class medications should be dose-adjusted in the context of moderate to severe hepatic impairment. Remember that liver function tests are not a reliable indicator of hepatic disease.

Consider Other Medications Your Patient Is Taking

Medications that are not water-soluble and therefore not eliminated by the kidneys must first be converted into more polarized, water-soluble compounds by the liver. The oxidative pathways known as the cytochrome P450 system metabolize environmental toxins and more

lipophilic medications. Several commonly prescribed antidepressants, including fluoxetine, paroxetine, and bupropion, are established inhibitors of the 2D6 isoenzymes, with fluoxetine and paroxetine known to be especially strong inhibitors. As a result, serum levels of medications metabolized preferentially by this enzyme, such as many antidepressants, HIV medications, and beta blockers, will increase. Tertiary TCAs such as amitriptyline may increase to toxic levels. While it is always unsafe to coadminister any SSRI with an MAOI due to the risk of serotonin syndrome, caution must also be used in combining any antidepressant with P450 inhibitory effects with another antidepressant metabolized by the same enzyme (Table 4-1).

Consider the Impact of Aging

Although the impact of aging on absorption is unclear, the impact on drug distribution is well established. Fat stores increase as muscle mass diminishes and so lipophilic agents are distributed more widely in older (and overweight) individuals. Since most psychotropic agents are highly lipophilic, this results in prolonged drug clearance and longer time to achieve a therapeutic effect, since equilibrium is not achieved until fat stores have been saturated. The net result is lower serum levels with a longer half-life. For water-soluble agents such as lithium, higher serum concentrations are likely as aging reduces total body water stores. For drugs that are highly protein bound, free drug levels increase as albumin levels decline. This means higher levels of unbound bioactive drug and more CNS penetration of drugs such as valproate.

Metabolism of drugs is also affected by the aging process.[179] Demethylation and to a moderate degree, acetylation and glucuronidation are impaired. While hepatic disease impacts P450 systems, the cytochrome system is relatively spared by aging with the exception of isoenzyme 2D6, which is moderately impaired. However, hepatic circulation diminishes and so lower dosing is warranted given the longer half-life of hepatically metabolized drugs. Renal function declines by an estimated 1% per year starting at age 30 and so renally excreted agents such as lithium, gabapentin, pregabalin, and topiramate should be adjusted accordingly.[179]

Receptor level changes occur as the body ages and thereby impact the pharmacodynamic impact of medications. For example, as estrogen levels decline during perimenopause, serotonin receptors appear to downregulate, which might play a role in declining sensitivity for women to serotonergic antidepressants postmenopausally (Chapter 8).

■ OTHER SOMATIC THERAPIES

Nonpharmacological somatic therapies can be a mainstay of treatment for the medically ill population. Electroconvulsive therapy (ECT) has been employed for more than 75 years. More recently, novel somatic therapies are being developed to noninvasively stimulate the brain using electrical or magnetic fields. These can be administered through the scalp (transcranial magnetic stimulation, magnetic seizure therapy [MST], and transcranial direct current stimulation [tDCS]), via stimulation of the vagus nerve, or with electrodes implanted directly into the brain (deep brain stimulation). These treatments are uniquely suited for the medical population as they can avert drug–drug interactions and/or systemic side effects. These somatic therapies are compared in **Table 4-4**.

Electroconvulsive Therapy

ECT, electrically induced therapeutic seizures, has remained the most effective antidepressant treatment in psychiatry. It is the most rapid treatment available for major depressive episodes with and without psychotic features,[180] critical for patients with medical illness whose morbidity and mortality is increased by comorbid depression. Remission rate after ECT is as high as 80% to 90% and

TABLE 4-4 Comparison of Somatic Therapies

	FDA Approved for Depression	Type of Stimulation	Seizure Induction	Unique Aspects
ECT	Yes	Electrical	Yes	Unmatched efficacy, significant side effects, newer delivery methods improve efficacy and tolerability
VNS	Yes (as adjunctive treatment in adults)	Electrical	No	Long-term treatment, not an acute treatment
rTMS	Yes	Magnetic	No	Noninvasive, focal Minimal side effects, no anesthesia
MST	No	Magnetic	Yes	Potential to retain therapeutic efficacy of ECT Focal stimulation Fewer cognitive side effects than ECT
DBS	No	Electrical	No	Target circuitry precisely, reaches deeper brain structures than magnetic fields or focal ECT
tDCS	No	Electrical	No	Noninvasive, portable, and inexpensive Few side effects

ECT, electroconvulsive therapy; VNS, vagus nerve stimulation; rTMS, repetitive transcranial magnetic stimulation; MST, magnetic seizure therapy; DBS, deep brain stimulation; tDCS, transcranial direct current stimulation (i.e., direct current polarization).

efficacy is largely equivalent in depressed patients with unipolar and bipolar mood disorders,[181] with bipolar patients responding more quickly.[182] ECT is more effective for psychotic depression, particularly with mood-congruent delusions,[183] and for primary depressive episodes as compared to those with other, comorbid psychiatric diagnoses.[184,185] Patients with medication-resistant depression have a lower remission rate with ECT,[184,186] as with other antidepressant interventions. Innovations over the past 30 years have improved ECT administration, safety, efficacy, and side effects, making it safe, effective, and life-saving. Right unilateral ECT is associated with better post-treatment medical quality-of-life than bilateral.[187]

Indications for ECT as a first-line treatment include: (1) urgent need (either psychiatric or medical) for a rapid response; (2) when treatment alternatives are associated with a higher risk than ECT; (3) a history of preferential response to ECT; or (4) patient preference for ECT. Most patients are referred for ECT on a *secondary* basis due to (1) lack of adequate response or demonstrated intolerance to treatment alternatives or (2) deterioration of the patient's condition to the point at which criteria for primary indications are met.

Contraindications and High-Risk Situations

Many patients with depression and medical illness are older, and although there is no age limit for ECT, the risks increase with age.[188] However, ECT has lower mortality for elderly patients than those treated with other modalities,[189] and elderly patients account for a greater fraction of overall ECT use.[190] Advanced age does alter ECT technique since anesthetic agents used with ECT are subject to age-dependent changes in tolerance and metabolism, and seizure threshold increases with age.

Although there are no "absolute" contraindications for ECT, specialty consultation is prudent for patients with significant cardiac, pulmonary, or cerebral disease. Space-occupying intracerebral lesions are a relative contraindication as ECT increases intracerebral pressure; however, there are reports of ECT being safely administered to depressed patients with slow-growing brain lesions.[191] Recent myocardial infarction may raise the risk of the ECT effect on the sympathetic and parasympathetic nervous system; the risk depends on the extent of the infarct, the degree of healing, and current cardiovascular status. Other high-risk conditions are unstable angina, poorly compensated congestive heart failure, severe valvular cardiac disease, unstable vascular aneurysm or malformation, recent cerebral infarction, severe pulmonary dysfunction, and other increased anesthesia risks.

Patients with hypertension have blood pressure stabilized before ECT and receive their routine antihypertensive medication before each treatment. Patients with coronary artery disease receive their antianginal agents before ECT with consideration given to the use of acute sympatholytics when ECT is delivered to avoid peri-ECT angina. Cardiac pacemakers and implantable defibrillators reduce the cardiac risk of pathological arrhythmias with ECT. Patients with diabetes mellitus and asthma require special management before, during, and after ECT. ECT has been safely administered to patients with a history of brain surgery, deep brain stimulators, cardiac pacemakers, implanted defibrillators, and vagus nerve stimulators.

Side Effects

ECT side effects are related to the physiological effects of the seizure in the setting of general anesthesia and muscular paralysis. Sympathetic and parasympathetic discharges typically produce transient benign disturbances in cardiac rate, rhythm, and blood pressure. These changes can be associated with arrhythmias or cardiac ischemia, but significant sequelae are rare.[192] Pharmacological prophylaxis may then be indicated.[180,193,194] More common and mild systemic side effects include headache, muscle pain, and nausea.

Amnesia is the most commonly discussed side effect of ECT. Memory difficulties increase over a course of treatments and diminish once ECT is stopped. Less often, memory function may actually improve following ECT, especially when depression-related cognitive deficits or frank pseudodementia are present. Amnestic effects with ECT are more prominent and last longer in patients with preexisting cerebral disease or with bilateral electrode placement.

Two types of memory deficits occur. Most prominent is *retrograde amnesia*, difficulty remembering information learned prior to ECT. This is greatest for more recent memories, that is, those occurring in the months before ECT. Retrograde amnesia is more marked for information of an impersonal nature,[195] and losses diminish following ECT.[196]

ECT can also induce *anterograde amnesia*, difficulty retaining newly learned information, most severe during the ECT course, and typically resolving days to weeks after ECT discontinuation. The likelihood, severity, and persistence of this amnesia are influenced by the type of ECT, including electrode placement (bilateral greater than right unilateral) and dosing.[197–199] Pharmacotherapy in conjunction with right unilateral ECT appears as effective as bilateral ECT alone with fewer cognitive side effects.[200] Amnesia during the ECT course can be diminished by increasing the interval between treatments or changing ECT type. New studies are underway to assess whether memory-enhancing cognitive therapies can diminish amnestic side effects.[201]

A period of postictal confusion, from 10 minutes to more than 1 hour after the seizure, is common. Interictal delirium, however, is far less common, occurring mostly in patients with preexisting cerebral impairment.[191] Structural brain changes do not occur with induced seizures.[202,203]

The risk of death with ECT is very low and is similar to that of other anesthetic procedures.[180,193] The most common cause of death with ECT is cardiovascular decompensation. Other causes include prolonged apnea, status epilepticus, and cerebral herniation (e.g., undiagnosed brain tumor).

Vagus Nerve Stimulation

Vagus nerve stimulation (VNS) is FDA-approved for adjunctive treatment of chronic or recurrent, medication-resistant depression. It entails the direct electrical stimulation of the left cervical vagus nerve via a pulse generator implanted in the left chest wall. VNS appears to have greater efficacy than pharmacologic treatment alone, though this is controversial.[204–208] In the first open label study,[205] response rates were 40% to adjunctive VNS treatment. Response rates have been sustained and remission rates increased over time, along with significant improvements in function.[206]

A randomized, controlled, multicenter trial comparing adjunctive VNS with sham treatment in depression failed to show a significant difference on the primary outcomes.[207] However, again, longer duration of treatment revealed progressively more improvement and remission. These results indicated that VNS was associated with greater improvement than pharmacological treatment alone.[208] In addition, reduced hospital visits, outpatient visits, and number of psychotropic medications were reported in one study,[209] especially important for the medically ill population.

Safety and Tolerability

VNS is generally well tolerated. Voice alteration, dyspnea, and neck pain are the most frequently reported side effects.[208] The surgical implantation of the stimulator carries a low risk of infection, vocal cord paralysis, and bradycardia or asystole.[208] In contrast to ECT, VNS does not have neurocognitive side effects,[210] and some of these deficits may even improve with VNS,[210] apparently as a result of the improvement in depression.

Contraindications

VNS is contraindicated in patients with bilateral or left cervical vagotomy, or various uses of diathermy. Since VNS has improved cardiac function in heart failure patients[211] and improves vagal tone, a known predictor of outcome in cardiac disease in depressed patients,[212] VNS may be especially useful in depressed patients with heart disease.

Transcranial Magnetic Stimulation

Repetitive transcranial magnetic stimulation (rTMS) provides noninvasive brain stimulation with magnetic pulses to induce neuronal depolarization in the cortex.[213] Unlike ECT, rTMS requires neither anesthesia nor seizure induction and is performed in the outpatient setting. It does not produce clinically apparent cognitive side effects, making it an excellent choice for patients with cognitive impairment. rTMS sessions typically last 40 minutes and are repeated daily, 5 days/week, for 4 to 6 weeks. Studies suggest that higher intensities, more pulses per session, and more pulses per course are

associated with superior outcome in depression.[214] Younger patients tend to have a better response.[215,216]

Many studies have shown that rTMS may be useful in the treatment of major depressive episodes.[217–221] In 2008, high-frequency rTMS to the left dorsolateral prefrontal cortex was approved by the FDA for the treatment of major depressive disorder. In one important trial, improvement was seen at week 4 and rates of response were about 24% and remission 14%.[222] Follow-up of patients found remission rates as high as 58%.[223] Three years later, 84% of patients who had relapsed were able to achieve remission again with adjunctive rTMS.[224] Fewer prior treatment failures, shorter duration of illness, and lack of comorbid anxiety disorder were strong predictors of response to TMS.[223]

The antidepressant efficacy of TMS may be comparable to that of ECT in nonpsychotic patients,[223,225,226] but true double-blinding of such comparisons remains evasive. Despite many placebo-controlled trials revealing significant difference between rTMS and sham, only a few more recent studies report substantial rates of response.[219,220] This may be due to the short duration of earlier trials (two weeks or less). More recent studies using longer durations of treatment are more encouraging.[227]

Contraindications

There are no medical contraindications to rTMS except prior seizure and having metal in the head near the stimulating coil.

Side Effects

rTMS has a favorable systemic and cognitive side-effect profile for medically ill patients. Headache and scalp pain are the main side effects of rTMS and patients return to their responsibilities immediately following each session. Patients may feel a tapping sensation at the site of stimulation and stimulation of superficial nerves and muscle under the stimulating coil can result in eye blinking and/or jaw clenching. rTMS has a risk of seizure when excessive levels of stimulation are used. Adherence to published safety guidelines for dosage and medical monitoring can ensure safety.[228,229]

Magnetic Seizure Therapy

MST is an investigational treatment that uses high-dose TMS to induce therapeutic seizures. MST requires anesthesia, but offers better control over the site of stimulation and current than ECT. Thus MST allows the targeting of specific brain regions implicated in depression while reducing spread electric current to brain areas responsible for cognitive side effects[230–232] MST seizures have shorter duration, lower ictal EEG amplitude, less postictal suppression, and faster orientation recovery.[233] Measures of attention, retrograde amnesia, and category fluency are superior in MST. Preliminary studies demonstrate equal efficacy for MST and RUL ECT,[234,235] and response in a bipolar depressed patient.[236] Since MST has the potential of retaining the efficacy of ECT with fewer cognitive side effects, it may be of use in patients who cannot tolerate the memory effects of ECT and in patients with cardiac disease, as animal studies suggest it has less cardiodepressant effects.[237]

Deep Brain Stimulation

Deep brain stimulation (DBS) chronically stimulates targeted brain areas and, unlike lesioning procedures, is believed to be fully reversible. DBS has been successfully used in treatment-refractory neurological disorders and is being studied for the treatment of psychiatric conditions, including depression. DBS has no known systemic side effects and improves cognition.[238] About 100 patients worldwide have received DBS for depression.

Multiple subcortical regions have been targeted.[239,240] These targets were selected from brain imaging studies of dysfunctional emotion processing in depression,[241-244] and reward circuits contributing to depressive symptoms.[240,245] All open-label studies have response rates in over 50% of patients. However, in a multicenter study of DBS, response rates were somewhat less promising.[246] Subsequent studies are needed to establish the safety, efficacy, and best targets of this most focal, though most invasive, treatment for depression.

Transcranial Direct Current Stimulation

Transcranial direct current stimulation (tDCS) is an experimental noninvasive means of electrically stimulating the cerebral cortex that may enhance verbal fluency and improve word recall in stroke[247] and depressed patients.[248-251] Recent double blind, randomized, sham-controlled trials of tDCS in depression had mixed results.[252-257] The optimal site of stimulation is yet to be determined.[254,256,257] Knotkova and colleagues found it reduced depressive symptoms in HIV-positive patients[258] and there is a case report of improved cognition and depressive symptoms in a post-stroke patient with depression.[259] The low cost and good safety profile of tDCS make it an attractive modality relative to more invasive and costly procedures.[260]

OUTCOMES

■ MEASUREMENT-BASED CARE

Measurement-based care (MBC) involves systematically collecting and recording data on treatment progress and outcomes to guide treatment choices and adjustments. This is essential to providing optimal mental health care[262,263] and results in better outcomes than pharmacotherapy without it.[264] The questionnaires used in MBC help to engage patients in their treatment by allowing them to track their own progress toward treatment goals. Monitoring progress and outcomes provides systematic feedback for the clinician,[265] which has been shown to improve treatment outcomes.[262] MBC also allows the provider to adjust the treatment if adequate progress is not observed[266] and, as such, serves as a structured feedback loop for continuously monitoring the effectiveness of the psychological and/or pharmacological intervention. For example, MBC can prompt treatment changes, the addition of other services or interventions, or conversely, the tapering of care after functioning has improved. A large RCT across 14 primary care sites evaluated MBC-based collaborative care for patients with depression, diabetes, coronary heart disease, or both. The care management intervention significantly improved control of depression and medical disease as compared with usual care. Furthermore, patients in the intervention group were more likely to initiate antidepressant medications, accept adjustments to those medications, and report better quality-of-life and greater satisfaction with their care.[267]

Continuous attention to outcomes also allows for assessing the progress of patient populations. This enables healthcare systems to continually improve clinical programs, and to monitor the performance of individual clinicians and administrative staff. MBC also allows systems to demonstrate performance to payors[262] and other external stakeholders.

MBC is typically used to measure depressive symptoms, adherence to the medication, and medication side effects.[263] Less commonly measured, but no less important, is patient functioning and/or quality-of-life as a nonsymptom-based indicator of treatment progress and outcomes. Standardized depression symptom rating scales provide more sensitive and accurate evaluation than global judgments by the clinician or patient.[263] Rather than clinicians merely asking patients "How are you feeling?" or "What changes have you noticed in your mood since we last met?" validated symptom measures provide a more accurate foundation for decision making and treatment planning.[263,267] Systematically measuring depression at treatment initiation provides a baseline level of depression severity against which to gauge progress. In addition,

by comparing a patient's initial depression severity level with the norms of other patient groups, this score can provide an indication of length of therapy and patient treatment response.[262]

Self-report Scales for Measurement of Depressive Symptoms, Treatment Response, and Outcome

As discussed in Chapter 3, the PHQ-9 is one of the most widely used self-report depression measures.[268] It captures all nine symptom domains of major depressive disorder, and assesses how often the patient has been bothered by each in the last 2 weeks.[263] It provides both a DSM-5 depression diagnosis and a continuous score reflecting depressive symptom severity.[14] The PHQ-9 is sensitive to change over time[269] and to treatment effects.[270,271] It is effective for depression screening across a range of medical settings, including primary care and specialty care settings.[272] The quick inventory of depressive symptomatology (QIDS-SR) is another self-report instrument that assesses the nine domains of major depression.[273] It is useful for evaluating symptom severity over time. The Beck depression inventory-II (BDI-II) is a self-report scale that measures depressive thoughts and attitudes as well as the somatic symptoms of depression, and is sensitive to change over time.[97,274]

Self-report Scales for Measurement of Medication Side Effects and Medication Adherence

The brief medication questionnaire (BMQ) provides an estimate of adherence to the medical regimen and the reasons for nonadherence.[263,275,276] The widely used medication adherence questionnaire (MAQ), also known as Morisky 4, is composed of four items and has been validated in a wide range of medical conditions.[276]

Self-Report Scales for Measurement of Quality-of-Life and Functioning

Quality-of-life and life functioning may improve with depression treatment somewhat independently of symptom improvement. They are, therefore, important outcome variables. A well-established and widely used health-related quality-of-life measure is the medical outcomes scale-short form (SF) general health survey. There are 36-, 12-, and 8-item versions. All versions of this questionnaire assess eight health-related quality-of-life domains: physical functioning, role limitations due to physical health, bodily pain, general health perceptions, vitality, social functioning, and role limitations due to emotional problems and mental health.[277] One advantage of the MOS-SF is the existence of norms for many different populations. A potentially useful measure of functioning is the disruption of functioning index (DFI), which is adapted from the pain disability index.[278,279] This scale includes seven items capturing the degree to which aspects of life are disrupted by a specific problem (e.g., depression and/or medical illness).

Scheduling Assessments and Decision Points

MBC should include an established clinic visit schedule; regular measurement and monitoring of depressive symptoms, medication side effects, and medication adherence; and use of a treatment algorithm. Response to medications should be measured every 2 weeks for the first 6 weeks after each change in the regimen. After 6 weeks, measurement should be conducted every 3 weeks until remission is achieved or a treatment change is made. Once remission is achieved, assess patients every 3 months.[263] Critical decision points in the treatment algorithm provide a timetable for evaluating patients' treatment response, tolerance of side effects, and functioning[263] Use assessments to make treatment decisions at the critical decision points of weeks two, four, six, nine, and twelve. Treatment algorithms include options for partial response and nonresponse.[263,280,281] This continuous and regular measurement of treatment progress is inherent in CBT for depression. To measure treatment progress from psychotherapy in general, set collaborative and measurable treatment goals with the patient (e.g., a 50% reduction in depressive symptoms by mid-treatment), monitor treatment process and outcomes bi-weekly for the first month and then at least monthly thereafter, and make adjustments accordingly.[282]

CONCLUSION

Effectively treating depression in medically ill patients is fundamental to optimizing the overall health of this population. Depression treatment is also key in lowering healthcare costs. Although more research is needed to achieve better targeting and more rapid initiation of treatments, effective treatment also depends on a thorough clinical assessment (Chapter 3) and careful measurement of progress and care delivery (Chapter 23). Engaging patients and their significant others, as well as the entire healthcare team, in this process is critical.

REFERENCES

1. Kwana BM, Dimidijiana S, Rizvib SL. Treatment preference, engagement, and clinical improvement in pharmacotherapy versus psychotherapy for depression. *Behav Res Ther.* 2010;48(8):799–804.

2. Judd LL, Paulus MJ, Schettler PJ, et al. Does incomplete recovery from first lifetime major depressive episode herald a chronic course of illness? *Am J Psychiat.* 2000;157:1501–1504.

3. Ramasubbu R, Patten SB. Effect of depression on stroke morbidity and mortality. *Can J Psychiatry.* 2003;48:250–257.

4. Lustman PJ, Anderson RJ, Freedland KE, de Groot M, Carney RM, Clouse RE. Depression and poor glycemic control: a meta-analytic review of the literature. *Diabetes Care.* 2000;23:934–942.

5. Unutzer J, Schoenbaum M, Katon WJ, et al. Healthcare costs associated with depression in medically Ill fee-for-service medicare participants. *J of Am Geriatr Soc.* 2009;57(3):506–510.

6. Center for Disease Control (CDC) and Prevention Weekly Morbidity and Mortality Report. May 3, 2013. http://www.cdc.gov/mmwr/pdf/wk/mm6217.pdf

7. CDC Promotes Public Health Approach to Address Depression Among Older Adults. http://www.cdc.gov/aging/pdf/CIB_mental_health.pdf

8. Unutzer J, Katon WJ, Fan MY, et al. Long-term cost effects of collaborative care for late-life depression. *Am J Manag Care.* 2008;14:95–100.

9. Arkowitz H, Westra HA, Miller WR, et al., eds. *Motivational Interviewing in the Treatment of Psychological Problems (Applications of Motivational Interviewing).* New York, NY: The Guillford Press; 2008.

10. Eaddy MT, Cook CL, O'Day K, Burch SP, Cantrell CR. How patient cost-sharing trends affect adherence and outcomes: A literature review. *PT.* 2012;37(1):45–55.

11. Weiden PJ, Rao N. Teaching medication compliance to psychiatric residents: placing an orphan topic into a training curriculum. *Acad Psychiatry.* 2005;29:203–210.

12. Kaslow NJ, Racusin GR. Family therapy for depression in young people. In: Reynolds WM, Johnston HF, eds. *Handbook of Depression in Children and Adolescents.* New York, NY: Plenum Press; 1994:345–363.

13. Keitner GL, Miller IW. Family functioning and major depression: an overview. *Am J Psychiat.* 1990;147(9):1128–1137.

14. Yeung A, Shyu I, Fisher L, Wu S, Yang H, Fava M. Culturally sensicollaborative treatment for depressed Chinese Americans in primary care. *Am J Public Health.* 2010;100:2397–2402.

15. Yeung A, Trinh NH, Chang TE, Fava M. The Engagement Interview Protocol (EIP): Improving the acceptance of mental health treatment among Chinese immigrants. *Int J Cult Ment Health.* 2011;4:91–105.

16. Yeung A, Chang D, Gresham RL Jr, Nierenberg AA, Fava M. Illness beliefs of depressed Chinese American patients in primary care. *J Nerv Ment Dis.* 2004;192(4):324–327.

17. Leng JC, Changrani J, Tseng CH, Gany F. Detection of depression with different interpreting methods among Chinese and Latino primary care patients: a randomized controlled trial. *J Immigr Minor Health.* 2010;12:234–241.

18. Alegria M, Canino G, Shrout PE, et al. Prevalence of mental illness in immigrant and non-immigrant U.S. Latino groups. *Am J Psychiatry.* 2008;165(3):359–369.

19. González HM, Vega WA, Williams DR, Tarraf W, West BT, Neighbors HW. Depression care in the United States: too little for too few. *Arch Gen Psychiatry.* 2010;67(1):37–46.

20. Karasz A, Garcia N, Ferri L. Conceptual models of depression in primary care patients: A comparative study. *J Cross Cult Psychol.* 2009;40(6):1041–1059.

21. Yeung A, Fung F, Yu SC, et al. Validation of the patient health questionnaire-9 for depression screening among Chinese Americans. *Compr Psychiatry.* 2008,49(2):211–17.

22. Bao Y, Alexopoulos GS, Casalino LP, et al. Can Collaborative Depression Care Management Reduce Disparities in Depression Treatment and Outcomes. *Arch Gen Psychiatry.* 2011;68(6):627–36.

23. Cooper LA, Ghods Dinoso BK, Ford DE, et al. Comparative effectiveness of standard versus patient-centered collaborative care interventions for depression among African Americans in primary care settings: the BRIDGE Study. *Health Serv Res.* 2013;48(1):150–174.

24. Hails K, Brill CD, Chang T, Yeung A, Fava M, Trinh NH. Cross-cultural aspects of depression management in primary care. *Curr Psychiatry Rep.* 2012;14(4):336–344.

25. Lewis-Fernández R, Balán IC, Patel SR, et al. Impact of motivational pharmacotherapy on treatment retention among depressed Latinos. *Psychiatry.* 2013 Fall;76(3):210–222.

26. Interian A, Lewis-Fernández R, Gara MA, Escobar JI. A randomized-controlled trial of an intervention to improve antidepressant adherence among Latinos with depression. *Depress Anxiety.* 2013;30(7):688–996.

27. Trinh NH, Hagan PN, Flaherty K, et al. Evaluating patient acceptability of a culturally focused psychiatric consultation intervention for Latino Americans with depression. *J Immigr Minor Health.* 2014;16(6):1271–1277.

28. Garcia-Toro M, Ibarra O, Gili M, et al. Four hygienic-dietary recommendations as add-on treatment in depression: a randomized-controlled trial. *J Affect Disorders.* 2012;40:200–203.

29. Conn DK, Madan R. Use of sleep-promoting medications in nursing home residents : risks versus benefits. *Drugs Aging.* 2006; 23(4):271–287.

30. Foley D, Ancoli-Israel S, Britz P, Walsh J. Sleep disturbances and chronic disease in older adults: results of the 2003 National Sleep Foundation Sleep in America Survey. *J Psychosom Res.* 2004; 56:497–502.

31. Naismith SL, Rogers NL, Lewis SJ, et al. Sleep disturbance relates to neuropsychological functioning in late-life depression. *J Affect Disord.* 2011;132:139–145.

32. Gangwisch JE, Malaspina D, Boden-Albala B, Heymsfield SB. Inadequate sleep as a risk factor for obesity: analyses of the NHANES I. *Sleep.* 2005;28(10):1289–1296.

33. Gangwisch JE, Heymsfield SB, Boden-Albala B, et al. Short sleep duration as a risk factor for hypertension: analyses of the first National Health and Nutrition Examination Survey. *Hypertension.* 2006;47:833–839.

34. Ayas NT, White DP, Manson JE, et al. A prospective study of sleep duration and coronary heart disease in women. *Arch Intern Med.* 2003;163:205–209.

35. Gangwisch JE, Malaspina D, Babiss LA, et al. Short sleep duration as a risk factor for hypercholesterolemia: analyses of the National Longitudinal Study of Adolescent Health. *Sleep.* 2010;33(7):956–961.

36. Gangwisch JE, Heymsfield SB, Boden-Albala B, et al. Sleep duration as a risk factor for diabetes incidence in a large U.S. sample. *Sleep.* 2007;30(12):1667–1673.

37. Ferrie JE, Shipley MJ, Cappuccio FP, et al. A prospective study of change in sleep duration: associations with mortality in the Whitehall II cohort. *Sleep.* 2007;30(12):1659–1666..

38. Kripke DF, Garfinkel L, Wingard DL, Klauber MR, Marler MR. Mortality associated with sleep duration and insomnia. *Arch Gen Psychiat.* 2002;59:131–136.

39. Kripke DF, Langer RD, Kline LE. Hypnotics' association with mortality or cancer: a matched cohort study. *BMJ Open.* 2012;2(1): e000850.

40. Paterniti S, Dufouil C, Alperovitch A. Long-term benzodiazepine use and cognitive decline in the elderly: the Epidemiology of Vascular Aging Study. *J Clin Psychopharm.* 2002;22(3):285–293.

41. Weich S, Pearce HL, Croft P, et al. Effect of anxiolytic and hypnotic drug prescriptions on mortality hazards: retrospective cohort study. *BMJ.* 2014;348:g1996..

42. Roth T. Hypnotic use for insomnia management in chronic obstructive pulmonary disease. *Sleep Med.* 2009;10:19–25.

43. Substance Abuse and Mental Health Services Administration. The Dawn Report, Emergency Department Visits for Adverse Reactions Involving the Insomnia Medication Zolpidem. May 1, 2013. http://www.samhsa.gov/data/2k13/DAWN079/sr079-Zolpidem.htm

44. Coupland C, Dhiman P, Morriss R, Arthur A, Barton G, Hippisley-Cox J. Antidepressant use and risk of adverse outcomes in older people: population based cohort study. *BMJ.* 2011;343:d4551.

45. Wenzel-Seifert K, Wittmann M, Haen E. QTc prolongation by psychotropic drugs and the risk of Torsade de Pointes. *Dtsch Arztebl Int.* 2011;108(41):687–693.

46. Coe HV, Hong IS. Safety of low doses of quetiapine when used for insomnia. *Ann Pharmacother.* 2012;46(5):718–722.

47. Ray WA, Meredith S, Thapa PB, Meador KG, Hall K, Murray KT. Antipsychotics and the risk of sudden cardiac death. *Arch Gen Psychiat.* 2001;58:1161–1167.

48. Agostini JV, Leo-Summers LS, Inouye SK. Cognitive and other adverse effects of diphenhydramine use in hospitalized older patients. *Arch Intern Med.* 2001;161:2091–2097.

49. Sack RL, Hughes RJ, Edgar DM, Lewy AJ. Sleep-promoting effects of melatonin: at what dose, in whom, under what conditions, and by what mechanisms? *Sleep.* 1997;20(10):908–915.

50. Liu J, Wang LN. Ramelteon in the treatment of chronic insomnia: systematic review and meta-analysis. *Int J Clin Practice.* 2012;66(9):867–873.

51. Scheer FA, Morris CJ, Garcia JI, et al. Repeated melatonin supplementation improves sleep in hypertensive patients treated with beta-blockers: a randomized controlled trial. *Sleep* 2012;35(10):1395–1402.

52. Wirz-Justice A, Graw P, Krauchi K, et al. 'Natural' light treatment of seasonal affective disorder. *J Affect Disord.* 1996;37:109–120.

53. Golden RN, Gaynes BN, Ekstrom RD, et al. The efficacy of light therapy in the treatment of mood disorders: a review and meta-analysis of the evidence. *Am J Psychiat.* 2005;162:656–662.

54. Terman M. Evolving applications of light therapy. *Sleep Med Rev* 2007;11:497–507.

55. Anderson JL, Glod CA, Dai J, Cao Y, Lockley W. Lux vs. wavelength in light treatment of seasonal affective disorder. *Acta Psychiatr Scand.* 2009:120;203–212.

56. Terman M, Terman JS. Bright light therapy: side effects and benefits across the symptom spectrum. *J Clin Psychiat.* 1999; 60(11):799–808; quiz 809.

57. Faith MS, Butryn M, Wadden TA, Fabricatore A, Nguyen AM, Heymsfield SB. Evidence for prospective associations among depression and obesity in population-based studies. *Obes Rev.* 2011;12:e438–e453.

58. Sanchez-Villegas A, Delgado-Rodriguez M, Alonso A, et al. Association of the Mediterranean dietary pattern with the incidence of depression: the Seguimiento Universidad de Navarra/ University of Navarra follow-up (SUN) cohort. *Arch Gen Psychiat.* 2009;66(10):1090–1098.

59. Akbaraly TN, Brunner EJ, Ferrie JE, Marmot MG, Kivimaki M, Singh-Manoux A. Dietary pattern and depressive symptoms in middle age. *Brit J Psychiat.* 2009;195:408–413.

60. Jacka FN, Pasco JA, Mykletun A, et al. Association of Western and traditional diets with depression and anxiety in women. *Am J Psychiat.* 2010;167:1–7.

61. Davison KM, Kaplan BJ. Nutrient intakes are correlated with overall psychiatric functioning in adults with mood disorders. *Can J Psychiat.* 2012;57(2):85–92.

62. Sanchez-Villegas A, Galbete C, Martinez-Gonzalez MA, et al. The effect of the Mediterranean diet on plasma brain-derived neurotrophic factor (BDNF) levels: the PREDIMED-NAVARRA randomized trial. *Nutr Neurosci.* 2011;14(5)195–201.

63. Sublette ME, Ellis SP, Geant AL, Mann JJ. Meta-analysis of the effects of eicosapentaenoic acid (EPA) in clinical trials in depression. *J Clin Psychiat.* 2011;72(12):1577–1584.

64. Kjaergaard M, Waterloo K, Wang CE, et al, Effect of vitamin D supplement on depression scores in people with low levels of serum 25-hydroxyvitamin D: nested case-control study and randomised clinical trial. *Brit J Psychiat.* 2012;201(5):360–368.

65. Guowei L, Lawrence M, Zainab S, et al. Efficacy of vitamin D supplementation in depression in adults: a systematic review. *J Clin Endocrinol Metab.* 2014;99(3):757–76.

66. Sepehrmanesh Z, Kolahdooz F, Abedi F, et al. Vitamin D supplementation affects the beck depression inventory, insulin resistance, and biomarkers of oxidative stress in patients with major depressive disorder: a randomized, controlled clinical trial. *J Nutr.* 2016;146(2):243–8.

67. Morris DW, Trivedi M, Rush AJ. Folate and unipolar depression. *J Altern Complement Med.* 2008;14(3):277–285.

68. Papakostas GI, Peterson T, Mischoulon D, et al. Serum folate, vitamin B12, and homocysteine in major depressive disorder, Part 1: predictors of clinical response in fluoxetine-resistant depression. *J Clin Psychiat.* 2004;65:1090–1095.

69. Arinami T, Yamada N, Yamakawa-Kobayashi K, et al. Methylenetetrahydrofolate reductase variant and schizophrenia/depression. *Am J Med Genet.* 1997;74:526–528.

70. Papakostas GI, Shelton RC, Zajecka JM, et al. L-methylfolate as adjunctive therapy for SSRI-resistant major depression: results of two randomized, double-blind, parallel-sequential trials. *Amer J Psychiat.* 2012;169:1267–1274.

71. Coppen A, Bailey J. Enhancement of the antidepressant action of fluoxetine by folic acid: a randomised, placebo controlled trial. *J Affect Disorders*. 2000;60:121–113.

72. Rayman M, Thompson A, Warren-Perry M, et al. Impact of selenium on mood and quality of life: a randomized, controlled trial. *Biol Psychiat*. 2006;59:147–154.

73. Docherty JP, Sack DA, Roffman M, Finch M, Komorowski JR. A double-blind, placebo-controlled, exploratory trial of chromium picolinate in atypical depression: effect on carbohydrate craving. *J Psychiatr Pract*. 2005;11(5):302–314.

74. Kim K, Frongillo EA. Participation in food assistance programs modifies the relation of food insecurity with weight and depression in elders. *J Nutr*. 2007;137(4):1005–1010.

75. Song MR, Lee Y, Baek J, Miller M. Physical activity status in adults with depression in the National Health and Nutrition Examination Survey, 2005-2006. *Public Health Nurs*. 2011;29(3):208–217.

76. Chalder M, Wiles NJ, Campbell J, et al. A pragmatic randomised controlled trial to evaluate the cost-effectiveness of a physical activity intervention as a treatment for depression: the treating depression with physical activity (TREAD) trial. *Health Technol Assess*. 2012;16(10):1–164.

77. Rozanski A. Exercise as medical treatment for depression. *J Am Coll Cardiol*. 2012;60(12):1064–1066.

78. Josefsson T, Lindwall M, Archer T. Physical exercise intervention in depressive disorders: meta-analysis and systematic review. *Scand J Med Sci Sports*. 2014;24(2):259–272.

79. Hoffman SG, Sawyer AT, Witt AA, Oh D. The effect of mindfulness-based therapy on anxiety and depression: A meta-analytic review. *J Consult Clin Psychology*. 2010;78(2):169–183.

80. Benson H, Beary JF, Carol MP. The relaxation response. *Psychiatry*. 1974;37(1):37–46.

81. Samuelson M, Foret M, Baim M, et al. Exploring the effectiveness of a comprehensive mind-body intervention for medical symptom relief. *J Altern Complement Med*. 2010;16(2):187–192.

82. Wang F, Man JK, Lee EO, et al. The effects of qigong on anxiety, depression, and psychological well-being: a systematic review and meta-analysis. *Evid Based Complement Alternat Med*. 2013;2013:152738.

83. Whooley MA, Simon GE. Managing depression in medical outpatients. *N Eng J Med*. 2000;343:1942–1950.

84. Evans DL, Charney DS, Lewis L, et al. Mood disorders in the medically ill: Scientific review and recommendations. *Biol Psychiatry*. 2005;58:175–189.

85. Robinson R, Krishnan K. Depression and the medically ill. In: Davis KL, Charney D, Coyle JT, et al., eds. *Neuropsychopharmacology: The Fifth Generation of Progress*. American College of Neuropsychopharmacology; 2002:1179–1185.

86. Caron A, Weissman MM. Interpersonal psychotherapy in the treatment of depression in medical patients. *Prim psychiatry*. 2006;13:43–50.

87. Hopko DR, Lejuez CW, Ruggiero KJ, Eifert GH. Contemporary behavioral activation treatments for depression: Procedures, principles, and progress. *Clin Psychol Rev*. 2003;23:699–717.

88. Hopko DR, Bell JL, Armento M, et al. Cognitive-behavior therapy for depressed cancer patients in a medical care setting. *Behav Ther*. 2008;39:126–136.

89. Bohlmeijer E, Prenger R, Taal E, Cuijpers P. The effects of mindfulness-based stress reduction therapy on mental health of adults with a chronic medical disease: a meta-analysis. *J Psychosom Res*. 2010;68:539–544.

90. Lespérance F, Frasure-Smith N, Koszycki D, et al. CREATE Investigators. Effects of citalopram and interpersonal psychotherapy on depression in patients with coronary artery disease: the Canadian Cardiac Randomized Evaluation of Antidepressant and Psychotherapy Efficacy (CREATE) trial. *JAMA*. 2007;297:367—379.

91. Schulberg HC, Raue PJ, Rollman BL. "The effectiveness of psychotherapy in treating depressive disorders in primary care practice: clinical and cost perspectives." *Gen Hosp Psychiatry*. 2002;24(4):203–212.

92. Koszycki D, Lafontaine S, Frasure-Smith N, Swenson R, Lesperance F. An open-label trial of interpersonal psychotherapy in depressed patients with coronary disease. *Psychosomatics*. 2004;45(4):319–324.

93. Markowitz JC, Kocsis JH, Fishman B, et al. Treatment of depressive symptoms in human immunodeficiency virus-positive patients. *Arch Gen Psychiatry*. 1998;55(5):452–457.

94. Donnelly JM, Kornblith AB, Fleishman S, et al. A pilot study of interpersonal psychotherapy by telephone with cancer patients and their partners. *Psychooncology*. 2003;9(1):44–56.

95. Wiessman MM. Recent non-medication trials of interpersonal psychotherapy for depression. *Int J Neuropsychopharmacol*. 2007; 10:117–122.

96. Markowitz JC, Weissman MM. Interpersonal psychotherapy: Principles and applications. *World Psychiatry*. 2004;3(3):136–139.

97. Beck AT, Steer RA, Brown GK. *Manual for the Beck Depression Inventory-II*. San Antonio, TX: Psychological Corporation;1996.

98. Sandoval GA, Brown AD, Sullivan T, Green E. Factors that influence cancer patients' overall perceptions of the quality of care. *Int J Qual Health Care*. 2006;18:266–274.

99. Klerman GL, Weissman MM, Rounsaville B, Chevron E. *Interpersonal Psychotherapy of Depression*. New York, NY: Basic Books; 1984.

100. Weissman MM, Markowitz JC, Klerman GL *Comprehensive Guide to Interpersonal Psychotherapy*. New York, NY: Basic Books; 2000.

101. Mello MF, Mari JJ, Bacaltchuk J, Verdeli H, Neugebauer R. A systematic review of research findings on the efficacy of IPT for depressive disorders. *Eur Arch Psychiatry Clin Neurosci*. 2005;255:75–82.

102. Cape J, Whittington C, Buszewicz M, Wallace P, Underwood L. Brief psychological therapies for anxiety and depression in primary care: meta-analysis and meta-regression. *BMC Med*. 2010;8:38.

103. Safren SA, Gonzalez JS, Wexler DJ, et al. A randomized controlled trial of CBT for adherence and depression (CBT-AD) in patients with uncontrolled type 2 diabetes. *Diabetes Care*. 2014;37(3):625–633.

104. Baumeister H. Psychological and pharmacological interventions for depression in patients with diabetes mellitus and depression. *Cochrane Database of Systematic Reviews*. 2012;(12):CD008381. Available from Cochrane Database of Systematic Reviews, Ipswich, MA. Accessed April 21, 2014.

105. Safren SA, O'Cleirigh C, Tan JY, et al. A randomized controlled trial of cognitive behavioral therapy for adherence and depression (CBT-AD) in HIV-infected individuals. *Health Psychol*. 2009; 28(1):1–10.

106. Ramasubbu R, Beaulieu S, Taylor V, Schaffer A, McIntyre R. The CANMAT task force recommendations for the management of patients with mood disorders and comorbid medical conditions: Diagnostic, assessment, and treatment principles. *Ann Clin Psychiatry*. 2012;24(1):82–90.

107. Cully JA, Stanley MA, Deswal A, Hanania NA, Phillips LL, Kunik ME. Cognitive-behavioral therapy for chronic cardiopulmonary

conditions: preliminary outcomes from an open trial. *Prim Care Companion J Clin Psychiatry.* 2010;12(4):pii: PCC.09m00896.

108. Rutledge T, Reis V, Linke SE, Greenberg BH, Mills PJ. Depression in heart failure. A meta-analytic review of prevalence, intervention effects, and associations with clinical outcomes. *J Am Coll Cardiol.* 2006;48:1527–1537.

109. Dobkin RD, Menza M, Allen LA, et al. Cognitive-behavioral therapy for depression in Parkinson's disease: a randomized controlled trial. *Am J Psychiatry.* 2011;168(10):1066–1074.

110. Hind D, Cotter J, Thake A, et al. "Cognitive behavioural therapy for the treatment of depression in people with multiple sclerosis: a systematic review and meta-analysis." *BMC psychiatry.* 2014;14:5.

111. Mohr DC, Goodkin DE. Treatment of depression in multiple sclerosis: review and meta-analysis. *Clin Psychol Sci Prac.* 1999;6:1–9.

112. Diaz Sibaja MA, Comeche Moreno MI, Mas Hesse B. [Protocolized cognitive–behavioural group therapy for inflammatory bowel disease]. *Rev Esp Enferm Dig.* 2007;99(10):593–598.

113. Schwarz SP, Blanchard EB. Evaluation of a psychological treatment for inflammatory bowel disease. *Behav Res Ther.* 1991; 29(2):167–177.

114. Zautra AJ, Davis MC, Reich JW, et al. Comparison of cognitive behavioral and mindfulness meditation interventions on adaptation to rheumatoid arthritis for patients with and without history of recurrent depression. *J Consult Clin Psychol.* 2008;76:408–421.

115. Hedayati S, Yalamanchili V, Finkelstein FO. "A practical approach to the treatment of depression in patients with chronic kidney disease and end-stage renal disease." *Kidney Int.* 2012;81(3).247–255.

116. Cukor D. "Use of CBT to treat depression among patients on hemodialysis." *Psychiatr Serv.* 2007;58(5):711–712.

117. Savard J, Simard S, Giguere I, et al. Randomized clinical trial on cognitive therapy for depression in women with metastatic breast cancer: psychological and immunological effects. *Palliat Support Care.* 2006;4:219–237.

118. Pitceathly C, Maguire P, Fletcher I, et al. Can a brief psychological intervention prevent anxiety or depressive disorders in cancer patients? A randomised controlled trial. *Ann Oncol.* 2009;20:928–934.

119. Fawzy FI, Fawzy NW, Canada AL. Psychoeducational intervention programs for patients with cancer. In: Baum A, Andersen BL, eds. *Psychosocial Interventions for Cancer.* Washington, DC: American Psychological Association; 2001:235–267.

120. Nezu AM, Nezu CM, Felgoise SH, McLure KS, Houts PS. Project Genesis: assessing the efficacy of problem-solving therapy for distressed adult cancer patients. *J Consult Clin Psychol.* 2003; 71(6):1036–1048.

121. Butler AC, Beck AT. Cognitive therapy for depression. *Clin Psycholo.* 1995;48(3):3–5.

122. Nezu A, Maguth-Nezu C, D'Zurilla TJ. Problem-solving therapy. In Kazantzis N, Reinecke MA, Freeman A, eds. *Cognitive and Behavioral Theories in Clinical Practice.* New York, NY: The Guilford Press;2010:76–114.

123. Malouff J, Thorsteinsson E, Schutte N. The efficacy of problem solving therapy in reducing mental and physical health problems: A meta-analysis. *Clin Psychol Rev.* 2007;27:46–57.

124. D'Zurilla TJ, Nezu AM. Problem-solving therapy. In: Dobson KS, ed. *Handbook of Cognitive Behavioral Therapies.* New York, NY: Guilford Press; 2010:197–225.

125. Hopko DR, Armento ME, Roberston SM, et al. Brief behavioral activation and problem-solving therapy for depressed

breast cancer patients: randomized trial. *J Consult Clin Psychol.* 2011;79(6):834–849.

126. Ell K, Xie B, Quon B, Quinn DI, Dwight-Johnson M, Lee PJ. Randomized controlled trial of collaborative care management of depression among low-income patients with cancer. *J Clin Oncol.* 2008;26(27):4488–4496.

127. Gellis ZD, Bruce ML. Problem-solving therapy for subthreshold depression in home healthcare patients with cardiovascular disease. *Am J Geriatr Psychiatry.* 2010;18(6):464–474.

128 Katon WJ, Lin E, Von Korff M, et al. Collaborative care for patients with depression and chronic illnesses. *N Engl J Med.* 2010;363(27):2611–2620.

129. Ell K, Katon W, Xie B, et al. Collaborative care management of major depression among low-income, predominantly Hispanic subjects with diabetes A randomized controlled trial. *Diabetes Care.* 2010;33(4):706–713.

130. Nezu AM. Problem solving and behavior therapy revisited. *Behav Ther.* 2004;35:1–33.

131. Kabat-Zinn J. *Full Catastrophe Living: Using the Wisdom of Your Body and Mind to Face Stress, Pain, and Illness.* New York, NY: Delacorte Press; 1990.

132. Pradhan EK, Baumgarten M, Langenberg P, et al. "Effect of Mindfulness-Based stress reduction in rheumatoid arthritis patients." *Arthritis Rheum* 2007;57(7):1134–1142.

133. Gregg JA, Callaghan GM, Hayes SC, Glenn-Lawson JL. Improving diabetes self-management through acceptance, mindfulness, and values: a randomized controlled trial. *J Consult Clin Psychol.* 2007;75:336–343.

134. Segal Z, Teasdale JD. *Mindfulness-Based Cognitive Therapy for Depression: a New Approach to Preventing Depression Relapse.* New York, NY: Guilford Press; 2002.

135. Gonzalez-Garcia M, Ferrer MJ, Borras X, et al. Effectiveness of mindfulness-based cognitive therapy on the quality of life, emotional status, and CD4 cell count of patients aging with HIV infection. *AIDS Behav.* 2014;18:676–685.

136. Abbott RA, Whear R, Rodgers LR, et al. "Effectiveness of mindfulness-based stress reduction and mindfulness based cognitive therapy in vascular disease: A systematic review and meta-analysis of randomised controlled trials." *J Psychosom Res.* 2014;76(5):341–351.

137. Foley E, Huxter M, Baillie A, Price M, Sinclair E. Mindfulness-based cognitive therapy for individuals whose lives have been affected by cancer: A randomized controlled trial. *J of Consult Clin.* 2010; 78(1):72–79.

138. Bédard M, Felteau M, Marshall S, et al. "Mindfulness-based cognitive therapy reduces symptoms of depression in people with a traumatic brain injury: Results from a randomized controlled trial." *J Head Trauma Rehabil.* 2013;29(4):E13–E22.

139. Moustgaard A, Bedard M, Felteau M. Mindfulness-based cognitive therapy (MBCT) for individuals who had a stroke: results from a pilot study. *J Cogn Rehabil.* 2007;25:1–10.

140. Ramasubbu R, Taylor VH, Samaan Z. The Canadian Network for Mood and Anxiety Treatments (CANMAT) task force recommendations for the management of patients with mood disorders and select comorbid medical conditions. *Ann Clin Psychiatry.* 2012;24:91–109.

141. Driessen E, Cujpers P, de Maat SC, et al. The efficacy of short-term psychodynamic psychotherapy for depression: a meta-analysis. *Clin Psychol Rev.* 2010;30(1):25–36.

142. Mitchell AJ, Vaze A, Rao S. Clinical diagnosis of depression in primary care: a meta-analysis. *Lancet.* 2009;374:609–619.

143. *American Psychiatric Association Practice Guideline for the Treatment of Patients with Major Depressive Disorder.* 3rd ed. Available at http://psychiatryonline.org/pdfaccess.ashx?ResourceID = 243261&PDFSource = 6

144. *National Institute for Clinical Excellence.* Available at http://guidance.nice.org.uk/CG90/NICEGuidance/pdf

145. *Veterans Administration/Department of Defense, Clinical Practice Guideline for Management of Major Depressive Disorder.* 2009. Available at http://www.healthquality.va.gov/mdd/mdd_full09_c.pdf

146. MacGillivray S, Arroll B, Hatcher S, et al. Efficacy and tolerability of selective serotonin reuptake inhibitors compared with tricyclic antidepressants in depression treated in primary care: systematic review and meta-analysis. *BMJ.* 2003;326(7397):1014.

147. Thase ME, Larsen KG, Kennedy SH. Assessing the 'true' effect of active antidepressant therapy v. placebo in major depressive disorder: use of a mixture model. *Brit J Psychiatry.* 2011;199:501–507.

148. Ionescu DF, Niciu MJ, Richards EM, Zarate CA. Pharmacologic treatment of dimensional anxious depression: A review. *Prim Care Companion CNS Disord.* 2014;16(3):pii: PCC.13r01621pii: PCC.13r01621.

149. Carpenter DJ. St. John's wort and S-adenosyl methionine as "natural" alternatives to conventional antidepressants in the era of the suicidality boxed warning: what is the evidence for clinically relevant benefit? *Alternat Med Rev.* 2011;16(1):17–39.

150. Kasper S, Gastpar M, Muller WE, et al. Efficacy of St. John's wort extract WS 5570 in acute treatment of mild depression: a reanalysis of data from controlled clinical trials. *Eur Arch Psychiatry Clin Neurosci.* 2008;258(1):59–63.

151. Sarris J. St. John's wort for the treatment of psychiatric disorders. *Psychiatr Clin North Am.* 2013;36(1):65–72.

152. Papakostas GI, Micholoun D, Shyu I, Alpert JE, Fava M. S-adenosyl methionine (SAMe) augmentation of serotonin reuptake inhibitors for antidepressant nonresponders with major depressive disorder: a double-blind, randomized clinical trial. *Am J Psychiatry.* 2010;167(8):942–948.

153. Borrelli F, Izzo AA. Herb-drug interactions with St John's wort (Hypericum perforatum): an update on clinical observations. *AAPS J.* 2009;11(4):710–727.

154. Papakostas GI, Alpert JE, Fava M. S-adenosyl-methionine in depression: a comprehensive review of the literature. *Curr Psychiatry Rep.* 2003;5(6):460–466.

155. Iruela LM, Minquex L, Merino J, Monedero G. Toxic interaction of S-adenosylmethionine and clomipramine. *Am J Psychiatry.* 1993;150(3):522.

156. Jindal RD. Insomnia in patients with depression: some pathophysiological and treatment considerations. *CNS Drugs.* 2009;23(4):309–329.

157. Jann MW, Slade JH. Antidepressant agents for the treatment of chronic pain and depression. *Pharmacotherapy.* 2007;27(11):1571–1587.

158. Foley KF, DeSanty KP, Kast RE. Bupropion: pharmacology and therapeutic applications. *Expert Rev Neurother.* 2006;6(9):1249–1265.

159. Wenzel-Seifert K, Wittmann M, Haen E. QTc prolongation by psychotropic drugs and the risk of Torsade de Pointes. *Dtsch Arztebl Int.* 2011;108(41):687–693.

160. Jeon SH, Jaekal J, Lee SH, et al. Effects of nortriptyline on QT prolongation: a safety pharmacology study. *Hum Exp Toxicol.* 2011;30:1649–1656.

161. *FDA Drug Safety Communication: Revised recommendations for Celexa (citalopram hydrobromide) related to a potential risk of abnormal heart rhythms with high doses.* Available at http://www.fda.gov/Drugs/DrugSafety/ucm297391.htm

162. Castro VM, Clements CC, Murphy SN, et al. QT interval and antidepressant use: a cross sectional study of electronic health records. *BMJ.* 2013;346:f288.

163. Humphries JE, Wheby MS, VandenBerg SR. Fluoxetine and the bleeding time. *Arch Pathol Lab Med.* 1990;114:727–728.

164. Hackam DG, Mrkobrada M. Selective serotonin reuptake inhibitors and brain hemorrhage: a meta-analysis. *Neurology.* 2012;79(18):1862–1865.

165. Auerbach AD, Vittinghoff E, Maselli J, Pekow PS, Young JQ, Lindenauer PK. Perioperative use of selective serotonin reuptake inhibitors and risks for adverse outcomes of surgery. *JAMA Intern Med.* 2013;173(12):1075–1081.

166. Maschino F, Hurault-Delarue C, Chebbane L, Fabry V, Montastruc JL, Bagheri H; French Association of Regional Pharmacovigilance Centers. Bleeding adverse drug reactions (ADRs) in patients exposed to antiplatelet plus serotonin reuptake inhibitor drugs: analysis of the French Spontaneous Reporting Database for a controversial ADR. *Eur J Clin Pharmacol.* 2012;68(11):1557–1560.

167. Andrade C, Sandarsh S, Chethan KB, Nagesh KS. Serotonin reuptake inhibitor antidepressants and abnormal bleeding: a review for clinicians and a reconsideration of mechanisms. *J Clin Psychiatry.* 2010;71(12):1565–1575.

168. Rizzoli R, Cooper C, Reginster JY. Antidepressant medications and osteoporosis. *Bone.* 2012;51(3):606–613.

169. Fava M. Weight gain and antidepressants. *J Clin Psychiatry.* 2000;61Suppl 11:37–41.

170. Sussman N, Ginsberg DL, Bikoff J. Effects of nefazodone on body weight: a pooled analysis of selective serotonin reuptake inhibitor- and imipramine-controlled trials. *J Clin Psychiatry.* 2001;62(4):256–260.

171. Schwartz TL, Nihalani N, Jindal S, Kirk S, Jones N. Psychiatric medication-induced obesity: a review. *Obesity Reviews.* 2004;5:115–121.

172. Zoellner H. Dental infection and vascular disease. *Semin Thromb Hemost.* 2011;37(3):181–192.

173. Darowski A, Chambers SA, Chambers DJ. Antidepressants and falls in the elderly. *Drugs Aging.* 2009;26(5):381–394.

174. Kerse N, Flicker L, Pfaff JJ, et al. Falls, depression and antidepressants in later life: a large primary care appraisal. *PLoS One.* 2008;3:e2423.

175. Kallin K, Gustafson Y, Sandman PO, Karlsson S. Drugs and falls in older people in geriatric care settings. *Aging Clin Exp Res.* 2004;16:270–276.

176. Arfken CL, Wilson JG, Aronson SM. Retrospective review of selective serotonin reuptake inhibitors and falling in older nursing home residents. *Int Psychogeriatr.* 2001;13:85–91.

177. Spigset O, Hedenmalm K. Hyponatremia in relation to treatment with antidepressants: a survey of reports in the World Health Organization data base for spontaneous reporting of adverse drug reactions. *Pharmacotherapy.* 2012;17(2):348–352.

178. Verbeeck RK, Musuamba FT. Pharmacokinetics and dosage adjustment in patients with renal dysfunction. *Eur J Clin Pharmacol.* 2009;65:757–773.

179. Mangoni AA, Jackson SH. Age-related changes in pharmacokinetics and pharmacodynamics: basic principles and practical applications. *Br J Clin Pharmacol.* 2004;57(1):6–14.

180. Ramasubbu R, Beaulieu S, Taylor V, et al. Ann Clin Psychiatry, American Psychiatric Association: Task Force on Electroconvulsive Therapy. *The Practice of electroconvulsive Therapy: Recommendations for Treatment, Training, and Privileging*. Washington DC: American Psychiatric Association; 2001.

181. Bailine S, Fink M, Knapp R, et al. Electroconvulsive therapy is equally effective in unipolar and bipolar depression. *Acta Psychiatr Scand*. 2010;121(6):431–436.

182. Daly JJ, Prudic J, Devanand DP, et al. ECT in bipolar and unipolar depression: differences in speed of response. *Bipolar Disord*. 2001;3(2):95–104.

183. Sobin C, Prudic J, Devanand DP, et al. Who responds to electroconvulsive therapy? A comparison of effective and ineffective forms of treatment. *Br J Psychiatry*. 1996;169(3):322–328.

184. Prudic J, Haskett RF, Mulsant B, et al. Resistance to antidepressant medications and short-term clinical response to ECT. *Am J Psychiatry*. 1996;153(8):985–992.

185. Zorumski CF, Rutherford JL, Burke WJ, Reich T. ECT in primary and secondary depression. *J Clin Psychiatry*. 1986;47(6):298–300.

186. Dombrovski AY, Mulsant BH, Haskett RF, et al. Predictors of remission after electroconvulsive therapy in unipolar major depression. *J Clin Psychiatry*. 2005;66(8):1043–1049.

187. McCall WV, Rosenquist PB, Kimball J, et al. Health-related quality of life in a clinical trial of ECT followed by continuation pharmacotherapy: effects immediately after ECT and at 24 weeks. *J ECT*. 2011;27(2):97–102.

188. Coffey C, Kellner CH,. Electroconvulsive therapy in geriatric neuropsychiatry. In: Coffey CE, Cummings JL, eds.*American Psychiatric Press Textbook of Geriatric Neuropsychiatry*. 2nd ed. Washington, DC: American Psychiatric Press; 2000:829–859.

189. Philibert RA, Richards L, Lynch CF, Winokur G. Effect of ECT on mortality and clinical outcome in geriatric unipolar depression. *J Clin Psychiatry*. 1995;56(9):390–394.

190. Thompson JW, Weiner RD, Myers CP. Use of ECT in the United States in 1975, 1980, and 1986. *Am J Psychiatry*. 1994; 151(11):1657–1661.

191. Krystal AD, Coffey CE. Neuropsychiatric considerations in the use of electroconvulsive therapy. *J Neuropsychiatry Clin Neurosci*. 1997;9(2):283–292.

192. Weiner RD. Retrograde amnesia with electroconvulsive therapy: characteristics and implications. *Arch Gen Psychiatry*. 2000;57(6):591–592.

193. Abrams R. Stimulus titration and ECT dosing. *J Ect*. 2002;18(1):3–9; discussion 14–15.

194. Zielinski RJ, Roose SP, Devanand DP, Woodring S, Sackeim HA. Cardiovascular complications of ECT in depressed patients with cardiac disease.*Am J Psychiatry*. 1993;150(6):904–909.

195. Lisanby SH, Maddox JH, Prudic J, Devanand DP, Sackeim HA. The effects of electroconvulsive therapy on memory of autobiographical and public events. *Arch Gen Psychiatry*. 2000;57(6):581–590.

196. McElhiney M, Moody BJ, Steif BL, et al. Autobiographical memory and mood: effects of electroconvulsive therapy. *Neuropsychology*. 1995;9:501–517.

197. Sackeim HA, Prudic J, Devanand DP, et al. A prospective, randomized, double-blind comparison of bilateral and right unilateral electroconvulsive therapy at different stimulus intensities. *Arch Gen Psychiatry*. 2000;57(5):425–434.

198. Sackeim HA, Prudic J, Devanand DP, et al. Effects of stimulus intensity and electrode placement on the efficacy and cognitive effects of electroconvulsive therapy. *N Engl J Med*. 1993;328(12):839–846.

199. Sobin C, Sackeim HA, Prudic J, et al. Predictors of retrograde amnesia following ECT. *Am J Psychiatry*. 1995;152(7):995–1001.

200. Sackeim HA, Dillingham EM, Prudic J, et al. Effect of concomitant pharmacotherapy on electroconvulsive therapy outcomes: short-term efficacy and adverse effects. *Arch Gen Psychiatry*. 2009;66(7):729–737.

201. Choi J, Lisanby SH, Medalia A, Prudic J: A conceptual introduction to cognitive remediation for memory deficits associated with right unilateral electroconvulsive therapy. *J ECT*. 2011;27(4):286–291.

202. Devanand DP, Dwork AJ, Hutchinson ER, et a;. Does ECT alter brain structure? *Am J Psychiatry*. 1994;151(7):957–970.

203. Coffey CE, Weiner RD, Djang WT, et al. Brain anatomic effects of electroconvulsive therapy. A prospective magnetic resonance imaging study. *Arch Gen Psychiatry*. 1991, 48(11):1013–1021.

204. George MS, Sackeim HA, Rush AJ, et al. Vagus nerve stimulation: a new tool for brain research and therapy. *Biol Psychiatry*. 2000;47(4):287–295.

205. Rush AJ, George MS, Sackeim HA, et al. Vagus nerve stimulation (VNS) for treatment-resistant depressions: a multicenter study. *Biol Psychiatry*. 2000;47(4):276–286.

206. Sackeim HA, Rush AJ, George MS, et al. Vagus nerve stimulation (VNS) for treatment-resistant depression: efficacy, side effects, and predictors of outcome. *Neuropsychopharmacology*. 2001;25(5):713–728.

207. Rush AJ, Marangell LB, Sackeim HA, et al. Vagus nerve stimulation for treatment-resistant depression: a randomized, controlled acute phase trial. *Biol Psychiatry*. 2005, 58(5):347–354.

208. George MS, Rush AJ, Marangell LB, et al. A one-year comparison of vagus nerve stimulation with treatment as usual for treatment-resistant depression. *Biol Psychiatry*. 2005;58(5):364–373.

209. Sperling W, Reulbach U, Kornhuber J. Clinical benefits and cost effectiveness of vagus nerve stimulation in a long-term treatment of patients with major depression. *Pharmacopsychiatry*. 2009;42(3):85–88.

210. Sackeim HA, Keilp JG, Rush AJ, et al. The effects of vagus nerve stimulation on cognitive performance in patients with treatment-resistant depression. *Neuropsychiatry Neuropsychol Behav Neurol*. 2001;14(1):53–62.

211. Schwartz PJ, De Ferrari GM, Sanzo A, et al. Long term vagal stimulation in patients with advanced heart failure: first experience in man. *Eur J Heart Fail*. 2008;10(9):884–891.

212. Sperling W, Reulbach U, Bleich S, Padberg F, Kornhuber J, Mueck-Weymann M. Cardiac effects of vagus nerve stimulation in patients with major depression. *Pharmacopsychiatry*. 2010, 43(1):7–11.

213. Barker AT, Jalinous R, Freeston IL. Non-invasive magnetic stimulation of human motor cortex. *Lancet*. 1985;1(8437):1106–1107.

214. Gershon AA, Dannon PN, Grunhaus L. Transcranial magnetic stimulation in the treatment of depression. *Am J Psychiatry*. 2003;160(5):835–845.

215. Fitzgerald PB, Hoy K, McQueen S, et al. A randomized trial of rTMS targeted with MRI based neuro-navigation in treatment-resistant depression. *Neuropsychopharmacology* 2009;34(5):1255–1262.

216. Aguirre I, Carretero B, Ibarra O, et al. Age predicts low-frequency transcranial magnetic stimulation efficacy in major depression. *J Affect Disord*. 2011;130(3):466–469.

217. Aarre TF, Dahl AA, Johansen JB, Kjonniksen I, Neckelmann D. Efficacy of repetitive transcranial magnetic stimulation in depression: a review of the evidence. *Nord J Psychiatry*. 2003;57(3): 227–232.

218. Burt T, Lisanby SH, Sackeim HA. Neuropsychiatric applications of transcranial magnetic stimulation: a meta analysis. *Int J Neuropsychopharmacol*. 2002;5(1):73–103.

219. Holtzheimer PE 3rd, Russo J, Avery DH. A meta-analysis of repetitive transcranial magnetic stimulation in the treatment of depression. *Psychopharmacol Bull*. 2001;35(4):149–169.

220. Kozel FA, George MS. Meta-analysis of left prefrontal repetitive transcranial magnetic stimulation (rTMS) to treat depression. *J Psychiatr Pract*. 2002;8(5):270–275.

221. Loo CK, Mitchell PB. A review of the efficacy of transcranial magnetic stimulation (TMS) treatment for depression, and current and future strategies to optimize efficacy. *J Affect Disord*. 2005;88(3):255–267.

222. O'Reardon JP, Solvason HB, Janicak PG, et al. Efficacy and safety of transcranial magnetic stimulation in the acute treatment of major depression: a multisite randomized controlled trial. *Biol Psychiatry*. 2007;62(11):1208–1216.

223. Mantovani A, Pavlicova M, Avery D, et al. Long-term efficacy of repeated daily prefrontal transcranial magnetic stimulation (TMS) in treatment-resistant depression. *Depress Anxiety*. 2012;29(10):883–890.

224. Janicak PG, Nahas Z, Lisanby SH, et al. Durability of clinical benefit with transcranial magnetic stimulation (TMS) in the treatment of pharmacoresistant major depression: assessment of relapse during a 6-month, multisite, open-label study. *Brain Stimul*. 2010;3(4):187–199.

225. George MS, Lisanby SH, Avery D, et al. Daily left prefrontal transcranial magnetic stimulation therapy for major depressive disorder: a sham-controlled randomized trial. *Arch Gen Psychiatry*. 2010;67(5):507–516.

226. Lisanby SH, Husain MM, Rosenquist PB, et al. Daily left prefrontal repetitive transcranial magnetic stimulation in the acute treatment of major depression: clinical predictors of outcome in a multisite, randomized controlled clinical trial. *Neuropsychopharmacology* . 2009;34(2):522–534.

227. Allan CL, Herrmann LL, Ebmeier KP. Transcranial magnetic stimulation in the management of mood disorders. *Neuropsychobiology*. 2011;64(3):163–169.

228. Wassermann EM. Risk and safety of repetitive transcranial magnetic stimulation: report and suggested guidelines from the International Workshop on the Safety of Repetitive Transcranial Magnetic Stimulation, June 5–7, 1996. *Electroencephalogr Clin Neurophysiol*. 1998;108(1):1–16.

229. Belmaker B, Fitzgerald P, George MS, et al. Managing the risks of repetitive transcranial stimulation. *CNS Spectr*. 2003;8(7):489.

230. Lisanby SH, Luber B, Schlaepfer TE, Sackeim HA. Safety and feasibility of magnetic seizure therapy (MST) in major depression: randomized within-subject comparison with electroconvulsive therapy. *Neuropsychopharmacology* 2003;28(10):1852–1865.

231. Kosel M, Frick C, Lisanby SH, Fisch HU, Schlaepfer TE. Magnetic seizure therapy improves mood in refractory major depression. *Neuropsychopharmacology*. 2003;28(11):2045–2048.

232. Lisanby SH, Schlaepfer TE, Fisch HU, Sackeim HA. Magnetic seizure therapy of major depression. *Arch Gen Psychiatry*. 2001;58(3):303–305.

233. Kirov G, Ebmeier KP, Scott AI, et al. Quick recovery of orientation after magnetic seizure therapy for major depressive disorder. *Br J Psychiatry*. 2008;193(2):152–155.

234. Fitzgerald PB, Hoy KE, Herring SE, Clinton AM, Downey G, Daskalakis ZJ. Pilot study of the clinical and cognitive effects of high-frequency magnetic seizure therapy in major depressive disorder. *Depress Anxiety*. 2013;30(2):129–136.

235. Kayser S, Bewernick BH, Grubert C, Hadrysiewicz BL, Axmacher N, Schlaepfer TE. Antidepressant effects, of magnetic seizure therapy and electroconvulsive therapy, in treatment-resistant depression. *J Psychiatr Res*. 2011;45(5):569–576.

236. Kayser S, Bewernick B, Axmacher N, Schlaepfer TE. Magnetic seizure therapy of treatment-resistant depression in a patient with bipolar disorder. *JECT*. 2009;25(2):137–140.

237. Rowny SB, Cycowicz YM, McClintock SM, Truesdale MD, Luber B, Lisanby SH. Differential heart rate response to magnetic seizure therapy (MST) relative to electroconvulsive therapy: a nonhuman primate model. *Neuroimage*. 2009;47(3):1086–1091.

238. Grubert C, Hurlemann R, Bewernick BH, et al. Neuropsychological safety of nucleus accumbens deep brain stimulation for major depression: effects of 12-month stimulation. *World J Biol Psychiatry*. 2011;12(7):516–527.

239. Anderson RJ, Frye MA, Abulseoud OA, et al. Deep brain stimulation for treatment-resistant depression: efficacy, safety and mechanisms of action. *Neurosci Biobehav Rev*. 2012;36(8):1920–1933.

240. Schlaepfer TE, Bewernick BH, Kayser S, Madler B, Coenen VA. Rapid effects of deep brain stimulation for treatment-resistant major depression. *Biol Psychiatry*. 2013;73(12):1204–1212.

241. Mayberg HS, Lozano AM, Voon V, et al. Deep brain stimulation for treatment-resistant depression. *Neuron*. 2005;45(5):651–660.

242. Jimenez F, Velasco F, Salin-Pascual R, et al. A patient with a resistant major depression disorder treated with deep brain stimulation in the inferior thalamic peduncle. *Neurosurgery*. 2005;57(3):585–593; discussion 585–593.

243. Jimenez F, Nicolini H, Lozano AM, Piedimonte F, Salin R, Velasco F. Electrical Stimulation of the Inferior Thalamic Peduncle in the Treatment of Major Depression and Obsessive Compulsive Disorders. *World neurosurgery*. 2013;80(3–4):S30.e17–e12.

244. Malone DA Jr, Dougherty DD, Rezai AR, et al. Deep brain stimulation of the ventral capsule/ventral striatum for treatment-resistant depression. *Biol Psychiatry*. 2009;65(4):267–275.

245. Schlaepfer TE, Cohen MX, Frick C, et al. Deep brain stimulation to reward circuitry alleviates anhedonia in refractory major depression. *Neuropsychopharmacology*. 2008;33(2):368–377.

246. Lozano AM, Giacobbe P, Hamani C, et al. A multicenter pilot study of subcallosal cingulate area deep brain stimulation for treatment-resistant depression. *J Neurosurg* 2012;116(2): 315–322.

247. Hummel F, Celnik P, Giraux P, et al. Effects of non-invasive cortical stimulation on skilled motor function in chronic stroke. *Brain*. 2005;128(Pt 3):490–499.

248. Wolkenstein L, Plewnia C. Amelioration of cognitive control in depression by transcranial direct current stimulation. *Biological Psychiatry*. 2013;73(7):646–651.

249. Brunoni AR, Zanao TA, Ferrucci R, et al. Bifrontal tDCS prevents implicit learning acquisition in antidepressant-free patients with major depressive disorder. *Prog Neuropsychopharmacol Biol Psychiatry*. 2013;43:146–150.

250. Oliveira JF, Zanao TA, Valiengo L, et al. Acute working memory improvement after tDCS in antidepressant-free patients with major depressive disorder. *Neurosci Lett*. 2013;537:60–64.

251. Boggio PS, Bermpohl F, Vergara AO, et al. Go-no-go task performance improvement after anodal transcranial DC stimulation of the left dorsolateral prefrontal cortex in major depression. *J Affect Disord*. 2007;101(1–3):91–98.

252. Fregni F, Boggio PS, Nitsche M, Pascual-Leone A. Transcranial direct current stimulation. *Br J Psychiatry*. 2005;186:446–447.

253. Palm U, Schiller C, Fintescu Z, et al. Transcranial direct current stimulation in treatment resistant depression: a randomized double-blind, placebo-controlled study. *Brain Stimul*. 2012;5(3):242–251.

254. Martin DM, Alonzo A, Mitchell PB, Sachdev P, Galvez V, Loo CK. Fronto-extracephalic transcranial direct current stimulation as a treatment for major depression: an open-label pilot study. *J Affect Disord*. 2011;134(1–3):459–463.

255. Brunoni AR, Ferrucci R, Bortolomasi M, et al. Transcranial direct current stimulation (tDCS) in unipolar vs. bipolar depressive disorder. *Prog Neuropsychopharmacol Biol Psychiatry*. 2011;35(1):96–101.

256. Berlim MT, Van den Eynde F, Daskalakis ZJ. Clinical utility of transcranial direct current stimulation (tDCS) for treating major depression: a systematic review and meta-analysis of randomized, double-blind and sham-controlled trials. *J Psychiatr Res*. 2013;47(1):1–7.

257. Kalu UG, Sexton CE, Loo CK, Ebmeier KP. Transcranial direct current stimulation in the treatment of major depression: a meta-analysis. *Psychol Med*. 2012; 42(9):1791–1800.

258. Knotkova H, Rosedale M, Strauss SM, et al. Using transcranial direct current stimulation to treat depression in HIV-infected persons: The outcomes of a feasibility study. *Front Psychiatry*. 2012;3:59.

259. Bueno VF, Brunoni AR, Boggio PS, Bensenor IM, Fregni F. Mood and cognitive effects of transcranial direct current stimulation in post-stroke depression. *Neurocase*. 2011;17(4):318–322.

260. Nitsche MA. Transcranial direct current stimulation: a new treatment for depression? *Bipolar Disord*. 2002;4Suppl 1:98–99.

261. Morin CM, Hauri PJ, Espie CA, Spielman AJ, Buysse DJ, Bootzin RR. Nonpharmacologic treatment of chronic insomnia. An American Academy of Sleep Medicine review. *Sleep*. 1999;22(8):1134–1156.

262. Trivedi MH. Tools and strategies for ongoing assessment of depression: A measurement-based approach to remission. *J Clin Psychiatry*. 2009;70(suppl 6):26–31.

263. Trivedi MH, Daly EJ. Measurement-based care for refractory depression: a clinical decision support model for clinical research and practice. *Drug Alcohol Depend*. 2007;88 Suppl 2:S61–S71.

264. Whipple J, Lambert M. Outcome measures for practice. *Ann Rev Clin Psychol*. 2011;7:87–111.

265. APA Presidential Task Force on Evidence-Based Practice US. Evidence-based practice in psychology. *Am Psychol*. 2006;61(4):271–285.

266. Zimmerman M. Using scales to monitor symptoms and treatment of depression (measurement based care). In: Roy-Byrne P, Solomon D, eds. *UpToDate*. 2013. Available at http://www.uptodate.com/contents/using-scales-to-monitor-symptoms-and-treatment-of-depression-measurement-based-care. Accessed April 24, 2013.

267. Lin EH, Von Korff M, Ciechanowski P, et al. Treatment adjustment and medication adherence for complex patients with diabetes, heart disease, and depression: A randomized controlled trial. *Ann Fam Med*. 2012;10:6–14.

268. Kroenke K, Spitzer RL, Williams JB. "The PHQ-9: validity of a brief depression severity measure." *J Gen Intern Med*. 2001;16(9):606–613.

269. Lowe B, Unutzer J, Callahan CM, Perkins AJ, Kroenke K. Monitoring depression treatment outcomes with the Patient Health Questionnaire-9. *Med Care*. 2004;42:1194–1201.

270. Löwe B, Kroenke K, Herzog W, Gräfe K. Measuring depression outcome with a brief self-report instrument: sensitivity to change of the Patient Health Questionnaire (PHQ-9). *J Affect Disord*. 2004;81(1):61–66.

271. Gilbody S, Richards D, Brealey S, Hewitt C. Screening for depression in medical settings with the patient health questionnaire (PHQ): A diagnostic meta-analysis. *J Gen Intern Med*. 2007;22(11):1596–1602.

272. Svarstad BL, Chewning BA, Sleath BL, Claesson C. The Brief Medication Questionnaire: a tool for screening patient adherence and barriers to adherence. *Patient Educ Couns*. 1999;37(2):113–124.

273. Rush AJ, Trivedi MH, Ibrahim HM, et al. "The 16-Item Quick Inventory of Depressive Symptomatology (QIDS), clinician rating (QIDS-C), and self-report (QIDS-SR): a psychometric evaluation in patients with chronic major depression." *Biol Psychiatry*. 2003;54(5):573–583.

274. Steer RA, Ball R, Ranieri WF, Beck AT. "Dimensions of the Beck depression inventory II in clinically depressed outpatients." *J Clin Psychology*. 1999;55(1):117–128.

275. Lavsa SM, Holzworth A, Ansani NT. Selection of a validated scale for measuring medication adherence. *J Am Pharm Assoc*. 2011;51(1):90–94.

276. Pollard AC. Preliminary validity study of the pain disability index. *Perceptual and Motor Skills*. 1984;59:974.

277. Trivedi MH, Kleiber BA. Using treatment algorithms for the effective management of treatment-resistant depression. *J Clin Psychiatry*. 2001;62(S18):25–29.

278. Tait R, Pollard A, Margols R, Duckro P, Kraus S. The pain disability index: Psychometric and Validity Data. *Arch Phys Med Rehabil*. 1987;68:438–441.

279. Ware J, Kosinski M, Dewey J, Gandek B. *How to Score and Interpret Single-Item Health Status Measures: A Manual for Users of the SF-8 Health Survey*. Boston, MA: QualyMetric; 2001.

280. Crimson M, Trivedi M, Pigott T, et al. The Texas Medication Algorithm Project: Report of the Texas consensus conference panel on medication treatment of major depressive disorder. *J Clin Psychiatry*. 1999;60:142–156.

281. Persons J, Roberts NA, Zalecki CA, Brechwald W. Naturalistic outcome of case formulation-driven cognitive-behavior therapy for anxious depressed outpatients. *Behav Res Ther*. 2006;44:1041–1051.

282. Katon WJ, Lin E, Von Korff M, et al. Collaborative care for patients with depression and chronic illnesses. *N Engl J Med*. 2010;363(27):2611–2620.

SECTION III

Depression in Medical Illness

CHAPTER 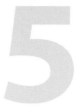5

Depression and Neurologic Illness

Laura Safar, MD

John Sullivan, MD

Gaston Baslet, MD

Jessica Harder, MD

Laura Morrissey, MSW

Shreya Raj, MD

Kirk Daffner, MD

David Silbersweig, MD

INTRODUCTION

Depression is the most highly prevalent neuropsychiatric syndrome across all neurologic illnesses (**Fig. 5-1**). The relationship between depression and neurologic illness is complex in several aspects, including pathophysiology, clinical presentation, and response to treatment. Depression may sometimes be the direct result of brain pathology, very much like other neurological manifestations, such as cognitive or motor disturbances. In other cases, a more complex interplay of neurobiological, environmental, and coping mechanisms appears responsible for the development of depressive symptoms (**Box 5-1**). Neurologic illness may produce signs and symptoms that mimic depression, such as psychomotor retardation, apathy, concentration deficits, and sleep disorders, making the diagnosis of depression in the context of neurologic illness challenging. However, the identification and treatment of depression in these individuals is of fundamental importance, as this tends to improve the prognosis of the neurological disease.

This chapter covers depression in the context of specific neurological disorders, such as dementia, cerebrovascular disease, Parkinson disease (PD) and other movement disorders, multiple sclerosis, traumatic brain illness, and epilepsy. Depression in the context of pain is covered in Chapter 21 and depression in the context of a sleep disorder is covered in chapter 22.

See Figure 5-1 and Box 5-1 for prevalence and risk factors of depression in different neurological illnesses.

DEMENTIA

"Dementia" refers to a syndrome characterized by cognitive deterioration, behavioral abnormalities, and possible personality changes that significantly affect daily functioning. A dementia syndrome can be caused by myriad etiologies, including neurodegenerative processes, such as Alzheimer disease (AD), dementia with Lewy bodies, and frontotemporal dementia, cerebrovascular disease, traumatic brain injury (TBI), infectious illnesses such as HIV, and other neurologic disturbances. This section covers depression in dementia secondary to a neurodegenerative process, with emphasis on depression in AD. Depression refers to clinically significant depressive symptoms, rather than particular subtypes as defined by Diagnostic and Statistical Manual of Mental Disorders (DSM) unless otherwise noted. Cerebrovascular depression and depression associated with PD are addressed later in this chapter.

■ EPIDEMIOLOGY

Neuropsychiatric symptoms are common in dementia, and depression is one of the most frequent manifestations.[1,2] Much of the research in this area has focused on the relationship between depression and AD. The reported prevalence of depression in the AD population (dAD) varies widely. This heterogeneity is in part due to differences in depression criteria, depressive subtypes included, study settings, and assessment methods used in various studies.[3] Estimates range between 1% and 90%, but the majority fall between 30% and 50%[3-5]

There is very little published data on depressive subtypes within the dementia population. A 2010 study[6] categorized patients with dementia into one of three groups by etiology: AD, vascular dementia, or unidentified dementia. Approximately 18.5% of patients with AD were depressed; 5.05% of that group met ICD-9 criteria for major depressive disorder (MDD), 1.93% for dysthymic disorder, 0.71%

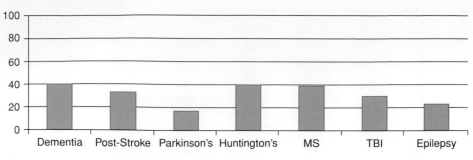

Figure 5-1 *Mean risk of depression for selected illnesses (% prevalence for particular disease.)*

for adjustment disorder with depressive symptoms, and 0.20% depressive psychosis. An additional 12.8% were diagnosed with depressive disorder not otherwise specified.

■ PATHOPHYSIOLOGY

In AD, the pathophysiological process is thought to begin many years before the clinical symptoms. In an initial stage, there may be asymptomatic cerebral amyloidosis without evidence of neurodegeneration. Later on, markers of neuronal injury, such as elevated CSF tau, cortical thinning/gray matter loss, and cortical hypometabolism may be present. After the preclinical stage, often a period termed mild cognitive impairment (MCI) during which a person experiences a subjective sense of intellectual decline without a change in functional ability precedes diagnosis. Ample evidence suggests that depression and dementia are inextricably linked. Whether depression is a risk factor, prodrome, or consequence of AD is an ongoing area of research. Several studies suggest a history of depression earlier in life approximately doubles the risk of developing dementia.[7–11] On the other hand, late-life depression (usually defined as presenting at age 60 or older) may represent a prodrome of incipient dementia. Although a definitive pathophysiological link between depression and dementia has yet to be established, several theories have been proposed.[12,13] These include dysregulation of the hypothalamic–pituitary–adrenal (HPA) axis, sequelae of chronic inflammation, and nerve growth factor derangements. See **Box 5-2** for possible mechanisms for depression in neurological illnesses.

Dysregulation of the Hypothalamic–Pituitary–Adrenal Axis

Major depression is associated with elevated cortisol levels, mediated by increased cortisol release and lack of sensitivity to normal negative feedback mechanisms. Excess cortisol is linked to hippocampal atrophy in animal models and human studies, an anatomical change that also occurs in AD.[14] In addition, longitudinal studies suggest that chronically elevated glucocorticoids levels can adversely affect memory.[15] Glucocorticoids can trigger apoptotic death in hippocampal neurons via activation of the glucocorticoid receptors.[16] In animal models of AD, stress level glucocorticoid administration promotes beta-amyloid deposition.[17]

Chronic Inflammation

Both depression and cognitive decline may be mediated through inflammation. Depression is considered a proinflammatory state, with increased levels of cytokines, such as interleukin-6 (IL-6) and tumor necrosis factor (TNF). These cytokines can (through a series of intermediary steps) reduce synaptic plasticity and hippocampal neurogenesis. Proinflammatory cytokines can also promote neurodegeneration by inducing neuronal apoptosis.[18] Amyloid-β (Aβ) can activate microglia to release proinflammatory cytokines. Microglia activation can be found in patients even at the earliest stages of cognitive decline, such as MCI.[19]

Nerve Growth Factors

Neurotrophins are essential in modulating synaptic plasticity and maintenance of neuronal health.[20] Levels of certain neurotrophins, such as brain-derived neurotrophic growth factor (BDNF) and transforming growth factor (TGF), are reduced in both dementia and depression. Impaired BNDF signaling occurs in animal models of stress-induced depression, humans with depression, and individuals with AD. BDNF is essential in regulating hippocampal plasticity, and therefore likely involved in maintaining cognition and memory.

It bears mentioning that simply being aware of cognitive deficits, or being diagnosed with a neurodegenerative disorder, do not seem to necessarily result in a "reactive" depression. Several studies

---

BOX 5-1
IMPORTANT RISK FACTORS FOR DEPRESSION IN NEUROLOGICAL DISEASE

Sociodemographic
Living alone
Social stress
Clinical
Personal or family history of depression
Physical impairment
Cognitive impairment
Alcohol and substance use disorders
Medical
Dementia
Cerebrovascular disease
Cortical and subcortical atrophy
Lesions of left frontal lobe, basal ganglia
Frontal and temporal lesions; atrophy and hypointense lesion burden (MS)
Other specific lesions (see **Fig. 5-2**)

BOX 5-2
POSSIBLE MEDIATORS BETWEEN NEUROLOGICAL ILLNESSES AND DEPRESSION

Dysregulation of HPA axis
Chronic inflammation
Nerve growth factor derangements
Direct brain insults
Depletion of neurotransmitters
Microvascular disease
Reaction to serious illness
Learned helplessness (e.g., epilepsy)

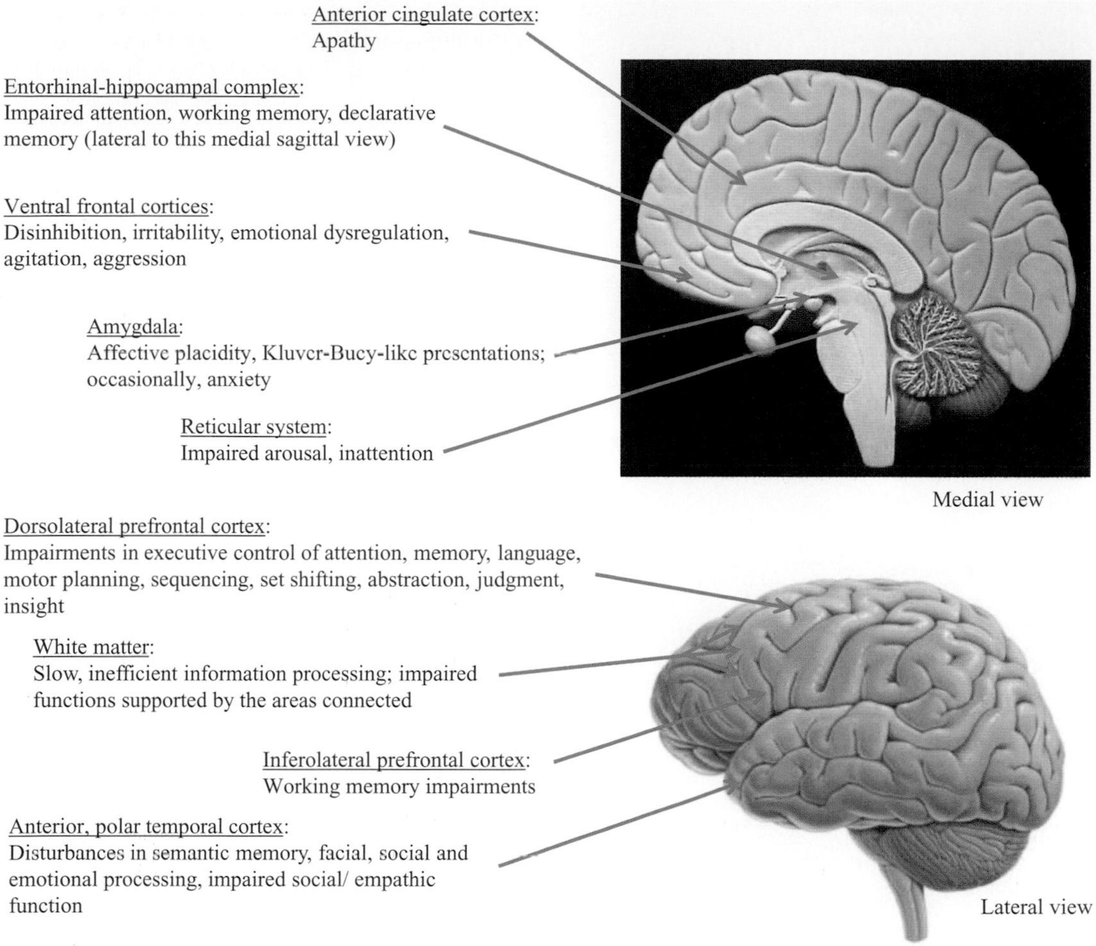

Anterior cingulate cortex:
Apathy

Entorhinal-hippocampal complex:
Impaired attention, working memory, declarative
memory (lateral to this medial sagittal view)

Ventral frontal cortices:
Disinhibition, irritability, emotional dysregulation,
agitation, aggression

Amygdala:
Affective placidity, Kluver-Bucy-like presentations;
occasionally, anxiety

Reticular system:
Impaired arousal, inattention

Dorsolateral prefrontal cortex:
Impairments in executive control of attention, memory, language,
motor planning, sequencing, set shifting, abstraction, judgment,
insight

White matter:
Slow, inefficient information processing; impaired
functions supported by the areas connected

Inferolateral prefrontal cortex:
Working memory impairments

Anterior, polar temporal cortex:
Disturbances in semantic memory, facial, social and
emotional processing, impaired social/ empathic
function

Medial view

Lateral view

Figure 5-2 *Localization-based clinical phenomena underlying brain-behavior relationships in traumatic brain injury.*

showed no correlations between awareness of cognitive deficits or diagnosis of cognitive impairment and depression scores.[21–24]

■ CLINICAL PRESENTATION

In general, depression in dementia presents similarly to major depression in the nondemented population. Regarding depression in the setting of earlier and milder cognitive deficits, the most common symptoms of depression in MCI may be excessive worrying, hopelessness, and crying spells.[25,26] See **Box 5-3** for symptoms commonly associated with depression in the different neurological illnesses.

Depression in AD is notable for a higher frequency of motivational disturbances such as psychomotor slowing and fatigue, whereas geriatric depression without cognitive impairment has a higher frequency of mood symptoms, such as depressed mood, anxiety, suicidality, and sleep and appetitive disturbances.[27] Studies have also found that depression with AD is associated with higher rates of delusions and other psychotic symptoms than general geriatric depression.[27,28] A 2011 study of AD patients found that within those with depression, sadness, loss of interest, and agitation/retardation were the most common among the depressive symptoms.[29] Sadness, anxiety, suicidal thoughts, poor self-esteem, multiple physical complaints, and pessimism best distinguished the depressed patients from the nondepressed.

Depression is considered part of the behavioral and psychological symptoms of dementia (BPSD) spectrum, and is frequently found with other comorbid neuropsychiatric symptoms. These may include anxiety, apathy, psychotic symptoms, mood lability, agitation, or some combination thereof.[30] In a 2013 study, Van der Mussele et al.[31] found that a number of behavioral symptoms such

as delusions, hallucinations, psychosis, activity disturbances, aggressiveness, diurnal rhythm disturbances, affective disturbances, and anxiety/phobia were more prevalent in depressed AD patients than nondepressed AD patients.

■ COURSE AND NATURAL HISTORY

Longitudinal studies of depression in patients with dementia suggest that mood symptoms may have an episodic, rather than chronic, course and that in a significant percentage of these patients symptoms may improve or remit in subsequent assessments.[32–34] In each of these studies, patients with depression would have had access to, and in some cases received, antidepressant treatment. The prevalence of depression and associated complaints (sadness, suicidal ideation, low self-esteem, guilt, anxiety, crying, and hopelessness) in patients with Alzheimer dementia has been found to be highest in the moderately demented population, followed by the mild dementia population.[35] Severe dementia is associated with the lowest prevalence of depressive symptoms. As dementia progresses from moderate to severe stages, patients may lose the ability to experience and communicate their psychological state. In addition, they may display other behavioral symptoms such as agitation, aggression, or anxiety, interfering with the identification of depressive symptoms.

■ ASSESSMENT

While individuals with MCI and mild to moderate dementia may underestimate their cognitive deficits, they remain key informants on their subjective mood state.[36] Caregiver input is needed on standard measures of depression, which require recall of sleep and

BOX 5-3
DEPRESSION IN NEUROLOGICAL ILLNESSES: IMPORTANT ASSOCIATED SYMPTOMS

More typical in depression associated with cognitive impairment

Confounding

Worrying

Hopelessness

Crying and affective lability

Motivational disturbances

Psychomotor slowing and fatigue

Delusions

Neurovegetative symptoms

More typical in depression associated with cerebrovascular disease

Anhedonia

Executive dyscontrol

More typical in Parkinson disease

Bradyphrenia

Apathy

More typical in MS

Fatigue

Insomnia, other sleep disorders

Cognitive deficits

Irritability and mood lability

More typical in TBI

Fatigue

Frustration

Poor concentration

Sleep disturbance

More typical in epilepsy

Short lived symptoms associated with particular phase of the seizure (i.e., pre or post ictal)

eating patterns and engagement in activities; caregivers also have important observations on affect and behavioral manifestations, such as tearfulness and withdrawal. Although caregivers' reports may be influenced by their own level of distress, studies still show high concordance between clinician-rated, caregiver-observed, and patient-reported mood.[36] The best practice for assessment is a clinical interview with both patient and caregiver.

Diagnostic Criteria

There is substantial overlap between some of the depression criteria and symptoms of dementia (e.g., difficulties with concentration and memory, apathy, and fatigue). In 2001, using the existing criteria for major depression as laid out in the DSM-IV, an expert panel convened by the National Institute for Mental Health (NIMH) created a provisional set of diagnostic criteria for depression in patients with AD: the NIMH-dAD (Table 5-1).

The minimum number of symptoms required to diagnose depression in AD was decreased from 5 to 3 and the requirement that symptoms be present "most of the day, nearly every day" was eliminated in favor of relevant symptoms being present "during the same 2-week period." Anhedonia, or decreased ability to take pleasure in normally enjoyable activities, was expanded to include loss of pleasurable affect or pleasure associated with social and other activities. In addition, "Markedly diminished interest in... activities" was thought to correspond too closely to apathy, a separate neuropsychiatric symptom seen in dementia, and was removed from the

criteria. Finally, there were two additional criteria added: social isolation/withdrawal and irritability. The NIMH-dAD has been validated in a small cohort study[37] where it is seen to have higher sensitivity and specificity for depression than the DSM criteria.

While much research continues to use DSM criteria for depression in dementia, the NIMH-dAD criteria may be more clinically useful when differentiating depression from age-related physiologic and cognitive changes.

Rating Scales

There are several rating scales used to evaluate dementia in depression. Each has its benefits and drawbacks. The Cornell Scale for Depression in Dementia (CSDD) was designed specifically for assessing depression in patients who have cognitive impairments that may hamper answering questions about depressive symptoms. It comprises 19 caregiver and clinician-rated items, a strength as individuals with dementia may not be able to accurately describe their own mood or symptoms. The Geriatric Depression Scale (GDS) is commonly used in the clinical setting. There are 15-item and 30-item versions and the former generally takes 5 to 7 minutes to fill out. The GDS focuses on cognitive and affective aspects of depression, avoiding somatic and sexual symptoms that may return false positive in an older population. The Hamilton Depression Scale's (HDS) longer length and complexity renders it more useful for clinical studies than office use. It is interviewer-administered questionnaire better suited to monitor depressive symptoms and treatment efficacy, than to be used as a screening device (**Table 5-2**).[13]

Comorbidities

Any evaluation of mood in dementia requires careful assessment of contributing medical comorbidities, medications with sedating or cognitively dulling side effects, inadequately addressed pain, and metabolic disturbances. Relevant tests include chemistry profile, complete blood count (**Box 5-4**), liver function tests, thyroid panel, vitamin B12 and folate levels. Additional workup to be considered includes a urinalysis, chest x-ray, electrocardiogram, and neuroimaging. In cases where a patient has episodic changes in mood or alertness, an electroencephalogram may be useful.

■ DIFFERENTIAL DIAGNOSIS

The reversible dementia of depression (formally termed "pseudodementia") presents almost identically to a dementia caused by neurodegenerative processes. It is often diagnosed retrospectively, after successful treatment for mood symptoms results in resolution of cognitive deficits as well. Neuropsychological testing is considered the gold standard in distinguishing between the entities,[38] although "poor effort" on testing in the severely depressed may limit its usefulness. Apathy is a common finding in AD, and can present early in the course of the disease. Apathetic patients may appear disinterested in activities they used to enjoy, resist participation in social or family events, and remain inactive for extended periods of time. While apathetic patients have many of the same motivational deficits seen in depression, the syndromes are dissociable.[39,40] There are several scales designed to assess for apathy; these include, but are not limited to, the Starkstein Apathy Scale, the Lille Apathy Rating Scale and the Apathy Evaluation Scale. Another important differential diagnosis of dAD is pathological affective display.[41] Individuals may present with sudden episodes of laughing or crying. The emotional reaction may be completely unrelated to the individual's state of mind or the current situation. At other times, it may be congruent with the individual's mood but out of proportion to the situation. It is important to note that while the crying may be a pathological display of affect, studies have found significantly higher

TABLE 5-1 Criteria for NIMH Depression of AD as Compared to MDD Criteria

MDD	Depression of AD
≥ 5 of the following symptoms, **present most of the day, nearly every day** during a 2-week period and representing change from baseline functioning	≥3 of the following symptoms, **present during a 2-week period** and representing change from baseline functioning
1. Depressed mood most of the day, as either indicated by subjective report or observation of others 2. **Markedly diminished interest or pleasure in all, or almost all, activities** (either 1 or 2 are required) 3. Significant weight loss when not dieting or weight gain, or decrease or increase in appetite 4. Insomnia or hypersomnia 5. Psychomotor agitation or retardation 6. Fatigue or loss of energy 7. Feelings of worthlessness or excessive or inappropriate guilt 8. Diminished ability to think or concentrate 9. Recurrent thoughts of death, recurrent suicidal ideation without a specific plan, or a suicide attempt or a specific plan for committing suicide	1. Clinically significant depressed mood (e.g., depressed, sad, hopeless, discouraged, tearful) 2. **Decreased positive affect** or pleasure in response to social contacts and usual activities (either 1 or 2 are required) 3. Disruption in appetite 4. Disruption in sleep 5. Psychomotor changes (e.g., agitation or retardation) 6. Fatigue or loss of energy 7. Feelings of worthlessness, hopelessness, or excessive or inappropriate guilt 8. Diminished ability to think or concentrate 9. Recurrent thoughts of death, suicidal ideation, plan, or attempt 10. **Social isolation or withdrawal** 11. **Irritability**
Does not meet criteria for a Mixed Episode. The symptoms are **not better accounted for by bereavement.**	All criteria are met for **dementia of the Alzheimer type (DSM-IV-TR).** Symptoms are **not better accounted for by other conditions, such as major depressive disorder, bipolar disorder, bereavement, schizophrenia, schizoaffective disorder, psychosis of Alzheimer disease, anxiety disorders, or substance-related disorder.**
The symptoms cause clinically significant distress **or impairment in social, occupational, or other important areas of functioning.**	The symptoms cause **clinically significant distress or disruption in functioning.**

levels of depression and anxiety in patients with pathological affect than in those without it.[42] Thus, any individuals in whom pathological display of affect is suspected should be carefully screened for concomitant depressive symptoms (**Box 5-5**).

■ TREATMENT

There are compelling reasons to treat depression in patients with dementia as soon as possible. It has been demonstrated that depression is associated with earlier placement into a nursing home and a greater likelihood of being discharged earlier from an assisted living facility to a nursing home.[43,44] It is also associated with greater rates of physical aggression toward caregivers.[45] Finally, the caregivers for people with dementia and depression are at higher risk for depression themselves.[46] Promptly identifying and treating depressive symptoms results in better outcomes for both dementia patients and their caregivers.[47,48] Treatment may involve biological

and psychosocial interventions. **Box 5-6** summarizes treatment alternatives for depression in neurological illnesses.

■ PSYCHOPHARMACOLOGICAL TREATMENT
Antidepressants

Healthcare providers selecting a pharmacological intervention must take several factors into account, including medication's mechanism of action, side effect profile, interactions, cost and dosing schedule. Serotonin reuptake inhibitors (SSRIs) are generally well tolerated, but may induce agitation, worsening apathy, tremor or sleep disturbances. In addition, it is particularly important to monitor interactions due to the heightened risk for serotonin syndrome, and EKG due to risk for QTc prolongation. SNRIs are an alternative with the potential added benefit of their noradrenergic action, although there are no controlled studies for its use in this population. Tricyclic antidepressants (TCA) carry cardiac risks, including conduction

TABLE 5-2 Depression Rating Scales

	Cornell Scale for Depression in Dementia	Geriatric Depression Scale	Hamilton Depression Scale
Description	19 caregiver and clinician rated items	15-item version and 30-item version	21 item (although score based on first 17 items only), clinician administered scale
Strengths	Designed for patients whose cognitive impairments interfere with answering questions about mood	Less emphasis on sexual and somatic symptoms that may lead to false positives in geriatric population 15-item version is short; can be completed easily during clinical appointments	Can be used to track symptom severity over time and monitor treatment efficacy
Drawbacks			Clinician needs to administer test Length can make it unwieldy to administer in clinical visits

problems and potential heart block. They can also have anticholinergic side effects that interfere with cognition, worsen confusion or cause delirium. Other side effects include orthostatic hypotension, dizziness, dry mouth, constipation, sedation, and urinary retention.[41] TCAs should be avoided in patients with closed angle glaucoma. If a TCA must be used, nortriptyline and desipramine have the least severe anticholinergic side effects and one can follow plasma levels to avoid toxicity. Monamine oxidase inhibitors (MAOI) have the benefit of little anticholinergic side effects. They are generally quite well tolerated, but require adherence to a restrictive diet, as ingesting tyramine-rich foods while on an MAOI can cause a hypertensive crisis. One way to circumvent this risk is by using the selegiline patch at its lowest dose of 6 mg/24 hours.[13]

Research studies have not provided clear direction about which medications confer greatest benefit to depressed individuals with dementia. A 2007 meta-analysis reviewed dAD treatment with TCAs and selective SSRIs. Overall, antidepressant treatment was superior to placebo.[48] However, a recent large community-based, multicenter, randomized/placebo-controlled controlled trial in patients with mild to moderate depression in AD showed no difference in patients treated with sertraline or mirtazapine as compared to placebo.[49] The Work Group on AD and other dementias (convened by the American Psychiatric Association) suggests SSRIs as the first-line treatment. This is mainly due to SSRIs being better tolerated than other antidepressant classes. There is no clear consensus on which SSRI works best in the dAD population, but paroxetine should be avoided for its relatively greater anticholinergic effects. If patients with dementia develop intolerable side effects or fail to achieve remission, one can consider substituting bupropion, an SNRI such as venlafaxine, or mirtazapine.[50]

Antipsychotics

The use of antipsychotics in persons with dementia remains controversial. They do not have an indication for depression per se, but may be helpful in addressing comorbid agitation, aggression or psychotic symptoms. Conventional antipsychotics are generally avoided as older patients and those with neurodegenerative disorders may be especially vulnerable to side effects, such as tardive dyskinesias, parkinsonism, and increased risk of falling.[51] Second-generation, or atypical, antipsychotics are better tolerated but several well-documented studies have shown that they may carry an increased risk of adverse cerebrovascular events and a higher rate of all-cause death in individuals with dementia.[52] However, as most seasoned geriatric psychiatrists and behavioral neurologists can attest, these concerns must be balanced with the need to manage the neuropsychiatric symptoms of dementia that may be dangerous to the patient or their caregivers. In 2008, the American

College of Neuropsychopharmacology (ACNP) published a white paper reviewing available evidence on antipsychotic drug use in the elderly with dementia.[53] They provided several clinical recommendations, which included: ruling out medical etiologies of BPSD (e.g., delirium or pain), utilizing nonpharmacologic interventions, and involving caregivers and family members in informed decision making about when to use antipsychotics and the potential risks. If antipsychotic use is unavoidable, the authors recommended identifying target symptoms, monitoring for efficacy and side effects frequently, and discontinuing the medication if target symptoms did not decrease or resolve.

In regard to medication choice, the authors felt that there was not enough evidence to suggest one atypical over another. Whatever agent was used, they advocated for the lowest required doses for the shortest time possible.

Other Psychopharmacotherapy

Studies that looked at the efficacy of cholinesterase inhibitors for neuropsychiatric symptoms in dementia have demonstrated improvement in various mood symptoms (e.g., anxiety, apathy) but not depression.[54–56] Similarly, randomized control trials of anticonvulsant mood stabilizers have provided mixed results at best.[57] Stimulants have also failed to show conclusive effects on depression of dementia: while one study found improvement in depression scores in a small group of AD patients treated with methylphenidate,[58] another suggests that this may be due to a reduction in negative symptoms rather than true remission of depressive symptoms.[59]

■ BRAIN STIMULATION THERAPIES

ECT can be considered to address depressive symptoms in dementia.[60] In the elderly without dementia, it can be quite useful in treating depression with psychotic features. However, dementia patients are at heightened risk for adverse cognitive effects of ECT, especially those at later stages of a neurodegenerative process or with a heavy cerebrovascular burden. Often times, dementia patients have medical comorbidities rendering them vulnerable to anesthetic agents. Thus, ECT should be reserved for medication refractory cases, and the patient and/or family must be intensively counseled on the risks and benefits of ECT before providing consent.

There are a limited number of studies looking at other brain stimulation therapies' effects on depression in dementia. There is no consensus as to whether deep brain stimulation (DBS) has any effect on neuropsychiatric symptoms of AD, although its effects in PD are discussed later in this chapter. Vagus nerve stimulation (VNS) appears to be well tolerated in the Alzheimer population but has yet to demonstrate robust effects on mood symptoms.[61,62] Transcranial magnetic stimulation (TMS) may have a mild antidepressant effect in depressed patients with AD[63,64] and dementia with Lewy bodies.[65]

■ PSYCHOSOCIAL TREATMENT

The psychosocial treatment of depression in dementia is discussed in a separate section below.

■ SUMMARY

In summary, first-line pharmacologic treatment of depression in dementia should be an antidepressant. Among the various classes, SSRIs offer the best risk/benefit ratio, given their relatively benign side effect profile and lack of diet restrictions. SNRIs can be a useful alternative. If depressive symptoms are refractory, one can consider TCAs or MAOIs with careful patient and caregiver education. ECT remains an option for severe depression when medication truly cannot be tolerated or is ineffective. While newer brain stimulation therapies such as VNS and TMS appear to be well tolerated, they have yet to build a robust body of evidence to support their use in treatment depression in dementia.

■ PSYCHOSOCIAL TREATMENT OF DEPRESSION IN DEMENTIA AND OTHER NEUROLOGICAL DISEASES

While the main focus of this section is psychosocial treatment of depression in Dementia, many of the general principles discussed here can be applied to depression in other neurological conditions; this includes depression in the context of other neurodegenerative illnesses such as PD, and depression related to brain vascular illness. Often it is family members and not the patient him- or herself who request help with dementia diagnosis and treatment. It is important to help families understand that anosognosia represents impairment in the cognitive processes that support insight; in other words, "denial" is not purely a psychological defense.[66] While there is variability in the response to dementia diagnosis, an overarching theme is the tension between preserving key aspects of identity and accommodating change; for people with dementia and their caregivers, dynamics of autonomy and independence are salient with conflicts often emerging around safety.[67]

Consensus has emerged in favor of "telling the truth in dementia" and current guidelines warn against providers' fear of inflicting harm and caregiver-expressed concerns about impact of diagnosis on patients; instead, the recommendation is for an early dialogue with the patient to elicit his or her preferences for information on diagnosis and prognosis and involvement in treatment decision-making.[68] As preferences may change over time it is important to continue this conversation longitudinally, timing and tailoring the referrals according to the clinical needs and the range of resources available.

The majority of people with dementia live in the community with family caregivers who themselves are at risk for psychiatric morbidity (see **Box 5-7**).[69] Rates of depression in dementia caregivers

range from 23% to 85% in developed countries.[69] The burden of care is highest in the presence of BPSD and neuropsychiatric symptoms, rather than cognitive impairment and needs for direct physical care, are more likely to prompt institutionalization (see Text **box 5-7**).[70–72]

While there is evidence that support and counseling for caregivers reduces depression[73] the most effective interventions add cognitive restructuring techniques[74] and individually tailored behavioral management training.[71,75]

Given risk of MCI advancing to dementia, MCI caregivers are ideal targets for skill- and resource-building interventions.[76] Spouse caregivers of people with early-onset Alzheimer's and frontotemporal degeneration are hard-hit as they are often raising young children and suffer financial losses during wage-earning years[70]; they are in need of more specialized information and support which may best be delivered by telephone and internet in remote areas where more specialized services are not available.[77] Technology-based formats may also better reach caregivers in cultural minorities who have lower rates of resource use.[78]

The loss of language, memory, and insight inherent to dementia may be obstacles to the use of traditional psychotherapy. The number of randomized controlled trials of psychotherapy for depression in MCI and dementia is limited and the sample size in existing studies is small; however, research shows that psychotherapy can be adapted and is acceptable to people with MCI and early dementia.[79–82] There is some evidence that long-term interpersonal psychotherapy protects against depression recurrent in older people with mild to moderate cognitive impairment.[80] Even when adapted to include caregiver, short-term psychodynamic psychotherapy does not seem to produce measurable benefit.[83] More research is needed to determine which specific cognitive abilities predict or preclude psychotherapy.

Problem-solving therapy (PST), an approach of inculcating skills to cope with everyday problems, has been adapted to the treatment of depression in elderly people with dementia and executive dysfunction, and is more effective that more emotionally oriented supportive psychotherapy in treating depression and reducing disability.[84,85] It is important to note, however, that supportive therapy is a highly flexible approach that includes aspects of problem solving.[86] Problem-solving and behavioral therapy have been adapted for intervention with caregivers of people with dementia. The caregiver is trained to initiate pleasant events, distract from negative thoughts, and alter the environment/routine. In two randomized controlled trials, problem-focused therapy with the patient and caregiver in the home was more effective than supportive therapy in reducing symptoms of depression in the person with dementia.[87,88]

The Alzheimer's association offers community-based support and education programs for patients and caregivers, especially in the vulnerable period after initial diagnosis.[89] Participants meet with other newly diagnosed individuals in their community to share experiences and concerns, learn more about the disease, reduce feelings of isolation, and receive assistance in coping with lifestyle changes and developing long-term care plans. While some researchers caution that providing too much information too soon can increase depression for newcomers to groups,[90] a waitlist-controlled clinical trial of an Alzheimer's Association Early Stage Memory Loss Support Group found significant reduction in depression symptoms for those enrolled in the group.[91] A large-scale randomized controlled Danish trial of 12-month structured psychosocial intervention of counseling, education, and support to people with Alzheimer's and their caregivers found only a small positive effect on mood which was not sustained 24 months after the intervention ended.[92,93] A similar Norwegian study found no effect.[94] The lack of findings may be attributed to a floor effect as patients had minimal depression symptoms at the outset.[92,93] These studies suggest that it is important to assess need and adjust level

---

BOX 5-7
RISK FACTORS FOR CAREGIVER STRAIN AND PSYCHOLOGICAL MORBIDITY

Neuropsychiatric symptoms of patient
Lack of financial resources
Poor relationship quality and low levels of past/current intimacy
Caregiver perception of "role captivity"
Emotion-based or confrontational coping/communication style

of intervention accordingly; doing so requires regular follow-up and the ability of providers to "prescribe interventions"[95]

Although mood is not the primary target of cognitive rehabilitation, training, and remediation, these interventions have secondary benefits likely mediated by increasing experiences of competence and decreasing experiences of frustration in everyday life.[96,97] Incorporating cognitive behavioral interventions and motivational interviewing techniques may improve engagement and outcomes.[98] A waitlist-controlled study combining activity planning, assertiveness training, relaxation techniques, stress management, motor exercise, use of memory aids, and motor exercise in group format for people with MCI showed improvement in mood.[99] A randomized control trial of a cognitive-motor intervention consisting of reality orientation, ADL training, and psychosocial support produced mood and cognitive benefits in a people with Alzheimer's compared with patients treated with psychosocial support alone.[100] Some of the highest-quality studies producing the most significant results combine different categories of intervention; this makes it difficult to determine the active ingredient but also suggests that a combination of interventions produces important synergies. Examples include a randomized controlled trial of 153 community dwelling people with AD which combined a home-based exercise program with caregiver training in behavioral management techniques and found significantly reduced rates of depression and delayed institutionalization.[101] Psychosocial interventions can also be used in the treatment of depression and apathy in more advanced dementia and long-term care settings; these include multisensory stimulation, a variety of activities (music, dance, exercise), therapeutic conversation/reminiscence, pet therapy, cognitive stimulation (as distinct from rehabilitation)/reality orientation, and models of care. Individualized interventions that take into account characteristics and interests of the person with dementia and provide opportunities for meaningful activity are most effective in reducing symptoms of depression and apathy.[102–107] Music may be most effective in more advanced dementia.[104,108]

■ SUMMARY

There are various challenges to interpreting the robust meta-analytic literature on psychosocial interventions.[72,75,79,81,109,110] Researchers use different terminology to label interventions, making it difficult to directly compare individual referenced studies. Inclusion criteria vary among the reviews, especially for control conditions, raising concern about the placebo effect of receiving stimulation and human contact regardless of the effectiveness of any specific method.[111] Conversely, a finding of lack of effectiveness for a specific intervention may represent an artifact of difficulty validating an intervention.[106]

Despite equivocation about the effectiveness of specific interventions and various over-arching approaches, comparison of the meta-analytic literature yields strong support for interventions that are individually tailored, use multiple treatment components, include the caregiver, and include follow-up.[72,75,111] There is particularly strong evidence for problem-solving approaches and modified cognitive behavioral therapy (CBT) intervening directly with a patient with MCI or early dementia or by training the family caregiver to deliver the interventions.[109,110] In line with the correlation between neuropsychiatric symptoms (see Text **box 5-8**) and caregiver stress, improving caregiver skills to manage behaviors also benefits caregiver mood.

CEREBROVASCULAR DISEASE

Cerebrovascular disease is a significant contributor to late-life depression. The terminology in this section follows current usage in distinguishing poststroke depression from "vascular depression," a term which in the past has been used to refer to depression related to both discrete infarcts and to the accumulation of subcortical

microvascular ischemic changes. Poststroke depression is diagnosed based on the temporal relationship between a clinically apparent stroke and the onset of depression. Vascular depression is an evolving concept that arose from the observation of the correlation of depression and subcortical microvascular disease, which has become more widely appreciated in the age of increasingly available MRI. Unlike idiopathic MDD, poststroke and vascular depression primarily have onset late in life. They have modifiable risk factors, which coincide with the risk factors for cerebrovascular disease itself. Anticipation, recognition, and treatment of depression associated with cerebrovascular disease can reduce its morbidity, and improve outcomes related to vascular disease itself (see Text **box 5-9** for a review of Anxiety and Cerebrovascular disease).[112]

BOX 5-8
ANXIETY IN DEMENTIA

- In patients with dementia and anxiety, restlessness, or agitation, important differential diagnoses to consider include discomfort due to pain or other somatic symptoms the patient cannot communicate, delirium and psychosis.
- Patients with dementia may develop paradoxical anxiety as a reaction to benzodiazepines, antihistaminergic medications, and agents with anticholinergic properties. Rule out akathisia in patients on antipsychotics.
- Anxiety is a common response to cognitive deficits. For instance, patients may feel anxious when they cannot communicate due to aphasia, or when they experience loss of control of their basic daily activities due to executive dysfunction or amnesia.
- Anxiety can exacerbate cognitive deficits as it may negatively affect attention, executive function, encoding and retrieval of information.
- Behavioral interventions such as reassurance, use of cognitive compensatory strategies such as calendars and notebooks, and clear and firm communications from trusted caregivers can be of help. Caregivers may benefit from psychoeducation and modeling by healthcare providers to effectively intervene in these situations. CBT interventions including relaxation training can be effective, preferably modified to allow for caregiver participation in treatment.
- Medications that can help anxiety include SSRIs, SNRIs, buspirone, mirtazapine.
- Avoid benzodiazepines and medications with high anticholinergic activity as they may worsen cognitive deficits.

BOX 5-9
ANXIETY AND CEREBROVASCULAR DISEASE

- Anxiety after stroke occurs frequently, both independently and comorbid with depression.
- Symptoms may include excessive worries and fears, somatic symptoms such as palpitations, muscle tension, restlessness, and insomnia.
- Anxiety can worsen poststroke cognitive deficits and rehabilitation outcomes.
- Pharmacological treatment options include SSRIs, SNRIs, buspirone, mirtazapine. Nortriptyline can also be of help, although it is not considered a first line of treatment due to its potential anticholinergic and other side effects.
- Avoid benzodiazepines and medications with high anticholinergic activity as they may worsen cognitive deficits.

POSTSTROKE DEPRESSION

■ EPIDEMIOLOGY

Stroke is the fourth leading cause of death in the United States, and it is estimated that 6.8 million Americans over the age of 20 have suffered a stroke, with an annual incidence of approximately 795,000[113] Among the approximately 75% who survive a stroke, one-third will experience poststroke depression, with the greatest risk in the first year after the stroke.[114] See Figure 5-1 for a comparison of the prevalence of depression in different neurological illnesses and Box 5-1 for risk factors for depression in neurological disease. The factors that increase the risk of depression after stroke include: personal or family history of depression, degree of subcortical atrophy prior to the stroke, and degree of physical or cognitive impairment after the stroke. Confounding the last factor, however, is the observation that the presence of poststroke depression worsens outcomes and increases the degree of residual disability after stroke.[115]

■ PATHOPHYSIOLOGY

Several factors may mediate the development of depression in neurological illnesses (Box 5-2). The experience of stroke as a sudden loss of physical, verbal, or cognitive function, and the immediate onset of significant disability is a traumatic experience, and poststroke depression shares some of its origins in the reactive nature of depression that emerges in the wake of any significant medical diagnosis or illness. The fact that stroke is itself a brain injury, however, suggests that depression may arise from the infarction itself. This hypothesis has been borne out in the observation that the risk of poststroke depression is related to the location of the lesion. The ability of lesion location to predict poststroke depression remains debatable, but evidence suggests that infarcts in the left frontal lobe and basal ganglia are more likely to precipitate depression. Poststroke depression may correlate with the proximity of the infarct to the anterior pole of the left frontal lobe[116] though this is not consistently observed, and may be more significant in the early phases of stroke recovery (2–6 months after the event).[117]

A depletion of monoamine neurotransmitters may also be involved in the development of poststroke depression. Multiple rodent models of stroke have shown ipsilateral depletion of serotonin, norepinephrine, and dopamine after stroke, and reduction of monoamine metabolites has been demonstrated in the CSF of human patients with poststroke depression. PET imaging of 5-HT2 receptors shows evidence of greater upregulation of serotonin receptors in the right hemisphere compared to the left in patients with poststroke depression. This difference in receptor expression after stroke may represent hemispheric differences in response to injury, and correlate with the lateralization of depression risk after stroke, as well as support the hypothesis of monoamine depletion leading to poststroke depression.[118]

■ CLINICAL PRESENTATION

Symptoms of poststroke depression do not significantly differ from those of idiopathic major depressive disorder. Because of overlapping symptoms of stroke and depression (e.g., changes in energy, sleep, appetite, libido, and cognition), several studies have examined the validity of DSM criteria for major depression in the setting of stroke. Adjusting diagnostic criteria, however, to account for the origin of neurovegetative symptoms (i.e., attempts to exclude symptoms judged to be direct sequelae of the stroke) does not improve the sensitivity or specificity of DSM criteria for major depressive disorder in the setting of stroke.[119]

DSM criteria for MDD are sensitive and specific for poststroke depression as well. The symptoms of poststroke depression do not differentiate it from other forms of late-life depression. The particular presentation of individual cases likely depends on the lesion location and the extent of disability, combined with the individual's reaction to the stroke due to the new and potentially traumatic onset of functional impairment.

■ COURSE AND NATURAL HISTORY

The course of poststroke depression has been examined in several longitudinal studies, but the conclusions have been inconsistent and the degree of treatment in most case series has not been clearly delineated. There is some consensus, however, that depressive symptoms that emerge rapidly, within hours to days of stroke, tend to peak within 3 to 6 months of onset and approximately 50% experience remission by 1 year. Patients who experience onset of depression 2 months after stroke or later, however, typically have a more protracted course, and up to 50% remain depressed 2 years after their stroke. One confounding factor is the degree of physical disability, which correlates with risk of depression; patients with greater disability tend to be overrepresented in the hospital and rehab settings where patients have been recruited for many of these studies.[120]

■ ASSESSMENT AND DIFFERENTIAL DIAGNOSIS

Lack of awareness of the high prevalence of poststroke depression, misattribution of depressive symptoms to physical consequences of the stroke, and perception that the patient's distress may be an "appropriate" reaction to stroke all likely lead to the underdiagnosis of poststroke depression. Recognition of this entity, however, is important, because appropriate treatment of depression can alleviate the suffering of the depressed patient as well as improve rehabilitation outcomes. As discussed, DSM criteria for MDD are sensitive and specific for poststroke depression. The defining characteristic of this entity is onset after a clinically apparent stroke. Other symptoms can emerge after stroke, however, that can complicate or confound the diagnosis of depression. The most common poststroke symptom that mimics depression is apathy. By definition, apathy is a reduction of motivation not attributable to emotional distress, cognitive impairment, or level of consciousness.[121] Apathy is also a common feature of depression, and is included on the Hamilton Rating Scale for Depression. However, several studies and reviews demonstrate that apathy and depression are not always correlated and can be differentiated.[122] A case series[123] compared apathy and depression levels across stroke, AD, and idiopathic major depression. While the relationship between apathy and depression varied among the groups, patients with major depression or left-hemisphere stroke tended to higher depression scores and lower apathy scores. Patients with right hemisphere stroke had high levels of both apathy and depression, although these symptoms did not correlate with each other in this group. A longitudinal study of patients with poststroke depression found that within 3 months of a stroke, levels of apathy and depression did not correlate, but that a correlation emerged over time and was significant at 1 year. Both apathy and depression were predicted by the presence of dementia, but depression was independently predicted by psychosocial factors, such as not living with a family member. Although the correlation increased, there were a significant number of patients at 1 year who demonstrated apathy or depression, but not both.[124]

Although apathy likely shares with depression an origin in the disruption of frontal subcortical networks, distinguishing the two phenomena has treatment implications: failure to distinguish them can lead to treatment failure. Primarily studied in dementia, apathy has not been found to be responsive to antidepressants,[125] whereas poststroke depression has (discussed below). When apathy occurs after stroke, careful assessment for other symptoms of depression is required to differentiate the two syndromes. If apathy coexists with depression, the treatment of both syndromes may be indicated.

■ TREATMENT

Treatment of poststroke depression is important, as degree of depressive symptoms negatively correlates with rehabilitation potential[112] and poststroke outcomes. See Box 5-6 for a summary of treatment of depression in neurological disorders.

■ PSYCHOPHARMACOLOGICAL TREATMENT

Numerous studies comparing antidepressants against alternate agents or placebo have demonstrated widely varying efficacy in antidepressant treatment for poststroke depression. The range of study types, enrollment criteria, and means of assessment make it difficult to draw firm conclusions, but several studies have demonstrated efficacy of antidepressant agents in this population. The most commonly studied agents are SSRI and TCAs. In general, antidepressants from either class outperform placebo, although placebo response is high, which is typical for antidepressant trials. Nortriptyline has been shown to significantly outperform both fluoxetine and placebo.[120] Use of tricyclic agents, while possibly more effective than SSRIs or SNRIs, is limited by their adverse effects. Patients with poststroke depression tend to be elderly and are more likely to have vascular disease. Anticholinergic effects and risk of cardiac arrhythmias may lead most clinicians to reject these agents in favor of SSRI antidepressants.

Several case series and chart reviews have demonstrated the safety and tolerability of psychostimulants in poststroke depression, but have not demonstrated efficacy. Nonetheless, the potential of stimulants to increase energy and physical activity level has led to their empiric use, particularly in the rehab environment.

■ BRAIN STIMULATION THERAPIES

Two retrospective chart reviews have demonstrated the safety and efficacy of ECT for poststroke depression, with some patients receiving treatment within 1 month of stroke.[126] Repetitive transcranial magnetic stimulation (rTMS) has growing evidence for use in recovery of motor and cognitive stroke symptoms, but no published evidence to date addresses its use for poststroke depression.

■ PSYCHOSOCIAL TREATMENT

Several of the principles discussed above, regarding the psychosocial treatment of depression in dementia, also apply to poststroke depression. Poststroke patients also struggle with issues of loss of function and many times loss of independence. They may depend from caregivers and the inclusion of caregivers in treatment may increase effectiveness of the interventions. On the other hand, in the context of a static brain lesion, the potential for rehabilitation changes the prognosis and the dynamics of the relationship with caregivers. Different approaches including cognitive behavioral therapy, mindfulness-based interventions, and acceptance and commitment therapy have been used. Unfortunately the evidence of benefit of psychotherapy in this population has been limited.[127]

■ SUMMARY

In addition to significant physical disability stroke can also lead to depression, which can be an independent cause of disability and also exacerbate the residual physical symptoms of a stroke. Particularly in frontal lobe strokes, the lesion itself may injure regions of the brain involved in emotional regulation, leading directly to depression. Poststroke depression has been associated more with infarcts of the left frontal lobe than with other brain regions, but depression can emerge after an infarct in any location. The sudden onset of significant disability and loss of independence after a stroke can trigger a depressive episode. Patients with personal and family histories of depression are at higher risk. Recognition and treatment of depression in the wake of a stroke, particularly in the acute phase, can improve rehabilitation participation and outcomes. Although TCAs have more evidence for efficacy in poststroke depression their side effects may limit their use, particularly in elderly patients. SSRIs have demonstrated efficacy as well, and ECT has been used successfully used in severe and refractory depression.

VASCULAR DEPRESSION

Although cases of depressed elderly patients with atherosclerosis were described prior, "vascular depression" was first hypothesized as a distinct syndrome when Alexopoulos et al. described an association of late-life depression with impaired executive function and white matter hyperintensities on T2-weighted MRI.[128] This suggested areas for further investigation including involvement of frontal subcortical circuits in idiopathic depression, and also evolved into a recognizable subtype of depression. However, there is not yet a consensus for criteria defining vascular depression, which complicates attempts to investigate the syndrome. Some investigators prefer the term "subcortical ischemic depression," and others refer to "depression executive dysfunction," which describes the syndrome symptomatically allowing for other causes. Despite terminology differences, most investigators agree that the triad of depression onset after sixth decade, white matter hyperintensities found on MRI, and executive dysfunction comprises the core features of vascular depression.

■ EPIDEMIOLOGY

Estimating the prevalence of vascular depression is complicated by the general under-recognition of late-life depression and the requirement of imaging and cognitive assessment for diagnosis. In a large cross-sectional study vascular depression prevalence is estimated at 3.4% of Americans aged 50 and older, approximately 2.64 million people.[129] However, the criteria in this study do not include imaging findings or measures of cognitive impairment, and include poststroke depression. Other salient findings include evidence of late-life depression under-treatment and increased morbidity of cerebrovascular disease-associated depression in which only 40% of the depressed respondents reported current treatment, and only 10% reported treatment considered adequate to guidelines. Respondents with cerebrovascular disease or risk factors reported significantly higher functional limitations across several domains, including cognitive, mobility, social, and overall role impairments.

■ PATHOPHYSIOLOGY

See Boxes 5-1 and 5-2 for a summary of factors relevant to the development of vascular depression. Studies on the mechanism of vascular depression have centered on the white matter hyperintensities which represent microvascular disease. The amount of white matter hyperintensities correlates with age, regardless of the presence of depression. There is a correlation between the white matter disease burden in the frontal lobes and the incidence of depression. Periventricular hyperintensities appear equally prevalent in depressed and nondepressed subjects. Deep white matter hyperintensities, however, have consistently been found to be more prevalent in depressed subjects, and with late-onset depression in particular.[130] These deep white matter lesions are thought to be disruptive to frontal-subcortical and to a lesser extent temporal lobe function in vascular depression.

The correlation of executive dysfunction with white matter disease and depression suggests disruption of dorsolateral prefrontal striatal circuits. Postmortem tissue analysis demonstrates that subcortical ischemia preferentially affects the dorsolateral prefrontal cortex in patients with late-life depression[131] and that white matter hyperintensities in vascular depression are ischemic, rather than inflammatory.[132]

■ CLINICAL PRESENTATION

Vascular depression differs from other forms of depression in several ways, although there is significant overlap.[133] Anhedonia as a major symptom is more common in vascular depression than subjectively depressed or low mood (Box 5-3). Vascular depression shares characteristics with frontal lobe syndromes, particularly those arising from dysfunction of medial or dorsolateral prefrontal cortices. Executive dysfunction, commonly seen in dysfunction of the dorsolateral prefrontal cortex or its connections, is a defining characteristic of vascular depression. Family history of mood disorder is less common in vascular depression than in idiopathic depression.

■ COURSE AND NATURAL HISTORY

The clinical course of vascular depression is similar to that of refractory major depression in that it generally becomes a chronic condition and tends not to respond to antidepressant treatment. Progression of white matter disease is a risk factor for the onset of vascular depression[134] but it is not known whether progression of subcortical vascular disease in an individual patient correlates with worsened depression. Vascular depression is often comorbid with dementia, as microvascular disease causes subcortical vascular depression and also exacerbates dementia from other etiologies, such as AD.

■ ASSESSMENT AND DIFFERENTIAL DIAGNOSIS

The presence of executive dysfunction in vascular depression may lead to some confusion over whether a given patient's symptoms represent depression or dementia. The syndrome of "reversible dementia of depression," also known as "pseudodementia," has long been described, with deficits not only of memory but also of executive dysfunction (Box 5-5). Concern over this syndrome has been that clinicians often overlook depressive symptoms in the presence of cognitive impairment in elderly patients. Awareness of the entity of vascular depression, however, introduces a third consideration in addition to the possible diagnoses of idiopathic depression and dementia due to neurodegenerative process. Vascular depression comprises symptoms of both depression and executive dysfunction and shares features with depression and dementia of other etiologies. Diagnosis of vascular depression, however, implies the presence of microvascular disease, demonstrated by subcortical white matter hyperintensities on T2-weighted MRI. Brain imaging in this setting may help distinguish among idiopathic depression and vascular depression in elderly patients or patients with significant vascular risk factors.

The syndrome of apathy can also present a diagnostic challenge. Apathy and executive dysfunction may present as features of vascular depression, but also can signify the emergence of a neurodegenerative disorder or the sequelae of a stroke or other structural lesion. Differentiation of apathy from depression has been previously covered in the discussion of poststroke depression, and similar considerations apply with vascular depression.

■ TREATMENT
Psychopharmacological Treatment

Given its likely distinct psychopathology, it seems intuitive that the treatment profile of vascular depression would differ from idiopathic depression. Several studies have demonstrated variable response to SSRIs. Response to these medications seems to inversely correlate with the progression of white matter hyperintensities[134] and degree of neuropsychological impairment. In a nonrandomized trial 33% of patients achieved remission over 12 weeks with SSRI treatment. The likelihood of remission, assessed by MADRS score, diminished with increasing deficits in overall executive function, language processing, episodic memory, and processing speed.[135] A

placebo-controlled trial of sertraline in elderly patients with depression (but not specifically with vascular depression) found that sertraline performed worse than placebo in patients with impaired executive function, as measured by response inhibition.[136] This suggests that patients with executive dysfunction and depression, including vascular depression, may be subject to the side effects of antidepressants but not their benefits.

Brain Stimulation Therapies

A study comparing rTMS of the prefrontal cortex to sham rTMS found a response rate of 39% and a remission rate of 27%,[137] which are comparable to rates seen with antidepressants. Unlike antidepressants, however, response to treatment did not correlate with degree of cognitive impairment or executive dysfunction. There was a decreasing response to rTMS with increasing age and also with decreased volume of frontal gray matter. There is limited evidence regarding use of electroconvulsive therapy (ECT) in vascular depression, but one small series and several case reports suggest it is effective and generally well tolerated, although perhaps with increased risk of delirium compared to ECT in idiopathic depression.[138]

Psychosocial Treatment

Given its usual age of onset, psychotherapy with patients with vascular depression shares characteristics with psychotherapy with the ill, elderly patient; please refer to Chapter 17 for discussion of this topic. An important role of psychotherapy with this population is to support the work patients need to do in sustaining positive health behaviors, to help decrease their vascular risk factors. Several of the aspects of psychotherapy in the context of dementia, discussed above, apply to this population as well; importantly, the inclusion of caregivers in the plan of care may augment treatment results.

■ SUMMARY

Vascular depression is an increasingly recognized etiology of late-onset depression, often presenting with cognitive symptoms characteristic of subcortical dementia. The correlation of depression severity and cognitive dysfunction with the extent of subcortical microvascular disease seen on MRI suggests that disruption of subcortical networks is the common cause of both the depression and cognitive symptoms. Response to antidepressants appears to be poor in vascular depression. Attention, therefore, should turn to prevention. Although not proven, prevention of cerebral microvascular disease through blood pressure control, management of hyperlipidemia, and other vascular risk factors, may offer protection against vascular depression in addition to its known other cerebrovascular and cardiovascular benefits.

PARKINSON DISEASE

■ EPIDEMIOLOGY

PD is a neurodegenerative illness resulting from deterioration and loss of dopamine-producing neurons in the substantia nigra of the midbrain. This results in decreased dopaminergic input to the basal ganglia, producing the characteristic motor symptoms of rigidity, bradykinesia, tremor, and postural instability. It is the second most common neurodegenerative disease after AD. Estimated prevalence in developed countries is 0.3% of the population and 1% of those 60 and older. Prevalence increases with age up to about 4% in the oldest cohorts,[139] and nearly 1 million Americans have PD.

In addition to motor manifestations, psychiatric symptoms are common, with depression being the most frequent (Fig. 5-1). Estimates of depression rates in PD vary widely, but it is estimated that 17% of patients with PD meet DSM-5 criteria for MDD, with an additional 35% meeting criteria for dysthymic or subsyndromal depression.[140]

Rates of depression in patients who are ultimately diagnosed with PD are about double that of the general population.[141,142] Mood symptoms can precede clinical motor parkinsonism for up to 20 years, but the peak is 3 to 6 years prior to onset of motor symptoms and PD diagnosis.[143] It should be noted that most reports of depression onset rely in part upon patients' recall and thus are subject to some degree of reporting bias. However, an association between depression and PD is upheld by a retrospective cohort study of patients with depression that[144] found a hazard ratio for developing PD of 3.13 among patients diagnosed with depression using International Classification of Primary Care (ICPC) criteria.

■ PATHOPHYSIOLOGY

It is likely that some cases of depression associated with PD are reactions to the diagnosis and long-term prognosis of progressive disability (see Box 5-2). However, prevalence of depression in PD is as much as twice that seen in other conditions that produce equivalent disability[145] suggesting that the pathophysiology underlying PD contributes to the development of depressive symptoms.

There is a correlation between depressive symptoms and certain motor symptoms, which supports the idea of a common pathophysiologic pathway. For example, there is a higher prevalence of depression in patients with predominantly akinetic-rigid motor symptoms versus tremor-rigid-bradykinetic symptoms.[146]

The primary pathophysiological process in PD is regression and loss of dopamine-producing neurons in the substantia nigra. The downstream effects of this include motor symptoms due to loss of dopaminergic input to the basal ganglia. The basal ganglia, in particular the ventral striatum, also have significant function in emotional processing, as part of the prefrontal-striatal-thalamic circuits. PET imaging of dopamine and norepinephrine transport receptors in patients with PD and depression[147] shows that depression symptom severity, measured by Beck Depression Inventory (BDI), correlates with decreased dopamine and norepinephrine receptor binding in the ventral striatum. Patients with PD and depression have reduced binding in the locus coeruleus, mediodorsal and inferior thalamus, left ventral striatum, and right amygdala when compared to patients with PD and without depression. The latter group shows less binding in these areas compared to healthy controls. This suggests that depression in PD may be a consequence of a subset of the pathological processes of PD itself. It is not clear whether this is related to an underlying predisposition or vulnerability, or from idiosyncratic disease progression.

Structural and functional imaging studies further highlight the involvement of the mediodorsal, or "limbic" thalamus. In an fMRI and voxel-based morphometry study comparing patients with PD with or without depression, there is increased volume in bilateral mediodorsal thalami and reduced activation in the left mediodorsal thalamus and in the left medial prefrontal cortex in the depressed patients.[148]

■ CLINICAL PRESENTATION

Depression may emerge before diagnosis or in the early or late stages after diagnosis of PD. Somatic symptoms of depression may be masked or confounded by parkinsonian motor symptoms, such as bradykinesia and hypomimia (Box 5-3). Many patients with PD who do not have depression experience early waking and decreased energy, and psychomotor retardation is nearly universal. Other symptoms, however, such as decreased appetite and libido, increased sleep latency and overnight waking, and nonsomatic depression symptoms such as low mood, anhedonia, feelings of guilt, and preoccupation with death are generally attributable to depression.[149] PD patients on levodopa may experience dysphoria and/or anxiety, combined with their motor fluctuations, as part of the "on/off" cycle: In most cases the effect of levodopa gradually wears off a few hours after each dose. During this "off" period the patient experiences exacerbation of the PD motor symptoms, and may also become more depressed and anxious. After the following levodopa dose, in the "on" period, the patient's mobility increases—possibly with added dyskinesia—and the mood improves.

■ COURSE AND NATURAL HISTORY

Evolution of depressive symptoms in PD tends to mirror the motor symptoms. A longitudinal study of nonmotor symptoms[150] shows that depressive symptoms decrease over the first 2 years after PD diagnosis as dopaminergic therapy is initiated and titrated. As neurodegeneration progresses, however, depressive symptoms return and become more refractory, as do the motor and autonomic symptoms.

Depression in PD can exacerbate the disability produced by motor symptoms, and itself can be considered a marker of disease severity. Depression is independently correlated with degree of disability in PD, and in a cross-sectional study[151] nonmotor symptoms (primarily depression and cognitive impairment) account for 37% to 54% of the total variance in disability among patients.

Patients recognize the morbidity associated with depression in PD. In a patient survey,[152] patients with early (<6 years) PD rate "mood" as the sixth most bothersome symptom. Patients with more advanced illness (>6 years) however, rate "mood" as the second most bothersome symptom, behind medication-related symptom fluctuations.

■ ASSESSMENT AND DIFFERENTIAL DIAGNOSIS

There are no specific criteria for diagnosis of depression in PD, and DSM criteria are generally used. Marsh[149] has suggested modifying DSM criteria somewhat to be more inclusive of the range of depressive symptoms found in PD. She recommends disregarding the "etiologic" criteria of DSM and considering symptoms based on observation rather than presumed etiology. Another recommendation is to carefully assess anhedonia to distinguish it from apathy, which may appear in patients with PD who are not depressed. Last, diagnosis of minor depression or dysthymia in PD is encouraged, as these "subsyndromal" depressive symptoms can cause significant distress and functional impairment in PD, without rising to the level of major depression.

Depression scales may be useful in PD to monitor the progression of symptoms or to screen for unreported or difficult-to-detect depression. The BDI[153] and the Hamilton and Montgomery–Asberg rating scales[154] are valid instruments for diagnosing and assessing severity of depression in PD, although the cutoffs for clinical significance tend to slightly overdiagnose depression because of the confounding effect of motor symptoms.

Because of its inherent morbidity and association with greater functional impairment, diagnosis of depression in PD is as important as it can be difficult. The overlap of motor symptoms with depression symptoms can easily lead to depression being overlooked. In one prospective study, diagnostic accuracy of the treating neurologist was 35%.[155] Routine screening of PD patients for depression and other nonmotor symptoms should be commonplace and is effectively done using self-report checklists, such as the BDI.

■ TREATMENT
Psychopharmacologic Treatment

Treatment of depression in PD has evolved in recent years (Box 5-6). Even in the absence of controlled trials, clinicians have used antidepressants to treat the observed symptoms of depression in patients with PD, with some anecdotally encouraging results. As most psychiatrists switched from TCAs to the better-tolerated SSRIs, most neurologists and neuropsychiatrists also switched to SSRIs for their patients with PD who were depressed. There have been limited controlled trials of antidepressants in this population and results have been inconsistent. A study in 2009 that compared nortriptyline with paroxetine for depression in PD shows significant advantage of nortriptyline,[156] although this study had several limitations including its brief duration, relatively small size, and a high dropout rate.[157]

There is some concern over the potential exacerbation of motor symptoms by SSRIs, however the evidence remains inconclusive.[158,159] A randomized, double-blind, placebo-controlled study demonstrates that both the SNRI venlafaxine and the SSRI paroxetine may improve depression in subjects with PD.[160] The use of another SNRI medication, duloxetine, has benefit in a small series.[161] The positive effects of SNRIs are not surprising, as the increase in both serotonergic and noradrenergic tone produced by these medications is similar to the actions of TCAs. Bupropion, an antidepressant which inhibits reuptake of norepinephrine and dopamine (NDRI), should theoretically be of benefit in PD, given its dopaminergic mechanism of action. It has been reported effective anecdotally and in a single published case report, and recommended for further study because of its low likelihood of worsening, and potential for ameliorating, motor symptoms.[162,163]

Treatment of PD itself, with dopaminergic medications, can also treat concomitant depression. MAO inhibitors, while they have fallen out of fashion as antidepressants, continue to be used to treat PD, typically providing benefits in reducing "on/off" motor fluctuations. Most commonly used are the selective MAO-B inhibitors selegiline and rasagiline. One trial comparing two doses of rasagiline in 22 patients with PD and depression shows significant improvement in motor symptoms, without significant differences between patients receiving 1 or 2 mg/d. All patients also showed improvement in depression symptoms, however, the patients receiving the higher dose show significantly greater improvement in depression as measured by the Hamilton Depression Rating Scale.[164] This suggests that the antidepressant benefits of rasagiline are independent of its motor benefits, and that this medication may be particularly useful in patients with PD who are depressed. Dopamine agonists such as pramipexole, commonly used to treat PD's motor symptoms, may also benefit PD depression. The evidence from controlled studies is still insufficient to recommend these agents as a first line of treatment.

Brain Stimulation Therapies

While there has not been a randomized controlled trial of ECT for depression in PD, there are numerous noncontrolled studies reporting efficacy and tolerability. ECT should certainly be considered as a treatment for medication-refractory or severe depression in patients with PD. rTMS has shown promising results in patients with PD and depression. In addition, beneficial effects on motor and cognitive symptoms have also been reported.[165]

DBS has emerged as an important treatment option for PD, particularly in patients with advanced disease or with side effects that limit the usefulness of dopaminergic medications. The most common sites for stimulator placement in PD are the subthalamic nucleus (STN) and the globus pallidus interna (GPi). The effects of DBS for PD are most clearly seen in the improvement of motor symptoms, but changes in mood have been observed as well. The evidence has been mixed, with some early reports of increased incidence of depression following DBS surgery and subsequent larger randomized trials showing little difference in mood outcomes of DBS versus medical management of PD.[166] Although some reports have suggested greater risk of depression following DBS placement in the STN as compared with GPi, a study designed to compare these sites using mood and cognitive measures as primary endpoints failed to find a significant difference.[167] Stimulation of STN often allows

for reduction of dopaminergic medication due to less prominent motor symptoms, but dose reduction of levodopa or dopamine agonists may exacerbate underlying depressive symptoms which these medications had been treating as well. Although premorbid well-controlled depression is not a contraindication to DBS, surgery can be associated with a relapse of depression, and all DBS patients should be monitored postsurgically for emergence or evolution of depressive symptoms.[168]

Psychosocial Treatment

Nonpharmacological treatments appear useful for depression in PD as well. A randomized controlled trial of CBT for depression in PD adapts CBT to the unique needs of patients with PD to include exercise, behavioral activation, thought monitoring and restructuring, relaxation training, worry control, and sleep hygiene. CBT for patients with PD was supplemented with individual caregiver sessions designed to equip caregivers with the skills necessary to facilitate practice of CBT at home.[169] In comparison with the control group, which received clinical monitoring alone, the treatment group shows significant improvement in measures of depression. Further, this study reveals that caregiver participation rather than patient factors (motor disability, psychiatric comorbidity, and executive function) predicts treatment response.[170]

There is some evidence for group therapy in the treatment of depression in PD. A small-scale randomized waitlist controlled trial of group therapy demonstrated a significant reduction in depression in group participants; the group therapy used psychodrama methods (e.g., role play; emotional expression) in 12 sessions, also providing education on Parkinson's and information on coping skills and adaptive resources.[171] Patient Education Program Parkinson (PEPP) which is a standardized program using CBT techniques administered to small groups of patients and caregivers also shows that mood improves significantly for the treatment group.[172]

A review of psychosocial treatments for depression and anxiety in PD points out that interventions that primarily target symptoms of PD have secondary mood benefits.[173] A study of multidisciplinary rehabilitation including individually administered physical, occupational, and speech therapies, group relaxation exercises, expert lectures, and caregiver groups showed significant improvement in mood, although the benefits were not sustained 6 months after termination.[174,175] This suggests the need for longer-term interventions or maintenance sessions to address the continuing needs of patients and the progressive nature of PD itself.

■ SUMMARY

PD is a neurodegenerative illness whose core pathology is loss of dopaminergic neurons in the nigrostriatal pathway. The reduction in dopaminergic tone in the ventral striatum is associated with emergence of depression in patients with PD. The diagnosis of, and the progressive symptoms and disability from, a neurodegenerative process also can be psychologically destabilizing and trigger depression symptoms or a major depressive episode. Depression, therefore, is prevalent among patients with PD and can lead to significant additional morbidity. Recognition of depression in PD can be challenging, due to the overlap of neurovegetative symptoms of depression and motor symptoms of PD. Because the effects of depression can exacerbate functional deterioration of patients with PD, routine screening of this population for depression is important. Multiple treatment modalities are beneficial, including TCAs, SSRIs, SNRIs, bupropion, and nonpharmacological treatments such as individual and group CBT for both patients and caregivers. Treatment of PD with levodopa and dopamine agonists will often ameliorate depression. In addition, MAO-B inhibitors, such as rasagiline, can be used to treat both depression and motor symptoms in patients with both PD and depression.

BOX 5-10
ANXIETY IN PARKINSON DISEASE

- Anxiety symptoms are common in Parkinson disease (PD), both independently and comorbid with depression.
- Patients may experience any of the classic anxiety symptoms typical of primary anxiety disorders.
- In addition, anxiety symptoms more typical of PD include fear of falling and "freezing," and anticipatory anxiety about the "wearing off" of the anti-parkinsonian drugs.
- Anxiety symptoms may fluctuate during the day, in correlation with fluctuations in the individual's dopaminergic state. PD patients on levodopa may experience anxiety, usually combined with dysphoria, when the effect of levodopa wears off. Mood and anxiety (as well as mobility) tend to improve with the subsequent levodopa dose.
- PD patients may also experience anxiety about social situations where their motor and cognitive symptoms become evident
- Pharmacological treatment options include SSRIs, SNRIs, and Nortriptyline. Judicious use of benzodiazepines in cases of severe anxiety resistant to monotherapy with these agents can be also considered, with attention to their potential side effects.
- Working in collaboration with the patient's neurologist, focusing on reducing the on–off fluctuations may address many of the anxiety symptoms. This can be accomplished through different strategies, including the addition of dopaminergic agonist or COMT inhibitors.
- CBT may be effective as well for management of anxiety in patients with PD.

ECT should be considered for severe or medication-refractory depression (see **box 5-10** for a review of Anxiety in Parkinson's Disease).

HUNTINGTON DISEASE

■ EPIDEMIOLOGY

Huntington disease (HD) is a genetic, autosomal dominant, progressive, neurodegenerative disease with motor and psychiatric features. Although the movement disorder associated with HD has been considered its core feature and the disease was previously known as Huntington chorea,[176] its psychiatric symptoms have been observed and reported since its initial description.[177] Psychiatric disturbances, including depression, anxiety, mania, and psychosis are now considered one of the triad of core symptoms of HD, along with movement disorder and cognitive decline. HD is progressive, with a uniformly poor prognosis. Mean survival after diagnosis ranges from 10 to 15 years, typically with an extended period of severe disability and loss of independent function.

The prevalence of HD varies by ethnicity and geographic location. It is estimated to occur in 5.7 per 100,000 in people of Northern European ancestry, and is less prevalent in populations with non-European roots.[177] Diagnosis is most often made after the emergence of motor symptoms, although genetic testing can identify the disease before any symptoms are apparent. The movement symptoms of HD typically have onset in the fourth or fifth decade, although earlier and even juvenile onset cases are seen. There is some evidence that psychiatric symptoms, particularly depression, and cognitive impairment can precede motor symptoms for years. Most attempts to quantify the length of prodromal mood symptoms are hampered by recall bias and a retrospective approach. A cross-sectional study comparing 55 HD gene carriers without motor symptoms, 85 gene carriers with motor symptoms, and 56 noncarrier first-degree relatives of HD carriers with the general population[178] shows that gene carriers, both symptomatic and presymptomatic, have a significantly increased prevalence of MDD. The evidence for depression in clinically evident HD is unequivocal (Fig. 5-1). MDD affects up to 40% of patients, increasing up to 60% when subsyndromal depression is included.[179]

■ PATHOPHYSIOLOGY

HD[180] results from a mutation on the short arm of chromosome 4, in a gene for the protein product huntingtin. This gene contains a series of CAG repeats of variable length, whereas the normal allele contains 10 to 35 repeats. Alleles carrying 40 or more repeats are considered positive for the mutation, whereas carriers with 36 to 39 repeats are considered "indeterminate" and may show some symptoms due to incomplete penetrance, or remain asymptomatic. As in other trinucleotide repeat disorders, an increased number of repeats does not clearly correlate with severity of symptoms but does correlate with earlier age of onset.

The role of the huntingtin protein in normal neuronal function is unclear, but the abnormal protein forms intranuclear and cytosolic inclusions. This leads to impaired neuronal function and cell death.[181] The striatum is preferentially affected and structural imaging shows caudate atrophy with increasing severity as the disease progresses. The damage to the striatum causes the movement symptoms of HD, and likely also contributes to the depressive symptoms. The caudate has connections with multiple frontal-subcortical circuits, important for emotional regulation. The medial caudate has rich limbic connections as well. Downstream effects from damage to the caudate affect function of orbitofrontal and prefrontal cortices, demonstrated by reduced glucose metabolism in these areas in depressed patients, including depressed patients with HD.[182] Evidence that the pathophysiology is itself a cause of depression, rather than a reactive or adjustment response to a neurodegenerative disorder, is demonstrated by the increased prevalence of depression in HD as compared with AD.[183]

■ CLINICAL PRESENTATION

Depression and other psychiatric symptoms often predate the emergence of motor symptoms, and the diagnosis of HD. In a prodromal analysis, 42% of presymptomatic carriers were taking psychiatric medication at the time of the study, compared to 5% of noncarrier relatives.[168] Despite the elevated index of suspicion for depression among clinicians treating patients with HD, depression may still be challenging to diagnose. Bradyphrenia, apathy, and constitutional symptoms such as sleep disturbance and weight loss are features of HD seen even in the absence of depression.

Other psychiatric symptoms can emerge in HD, sometimes in addition to depression. Anxiety is common, notably obsessive-compulsive disorder.[184] Psychosis, primarily paranoia or delusions and less commonly hallucinations, is seen at times, with up to 11% reporting at least one psychotic symptom during the course of illness.[185] Irritability is a common feature early in the course of HD, and this can progress along with motor and cognitive symptoms. Impaired impulse control and behavioral disinhibition can also occur.

■ COURSE AND NATURAL HISTORY

Left untreated, depression can become chronic in HD, particularly given the inevitable increase in physical and cognitive disability of this illness. The presence of depressive symptoms at baseline is a predictor of more rapid functional decline.[186] In one small study, severity of depression does not appear to advance in correlation with severity of motor symptoms, and does not correlate with number of CAG repeats.[187] Suicide attempts are a significant source of morbidity and mortality. An increase in the rate of death by suicide has been observed in HD patients for decades, and was noted in the original description of the illness. Analysis of records from one registry of patients with HD[188] reveals that suicide was the proximate cause of death in 5.7% of patients, roughly four times the rate in the general population. In addition, 27.6% of patients report or were recorded as attempting suicide at least once. Identified risk factors for suicide in this population are prior suicide attempt and family history of suicide. It has not been determined whether the presence or severity of comorbid depression confers additional risk. It is clear, however, that screening for suicidal ideation is required during the treatment of these patients and of patients at risk for HD. There has been much debate over the ethics and consequences of testing asymptomatic patients for the Huntington gene. Up to one-third of patients at risk for HD reported suicide as a concern when approached with the option for testing. Approximately 10% to 20% of patients at risk for HD opt to receive genetic testing.[189] Several studies have shown an increase in depressive symptoms experienced by patients receiving a positive test result (indicating they will develop HD) compared to those who receive a negative result. These differences, however, largely disappear when reassessed at 12 months.

■ ASSESSMENT AND DIFFERENTIAL DIAGNOSIS

As mentioned above, depression and HD have common symptoms. This presents a challenge both for the study of depression in HD and also for diagnosis and treatment. The BDI-II includes somatic symptoms that also can arise in patients with HD without depression such as loss of appetite, sleep disturbance, fatigue, and reduced libido. Because of this, it presents a lower specificity of 66% which renders it an appropriate screening tool, but not sufficiently accurate to distinguish the presence of depression in patients with HD. Two alternative self-report scales, the Hospital Anxiety and Depression Scale (HADS: sensitivity 100%, specificity 70%) and the Depression Intensity Scale Circles (DISCs: sensitivity 92%, specificity 82%) show adequate validity.[190] Items on the BDI-II and the Hamilton Rating Scale for Depression (HAM-D) that refer to emotional rather than somatic symptoms correlate better with depression. Specific items include "Feel sad," "discouraged about future," "disappointed in self" and "feel like a failure"[191] When using self-report depression inventories for patients with HD, the astute clinician will be able to make the diagnosis by reviewing the responses to individual items, rather than simply relying on the overall total score.

■ TREATMENT
Psychopharmacological Treatment

Though it is likely that pathophysiology of depression in HD differs from idiopathic major depression, specific treatments targeting depression in HD have not yet resulted. The list of treatments of depression in neurological illnesses shown in Box 5-6 may be useful in HD.

Several open label trials and case series and reports suggest the utility of antidepressant medications. One series of 26 patient reports significant improvement of depressive symptoms with venlafaxine.[192] Published cases report positive results with fluoxetine[193] and MAO inhibitors.[194] There are few effective treatments for the motor symptoms of HD. The only agent approved by the United States Food and Drug administration is tetrabenazine, a presynaptic dopamine deplete which may provoke depression as a side effects. Other antidopaminergic agents that have been used to reduce chorea in HD include typical and atypical antipsychotics. Among these agents, the dopamine partial agonist aripiprazole may be the most beneficial in patients with significant motor symptoms and comorbid depression.[195]

Brain Stimulation Therapies

Severe depression in HD has also been shown to respond to ECT,[196] although the cognitive impairment of advanced HD may predispose patients to post-ECT delirium. While no randomized controlled trials have been published, the existing case reports and series suggest that ECT in HD is as effective and well-tolerated as it is in idiopathic major depression.

rTMS has been used as an investigative tool to study cortical excitability in HD. There are a small number of case reports with mixed results using rTMS for motor symptoms in HD.[197] At present, there is no evidence for or against the use of rTMS for depression in HD.

Psychosocial Treatment

While not focused on treatment of depression, one published case series of group therapy reports improved level of function and decreased behavioral outbursts in chronically hospitalized HD patients with Remotivation therapy. This therapy was designed to "motivate and engage nonverbal, withdrawn, and apathetic patients" in a hospital setting.[198] It shows improvements in ADLs, level of interpersonal engagement, and participation in family and group activities.

■ SUMMARY

Depression is a highly prevalent psychiatric symptom in HD. Because HD manifests with somatic symptoms that resemble neurovegetative symptoms of depression, misattribution of symptoms can occur and render the diagnosis of depression challenging. The pathogenesis of HD itself, with progressive neuronal dysfunction and loss that preferentially affects the striatum, may also cause depression more directly by disruption of frontal-striatal networks involved in mood regulation. Depression is associated with more rapid functional decline in HD. There are no randomized controlled trials of medications for depression in HD. Multiple published cases and anecdotal reports suggest some benefit in traditional antidepressants, including SSRIs, SNRIs, and MAO inhibitors. Aripiprazole, an atypical antipsychotic and dopamine partial agonist, may have benefits for both motor and nonmotor symptoms of HD, including depression. ECT remains an option for severe or refractory depression (see Text **box 5-11** for a review of Anxiety in Huntington's Disease).

MULTIPLE SCLEROSIS

■ EPIDEMIOLOGY

Depression is a frequent component of the clinical presentation of Multiple Sclerosis (MS) (See Fig. 5-1). Unfortunately, it is often unrecognized and undertreated.[199,200] Its detection and treatment may bring substantial improvement to adherence to MS treatment, illness prognosis, and quality of life of patients with MS.[201] MS most commonly affects young adults, and is more common in women. The lifetime prevalence of MDD in MS patients is 23% to 54%.[202–205] In a community based sample, the 12-month period prevalence of MD in MS was 25.7% for those in the 18- to 45-year range.[206] This was significantly higher than the rate of MD in both

---

BOX 5-11
ANXIETY IN HUNTINGTON DISEASE

- Anxiety symptoms are common in Huntington disease and can be part of the prodromal phase of this illness.
- Patients may experience any of the anxiety symptoms typical of primary anxiety disorders.
- Fear of onset, preoccupation about illness progression, and fear of losing one's capabilities and independence are common.
- Patients may discuss their preoccupation about other relatives, especially their children, developing the illness. Genetic counseling including the patient's family members is important aspect of treatment.

patients with other chronic illnesses and the general population. The point prevalence of depressive symptoms (as opposed to MD) ranges from 31.4% to 79% of MS patients[207–210,] Early onset of MS[210] and severity of illness and resulting disability[209] are both associated with increased depression risk. Adjusted for severity of illness, course of illness (relapsing-remitting, primary progressive, secondary progressive) does not seem associated with differences in the severity of depression. The presence of cognitive difficulties, lower education level, younger age, and lack of social support are all significantly associated with depression.

Patients with MS present an increased rate of completed suicide compared with the age-matched general population and with other neurological illnesses.[211] A quarter of patients with MS may have lifetime suicidal intent.[212] Risk factors for suicide intent in patients with MS include:

- lifetime diagnoses of major depression or anxiety disorders
- prior suicidal ideation or intent
- comorbid depression and anxiety disorder
- alcohol abuse
- living alone
- social stress
- family history of mental illness

Males with MS are at higher risk of completed suicide than females. For males with MS, the factors associated with increased suicide risk include[213,214]:

- early illness onset and diagnosis
- less than 5 years since diagnosis
- recent worsening of disease
- significant level of disability
- access to violent means of suicide

■ PATHOPHYSIOLOGY

The pathophysiology of depression in MS is multifactorial (see Boxes 5-1 and 5-2). Premorbid factors, illness-related biological and clinical characteristics, the individual's response, and elements of the social environment all have a role and interact in the development and course of depression. The prevalence of major depression in individuals with MS is higher in those with a family history of major depression[208] although this factor has less relative weight than in primary MD.[215] Several studies evaluate the relationship between structural and functional brain changes in MS and depression. A study evaluating the potential negative effect of demyelination on mood found that the presence of lesions in the left arcuate fasciculus region is associated with depressive symptoms.[216] Superior frontal and superior parietal hypointense T1 lesions predict the presence of depression, while superior frontal, superior parietal and temporal T1 lesions, third and lateral ventricles enlargement, and frontal atrophy predict the severity of depression in one study.[217] Greater lesion volume in the left medial inferior prefrontal cortex, anterior temporal atrophy,[218] and hippocampal atrophy—which may be concurrent with higher cortisol levels[219,220]—may also be associated with depression in MS. In summary, studies highlight the importance of frontal and temporal lesion volume—especially hypointense lesions—and atrophy in the development of MS depression. The global burden of brain lesion volume and atrophy also seems important. A potential conclusion is that atrophy and cortical-subcortical disconnection due to frontal, temporal, and parietal white matter destructive lesions may contribute to depression in MS. Depression does not appear to be related to hyperintense lesions. Hyperintense areas may be nonspecific for the extent of tissue injury and neuronal pathways may function sufficiently in the presence of less severe insults, while persistent mood changes are more likely due to chronic destructive brain changes represented by the hypointense lesions. The use of diffusion tensor imaging

(DTI) highlights the importance of more subtle brain changes[221] as reduced fractional anisotropy and higher mean diffusivity in left anterior temporal normal—appearing white and gray matter—as well as higher mean diffusivity in right inferior frontal hyperintense lesions-correlate with depression. The contributions from functional neuroimaging techniques include an early PET study where increased perfusion in limbic areas significantly correlated with depression.[222] In a functional MRI study, nondepressed patients with MS show increased activity in the ventrolateral Pre Frontal Cortex (vl PFC) and lack of connectivity between the amygdala and PFC when processing emotional stimuli.[223] These findings may suggest that patients with MS are particularly vulnerable to developing a mood disorder and that they may have an ongoing compensatory mechanism at work to maintain euthymic mood.

Immunological and inflammatory factors and dysfunction of the HPA have a role in MS-related depression.[224] The increase in proinflammatory cytokines, activation of the HPA, and reduction in neurotrophic factors that occur in MS may each account for the increased rate of depression in this illness.[225] Evidence supporting the role of a HPA axis dysfunction in MS-related depression includes the finding that evening cortisol concentrations do not decline in MS patients with depression.[226] Raised cortisol levels may not be suppressed with exogenous steroids administration in these patients, finding which may correlate with enhanced brain lesions.[227] The corticosteroids used to treat MS may contribute to depressive symptoms; some of the immune-modulatory agents used in MS treatment may also have a role in the development of depression, such as interferon beta-1b and Natalizumab.[228–231] Of the first-line oral drugs used to treat MS, Teriflunomide, and Dimethyl fumarate do not appear to affect depression, while initial data suggests that Fingolimod may have potential benefits for depression.

From a psychosocial perspective, a stress and coping strategies model is useful in understanding the pathophysiology of depression in MS. Predictors of depression include stress, limited social support, loss of hope, uncertainty about prognosis, and use of emotion-focused coping strategies.[205,232,233] Cognitively impaired patients with MS are more likely to use high levels of avoidance as a coping strategy, which also renders them at increased risk for depression.[234] Decreased use of active coping strategies and increased avoidance may increase depression risk; increased use of active coping strategies may result in decreased depressed mood longitudinally.[235]

■ CLINICAL PRESENTATION

The phenomenology of major depression in patients with MS is similar to that described for this disorder in the general population. There is a significant overlap between several MS symptoms such as fatigue, sleep, and cognitive disturbances, and symptoms of depression (Box 5-3). As discussed in the assessment section, different strategies can assist in the diagnosis of depression in this context. Fatigue may be the most frequent symptom in MS with a prevalence of up to 80% of MS patients. It has a reciprocal relationship with physical disability and depression.[236] Factors involved in its pathogenesis may include neuroconduction delay, monoamine disturbances, lesion localization, and immunomodulatory and inflammatory factors. Amantadine, modafinil and related agents, stimulants, and exercise programs are used for its treatment. Fatigue can also be secondary to sleep disturbances and to anxiety and depression, in which case addressing the primary disorder is important. Sleep disorders as a group may present in about 50% of patients with MS. These may include insomnia, nocturnal movement disorders, sleep-disordered breathing, narcolepsy, and REM behavior disorder. Sleep disturbances may be secondary to other MS symptoms such as pain, spasticity, and nocturia; they may be side effects of medications or secondary to neuropsychiatric disorders, such as depression and anxiety. Their management warrants a thorough clinical assessment with possible addition of a polysomnogram, and treatment according to the etiology. (see also Chapter 22).[237] Cognitive deficits can occasionally be the initial presentation of MS.[238] They may contribute to the development of depression, and in turn depression may worsen cognition further.[239–242] Other commonly comorbid symptoms include apathy and anxiety, which may occur in about 30% and 20% of MS patients, respectively. Anxiety symptoms may present in the form of generalized anxiety disorder, panic, OCD, and social anxiety symptoms.

Patients with MS may present a wide range of mood and affect symptoms, many times in combination with depression. These manifestations may take the form of pathological or pseudobulbar affect, which is present in about 10% of patients with MS. Bipolar disorder, or related symptoms without the full bipolar syndrome, can be present. Anger, agitation, irritability, euphoria, and disinhibition may co-occur with depression at higher rates than in primary major depressive disorder, and without other associated bipolar symptoms.[204,207,208]

Some of these symptoms, including irritability, disinhibition, emotional lability, and apathy, may be sustained and become new personality traits secondary to the illness.

Patients with MS present an increased rate of suicide ideation and attempts; it is important to screen and monitor for suicidal risk in MS patients, including evaluation of the risk factors detailed above. Somatic pain is rated by as many as 32% of MS patients as one of their worst symptoms. Depression and pain may reciprocally potentiate each other and it is important to address both in the management of these patients.

■ COURSE AND NATURAL HISTORY

The heterogeneity of MS makes the course of this illness very variable. There are several patterns of progression: relapsing remitting, secondary progressive, primary progressive, and progressive relapsing. Illness exacerbations and progression contribute to the development of depression.[243,244] The Kurtzke Expanded Disability Status Scale (EDSS) quantifies MS-related disability in eight functional systems (pyramidal, cerebellar, brainstem, sensory, bowel and bladder, visual, cerebral, other) and allows neurologists to assign a functional system score (FSS) in each of these. Higher levels of disability may be associated with higher levels of depression.[209,245] Untreated depression, in turn, may negatively affect the course of MS. It can negatively affect the physical outcome and disease exacerbations, cognitive function, adherence to treatment, suicide risk, and quality of life of patients and their caregivers.[201,246] MS can significantly affect families: Children whose parents have MS may present greater emotional and behavioral problems than children of parents in the general population.[247] In turn, this may contribute to feelings of inadequacy and guilt in depressed MS patients.

■ ASSESSMENT AND DIFFERENTIAL DIAGNOSIS

Depression in MS is underdiagnosed and undertreated.[200] Patients should be encouraged to report symptoms of depression and clinicians should screen for them.

To assist with the diagnostic challenge that several symptoms are shared by depression and a medical illness, some scales assign more weight to the presence of depressive beliefs. One of these self-administered scales, the BDI, is validated for use in MS patients.[248] The 9-item self-administered patient health questionnaire (PHQ-9) may be useful in this population.[249] The SCID-IV 2-Question can be used to screen for depression, and the center for Neurologic Study Emotional Lability Scale to screen for pathological or pseudobulbar affect. The 28-items General Health Questionnaire may be useful to screen for depression and other emotional disturbances.[229]

■ TREATMENT

The treatment of depression in MS patients should be interdisciplinary and use an integrated biopsychosocial approach. (Box 5-6).[250] Treating depression may bring several benefits to patients and caregivers, including enhancement of adherence to disease-modifying agents.[231]

Psychopharmacological Treatment

There are limited quality studies evaluating pharmacologic options. One shows that sertraline and CBT are equally effective and superior to supportive group therapy.[251] Desipramine shows a trend toward efficacy in a small, nonrandomized study.[252] A study comparing paroxetine with placebo shows no significant differences in primary outcomes.[253] Moclobemide and duloxetine may be effective according to evidence from small open trials.[254,255] As discussed in pathophysiology, one of the MS disease-modifying drugs (DMA), fingolimod, may have benefits for depression; still, further research is needed for further characterization of the effects of DMAs in mood. Pathologic or pseudobulbar affect may be comorbid with depression. Different antidepressants including SSRIs and tricyclics may be effective. A combination of dextromethorphan and quinidine may be useful.[256] as well.

Brain Stimulation Therapies

ECT appears as an effective treatment for depression in MS according to the limited evidence available, which includes several case reports. It should be especially considered for patients with severe depression, acute suicidal risk, and those who have failed other first-line approaches.[257,258] There has been concern, based on isolated case reports, that some patients with MS may suffer neurological deterioration after ECT. The presence of contrast-enhanced lesions may be a risk factor for disease exacerbation with ECT and the possible value of gadolinium-enhanced MRI for identifying high-risk patients has been discussed.[259] A small randomized, sham-controlled study of the safety and efficacy of deep rTMS on fatigue and depression in patients with MS showed potential benefits.[260]

Psychotherapy

CBT may be effective for patients with MS and depression delivered in group[261] or individual format[251] and also when administered by phone.[262] A computerized form of CBT may have low acceptability among MS users for several reasons including the logistics of computer use, the perpetuation of social isolation and the lack of human input during the intervention.[263] A randomized trial shows that mindfulness training is effective to reduce depression and fatigue and improve quality of life.[264]

■ SUMMARY

Depression is highly prevalent in MS. It affects the quality of life of individuals with MS and their families. It is associated with increased morbidity and mortality, and decreased adherence to MS treatment. The pathophysiology is multifactorial. Its biological components include the load and localization of brain lesions, degree of brain atrophy, inflammatory and immunological factors. Its psychosocial elements include levels of stress, lack or limited social support, and coping style. Its clinical presentation may be the same as that of primary major depression. Certain overlapping symptoms between depression and MS such as fatigue, sleep, and cognitive disorders may make the diagnosis challenging. Associated and comorbid symptoms may include apathy, anxiety, pain, irritability and pathological affect. Individuals with MS and depression have higher risk for suicide. It is important to proactively screen and treat depression in MS as it has a significant impact on the prognosis of this illness. The treatment should be multidisciplinary and address

BOX 5-12
ANXIETY IN MULTIPLE SCLEROSIS[274]

- Although less well studied than depression, anxiety disorders are very prevalent in multiple sclerosis (MS).
- Anxiety is common early after diagnosis due to adjustment difficulties and fears about the potential changes this illness will bring to the patient's life.
- It is also commonly present in acute MS relapses as the symptoms cause disruption to the individual's routine.
- Uncertainty about the illness' potential course and prognosis is one of the factors involved in the development of anxiety.
- Among the disease-modifying drugs, Glatiramer is most likely associated with anxiety as a side effect.
- Patients may experience any of the anxiety symptoms typical of primary anxiety disorders.
- Anxiety may be associated with increased somatic complaints. Collaboration with the patient's neurologist is important in situations where it is unclear if somatic symptoms are due to anxiety or represent an MS relapse.
- There is limited specific information about treatment of anxiety disorders in MS. As in primary anxiety disorders, treatment may involve medications such as SSRIs and SNRIs, and psychotherapy approaches including CBT.

biological and psychosocial factors. There are limited quality studies supporting the use of specific antidepressants in MS, but antidepressants may be as effective as in primary depression. Different types of psychotherapy including CBT and mindfulness training may be effective. ECT should be considered in cases of severe and treatment-resistant depression (see Text **box 5-12** for a review of Anxiety in Multiple Sclerosis).

TRAUMATIC BRAIN INJURY

■ EPIDEMIOLOGY

MDD is recognized as the most common psychiatric complication after TBI.[265,266] The prevalence and incidence rates of MDD after TBI range from 18% to 61% and from 15% to 33%, respectively (see Fig. 5-1).[267] The methodology of prevalence and incidence studies is varied. The postinjury time points at which prevalence is measured and the use of different instruments to assess for the presence of MDD make such investigations difficult to compare.

One of the largest studies to date reports 53% of patients meeting criteria for MDD at some point during the first year after TBI. Of the total sample, 23% experience depression for the first time after their TBI, while others with post-TBI depression were depressed at the time of the injury or experienced a recurrence of a primary preinjury MDD. The highest point prevalence is at 1 month following the injury (31%).[268] Another study identifies 42% of subjects meeting criteria for MDD at some point during the first-year post-TBI.[269] Of those, 26% present MDD during initial hospital admission for TBI, while 17% have a delayed presentation. Other studies report new onset of depression in 18 to 33% of subjects within the first-year post-TBI.[270–272]

Studies also measure prevalence of MDD beyond the first-year post-TBI. An evaluation done on an average of 32.5 months post-TBI identifies 26% of patients with MDD at the time of the evaluation and an additional 28% with an already resolved post-TBI MDD episode.[273] From 10 to 126 months post-TBI, 27% of patients meet five or more of the nine DSM MDD criteria.[274] When the average time postinjury is 2.5 years, the prevalence rate is 42% at the time of the evaluation.[267] When the average time postinjury is 8 years (range 1–37 years), 61% of the subjects meet MDD criteria at some point after TBI.[275]

Longer-term studies evaluate prevalence of MDD decades after TBI. A 30-year follow-up study[265] identifies a MDD lifetime prevalence of 27%, with 10% meeting criteria at the time of the assessment. A MDD lifetime prevalence of 18.5% is reported in World War II veterans 50 years after a TBI, with 11% meeting criteria at the time of the evaluation. The lifetime risk of developing MDD in the veterans TBI group compared to a non-TBI one is 1.5-fold.[276]

A very large National Survey of Children's Health of 12 to 17 years old identifies a 3.3-fold greater risk of depression in those with a history of concussion.[277] For retired football players, a history of three or more concussions is associated with a 3-fold increase in the development of lifetime depression, versus those with one or two concussions who have a 1.5-fold increased risk.[278] In summary, MDD is a common occurrence after TBI. The highest prevalence is in the first year after injury, but high rates of depression continue several months or even decades after the TBI.

■ PATHOPHYSIOLOGY

TBI is defined as an insult to the brain caused by an external force that produces one of the following: alteration of consciousness, altered mental state, any loss of memory of events surrounding the accident and/or focal neurological deficits. The biomechanical forces applied to the brain during the trauma can be either contact forces or inertial forces. Contact forces most commonly cause impact or contusions in the anterior and inferior frontal and temporal areas. Inertial forces, on the contrary, refer to acceleration and deceleration forces causing a stretch and strain of white matter tracks throughout the central nervous system (CNS), including the upper brainstem, corpus callosum and gray-white matter junctions of the cerebral cortex. The latter described process is termed diffuse axonal injury. Blast-related injuries directly affect air-filled organs, and it remains unclear if they can directly affect the brain, but may secondarily cause TBI effects through contact or inertial forces. Coupled with the mechanisms described, a cytotoxic cascade (calcium and magnesium dysregulation, calcium-regulated protein activation, mitochondrial dysfunction, free-radical formation) and neurotransmitter disturbances (dysfunctional elevations in cerebral glutamate, acetylcholine, dopamine, and norepinephrine) usually accompany the immediate effects following the injury.[279]

Injury to specific brain regions and the pathways connecting these regions may translate into specific clinical symptoms of TBI. Figure 5-2 illustrates the clinical phenomena that commonly occur with localized injuries.[279]

Few studies have looked at lesion localization in TBI and its association with depression. During the preimaging era information from neurosurgical notes establishes that right frontal damage is commonly associated to mood disturbance.[280] A study on Vietnam War veterans with penetrating brain injuries identifies right orbitofrontal lesions as more likely to be associated with edginess, anxiety and depressive symptoms, while left dorsolateral prefrontal lesions are associated with greater anger and hostility.[281] Left frontal lateral and left basal ganglia lesions are associated with higher rates of depression,[282,283] with the difference between lateral and medial regions being more likely to distinguish depression during the first 3 months after the injury.[283] A hypothesis based on a structural MRI study[284] proposes that an imbalance of negative valence (mediated by frontal lobes) and arousal (mediated by right parietal lobe) may play a role in the pathogenesis of depression, with another study signaling a similar imbalance between right versus left and anterior versus posterior regions in post-TBI depression.[285]

Functional neuroimaging studies reveal altered functionality and connectivity between different brain regions in post-TBI neuropsychiatric disorders. An fMRI study of veterans with blast-related concussions shows that those with post-TBI depression have more heightened amygdala reactivity, lower activation of prefrontal cortex, and lower fractional anisotropy (FA), which signals disruption of white matter tracts, in several tracts including the superior longitudinal fasciculus compared to nondepressed patients.[286] During an error-monitoring task, patients with post-TBI depression and a history of suicidal ideation show more activation of the anterior cingulate and prefrontal cortices.[287] Magnetic resonance spectroscopy imaging (MRS) detects reduced N-acetylaspartate/creatine ratio and reduced choline/creatine in the right basal ganglia in patients with post-TBI depression compared to patients after TBI who were not depressed, signaling neuronal and axonal alteration in that area.[285]

Chronic traumatic encephalopathy (CTE) refers to the neurodegenerative disease associated with repeated concussive and subconcussive head injuries, and it was formerly known as dementia pugilistica given its former association to boxers. Pathological findings that characterize CTE include frontal and temporal atrophy, axonal degeneration, and hyperphosphorylated tau and TAR DNA-binding protein (TDP-43) pathology.[288] CTE is clinically associated to depression and other psychiatric symptoms such as irritability, impulsivity, aggression, short-term memory loss and heightened suicidality, with onset after experiencing repetitive mild TBI 8 to 10 years before. The stages in CTE refer to the spread of p-tau pathology that goes from discrete foci in certain cortical regions (stage I) to most regions of the cerebral cortex and the medial temporal lobe (stage IV). Depression is described in all four pathology-confirmed stages of CTE.[289]

Other physiological consequences associated with TBI include posttraumatic epilepsy[290] and pituitary injury[291]; they can both contribute to depression pathogenesis.

Most studies demonstrate that injury severity does not predict development of MDD[268,292] although course may differ per severity subgroups.[293]

Psychosocial factors such as premorbid personality and psychiatric conditions, emotional reaction to the injury, inability to have a functional reintegration, environmental factors and compensation or litigation, can all have a significant impact in the development of post-TBI depression.[280]

History of premorbid depression is more common in patients with post-TBI depression compared to those who do not develop depression after their injury.[268,292] Older age seems to be protective against post-TBI depression[268,294] although contradictory results have also been reported.[295,296] Lifetime history of alcohol abuse,[268] fear of job loss, dissatisfaction with work situation,[297] unemployment and poverty[274] have been linked to the development of depression following TBI.

In sum, the development of post-TBI depression depends on the potential interactions of several biological and psychosocial factors, as illustrated in **Figure 5-3**.

Development of post-TBI depression is dependent on a number of preinjury biological and psychosocial factors as well as injury factors. Postinjury factors also play a role in the development and perpetuation of depression. These same factors may play a role in the development of other cognitive, somatic or associated behavioral syndromes. Symptomatic presentation in post-TBI depression can be pleomorphic, involving cognitive, somatic, and accompanying behavioral symptoms. These need to be distinguished as either part of the diagnosis of depression or as separate clinical entities.

■ **CLINICAL PRESENTATION**

Most studies on post-TBI depression utilize the criteria listed by DSM to confirm the diagnosis. Usually the category of "mood disorder due to a general condition" with either "depressive features" (for those not meeting full MDD criteria) or "major depressive features" (for those meeting full criteria) is selected in clinical scenarios. A number of somatic, behavioral, and motivation symptoms can be present in post-TBI patients with or without depression, at times making the diagnosis of depression challenging.[267] Still, DSM criteria are considered to have good sensitivity and specificity for the diagnosis of depression in patients after TBI.[298]

Fatigue, frustration, poor concentration, and sleep disturbance are some of the most commonly symptoms reported in post-TBI depressed patients, although they are not specific (Box 5-3).[275] Other postconcussive symptoms, such as headaches, dizziness, and

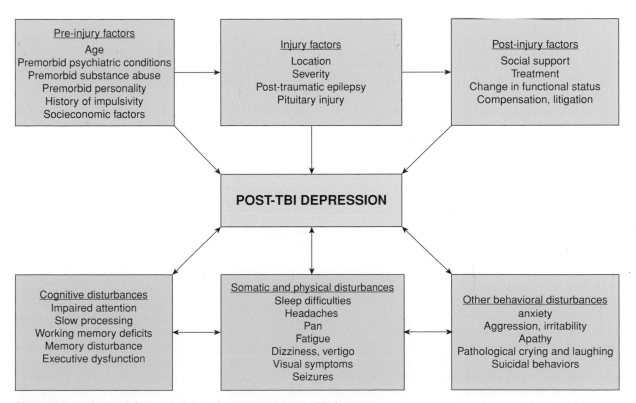

Figure 5-3 *Multiple risk factors and clinical presentation in post-TBI depression.*

TABLE 5-3 Classification of Traumatic Brain Injury Severity

Severity of TBI	Mild	Moderate	Severe
Period of loss of consciousness	30 min or less	30 min to 1 week	More than 1 week
Glasgow Coma Scale score	13–15	9–12	8 or less
Posttraumatic amnesia	<24 hours	24 hours-1 week	> 1 week
Approximate % of all TBIs	80	10	10
% that experience full recovery	80	20	Almost none

TBI, traumatic brain injury.

blurred vision are reported in increased number and severity by depressed patients.[299] The Neurobehavioral Functioning Index has been used to detect depression in patients after TBI, and identifies specific symptoms that distinguish patients with depression. These symptoms include feeling sad or blue, feeling hopeless, frustrated, easily irritated, having difficulty enjoying activities, feeling uncomfortable around others, loss of interest in sex, and feelings of worthlessness. Somatic symptoms (poor appetite, trouble falling asleep) and cognitive ones (cannot get mind off certain thoughts, forget if done things, forget to do chores) can also identify patients with depression after TBI.[300]

Objective testing of cognitive function demonstrates more pronounced impairment in patients with post-TBI with depression, specifically in the domain of executive function.[272,273] Verbal memory and processing speed may be more impaired in patients after TBI with depression versus patients after TBI without depression.[272,273] It is noteworthy that roughly 50% of mild and moderate TBI patients without MDD still present objective evidence of impairment in at least one cognitive domain.[260]

While many symptoms listed in the MDD criteria may exist independently in patients after TBI, they should still be included in the DSM criteria used to diagnose post-TBI depression, as their report is usually elevated due to mood factors.

Anxiety is comorbid in up to 77% and aggression in up to 57% of patients after TBI who are depressed.[272] Anxiety occurs eight times more commonly in patients after TBI with depression than those after TBI who are not depressed.[268] Concurrent rather than sequential treatment of these comorbid conditions is recommended.

A history of TBI increases the risk of suicide attempt.[301,302] TBI-related completed suicide is associated with a history of comorbid psychiatric and alcohol disorders,[293] but increased risk of suicide attempt still exists when controlling for psychiatric comorbidities.[302] Later stages of pathology-confirmed CTE are associated with higher rates of suicide.[289] Aggression and hostility are predictors of suicide attempt and should always be screened for in patients after TBI as potential risk factors for depression and suicidality.[301]

Involuntary emotional expressions[303] and apathy[304] can exist comorbidly with post-TBI depression and should be distinguished as either separate or comorbid clinical entities.

Figure 5-1 illustrates the range of cognitive, somatic and behavioral disturbances that may be associated with post-TBI depression or may present as independent entities in the post-TBI population.

■ COURSE AND NATURAL HISTORY

Over the course of the first-year post-TBI, depression has an estimated mean duration of 4.7 months[269] with the highest prevalence of post-TBI depression at 1 month after the injury.[268]

Individuals with mild TBI and prior psychiatric history tend to present with more persistent psychiatric problems, including affective disorders, than those with moderate and severe TBI with or without a prior psychiatric history. For those with moderate and severe TBI, the risk of psychiatric difficulties tends to be higher

immediately following the insult with a following decline in symptom prevalence.[305] See **Table 5-3** for classification of TBI based on severity.

Sleep difficulties soon after TBI predict severity of depression 1 year after the injury.[306]

Depression is associated with more pronounced psychosocial dysfunction and a stronger perception of disability.[273,299] Post-TBI depression lasting more than 6 months is associated with deterioration in social functioning and activities of daily living during the first-year post-injury.[292] The individual's perception of changes in daily functioning may impact the onset of depression.[307] Severity of depression and anxiety is a strong predictor of health-related quality of life 12 months after a severe TBI.[308]

The return-to-work rate in TBI is low, with post-TBI unemployment rates of up to 70%[309] A study finds no difference in the return-to-work rate between patients post TBI with and without depression,[299] and another finds fatigue but not depression to predict the number of days to return-to-work.[310]

The presence of depression with or without head injury may account for the individual's report of postconcussive symptoms, including cognitive complaints.[311] Treatment with the antidepressant sertraline shows improvement in cognitive measures and subjective perception of cognitive and health status in patients after TBI with depression.[312]

Post-TBI depression can evolve into a chronic condition for a subgroup of patients and its presence signals a decline in functional status. Appropriately addressing depression improves perception of health status and may also influence functional recovery. Figure 5-2 highlights the role of postinjury factors in both the development and perpetuation of depressive symptoms after TBI.

■ ASSESSMENT AND DIFFERENTIAL DIAGNOSIS

As previously mentioned DSM criteria are appropriate for diagnosis of post-TBI depression.[298] Different instruments can be used to assess for the presence of MDD diagnostic criteria, including the Structured Clinical Interview for DSM-IV (SCID), or the Schedules for Clinical Assessment in Neuropsychiatry,[313] although these are more commonly used in research settings. The BDI is a self-report measure that can be helpful to assess and monitor treatment progress of depression in the TBI population.[314,315] However, its score may be influenced by nondepression-related problems and astute clinical correlation is recommended.[316] The PHQ-9 is a valid and reliable self-report screening tool for post-TBI depression and is very easy to administer.[317] The Neurobehavioral Functioning Index is another self-report measure that can be used in patients after TBI for the assessment of multiple problems or symptoms and can accurately distinguish depressed from nondepressed patients.[300] Given the frequent comorbidity with anxiety, self-report measures that combine depression and anxiety ratings are useful. The Depression, Anxiety and Stress Scale (DASS) and Hospital Anxiety and Depression Scale (HADS) are validated in the post-TBI population.[318] Because of the potential discrepancy found in TBI patients between self-report and objective measures[319,320] use of clinician-rated measures, such as the Hamilton Depression Rating Scale (HDRS), may be useful for the assessment of depression.

Cognition and level of functioning should be assessed periodically in patients after TBI, as the severity of cognitive and functional impairment may fluctuate over time and may inform treatment course. Within the first-year postinjury, the Rancho Los Amigos Levels of Cognitive Functioning Scale is a widely accepted measure of the clinical, cognitive and functional impact of the TBI and helps identify those patients that will most likely benefit from rehabilitation services.[321]

A number of clinical conditions that present with affective symptoms need to be distinguished from post-TBI depression. Pathological laughing and crying (PLC), defined as uncontrollable episodes of laughing or crying triggered by a stimulus that would not normally cause such a response, has a prevalence of 10.9% during the first year following a TBI.[303] PLC is associated with higher severity of depression, which calls for a careful assessment and distinction of both conditions. Another important distinction is the presence of apathy. One study assessing post-TBI affective changes reports 11% of subjects with apathy without depression, 11% with depression without apathy, 60% with both depression and apathy and 18% with neither syndrome.[304] The Apathy Evaluation Scale can distinguish apathy from depression and anxiety.

Anxiety should always be screened for. In addition to comorbid depression and anxiety, an anxiety disorder may be present in about 20% of nondepressed post-TBI patients.[272] Generalized anxiety disorder, panic disorder and posttraumatic stress disorder (PTSD) are the most common anxiety disorders present in post-TBI depression.

PTSD following TBI should be considered as part of the differential diagnosis and as a comorbid condition in post-TBI depression. Although there may not be a PTSD prevalence difference between those individuals sustaining a closed head injury versus those being exposed to other traumas,[322] PTSD occurs in post-TBI patients, even without a cohesive recall of the event, and is associated with higher depression scores.[268,323]

Post-TBI aggressive behaviors occur in 57% of post-TBI depressed patients versus in 23% of post-TBI nondepressed patients.[272] Aggression is present in 34% of post-TBI patients during the first 6 months postinjury and its presence is correlated with depression.[324] In a cohort of aggressive versus nonaggressive men, aggression is significantly associated with a prior history of closed head injury.[325] As previously stated, aggression may increase the risk for suicidality.

History or presence of mania or hypomania that may signal a premorbid or post-TBI bipolar disorder, comorbid substance abuse and of other medical conditions should always be part of a comprehensive assessment in patients after TBI. Post-TBI mania has been identified in 9.1% of patients during the first year following the insult.[326]

Some self-report instruments are validated in the post-TBI population, but objective corroboration is always necessary for an accurate diagnosis. A solid clinical assessment of depression relies on the clinician's expertise and ability to distinguish and identify comorbid conditions, such as PLC, apathy, anxiety, aggression and others as discussed above. The post-TBI population is particularly susceptible to suicidality, which should be screened for regardless if depression is deemed present or not.

■ TREATMENT

See Box 5-6 for a summary of treatments of depression in neurological illnesses.

■ PSYCHOPHARMACOLOGICAL TREATMENT

Given that the onset of post-TBI depression tends to occur soon after the traumatic event and may evolve into a chronic illness, it is always recommended that treatment takes place immediately after mild depressive symptoms are recognized, even if this occurs during the recovery from TBI's physical sequelae. See **Table 5-4** for a summary of studies conducted on psychopharmacologic treatment of post-TBI depression. One study evaluating the role of early administration of the antidepressant sertraline in patients after TBI without depression as a prophylactic treatment[327] finds a significant reduction of depressive symptomatology in those receiving sertraline compared to placebo; however, the effects were not sustained when the drug was discontinued at 3 months.

There is no psychotropic agent that carries an FDA approval for use in patients after TBI with depression. A randomized, double-blind, placebo-controlled study shows that both sertraline and placebo may improve mood, anxiety and quality of life measures, but there was no statistically significant difference between the groups.[328] Another randomized, double-blind trial comparing the efficacy of sertraline, methylphenidate and placebo finds reduction in HDRS for both patients treated with methylphenidate and sertraline compared to those treated with placebo. Both methylphenidate and placebo treatment significantly improves measures of cognitive function, specifically reaction time, and postconcussive symptoms, though sertraline treatment does not.[329]

A nonrandomized, placebo run-in trial of sertraline for 8 weeks in 15 patients after mild TBI shows improvement in depression severity, psychological distress, postconcussive symptoms, cognitive functioning and quality of life.[330] Other SSRIs with efficacy in open trials include citalopram, either as monotherapy,[331] or in combination with carbamazepine,[332] and fluoxetine.[333] The use of the TCA desipramine is supported by a study with a placebo cross-over design.[334] Amitriptyline seems less effective in treating depression in this population.[335,336] The efficacy of other antidepressants, including the serotonin-norepinephrine reuptake inhibitor milnacipran,[337] and the selective monoamide oxidase inhibitor moclobemide,[338] as well as the cholinesterase inhibitor donepezil[339] for post-TBI depression in open trials is summarized in Table 5-4[340] Citalopram does not seem to provide protection toward depression relapse for post-TBI patients with depression in remission.[341]

■ BRAIN STIMULATION THERAPIES

ECT may be effective for patients after TBI with depression.[342] While ECT is not contraindicated in post-TBI patients, when indicated and administered, the use of the lowest effective energy and nondominant unilateral currents are recommended given the potential for cognitive side effects.

■ PSYCHOSOCIAL TREATMENT

A randomized controlled trial of individual CBT plus cognitive remediation compared to a wait list group shows significant improvement in depression severity. Improvements are more pronounced one and 3 months after treatment.[343]

CBT delivered in groups or by phone may reduce depression and anxiety[344] with sustained benefits 6 months following treatment.[345] The CBT protocol was adapted to the specific needs of patients after TBI, including their cognitive impairment.

A 6-week Internet-based online CBT program for patients after TBI shows improvement in mood symptoms, but with poor adherence, likely influenced by the sample's cognitive impairment.[346] A controlled 10-week mindfulness-based cognitive therapy (MBCT) study shows improvement in depression severity, which is maintained after 3 months.[347]

In contrast, a noncontrolled CBT-based coping skills group intervention for 5 weeks shows improvement in adaptive coping, but no changes in depression severity compared to baseline.[348]

Exercise, including swimming, has positive results in the treatment of depressive symptoms in patients after TBI, in small or uncontrolled

Table 5–4   Summary of Psychopharmacological Studies in Post-TBI Depression

Authors	AAN Evidence Level	N	TBI Sample Severity Level	Depression Instruments	Design and Intervention	Results and Conclusions
Ashman et al. (2009)	I	52	Different severities of TBI 17 ± 14 yr post-injury	HDRS	DB, RCT of sertraline (25–200 mg/d) or PB for 10 wks	Significant improvement from pre- to post-treatment in depression, anxiety, and QOL measures, but no group differences.
Lee et al. (2005)	II	30	Mild to moderate TBI	HDRS BDI	DB, RCT of MPH (5–20 mg/d), sertraline (25–100 mg/d), or PB for 4 wks	Both drugs improved HDRS scores more than PB; MPH improved cognition and alertness more than sertraline.
Dinan and Moyabed (1992)	II	26	13 mild TBI depressed patients vs. 13 non-TBI depressed controls	HDRS	Open trial of amitriptyline (up to 250 mg/d) for 6 wks	4/13 persons with mild TBI vs. 11/13 non-TBI depressed controls showed significantly improvement.
Saran (1985)	III	22	10 mild TBI patients vs. 12 non-TBI depressed controls	HDRS	Open trial of amitriptyline (200–300 mg/d) for 4 wks; nonresponders had trial of phenelzine (60–90 mg/d) after 3–7 day washout	No response with either drug in TBI subjects; all depressed controls improved on amitriptyline.
Wroblewski et al. (1996)	III	10	Severe TBI	DSM-IIIR 9-item symptom checklist	Blinded, randomized crossover study of desipramine (150–300 mg/d) vs. PB.	Six of 7 study completers on desipramine had significant improvement.
Fann et al. (2000)	III	15	Mild TBI Mean 10.6 mo post-TBI	HDRS	Nonrandomized, single-blind trial of sertraline (15–150 mg/d) vs. placebo for 8 wks	Significant improvements in depression, psychological distress, post-concussive symptoms by week 8 of sertraline.
Horsefield et al. (2002)	IV	5	Different severities of TBI	HDRS	Open trial of fluoxetine (20–60 mg/d) for 8 mo	Significant reduction in mood and cognitive measures.
Khateb et al. (2005)	IV	10	Moderate to severe TBI	HADS	Open trial of donepezil for 3 mo	Nonsignificant reduction in HADS depression scores; significant improvement in processing speed, learning and attention.
Kanetani et al. (2003)	IV	10	Mild to moderate TBI	HDRS	Open trial of milnacipran (30–150 mg/d) for 6 wks	Response rate was 66.7% and remission rate was 44.4%; significant improvement in cognition on MMSE
Newburn et al. (1999)	IV	26	TBI severity not noted	HDRS	Open trial of moclobemide (450–600 mg/d)	HDRS reduction was 81%; irritability scores dropped by 57% and pain scores dropped by 39%
Perino et al. (2001)	IV	20	Severe TBI	BPRS CGI	Open trial of citalopram (20 mg/d) plus carbamazepine (600 mg/d) for 12 wks	Significant reductions in depression and behavioral disorders.
Rapoport et al. (2008)	IV	54	Mild to moderate TBI	HDRS	Open trial of citalopram (20–50 mg/d) for 6 and 10 wks	Similar response rate as seen in patients with major depression without TBI: at 10 wks, 27% remission and 46% response.

AAN, American Academy of Neurology; TBI, traumatic brain injury; yr, years; DB, double-blind; wks, weeks; PB, placebo; mo, months; DSM-IIIR, Diagnostic and Statistical Manual of Mental Disorders, Third Edition, Revised; MDD, major depressive disorder; BDI, Beck Depression Inventory; MPH, methylphenidate; BPRS, Brief Psychiatric Rating Scale; CGI, Clinical Global Impressions Scale; HADS, Hospital Anxiety and Depression Scale; HDRS, Hamilton Depression Rating Scale; MMSE, mini-mental state examination; PCS, post-concussive symptoms; QOL, quality of life; RCT, randomized controlled trial.

Reproduced with permission from Plantier D, Luauté J. SOFMER group: Drugs for behavior disorders after traumatic brain injury: Systematic review and expert consensus leading to French recommendations for good practice. Ann Phys Rehabil Med. *2016;59(1):42–57.*

trials.[349,350] A large trial comparing aerobic exercise to relaxation training for 12 weeks in patients with recent and severe TBI shows no difference between the groups, but does show reduction of depression and anxiety in both groups.[351] A randomized controlled trial of light therapy for treatment of fatigue in patients after TBI shows no effect of this intervention in depression severity, a secondary outcome measure.[352]

Meta-analyses of depression treatment in patients with TBI shows an overall effect size of 1.89 (95%CI = 1.20–2.58) for pre- and post-treatment comparisons of psychopharmacological and nonpsychopharmacological interventions. However, meta-analysis evaluating only controlled studies identifies an overall effect size of 0.46 (95% CI = −0.44–1.36), favoring the control interventions.[353]

■ SUMMARY

Depression is the most common psychiatric complication after TBI. Preinjury history of depression and alcohol abuse are risk factors for the development of post-TBI depression, as are other premorbid environmental factors, such as unemployment, poverty, and dissatisfaction with work situation. Contusions in the frontal and temporal areas and diffuse axonal injury are mechanisms commonly associated with TBI. Repetitive trauma can evolve into a neurodegenerative process highly associated to depression. Structural and functional alterations specifically associated to post-TBI depression have been detected in studies, with alterations in the structure and function of the prefrontal cortex and its connectivity being the most consistent findings. The clinical presentation of post-TBI depression can be challenging, as a number of somatic, behavioral and motivational symptoms tend to be present. DSM-5 criteria should continue to be used to establish the diagnosis clinically, and a number of screening instruments such as the PHQ-9 and BDI are validated in post-TBI depression. Frequently comorbid conditions should be considered when evaluating post-TBI depression, and these include anxiety, apathy, pathological affect, aggressive behaviors and cognitive deficits. The highest prevalence of post-TBI depression occurs within the first year of the injury, but delayed presentations beyond the first year are not uncommon. Mild severity of the injury and prior psychiatric history seems to increase the risk of persisting post-TBI psychiatric difficulties. Evidence-based treatments for depression in patient's post-TBI include the use of antidepressants, cognitive-behavioral therapy, and MBCT. The use of exercise, which many times is part of the rehabilitation process, can exert a positive effect on mood (see Text **box 5-13** for a review of Anxiety and Traumatic Brain Illness).

BOX 5-13
ANXIETY AND TRAUMATIC BRAIN ILLNESS

- Anxiety is comorbid in up to 77% of patients who have depression after traumatic brain illness (TBI). It occurs eight times more commonly in patients with post-TBI depression compared to those who are not depressed.

- In addition to their comorbidity with depression, anxiety disorders may be present in about 20% of nondepressed patients.

- Patients may experience any of the anxiety symptoms typical of primary anxiety disorders.

- Generalized anxiety disorder, panic disorder, and post-traumatic stress disorder are the most common anxiety disorders post-TBI. Obsessive-compulsive disorder and phobias may also develop post-TBI.

- PTSD may occur even in patients without a cohesive recall of the traumatic event.

- Anxiety may be present as part of a postconcussion syndrome.

- Screening for and treating anxiety in patients with TBI may markedly improve their prognosis.

EPILEPSY

■ EPIDEMIOLOGY

Depression is common among patients with epilepsy (Fig. 5-1), and patients with both epilepsy and depression are at risk for developing a more severe seizure disorder.[354] Recent meta-analyses demonstrate a pooled prevalence of active depression (within the last 12 months) in persons with epilepsy (PWE) of just over 23% (range 13.2–36.5%) and a lifetime pooled prevalence of 13.0% (range 4.1–32.5%). Odds ratio (OR) of active depression in PWE relative to persons without epilepsy is estimated at 2.77 pooled, with the range of individual adjusted OR models varying from 1.1 to 3.49, and overall OR for lifetime depression of 2.2 with a range of 1.48 to 3.96[355] Heterogeneity in individual study prevalence estimates is likely driven by variations in the method of diagnosing depression.[355] The increased risk for depression in PWE is not accounted for solely by the presence of chronic disease: a population-based analysis comparing rates of neuropsychiatric comorbidities accompanying epilepsy versus other conditions (asthma, diabetes, migraine) finds the highest prevalence rates for depression in epilepsy (9.6%) with an adjusted OR of 2.7[356] Despite significant heterogeneity in epilepsy subtypes in this discussion they are treated as one entity, except where noted.

Additionally, depression and suicide attempt independently increase incident risk of developing epilepsy.[357] Conversely, a diagnosis of epilepsy increases the incidence risk ratio for depression and suicidality both before and after diagnosis.[358] Thus, depression appears to be both a risk factor for developing epilepsy and, frequently, comorbid with it. In addition, comorbid depression is associated with diminished treatment-responsiveness.[359]

There is relatively little data regarding the contribution of family history to depression in epilepsy, but at least one study of children and adolescents with epilepsy finds family history to be highly statistically significant in contributing to depression.[360]

Genetics may play a role as well. There is a rat model of hereditary absence epilepsy with comorbid behavioral correlates to human depression.[361] Future study may reveal genes conferring a high risk for both conditions. Population-based study of the genetics of epilepsy is demonstrating that specific gene dysregulation can have pleiotropic effects: copy number variation (CNV) is a form of genetic variability that arises when segments of DNA are duplicated or deleted during meiosis or recombination. Certain recurrent CNVs are associated with epilepsy as well as with neuropsychiatric conditions, such as autism, schizophrenia, and ADHD. That is, these CNVs convey an increased risk for a range of neuropsychiatric disorders including epilepsy.[362] Future research may also shed more light on the genetic underpinnings of epilepsy and depression, whether by way of a common CNV leading to increased risk for both conditions or via some other mechanism.

■ PATHOPHYSIOLOGY

The neuropsychiatric origins of depression in epilepsy are likely multi-factorial (Box 5-2) and reflect both diathesis and stress contributors. Etiology can then be understood at the levels of both psychological mechanism and neurobiological pathophysiology. Among the contributing psychological mechanisms, special attention should be paid to the ways in which living with epilepsy parallels a "learned helplessness" experimental model for inducing depressive behavior: recurrent seizures are aversive events that occur at unpredictable intervals largely outside the control of the individual experiencing them.[363] In addition, the burden of living with a chronic illness with its associated injuries, effects on functioning, and social stigma create chronically high levels of psychological distress in epilepsy patients that are known to contribute to depression.[364] That said, it is not the burden of chronic illness alone that raises depression risk in PWE: epilepsy is associated with a risk of depression and other neuropsychiatric disorders that exceeds the risk associated with other chronic illnesses (both asthma and diabetes).[356]

On a neurobiological level, epileptic seizures are marked by paroxysmal hypersynchronous neural discharges that result from cortical hyperexcitability. Shared pathophysiology may be related to alterations in cortical excitability. There are several leading mechanisms by which underlying pathophysiology has been hypothesized to predispose to both depression and epilepsy, including (1) a hyperactive HPA, (2) structural and functional abnormalities of cortical structures, (3) increased glutamatergic and decreased GABAergic and serotonergic activity, and (4) immunological abnormalities.[351]

Alterations in hormonal milieu, especially over-activation of the HPA axis, appear to be one shared contributing mechanism. In rats, treatment with high-dose corticosteroids prior to epileptogenic kindling accelerates seizure appearance and leads to higher amplitude hippocampal cell spiking even when serum corticosteroid levels are no longer elevated.[365] Chronic low-dose corticosteroid supplementation, perhaps more akin to the physiological elevations seen with chronic depression, also leads to accelerated kindling in rats, albeit in an amygdala model of epilepsy.[366] Blocking the glucocorticoid receptor prevents amygdalar kindling in these rats,[367] indicating that the corticosteroid supplementation is critically involved in the development of epilepsy in this setting. It is thought that perhaps the elevated cortisol contributes to cortical hyperexcitability via neurotransmitter effects, for example by producing excessive synaptic glutamate and decreasing serotonin activity.[364]

Changes in hippocampal volume and neurogenesis are noted in animal models of both persistent temporal lobe epilepsy (TLE) and enduring depression.[364] In addition, functional changes (decrements) in serotonin receptor binding in limbic regions, as seen on PET scanning, are much more pronounced in patients with both depression and TLE than in those with TLE alone,[368] pointing toward a possible shared mechanism.

Abnormal neurotransmitter levels appear to be involved in the common pathophysiology of depression and epilepsy. Adequate serotonin levels in the hippocampus protected an animal model from pilocarpine-induced seizures[369] perhaps via neuronal hyperpolarization mediated by the 5-HT1A receptor.[370] Insufficient synaptic serotonin seen in both depression and epilepsy may therefore represent a common mechanism and a model by which they each can exacerbate the other. Enhanced CSF glutamate, on the other hand, is seen in depression associated with a failure of glutamate transporter proteins and resultant neuronal hyperexcitability and death,[364] and NMDA antagonism has been associated with therapeutic effects on amygdalar kindling and status epilepticus as well as stress-induced depression phenotypes in animal models,[371] supporting a role for excessive glutamate in common pathophysiology. Diminished region-specific GABAergic activity occurs in both animal and human models of depression and seizure disorders, and enhanced GABA functioning produces both antidepressant and anticonvulsant effects.[364,371] Alterations in the acetylcholine, norepinephrine, and dopamine systems may contribute to common pathogenesis of epilepsy and depression as well.[371]

Release of proinflammatory cytokines in depression may be a further contributor to exacerbation of seizure risk: IL-1β has proconvulsant properties by promoting extracellular glutamate.[364]

Based on animal models of postictal depressive symptoms (e.g., reactive aggression) mitigated by morphine pretreatment and exacerbated by naloxone pretreatment, endogenous opioids released during seizures are thought to play a role in the mood-elevating effects of ECT, and postictal aggressive behavior is postulated to represent endogenous opioid withdrawal.[372,373] As such, there may

be a role for seizure-related fluctuations in endogenous opioids in the pathogenesis of depressive disturbances in humans with epilepsy as well.

It is also possible that seizure focus has an influence on depression risk in epilepsy. Of particular interest is the distinction between temporal lobe and non-TLE. Mesial temporal sclerosis (MTS), gliosis, and volume loss associated with mesial TLE is a risk factor for depression with inconsistent findings. One study[374] finds that MTS significantly increases the risk for depression over nonlesional epilepsy or epilepsy with lesions elsewhere in the brain. This is in contrast with prior data indicating that nonlesional epilepsy poses a significantly greater risk for depression over lesional, including epilepsy associated with MTS.[375] Diagnostic methods, inclusion criteria, and analysis of confounding variables may be contributing to the discrepancies in the data; clearly more research is needed to clarify the relationships between lesions, location of epileptic focus, and depression.

Paradoxically, although seizures and depression appear to have common pathophysiological mechanisms, and in some respects each disorder can potentiate the other, ECT, which is seizure induced with an externally applied electrical stimulus, has long been used as an effective treatment for depression. Moreover, seizures can be anticonvulsant.[376]

ECT may act via a number of potential mechanisms, including the inhibitory and monoamine neurotransmitter systems, neurogenesis, and the endocrine system.[377] Depletion of cortical gamma-aminobutyric-acid (GABA) during ECT, leading to a compensatory increase in the function of inhibitory (GABA) neurotransmission, is proposed as one source of the treatment's antidepressant and anticonvulsant properties. ECT enhances serotonergic (5-HT1A) receptor function and striatal dopamine receptor (D1 and D3) binding and decreases the number of alpha-2 receptors in noradrenergic neurons in the locus coeruleus, suggesting that effects on these neurotransmitter systems may contribute to the effects of ECT.[377]

ECT also increases proliferation of precursor cells in the monkey hippocampus; neurogenesis is thus also postulated as a mechanism for the antidepressant effects of seizures.[377]

Electrically induced seizures are accompanied by marked acute changes in endocrine function: prolactin, oxytocin, and growth hormone all increase. However, there is no evidence suggesting these alterations are a mechanism for clinical improvement.[377] On the other hand, normalization of derangements in the HPA axis correlates with clinical response, suggesting this too may represent a mechanism of antidepressant action for ECT.[378] Additional research will help to elucidate the complex pathophysiological mechanisms involved in epilepsy and depression and to clarify the seemingly contradictory effect of seizures on mood disorders.

■ CLINICAL PRESENTATION

Depression is a syndrome affecting mood, activity level, and somatic rhythms. In addition to major depression, depressive disorders in epilepsy can include a range of presentations: less pervasive symptomatology (minor depression, or depressive disorder not otherwise specified), less severe symptoms combined with longer duration of disturbance (persistent depressive disorder, formerly dysthymic disorder), and symptoms that interleave with periods of mania or hypomania (bipolar spectrum disorders). Appropriate and self-limiting reactive symptoms (e.g., to a failed temporal lobectomy) must be attended to and distinguished from a disorder of affect. In addition, patients with epilepsy (PWE) can be affected by a range of peri-ictal depressive symptoms (Box 5-3).

Preictal depressive symptoms may present as prodromal dysphoria, irritability, and low frustration tolerance beginning hours to days before seizure onset.[379] Self-reported low mood and negative life events prior to seizure events are both independently associated with the occurrence of seizure, suggesting that depressed mood may represent a prodromal aspect of seizure.[380] A boost in mood may occur following seizure events.[380]

Ictal depressive symptoms—those that represent actual manifestation of seizure activity itself—are the second most common ictal affect after fear and are associated with both temporal and diffuse epileptic localizations.[381] Distinguishing characteristics of ictal depressive symptoms include a stereotyped depressive reaction, short-lived experience, lack of contextualizing factors for the low mood, and association with other clearly ictal phenomena including evolution to altered consciousness. Unfortunately frequency of this seizure semiology has not been definitively studied and so prevalence data are limited.[379]

Postictal depressive symptoms may represent the appearance of affective symptoms in the postseizure period (in 5–7 days after) or the exacerbation of a preexisting affective disturbance; indeed these symptoms appear to be more common in those with a prior history of depression or anxiety.[373] A study of postictal depressive symptoms in patients with refractory partial epilepsy found that these lasted a median of 24 hours and were quite prevalent (>20% for each symptom)[382]; the symptoms reported were the same as those reported for major depression.

Interictal symptoms may meet criteria for one of the standard depressive disorder diagnoses referenced above; however, some find that these criteria incompletely describe the clinical affective syndromes seen interictally. The interictal dysphoric disorder (IDD), an entity described as having eight key components including depressed mood, anergia, pain, sleep disturbance, irritable explosive affect, sudden euphorias, fear, and anxiety[383] is put forth as one alternative diagnostic category to capture these clinical syndromes, with an emphasis on the chronicity of the dysthymia and the paroxysmal nature of the other components.

A description of the clinical presentation of depression in epilepsy would not be complete without mentions of the other comorbid psychiatric conditions that frequently present along with it: these include anxiety, psychosis, and elevated mood states (See Box 5-14).

■ COURSE AND NATURAL HISTORY

The presence of depression, current or prior, negatively impacts the course of epilepsy, and is associated with a higher likelihood of treatment resistance. There is an odds ratio of 2.26 for psychiatric diagnosis (of which depression accounted for 85%) and refractory epilepsy.[359] Depressive symptoms and seizure frequency mutually influence each other over time.[384] Older work on the effect of psychotropic treatment on seizure frequency suggested that improvement in psychiatric symptomatology is associated with improvement in epilepsy control.[385] However, more recent analyses[386] show that changes in the course of epilepsy during antidepressant treatment could be related to effects on the underlying processes involved in epileptogenesis. Additional data on the effect that course of depression has on prognosis in epilepsy will help to clarify whether both depression course and neurobiological treatment are independent predictors.

The management of epilepsy, regardless of effectiveness of outcome, may also affect the prognosis of depressive illness. Patients with epilepsy have an increased risk of suicide (up to 10-fold) when compared with a general population and a high lifetime prevalence of suicidal thoughts, plans, and attempts.[363] There is increased risk for suicide in a number of epilepsy sub-groups, including newly diagnosed epilepsy, tertiary care settings or epilepsy institutions, TLE, and postsurgical treatment for epilepsy including temporal lobectomy.[387] Interestingly, resective epilepsy surgery may be associated with a higher risk of death by suicide than nonsurgical epilepsy management, even when good seizure control is achieved.[388] It may be that the burden of adjusting to life unencumbered by seizures produces a host of new stresses that could prove intolerable

and lead to suicide.[389] Conversely, failed epilepsy surgery may provoke a feeling of hopelessness in that the last resort has been tried, and thereby lead to suicide.[363]

■ ASSESSMENT AND DIFFERENTIAL DIAGNOSIS

Depression in patients with epilepsy can be assessed clinically using the standard criteria outlined in the Diagnostic and Statistic Manual of Mental Disorders and some combination of observation, clinical interview, or a depression checklist such as the Hamilton Depression Rating Scale (HAM-D). Self-administered screening tools such as BDI or PHQ-9 can circumvent the issue of time limitations in brief clinical encounters and enable assessment of depressive symptoms in more patients. However, some depression screening instruments rely heavily on somatic symptoms, which in patients with epilepsy can be associated with the disease itself or with antiepileptic medications. A brief (6-item) neurological disorders depression inventory for epilepsy (NDDI-E) minimizes these confounding sources and demonstrates high specificity for a diagnosis of major depression as well as a better positive predictive value than either the BDI or the PHQ-2.[390]

Clinically, it can be difficult to differentiate neurovegetative and cognitive symptoms of depression from side effects of some antiepileptic drugs (AEDs), which can include lethargy, weight changes, and poor concentration. In these cases, the presence or absence of anhedonia can help clarify whether a depressive disorder is present.[391]

While some recommend that practitioners disregard the presence of epilepsy in making a depression diagnosis,[363] it is a questionable practice given seizure-related effects on mood and affect regulation. In particular it may prove important to distinguish premorbid or interictal depressive disorders from postictal mood disturbance given that the latter may not respond to pharmacotherapy, even though the two may only be distinguishable based on the shorter duration of postictal mood phenomena.[373] Blumer et al.[383] advocate for the use of an 8-item subset from the Seizure Questionnaire assessing aspects of mood, irritability, pain, euphoria, anxiety/fear, energy, and sleep to establish a diagnosis of IDD.

Given the risks of suicidal behavior in patients with epilepsy, there is also interest in specific screening tools for suicidality in epilepsy. A comparison of three instruments—the MINI International Neuropsychiatric Interview (MINI), Columbia Suicide Severity Rating Scale (C-SSRS), and Interactive Voice Response System CSSRS (E-CSSRS)—finds that slightly more suicidal behavior was reported with the E-CSSRS than C-SSRS, suggesting the E-CSSRS may be optimal for detection of suicidality in epilepsy.[392]

■ TREATMENT

Treatment of depression in people with epilepsy needs to take into account the possible risks of depression and suicidality associated with medical and surgical management of epilepsy, the possible risks of lowered seizure threshold associated with some antidepressants, and the psychosocial factors unique to this population (Box 5-6).

As stated above, surgical management of epilepsy, even when successful, is associated with a risk of suicide even with excellent postoperative seizure control. This could be related to new or compounded deficits associated with the surgery, but may be related to the "burden of normality," the sudden pressure of adjusting to life as a well person. Thorough psychosocial assessment to understand the meaning of the patient's epilepsy to the patient, identify postcure expectations, and otherwise assist with transition to a well state is proposed as one way to reduce that risk.[393]

■ PSYCHOPHARMACOLOGICAL TREATMENT

Medical management of epilepsy may carry its own risks of behavioral disturbances. In 2008 the FDA issued an alert regarding a

1.8-fold increased risk of suicidality in patients on all AEDs for different indications, including epilepsy, based on data from a meta-analysis of 199 clinical trials of 11 AEDs involving over 43,000 patients. Patients with epilepsy were found to have a higher risk of suicidality on AEDs than patients with psychiatric or other disorders who were taking AEDs. However, as several authors have noted,[354,393] trials without suicidality—that is, two-thirds of them—were excluded from the analysis and the suicidality data were not prospectively collected, increasing the risk of reporting bias. Moreover, the risk was assumed to apply to the entire class of AEDs despite very varied mechanisms of action rather than focusing on the AEDs (lamotrigine and topiramate) with a statistically significant increase in suicidality risk or noting that some AEDs (carbamazepine and valproate) had a nonsignificant protective effect on suicidality.[394] A recent case-control study of 44,300 epilepsy patients treated with AEDs attempted to account for these variables by studying suicidal behavior prospectively and by class of AEDs. The results show that newer AEDs with a high risk for causing depression (levetiracetam, tiagabine, topiramate, and vigabatrin) are associated with an increased risk of self-harm/suicidal behavior but others, including the barbiturates, valproate, lamotrigine, carbamazepine, oxcarbazepine, gabapentin, phenytoin, and ethosuximide, are not.[395] A massive cohort study involving 5.13 million patients examines associations between AED use, epilepsy, depression, bipolar disorder, and suicide or suicide attempt. In the subgroup analysis, while some subgroups' use of AEDs is significantly associated with suicide-related events, the subgroup of patients with both epilepsy and depression shows no significant increase in suicide-related events.[396] Given these contradictory findings, an expert consensus reminds practitioners of the multivariable nature of suicidality in epilepsy, the significant morbidity and mortality associated with failing to treat epilepsy with AEDs, and appropriate strategies for risk management in these patients including screening, psychiatric referral, adjustments to AED regimen, and close communication regarding emergent suicidality.[397] Awareness of specific antiepileptic medications' propensity to cause depression and suicidality, along with attention to enzyme induction and inhibition properties of specific antidepressants and antiepileptics to maintain appropriate serum levels, should guide selection of drug regimen but not prevent appropriate management of seizures out of concern for inducing suicidality.

Many clinicians have avoided treating patients with epilepsy and depression with antidepressants because of concerns that these medications may lower seizure threshold. TCAs, and to a lesser extent SSRIs, were thought to be proconvulsant, but more recent data suggests that seizure frequency is not negatively affected, and may even be helped, by the addition of antidepressant therapy. With the notable exceptions of clomipramine and bupropion, antidepressants appear to be safe for use in epilepsy (**Table 5-5**).[379,398,399,400–402]

An analysis of seizure incidence in clinical trials demonstrates increased risk for seizures associated with bupropion and clomipramine, as well as with some antipsychotic medications (clozapine,

quetiapine, olanzapine) but an overall lower risk for seizures among those taking antidepressants compared to placebo.[399] Evaluation of the effects of extracellular hippocampal serotonin and dopamine in an animal model shows anticonvulsant effects of both neurotransmitters within a range many times above baseline levels; however, elevation above this protective range, as well as D-2 and HT-1 receptor blockade, is associated with proconvulsant effects.[369] This is consistent with the observation that antidepressants tend to be associated with seizures primarily in overdose, and even raises the question of whether pro-serotonergic antidepressants should be given a trial as antiepileptic medications in their own right.[389] That even relatively safe antidepressants can represent a proconvulsant risk in overdose does bear on treatment recommendations for those patients with epilepsy thought to be at high risk for suicide attempts: one clinical resource indicates elevated risk for seizures in overdoses of some tricyclics (desipramine, nortryptiline, imipramine) as well as other drugs (amoxapine, maprotiline).[400] SSRIs remain the first-line treatment for depression in epilepsy given their superior safety profile even in overdose and their efficacy in treating irritability and other atypical depressive symptoms; those with minimal effect on the CYP450 enzymes such as citalopram and sertraline are preferred in patients taking hepatically metabolized AEDs in order to minimize pharmacokinetic interactions.[379]

As with any attempt to treat a depressive disorder, assessment for propensity to mania or hypomania is a necessity. If mood stabilizing treatment is indicated, it is essential to attend to the properties of the mood stabilizing agents considered. Lithium, for example, can be proconvulsant even at therapeutic doses and normal serum concentrations.[379,401,402] Several AEDs including valproate, lamotrigine, carbamazepine, and oxcarbazepine have mood stabilizing properties and should be considered as a first line of treatment in those cases.

■ BRAIN STIMULATION THERAPIES

ECT holds some potential as a treatment for depression in patients with epilepsy, but limited supporting data have been gathered so far. Case reports have demonstrated safety and efficacy.[403–405] A small retrospective chart review of patients with epilepsy and depression who underwent ECT, most of whom were on antiepileptic medication, shows mean seizure length commensurate with published norms for nonepileptic patients and that ECT is an effective treatment for depressive symptoms.[406] The authors note two challenges associated with use of ECT in patients with epilepsy: first, the risk of inducing spontaneous seizure activity, especially if antiepileptic doses are lowered to allow planned seizure induction, and second, that of seizures being difficult to induce or of inadequate length. They concluded that epilepsy was not a contraindication to treatment with ECT, and that treatment can proceed with existing AED regimen in place, albeit with ongoing discussion with managing neurologists about how to proceed if seizure induction proves difficult and ongoing monitoring for spontaneous seizures. If AED dose reductions prove necessary to complete ECT, AEDs should be returned to pretreatment regimen following ECT.[406] Others recommend holding AEDs on the morning of ECT treatment except in those patients with recent generalized seizures or at high risk for status epilepticus.[407]

TMS, which uses brief, rapidly changing magnetic field induction over the scalp to induce a focal electrical current in the underlying cortex, appears to be potentially useful in the treatment of mild to moderate treatment resistant depression, and it has the advantage of being noninvasive and well tolerated.[408] While definitive studies demonstrating benefit have not been done, it is speculated that the ability of TMS to decrease cortical excitability might make it beneficial in epilepsy if the seizure focus is sufficiently close to the brain surface. It is further hypothesized that TMS of an epileptic

---

TABLE 5-5 Seizure Risk by Antidepressant (for Doses Within the Therapeutic Range)

Seizure risk	Antidepressant
Low to moderate	bupropion SR, citalopram, escitalopram, duloxetine, fluoxetine, nefazodone, mirtazapine, venlafaxine, phenelzine, tranylcypromine, fluoxetine, paroxetine, sertraline, and trazodone
High	clomipramine, bupropion IR, maprotiline, amoxapine

focus could reduce its inhibitory inputs to other areas, such as the prefrontal cortex, and thereby improve mood.[409] More research will be needed to see whether these hypothetical benefits for depression in epilepsy are borne out.

DBS utilizes intracerebrally implanted electrodes attached to a neurostimulator to stimulate nearby neurons. A Cochrane review of randomized controlled trials of deep brain or cortical stimulation for epilepsy found that anterior thalamic DBS, responsive ictal onset zone stimulation, and hippocampal DBS were all associated with a moderate reduction in seizure frequency in refractory epilepsy patients, but that anterior thalamic DBS was associated with higher rates of depression.[410] Although there have been some limited reports of efficacy of DBS for the treatment of depression, placebo-controlled trial data are lacking. As such, it is too early to say whether DBS will be a beneficial treatment for patients with epilepsy and depression, have no effect, or do harm, but target site will likely have an impact and differential effects based on DBS target will need to be carefully characterized.

VNS uses an electrical stimulator attached to a programmable pulse generator to stimulate the patient's left vagus nerve. A randomized, open-label study of best medical practices for pharmacoresistant focal epilepsy versus best medical practices plus VNS found that seizure frequency was significantly improved in the group getting VNS, but depression scores did not change (as measured by the Centre for Epidemiologic Studies Depression scale and the Neurological Disorders Depression Inventory in Epilepsy).[411] These results are suggestive of benefit for VNS in epilepsy but not in associated depressive symptoms, though not conclusive.

Transcutaneous vagus nerve stimulation (tVNS), in which the vagus nerve is stimulated noninvasively via the ear (somatic sensory territory of the vagus nerve), has been proposed as a treatment for treatment-refractory epilepsy that avoids the risks of invasive nerve stimulators.[412] A randomized controlled trial of tVNS versus sham stimulation (in a region not part of the vagus nerve territory) for treatment-refractory epilepsy patients found statistically significant reductions in seizure frequency with tVNS treatment. In addition, statistically significant improvements in depression (as measured by the Self-Rating Depression Scale) were found in the treatment but not the control group patients. A review of the use of tVNS for neuropsychiatric disorders found benefit for major depression compared with sham-stimulated patients as well as benefit in pharmacoresistant epilepsy[413] but was limited by small numbers of existing trials and their inherent biases. In summary, tVNS appears promising for the treatment of epilepsy and depression, as well as their comorbid appearance, but more research needs to be done to establish benefit.

■ PSYCHOSOCIAL TREATMENT

Given the ways in which living with epilepsy parallels a "learned helplessness" model for depression, therapies aimed at altering cognitions, especially those concerning locus of control, may be helpful. CBT, behavioral activation, and acceptance and commitment therapy (ACT) are all helpful, with only a few hours of ACT showing a benefit to quality of life measures.[363] CBT seems to help prevent depression in adolescents with a new diagnosis of epilepsy, and is demonstrated on MRI to improve neural activation in regions showing reduced activity in patients with depression and epilepsy.[363] However, high-quality data are mixed.

A review[414] of existing randomized controlled trials of CBT for depression in epilepsy (6 trials involving 247 patients) shows mixed results; it seems that a focus on coping and reducing depression accounts for the positive efficacy trials whereas a focus on seizure control is more associated with a lack of efficacy. Individual therapy rather than group treatments as well as therapy "booster" sessions to revise and practice CBT skills are associated with the trials finding

---

> ## BOX 5-14
> ## ANXIETY AND EPILEPSY
>
> - The prevalence of anxiety disorders is high in patients with epilepsy, both comorbid with depression and standing alone.
> - Patients may experience any of the anxiety symptoms typical of primary anxiety disorders.
> - Importantly, anxiety symptoms may overlap with those of a seizure disorder. For instance fear, feelings of depersonalization and derealization, dizziness and paresthesias may be present as manifestations of a panic attack or represent ictal phenomena.
> - The clinical differential diagnosis between "primary" anxiety symptoms and those secondary to seizures may be challenging. Anxiety symptoms secondary to ictal activity tend to be stereotypic (occur the same way or similar each time); they are more likely to present with alterations in consciousness and automatisms. EEG including long-term monitoring may be needed to reach an accurate diagnosis in the most challenging cases.
> - Patients with epilepsy may experience anxiety about the unpredictability of seizure recurrence, especially in situations that would imply danger (driving; holding a baby) and in situations that may cause embarrassment.
> - Treating anxiety in patients with epilepsy may markedly improve their prognosis and quality of life.
> - As in primary anxiety disorders, the treatment tools include SSRIs, SNRIs, and psychotherapy including CBT.
> - Benzodiazepines are not a preferred treatment for these patients. In addition to their known side effects, patients with epilepsy may be at increased risk for seizures caused by withdrawal. Furthermore, patients with epilepsy who develop tolerance to benzodiazepine may be less likely to respond to these agents when used as "rescue" medications to terminate an acute seizure episode.

in favor of CBT efficacy,[414] suggesting a focus for implementation. These data must be interpreted cautiously however, taking note of RCT limitations such as small sample size and unclear or inconsistent diagnostic and outcome measures.

■ SUMMARY

Depression is a risk factor for epilepsy, and vice versa. The presence of one also exacerbates the course of the other. Taking into account specific treatment considerations, including future information on the effects of AEDs on depression and suicidality as it becomes available, depression in epilepsy should be aggressively treated. Further research clarifying neurobiological predispositions to both conditions will be essential in clarifying the bidirectionality of the depression and epilepsy link (see Text **box 5-14** for a review of Anxiety and Epilepsy).

REFERENCES

1. Assal F, Cummings JL. Neuropsychiatric symptoms in the dementias. *Curr Opin Neurol.* 2002;15(4):445–450.

2. Lyketsos CG, Lopez O, Jones B, Fitzpatrick AL, Breitner J, DeKosky S. Prevalence of neuropsychiatric symptoms in dementia and mild cognitive impairment: results from the cardiovascular health study. *JAMA.* 2002;288(12):1475–1483.

3. Olin JT, Katz IR, Meyers BS, Schneider LS, Lebowitz BD. Provisional diagnostic criteria for depression of Alzheimer disease: rationale and background. *Am J Geriatr Psychiatry.* 2002;10(2):129–141.

4. Lee HB, Lyketsos CG. Depression in Alzheimer's disease: heterogeneity and related issues. *Biol Psychiatry*. 2003;54(3):353–362. Review.

5. Lyketsos CG, Steinberg M, Tschanz JT, Norton MC, Steffens DC, Breitner JC. Mental and behavioral disturbances in dementia: findings from the Cache County Study on Memory in Aging. *Am J Psychiatry*. 2000;157(5):708–714.

6. Castilla-Puentes RC, Habeych ME. Subtypes of depression among patients with Alzheimer's disease and other dementias. *Alzheimers Dement*. 2010;6(1):63–69.

7. Byers AL, Yaffe K. Depression and risk of developing dementia. *Nat Rev Neurol*. 2011;7(6):323–331.

8. Dotson VM, Beydoun MA, Zonderman AB. Recurrent depressive symptoms and the incidence of dementia and mild cognitive impairment. *Neurology*. 2010;75:27–34.

9. Barnes DE, Yaffe K, McCormik M, et al. Mid-life versus late-life depression and risk of dementia: differential effects for vascular dementia and Alzheimer's disease [abstract]. *Alzheimers Dement*. 2010;6(Suppl. 1):S109.

10. Green RC, Cupples LA, Kurz A, et al. Depression as a risk factor for Alzheimer disease: the MIRAGE Study. *Arch Neurol*. 2003;60:753–759.

11. Dal Forno G, Palermo MT, Donohue JE, Karagiozis H, Zonderman AB, Kawas CH. Depressive symptoms, sex, and risk for Alzheimer's disease. *Ann Neurol*. 2005;57:381–387.

12. Caraci F, Copani A, Nicoletti F, Drago F. Depression and Alzheimer's disease: neurobiological links and common pharmacological targets. *Eur J Pharmacol*. 2010;626(1):64–71.

13. Ellison JM, Kyomen HH, Harper DG. Depression in later life: an overview with treatment recommendations. *Psychiatr Clin North Am*. 2012;35(1):203–229.

14. McEwen BS. Physiology and neurobiology of stress and adaptation: central role of the brain. *Physiol Rev*. 2007;87(3):873–904.

15. Lupien SJ, Maheu F, Tu M, Fiocco A, Schramek TE. The effects of stress and stress hormones on human cognition: Implications for the field of brain and cognition. *Brain Cogn*. 2007;65(3):209–237.

16. Crochemore C, Lu J, Wu Y, Liposits Z, Sousa N, Holsboer F, Almeida OF. Direct targeting of hippocampal neurons for apoptosis by glucocorticoids is reversible by mineralocorticoid receptor activation. *Mol Psychiatry*. 2005;10(8):790–798.

17. Green KN, Billings LM, Roozendaal B, McGaugh JL, LaFerla FM. Glucocorticoids increase amyloid-beta and tau pathology in a mouse model of Alzheimer's disease. *J Neurosci*. 2006; 26(35):9047–9056.

18. Rojo LE, Fernández JA, Maccioni AA, Jimenez JM, Maccioni RB. Neuroinflammation: implications for the pathogenesis and molecular diagnosis of Alzheimer's disease. *Arch Med Res*. 2008;39(1):1–16.

19. Okello A, Edison P, Archer HA, et al. Microglial activation and amyloid deposition in mild cognitive impairment: a PET study. *Neurology*. 2009;72(1):56–62.

20. Fumagalli F, Molteni R, Calabrese F, Maj PF, Racagni G, Riva MA. Neurotrophic factors in neurodegenerative disorders : potential for therapy. *CNS Drugs*. 2008;22(12):1005–1019.

21. Wilson RS, Arnold SE, Beck TL, Bienias JL, Bennett DA. Change in depressive symptoms during the prodromal phase of Alzheimer disease. *Arch Gen Psychiatry*. 2008;65(4):439–445.

22. Ballard CG, Cassidy G, Bannister C, Mohan RN. Prevalence, symptom profile, and aetiology of depression in dementia sufferers. *J Affect Disord*. 1993;29:1–6.

23. Cummings JL, Ross W, Absher J, Gornbein J, Hadjiaghai L. Depressive symptoms in Alzheimer disease: assessment and determinants. *Alzheimer Dis Assoc Disord*. 1995;9:87–93.

24. Verhey FR, Rozendaal N, Ponds RW, Jolles J. Dementia, awareness and depression. *Int J Geriatr Psychiatry*. 1993;8:851–856.

25. Forsell Y, Palmer K, Fratiglioni L. Psychiatric symptoms/syndromes in elderly persons with mild cognitive impairment. Data from a cross-sectional study. *Acta Neurol Scand Suppl*. 2003;179:25–28.

26. Lopez OL, Becker JT, Sweet RA. Non-cognitive symptoms in mild cognitive impairment subjects. *Neurocase*. 2005;11:65–71.

27. Janzing JG, Hooijer C, van 't Hof MA, Zitman FG. Depression in subjects with and without dementia: a comparison using GMS-AGECAT. *Int J Geriatr Psychiatry*. 2002;17(1):1–5.

28. Zubenko GS, Zubenko WN, McPherson S, et al. A collaborative study of the emergence and clinical features of the major depressive syndrome of Alzheimer's disease. *Am J Psychiatry*. 2003;160(5):857–866.

29. Engedal K, Barca ML, Laks J, Selbaek G. Depression in Alzheimer's disease: specificity of depressive symptoms using three different clinical criteria. *Int J Geriatr Psychiatry*. 2011;26(9):944–951.

30. Even C, Weintraub D. Case for and against specificity of depression in Alzheimer's disease. *Psychiatry Clin Neurosci*. 2010;64(4):358–366.

31. Van der Mussele S, Bekelaar K, Le Bastard N, et al. Prevalence and associated behavioral symptoms of depression in mild cognitive impairment and dementia due to Alzheimer's disease. *Int J Geriatr Psychiatry*. 2013;28(9):947–958.

32. Aalten P, de Vugt ME, Jaspers N, Jolles J, Verhey FR. The course of neuropsychiatric symptoms in dementia. Part I: findings from the two-year longitudinal Maasbed study. *Int J Geriatr Psychiatry*. 2005;20(6):523–530.

33. Ballard CG, Margallo-Lana M, Fossey J, et al. A 1-year follow-up study of behavioral and psychological symptoms in dementia among people in care environments. *J Clin Psychiatry*. 2001;62(8):631–636.

34. Payne JL, Sheppard JM, Steinberg M, et al. Incidence, prevalence, and outcomes of depression in residents of a long-term care facility with dementia. *Int J Geriatr Psychiatry*. 2002;17:247–253.

35. Lopez O, Becker J, Sweet RA, et al. Psychiatric symptoms vary with the severity of dementia in probable Alzheimer's disease. *J Neuropsychiatry Clin Neurosci*. 2003;15(3):346–353.

36. Arlt S, Hornung J, Eichenlaub M, Jahn H, Bullinger M, Petersen C. The patient with dementia, the caregiver and the doctor: cognition, depression and quality of life from three perspectives. *Int J Geriatr Psychiatry*. 2008;23(6):604–610.

37. Teng E, Ringman JM, Ross LK, et al.; Alzheimer's Disease Research Centers of California-Depression in Alzheimer's Disease Investigators. Diagnosing depression in Alzheimer disease with the national institute of mental health provisional criteria. *Am J Geriatr Psychiatry*. 2008;16(6):469–477.

38. Kabasakalian A, Finney GR. Reversible dementias. *Int Rev Neurobiol*. 2009;84:283–302.

39. Starkstein SE, Petracca G, Chemerinski E, Kremer J. Syndromic validity of apathy in Alzheimer's disease. *Am J Psychiatry*. 2001;158(6):872–877.

40. de Jonghe JF, Goedhart AW, Ooms ME, et al. Negative symptoms in Alzheimer's disease: a confirmatory factor analysis. *Int J Geriatr Psychiatry*. 2003;18(8):748–753.

41. Starkstein SE, Mizrahi R, Power BD. Depression in Alzheimer's disease: phenomenology, clinical correlates and treatment. *Int Rev Psychiatry*. 2008;20(4):382–388.

42. Teng E, Lu PH, Cummings JL. Neuropsychiatric symptoms are associated with progression from mild cognitive impairment to Alzheimer's disease. *Dement Geriatr Cogn Disord.* 2007;24(4):253–259.

43. Steele C, Rovner B, Chase GA, Folstein M. Psychiatric symptoms and nursing home placement of patients with Alzheimer's disease. *Am J Psychiatry.* 1990;147(8):1049–1051.

44. Kopetz S, Steele CD, Brandt J, et al. Characteristics and outcomes of dementia residents in an assisted living facility. *Int J Geriatr Psychiatry.* 2000;15(7):586–593.

45. Lyketsos CG, Lindell Veiel L, Baker A, Steele C. A randomized, controlled trial of bright light therapy for agitated behaviors in dementia patients residing in long-term care. *Int J Geriatr Psychiatry.* 1999;14(7):520–525.

46. González-Salvador MT, Arango C, Lyketsos CG, Barba AC. The stress and psychological morbidity of the Alzheimer patient caregiver. *Int J Geriatr Psychiatry.* 1999;14(9):701–710.

47. Levy K, Lanctôt KL, Farber SB, Li A, Herrmann N. Does pharmacological treatment of neuropsychiatric symptoms in Alzheimer's disease relieve caregiver burden? *Drugs Aging.* 2012;29(3):167–179.

48. Thompson S, Herrmann N, Rapoport MJ, Lanctôt KL. Efficacy and safety of antidepressants for treatment of depression in Alzheimer's disease: a metaanalysis. *Can J Psychiatry.* 2007;52(4):248–255.

49. Banerjee S, Hellier J, Dewey M, et al. Sertraline or mirtazapine for depression in dementia (HTA-SADD): a randomised, multicentre, double-blind, placebo-controlled trial. *Lancet.* 2011;378(9789):403–411.

50. APA Work Group on Alzheimer's Disease and other Dementias, Rabins PV, Blacker D, Rovner BW, et al. American Psychiatric Association practice guideline for the treatment of patients with Alzheimer's disease and other dementias. Second edition. *Am J Psychiatry.* 2007;164(12 Suppl):5–56.

51. Lawlor BA. Behavioral and psychological symptoms in dementia: the role of atypical antipsychotics. *J Clin Psychiatry.* 2004;65(Suppl 1):5–10.

52. Gareri P, De Fazio P, Manfredi VG, De Sarro G. Use and safety of antipsychotics in behavioral disorders in elderly people with dementia. *J Clin Psychopharmacol.* 2014;34(1):109–123.

53. Jeste DV, Blazer D, Casey D, et al. ACNP White Paper: update on use of antipsychotic drugs in elderly persons with dementia. *Neuropsychopharmacology.* 2008;33(5)957–970.

54. Cummings JL, Schneider L, Tariot PN, Kershaw PR, Weiying Y. Reduction of behavioural disturbances and caregiver distress by galantamine in patients with Alzheimer's disease. *Am J Psychiatry.* 2004;161:532–538.

55. Gauthier S, Feldman H, Hecker J, Vellas B, Emir B, Subbiah P; Donepezil MSAD study investigators group. Functional, cognitive, and behavioral effects of donepezil in patients with moderate Alzheimer's disease. *Curr Med Res Opin.* 2002;18:347–354.

56. Mega MS, Masterman DM, O'Connor SM, Barclay TR, Cummings JL. The spectrum of behavioral responses to cholinesterase inhibitor therapy in Alzheimer disease. *Arch Neurol.* 1999;56:1388–1393.

57. Pinheiro D. Anticonvulsant mood stabilizers in the treatment of behavioral and psychological symptoms of dementia (BPSD). *Encephale.* 2008;34(4):409–415.

58. Padala PR, Burke WJ, Shostrom VK, et al. Methylphenidate for apathy and functional status in dementia of the Alzheimer type. *Am J Geriatr Psychiatry.* 2010;18(4):371–374.

59. Galynker I, Ieronimo C. Methylphenidate treatment of negative symptoms in patients with dementia. *J Neuropsychiatry Clin Neurosci.* 1997;9(2):231–239.

60. Oudman E. Is electroconvulsive therapy (ECT) effective and safe for treatment of depression in dementia? A short review. *J ECT.* 2012;28(1):34–38.

61. Merrill C, Jonsson MA, et al. Vagus nerve stimulation in patients with Alzheimer's disease: Additional follow-up results of a pilot study through 1 year. *J Clin Psychiatry.* 2006;67:1171–1178.

62. Sjogren MJ, Hellstrom PT, Jonsson MA, Runnerstam M, Silander HC, Ben-Menachem E. Cognition-enhancing effect of vagus nerve stimulation in patients with Alzheimer's disease: a pilot study. *J Clin Psychiatry.* 2002;63:972–980.

63. Ahmed MA, Darwish ES, Khedr EM, El Serogy YM, Ali AM. Effects of low versus high frequencies of repetitive transcranial magnetic stimulation on cognitive function and cortical excitability in Alzheimer's dementia. *J Neurol.* 2012;259:83–92.

64. Bentwich J, Dobronevsky E, Aichenbaum S, et al. Beneficial effect of repetitive transcranial magnetic stimulation combined with cognitive training for the treatment of Alzheimer's disease: a proof of concept study. *J Neural Transm Vienna.* 2011;118:463–471.

65. Takahashi S, Mizukami K, Yasuno F, Asada T. Depression associated with dementia with Lewy bodies (DLB) and the effect of somatotherapy. *Psychogeriatrics.* 2009;9:56–61.

66. Ecklund-Johnson E, Torres I. Unawareness of deficits in Alzheimer's disease and other dementias: operational definitions and empirical findings. *Neuropsychol Rev.* 2005;15(3):147–166.

67. Bunn F, Goodman C, Sworn K, et al. Psychosocial factors that shape patient and carer experiences of dementia diagnosis and treatment: a systematic review of qualitative studies. *PLoS Med.* 2012;9(10):1–12.

68. Werner P, Karnieli-Miller O, Eidelman S. Current knowledge and future directions about the disclosure of dementia: a systematic review of the first decade of the 21st century. *Alzheimers Dement.* 2013;9(2):74–88.

69. Brodaty H, Donkin M. Family caregivers of people with dementia. *Dialogues Clin Neurosci.* 2009;11(2):217–228.

70. van Vliet D, de Vugt ME, Bakker C, Koopmans RT, Verhey FR. Impact of early onset dementia on caregivers: a review. *Int J Geriatr Psychiatry.* 2010;25(11):1091–1100.

71. Black W, Almeida OP. A systematic review of the association between the behavioral and psychological symptoms of dementia and burden of care. *Int Psychogeriatr.* 2004;16(3):295–315.

72. Brodaty H, Arasaratnam C. Meta-analysis of nonpharmacological interventions for neuropsychiatric symptoms of dementia. *Am J Psychiatry.* 2012;169(9):946–953.

73. Mittelman MS, Brodaty H, Wallen AS, Burns A. A three-country randomized controlled trial of a psychosocial intervention for caregivers combined with pharmacological treatment for patients with Alzheimer disease: effects on caregiver depression. *Am J Geriatr Psychiatry.* 2008;16(11):893–904.

74. Vernooij-Dassen M, Draskovic I, McCleary J, Downs M. Cognitive reframing for carers of people with dementia. *Cochrane Database Syst Rev.* 2011;11:1–37.

75. Olazarán J, Reisberg B, Clare L, et al., Nonpharmacological therapies in Alzheimer's disease: a systematic review of efficacy. *Dement Geriatr Cogn Disord.* 2010;30:161–178.

76. Garand L, Dew MA, Eazor LR, DeKosky ST, Reynolds CF 3rd. Caregiving burden and psychiatric morbidity in spouses of persons with mild cognitive impairment. *Int J Geriatr Psychiatry*. 2005;20(6):512–522.

77. Diehl-Schmid J, Schmidt EM, Nunnemann, et al. Caregiver burden and needs in frontotemporal dementia. *J Geriat Psychiary Neurol*. 2013;26(4):221–229.

78. Czaja SJ, Loewenstein D, Schulz R, Nair SN, Perdomo D. A videophone psychosocial intervention for dementia caregivers. *Am J Geriatr Psychiatry*. 2013;21(11):1071–1081.

79. Orgeta V, Qazi A, Spector AE, Orrell M. Psychological treatments for depression and anxiety in dementia and mild cognitive impairment. *Cochrane Database Syst Rev*. 2014;1:1–59.

80. Carreira K, Miller M, Reynolds C, et al. A controlled evaluation of monthly maintenance interpersonal psychotherapy in late-life depression with varying levels of cognitive function. *Int J Geriatr Psychiatry*. 2008;23(11):1110–1113.

81. Regan B, Varanelli L. Adjustment, depression, and anxiety in mild cognitive impairment and early dementia: a systematic review of psychological intervention studies. *Int Psychogeriatr*. 2013;25(12):1963–1984.

82. Burns A, Guthrie E, Byrne J, et al. Brief psychotherapy in Alzheimer's disease: randomised controlled trial. *Br J Psychiatry*. 2005;187(2):143–147.

83. Bharucha AJ, Dew MA, Miller MD, Borson MD, Reynolds C III. Psychotherapy in long-term care: a review. *J Am Med Dir Assoc*. 2006;7(9):568–580.

84. Alexopoulos GS, Raue P, Areán P. Problem-solving therapy versus supportive therapy in geriatric major depression with executive dysfunction. *Am J Geriatr Psychiatry*. 2003;11(1):46–52.

85. Alexopoulos GS, Raue PJ, Kiosses DN, et al. Problem solving therapy and supportive therapy in older adults with major depression and executive dysfunction: effect on disability. *Arch Gen Psychiatry*. 2011;68(1):33–41.

86. Junaid O, Hegde S. Supportive psychotherapy in dementia. *Adv Psychiatr Treatment*. 2007;13:17–23.

87. Kiosses DN, Arean PA, Teri L, Alexopoulos GS. Home-delivered problem adaptation therapy (PATH) for depressed, cognitively impaired, disabled elders: A preliminary study. *Am J Geriatr Psychiatry*. 2010;18(11):988–998.

88. Teri L, Logsdon RG, Uomoto J, McCurry SM. Behavioral treatment of depression in dementia patients: a controlled clinical trial. *Gerontol B Psychol Sci Soc Sci*. 1997;53:159–166.

89. Burgener SC, Buettner LL, Beattie E, Rose KM. Effectiveness of community-based, nonpharmacological interventions for early-stage dementia: conclusions and recommendations. *J Gerontol Nurs*. 2009;35(3):50–57.

90. Cheston R, Jones R. A small-scale study comparing the impact of psycho-education and exploratory psychotherapy groups on newcomers to a group for people with dementia. *Aging Ment Health*. 2009;13(3):420–425.

91. Logsdon RG, Pike KC, McCurry SM, et al. Early-stage memory loss support groups: outcomes from a randomized controlled clinical trial. *J Gerontol B Psychol Sci Soc Sci*. 2010;65B(6):691–697.

92. Waldorff FB, Buss DV, Eckermann A, et al. Efficacy of psychosocial intervention in patients with mild Alzheimer's disease: the multicentre, rater blinded, randomised Danish Alzheimer Intervention Study (DAISY). *BMJ*. 2012;345:1–14.

93. Phung KT, Waldorff FB, Buss DV, et al. A three-year follow-up on the efficacy of psychosocial interventions for patients with mild dementia and their caregivers: the multicentre, rater-blinded, randomised Danish Alzheimer Intervention Study (DAISY). *BMJ Open*. 2013;3(11):e003584.

94. Bruvik FK, Allore HG, Ranhoff AH, Engedal K. The effect of psychosocial support intervention on depression in patients with dementia and their family caregivers: an assessor-blinded randomized controlled trial. *Dement Geriatr Cogn Dis Extra*. 20133(1):386–397.

95. Brodaty H, Green A, Koschera A. Meta-analysis of psychosocial interventions for caregivers of people with dementia. *J Am Geriatr Soc*. 2003;51(5):657–664.

96. Woods B, Aguirre E, Spector AE, Orrell M. Cognitive stimulation to improve cognitive functioning in people with dementia (Review). *Cochrane Database Syst Rev*. 2012;2:1–80.

97. Clare L, Woods RT, Moniz Cook ED, Orrell M, Spector A. Cognitive rehabilitation and cognitive training for early-stage Alzheimer's disease and vascular dementia. *Cochrane Cochrane Database Syst Rev*. 2003;(4):1–39.

98. Choi J, Twamly EW. Cognitive rehabilitation therapies for Alzheimer's disease: a review of methods to improve treatment engagement and self-efficacy. *Neuropsychol Rev*. 2013;23:48–62.

99. Kurz A, Pohl C, Ramsenthaler M, Sorg C. Cognitive rehabilitation in patients with mild cognitive impairment. *Int J Geriatr Psychiatry*. 2009;24:163–168.

100. Olazarán J, Muñiz R, Reisberg B, et al. Benefits of cognitive-motor intervention in MCI and mild to moderate Alzheimer disease. *Neurology*. 2004;63(12):2348–2353.

101. Teri L, Gibbons LE, McCurry SM. Exercise plus behavioral management in patients with Alzheimer disease: a randomized controlled trial. *JAMA*. 2003;290(15):2015–2022.

102. Sitzer DI, Twamley EW, Jeste DV. Cognitive training in Alzheimer's disease: a meta-analysis of the literature. *Acta Psychiatr Scand*. 2006;114:75–90.

103. Lawrence V, Fossey J, Ballard C, Moniz-Cook E, Murray J. Improving quality of life for people with dementia in care homes: making psychosocial interventions work. *Br J Psychiatry*. 2012;201(5):344–351.

104. Gitlin LN, Kales HC, Lyketsos CG. Managing behavioral symptoms in dementia using nonpharmacologic approaches: an overview. *JAMA*. 2012;308(19):2020–2029.

105. Vernooij-Dassen M, Vasee E, Zuidema S, Cohen-Mansfield J, Myle W. Psychosocial interventions for dementia patients in long-term care. *Int Psychogeriatr*. 2010;22(7):1121–1128.

106. Brodaty H, Burns K. Nonpharmacological management of apathy in dementia: a systematic review. *Am J Geriatr Psychiatry*. 2012;20(7):549–564.

107. Van Haitsma KS, Curyto K, Abbott KM, Towsley GL, Spector A, Kleban M. A randomized controlled trial for an individualized positive psychosocial intervention for the affective and behavioral symptoms of dementia in nursing home residents. *J Gerontol B Psychol Sci Soc Sci*. 2013;70(1):35–45.

108. Ferrero-Arias J, Goñi-Imízcoz M, González-Bernal J, Lara-Ortega F, da Silva-González A, Díez-Lopez M. The efficacy of nonpharmacological treatment for dementia-related apathy. *Azheimer Dis Assoc Disord*. 2011;25(3):213–219.

109. Teri L, McKenzie G, LaFazia D. Psychosocial treatment of depression in older adults with dementia. *Clin Psychol Sci Pract*. 2005;12(3):303–316.

110. Verkaik R, van Weert J, Francke A. The effects of psychosocial methods on depressed, aggressive and apathetic behaviors of people with dementia: a systematic review. *Int J Geriatr Psychiatry*. 2005;20(4):301–314.

111. O'Connor DW, Ames D, Gardner B, King M. Psychosocial treatments of psychological symptoms in dementia: a systematic review of reports meeting quality standards. *Int Psychogeriatr*. 2009;21(2):241–251.

112. Gillen R, Tennen H, McKee TE, Gernert-Dott P. ScienceDirect.com—Archives of physical medicine and rehabilitation—depressive symptoms and history of depression predict rehabilitation efficiency in stroke patients. *Arch Phys Med Rehabil*. 2001;82(12):1645–1649.

113. Go AS, Mozaffarian D, Roger VL, et al. Heart disease and stroke statistics—2013 update: A report from the American Heart Association. *Circulation*. 2013;127(1):e6–e245.

114. Hackett ML, Yapa CC, Parag VV, Anderson CS. Frequency of depression after stroke: a systematic review of observational studies. *Stroke*. 2005;36(6):1330–1340.

115. Sinyor D, Amato P, Kaloupek DG, Becker R, Goldenberg M, Coopersmith H. Post-stroke depression: relationships to functional impairment, coping strategies, and rehabilitation outcome. *Stroke*. 1986;17(6):1102–1107.

116. Robinson RG, Szetela B. Mood change following left hemispheric brain injury. *Ann Neurol*. 1981;9(5):447–453.

117. Narushima K, Kosier JT, Robinson RG. A reappraisal of poststroke depression, intra- and inter-hemispheric lesion location using meta-analysis. *J Neuropsychiatry*. 2003;15(4):422–430.

118. Mayberg HS, Robinson RG, Wong DF. PET imaging of cortical S2 serotonin receptors after stroke: lateralized changes and relationship to depression. *Am J Psychiatry*. 1988;145:937–943.

119. Spalletta G, Ripa A, Caltagirone C. Symptom profile of DSM-IV major and minor depressive disorders in first-ever stroke patients. *Am J Geriatr Psychiatry*. 2012;13(2):108–115.

120. Whyte EM, Mulsant BH. Post stroke depression: epidemiology, pathophysiology, and biological treatment. *Biol Psychiatry*. 2002;52(3):253–264.

121. Marin RS. Differential diagnosis and classification of apathy. *Am J Psychiatry*. 1990;147(1):22–30.

122. Levy ML, Cummings JL, Fairbanks LA, et al. Apathy is not depression. *J Neuropsychiatry*. 1998;10(3):314–319.

123. Marin RS, Firinciogullari S, Biedrzycki RC. Group differences in the relationship between apathy and depression. *J Nerv Ment Dis*. 1994;182(4):235–239.

124. Withall A, Brodaty H, Altendorf A, Sachdev PS. A longitudinal study examining the independence of apathy and depression after stroke: the Sydney Stroke Study. *Int Psychogeriatr*. 2010;23(02):264–273.

125. Berman K, Brodaty H, Withall A, Seeher K. Pharmacologic treatment of apathy in dementia. *Am J Geriatr Psychiatry*. 2012;20(2):104–122.

126. Currier MB, Murray GB, Welch CC. Electroconvulsive therapy for post-stroke depressed geriatric patients. *J Neuropsychiatry Clin Neurosci*. 1992;4(2):140–144.

127. Hackett M, Anderson C, House A, Xia J. Interventions for treating depression after stroke. *Cochrane Database Syst Rev*. 2008;(4):CD003437.

128. Alexopoulos GS, Meyers BS, Young RC, Campbell S, Silbersweig D, Charlson M. "Vascular depression" hypothesis. *Arch Gen Psychiatry*. 1997;54(10):915–922.

129. González HM, Tarraf W, Whitfield K, Gallo JJ. Vascular depression prevalence and epidemiology in the United States. *J Psychiatr Res*. 2012;46(4):456–461.

130. O'Brien J, Desmond P, Ames D, Schweitzer I, Harrigan S, Tress B. A magnetic resonance imaging study of white matter lesions in depression and Alzheimer's disease. *Br J Psychiatry*. 1996;168:477–485.

131. Thomas AJ, Perry R, Kalaria RN, Oakley A, McMeekin W, O'Brien JT. Neuropathological evidence for ischemia in the white matter of the dorsolateral prefrontal cortex in late-life depression. *Int J Geriatr Psychiatry*. 2003;18(1):7–13.

132. Thomas AJ, O'Brien JT, Davis S, et al. Ischemic basis for deep white matter hyperintensities in major depression: a neuropathological study. *Arch Gen Psychiatry*. 2002;59(9):785–792.

133. Pimontel MA, Reinlieb ME, Johnert LC, Garcon E, Sneed JR, Roose SP. The external validity of MRI-defined vascular depression. *Int J Geriatr Psychiatry*. 2013;28(11):1189–1196.

134. Taylor WD, Steffens DC, MacFall JR, et al. White matter hyperintensity progression and late-life depression outcomes. *Arch Gen Psychiatry*. 2003;60(11):1090–1096.

135. Sheline YI, Barch DM, Garcia K, et al. Cognitive function in late life depression: relationships to depression severity, cerebrovascular risk factors and processing speed. *Biol Psychiatry*. 2006;60(1):58–65.

136. Sneed JR, Culang ME, Keilp JG, Rutherford BR, Devanand DP, Roose SP. Antidepressant medication and executive dysfunction: a deleterious interaction in late-life depression. *Am J Geriatr Psychiatry*. 2010;18(2):128–135.

137. Jorge RE, Moser DJ, Acion L. Treatment of vascular depression using repetitive transcranial magnetic stimulation. *Arch Gen Psychiatry*. 2008;65(3):268–276.

138. Coffey CE, Hinkle PE, Weiner RD, et al. Electroconvulsive therapy of depression in patients with white matter hyperintensity. *Biol Psychiatry*. 1987;22:629–636.

139. Alves G, Forsaa EB, Pedersen KF, Dreetz Gjerstad M, Larsen JP. Epidemiology of Parkinson's disease. *J Neurol*. 2008;255(S5):18–32.

140. Reijnders JS, Ehrt U, Weber WE, Aarsland D, Leentjens AF. A systematic review of prevalence studies of depression in Parkinson's disease. *Mov Disord*. 2008;23(2):183–189.

141. Ishihara L, Brayne C. A systematic review of depression and mental illness preceding Parkinson's disease. *Acta Neurol Scand*. 2006;113(4):211–220.

142. Noyce AJ, Bestwick JP, Silveira-Moriyama L, et al. Meta-analysis of early nonmotor features and risk factors for Parkinson disease. *Ann Neurol*. 2012;72(6):893–901.

143. Tolosa E, Compta Y, Gaig C. The premotor phase of Parkinson's disease. *Parkinsonism Relat Disord*. 2007;13:S2–S7.

144. Schuurman AG, van den Akker M, Ensinck KT, et al. Increased risk of Parkinson's disease after depression: A retrospective cohort study. *Neurology*. 2002;58(10):1501–1504.

145. Menza MA, Mark MH. Parkinson's disease and depression: the relationship to disability and personality. *J Neuropsychiatry*. 1994;6(2):165–169.

146. Starkstein SE, Petracca G, Chemerinski E, et al. Depression in classic versus akinetic-rigid Parkinson's disease. *Mov Disord*. 1998;13(1):29–33.

147. Remy P, Doder M, Lees AJ, Turjanski N, Brooks DJ. Depression in Parkinson's disease: loss of dopamine and noradrenaline innervation in the limbic system. *Brain*. 2005;128(6):1314–1322.

148. Cardoso EF, Maia FM, Fregni F, et al. Depression in Parkinson's disease: Convergence from voxel-based morphometry and functional magnetic resonance imaging in the limbic thalamus. *Neuroimage*. 2009;47(2):467–472.

149. Marsh L, McDonald WM, Cummings J, Ravina B, NINDS/NIMH Work Group on Depression and Parkinson's Disease. Provisional diagnostic criteria for depression in Parkinson's disease: Report of an NINDS/NIMH Work Group. *Mov Disord*. 2006;21(2): 148–158.

150. Erro R, Picillo M, Vitale C, et al. Non-motor symptoms in early Parkinson's disease: a 2-year follow-up study on previously untreated patients. *J Neurol Neurosurg Psychiatr*. 2013;84(1):14–17.

151. Weintraub D, Moberg PJ, Duda JE, Katz IR, Stern MB. Effect of psychiatric and other nonmotor symptoms on disability in Parkinson's disease. *J Am Geriatr Soc*. 2004;52(5):784–788.

152. Politis M, Wu K, Molloy S, G Bain P, Chaudhuri KR, Piccini P. Parkinson's disease symptoms: The patient's perspective. *Mov Disord*. 2010;25(11):1646–1651.

153. Leentjens AF, Verhey FR, Luijckx GJ, Troost J. The validity of the Beck depression inventory as a screening and diagnostic instrument for depression in patients with Parkinson's disease. *Mov Disord*. 2001;15(6):1221–1224.

154. Leentjens AF, Verhey FR, Lousberg R, Spitsbergen H, Wilmink FW. The validity of the Hamilton and Montgomery—Asberg depression rating scales as screening and diagnostic tools for depression in Parkinson's disease. *Int J Geriatr Psychiatry*. 2000;15(7):644–649.

155. Shulman LM, Taback RL, Rabinstein AA, Weiner WJ. Non-recognition of depression and other non-motor symptoms in Parkinson's disease. *Parkinsonism Relat Disord*. 2002;8(3):193–197.

156. Menza M, Dobkin RD, Marin H, et al. A controlled trial of anti-depressants in patients with Parkinson disease and depression. *Neurology*. 2009;72(10):886–892.

157. Okun MS, Fernandez HH. Will tricyclic antidepressants make a comeback for depressed Parkinson disease patients? *Neurology*. 2009;72(10):868–869.

158. Simons JA. Fluoxetine in Parkinson's disease. *Mov Disord*. 1996;11(5):581–582.

159. Kulisevsky J, Pagonabarraga J, Pascual-Sedano B, Gironell A, García-Sánchez C, Martínez-Corral M. Motor changes during sertraline treatment in depressed patients with Parkinson's disease. *Eur J Neurol*. 2008;15(9):953–959.

160. Richard IH, McDermott MP, Kurlan R, et al. A randomized, double-blind, placebo-controlled trial of antidepressants in Parkinson disease. *Neurology*. 2012;78(16):1229–1236.

161. Bonuccelli U, Meco G, Fabbrini G, et al. A non-comparative assessment of tolerability and efficacy of duloxetine in the treatment of depressed patients with Parkinson's disease. *Expert Opin Pharmacother*. 2012;13(16):2269–2280.

162. Raskin S, Durst R. Bupropion as the treatment of choice in depression associated with Parkinson's disease and its various treatments. *Med Hypotheses*. 2010;75(6):544–546.

163. Zaluska M, Dyduch A. Bupropion in the treatment of depression in Parkinson's disease. *Int Psychogeriatr*. 2011;(23):325–327.

164. Korchounov A, Winter Y, Rossy W. Combined beneficial effect of rasagiline on motor function and depression in de novo PD. *Clin Neuropharm*. 2012;35:121–124.

165. Aarsland D, Pahlhagen S, Ballard C, et al. Depression in Parkinson disease—epidemiology, mechanisms and management. *Nat Rev*. 2012;8:35–47.

166. Schuepbach WM, Rau J, Knudsen K, et al., EARLYSTIM Study Group. Neurostimulation for Parkinson's disease with early motor complications. *N Engl J Med*. 2013;368:610–622.

167. Okun MS, Fernandez HH, Wu SS, et al. Cognition and mood in Parkinson's disease in subthalamic nucleus versus globus pallidus interna deep brain stimulation: the COMPARE trial. *Ann Neurol*. 2009;65:586–595.

168. Okun MS, Wu SS, Foote KD, et al. Do stable patients with a premorbid depression history have a worse outcome after deep brain stimulation for Parkinson disease? *Neurosurgery*. 2011;69:357–360.

169. Dobkin RD, Menza M, Allen LA, et al. Cognitive-behavioral therapy for depression in Parkinson's disease: A randomized, controlled trial. *Am J Psychiatry*. 2011;168(10):1066–1074.

170. Dobkin RD, Rubino JT, Allen LA, et al. Predictors of treatment response to cognitive-behavioral therapy for depression in Parkinson's disease. *J Consult Clin Psychol*. 2012;80(4):694–699.

171. Sproeseer E, Viana MA, Quagliato EM, et al. The effect of psychotherapy in patients with PD: a controlled study. *Parkisonism Relat Disord*. 2010;16(4):89–95.

172. A'Campco LE, Wekking EM, Slpithoff-Kamminga NG, Le Cessie S, Roos RA. The benefits of a standardized patient education program for patients with Parkinson's disease and their caregivers. *Parkisonism Relat Disorder*. 2010;16(2):89–95.

173. Yang S, Sajatovic M, Walter B. Psychosocial interventions for depression and anxiety in Parkinson's disease. *J Geriatr Psychiatry Neurol*. 2012;25(2):113–121.

174. Trend P, Kaye J, Gage H, Owen C, Wade D. Short-term effectiveness of intensive multidisciplinary rehabilitation therapy for people with Parkinson's disease and their carers. *Clin Rehabil Relat Res*. 2002;16(7):717–725.

175. Wade DT, Gage H, Owen C, Wade D. Multidisciplinary rehabilitation for people with Parkinson's Disease: a randomized controlled study. *J Neurol Neurosurg Psychiatry*. 2003;74(2): 158–162.

176. Huntington G. On chorea. *Med Surg Rep Philadelphia*. 1872;26: 317–321.

177. Pringsheim T, Wiltshire K, Day L, et al. The incidence and prevalence of Huntington's disease: a systematic review and meta-analysis. *Mov Disord*. 2012;27:1083–1091.

178. Van Duijn E, Kingma EM, Timman R, et al. Cross-sectional study on prevalences of psychiatric disorders in mutation carriers of Huntington's disease compared with mutation-negative first-degree relatives. *J Clin Psychiatry*. 2008;69:1804–1810.

179. Paulsen JS, Ready RE, Hamilton JM, Mega MS, Cummings JL. Neuropsychiatric aspects of Huntington's disease. *J Neurol Neurosurg Psychiatry*. 2001;71:310–314.

180. Gusella J, Wexler NS, Conneally PM, et al. A polymorphic DNA marker genetically linked to Huntington's disease. *Nature*. 1983;306:234–238.

181. Zuccato C, Valenza M, Cattaneo E. Molecular mechanisms and potential therapeutical targets in Huntington's disease. *Physiol Rev*. 2010;90:905–981.

182. Mayberg HS, Starkstein SE, Peyser CE, et al: Paralimbic frontal lobe hypometabolism in depression associated with Huntington's disease. *Neurology*. 1992;42:1791–1797.

183. Mindham RH, Steele C, Folstein MF, Lucas J. A comparison of the frequency of major affective disorder in Huntington's disease and Alzheimer's disease. *J Neurol Neurosurg Psychiatry*. 1985; 48:1172–1174.

184. Anderson K, Louis ED, Stern Y, Marder KS. Cognitive correlates of obsessive and compulsive symptoms in Huntington's disease. *Am J Psychiatry*. 2001;158:799–801.

185. Paulsen JS, Ready RE, Hamilton JM, Mega MS, Cummings JL. Neuropsychiatric aspects of Huntington's disease. *J Neurol Neurosurg Psychiatry*. 2001;71:310–314.

186. Marder K, Zhao H, Myers RH. Rate of functional decline in Huntington's disease. Huntington Study Group. *Neurology*. 2000;54:452–458.

187. Zappacosta B, Monza D, Meoni C, et al. Psychiatric symptoms do not correlate with cognitive decline, motor symptoms, or CAG repeat length in Huntington's disease. *Arch Neurol*. 1996;53(6):493–497.

188. Farrer LA. Suicide and attempted suicide in Huntington's disease: implications for preclinical testing of persons at risk. *Am Med Genet*. 1986;24:305–311.

189. Meiser B, Dunn S. Psychological impact of genetic testing for Huntington's disease: an update of the literature. *J Neurol Neurosurg Psychiatry*. 2000;69:574–578.

190. De Souza J, Jones LA, Rickards H. Validation of self-report depression rating scales in Huntington's disease. *Mov Disord*. 2010;25:91–96.

191. Rickards H, DeSouza J, Crooks J, et al. Discriminant analysis of Beck depression inventory and Hamilton rating scale for depression in Huntington's disease. *J Neuropsychiatry Clin Neurosci*. 2011;23:399–402.

192. Holl AK, Wilkinson L, Painold A, Holl EM, Bonelli RM. Combating depression in Huntington's disease: effective antidepressive treatment with venlafaxine XR. *Int Clin Psychopharmacol*. 2010;25(1):46–50.

193. Patel SV, Tariot PN, Asnis J. L-Deprenyl augmentation of fluoxetine in a patient with Huntington's disease. *Ann Clin Psychiatry*. 1996;8:23–26.

194. Ford MF. Treatment of depression in Huntington's disease with monoamine oxidase inhibitors. *Br J Psychiatry*. 1986;149:654–656.

195. Ciammola A, Sassone J, Colciago C, et al. Aripiprazole in the treatment of Huntington's disease: a case series. *Neuropsychiatr Dis Treat*. 2009;5:1–4.

196. Cusin C, Franco FB, Fernandez-Robles C, DuBois CM, Welch CA. Rapid improvement of depression and psychotic symptoms in Huntington's disease: a retrospective chart review of seven patients treated with electroconvulsive therapy. *Gen Hosp Psychiatry*. 2013;35(6):678. e3–5.

197. Shukla A, Jayarajan RN, Muralidharan K, Jain S. Repetitive transcranial magnetic stimulation not beneficial in severe choreiform movements of Huntington disease. *J ECT*. 2013;29(2):e16–e17.

198. Sullivan FR, Bird ED, Alpay M, Cha JH. Remotivation therapy and Huntington's disease. *J Neurosci Nurs*. 2001;33:136–142.

199. Mohr DC, Hart SL, Fonareva I, Tasch ES. Treatment of depression for patients with multiple sclerosis in neurology clinics. *Mult Scler*. 2006;12(2):204–208.

200. McGuigan C, Hutchinson M. Unrecognized symptoms of depression in a community-based population with multiple sclerosis. *J Neurol*. 2006;253(2):219–223.

201. D'Alisa S, Miscio G, Baudo S, Simone A, Tesio L, Mauro A. Depression is the main determinant of quality of life in multiple sclerosis: A classification-regression (CART) study. *Disabil Rehabil*. 2006;28(5):307–314.

202. Joffe RT, Lippert GP, Gray TA, Sawa G, Horvath Z. Mood disorder and multiple sclerosis. *Arch Neurol*. 1987;44(4):376–378.

203. Sadovnick AD, Remick RA, Allen J, et al. Depression and multiple sclerosis. *Neurology*. 1996;46(3):628–632.

204. Minden SL, Orav J, Reich P. Depression in multiple sclerosis. *Gen Hosp Psychiatry*. 1987;9(6):426–434.

205. Patten SB, Metz LM, Reimer MA. Biopsychosocial correlates of lifetime major depression in a multiple sclerosis population. *Mult Scler*. 2000;6(2):115–120.

206. Patten SB, Beck CA, Williams JV, Barbui C, Metz LM. Major depression in multiple sclerosis: A population-based perspective. *Neurology*. 2003;61(11):1524–1527.

207. Figved N, Klevan G, Myhr KM, et al. Neuropsychiatric symptoms in patients with multiple sclerosis. *Acta Psychiatr Scand*. 2005;112(6):463–468.

208. Diaz-Olavarrieta C, Cummings JL, Velazquez J, Garcia de la Cadena C. Neuropsychiatric manifestations of multiple sclerosis. *J Neuropsychiatry Clin Neurosci*. 1999;11(1):51–57.

209. Chwastiak L, Ehde DM, Gibbons LE, Sullivan M, Bowen JD, Kraft GH. Depressive symptoms and severity of illness in multiple sclerosis: Epidemiologic study of a large community sample. *Am J Psychiatry*. 2002;159(11):1862–1868.

210. Beiske AG, Svensson E, Sandanger I, et al. Depression and anxiety amongst multiple sclerosis patients. *Eur J Neurol*. 2008;15(3):239–245.

211. Sadovnick AD, Eisen K, Ebers GC, Paty DW. Cause of death in patients attending multiple sclerosis clinics. *Neurology*. 1991;41(8):1193–1196.

212. Feinstein A. An examination of suicidal intent in patients with multiple sclerosis. *Neurology*. 2002;59(5):674–678.

213. Stenager EN, Koch-Henriksen N, Stenager E. Risk factors for suicide in multiple sclerosis. *Psychother Psychosom*. 1996;65(2): 86–90.

214. Stenager EN, Stenager E, Koch-Henriksen N, et al. Suicide and multiple sclerosis: An epidemiological investigation. *J Neurol Neurosurg Psychiatry*. 1992;55(7):542–545.

215. Joffe RT, Lippert GP, Gray TA, Sawa G, Horvath Z. Personal and family history of affective illness in patients with multiple sclerosis. *J Affect Disord*. 1987;12(1):63–65.

216. Pujol J, Bello J, Deus J, Marti-Vilalta JL, Capdevila A. Lesions in the left arcuate fasciculus region and depressive symptoms in multiple sclerosis. *Neurology*. 1997;49(4):1105–1110.

217. Bakshi R, Czarnecki D, Shaikh ZA, et al. Brain MRI lesions and atrophy are related to depression in multiple sclerosis. *Neuroreport*. 2000;11(6):1153–1158.

218. Feinstein A, Roy P, Lobaugh N, Feinstein K, O'Connor P, Black S. Structural brain abnormalities in multiple sclerosis patients with major depression. *Neurology*. 2004;62(4):586–590.

219. Gold SM, Kern KC, O'Connor MF, et al. Smaller cornu ammonis 2–3/dentate gyrus volumes and elevated cortisol in multiple sclerosis patients with depressive symptoms. *Biol Psychiatry*. 2010;68(6):553–559.

220. Kiy G, Lehmann P, Hahn HK, Eling P, Kastrup A, Hildebrandt H. Decreased hippocampal volume, indirectly measured, is associated with depressive symptoms and consolidation deficits in multiple sclerosis. *Mult Scler*. 2011;17(9):1088–1097.

221. Feinstein A, O'Connor P, Akbar N, Moradzadeh L, Scott CJ, Lobaugh NJ. Diffusion tensor imaging abnormalities in depressed multiple sclerosis patients. *Mult Scler*. 2010;16(2):189–196.

222. Sabatini U, Pozzilli C, Pantano P, et al. Involvement of the limbic system in multiple sclerosis patients with depressive disorders. *Biol Psychiatry*. 1996;39(11):970–975.

223. Passamonti L, Cerasa A, Liguori M, et al. Neurobiological mechanisms underlying emotional processing in relapsing-remitting multiple sclerosis. *Brain*. 2009;132(Pt 12):3380–3391.

224. Michelson D, Stone L, Galliven E, et al. Multiple sclerosis is associated with alterations in hypothalamic–pituitary–adrenal axis function. *J Clin Endocrinol Metab*. 1994;79(3):848–853.

225. Pucak ML, Carroll KA, Kerr DA, Kaplin AI. Neuropsychiatric manifestations of depression in multiple sclerosis: Neuroinflammatory, neuroendocrine, and neurotrophic mechanisms in the pathogenesis of immune-mediated depression. *Dialogues Clin Neurosci*. 2007;9(2):125–139.

226. Gold SM, Kruger S, Ziegler KJ, et al. Endocrine and immune substrates of depressive symptoms and fatigue in multiple sclerosis patients with comorbid major depression. *J Neurol Neurosurg Psychiatry*. 2011;82(7):814—818.

227. Fassbender K, Schmidt R, Mossner R, et al. Mood disorders and dysfunction of the hypothalamic–pituitary–adrenal axis in multiple sclerosis: Association with cerebral inflammation. *Arch Neurol*. 1998;55(1):66–72.

228. Feinstein A, O'Connor P, Feinstein K. Multiple sclerosis, interferon beta-1b and depression A prospective investigation. *J Neurol*. 2002;249(7):815–820.

229. Minden SL, Feinstein A, Kalb RC, Miller D, et al. Evidence-based guideline: Assessment and management of psychiatric disorders in individuals with MS: Report of the Guideline Development Subcommittee of the American Academy of Neurology. *Neurology*. 2014;82:174–181.

230. Mohr DC, Likosky W, Dwyer P, Van Der Wende J, Boudewyn AC, Goodkin DE. Course of depression during the initiation of interferon beta-1a treatment for multiple sclerosis. *Arch Neurol*. 1999;56(10):1263–1265.

231. Mohr DC, Goodkin DE, Likosky W, Gatto N, Baumann KA, Rudick RA. Treatment of depression improves adherence to interferon beta-1b therapy for multiple sclerosis. *Arch Neurol*. 1997;54(5):531–533.

232. Pakenham KI. Adjustment to multiple sclerosis: Application of a stress and coping model. *Health Psychol*. 1999;18(4):383–392.

233. Lynch SG, Kroencke DC, Denney DR. The relationship between disability and depression in multiple sclerosis: the role of uncertainty, coping and hope. *Mult Scler*. 2001;7(6):411–416.

234. Arnett PA, Higginson CI, Voss WD, Randolph JJ, Grandey AA. Relationship between coping, cognitive dysfunction and depression in multiple sclerosis. *Clin Neuropsychol*. 2002;16(3):341–355.

235. Arnett PA, Randolph JJ. Longitudinal course of depression symptoms in multiple sclerosis. *J Neurol Neurosurg Psychiatry*. 2006;77(5):606–610.

236. Bakshi R, Shaikh ZA, Miletich RS, et al. Fatigue in multiple sclerosis and its relationship to depression and neurologic disability. *Mult Scler*. 2000;6(3):181–185.

237. Lunde HM, Bjorvatn B, Myhr K-M, Bo L. Clinical assessment and management of sleep disorders in multiple sclerosis: a literature review. *Acta Neurol Scand*. 2013;127(196):24–30.

238. Feinstein A, Kartsounis LD, Miller DH, Youl BD, Ron MA. Clinically isolated lesions of the type seen in multiple sclerosis: A cognitive, psychiatric, and MRI follow up study. *J Neurol Neurosurg Psychiatry*. 1992;55(10):869–876.

239. Arnett PA, Higginson CI, Voss WD, Bender WI, Wurst JM, Tippin JM. Depression in multiple sclerosis: Relationship to working memory capacity. *Neuropsychology*. 1999;13(4):546–556.

240. Arnett PA, Higginson CI, Voss WD, et al. Depressed mood in multiple sclerosis: Relationship to capacity-demanding memory and attentional functioning. *Neuropsychology*. 1999;13(3): 434–446.

241. Demaree HA, Gaudino E, DeLuca J. The relationship between depressive symptoms and cognitive dysfunction in multiple sclerosis. *Cogn Neuropsychiatry*. 2003;8(3):161–171.

242. Figved N, Benedict R, Klevan G, et al. Relationship of cognitive impairment to psychiatric symptoms in multiple sclerosis. *Mult Scler*. 2008;14(8):1084–1090.

243. Dalos NP, Rabins PV, Brooks BR, O'Donnell P. Disease activity and emotional state in multiple sclerosis. *Ann Neurol*. 1983;13(5):573–577.

244. Zabad RK, Patten SB, Metz LM. The association of depression with disease course in multiple sclerosis. *Neurology*. 2005;64(2):359–360.

245. Patten SB, Lavorato DH, Metz LM. Clinical correlates of CES-D depressive symptom ratings in an MS population. *Gen Hosp Psychiatry*. 2005;27(6):439–445.

246. Figved N, Myhr KM, Larsen JP, Aarsland D. Caregiver burden in multiple sclerosis: The impact of neuropsychiatric symptoms. *J Neurol Neurosurg Psychiatry*. 2007;78(10):1097–1102.

247. Diareme S, Tsiantis J, Kolaitis G, et al. Emotional and behavioural difficulties in children of parents with multiple sclerosis: A controlled study in Greece. *Eur Child Adolesc Psychiatry*. 2006;15(6):309–318.

248. Benedict RH, Fishman I, McClellan MM, Bakshi R, Weinstock-Guttman B. Validity of the Beck depression inventory-fast screen in multiple sclerosis. *Mult Scler*. 2003;9(4):393–396.

249. Sjonnesen K, Berzins S, Fiest KM, et al. Evaluation of the 9-item patient health questionnaire (PHQ-9) as an assessment instrument for symptoms of depression in patients with multiple sclerosis. *Postgrad Med*. 2012;124(5):69–77.

250. Goldman Consensus Group. The Goldman Consensus statement of depression in multiple sclerosis. *Mult Scler*. 2005;11:328–337.

251. Mohr DC, Boudewyn AC, Goodkin DE, Bostrom A, Epstein L. Comparative outcomes for individual cognitive-behavior therapy, supportive-expressive group psychotherapy, and sertraline for the treatment of depression in multiple sclerosis. *J Consult Clin Psychol*. 2001;69(6):942–949.

252. Schiffer RB, Wineman NM. Antidepressant pharmacotherapy of depression associated with multiple sclerosis. *Am J Psychiatry*. 1990;147(11):1493–1497.

253. Ehde DM, Kraft GH, Chwastiak L, et al. Efficacy of paroxetine in treating major depressive disorder in persons with multiple sclerosis. *Gen Hosp Psychiatry*. 2008;30(1):40–48.

254. Barak Y, Ur E, Achiron A. Moclobemide treatment in multiple sclerosis patients with comorbid depression: An open-label safety trial. *J Neuropsychiatry Clin Neurosci*. 1999;11(2):271–273.

255. Solaro C, Bergamaschi R, Rezzani C, et al. Duloxetine is effective in treating depression in multiple sclerosis patients: an open label multicenter study. *Clin Neuropharmacol*. 2013;36(4):114–116.

256. Panitch HS, Thisted RA, Smith RA, et al.; Pseudobulbar affect in multiple sclerosis study group. Randomized, controlled trial of dextromethorphan/quinidine for pseudobulbar affect in multiple sclerosis. *Ann Neurol*. 2006;59:780–787.

257. Rasmussen KG, Keegan BM. Electroconvulsive therapy in patients with multiple sclerosis. *J ECT*. 2007;23(3):179–180.

258. Pontikes TK, Dinwiddie SH. Electroconvulsive therapy in a patient with multiple sclerosis and recurrent catatonia. *J ECT*. 2010;26(4):270–271.

259. Mattingly G, Baker K, Zorumski CF, Figiel GS. Multiple sclerosis and ECT: Possible value of gadolinium-enhanced magnetic resonance scans for identifying high-risk patients. *J Neuropsychiatry Clin Neurosci*. 1992;4(2):145–151.

260. Schippling S, Tiede M, Lorenz I, et al. Deep transcranial magnet stimulation can improve depression and fatigue in multiple sclerosis—A clinical phase I/IIa study. *Neurology*. 2014;82(10):S33.007.

261. Larcombe NA, Wilson PH. An evaluation of cognitive-behaviour therapy for depression in patients with multiple sclerosis. *Br J Psychiatry*. 1984;145:366–371.

262. Mohr DC, Hart SL, Julian L, et al. Telephone-administered psychotherapy for depression. *Arch Gen Psychiatry*. 2005;62(9):1007–1014.

263. Hind D, O'Cathain A, Cooper CL, et al. The acceptability of computerised cognitive behavioural therapy for the treatment of depression in people with chronic physical disease: A qualitative study of people with multiple sclerosis. *Psychol Health*. 2010;25(6):699–712.

264. Grossman P, Kappos L, Gensicke H, et al. MS quality of life, depression, and fatigue improve after mindfulness training: A randomized trial. *Neurology*. 2010;75(13):1141–1149.

265. Hibbard MR, Uysal S, Kepler K, Bogdany J, Silver J. Axis I psychopathology in individuals with traumatic brain injury. *J Head Trauma Rehabil*. 1998;13(4):24–39.

266. Koponen S, Taiminen T, Portin R, et al. Axis I and II psychiatric disorders after traumatic brain injury: a 30-year follow-up study. *Am J Psychiatry*. 2002;159(8):1315–1321.

267. Kim E, Lauterbach EC, Reeve A, et al. Neuropsychiatric complications of traumatic brain injury: a critical review of the literature (a report by the ANPA Committee on Research). *J Neuropsychiatry Clin Neurosci*. 2007;19(2):106–127.

268. Bombardier CH, Fann JR, Temkin NR, et al. Rates of major depressive disorder and clinical outcomes following traumatic brain injury. *JAMA*. 2010;303(19):1938–1945.

269. Jorge RE, Robinson RG, Arndt SV, Starkstein SE, Forrester AW, Geisler F. Depression following traumatic brain injury: a 1 year longitudinal study. *J Affect Disord*. 1993;27(4):233–243.

270. Rao V, Bertrand M, Rosenberg P, et al. Predictors of new-onset depression after mild traumatic brain injury. *J Neuropsychiatry Clin Neurosci*. 2010;22(1):100–104.

271. Rapoport MJ, McCullagh S, Shammi P, Feinstein A. Cognitive impairment associated with major depression following mild and moderate traumatic brain injury. *J Neuropsychiatry Clin Neurosci*. 2005;17(1):61–65.

272. Jorge RE, Robinson RG, Moser D, et al. Major depression following traumatic brain injury. *Arch Gen Psychiatry*. 2004;61(1):42–50.

273. Fann JR, Katon WJ, Uomoto JM, Esselman PC. Psychiatric disorders and functional disability in outpatients with traumatic brain injuries. *Am J Psychiatry*. 1995;152(10):1493–1499.

274. Seel RT, Kreutzer JS, Rosenthal M, et al. Depression after traumatic brain injury: a National Institute on Disability and Rehabilitation research model systems multicenter investigation. *Arch Phys Med Rehabil*. 2003;84(2):177–184.

275. Kreutzer JS, Seel RT, Gourley E. The prevalence and symptom rates of depression after traumatic brain injury: a comprehensive examination. *Brain Inj*. 2001;15(7):563–576.

276. Holsinger T, Steffens DC, Phillips C, et al: Head injury in early adulthood and the lifetime risk of depression. *Arch Gen Psychiatry*. 2002;59(1):17–22.

277. Chrisman SP, Richardson LP. Prevalence of diagnosed depression in adolescents with history of concussion. *J Adolesc Health*. 2013;54(5):582-586.

278. Guskiewicz KM, Marshall SW, Bailes J, et al. Recurrent concussion and risk of depression in retired professional football players. *Med Sci Sports Exerc*. 2007;39:903–909.

279. Silver JM, McAllister TW, Arciniegas DB. Depression and cognitive complaints following mild traumatic brain injury. *Am J Psychiatry*. 2009;166(6):653–661.

280. Lishman WA. Brain damage in relation to psychiatric disability after head injury. *Br J Psychiatry*. 1968;114(509):373–410.

281. Grafman J, Vance SC, Weingartner H, Salazar AM, Amin D. The effects of lateralized frontal lesions on mood regulation. *Brain*. 1986;109(Pt 6):1127–1148.

282. Fedoroff JP, Starkstein SE, Forrester AW, et al. Depression in patients with acute traumatic brain injury. *Am J Psychiatry*. 1992;149(7):918–923.

283. Paradiso S, Chemerinski E, Yazici KM, Tartaro A, Robinson RG. Frontal lobe syndrome reassessed: comparison of patients with lateral or medial frontal brain damage. *J Neurol Neurosurg Psychiatry*. 1999;67(5):664–667.

284. Schönberger M, Ponsford J, Reutens D, et al. The relationship between mood disorders and MRI findings following traumatic brain injury. *Brain Inj*. 2011;25(6):543–550.

285. Rao V, Munro CA, Rosenberg P, et al. Neuroanatomical correlates of depression in post traumatic brain injury: preliminary results of a pilot study. *J Neuropsychiatry Clin Neurosci*. 2010;22(2):231–235.

286. Matthews SC, Strigo IA, Simmons AN, et al. A multimodal imaging study in U.S. veterans of operations Iraqi and enduring freedom with and without major depression after blast-related concussion. *Neuroimage*. 2011;54(Suppl 1):S69–S75.

287. Matthews S, Spadoni A, Knox K, Strigo I, Simmons A. Combat-exposed war veterans at risk for suicide show hyperactivation of prefrontal cortex and anterior cingulate during error processing. *Psychosom Med*. 2012;74(5):471–475.

288. Mez J, Stern RA, McKee AC. Chronic traumatic encephalopathy: where are we and where are we going? *Curr Neurol Neurosci Rep*. 2013;13(12):407.

289. McKee AC, Stern RA, Nowinski CJ, et al. The spectrum of disease in chronic traumatic encephalopathy. *Brain*. 2013;136(Pt 1):43–64.

290. Ferguson PL, Smith GM, Wannamaker BB, et al. A population-based study of risk of epilepsy after hospitalization for traumatic brain injury. *Epilepsia*. 2010;51(5):891–898.

291. Bavisetty S, Bavisetty S, McArthur DL, et al. Chronic hypopituitarism after traumatic brain injury: risk assessment and relationship to outcome. *Neurosurgery*. 2008;62(5):1080–1093; discussion 1093–1094.

292. Jorge RE, Robinson RG, Starkstein SE, Arndt SV. Influence of major depression on 1-year outcome in patients with traumatic brain injury. *J Neurosurg*. 1994;81(5):726–733.

293. Mainio A, Kyllönen T, Viilo K, et al. Traumatic brain injury, psychiatric disorders and suicide: a population-based study of suicide victims during the years 1988–2004 in Northern Finland. *Brain Inj*. 2007;21(8):851–855.

294. Rapoport MJ, McCullagh S, Streiner D, Feinstein A. Age and major depression after mild traumatic brain injury. *Am J Geriatr Psychiatry*. 2003;11(3):365–369.

295. Levin HS, McCauley SR, Josic CP, et al. Predicting depression following mild traumatic brain injury. *Arch Gen Psychiatry*. 2005;62(5):523–528.

296. Glenn MB, O'Neil-Pirozzi T, Goldstein R, Burke D, Jacob L. Depression amongst outpatients with traumatic brain injury. *Brain Inj*. 2001;15(9):811–818.

297. Gomez-Hernandez R, Max JE, Kosier T, Paradiso S, Robinson RG. Social impairment and depression after traumatic brain injury. *Arch Phys Med Rehabil*. 1997;78(12):1321–1326.

298. Jorge RE, Robinson RG, Arndt S. Are there symptoms that are specific for depressed mood in patients with traumatic brain injury? *J Nerv Ment Dis*. 1993;181(2):91–99.

299. Rapoport MJ, McCullagh S, Streiner D, Feinstein A. The clinical significance of major depression following mild traumatic brain injury. *Psychosomatics*. 2003;44(1):31–37.

300. Kennedy RE, Livingston L, Riddick A, et al. Evaluation of the neurobehavioral functioning inventory as a depression screening tool after traumatic brain injury. *J Head Trauma Rehabil*. 2005; 20(6):512–526.

301. Oquendo MA, Friedman JH, Grunebaum MF, et al. Suicidal behavior and mild traumatic brain injury in major depression. *J Nerv Ment Dis*. 2004;192(6):430–434.

302. Silver JM, Kramer R, Greenwald S, Weissman M. The association between head injuries and psychiatric disorders: Findings from the New Haven NIMH Epidemiologic Catchment Area Study. *Brain Inj*. 2001;15(11):935–945.

303. Tateno A, Jorge RE, Robinson RG. Pathological laughing and crying following traumatic brain injury. *J Neuropsychiatry Clin Neurosci*. 2004;16(4):426–434.

304. Kant R, Duffy JD, Pivovarnik A. Prevalence of apathy following head injury. *Brain Inj*. 1998;12(1):87–92.

305. Fann JR, Burington B, Leonetti A, Jaffe K, Katon WJ, Thompson RS. Psychiatric illness following traumatic brain injury in an adult health maintenance organization population. *Arch Gen Psychiatry*. 2004;61(1):53–61.

306. Rao V, McCann U, Han D, Bergey A, Smith MT. Does acute TBI-related sleep disturbance predict subsequent neuropsychiatric disturbances? *Brain Inj*. 2014;28(1):20–26.

307. Pagulayan KF, Hoffman JM, Temkin NR, Machamer JE, Dikmen SS. Functional limitations and depression after traumatic brain injury: examination of the temporal relationship. *Arch Phys Med Rehabil*. 2008;89(10):1887–1892.

308. Soberg HL, Røe C, Anke A, et al. Health-related quality of life 12 months after severe traumatic brain injury: a prospective nationwide cohort study. *J Rehabil Med*. 2013;45(8):785–791.

309. Yasuda S, Wehman P, Targett P, Cifu D, West M. Return to work for persons with traumatic brain injury. *Am J Phys Med Rehabil*. 2001;80(11):852–864.

310. Wäljas M, Iverson GL, Lange RT, et al. Return to work following mild traumatic brain injury. *J Head Trauma Rehabil*. 2013;29(5): 443–450.

311. Suhr JA, Gunstad J. Postconcussive symptom report: the relative influence of head injury and depression. *J Clin Exp Neuropsychol*. 2002;24(8):981–993.

312. Fann JR, Uomoto JM, Katon WJ. Cognitive improvement with treatment of depression following mild traumatic brain injury. *Psychosomatics*. 2001;42(1):48–54.

313. Alderfer BS, Arciniegas DB, Silver JM. Treatment of depression following traumatic brain injury. *J Head Trauma Rehabil*. 2005;20(6):544–562.

314. Green A, Felmingham K, Baguley IJ, Slewa-Younan S, Simpson S. The clinical utility of the Beck depression inventory after traumatic brain injury. *Brain Inj*. 2001;15(12):1021–1028.

315. Turner-Stokes L, Hassan N, Pierce K, Clegg F. Managing depression in brain injury rehabilitation: the use of an integrated care pathway and preliminary report of response to sertraline. *Clin Rehabil*. 2002;16(3):261–268.

316. Sliwinski M, Gordon WA, Bogdany J. The Beck depression inventory: is it a suitable measure of depression for individuals with traumatic brain injury? *J Head Trauma Rehabil*. 1998;13(4): 40–46.

317. Fann JR, Bombardier CH, Dikmen S, et al. Validity of the patient health questionnaire-9 in assessing depression following trau matic brain injury. *J Head Trauma Rehabil*. 2005;20(6): 501–511.

318. Dahm J, Wong D, Ponsford J. Validity of the Depression Anxiety Stress Scales in assessing depression and anxiety following traumatic brain injury. *J Affect Disord*. 2013;151(1):392–396.

319. Gordon WA, Haddad L, Brown M, Hibbard MR, Sliwinski M. The sensitivity and specificity of self-reported symptoms in individuals with traumatic brain injury. *Brain Inj*. 2000;14(1):21–33.

320. Kalpakjian CZ, Lam CS, Leahy BJ. Conceptualization and identification of depression in adults with brain damage by clients and rehabilitation clinical staff. *Brain Inj*. 2002;16(6):501–507.

321. Rappaport M, Hall KM, Hopkins K, Belleza T, Cope DN. Disability rating scale for severe head trauma: coma to community. *Arch Phys Med Rehabil*. 1982;63(3):118–123.

322. Bryant RA, Harvey AG. Postconcussive symptoms and posttraumatic stress disorder after mild traumatic brain injury. *J Nerv Ment Dis*. 1999;187(5):302–305.

323. Bryant RA. Posttraumatic stress disorder and mild brain injury: controversies, causes and consequences. *J Clin Exp Neuropsychol*. 2001;23(6):718–728.

324. Tateno A, Jorge RE, Robinson RG: Clinical correlates of aggressive behavior after traumatic brain injury. *J Neuropsychiatry Clin Neurosci*. 2003;15(2):155–160.

325. Rosenbaum A, Hoge SK, Adelman SA, et al. Head injury in partner-abusive men. *J Consult Clin Psychol*. 1994;62(6):1187–1193.

326. Jorge RE, Robinson RG, Starkstein SE, et al: Secondary mania following traumatic brain injury. *Am J Psychiatry*. 1993;150:916–921.

327. Novack TA, Baños JH, Brunner R, Renfroe S, Meythaler JM. Impact of early administration of sertraline on depressive symptoms in the first year after traumatic brain injury. *J Neurotrauma*. 2009;26(11):1921–1928.

328. Ashman TA, Cantor JB, Gordon WA, et al. A randomized controlled trial of sertraline for the treatment of depression in persons with traumatic brain injury. *Arch Phys Med Rehabil*. 2009;90(5):733–740.

329. Lee H, Kim SW, Kim JM, et al. Comparing effects of methylphenidate, sertraline and placebo on neuropsychiatric sequelae in patients with traumatic brain injury. *Hum Psychopharmacol*. 2005;20(2):97–104.

330. Fann JR, Uomoto JM, Katon WJ. Sertraline in the treatment of major depression following mild traumatic brain injury. *J Neuropsychiatry Clin Neurosci*. 2000;12(2):226–232.

331. Rapaport MJ, Chan F, Lanctot K, et al. An open-label study of citalopram for major depression following traumatic brain injury. *J Psychopharmacol*. 2008;22(8):860–864.

332. Perino C, Rago R, Cicolini A, Torta R, Monaco F. Mood and behavioural disorders following traumatic brain injury: Clinical evaluation and pharmacological management. *Brain Inj.* 2001;15(2):139–148.

333. Horsfield SA, Rosse RB, Tomasino V, et al. Fluoxetine's effects on cognitive performance in patients with traumatic brain injury. *Int J Psychiatry Med.* 2002;32(4):337–344.

334. Wroblewski BA, Joseph AB, Cornblatt RR. Antidepressant pharmacotherapy and the treatment of depression in patients with severe traumatic brain injury: A controlled, prospective study. *J Clin Psychiatry.* 1996;57(12):582–587.

335. Saran AS. Depression after minor closed head injury: Role of dexamethasone suppression test and antidepressants. *J Clin Psychiatry.* 1985;46(8): 335–338.

336. Dinan TG, Mobayed M. Treatment resistance of depression after head injury: A preliminary study of amitriptyline response. *Acta Psychiatr Scand.* 1992;85(4):292–294.

337. Kanetani K, Kimura M, Endo S. Therapeutic effects of milnacipran (serotonin noradrenaline reuptake inhibitor) on depression following mild and moderate traumatic brain injury. *J Nippon Med Sch.* 2003;70(4):313–320.

338. Newburn G, Edwards R, Thomas H, Collier J, Fox K, Collins C. Moclobemide in the treatment of major depressive disorder (DSM-3) following traumatic brain injury. *Brain Inj.* 1999;13(8):637–642.

339. Khateb A, Ammann J, Annoni JM, Diserens K. Cognition-enhancing effects of donepezil in traumatic brain injury. *Eur Neurol.* 2005;54(1):39–45.

340. Plantier D, Luaute J, the SOMFER group. Drugs for behavior disorders after traumatic brain injury: Systematic review and expert consensus leading to French recommendations for good practice. *Ann Phys Rehabil Med.* 2016;59(1):42–57.

341. Rapoport MJ, Mitchell RA, McCullagh S, et al. A randomized controlled trial of antidepressant continuation for major depression following traumatic brain injury. *J Clin Psychiatry.* 2010;71(9):1125–1111 30.

342. Kant R, Coffey CE, Bogyi AM. Safety and efficacy of ECT in patients with head injury a case series. *J Neuropsychiatry Clin Neurosci.* 1999;11(1):32–37.

343. Tiersky LA, Anselmi V, Johnston MV, et al. A trial of neuropsychologic rehabilitation in mild-spectrum traumatic brain injury. *Arch Phys Med Rehabil.* 2005;86(8):1565–1574.

344. Bradbury CL, Christensen BK, Lau MA, et al. The efficacy of cognitive behavior therapy in the treatment of emotional distress after acquired brain injury. *Arch Phys Med Rehabil.* 2008;89(12 Suppl):S61–S68.

345. Arundine A, Bradbury CL, Dupuis K, et al. Cognitive behavior therapy after acquired brain injury: maintenance of therapeutic benefits at 6 months posttreatment. *J Head Trauma Rehabil.* 2012;27(2):104–112.

346. Topolovec-Vranic J, Cullen N, Michalak A, et al. Evaluation of an online cognitive behavioural therapy program by patients with traumatic brain injury and depression. *Brain Inj.* 2010;24(5):762–772.

347. Bédard M, Felteau M, Marshall S, et al. Mindfulness-based cognitive therapy reduces symptoms of depression in people with a traumatic brain injury: results from a randomized controlled trial. *J Head Trauma Rehabil.* 2013;29(4):E13–E22.

348. Anson K, Ponsford J. Evaluation of a coping skills group following traumatic brain injury. *Brain Inj.* 2006;20(2):167–178.

349. Driver S, Ede A. Impact of physical activity on mood after TBI. *Brain Inj.* 2009;23(3):203–212.

350. Wise EK, Hoffman JM, Powell JM, Bombardier CH, Bell KR. Benefits of exercise maintenance after traumatic brain injury. *Arch Phys Med Rehabil.* 2012;93(8):1319–1323.

351. Bateman A, Culpan FJ, Pickering AD, et al. The effect of aerobic training on rehabilitation outcomes after recent severe brain injury: a randomized controlled evaluation. *Arch Phys Med Rehabil.* 2001;82(2):174–182.

352. Sinclair KL, Ponsford JL, Taffe J, Lockley SW, Rajaratnam SM. Randomized controlled trial of light therapy for fatigue following traumatic brain injury. *Neurorehabil Neural Repair.* 2013;28(4):303–313.

353. Barker-Collo S, Starkey N, Theadom A. Treatment for depression following mild traumatic brain injury in adults: a meta-analysis. *Brain Inj.* 2013;27(10):1124–1133.

354. Rudzinski LA, Meador KJ. Epilepsy: five new things. *Neurology.* 2011;76(7 Suppl 2):S20–S25.

355. Fiest KM, Dykeman J, Patten SB, et al. Depression in epilepsy: A systematic review and meta-analysis. *Neurology.* 2013;80(6):590–599.

356. Rai D, Kerr MP, McManus S, Jordanova V, Lewis G, Brugha TS. Epilepsy and psychiatric comorbidity: a nationally representative population-based study. *Epilepsia.* 2012;53(6):1095–1103.

357. Hesdorffer DC, Hauser WA, Olafsson E, Ludvigsson P, Kjartansson O. Depression and suicide attempt as risk factors for incident unprovoked seizures. *Ann Neurol.* 2006;59(1):35–41.

358. Hesdorffer DC, Ishihara L, Mynepalli L, Webb DJ, Weil J, Hauser WA. Epilepsy, suicidality, and psychiatric disorders: a bidirectional association. *Ann Neurol.* 2012;72(2):184–191.

359. Hitiris N, Mohanraj R, Norrie J, Sills GJ, Brodie MJ. Predictors of pharmacoresistant epilepsy. *Epilepsy Res.* 2007;75(2–3):192–196.

360. Thome-Souza S, Kuczynski E, Assumpção F Jr, et al. Which factors may play a pivotal role on determining the type of psychiatric disorder in children and adolescents with epilepsy? *Epilepsy Behav.* 2004;5(6):988–994.

361. Sarkisova K, van Luijtelaar G. The WAG/Rij strain: a genetic animal model of absence epilepsy with comorbidity of depression [corrected]. *Prog Neuropsychopharmacol Biol Psychiatry.* 2011;35(4):854–876.

362. Johnson MR, Shorvon SD. Heredity in epilepsy: neurodevelopment, comorbidity, and the neurological trait. *Epilepsy Behav.* 2011;22(3):421–427.

363. Hoppe C, Elger CE. Depression in epilepsy: a critical review from a clinical perspective. *Nat Rev Neurol.* 2011;7(8):462–472.

364. Kanner AM. Can neurobiological pathogenic mechanisms of depression facilitate the development of seizure disorders? *Lancet Neurol.* 2012;11(12):1093–1102.

365. Karst H, de Kloet ER, Joëls M. Episodic corticosterone treatment accelerates kindling epileptogenesis and triggers long-term changes in hippocampal CA1 cells, in the fully kindled state. *Eur J Neurosci.* 1999;11:889–898.

366. Taher TR, Salzberg M, Morris MJ, Rees S, O'Brien TJ. Chronic low-dose corticosterone supplementation enhances acquired epileptogenesis in the rat amygdala kindling model of TLE. *Neuropsychopharmacology.* 2005;30:1610–1616.

367. Kumar G, Couper A, O'Brien TJ, et al. The acceleration of amygdala kindling epileptogenesis by chronic low-dose corticosterone involves both mineralocorticoid and glucocorticoid receptors. *Psychoneuroendocrinology.* 2007;32(7):834–842.

368. Hasler G, Bonwetsch R, Giovacchini G, et al. 5-HT1A receptor binding in temporal lobe epilepsy patients with and without major depression. *Biol Psychiatry*. 2007;62(11):1258–1264.

369. Clinckers R, Smolders I, Meurs A, Ebinger G, Michotte Y. Anticonvulsant action of hippocampal dopamine and serotonin is independently mediated by D and 5-HT receptors. *J Neurochem*. 2004;89(4):834–843.

370. Gilling KE, Oltmanns F, Behr J. Impaired maturation of serotonergic function in the dentate gyrus associated with epilepsy. *Neurobiol Dis*. 2013;50:86–95.

371. Epps SA, Weinshenker D. Rhythm and blues: animal models of epilepsy and depression comorbidity. *Biochem Pharmacol*. 2013;85(2):135–146.

372. Engel J Jr, Bandler R, Griffith NC, Caldecott-Hazard S. Neurobiological evidence for epilepsy-induced interictal disturbances. *Adv Neurol*. 1991;55:97–111.

373. Kanner AM, Trimble M, Schmitz B. Postictal affective episodes. *Epilepsy Behav*. 2010;10:156–158.

374. Sanchez-Gistau V, Sugranyes G, Baillés E, et al. Is major depressive disorder specifically associated with mesial temporal sclerosis? *Epilepsia*. 2012;53(2):386–392.

375. Adams SJ, O'Brien TJ, Lloyd J, Kilpatrick CJ, Salzberg MR, Velakoulis D. Neuropsychiatric morbidity in focal epilepsy. *Br J Psychiatry*. 2008;192(6):464–469.

376. Sackeim HA. The anticonvulsant hypothesis of the mechanisms of action of ECT: current status. *J ECT*. 1999;15(1):5–26.

377. Merkl A, Heuser I, Bajbouj M. Antidepressant electroconvulsive therapy: mechanism of action, recent advances and limitations. *Exp Neurol*. 2009;219(1):20–26.

378. Kunugi H, Ida I, Owashi T, et al. Assessment of the dexamethasone/CRH test as a state-dependent marker for hypothalamic–pituitary–adrenal (HPA) axis abnormalities in major depressive episode: a Multicenter Study. *Neuropsychopharmacology*. 2006;31(1):212–220.

379. LaFrance WC Jr, Kanner AM, Hermann B. Psychiatric comorbidities in epilepsy. *Int Rev Neurobiol*. 2008;83:347–383.

380. Blanchet P, Frommer GP. Mood change preceding epileptic seizures. *J Nerv Ment Dis*. 1986;174(8):471–476.

381. Williams D. The structure of emotions reflected in epileptic experiences. *Brain*. 1956;79(1):29–67.

382. Kanner AM, Soto A, Gross-Kanner H. Prevalence and clinical characteristics of postictal psychiatric symptoms in partial epilepsy. *Neurology*. 2004;62(5):708–713.

383. Blumer D, Montouris G, Davies K. The interictal dysphoric disorder: recognition, pathogenesis, and treatment of the major psychiatric disorder of epilepsy. *Epilepsy Behav*. 2004;5(6):826–840.

384. Thapar A, Roland M, Harold G. Do depression symptoms predict seizure frequency–or vice versa? *Psychosom Res*. 2005;59(5):269–274.

385. Ojemann LM, Baugh-Bookman C, Dudley DL. Effect of psychotropic medications on seizure control in patients with epilepsy. *Neurology*. 1987;37(9):1525–1527.

386. Cardamone L, Salzberg M, O'Brien T, Jones N. Antidepressant therapy in epilepsy: can treating the comorbidities affect the underlying disorder? *Br J Pharmacol*. 2013;168(7):1531–1554.

387. Bell GS, Gaitatzis A, Bell CL, Johnson AL, Sander JW. Suicide in people with epilepsy: how great is the risk? *Epilepsia*. 2009; 50(8):1933–1942.

388. Bell GS, Sander JW. Suicide and epilepsy. *Curr Opin Neurol*. 2009; 22(2):174–178.

389. Hamid H, Kanner AM. Should antidepressant drugs of the selective serotonin reuptake inhibitor family be tested as antiepileptic drugs? *Epilepsy Behav*. 2013;26(3):261–265.

390. Gilliam FG, Barry JJ, Hermann BP, Meador KJ, Vahle V, Kanner AM. Rapid detection of major depression in epilepsy: a multicentre study. *Lancet Neurol*. 2006;5(5):399–405.

391. Ettinger AB, Kanner AM, eds. *Psychiatric Issues in Epilepsy*. 2nd ed. Philadelphia, PA: Wolters Kluwer/ Lippincott Williams & Wilkins; 2007.

392. Hesdorffer DC, French JA, Posner K, et al. Suicidal ideation and behavior screening in intractable focal epilepsy eligible for drug trials. *Epilepsia*. 2013;54(5):879–887.

393. Wilson SJ, Bladin PF, Saling MM. The burden of normality: a framework for rehabilitation after epilepsy surgery. *Epilepsia*. 2007;48(Suppl 9):13–16.

394. Hesdorffer DC, Kanner AM. The FDA alert on suicidality and antiepileptic drugs: Fire or false alarm? *Epilepsia*. 2009;50(5):978–986.

395. Andersohn F, Schade R, Willich SN, Garbe E. Use of antiepileptic drugs in epilepsy and the risk of self-harm or suicidal behavior. *Neurology*. 2010;75(4):335–340.

396. Arana MD, Charles E, Wentworth MS, José L, Ayuso-Mateos MD, Felix M. Arellano. Suicide-Related Events in Patients Treated with Antiepileptic Drugs. *N Engl J Med*. 2010;363:542–551.

397. Mula M, Kanner AM, Schmitz B, Schachter S. Antiepileptic drugs and suicidality: an expert consensus statement from the Task Force on Therapeutic Strategies of the ILAE Commission on Neuropsychobiology. *Epilepsia*. 2013;54(1):199–203.

398. Kondziella D, Asztely F. Don't be afraid to treat depression in patients with epilepsy! *Acta Neurol Scand*. 2009;119(2):75–80.

399. Alper K, Schwartz KA, Kolts RL, Khan A. Seizure incidence in psychopharmacological clinical trials: an analysis of Food and Drug Administration (FDA) summary basis of approval reports. *Biol Psychiatry*. 2007;62:345–354.

400. Judge BS, Rentmeester LL. Antidepressant overdose-induced seizures. *Neurol Clin*. 2011;29(3):565–580.

401. Bell AJ, Cole A, Eccleston D, Ferrier IN. Lithium neurotoxicity at normal therapeutic levels. *Br J Psychiatry*. 1993;162:689–692.

402. Lee KC, Finley PR, Alldredge BK. Risk of seizures associated with psychotropic medications: emphasis on new drugs and new findings. *Expert Opin Drug Saf*. 2003;2(3):233–247.

403. Kucia KA, Stepa?czak R, Tredzbor B. Electroconvulsive therapy for major depression in an elderly person with epilepsy. *World J Biol Psychiatry*. 2009;10(1):78–80.

404. Marchetti RL, Fiorre LA, Peluso MA, Rigonatti SP. Safety and efficacy of ECT in mental disorders associated with epilepsy: report of three cases. *J ECT*. 2003;19:173–176.

405. Regenold WT, Weintraub D, Taller A. Electroconvulsive therapy for epilepsy and major depression. *Am J Geriat Psychiatry*. 1998;6:180–183.

406. Lunde ME, Lee EK, Rasmussen KG. Electroconvulsive therapy in patients with epilepsy. *Epilepsy Behav*. 2006;9(2):355–359.

407. Harden CL. The co-morbidity of depression and epilepsy: epidemiology, etiology, and treatment. *Neurology*. 2002;59(6 Suppl 4): S48–S55.

408. Holtzheimer PE III, Kosel M, Schlaepfer T. Brain stimulation therapies for neuropsychiatric disease. In: Schlaepfer TE, Nemeroff CB, eds.

Handbook of Clinical Neurology. Vol. 106. 3rd series. *Neurobiology of Psychiatric Disorders*; Amsterdam, NL; Elsevier: 2012.

409. Fregni F, Schachter SC, Pascual-Leone A. Transcranial magnetic stimulation treatment for epilepsy: can it also improve depression and vice versa? *Epilepsy Behav*. 2005;7(2):182–189.

410. Sprengers M, Vonck K, Carrette E, Marson AG, Boon P. Deep brain and cortical stimulation for epilepsy. *Cochrane Database Syst Rev*. 2014;Issue 6:CD008497.

411. Ryvlin P, Gilliam FG, Nguyen DK, et al. The long-term effect of vagus nerve stimulation on quality of life in patients with pharmacoresistant focal epilepsy: the PuLsE (Open Prospective Randomized Long-term Effectiveness) trial. *Epilepsia*. 2014;55(6):893–900.

412. Aihua L, Lu S, Liping L, Xiuru W, Hua L, Yuping W. A controlled trial of transcutaneous vagus nerve stimulation for the treatment of pharmacoresistant epilepsy. *Epilepsy Behav*. 2014;39C: 105–110.

413. Shiozawa P, da Silva ME, de Carvalho TC, Cordeiro Q, Brunoni AR, Fregni F. Transcutaneous vagus and trigeminal nerve stimulation for neuropsychiatric disorders: a systematic review. *Arq Neuropsiquiatr*. 2014;72(7):542–547.

414. Gandy M, Sharpe L, Perry KN. Cognitive behavior therapy for depression in people with epilepsy: a systematic review. *Epilepsia*. 2013;54(10):1725–1734.

CHAPTER 6

Cancer and Depression

Fremonta Meyer, MD
Elizabeth Alfson, MD
John Peteet, MD
Rachel Yung, MD
Ilana Braun, MD

INTRODUCTION

A diagnosis of cancer is a significant life threat and psychosocial stressor, often leading to emotional distress in vulnerable individuals. Frequently, depressive syndromes are under-recognized in cancer patients; this is partly due to the difficulty of distinguishing depressive syndromes from adjustment disorders in response to cancer, and also because the neurovegetative and cognitive symptoms of depression may be considered normative in the context of cancer and its treatment. Conversely, dysphoric or apathetic cancer patients are sometimes misdiagnosed as depressed when they are in fact delirious.

EPIDEMIOLOGY

■ DEPRESSION AND RELATED DISORDERS

Cancer increases prevalence of certain psychiatric symptoms and syndromes, including depressive disorders, above baseline population levels. Historically, highly variable rates of depressive disorders were noted in cancer patients, primarily due to lack of diagnostic and methodologic standardization. A recent high-quality meta-analysis found prevalence of 16% for major depression, 19% for minor depression (a mood disorder that does not meet full criteria for major depression, but features at least two depressive symptoms for 2 weeks), and 19% for adjustment disorder.[1] This prevalence of major depression appears to be three to four times higher than that in the general population, whereas rates of dysthymia are relatively similar (**Fig. 6-1**).[2] Review of specific studies suggests an association between year of publication and prevalence, with higher rates of depression reported in earlier studies. It is possible that prevalence of depression in cancer has in fact decreased in recent years; if true, this may be a result of improved oncologic outcomes, decreased cancer-associated stigma, availability of palliative care, and increased attention to screening.[3] Alternatively, it may be that more recent studies employ more rigorous methods and therefore report more accurate rates; this hypothesis is supported by the finding that studies with more rigorous methods tend to report lower prevalence rates.[1]

Young age and low levels of social support are consistent risk factors for depression in cancer patients (**Box 6-1**).[4] Personal and family history of depression likely play roles as well.[5] In contrast to findings in the general population, women with cancer are not at higher risk for depression than men with cancer.[6,7] Ethnicity (particularly Latino) and lower income may be risk factors for depression in cancer.[8] Anemia[9] and hypogonadism may also be risk factors for depression in cancer patients, although confirmatory studies are needed. Although there is no consistent association between cancer type and incidence of depression, one large study found that patients with Hodgkin's lymphoma and lung, pancreatic, brain, and head and neck cancers had more distress than patients with other types of cancer.[10] In particular, early reports suggest depression more often precedes the diagnosis of pancreatic cancer than other types of cancer. However, the specificity of this association is unclear, and may be confounded by associated pain disorders and the poor clinical and functional status of many patients with pancreatic cancer at the time of diagnosis. Alternatively, there may be a shared pathophysiological mechanism that has not yet been determined.

■ SUICIDE AND DESIRE FOR HASTENED DEATH

Thoughts of suicide may be present in up to 17% of cancer patients.[11] In instances of suicidal ideation, hopelessness is at least

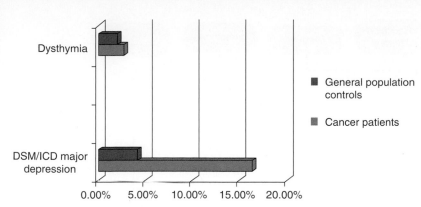

Figure 6-1 *Comparative point prevalence of mood disorders in cancer.*

as strong a contributor as depression.[12] More common than active suicidal ideation is some form of desire for hastened death, found in between 10% and 30% of patients who are terminally ill with cancer. Of note, the desire for hastened death is a unifying construct which encompasses passive wishes to die sooner than would occur naturally, active plans to commit suicide, and requests for euthanasia or assisted suicide.[13] Similarly, depression and hopelessness are strong yet independent contributors to the desire for hastened death.[13] An unknown but substantial frequency of cancer patients demonstrate contingent suicidality, linking their suicidal intent to a future time point or particular life circumstance (e.g., severe pain or dyspnea as natural death approaches).[14] There is a case report suggesting that some family members of cancer patients also struggle with severe anticipatory grief and are at risk for contingent suicide upon the death of their loved one.[15]

A case–control study of the suicide risk associated with medical illness among older Americans found that cancer was the only non-psychiatric medical condition independently associated with completed suicide (OR 2.3), and that metastatic disease further increased the suicide risk.[16] Adjusted rates of suicide are 31.4/100,000 person-years among those with cancer, compared with 16.7 in the general population.[17] Nonetheless, completed suicide is rare, particularly in the setting of adequate supportive treatment. In a study of over 17,000 patients cared for at home by palliative care teams, only 0.03% of deaths occurred due to suicide.[18] Another population-based study found that only 0.2% of all deaths in cancer patients resulted from suicide, with the highest risk in the first 6 months after diagnosis.[19] More recent work has confirmed that the relative risk of suicide as compared to cancer-free controls is very high in the

acute phase following a cancer diagnosis (RR 12.6 in the first week after diagnosis, RR 3.1 in the first year after diagnosis).[20] This finding suggests the need for early psychiatric assessment and intervention for at-risk patients, as well as communication training for primary care providers, emergency room physicians, oncologists and other providers who may be most likely to see patients during this time period. Risk factors for suicide among patients with cancer include male sex, white race, and unmarried status; lung cancer carries the highest rates, followed by stomach and oropharyngeal/laryngeal cancers.[17] Notably, these types of cancer are often associated with underlying alcohol or substance abuse, which are also risk factors for suicide. The risk is highest in the first 5 years after the diagnosis of cancer, but remains elevated for at least 15 years.[17] Mood disorders are present in 80% of patients with cancer who commit suicide.[21]

PATHOPHYSIOLOGY

Cancer activates many inflammatory pathways that may potentiate depression (**Fig. 6-2**), and the tumor burden may extend to the CNS (e.g., primary brain tumors, brain metastases, and leptomeningeal disease) where it may directly disrupt mood (**Box 6-2**). Surgery, chemotherapy, and radiation, which are often administered sequentially and repetitively, particularly in patients with advanced disease, may result in tissue damage and destruction and thus activate an innate immune response. Several chemotherapeutic agents (cyclophosphamide, 5-fluorouracil) are known to cross the blood–brain barrier. In animal models, these as well as other chemotherapeutic agents that do not cross the blood-brain barrier decrease cell proliferation in the hippocampal dentate gyrus, an area of the brain implicated in the pathogenesis of mood disorders.[22] In addition, chemotherapy and radiation may directly induce nuclear factor κ B (NFκB) and its downstream inflammatory gene products.[23] Circulating IL-6 levels are increased in patients with cancer and major depression as compared to healthy comparison subjects and cancer patients without depression.[24,25] There are other neuroendocrine alterations present that might increase the inflammatory response, including dexamethasone nonsuppression[24,26] and flattening of the diurnal cortisol curve.[25] In patients receiving injectable IFN-alpha for treatment of melanoma, exaggerated secretion of ACTH and cortisol in response to the first injection is associated with subsequent development of depression.[27]

BOX 6-1
IMPORTANT RISK FACTORS FOR DEPRESSION IN CANCER PATIENTS

Sociodemographic
Young age
Low levels of social support
Ethnicity (Latino)
Lower SES
Clinical
Personal history of depression
Family history of depression
Medical
Anemia
Hypogonadism
Possibly certain cancers (Hodgkin's, lung, pancreatic, brain, head and neck)
Pain

BOX 6-2
POSSIBLE MEDIATORS BETWEEN CANCER AND DEPRESSION

Inflammation
Neuroendocrine responses
Direct effects (of tumor on brain)
Treatments: Surgery, chemotherapy, radiation
Psychological distress

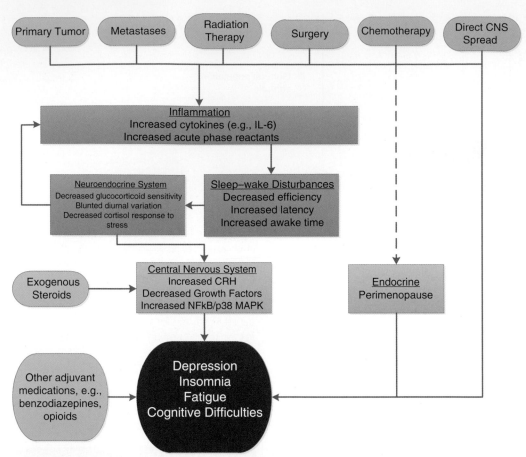

Figure 6-2 *Pathophysiology of depression and related comorbidities in the cancer setting.*

These physiologic factors coexist with profound psychological stress from the diagnosis of cancer, which is often followed by ongoing suffering, worry about recurrence and mortality, regardless of cancer stage. Given the known contribution of stress to inflammatory responses, it is probable that both physical and psychosocial challenges contribute to the biological mechanisms underlying depression in cancer patients. Still, there is a relative lack of data on biomarkers in cancer patients with major depression, as compared to a more ample literature on the biological parameters associated with cancer fatigue.[28]

CLINICAL PRESENTATION

There is little evidence of unique phenomenological distinctions among major depression, minor depression, and adjustment disorder with depressed mood in patients with cancer. However, approximately 30% of advanced cancer patients may ultimately cross over between major depressive disorder (MDD) and adjustment disorders (generally from adjustment disorder to MDD), reinforcing the importance of early intervention and longitudinal follow up.[29] Notably, several diagnostic criteria for MDD are confounded by symptoms resulting from cancer or its treatment, specifically low energy, poor appetite, altered psychomotor activity, and impaired concentration. In assessing major depression in patients with cancer, criteria of particular assistance in the differential diagnosis include anhedonia, early morning awakening, disability out of proportion to condition, guilt, suicidal ideation, and somatic symptoms out of proportion to known organic disease processes. Further, fatigue that is already present early in the morning, as opposed to fatigue that sets in gradually over the course of the day, may suggest depression as opposed to the expected effects of cancer and cancer treatment. Although controversy continues over how to weigh somatic versus

psychological symptoms in patients with cancer and comorbid depression, most clinicians favor an inclusive approach (in which somatic symptoms are counted toward a diagnosis of MDD), especially given that proinflammatory cytokines may contribute both to depression and somatic symptoms, such as pain and fatigue. Other non-DSM criteria may support a diagnosis of MDD (**Box 6-3**).

Suicidal ideation and/or requests for physician-assisted suicide often support a diagnosis of MDD, and require careful psychiatric evaluation. After assessment of any suicide risk factors other than medical illness, followed by decisive action to assure safety, patients

---

**BOX 6-3
IMPORTANT SYMPTOMS**

Confounding (symptoms that may result from cancer or cancer treatment as opposed to depression)
Poor sleep (early morning awakening more typical of depression)
Low energy (cancer more waxing and waning)
Decreased appetite
Psychomotor slowing (rule out akathisia from antiemetics)
Poor concentration
More typical in depression
Anhedonia
Guilt
Increased appetite (unless on steroids)
Suicidal ideation
Irritability
Hopelessness

TABLE 6-1 Particular Stressors Associated with Depression by Cancer Type

Cancer Type	Particular Stressors Contributing to Depression
Lung	Grave prognosis, dyspnea, pain, premorbid risk factors for mental disorders (e.g., smoking)
Head and neck	Difficulty eating/swallowing due to surgery and/or radiation, pain, premorbid risk factors for mental disorders (e.g., smoking, alcohol dependence)
Brain	Direct CNS effects, cognitive impairment, personality change, seizures/inability to drive, chronic corticosteroids, caregiver burden, grave prognosis
Breast	Body image and female identity (breast surgery +/− BSO), marital concerns, adjuvant hormonal therapies; patients may view the social context ("pink ribbons" in the mass media) as a relentlessly positive and/or trite celebration of breast cancer that doesn't correspond with their adverse personal experiences (particularly the case for stage IV patients)
Gynecologic	Body image and female identity (TAH/BSO), side effects from pelvic radiation (e.g., vaginal stenosis), grave prognosis (especially for ovarian cancer), fixation on CA125 values, frequent bowel obstructions, inability to eat often for several months at end-of-life
Hematologic	"Life or death" situation at diagnosis often with little time to prepare emotionally for intense course of treatments, long hospitalizations, multiple complications of stem cell transplant (infections, including CNS), long isolation period after transplant, possibility of disfiguring graft-versus-host disease
Gastrointestinal	Ostomy adjustment; chronic diarrhea, nausea, abdominal pain; sometimes, premorbid risk factors for depression (alcohol dependence in esophageal cancer)
Genitourinary	Urinary retention and/or incontinence, nocturia, management of chronic Foley or ileal loop with permanent stoma, erectile dysfunction and other sexual side effects, fixation on PSA values (prostate), emotional implications of "medical castration" with hormonal treatments
Sarcoma	Amputation, pain, social context ("rare cancer"), often affects young adults
Melanoma	Guilt about sun and tanning bed exposure, management of risk for family members, neuropsychiatric side effects of interferon-alpha, high risk of CNS metastases (often hemorrhagic)
All types	Chemotherapy-induced menopause, possible infertility, hair loss in setting of chemotherapy or brain radiation, intense treatment schedules interfering with work and travel

may benefit from gentle exploration of the meaning behind their request. Contributing psychodynamic factors may include a need for control, ambivalence (i.e., communicating desires to the physician reflects an underlying wish for rescue), or a split in the experience of the self, in which the medically ill self is experienced as an intrusive entity that needs to be eradicated for the good self to survive. Other possibilities include suicide as a means of revenge against loved ones, atonement for guilt (especially if the cancer was initially attributed to bad deeds, for instance smoking of tobacco, and unacceptable emotions), and actualizing a "felt experience" of already being dead.[30]

Patients with cancer experience many losses, including vitality, bodily integrity, independence, mental clarity, fertility, virility, and others in the course of their illness that may predispose them to depression. Specific stressors vary according to cancer type (**Table 6-1**).

Depression is associated with various psychiatric comorbidities in cancer patients, including anxiety disorders which may include symptoms of posttraumatic stress, though full syndromal PTSD is uncommon (**Box 6-4**).[31]

COURSE AND NATURAL HISTORY

Depressive symptoms appear to be most prominent at specific points in the course of the illness: at diagnosis, completion of active

---

BOX 6-4
COMMON COMORBIDITIES

Anxiety disorders
Type D personality (tendency toward negative affectivity and social inhibition)
Cognitive dysfunction

---

treatment when patients are confronted with existential angst and fears of recurrence in the setting of less active follow-up with medical providers, and at diagnosis of recurrence or metastasis. In patients with breast cancer, there is a nonlinear decline in the point prevalence of depression and anxiety in the years following diagnosis (50% in the first year; 25% in years 2–4; 15% in year 5), with an increase to 45% within 3 months of diagnosis of a recurrence.[32] In general, however, longitudinal studies using DSM-based criteria for caseness (as opposed to scores on depression scales) are lacking. Progressive disease may not cause substantially greater rates of depression than less symptomatic disease, a finding particularly robust in breast cancer.[33] However, metastasis is associated with elevated rates of depression, although the direction of causality remains to be determined.[34,35] Depression in patients with metastasis increases with increased physical and psychosocial symptom burden, though not with closeness to death per se.[36] Long-term cancer survivors (>5 years from diagnosis) who are in remission do not appear to have higher rates of major depression than the general population.[37]

Cancer patients with depression often exhibit maladaptive thoughts and behaviors, such as irritability, amplification of somatic symptoms, blaming themselves for their illness, withdrawing from family and professional caregivers, and limiting their travel and activities outside the home. These issues often result in reduced satisfaction with medical care, less effective communication with caregivers and physicians, reduced adherence to medical treatment plans, and longer hospitalizations.[38,39] They also demonstrate higher rates of complementary and alternative medication utilization.[40]

Importantly, even after adjusting for clinical factors affecting prognosis, depression has been shown to adversely affect quality of life and overall survival (i.e., all-cause mortality) in advanced cancer patients.[41–43] It does not, however, affect cancer progression.[43]

ASSESSMENT AND DIFFERENTIAL DIAGNOSIS

The primary differential diagnosis for depression in patients with cancer includes grief and adjustment disorders, substance-induced mood disorders, and hypoactive delirium (**Box 6-5**). Assessing the quality of tearfulness may be clinically useful in distinguishing adjustment disorders and grief from that of major depression: cathartic crying is more characteristic of adjustment disorders and grief, while draining or unrelieving crying may accompany a major depression. Grief reactions may include intense sadness, appetite loss, and sleep disturbance, but usually do not include the pervasive guilt and loss of self-esteem that accompanies major depression. In addition, grief-related emotions tend to come in waves interspersed with periods of time when the patient is able to enjoy activities; by contrast, depression is usually characterized by persistent anhedonia. Adjustment disorders also tend to be less severe and less functionally impairing than major depression. Obtaining collateral history from family members can help clarify the extent of impairment in day-to-day activities. It is also important to obtain a careful medication history, including any recent changes that would suggest a substance-induced depressive disorder.

Similarly, patients may appear withdrawn or dysphoric if they are using alcohol or illicit substances or misusing prescribed psychoactive medications, such as benzodiazepines or opioids for "chemical coping." Although chronic daily marijuana use may contribute to depressive symptoms, patients utilizing cannabis for medicinal purposes may report improvements in mood and sleep as well as pain relief.[44] Other patients with alcohol or substance abuse histories opt to turn over a new leaf after a cancer diagnosis, which occasionally results in full withdrawal.

Patients with occult hypoactive delirium may demonstrate flat affect, psychomotor slowing, decreased engagement, and suicidal ideation; this necessitates careful cognitive examination when evaluating the patient with cancer for depression. Differential diagnosis of suicidal ideation in this population must always include encephalopathic conditions; the presence of hallucinations or delusions is a risk factor for suicide attempts.[45] Finally, a complete differential diagnosis may include several other constructs (demoralization and conservation-withdrawal) that have been proposed to describe psychological symptoms of low mood, interest, or rumination. Demoralization syndrome includes existential distress, hopelessness, helplessness, isolation, and potential suicidality, but is differentiated from major depression by the lack of generalized anhedonia.[46] Conservation–withdrawal is a construct proposed to explain behavioral disengagement and inactivity as a means of conserving energy while fighting a serious illness; patients may display diminished speech and movement and withdrawal from usual activities, but usually lack depressed mood per se.[47]

■ SCREENING

There is an enhanced emphasis on depression screening in cancer settings as a result of the National Cancer Institute's recent mandate that all comprehensive cancer centers should screen oncology patients for emotional distress. Clinicians have historically underestimated the severity of depressive illness in the cancer population. One large study found a concordance of only 13% between oncologist and patient ratings in patients with severe depressive symptoms; nursing staff ratings had no greater concordance[48,49] with patient scales. The six-item Brief Edinburgh Depression Scale, initially developed for post-partum settings, may be useful as a screening tool for oncology practices; other options include the Patient Health Questionnaire-Depression Module (PHQ-9) and the Beck Depression Inventory (BDI). Although the Hospital Anxiety and Depression Scale (HADS) is the most extensively validated screening tool for emotional distress in cancer patients, thresholds for clinically significant distress are widely variable across studies.[50] Although there is no clear evidence that depression screening alone improves outcomes compared to usual care,[51] screening that is linked to collaborative care interventions in cancer patients shows promise in early trials.[52]

■ CANCER TREATMENTS OR ADJUVANT MEDICATIONS WHICH MAY LEAD TO DEPRESSION

Opioids, corticosteroids, interferon, adjuvant hormonal treatments, and several chemotherapeutic agents, including tyrosine kinase inhibitors,[53] are medications used in treating cancer that are also implicated in substance-induced depression (**Box 6-6**). Recognition of depression as a potential side effect can help clinicians tailor treatment when appropriate, for example, by minimizing steroid use, or to identify and treat any resulting depression in a timely fashion if it occurs.

Interferon

After high-risk early-stage or metastatic melanoma a year-long course of interferon alpha may be given. Among its many constitutional and neuropsychiatric side-effects, this recombinant cytokine can gradually trigger a depressive syndrome that, in instances, necessitates dose reduction or even discontinuation. Thus, mental health management for patients receiving interferon is especially important.

A small body of research supports use of antidepressants in patients receiving interferon alpha, both in resolving interferon-related depressive symptoms and allowing patients to successfully complete the interferon course.[54] Pretreatment with a serotoninergic antidepressant (in one small RCT, paroxetine) may delay or prevent onset of interferon-related depression in melanoma patients.[55] However, pretreatment is best reserved for patients who, at time of interferon initiation, are either already on an antidepressant regimen or report prominent depressive symptoms.[56] Interferon occasionally

---

BOX 6-5
DIFFERENTIAL DIAGNOSIS

Grief

Adjustment disorder

Alcohol or other substance use disorders

Delirium

Demoralization

Conservation-withdrawal

BOX 6-6
DRUGS THAT CAN CAUSE DEPRESSIVE SYMPTOMS

Corticosteroids

Interferon

Interleukin-2

Opioids

Tamoxifen (+/−)

Aromatase Inhibitors (+/−)

Paclitaxel (+/−)

Docetaxel (+/−)

Vincristine

Vinblastine

Procarbazine

L-asparaginase

Amphotericin B

Imatinib

Dasatinib

precipitates mania, hypomania, or a mixed state,[56,57] and this ill-effect may be fostered by antidepressants.

Although the SSRIs have been most widely studied for the treatment of interferon-related depression, other classes of antidepressants may deserve consideration. Anecdotally, bupropion may have utility in treating depressive symptoms associated with interferon[58] and one can posit that its energizing effects may help to stave off interferon-related fatigue.

Tamoxifen

Tamoxifen is used as adjuvant therapy for breast cancer and placebo-controlled trials show it does not increase rates of MDD.[59] Case reports of tamoxifen-induced major depression may be confounded by chemotherapy-induced amenorrhea. In addition, some literature suggests that chemotherapy and estrogen receptor positivity are independent risk factors for depression after a diagnosis of breast cancer diagnosis.[60] Tamoxifen is a protein kinase C inhibitor, similar to lithium and valproate, and has antimanic effects.[61] Despite the lack of group data, tamoxifen may contribute to depressive symptoms in a small subgroup of patients who are sensitive to hormonal fluctuations. If depressive symptoms are temporally correlated with tamoxifen and resolve after discontinuing it, and in addition do not respond to concomitant antidepressant therapy, oncologists can reduce the breast cancer recurrence risk by switching to aromatase inhibitors in postmenopausal women, or to ovarian suppression (leuprolide) plus an aromatase inhibitor in premenopausal women. However, some patients may continue to experience mood lability on ovarian suppression and/or aromatase inhibitors.

TREATMENT

Treatment of depression in cancer patients is effective at reducing key symptoms[62] as well as prevalence of the desire for hastened death,[63] and improves quality of life (**Boxes 6-7**) and (**6-8**).[52] Tricyclic antidepressants, selective serotonin reuptake inhibitors, and psychosocial interventions are all evidence-supported interventions for depression in patients with cancer.[62,64] However, there is little evidence to suggest that one antidepressant is more effective than another, and so far no difference has been found between the effectiveness of psychotherapeutic and pharmacologic interventions.

■ PHARMACOLOGIC INTERVENTIONS
SSRIs and SNRIs

Serotonin reuptake inhibitors (SSRIs and SNRIs) are among the first-line antidepressants in cancer patients because of safety and tolerability.

BOX 6-7
TREATMENTS FOR DEPRESSION IN PATIENTS WITH CANCER

SSRIs (note risk for discontinuation syndrome in SSRIs with short half-lives)

SNRIs (watch for dose-dependent hypertension)

Bupropion (may help fatigue)

Mirtazapine (may also help nausea)

TCAs (may help neuropathic pain)

Antipsychotics (as augmenting agent; may help nausea and insomnia)

Stimulants (fast onset of effect, help energy)

Cognitive behavioral therapy

Meaning-centered therapy

Group therapy

Supportive-expressive therapy

BOX 6-8
IMPORTANT DRUG–DRUG INTERACTIONS BETWEEN ANTIDEPRESSANTS AND CHEMOTHERAPY TREATMENTS

Tamoxifen (see Table 6-2)
Antiemetics (may have additive side effects)

All have approximately equal efficacy, and take effect after a trial of 2 to 6 weeks at an adequate dose. In addition to improving depression and anxiety, they reduce hot flashes by approximately 50% in breast cancer survivors.[65] Notably, prior randomized controlled trials of antidepressants in patients with cancer have tested fluoxetine, paroxetine, and mianserin rather than theoretically preferred antidepressants (discussed below). As antidepressants are more widely prescribed for mood symptoms in cancer, accrual to randomized placebo-controlled clinical trials has become increasingly difficult because many cancer patients are no longer willing to accept the possibility of receiving placebo. More recently, prevention studies have been conducted, including a recent randomized controlled trial in which prophylactic escitalopram was found to reduce the risk of developing depression by more than 50% in nondepressed patients undergoing treatment for head and neck cancer.[66]

Common side effects of SSRIs and SNRIs include gastrointestinal distress, activation, headache, dizziness, and sexual dysfunction, many of which resolve within a few weeks of starting therapy. Patients with severe cancer-induced gastrointestinal symptoms or significant chemotherapy-related nausea may require additional reassurance or consideration of alternative agents. Other side effects that warrant caution in patients with cancer are antidepressant-related hyponatremia (SIADH) and increased risk of gastrointestinal bleeding especially in light of the high prevalence of comorbid pulmonary conditions (which may themselves present a risk for SIADH) and chemotherapy- and disease-related thrombocytopenia. However, these side effects are uncommon and should not deter use.

Antidepressants with short half-lives (paroxetine, venlafaxine) may produce increased risk of discontinuation syndrome featuring flu-like symptoms, psychiatric symptoms (depression/anxiety/agitation), and dizziness; this affects patients at risk for bowel obstruction or other surgeries who may not be able to take oral medications for extended periods postoperatively. For example, patients with advanced ovarian cancer often experience sudden obstructions which necessitate NPO status, including discontinuation of all oral medications, placing them at risk for antidepressant discontinuation syndrome. Thus, they may benefit from antidepressants with longer half-lives, such as fluoxetine. Conversely, fluoxetine with its long half-life and P450 interactions may not be advisable for patients whose treatment regimens interact with it. For these reasons, medications with intermediate half-lives and few P450 interactions, for instance, citalopram, escitalopram, and sertraline, are often used in the cancer setting to avoid these issues.

The SNRIs (venlafaxine, duloxetine), though carrying the additional risk of dose-dependent hypertension, may have some advantage over SSRIs in augmenting pain management and menopausal symptoms, which may be acutely triggered by surgery or chemotherapy.

■ ATYPICAL ANTIDEPRESSANTS

Bupropion is a dual norepinephrine and dopamine reuptake inhibitor that improves fatigue and sexual dysfunction in patients with cancer[67] and also aids in smoking cessation. Because bupropion does not cause weight gain and may even promote weight loss, it may not be a first-line agent in cachectic patients. The metabolites of bupropion inhibit CYP2D6 and so it is not a preferred agent for patients receiving tamoxifen; in addition, bupropion has no beneficial effects on hot flashes. Because of its dose dependent effect on seizure threshold, bupropion should be avoided in patients who have had seizures due to primary brain tumors or metastases.

Mirtazapine is a noradrenergic agent and 5-HT2, 5-HT3, and H1 antagonist, that simultaneously targets depression and other symptoms common in patients with cancer, including insomnia, poor appetite, weight loss, and nausea. Mirtazapine has a more rapid onset of action than most antidepressants, with improvement seen within a week in studies of noncancer-related depression. The action of mirtazapine at 5-HT3 receptors is similar to that of the setron class of antiemetics, and mirtazapine may be effective for chemotherapy-induced nausea and vomiting.[68] Compared to SSRIs, mirtazapine has a low rate of sexual side effects.

Mirtazapine may theoretically retard the growth of some cancers. It, and other H1 antagonists, decrease levels of IL-6,[69,70] a growth factor for multiple forms of cancer. Thus, some advocate the use of mirtazapine in patients with IL-6-responsive cancers based on the theoretical benefit of downstream blocking of IL-6.[71] However, it should be noted that no study has documented that H1 antagonism slows cancer growth in vivo.

Side effects of mirtazapine include increased appetite, weight gain, sedation, constipation, dry mouth, dizziness and (rarely) neutropenia, agranulocytosis and hyponatremia. Sedation is more prominent in doses less than 15 mg/day, when antihistaminergic effects are greater, but may wane within days in some individuals. Mirtazapine may be less appropriate for treatment of depression in patients who are relatively well or who have gained weight from steroids or chemotherapy, for whom weight gain and increased appetite may not be desirable.

■ TRICYCLIC ANTIDEPRESSANTS

Tricyclic agents have anticholinergic side effects, muscarinic and alpha blockade, and drug interactions that limit their use to second-line agents, especially in the elderly. They may be helpful in neuropathic pain, as well as insomnia, due to histaminic blockade; constipation may be a helpful side effect to harness in a patient with diarrhea due to cancer or chemotherapy. Often, low doses are effective.

■ ANTIPSYCHOTICS

Olanzapine, quetiapine, and other antipsychotics may be useful as augmentation agents for standard antidepressants. They are also very useful for chemotherapy-related nausea and vomiting, insomnia, and anxiety in patients with cognitive impairment (where benzodiazepines are relatively contraindicated), and may counteract steroid-induced mood lability. Side effects that are a concern with long term use in the general population, such as tardive dyskinesia, diabetes, and metabolic syndrome, may be less of a concern in patients with life-limiting oncologic illness.

■ STIMULANTS

Studies of methylphenidate and dextroamphetamine have shown response rates of over 70% in patients with cancer and depression.[72–74] As patients near the end of life, and the weeks it may take a typical antidepressant to become effective are not available, methylphenidate and dextroamphetamine may be agents of choice for low energy and withdrawal; onset of effect for these can be 1 to 2 days. One option is to start psychostimulants at the same time as a typical antidepressant, then taper the psychostimulant as the typical agent becomes effective. Stimulants decrease fatigue and improve arousal, cognition,[75] and symptoms of hypoactive delirium,[76] all of which are particularly beneficial for patients with cancer. While decreased appetite is a known side effect, appetite actually improves in some depressed cancer patients treated with

stimulants.[73,74,77] Stimulants also appear to lessen opioid-related sedation to some degree, which may permit increasing doses of opioids for more effective pain relief.

Stimulants are very well-tolerated in patients with cancer, with rates of discontinuation consistently below 20%.[72,74,77] The most common side effects of methylphenidate, and those most likely to lead to treatment discontinuation, are agitation and insomnia; others include dry mouth, tremors, nausea, decreased appetite, headache, palpitations, and vomiting. There appears to be minimal risk of dependence, misuse, tolerance, or cardiac side effects in patients with cancer.[78]

The majority of studies in cancer patients have used immediate-release methylphenidate, although dextroamphetamine appears to be equally efficacious.[74] Methylphenidate is quite affordable, and a transdermal form of the drug has recently become available, which may be advantageous for patients who are unable to swallow.

■ MODAFINIL

Modafinil, a nonamphetamine-based stimulant approved for narcolepsy, is also well tolerated and has a similar side effect profile, including nausea, headache, diarrhea, nervousness, and dry mouth. Although modafinil has not been studied in depression associated with cancer, it appears to be a beneficial adjunctive treatment in cancer-related fatigue.[79] Unlike methylphenidate, modafinil is a CYP450 inducer and may accelerate metabolism of tricyclic antidepressants, warfarin, and other medications.

■ KETAMINE

Ketamine is a classic anesthetic agent and noncompetitive NMDA antagonist that, in subanesthetic doses, has robust and rapid therapeutic effects on depression, especially for patients who are resistant to conventional antidepressants.[80] Likewise, ketamine may ameliorate pain and depression in patients with advanced cancer; however, controlled trials are lacking. In addition, antidepressant effects of ketamine may result from upregulation of rapamycin (mTOR), which in turn could theoretically cause accelerated tumor growth.[81] In that context, controlled studies examining ketamine's effects on cancer outcomes as well as depression are needed.

■ ELECTROCONVULSIVE THERAPY

Electroconvulsive therapy (ECT), though highly effective in older adults with other medical conditions, has never been specifically studied in oncologic settings.[82] Space-occupying intracranial lesions are a relative contraindication, though the literature suggests that safe ECT is possible even in this setting.[83]

■ SPECIAL TOPICS
Managing Depression-Related Insomnia in Cancer

For both psychological and physical reasons, nearly half of cancer patients suffer sleep disruption.[84] Insomnia related to depression is frequently exacerbated by physical symptoms tied to tumor invasion or treatment side-effects. Pain, itchiness, urinary urgency, shortness of breath, and draining lesions can all contribute to a poor night's sleep. A steroid taper to quell chemotherapy-associated nausea, or stimulants targeting cancer fatigue, can also negatively impact sleep patterns.

Benzodiazepines act through the inhibitory gamma-aminobutyric acid (GABA) neurotransmitter system to rapidly promote sleep and quell anxiety, and can be useful adjuncts to antidepressants. One such medication, lorazepam, is ubiquitous in cancer treatment. Oncology providers often prescribe this medication on an as-needed basis for broad ranging symptom management, including insomnia, nausea, muscular discomfort, seizure control, and anxiety (for instance, in anticipation of chemotherapy or, in patients with claustrophobia, during magnetic resonance imaging).

Despite this popularity of benzodiazepines, they should be used with caution. Central nervous system side effects include disorientation, sedation, irritability, ataxia, frequent falls, dizziness, and respiratory suppression. Patients with cancer tend to be of advanced age and may have neoplastic or paraneoplastic central nervous system involvement of their disease, rendering them more sensitive to benzodiazepine effects. For these reasons, the intervention of choice may be to wean benzodiazepines rather than add them, and to rely on safer interventions such as cognitive behavior therapy for sleep or hypnotics such as eszopiclone, zaleplon, and zolpidem (See Chapter 10, Patients with Sleep Disorders).

As described above, administration of mirtazapine to the depressed cancer patient with insomnia may avoid risks associated with benzodiazepine use while producing higher quality sleep than that induced by benzodiazepines. Another option is trazodone, a postsynaptic serotonin and alpha receptor blocker which is useful in the treatment of insomnia and depression, despite limited evidence for its benefit in nondepressed patients with insomnia.[85] Side effects include orthostasis and priapism.

Several other benign pharmacologic interventions deserve special mention: gabapentin, melatonin, and ramelteon. Like lorazepam, gabapentin is frequently prescribed in cancer treatment for broad-ranging symptom management, including neuropathic pain and menopausal symptoms triggered by chemotherapy. Scant literature supports use of this agent in primary insomnia[86]; however, gabapentin can be quite sedating, particularly initially, and one can occasionally harness this side-effect to advantage. As an example: the bulk of a standard regimen for menopausal symptoms (300 mg three times daily) can be shifted to bedtime (for instance, 300 in the morning and then 600 mg at bedtime) in the hopes of improving sleep quality.

Melatonin and ramelteon (a melatonin agonist) help to synchronize circadian rhythms in patients with sleep schedule disruptions and in patients with low melatonin, such as the elderly. Initial investigations suggest that ramelteon is more effective than placebo in modestly decreasing sleep latency and increasing sleep duration, with effects lasting up to 6 months. Although the utility of ramelteon as a sleep aid in cancer patients has not been evaluated, it has a strong safety profile and general tolerability, making use in this population attractive. Clinically, it appears to be effective, though more so in treating initial rather than middle or terminal insomnia. Preliminary evidence also suggests that high melatonin levels may help to slow growth of certain cancers.[87]

Tamoxifen and Antidepressant Interactions

Beyond merely theoretical considerations related to using antidepressants with P450 interactions in combination with chemotherapy,

TABLE 6-2 Considerations for Co-administration with Tamoxifen: Antidepressants Arranged In Order of CYP2D6 Inhibition

None to Limited	Moderate	Significant
Venlafaxine	Sertraline	Paroxetine
Escitalopram	Duloxetine	Fluoxetine
Mirtazapine	Trazodone	Bupropion
Citalopram	Most TCAs	

treatment decisions must be based on patient circumstances and the specific chemotherapeutic agent in question. Tamoxifen and SSRI/SNRI interactions provide a particularly instructive example of a decision-making algorithm in the oncology setting. Specifically, potent inhibitors of CYP P450 isoenzyme 2D6, such as paroxetine or fluoxetine, may hinder metabolism of tamoxifen into one of its most active metabolites, endoxifen (4-hydoxy-N-desmethyl-tamoxifen). One study suggested that breast cancer patients on paroxetine have an increased risk of recurrence compared to patients on no antidepressants or other antidepressants.[88] For this reason, it may be best to avoid paroxetine in patients with breast cancer patients receiving adjuvant therapy with tamoxifen. However, this association with recurrence is not seen with other antidepressants that also inhibit isoenzyme 2D6, such as fluoxetine and bupropion. Moreover, the discovery of new tamoxifen metabolites and the finding that other CYP isoenzymes such as 3A4 and 2C9 are also involved in tamoxifen metabolism calls into question the relative importance of endoxifen and CYP 2D6 status in mediating the clinical effects of tamoxifen on target tissues.[89] Thus, decisions regarding antidepressant therapy on tamoxifen should be individualized based on breast cancer recurrence risk, severity of depressive symptoms, and effect of depressive recurrence on overall health and quality of life. **Table 6-2** lists common antidepressants and their relative levels of CYP2D6 inhibition.

PSYCHOTHERAPEUTIC INTERVENTIONS

Psychotherapy is a crucial component of psychiatric care for patients with cancer and depression. Cancer is a life-transforming diagnosis and a traumatic stressor which presents numerous immediate threats—including but not limited to mortality, physical disintegration, financial strain, isolation from previous social networks, and treatments that often seem worse than the disease and undermine the patient's confidence in medical care. Cancer patients must confront the threat of death and learn to cope with their fears, revise their interpersonal relationships, and set priorities for whatever time they have remaining. Those cancer patients who develop depression face an even more difficult adjustment due to the anhedonia and executive dysfunction that can limit their ability to hope for the best while planning for the worst. Hence "psychiatric medication management" in the depressed cancer patient is a misnomer; pharmacological treatment must be liberally integrated with psychotherapeutic approaches in order to address the most relevant aspects of the crisis.

Psychotherapy can decrease physical symptoms and psychological and existential distress, help cancer survivors manage their fears of recurrence and transition successfully out of the "sick role," and help terminally ill cancer patients cope with disease progression and find meaning and purpose as the end of the life approaches. Patients often identify strongly with the idea that cancer results in multiple losses which must be grieved, similarly to how one would mourn the losses of family members or close friends. Some principles of grief therapy that are particularly useful in the psychotherapy of cancer patients include prioritizing self-care activities while also scheduling grieving time, as well as making a coping plan in advance for anniversaries of important losses (dates of diagnosis and of disfiguring surgeries; deaths of family members and friends, especially if cancer related). Notably, major milestones such as holidays and birthdays are difficult times for cancer patients at certain points in the disease course, especially shortly after diagnosis or recurrence; they often fear that this holiday or birthday will be their last. Emphasizing self-care and behavioral activation is critical for the grieving cancer patient who is also depressed. Basic supportive psychotherapeutic tactics such as normalization are also very useful in combating the role shifts and isolation that accompany a potentially terminal diagnosis.

Cognitive behavioral therapy (CBT), meaning-centered therapy, group therapy, and supportive-expressive therapy are of particular utility for patients with cancer. Perhaps most commonly utilized for individual therapy is an eclectic mixture of supportive-expressive and CBT techniques. A supportive-expressive approach in the cancer patient hinges upon obtaining the narrative of how the patient was diagnosed with cancer. Themes that are highly relevant to the psychotherapy usually emerge in the course of that narrative. Common examples include guilt over delaying evaluation for concerning symptoms; self-blame based on lifestyle choices that may have contributed to cancer; and mistrust and anger at medical providers whom they perceive contributed to diagnostic delay. Patients' descriptions of how they handled the time period immediately following their diagnosis often provide a window into the maturity of their coping style and defense mechanisms. It is useful to ask how the patient has coped with major life stressors that pre-dated the cancer diagnosis, and to determine whether they have benefitted from individual or group therapy in the past. Psychoeducation should be liberally incorporated into treatment for all patients. For example, since many patients have an underlying fear that life stressors caused their cancer and may contribute to its progression, it is important to tell patients that research does not support an association between stress and cancer diagnosis or recurrence. If the clinician has worked with other cancer patients, a well-timed example of how another patient coped with cancer-related concerns may be extremely helpful in normalizing common concerns, decreasing a sense of isolation, and building a therapeutic alliance. Another general goal of therapy is to help patients rebuild confidence in their instincts about their physical sensations and to achieve an appropriate balance between amplifying and minimizing somatic complaints. Encouraging patients to self-advocate in the setting of instinctively concerning symptoms can help patients regain a sense of control. In this vein, improving patient-oncologist communication is also a central goal of therapy. During therapy it can be helpful to discuss details of their last visit and then assist the patient in developing a priority-ordered list of questions to ask their oncologist during the next visit.

As shown by the above examples, supportive-expressive therapy in cancer patients often tends to occur closer to the supportive end of the continuum, given that extensive exploratory work may overwhelm fragile defenses or simply have less salience in the setting of a situational crisis. Still, exploratory tactics can be useful, particularly as the therapeutic alliance deepens. Tactics relevant to the cancer setting include fully exploring the specific admixture of emotions that underlie "anxiety" as well as directly analyzing transference issues pertaining to the patient-oncologist relationship. Patients can benefit from recognizing that their emotional responses to the oncologist parallel their responses to others in their lives, including their family of origin.

CBT can decrease both pain and distress in cancer patients, according to a meta-analysis.[90,91] CBT teaches patients to identify thoughts and feelings associated with their symptoms and to become aware of cognitive distortions and negative automatic thoughts that increase physical and psychological distress. Maladaptive adjustment styles (e.g., avoidance/denial, fatalism, helplessness/hopelessness, and anxious preoccupation) can magnify distress in patients with cancer.[92] Practically speaking, unemployment, body image concerns, and demanding treatment schedules can result in limited day structure and social contact, which fuels depression. For these issues, we recommend behavioral activation (e.g., walking 5 minutes each day and increasing this by 5 minutes each day as tolerated), activity scheduling (to mimic work schedules), and exposure hierarchies (for patients who socially isolate because they are anxious about how healthy people will perceive them). Relaxation techniques, such as diaphragmatic breathing, progressive muscle relaxation, and autogenic training, can decrease physiologic arousal and improve coping.[93] Changing the interpretation of symptoms and stresses and learning coping strategies improves adjustment to cancer.[92] Mindfulness meditation, a component of third-wave CBT, also helps decrease anxiety and distress.[94,95]

Group therapies for patients with cancer exist in a variety of formats. Support groups are a major source of social support that can mitigate pain, distress, depression, and anxiety.[96,97] Groups decrease feelings of isolation that accompany cancer diagnosis and provide patients with a forum in which to express painful emotions. Supportive-expressive group psychotherapy uses unstructured groups to focus on patients' concerns, particularly around existential issues of meaning, death, isolation, and freedom.[98] Supportive-expressive groups have been shown to reduce mood disturbance, maladaptive coping, and traumatic stress symptoms.[98,99] Unfortunately, early hopes that group therapy might prolong survival in metastatic patients have not been conclusively borne out.[100] Still, researchers continue to explore the potential effects of group therapy on cancer outcomes. Intriguingly, a recent randomized clinical trial testing a group-based psychological intervention in patients with regional breast cancer found that intervention patients had significantly reduced risks of breast cancer recurrence and death.[101]

Breitbart et al.'s meaning-centered therapy focuses on increasing perceived meaning, peacefulness, and sense of purpose in terminally ill cancer patients, and may be employed in either individual or group settings.[102,103] Meaning centered therapy is based on Viktor Frankl's logotherapy, which holds that creativity, attitude, and experience are the three primary sources of meaning in life.[104] Over seven 90-minute sessions, patients discuss the following themes: concepts and sources of meaning; cancer and meaning; meaning and historical context of life; storytelling and life project; limitations and finiteness of life; responsibility, creativity, and deeds; experience, nature, art, and humor; and termination, goodbyes, and hopes for the future. In patients with advanced cancer, meaning-centered group therapy improves spiritual well-being, increases sense of meaning, and decreases anxiety and desire for death.[105]

Finally, contingent suicidality can present a challenge in the psychiatric care of patients with cancer. Therapeutic tactics for contingent suicidality include exploring the motivation for the patient's death wish, sharing the patient's sense of helplessness, and avoiding power struggles or forcing the patient to renounce their threats too soon in the therapy.[30] Much contingent suicidality in oncology patients resolves with good access to palliative care, aggressive symptom management at the end of life, and a commitment to giving patients a sense of control over the location and circumstances of their death.

■ SPIRITUALITY

Depressive suffering in cancer frequently has a spiritual dimension. In one study, seventy-eight percent of patients with advanced cancer report that spirituality is important to their cancer experience.[106] Prominent spiritual themes include religious/spiritual (R/S) coping; R/S beliefs and practices, such as prayer; R/S transformation due to the cancer experience; and R/S community as a source of support. Spirituality may also be a source of distress. In the same study, 43% reported at least one negative religious coping theme, which include feeling abandoned or punished by God, questioning God's love or power, believing the devil caused the cancer, and feeling abandoned by one's spiritual community.[107,108] Spiritual distress is associated with decreased quality of life in advanced cancer patients[108] and the provision of spiritual care with improved quality of life near death.[109] The Joint Commission currently mandates a spiritual assessment of every patient, and palliative medicine includes spiritual care among its goals. Even so, clinicians often hesitate to address the spiritual dimension of their patients' experience because of their own unresolved spiritual conflicts, their unfamiliarity with spiritual traditions, or concerns about influencing patients with their own values.

Clinicians can incorporate spirituality into differential diagnosis and comprehensive formulation in order to facilitate spiritually integrated treatment.[110] Spiritually integrated treatment involves matching available resources to the most pressing of the patient's symptoms and to the patient's most important vulnerabilities through exploration of the patient's spiritual history in combination with the more traditional psychosocial history. Spiritually integrated treatment addresses core existential concerns about identity, hope, meaning, justice, and connection. For example, religious patients with concerns around identity may benefit from grounding their identity in their relationship with God. Patients who struggle to maintain hope could receive interpersonal therapy or spiritual direction focusing on their doubts about trusting God or the future. Understanding punishment and forgiveness from a spiritual perspective may help patients distressed by questions of morality or overwhelmed by guilt. Learning to feel accepted or loved by God can help patients who feel isolated or rejected when depressed. Many forms of spiritual care are best accomplished through referral to or collaboration with spiritual resources, such as hospital chaplains. Incorporating spiritual perspectives and interventions into psychiatric treatment raises ethical, transferential, and counter transferential issues that are beyond the scope of this chapter. Further research is needed to understand how to better assess and address the intertwined depressive and spiritual distress experienced by patients with cancer.

CONCLUSION

Depression is a common comorbidity in patients with cancer that impairs quality of life, causing suffering in patients and in caregivers as well, and erodes patients' ability to make meaningful emotional connections and treatment decisions in the setting of life-threatening illness. Adequate diagnosis and treatment is crucial, and the underpinnings of treatment can be extrapolated from studies in the general population as well as from the growing evidence base of psychosocial oncology (**Box 6-9**).

Several areas clearly require more study. These include the prevalence and phenomenology of adjustment disorders, and the longitudinal course of major depression across the phases of

illness, with a focus on caseness as opposed to symptom scores. Many of the existing treatment trials are single center trials that do not account for potentially confounding effects of concurrent psychotherapeutic, pharmacological, or complementary/alternative therapies that the subjects may have been utilizing.[111] Especially crucial are large, placebo-controlled trials of antidepressants with fewer drug–drug interactions that incorporate measurement of biomarkers. Subject accrual in such trials is particularly difficult because many patients with cancer and depression are unwilling to accept the possibility of receiving placebo.

A multimodal treatment approach is most effective in this population. Such a strategy tailors psychosocial interventions to patient preference and clinical features, including cancer type, stage, and comorbidities, and combine psychotherapy with pharmacotherapy for moderate to severe depressive disorders. Collaborative care models of depression management should evaluate these individually tailored psychopharmacologic and psychotherapeutic approaches. Controlled trials should be conducted in order to evaluate whether routine depression screening may reduce unmet needs in cancer patients and diminish the risk of severe and persistent depressive symptoms.

REFERENCES

1. Mitchell AJ, Chan M, Bhatti H, et al. Prevalence of depression, anxiety and adjustment disorder in oncological, hematological and palliative care settings: a meta-analysis of 94 interview-based studies. *Lancet Oncol.* 2011;12(2):160–174.

2. Waraich P, Goldner EM, Somers JM, Hsu L. Prevalence and incidence studies of mood disorders: a systematic review of the literature. *Can J Psychiatry.* 2004;49(2):124–138.

3. Spiegel D, Giese-Davis J. Depression and cancer: mechanisms and disease progression. *Biol Psychiatry.* 2003;54:269–282.

4. Wilson KG, Chochinov HM, Skirko MG, et al. Depression and anxiety disorders in palliative cancer care. *J Pain Symptom Manage.* 2007;33:118–129.

5. Hill J, Holcombe C, Clark L, et al. Predictors of onset of depression and anxiety in the year after diagnosis of breast cancer. *Psychol Med.* 2011;41:1429–1436.

6. Pirl WF. Evidence report on the occurrence, assessment, and treatment of depression in cancer patients. *J Natl Cancer Inst Monogr.* 2004;32:32–39.

7. Strong V, Waters R, Hibberd C, et al. Emotional distress in cancer patients: the Edinburgh cancer center symptom study. *Br J Cancer.* 2007;96:868–874.

8. Ell K, Sanchez K, Vourlekis B, et al. Depression, correlates of depression, and receipt of depression care among low-income women with breast or gynecologic cancer. *J Clin Oncol.* 2005;23: 3052–3060.

9. Skarstein J, Bjelland I, Dahl AA, Laading J, Fossa SD. Is there an association between haemoglobin, depression, and anxiety in cancer patients? *J Psychosom Res.* 2005;58:477–483.

10. Carlson LE, Angen M, Cullum J, et al. High levels of untreated distress and fatigue in cancer patients. *Br J Cancer.* 2004;90:2297–2304.

11. Schneider KL, Shenassa E. Correlates of suicide ideation in a population-based sample of cancer patients. *J Psychosoc Oncol.* 2008;26:49–62.

12. Chochinov HM, Wilson KG, Enns M, et al. Depression, hopelessness, and suicidal ideation in the terminally ill. *Psychosomatics.* 1998;39:366–370.

BOX 6-9
SUMMARY

- Depression is commonly comorbid in patients with cancer
- Differential diagnosis is challenging; however, it is important not to miss major depression given its impact on quality of life
- Large scale studies are lacking, available evidence suggests that standard treatments for depression are effective in this population

13. Breitbart W, Rosenfeld B, Pessin H, et al. Depression, hopeless-ness, and desire for hastened death in terminally ill patients with cancer. *JAMA*. 2000;284:2907–2911.

14. Gutheil TG, Schetky D. A date with death: management of time-based and contingent suicidal intent. *Am J Psychiatry*. 1998;155:1502–1507.

15. Peteet J, Maytal G, Rokni H. Unimaginable loss: contingent suicidal ideation in family members. *Psychosomatics*. 2010;51:166–70.

16. Miller M, Mogun H, Azrael D, et al. Cancer and the risk of suicide in older Americans. *J Clin Oncol*. 2008;26:4720–4724.

17. Misono S, Weiss NS, Fann JR, et al. Incidence of suicide in per-sons with cancer. *J Clin Oncol*. 2008;26:4731–4738.

18. Ripamonti C, Filiberti A, Totis A, De Conno F, Tamburini M. Suicide among patients with cancer cared for at home by pal-liative care teams. *Lancet*. 1999;354:1877–1878.

19. Crocetti E, Arniani S, Acciai S, Barchielli A, Buiatti E. High suicide mortality soon after diagnosis among cancer patients in central Italy. *Br J Cancer*. 1998;77:1194–1196.

20. Fang F, Fall K, Mittleman MA, et al. Suicide and cardiovascular death after a cancer diagnosis. *N Engl J Med*. 2012;366:1310–1318.

21. Ganzini L, Goy ER, Dobscha SK. Prevalence of depression and anxiety in patients requesting physicians' aid in dying: cross sectional survey. *BMJ*. 2008;337:a1682.

22. Janelsins MC, Roscoe JA, Berg MJ, et al. IGF-1 partially restores chemotherapy-induced reductions in neural cell proliferation in adult C57BL/6 mice. *Cancer Invest*. 2010;28:544–553.

23. Aggarwal BB, Shishodia S, Sandur SK, et al. Inflammation and cancer: how hot is the link? *Biochem Pharmacol*. 2006;72:1605–1621.

24. Musselman DM, Miller AH, Porter MR, et al. Higher than normal plasma IL-6 concentrations in cancer patients with major depres-sion: preliminary findings. *Am J Psychiatry*. 2001;158:1252–1257.

25. Jehn CF, Kuenhardt D, Bartholomae D, et al. Biomarkers of depression in cancer patients. *Cancer*. 2006;107:2723–2729.

26. Evans DL, McCartney CF, Nemeroff CB, et al. Depression in women treated for gynecological cancer: clinical and neuroen-docrine assessment. *Am J Psychiatry*. 1986;143:447–452.

27. Capuron L, Raison CL, Musselman DL, et al. Association of exag-gerated HPA axis response to the initial injection of IFN-alpha with development of depression during IFN-alpha therapy. *Am J Psychiatry*. 2003;160:1342–1345.

28. Miller AH, Ancoli-Israel S, Bower JE, et al. Neuroendocrine-immune mechanisms of behavioral comorbidities in patients with cancer. *J Clin Oncol*. 2008;26:917–982

29. Akechi T, Okuyama T, Sugawara Y, et al. Major depression, adjust-ment disorders, and PTSD in terminally ill cancer patients: asso-ciated and predictive factors. *J Clin Oncol*. 2004;22:1957–1965.

30. Muskin PR. The request to die: role for a psychodynamic perspective on physician-assisted suicide. *JAMA*. 1998;279:323–328.

31. Mols F, Oelemans S, Denollet J, et al. Type D personality is asso-ciated with increased comorbidity burden and health care utilization among 3080 cancer survivors. *Gen Hosp Psychiatry*. 2012;34:352–359.

32. Burgess C, Cornelius V, Love SH, Graham J, Richards M, Ramirez A. Depression and anxiety in women with early breast cancer: five year observational cohort study. *BMJ*. 2005;330(7493):702.

33. Miovic M, Block S. Psychiatric disorders in advanced cancer. *Cancer*. 2007;110:1665–1676.

34. Ciaramella A, Poli P. Assessment of depression among can-cer patients: the role of pain, cancer type and treatment. *Psychooncology*. 2001;10:156–165.

35. Evans DL, Staab JP, Petitto JM, et al. Depression in the medical setting: biopsychological interactions and treatment consider-ations. *J Clin Psychiatry*. 1999;60(Suppl 4):40–55.

36. Lichtenthal W, Nilsson M, Zhang B, et al. Do rates of mental disorders and existential distress among advanced stage can-cer patients increase as death approaches? *Psychooncology*. 2009;18:50–61.

37. Pirl WF, Greer J, Temel JS, Yeap BY, Gilman SE. Major depres-sive disorder in long-term cancer survivors: analysis of the National Comorbidity Survey Replication. *J Clin Oncol*. 2009;27:4130–4134.

38. Spiegel DD, Giese-Davis JJ. Depression and anxiety in meta-static cancer. *Minerva Psichiatrica*. 2008;49(1):61–70.

39. Prieto JM, Blanch J, Atala J, et al. Psychiatric morbidity and impact on hospital length of stay in hematologic cancer patients undergoing stem cell transplantation. *J Clin Oncol*. 2002;20(7):1907–1917.

40. Montazeri AM, Sajadian A, Ebrahimi M, Akbari ME. Depression and the use of complementary medicine among breast cancer patients. *Support Care Cancer*. 2005;13:339–342.

41. Pirl WF, Greer JA, Traeger L, et al. Depression and survival in metastatic non-small cell lung cancer: effects of early palliative care. *J Clin Oncol*. 2012;30(12):1310–1315.

42. Mystakidou K, Tsilika E, Parpa E, et al. The relationship between quality of life and levels of hopelessness and depression in pal-liative care. *Depress Anxiety*. 2008;25(9):730–736.

43. Satin JR, Linden W, Phillips MJ. Depression as a predictor of cancer progression and mortality in cancer patients: a meta-analysis. *Cancer*. 2009;115(22):5349–5361.

44. Ware MA, Doyle CR, Woods R. Cannabis use for chronic non-cancer pain: results of a prospective survey. *Pain*. 2003;102(1–2):211–216.

45. Block SD. Assessing and managing depression in the termi-nally ill patient. ACP-ASIM End-of-Life Care Consensus Panel. American College of Physicians—American Society of Internal Medicine. *Ann Intern Med*. 2000;132:209–218.

46. Kissane DW, Wein S, Love A, Lee XQ, Kee PL, Clarke DM. The Demoralization Scale: a report of its development and prelimi-nary validation. *J Palliat Care*. 2004;20:269–276.

47. Ironside W. Conservation-withdrawal and action engage-ment: on a theory of survivor behavior. *Psychosom Med*. 1980;42:163–175.

48. McDonald MV, Passik SD, Dugan W, et al. Nurses' recognition of depression in their patients with cancer. *Oncol Nurs Forum*. 1999;26:593–599.

49. Passik SD, Dugan W, McDonald MV, et al. Oncologists' recog-nition of depression in their patients with cancer. *J Clin Oncol*. 1998;16:1594–1600.

50. Vodermaier A, Millman RD. Accuracy of the HADS as a screening tool in cancer patients: a systematic review and meta-analysis. *Support Care Cancer*. 2011;19(12):1899–1908.

51. Meijer A, Roseman M, Milette K, et al. Depression screening and patient outcomes in cancer: a systematic review. *PLoS One*. 2011;6(11):e27181.

52. Strong V, Waters R, Hibberd C, et al. Management of depression for people with cancer (SMaRT oncology 1): a randomized trial. *Lancet*. 2008;372:40–48.

53. Quek R, Morgan JA, George S, et al. Small molecule tyrosine kinase inhibitor and depression. *J Clin Oncol*. 2009;27:312–313.

54. Galvao-de Almeida A, Guindalini C, Batista-Neves S, et al. Can antidepressants prevent interferon-alpha induced depression? A review of the literature. *Gen Hosp Psychiatry*. 2010;32:401–405.

55. Musselman DL, Lawson DH, Gumnick JF, et al. Paroxetine for the prevention of depression induced by high-dose interferon alpha. *N Engl J Med*. 2001;344:961–966.

56. Raison CL, Demetrashvili M, Capuron L, Miller AH. Neuropsychiatric adverse effects of interferon-alpha. *CNS Drugs*. 2005;19(2):105–123.

57. Greenberg DB, Jonasch E, Gadd MA, et al. Adjuvant therapy of melanoma with interferon-alpha-2b is associated with mania and bipolar syndromes. *Cancer*. 2000;89(2):356–966.

58. Malek-Ahmadi P, Ghandour E. Bupropion for treatment of interferon-induced depression. *Ann Pharmacother*. 2004;38(7–8):1202–1205.

59. Day R, Ganz PA, Constantino JP. Tamoxifen and depression: more evidence from the National Surgical Adjuvant Breast and Bowel Project's Breast Cancer Prevention (P-1) Randomized Study. *J Natl Cancer Inst*. 2001;93(21):1615–1623.

60. Lee KC, Ray GT, Hunkeler EM, Finley PR. Tamoxifen treatment and new onset depression in breast cancer patients. *Psychosomatics*. 2007;48:205–210.

61. Amrolhalli Z, Rezaei F, Salehi B, et al. Double-blind, randomized, placebo-controlled 6-week study on the efficacy and safety of the tamoxifen adjunctive to lithium in acute bipolar mania. *J Affect Disord*. 2011;129:327–331.

62. Lorenz KA, Lynn J, Dy SM, et al. Evidence for improving palliative care at the end of life: a systematic review. *Ann Intern Med*. 2008;148:147–159.

63. O'Mahony S, Goulet J, Kornblith A, et al. Desire for hastened death, cancer pain and depression: report of a longitudinal observational study. *J Pain Symptom Manage*. 2005;29:446–457.

64. Carr D, Goudas L, Lawrence D, et al. Management of cancer symptoms: pain, depression, and fatigue. *Evid Rep Technol Assess (Summ)*. 2002;(61):1–5.

65. Bordeleau L, Pritchard K, Goodwin P, Loprinzi C. Therapeutic options for the management of hot flashes in breast cancer survivors: an evidence-based review. *Clin Ther*. 2007;29:230–241.

66. Lydiatt WM, Bessette D, Schmid KK, Sayles H, Burke WJ. Prevention of depression with escitalopram in patients undergoing treatment for head and neck cancer: randomized double blind placebo-controlled clinical trial. *JAMA Otolaryngol Head Neck Surg*. 2013;139:678–686.

67. Moss EL, Simpson JS, Pelletier G, Forsyth P. An open-label study of the effects of bupropion SR on fatigue, depression, and quality of life of mixed-site cancer patients and their partners. *Psychooncology*. 2006;15:259–267.

68. Pae CU. Low dose mirtazapine may be successful treatment option for severe nausea and vomiting. *Prog Neuropsychopharmacol Biol Psychiatry*. 2006;30:1143–1145.

69. Altschuler EL, Kast RE. Anti-histamines as anti-interleukin-6 agents. *N Eng J Med*. 2005;352:1156–1157.

70. Altschuler EL, Kast RE. Using histamine (H1) antagonists, in particular atypical antipsychotics, to treat anemia of chronic disease via interleukin-6 suppression. *Med Hypothes*. 2005;65:65–67.

71. Kast RE, Altschuler EL. Current drugs available now for interleukin-6 suppression as treatment adjunct in glioblastoma: anakinra, aprepitant, mirtazapine, olanzapine. *Int J Cancer Res*. 2006;2:303–314.

72. Homsi J, Nelson KA, Sarhill N, et al. A phase II study of methylphenidate for depression in advanced cancer. *Am J Hosp Palliat Care*. 2001;18(6):403–407.

73. Homsi J, Walsh D, Nelson KA, LeGrand S, Davis M.. Methylphenidate for depression in hospice practice: A case series. *Am J Hosp Palliat Care*. 2000;17:393–398.

74. Olin J, Masand P. Psychostimulants for depression in hospitalized cancer patients. *Psychosomatics*. 1996;37(1):57–62.

75. Meyers CA, Weitzner MA, Valentine AD, Levin VA. Methylphenidate therapy improves cognition, mood and function of brain tumor patients. *J Clin Oncol*. 1998;16(7):2522–2527.

76. Gagnon B, Low G, Schreier G. Methylphenidate hydrochloride improves cognitive function in patients with advanced cancer and hypoactive delirium: a prospective clinical study. *J Psychiatry Neurosci*. 2005;30(2):100–107.

77. Lasheen W, Walsh D, Mahmoud F, Davis MP, Rivera N, Khoshknabi DS. Methylphenidate Side Effects in Advanced Cancer: A Retrospective Analysis. *Am J Hosp Palliat Care*. 2010;27(1):16–23.

78. Orr K, Taylor D. Psychostimulants in the treatment of depression: A review of the evidence. *CNS Drugs*. 2007;21(3):239–257.

79. Kumar R: Approved and investigational uses of modafinil : an evidence-based review. *Drugs*. 2008;68:1803–1839.

80. Murrough JW, Perez AM, Pillemer S, et al. Rapid and longer-term antidepressant effects of repeated ketamine infusions in treatment-resistant major depression. *Biol Psychiatry*. 2013;74:250–256.

81. Yang C, Zhou Z, Yang J. Be prudent of ketamine in treating resistant depression in patients with cancer. *J Pall Med*. 2011;14:537.

82. Rao A, Cohen HJ: Symptom management in the elderly cancer patient: fatigue, pain, and depression. *J Natl Cancer Inst Monogr*. 2004;(32):150–157.

83. Rasmussen KG, Perry CL, Sutor B, Moore KM. ECT in patients with intracranial masses. *J Neuropsychiatry Clin Neurosci*. 2007;19:191–193.

84. Beszterczey A, Lipowski ZJ. Insomnia in cancer patients. *Can Med Assoc J*. 1977;116(4):355.

85. Mendelson WB. A review of the evidence for the efficacy and safety of trazodone in insomnia. *J Clin Psychiatry*. 2005;66:469–476.

86. Lo HS, Yang CM, Lo HG, Lee CY, Ting H, Tzang BS. Treatment effects of gabapentin for primary insomnia. *Clin Neuropharmacol*. 2010;33(2):84–90.

87. Mediavilla MD, Sanchez-Barcelo EJ, Tan DX, Manchester L, Reiter RJ. Basic mechanisms involved in the anti-cancer effects of melatonin. *Curr Med Chem*. 2010;17(36):4462–4481.

88. Kelly CM, Juurlink DN, Gomes T, et al. Selective serotonin reuptake inhibitors and breast cancer mortality in women receiving tamoxifen: a population-based cohort study. *BMJ*. 2010;340:c693.

89. Binkhorst L, van Gelder T, Mathijssen RH. Individualization of tamoxifen treatment for breast carcinoma. *Clin Pharm Therapeutics*. 2012;92:431–433.

90. Graves KD. Social cognitive theory and cancer patients' quality of life: a meta-analysis of psychosocial intervention components. *Health Psychol.* 2003;22:210–219.

91. Tatrow K, Montgomery GH. Cognitive behavioral therapy techniques for distress and pain in breast cancer patients: a meta-analysis. *J Behav Med.* 2006;29:17–27.

92. Moorey S, Greer S. *Cognitive Behavioral Therapy for People with Cancer.* Oxford, UP: Oxford: 2002.

93. Chochinov HM, Breitbart W, Eds. *Handbook of Psychiatry in Palliative Care Medicine*, Second Edition. New York, NY: Oxford; 2009.

94. Carlson LE, Ursuliak Z, Goodey E, Angen M, Speca M. The effects of a mindfulness medication-based stress reduction program on mood and symptoms of stress in cancer outpatients: 6 months follow-up. *Support Care Cancer.* 2001;9:112–123.

95. Speca M, Carlson LE, Goodey E, Angen M. A randomized, wait-list controlled clinical trial: the effect of a mindfulness medication-based stress reduction program on mood and symptoms of stress in cancer outpatients. *Psychosom Med.* 2000;62:613–622.

96. Muzzin LJ, Anderson NJ, Figueredo AT, Gudelis SO. The experience of cancer. *Soc Sci Med.* 1994;38(9):1201–1208.

97. Bordeleau JH, Szalai JP, Ennis M, et al. Quality of life in a randomized trial of group psychosocial support in metastatic breast cancer: Overall effects of the intervention and an exploration of missing data. *J Clin Oncol.* 2003;21(1):1944–1951.

98. Classen C, Butler LD, Koopman C, et al. Supportive-expressive group therapy and distress in patients with metastatic breast cancer: A randomized clinical intervention trial. *Arch Gen Psychiatry.* 2001;58:494–501.

99. Spiegel D, Bloom JR, Yalom I. Group support for patients with metastatic cancer: a randomized outcome study. *Arch Gen Psychiatry.* 1981;38:527–533.

100. Spiegel D, Butler LD, Giese-Davis J, et al. Effects of supportive-expressive group therapy on survival of patients with metastatic breast cancer—A randomized prospective trial. *Cancer.* 2007;110: 1130–1138.

101. Andersen BL, Yang H, Farrar WB, et al. Psychologic intervention improves survival for breast cancer patients. *Cancer.* 2008;113:3450–3458.

102. Breitbart W. Spirituality and meaning in supportive care: spirituality- and meaning-centered group psychotherapy interventions in advanced cancer. *Support Care Cancer.* 2002;49:366–372.

103. Breitbart W, Gibson C, Poppito SR, Berg A. Psychotherapeutic interventions at the end of life: a focus on meaning and spirituality. *Can J Psychiatry.* 2004;49:366–372.

104. Frankl V. *Man's Search for Meaning.* Boston, MA: Beacon; 1963.

105. Breitbart W, Rosenfeld B, Gibson C, et al. Meaning-centered group psychotherapy for patients with advanced cancer: a pilot randomized controlled trial. *Psycho-Oncology.* 2010;19(1):21–28.

106. Alcorn SR, Balboni MJ, Prigerson HG, et al. "If God wanted me yesterday, I wouldn't be here today": Religious and spiritual themes in patients' experiences of advanced cancer. *J Palliative Med.* 2010;13(5):581–588.

107. Pargament KI. *The Psychology of Religion and Coping: Theory, Research, Practice.* New York, NY: Guilford Press; 1997

108. Tarakeshwar N, Vanderwerker LC, Paulk E, Pearce MJ, Kasl SV, Prigerson HG. Religious coping is associated with the quality of life of patients with advanced cancer. *J Palliat Med.* 2006;9:646–657.

109. Balboni TA, Paulk MA, Balboni MJ, et al. Provision of spiritual care to advanced cancer patients. Associations with aggressive medical care and quality of life near death. *J Clin Oncol.* 2010;28:445–452.

110. Peteet JR. *Depression and the Soul. A Guide to Spiritually-Integrated Treatment.* New York, NY: Routledge; 2010.

111. Williams S, Dale J. The effectiveness of treatment for depression/depressive symptoms in adults with cancer: a systematic review. *Br J Cancer.* 2006;94:372–390.

CHAPTER 7

Depression in Cardiovascular Disease

Meghan Kolodziej, MD

Jaya Padmanabhan, MD

Joshua Leo, MD, MPH

Howard Hartley, MD

Depression is frequently encountered in the context of many cardiovascular diseases. The epidemiology, pathophysiology, clinical presentation, and course of the depression vary in each of these medical conditions. They are therefore discussed separately in this chapter. However, the treatment of depression in the context of these various cardiovascular diseases differs very little and thus is covered in a single section at the end.

CORONARY HEART DISEASE AND MYOCARDIAL INFARCTION

■ EPIDEMIOLOGY

Coronary heart disease (CHD) results from narrowing of the arteries that supply blood to the heart, leading to acute myocardial infarction (MI), angina pectoris, and other ischemic heart disease. The American Heart Association estimates that 15 million Americans have CHD, a prevalence of 6.4% among adults aged 20 or older.[1] Approximately 700,000 Americans have a new or recurrent MI each year.[1] While rates of hospitalization and death due to MI decreased from 1999 to 2009, CHD was still the cause of one in six deaths in 2009.[1] The 5-year mortality rate following a first MI is 36% for men and 47% for women aged 45 and older. Additionally, CHD is estimated to cost $195 billion per year in the United States in direct and indirect costs (**Figs. 7-1** to **7-3**).[1]

CHD is associated with elevated rates of depression. Prevalence of major depressive disorder (MDD) is approximately 17% to 27% among patients with CHD,[2] compared to an estimated lifetime prevalence of 16% in the general population.[3] An additional 20% to 30% of patients with CHD experience minor depression or subsyndromal depressive symptoms following MI.[4–6] Patients undergoing coronary artery bypass graft surgery (CABG) due to CHD demonstrate rates of depression of about 20% to 25%, and rates as high as 38% are reported when minor depression is included.[7,8] CHD is also associated with an increased risk of suicide, particularly within the first month of an MI, although the elevated risk may persist for several years.[9]

In addition to co-occurrence in individuals with already established CHD, depression is also an independent risk factor for the subsequent development of initial and recurrent cardiovascular disease in healthy men and women.[2] A large prospective study of individuals with a history of depression but without prior CHD revealed a 2.7-fold increase in subsequent CHD mortality.[10] In a prospective study of women without prior CHD, depressive symptoms were correlated with increased risk of MI, fatal CHD, and sudden cardiac death.[11] Depression confers a relative risk of 1.64 for the development of CHD,[12] and relative risk of about 1.5 for death due to cardiovascular disease.[13,14]

The risk of developing depression in CHD is related to biological, social, and psychological factors (**Box 7-1a**). Family history of depression is a known risk factor for MDD,[15] as well as for depression in the setting of CHD,[16] and heritability studies in twins also indicate that there are genetic risk factors for MDD.[15] However, it is unclear if MDD and CHD share any genetic risk factors. One study did demonstrate that the co-occurrence of depression and cardiovascular disease was partly explained by shared genetic factors.[17]

A number of demographic factors are associated with risk of depression after MI (**Box 7-1b**). Depressed patients with CHD are younger than nondepressed CHD patients.[18–20] A proposed explanation for this interaction is that younger patients experience more

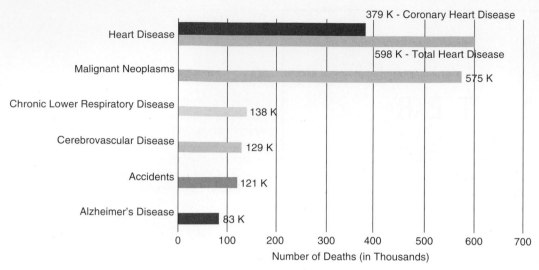

Figure 7-1 *Top six causes of death in the Unites States, 2010. (Data from NHLBI fact book (2012) and Murphy SL, Jiaquan X, Kochanek KD. Deaths: Final Data for 2010,* Natl Vital Stat Rep. *2013;61(4):1–117.)*

change in their physical mobility and lifestyle following MI than older patients.[2] Female gender is also associated with an increased rate of depression in CHD.[18,19,21,22] Women may also have an elevated risk of suicide after MI compared to men.[23] It is unclear whether depression imparts different risks for mortality or recurrent MI in women compared to men.[2]

Medical comorbidity may moderate the relationship between depression and CHD. The presence of other comorbidities, such as diabetes and obesity, are associated with depression in CHD.[24] These may in turn affect cardiovascular outcomes and partly account for the impact of depression on CHD risk.[2]

The role of social isolation has been studied in patients with depression and CHD.[25,26] Living alone is a risk factor for depression in the setting of MI,[27] and lack of social support in general predicts CHD mortality.[26] Social isolation also predicts persistent depression at 1 year follow-up for patients who were depressed at the time of MI.[25]

Psychological factors are also predictive of depression in CHD or following MI. Thus, "Type D" personality, a tendency toward negative affective states and social inhibition, predicts persistent depression over 1 year.[28] An individual's beliefs about heart disease may predict the development of post-MI depression; belief in the curability of heart disease is associated with reduced incidence of depression

after MI, while belief that one will have a lengthy illness is associated with increased incidence of depression after MI (**Fig. 7-4**).[29]

As with depression in medically healthy populations, a history of prior depressive episodes predicts recurrence of depression following acute MI, both in the hospital and after discharge.[27,30] Up to half of patients with post-MI depression have a history of depression before the MI.[31]

It is unclear whether increasing severity of CHD increases risk of depression. Most studies do not find correlations between the severity of depressive symptoms and measures of MI severity, including left ventricular ejection fraction,[7,8] serial CPKs, and Killip class (a classification of mortality risk following MI).[32–34] Likewise, significant associations have not been found between depressive symptoms and systolic and diastolic function, exercise-induced ischemia, and cardiac wall motion abnormalities.[33] However, a minority of studies have found that depression risk is correlated with CHD severity, specifically left ventricular dysfunction,[28] higher Killip class,[31,33,35] and poorer exercise tolerance.[27]

■ **PATHOPHYSIOLOGY**

Several pathophysiological mechanisms have been examined as biological mediators of the association between depression and

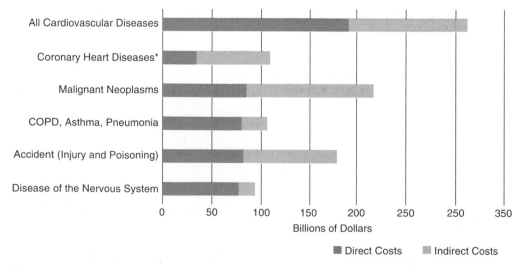

Figure 7-2 *Estimated total cost to the U.S. Economy, 2009. (Data from NHLBI fact book (2012) and Heidenreich PA, Trogdon JG, Khavjou OA, et al: Forecasting the future of cardiovascular disease in the United States: a policy statement from the American Heart Association,* Circulation. *2011;123(8):933–944.)*

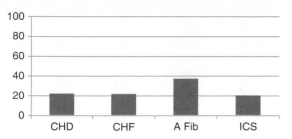

Figure 7-3 *Mean risk of depression for selected illnesses (% prevalence for particular disease).*

CHD (**Box 7-2**). Depression is accompanied by increased sympathetic nervous system activation and/or decreased parasympathetic function. Elevated levels of plasma norepinephrine, which may reflect increased sympathetic activity, are observed in depressed patients with CHD.[18,36] Resting heart rates are elevated in depressed CHD patients,[36,37] and elevated resting heart rate is associated with increased risk of MI and other cardiovascular diseases.[38] Additionally, depressed patients demonstrate decreased heart rate variability, another measure of cardiac autonomic function that is a risk factor for mortality following MI.[39] This finding is most consistent among patients with depression and CHD, but has also been observed among patients with depression and no medical comorbidities.[38]

Dysregulation of the hypothalamic–pituitary–adrenal (HPA) axis is another proposed biological mechanism to account for the association between depression and CHD. Elevated cortisol levels have been associated with depression, both in patients with CHD[40] and in medically healthy populations.[41] Elevated cortisol is also associated with CHD, and may impact release of vasodilators and vasoconstrictors from the endothelium.[40] It is unclear whether increased cortisol levels result from depression or cause depression. Patients with high levels of cortisol due to Cushing syndrome have elevated rates of depression and cardiovascular disease, suggesting that cortisol may have a causal influence on both of these disorders.[40]

Inflammation is proposed as an important mediator between depression and CHD. Levels of inflammatory cytokines, such as interleukin-1 beta (IL-1 beta), interleukin-6 (IL-6), C-reactive protein (CRP), and tumor necrosis factor (TNF) are elevated in patients with depression who are otherwise healthy.[42,43,44] These inflammatory markers are also associated with increased risk of CHD and MI.[42,45] They may contribute to the rupture of atherosclerotic plaques or impact myo-cardial contractility.[45] Interleukin-6, for example, is known to increase levels of CRP and to stimulate platelet aggregation.[45]

Altered platelet function may contribute to the association between depression and CHD. More than 99% of the body's serotonin is stored in platelets,[46] and platelets secrete serotonin upon activation, leading to platelet aggregation and coronary vasoconstriction.[47] There is increased sensitivity of platelets to serotonergic activation in patients with depression.[46] However, selective serotonin reuptake inhibitors have been found to reduce platelet aggregation,[48] perhaps by blocking signaling pathways in the clotting response that are mediated by serotonin transporters.[49]

A number of genetic factors may contribute to the connection between depression and CHD, although evidence is equivocal thus far. Recent research examining the 5-HTTLPR gene, a serotonin transporter gene promoter region finds that the short allele of this gene is associated with depressive symptoms and cardiac events.[42,50] Several other genes are also preliminary candidates for the link between depression and CHD. Single nucleotide polymorphisms in the gene for a clotting factor, the von Willebrand factor, are correlated with levels of depressive symptoms.[51] In addition, linkage studies identify several loci shared by depression and CHD.[52]

Reduced omega-3 levels may also link depression and CHD, though limited evidence is available. Patients with depression appear to have lower levels of serum omega-3 fatty acids, which are believed to be protective against CHD.[45] However, further studies are needed to determine whether omega-3 fatty acids have a causal role in the association between depression and CHD.

■ CLINICAL PRESENTATION

The clinical presentation of depression often differs in patients with CHD compared to medically healthy patients (**Box 7-3**). Patients with depression and CHD or a previous MI may be more likely to report the somatic symptoms of depression and less likely to report cognitive or affective symptoms.[53,54] Thus patients with depression and a recent MI had lower levels of cognitive/affective symptoms, including depressed mood, anhedonia, guilt, and concentration difficulties when compared to patients with depression and no MI, but had similar levels of somatic symptoms[55] including appetite/weight changes, sleep disturbances, psychomotor changes, and fatigue. Depressed patients with CHD may be more likely to report physical symptoms, such as shortness of breath and chest pain, and symptoms of irritability and anxiety.[5] Some research indicates that somatic symptoms of depression are more predictive of cardiovascular mortality and recurrent MI than cognitive/affective symptoms, but other studies have not confirmed this.[53,56]

Given the prominent somatic nature of depressive symptoms in CHD, it is often unclear to what degree these symptoms are due to depression itself and to what degree they result from CHD. Fatigue

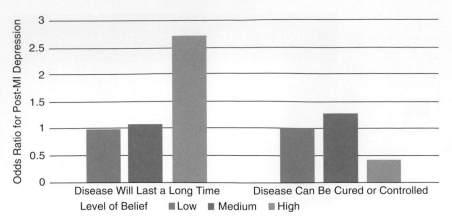

Figure 7-4 *Beliefs about illness and likelihood of development of depression 6 to 12 months after MI. (Data from Dickens C, McGowan L, Percival C, et al. Negative illness perceptions are associated with new-onset depression following myocardial infarction.* Gen Hosp Psychiatry. *2008;30(5):414–420.)*

and sleep disturbance are the primary symptoms shared by depression and CHD.[5] This overlap may make depression more difficult to identify in patients with CHD. Both patients and clinicians may attribute fatigue to the patient's medical condition, leading clinicians to overlook the possibility of depression. Similarly, reduced activity level could be due either to impaired cardiovascular function, or to depressive anhedonia. To distinguish these symptoms of depression from symptoms of cardiovascular disease, it may be helpful to focus on the presence of cognitive symptoms of depression, such as hopelessness, difficulty concentrating, or suicidal ideation. Routine medical evaluation for causes of fatigue and sleep disturbance may also assist in determining the etiology of a patient's somatic symptoms.

Qualitative studies have explored the emotional consequences of CHD. A recent study found that about half of male patients with depression and CHD felt that the two were related, and described feeling a loss of masculinity and shame over not being able to support their families financially.[57] In the year following an MI, about 25% of patients reported uncertainty about the future due to their medical condition and 20% reported reduced activity levels due to their cardiac condition.[20]

Depression also affects the experience and reporting of cardiac symptoms, such as chest pain. Post-MI patients with depressive symptoms have increased rates of angina compared to post-MI patients without depressive symptoms.[35,58,59]

Depression in CHD and following MI is associated with poorer quality of life, and greater physical limitations and disability.[35,60] Patients with post-MI depression have a four- to fivefold increase in rates of complete and partial disability compared to patients following MI without depression; this is true even after controlling for past history of depression and cardiac function.[61] Depression is also

associated with decrements in quality of life and lower satisfaction with cardiovascular care.[59]

■ COURSE AND NATURAL HISTORY

Depressive symptoms seem to be highest during hospitalization for MI and in the month following MI,[20,35] and then begin to remit over time. Approximately 30% to 65% of cases of depression may remit by 1 month following MI.[35,62] One study with a longer follow-up period found that approximately 31% of patients with recurrent MI were depressed at baseline, of whom 62% continued to be depressed at the 6-month time point.[20]

The preponderance of the evidence suggests that depression is associated with increased cardiovascular events and mortality in both patients with stable CHD and following MI.[18,22,63,64] Frasure-Smith and colleagues found that MDD was an independent risk factor for death within 6 months after MI.[22] In outpatients with stable CHD, the Heart and Soul Study reported that depressive symptoms were correlated with a 31% higher rate of cardiovascular events over an average follow-up period of 5 years.[18] A meta-analysis disclosed a twofold increase in mortality over a 2-year follow-up in depressed compared to nondepressed CHD patients (adjusted hazard ratio 1.76).[63] Although even mild levels of depressive symptoms may worsen outcome, the risk of mortality increases with severity of depression.[64] As noted, however, not all studies show an increase in mortality in patients with depression after MI.[62,65]

Depression is also associated with an increased frequency of cardiac interventions following MI, such as cardiac catheterization and angioplasty.[62] This may reflect a more complicated illness course or may result from higher reported symptom levels in patients with depression. Depression correlates with frequency of angina after MI[35] and frequency of chest pain is associated with increased risk

---

BOX 7-2
POSSIBLE MEDIATORS BETWEEN CHD AND DEPRESSION

Autonomic nervous system dysfunction
Sympathetic nervous system activation
HPA axis hyperactivity
Inflammation
Hypercoagulability
Cerebral gray matter loss
Medication nonadherence
Dietary nonadherence
Physical inactivity
Alcohol use
Tobacco use

BOX 7-3
IMPORTANT SYMPTOMS (DEPRESSION AND HEART DISEASE)

Confounding symptoms
Fatigue
Poor appetite
Weight changes
Impaired concentration
Dyssomnia
More typical in depression
Hopelessness
Poor concentration
Suicidal Ideation

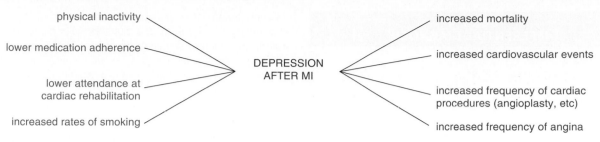

Figure 7-5 *Behavioral factors and outcomes associated with depression after MI. (For more information see reference numbers 18, 19, 22, 35, 62, 63, & 78.)*

of depression 1 year after MI.[25] The timing of depressive episodes is relevant for risk of recurrent cardiovascular events so that new-onset depressive episodes after MI may be particularly predictive of mortality and adverse cardiovascular events, whereas preexisting depression does not carry the same risk.[10,25,31,32] Patients whose first lifetime episode of MDD follows an MI may be at a greater risk of adverse cardiovascular outcomes than patients with a recurrent episode of MDD following MI.[66,67]

Certain depressive symptoms are more associated with poorer cardiovascular prognosis. The somatic symptoms of depression, but not cognitive/affective symptoms, predict worse cardiovascular outcomes and mortality rates, but the significance of this association is unclear, because somatic symptoms may reflect the presence of more severe cardiac disease rather than more severe depression.[53,68,69] One study specifically reports that anhedonia predicts adverse cardiovascular outcomes even after controlling for severity of depressive symptoms, while depressed mood does not.[70]

Adverse health-related behaviors, such as smoking, physical activity level, and medication adherence, may underlie some of the association between depression and poor outcomes in CHD (**Figs. 7-5** and **7-6**). When behavioral and biological risk factors for CHD are compared in depressed and nondepressed individuals, depressed patients differed more on behavioral risk factors than on biological risk factors.[71]

The interaction of smoking with depression and CHD has been closely examined. Depression is associated with increased rates of smoking and less success with smoking cessation in CHD patients[19] as well as in healthy populations.[2,24,72]

Depression is associated with lower levels of physical activity in both medically healthy populations[73,74] and patients with CHD,[19] and levels of physical inactivity do contribute to the association between depression and recurrent cardiovascular events following MI.[18] Depression also affects utilization of cardiac rehabilitation.[19,20,75] Persistently depressed patients with CHD are approximately 50% less likely to attend a cardiac rehabilitation program than nondepressed patients with CHD,[19] and complete fewer sessions even when they do enroll.[20] Depression may also diminish the level of cardiovascular benefit from rehabilitation.[75] This suggests that modifiable behavioral factors, such as activity level, could influence rates of cardiovascular events in patients with depression.[18]

Medication adherence is also affected by depression and has itself been linked to the risk of rehospitalization and mortality rates. Patients with CHD and depression are significantly less likely to adhere to baby aspirin prophylaxis than nondepressed CHD patients.[76,77] In patients with stable CHD, the rate of medication noncompliance is 14% in those with MDD compared to 5% in those without MDD.[78]

Depression may alter the CHD patient's perception of his/her illness, generating increased feelings of hopelessness or pessimism about recovery. Such feelings may in themselves predict poorer cardiovascular outcomes. Thus hopelessness is an independent predictor of mortality from cardiovascular events even after adjusting for depression.[79] Men with high levels of hopelessness are

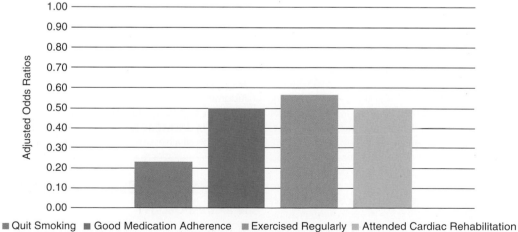

*Persistently depressed patients were defined as having Beck Depression Inventory > or = 10 at baseline and 3 months post-MI; persistently non-depressed patients had BDI < 10 at both timepoints.

Figure 7-6 *Adjusted Odds Ratios for Adherence to Preventive Behaviors Among Post-MI Patients. (Data from Kronish IM, Rieckmann N, Halm EA, et al. Persistent depression affects adherence to secondary prevention behaviors after acute coronary syndromes. J Gen Intern Med. 2006;21(11):1178–1183.)*

Hypothyroidism
Other endocrine disorders
Sleep disorders
Dementia
Delirium
Demoralization
Adjustment disorders
Post-traumatic stress disorder (ICD)

twice as likely to have a first MI and nearly four times as likely to die of cardiovascular causes compared to men with low levels of hopelessness.[79] Similarly, some evidence suggests that pessimistic expectations about recovery and return to normal life after MI are associated with increased mortality rates, even after controlling for cardiovascular disease severity and depressive symptoms.[80]

◼ ASSESSMENT AND DIFFERENTIAL DIAGNOSIS

Differential diagnosis of depression in patients with CHD can be broad (**Box 7-4**). Medically, it includes hypothyroidism and other endocrine disorders, sleep disorders, nutritional deficiencies, and medication reactions. Among psychiatric disorders, the differential includes MDD, minor depression or subsyndromal depression, bipolar disorder, dementia, delirium, and personality disorders. Two other conditions that deserve special consideration are demoralization and adjustment disorders.

Demoralization is a syndrome of existential distress that occurs in patients facing medical illness. It includes feelings of hopelessness, helplessness, and a loss of meaning or purpose in life.[81] Demoralization occurs in approximately 33% of cardiac patients, and frequently overlaps with major depression.[82] It is distinguished from depression in that demoralized patients may experience happiness and pleasure in other aspects of their lives but feel unable to cope with their medical situation and uncertainty about their future.[81] Adjustment disorders are also a common diagnosis in this medically ill population, and may be difficult to differentiate from depression. Adjustment disorders are characterized by an excessive or maladaptive response to a stressful life event, such as acute medical illness, and occur within 3 months of the stressor. Adjustment disorders are self-limited and resolve within 6 months of the stressor ending. Finally, individuals with adjustment disorders do not meet full criteria for a major depressive episode.

Routine depression screening is recommended in CHD patients,[83] and the American Heart Association recommends use of the Patient Health Questionnaire-2 (PHQ-2), an abbreviated form of the Patient Health Questionaire-9 (PHQ-9). This instrument has high sensitivity for depressive symptoms in cardiovascular disease although it lacks sensitivity for MDD.[42,84] The PHQ-2 consists of two questions: "During the past month, have you often been bothered by feeling down, depressed, or hopeless?" and "During the past month, have you often been bothered by little interest or pleasure in doing things?".[85] If a patient answers "yes" to either question, follow-up with a more comprehensive screening tool, such as the PHQ-9 or diagnostic clinical interview is recommended. A PHQ-9 score of 10 or greater can be used as a basis for initiating depression treatment.[85] (See "Treatment of Depression in the Context of Cardiovascular Disease" below).

It may be helpful to initiate depression assessment with open-ended questions about the level of interest in daily activities and social engagement, as some patients may deny feeling depressed due to fear of stigmatization.[5] Clinicians may also wish to guard against their tendency to consider a patient's depressive symptoms as a natural and understandable response to medical illness, thereby overlooking the possibility of a treatable major depression. Primary care physicians may sometimes normalize clinical depression as a perfectly natural response to a serious medical condition, which can lead to reduced exploration and assessment of depression as a treatment target.[86]

◼ SUMMARY

The prevalence of depression is higher among individuals with CHD or following MI than in the general population. Depression is both a risk factor for the onset of CHD, and also a predictor of poorer cardiovascular outcomes in individuals with pre-existing CHD. The extent to which this association is explained by shared pathophysiology versus behavioral factors remains unclear. Among CHD patients with depression, those with depressive episodes preceding the onset of their CHD may differ from those with no prior history of depression; additional research is needed to compare the clinical characteristics and cardiovascular prognosis of these two groups. Further studies are also needed to identify the most efficacious treatments for depression in CHD.

CASE 1

Myocardial Infarction Ms. K is a 60-year-old woman with a history of hyperlipidemia and obesity who was hospitalized for her first myocardial infarction (MI) 3 months ago. She received prompt and effective treatment with thrombolytic medication. Ms. K was working part-time as a personal care assistant prior to her MI, but lost her job after her hospitalization and has not sought other work. She is single and has one adult son who is financially supportive but does not live locally. Today, she presents to her primary care doctor for follow-up. She reports that she frequently experiences a feeling of heaviness in her chest and is worried about her heart. She endorses fatigue, difficulty sleeping, and difficulty completing errands due to lack of focus. When directly asked about depression, Ms. K is somewhat defensive, stating "I'm not losing my mind, life is just hard right now." She reports feeling overwhelmed by her team's dietary and lifestyle recommendations. She denies guilt, low self-worth, or suicidal intent, but states that "whenever my time's up, I'm ready."

Discussion: Ms. K has many risk factors for depression in CHD, including female gender, medical comorbidities, pessimistic beliefs about her prognosis, and social isolation. Her depressive presentation is typical, in that she endorses somatic symptoms but fewer affective or cognitive symptoms of depression. Although exhibiting many symptoms of depression, she is hesitant to admit that she is depressed. Her reluctance could be due to a lack of knowledge about symptoms of depression, her personal beliefs about mental illness, or a fear of stigma and judgment by her providers. Empathic validation of the patient's situation and education about depression may increase Ms. K's comfort in discussing her internal experience and may lead to the discussion of assessment and treatment options.

CONGESTIVE HEART FAILURE

◼ EPIDEMIOLOGY

In congestive heart failure (CHF), the heart is unable to pump enough blood to meet the body's demands. Currently, 5.7 million Americans are affected by CHF[87] and the prevalence is predicted to increase 25% over the next two decades as the population ages. Survival after heart failure diagnosis is improving; however, the mortality remains high and approximately 50% of heart failure patients die within 5 years of heart failure diagnosis.[88] Depression is a common comorbidity among CHF patients and carries important prognostic implications. Prevalence of depression in patients with CHF is between 9% and 60%, with an average of 21.5% in various studies.[89] Higher rates are reported in studies assessing depressive symptoms while lower rates are reported in patients assessed with a diagnostic clinical interview.[89]

The incidence of depression in CHF increases with severity of heart failure, correlating with higher New York Heart Association (NYHA) functional class[89] and with proxy measures of illness severity, such as disability and lack of independence.[90] Depression is also more common in younger CHF patients, women, and in those with prior history of depression.[90] CHF increases the risk of developing new-onset depression, with health status and social factors, such as living alone and alcohol abuse contributing to this risk.[91] Whether depression increases the risk of developing heart failure is less clear, though there may be some bidirectionality to this relationship. In patients 60 years or older with isolated systolic hypertension, depression is independently associated with development of heart failure over a 4.5-year follow-up.[92] In elderly individuals free from heart failure at baseline, depression emerged as an independent risk factor for development of heart failure among women, but not among men, over a 14-year period.[93]

■ PATHOPHYSIOLOGY

Potential mechanisms that link depression and CHF include autonomic nervous system dysfunction, inflammation, cardiac arrhythmias, hypercoagulability, and altered platelet functioning (Box 7-2). Sympathetic nervous system activation is increased in both major depression[36] and CHF,[94] norepinephrine levels are elevated in both conditions, and elevated plasma norepinephrine levels are an independent predictor of all-cause mortality in CHF.[94] Sympathetic activation from depression and heart failure may work synergistically to worsen outcome by increasing the risk for arrhythmia or sudden cardiac death. Little is known about whether treatment of depression reduces autonomic system dysfunction and impacts the course of CHF. In one trial, the antidepressant nefazodone not only improved depression scores, but reduced heart rate and plasma norepinephrine levels in patients with heart failure and depression.[95] In another trial, short-term treatment with sertraline significantly decreased norepinephrine appearance rates, correlating with a decrease in sympathetic nervous system activity.[96]

The hypothalamic-pituitary-adrenal (HPA) axis is another potential link between depression and heart failure. Elevated levels of the adrenal hormones cortisol and aldosterone are associated with heart failure progression and are independent predictors of death in heart failure patients.[97] Increased activation of the HPA axis occurs in depression, and thus elevated levels of these adrenal hormones in patients with depression and heart failure may result in greater severity of CHF and worsened outcomes.

Inflammatory cytokines, including interleukin 1 beta (IL-1 beta), interleukin 6 (IL-6), and tumor necrosis factor alpha (TNF-alpha) are elevated in both depression and heart failure.[98-101] In heart failure, proinflammatory cytokines may initially play a beneficial role in cardiac remodeling, but when overexpressed, contribute to worsening of heart failure.[101] It is unclear whether inflammation is a marker of depressed states or is a causal factor of depression. Depression may prospectively predict higher white blood cell count, which is a marker of systemic inflammation, in CHD patients.[102]

Behavioral mechanisms likely play a significant role in the relationship of depression and heart failure. Medication adherence in heart failure is challenging, requiring a large number of medications to be taken multiple times a day. Patients with depression are at threefold higher risk for nonadherence with medication compared with nondepressed individuals.[103] Nonadherence in turn is associated with heart failure related hospitalization and is an independent risk factor

for mortality.[104] Social supports also play a role, as family cohesion is positively associated with medication adherence[105] and patients with depression are less likely to have social supports. Depression is also associated with other adverse health-related behaviors, such as poor diet, physical inactivity, alcohol use, and tobacco use.

It has been suggested that there are areas of brain injury resulting from chronic heart failure that contribute to the pathogenesis of co-occurring depression. There appear to be differences in patterns of cerebral gray matter loss among patients with heart failure, including lateralized gray matter losses in the hippocampi, mammillary bodies, and frontal cortices.[106] Patients with heart failure and these patterns of gray matter loss were significantly more depressed and had poorer executive functioning than control subjects.[106]

■ CLINICAL PRESENTATION

Depression is underrecognized in CHF patients (**Box 7-3**). This may relate to lack of comfort by nonmental health specialists in diagnosing depression, time constraints, lack of support for management and follow-up, belief that depression is a normative response to the illness, and diagnostic difficulties posed by the overlap of depressive and heart failure symptoms. Symptoms of fatigue, poor appetite, weight gain or loss, impaired concentration, and sleep disturbance are common features of both depression and heart failure. Patients who have both conditions report more physical symptoms than patients with heart failure who are not depressed. In a study of elderly patients with both heart failure and depression, 68% report a loss of appetite and 79% report sleeping difficulties, as compared with 40% and 51%, respectively, of patients with heart failure who were not depressed.[107] Although the risk of depression increases along with severity of heart failure, patients with advanced heart failure also experience a greater burden of physical symptoms as their illness progresses. Thus depression inventories with high proportions of somatic symptoms may have a lower specificity in patients with heart failure than other cardiac conditions.[90]

Frequent psychiatric comorbidities in patients with heart failure include anxiety, panic disorder, alcohol abuse, and nicotine dependence. Anxiety and depression correlate highly with one another, with approximately 60% of depressed patients also having clinically significant levels of anxiety.[108] Rates of anxiety in CHF range from 20%

ANXIETY IN CARDIOVASCULAR DISEASE

- Anxiety is common in cardiovascular patients, with a prevalence of 10.9% in coronary heart disease patients,[1] 18.4% in heart failure patients,[2] and 28% to 38% in atrial fibrillation patients.[3]
- Post-traumatic stress disorder may occur following acute coronary syndromes (12%)[4] or after an out-of-hospital cardiac arrest (27%).[5]
- Anxiety worsens prognosis in patients with cardiovascular disease.
  - High levels of anxiety have been associated with increased risk of nonfatal MI or death among patients with coronary heart disease.[6]
  - Comorbid anxiety and depression have been associated with all-cause mortality and re-hospitalization in heart failure patients.[7]
  - Anxiety is associated with increased severity of atrial fibrillation symptoms.[8]
- Post-traumatic stress disorder has been found to increase long-term mortality among patients with implantable cardioverter-defibrillators.[9]
  - Anxiety may increase risk of developing cardiovascular disease.

- Anxiety[10] and post-traumatic stress disoder[11] in initially healthy individuals have been found to predict subsequent coronary heart disease events.
- Mechanisms linking anxiety and cardiovascular disease are unclear, but may include poor health behaviors, such as cigarette smoking, excessive alcohol consumption, and lower physical activity,[12] as well as activation of the hypothalamic–pituitary–adrenal axis, autonomic nervous system reactivity, inflammation, and endothelial dysfunction.

References

1. Tully PJ, Cosh SM. Generalized anxiety disorder prevalence and comorbidity with depression in coronary heart disease: A meta-analysis. *J Health Psychol.* 2012; 18(12):1601–1616.
2. Haworth JE, M oniz-Cook E, Clark AL, et al. Prevalence and predictors of anxiety and depression in a sample of chronic heart failure patients with left ventricular systolic dysfunction. *European J Heart Failure.* 2005; 7(5):803–808.
3. Thrall G, Lip GY, Carroll D, et al. Depression, anxiety and quality of life in patients with atrial fibrillation. *Chest.* 2007; 132(4):1259–1264.
4. Edmondson D, Richardson S, Falzon L, et al. posttraumatic stress disorder prevalence and risk of recurrence in acute coronary syndrome patients: A meta-analytic review. *PLoS One.* 2012; 7(6):e38915.
5. Gamper G, Willeit M, Sterz F, et al. Life after death: Posttraumatic stress disorder in survivors of cardiac arrest – prevalence, associated factors, and the influence of sedation and analgesia. *Crit Care Med.* 2004; 32(2): 378–383.
6. Woldecherkos A, Shibeshi MD, Yinong Y, et al. Anxiety worsens prognosis in patients with coronary artery disease. *J Am Coll Cardiol.* 2007; 49(20): 2021–2027.
7. Alhurani AS, Dekker RL, Abed MA, et al. The association of co-morbid symptoms of depression and anxiety with all-cause mortality and cardiac rehospitalization in patients with heart failure. *Psychosomatics.* 2015; 56(4):371–380.
8. Thompson TS, Barksdale DJ, Sears SF, et al. The effect of anxiety and depression on symptoms attributed to atrial fibrillation. *Pacing Clin Electrophysiol.* 2014; 37(4):439–446.
9. Ladwig KH, Schoefinius A, Dammann G, et al. Long-acting psychotraumatic properties of a cardiac arrest experience. *Am J Psychiatry.* 1999; 156(6): 912–919.
10. Janszky I, Ahnve S, Lundberg I, et al. Early-onset depression, anxiety, and risk of subsequent coronary heart disease. *J Am Coll Cardiol.* 2010; 56(1): 31–37.
11. Vaccarion V, Goldbert J, Rooks C, et al. Posttraumatic stress disorder and incidence of coronary heart disease: A twin study. *J Am Coll Cardiol.* 2013; 62(11): 970–978.
12. Strine TW, Chapman DP, Kobau R, et al. Associations of self-reported anxiety symptoms with health-related quality of life and health behaviors. *Soc Psychiatry Psychiatr Epidemiol.* 2005; 40(6): 432–438.

to 54%,[108–110] with women having higher rates of anxiety than men.[110] Panic disorder occurs in 9.3% of heart failure patients, of whom almost half have a comorbid depressive disorder. Although some studies show only depression predicts mortality in heart failure,[109] other studies suggest that anxiety is an independent risk, with the highest mortality risk carried by patients having both anxiety and depression.[108] Alcoholic cardiomyopathy is thought to be the cause of heart failure in 21% to 40% of patients with idiopathic dilated cardiomyopathy.[111,112] Although moderate consumption of alcohol is protective against heart failure, excessive alcohol intake is associated with cardiotoxicity. Mechanisms of alcoholic cardiomyopathy include myocyte loss, fibrosis, impaired cardiac contractility, altered calcium homeostasis, oxidative stress, and nutritional deficiencies. Alcohol use is common in depression, and in some individuals, may lead to a substance-induced depressive disorder. Alcohol use is associated with depression and unrecognized cognitive impairment in 58% of a population of veterans with CHF.[113]

■ COURSE AND NATURAL HISTORY

As heart failure worsens, depressive symptoms increase[114,115] and quality of life decreases.[116] Patients with heart failure and depression have a lower quality of life than patients with heart failure who are not depressed.[116, 117] Depression accelerates the progression of heart failure, leading to greater morbidity and mortality. During the first 6 months after discharge from the hospital for heart failure, severity of depression is associated with the degree of functional decline experienced.[118] In outpatients as well, depression predicts a decline in health status due to heart failure: outpatients who are depressed experience worsening of their heart failure symptoms, physical and social functioning, and quality of life.[117] This accelerated course in patients with heart failure and depression leads to more frequent hospitalization and increased healthcare expenditures.

Depression is also strongly associated with increased mortality in heart failure. Depressive symptoms on hospital admission are associated with increased mortality at 3 months,[119,120] 6 months,[118] and 1 year, independent of cardiac risk factors.[109] In a study of patients with comorbid depression and atrial fibrillation, depressive symptoms predict a 57% increase in mortality from cardiac causes over a follow-up of 39 months.[114] In the outpatient setting, depressive symptoms are associated with a 56% increase in the risk of death or cardiac hospitalization. Increased risks of hospitalization and death are not simply due to the greater cardiac morbidity among the depressed patients. Thus this relationship persists even after controlling for objective measures of heart failure severity and prognosis, such as left ventricular ejection fraction and N-terminal pro-B-type natriuretic peptide.[121]

In addition to increasing the rates of hospitalization for heart failure, depression increases the length of hospital stay.[120] Patients with CHF and a history of depression are also less likely to receive cardiac interventions during their hospitalization, be referred for outpatient heart failure management programs, or receive recommended heart failure education.[120] This suggests that patients with depression may differ in their hospital and post-discharge care, factors that may contribute to differing outcomes. These differences in care may also be related to depressed patients being medically sicker or having higher rates of medical comorbidity.

■ ASSESSMENT AND DIFFERENTIAL DIAGNOSIS

The American Heart Association issued a Science Advisory recommending that all patients with CHD be screened for depression. However it is not clear whether existing screening tools have adequate diagnostic sensitivity and specificity or whether identifying patients with depression actually improves outcomes. The prevalence rates of depression in CHF vary depending on the screening tools used, with rates highest using self-report questionnaires and lowest with diagnostic interviews.[89] The Beck Depression Inventory has good sensitivity for identifying depression in patients with heart failure, but a low specificity; only 55% of patients scoring as depressed by the Beck Depression Inventory have clinically significant depressive symptoms.[90] Despite these limitations, several self-report depression measures are predictive of heart failure morbidity and mortality, including the Beck Depression Inventory[115] and the two-question screening tool, PHQ-2.[122]

Assessment of depression in patients with heart failure must differentiate depression from demoralization, adjustment disorders, medical conditions (such as hypothyroidism and obstructive sleep apnea), and the effects of cardiac medications. Demoralization is a syndrome of existential distress, seen to occur in patients facing serious medical illness, that includes feelings of hopelessness, helplessness, and a loss of meaning or purpose in life.[81] Demoralization is reported in approximately 33% of cardiac patients. Although it frequently co-occurs with major depression,[82] demoralization is not synonymous with depression; not all depressed patients are demoralized and not all demoralized patients meet criteria for depression. Demoralization differs from depression in that demoralized patients may experience happiness and pleasure in daily life but still feel unable to cope with their medical situation and uncertainty about their future.[81]

Adjustment disorders are one of the most common diagnoses given to medically hospitalized patients and are characterized by an excessive or maladaptive response to a stressful life event, such as acute medical illness. Symptoms of an adjustment disorder are expected to be self-limited, resolving within 6 months of the stressor ending.

Depression in CHF patients may also be due to their cardiac medications. Historically, beta-blockers have carried a strong association with depression. Although they improve survival among patients with left ventricular systolic dysfunction, their use is limited by concerns about adverse effects in heart failure. This is particularly true of lipophilic beta-blockers that easily cross the blood–brain barrier, such as propranolol and metoprolol. However, current evidence suggests that associations between beta-blockers and depression may not be valid.[123] A review of beta-blockers in the management of cardiac patients, including those with CHF, found no increase in the risk of depression and only a small increase in fatigue and sexual dysfunction.[123] Higher doses or longer duration of treatment might be associated with an increased risk of depression, but this remains unclear at present.

■ SUMMARY

Depression is prevalent in CHF patients and has a strong impact on quality of life, functional decline, and mortality. Despite increasing recognition of this association, depression in patients with CHF remains underdiagnosed. Improving methods for identifying patients with CHF who have or are at risk for depression should allow earlier intervention and improve outcomes. New treatments for depression in heart failure are also needed as there are relatively few antidepressant and psychotherapy trials looking specifically at this patient population. Although there is a large body of research examining pathophysiologic mechanisms involved in both depression and heart failure, further studies are need to determine the pathways by which these conditions are linked, and to determine whether depression is merely a risk marker for heart failure mortality, or a causal risk factor.

CASE 2

HEART FAILURE

Ms. C is a 64-year-old widowed woman with viral cardiomyopathy, chronic renal impairment, and obstructive sleep apnea, who is admitted to the cardiology service of the hospital for the third time in 1 year for decompensated heart failure. Despite maximal medical therapy, she has had increasing frequency of hospitalizations and a declining functional status. She used to be an elementary school teacher, was an avid gardener, and enjoyed hiking and camping, but was forced to retire due to her health 3 years ago and is now receiving disability. Due to her fatigue and shortness of breath, she currently spends most of her time at home, watching television. She has two adult daughters who live nearby and are involved in her care, taking her to medical appointments and assisting with grocery shopping. Over the past 6 months she has found little enjoyment from her daily activities, worries about her health and her family at night, is not able to concentrate, has had a decreased appetite, and experienced weight gain in her abdomen and edema in her legs. At times she thinks that everyone would be better off without her and wishes that she would pass away in her sleep.

Discussion: This is a common presentation for major depressive disorder in heart failure. Ms. C's symptoms of depression have increased as the severity of her heart failure has increased, and many of her depressive symptoms overlap with her heart failure symptoms as well as the symptoms of her other comorbid medical conditions. Features that make a diagnosis of depression likely include the number of depressive symptoms she is reporting as well as the presence of anhedonia and passive suicidal ideation.

ATRIAL FIBRILLATION

■ EPIDEMIOLOGY

Atrial fibrillation (AF) is the most common sustained cardiac rhythm disorder and is associated with substantial morbidity and mortality related to heart failure, stroke, and other thromboembolic complications (**Fig. 7-7**). The primary risk factors for AF are hypertensive heart disease and CHD. Individuals with AF may experience symptoms of chest pain, palpitations, shortness of breath, fatigue, or lightheadedness. These symptoms may cause individuals considerable concern due to the unpredictable nature of AF, and cause worry about the meaning or significance of the symptoms. Interestingly the accuracy of the patient's awareness of AF is variable; 38% of patients with episodes lasting more than 48 hours are asymptomatic, and 40% of patients report AF-like symptoms in the absence of documented AF.[124]

The prevalence of depression in atrial fibrillation patients is not clear. Some reported rates are as high as 32%[114,125] to 42.7% of patients with AF,[126] well above the rates found in the general population. However, other studies found no increase in rates of depression in patients with AF; many of these studies, though, are limited by small sample sizes or by excluding patients with prior histories of depression or anxiety.

In studies of patients with atrial fibrillation and heart failure, risk factors for depression include female gender, nonwhite race, unmarried status, paroxysmal as opposed to persistent AF, history of previous treatment with antiarrhythmic agents, higher NYHA functional class, prior hospitalization for CHF,[114] more severe AF symptoms, and lower levels of education (**Box 7-1c**).[127]

■ PATHOPHYSIOLOGY

The pathophysiologic mechanisms linking depression to atrial fibrillation are similar to those proposed in other forms of cardiovascular disease: increased activation of the sympathetic nervous system, altered expression of cortisol and aldosterone, and systemic

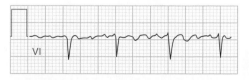
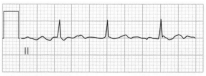

Figure 7-7 *Electrocardiogram of atrial fibrillation. (Reproduced with permission from Longo DL, Fauci AS, Kasper DL, et al. Harrison's Principles of Internal Medicine. 18th ed. New York: McGraw-Hill, Inc; 2012.)*

BOX 7-1C
IMPORTANT RISK FACTORS FOR DEPRESSION IN PATIENTS WITH ATRIAL FIBRILLATION

Sociodemographic
Female gender
Nonwhite race
Unmarried
Lower educational Level
Medical
Paroxysmal AF
Severe AF symptoms
History of prior treatment with antiarrhythmic drugs
Higher NYHA functional class of heart failure

---

inflammation (**Box 7-2**). These states are present in depressed patients, and associated with an increased risk of AF.[128–131] In addition, depression is associated with poor health behaviors, such as medication nonadherence, poor diet, physical inactivity, tobacco use, and alcohol use, all of which may affect the course of AF. Obstructive sleep apnea is also associated with both depression and AF (Chapter 21), and it is possible that disruption of sleep mediates the association of atrial fibrillation and depression. In patients with AF, untreated obstructive sleep apnea has been associated with recurrence of AF following ablation procedures.[132]

■ CLINICAL PRESENTATION

Depression is frequently comorbid with anxiety and somatization in patients with AF (**Boxes 7-5** and **7-6**). Seventy-one percent of patients with both AF and depression also have comorbid anxiety.[125] Anxiety sensitivity is a state in which individuals show heightened awareness and fear of the somatic symptoms of anxiety and over-interpret the significance of these symptoms. Studies have found that patients with AF and high anxiety sensitivity frequently have comorbid depression.[133] There is less information on somatoform disorders, though in one study somatization symptoms were present in 19.1% of patients with AF.[134] Evaluations of patients with AF should also include an assessment of alcohol use, as moderate to high levels of alcohol consumption is a precipitating factor for AF in both men and women.[135,136]

■ COURSE AND NATURAL HISTORY

Patients with AF have significantly poorer quality of life and are more symptomatic than healthy controls, the general population, and patients with CHD. Those with AF and more severe depression have an associated increase in the symptoms they attribute to their AF, regardless of AF severity.[134] Increased concern about AF symptoms not only impacts quality of life, but also leads to more frequent visits to healthcare providers and increased healthcare costs.

Without intervention, depression in patients with AF appears to persist over time, and rates of depression in these patients appear to be stable over 6 month follow-up.[125] Although there is limited information about the impact of depression on AF mortality, in patients with AF and CHF depressive symptoms are associated with increased mortality, even after adjustment for other prognostic factors.[114]

BOX 7-5
COMMON COMORBIDITIES

Anxiety disorders
Alcohol use disorders

BOX 7-6
TREATMENTS FOR DEPRESSION IN PATIENTS WITH CARDIOVASCULAR DISEASE

SSRs (may have preventive role)
Bupropion
Psychostimulants
ECT
Cognitive behavioral therapy
Interpersonal therapy
Exercise

Depression may impact the recurrence rates of AF following electric cardioversion or ablation therapies. Thus depression is an independent predictor of AF recurrence, which recurs in 85% of patients with comorbid depression compared with 39% of patients without depression, following successful electrical cardioversion.[137] Depression is also an independent risk factor for recurrence of AF after ablation. Interestingly, patients undergoing ablation experience improvements in depression and in quality of life following the intervention, suggesting that effective AF treatment has a beneficial effect on mood.[126,138]

■ ASSESSMENT AND DIFFERENTIAL DIAGNOSIS

When assessing depression in patients with AF, the differential diagnosis includes demoralization, adjustment disorders, generalized anxiety disorder, panic disorder, and somatoform disorders, such as hypochondriasis (Box 7-4). Patients with AF may have intermittent symptoms of dizziness, palpitations, fatigue, and shortness of breath. Although the symptoms themselves may be benign, patients may feel helpless because of the unpredictability of symptom recurrence. Some patients may worry that the symptoms are indicative of a more serious condition or that they are a forewarning of future catastrophic events, such as MI, heart failure, or stroke. Substance-induced mood disorders should also be considered in patients with moderate to heavy alcohol consumption given the potential contribution of alcohol to both mood disorders and AF.

■ SUMMARY

AF is highly prevalent in the general population and is associated with depression, anxiety, and impaired quality of life. Effective identification and treatment of depression may improve patient outcomes, increase medication adherence, reduce unnecessary utilization of medical care, and improve quality of life. Primary treatment strategies for AF are to control the heart rhythm or rate, and though neither is clearly superior in the general population, patients with high anxiety sensitivity have an improved prognosis with treatments that control heart rhythm.[133] It is not known whether the AF treatment strategy (rhythm control or rate control) leads to any differences in outcome in patients with both AF and depression. Finally, prospective studies are needed to clarify the ways in which biological and behavioral factors influence the pathogenesis and maintenance of AF.

CASE 3

ATRIAL FIBRILLATION

Ms. A is a 72-year-old woman with a history of anxiety, hypertension, and paroxysmal atrial fibrillation, diagnosed 5 years ago after she experienced an episode of racing heart, palpitations, dizziness, and shortness of breath, while she was playing with her grandchildren. Despite treatment with antiarrhythmic drugs, she continues to experience intermittent symptoms. When symptomatic, she worries that she could be having a heart attack or stroke, despite regular visits to her cardiologist and reassurance that her symptoms are not medically dangerous. As a result, Ms. A is afraid to drive to visit her children and grandchildren. At a routine visit to her cardiologist, she reports decreased enjoyment from life, feelings of helplessness and hopelessness about the future, restlessness, poor sleep, fatigue, and poor concentration.

Discussion: Ms. A's presentation is a typical one for depression in atrial fibrillation. Ms. A is not only experiencing symptoms of depression, but excessive worry about her physical symptoms in which she frequently misinterprets the significance of her symptoms, despite reassurance from her physician, as is commonly seen in somatization disorders, such as hypochondriasis.

SUDDEN CARDIAC DEATH

■ EPIDEMIOLOGY

Sudden cardiac death (SCD), defined as death within 1 hour of symptom onset, is caused by malignant arrhythmias, such as ventricular tachycardia or ventricular fibrillation (**Fig. 7-8**). SCD is responsible for more than half of all deaths from heart disease: ~450,000 deaths per year.[139] SCD rates are higher in the elderly, men, and in Blacks.[139] Psychological stress is known to increase ventricular arrhythmias in patients with ventricular ectopy[140] and depression increases the risk of ventricular arrhythmias in individuals with implantable cardioverter defibrillators.[141] Given these associations, depression is thought to be a possible risk factor for SCD.

■ PATHOPHYSIOLOGY

Pathophysiological mechanisms linking depression and SCD include sympathetic nervous system activation, increased resting heart rate, reduced heart rate variability, prolongation of the QT interval, susceptibility to ventricular arrhythmias, and decreased adherence with cardiovascular medications.

Antidepressant medications may also provide a link between depression and SCD. Tricyclic antidepressants (TCAs) cause QT prolongation and ventricular arrhythmias, and are associated with SCD risk in a dose-dependent manner.[142] Some SSRIs as well may cause QT prolongation and torsades de pointes at higher dosages. Antidepressants are a risk factor for SCD, even after controlling for the severity of depression.[11] Combined use of antidepressants and antipsychotics is associated with an increased incidence of SCD, with an odds ratio of 3.4.[143]

■ COURSE AND NATURAL HISTORY

Patients with depression are at increased risk for subsequent SCD though it is unclear whether the risk is mediated by depression itself and/or the use of antidepressants. Clinical depression is prospectively associated with a twofold higher risk for cardiac arrest and SCD after controlling for cardiovascular risk factors, tobacco, alcohol use, and antidepressant medications. Furthermore, the degree of that risk is correlated with the severity of depression.[144,145]

Other studies suggest that the risk of SCD in depression is mediated, at least in part, by the use of antidepressant medications. The Nurse's Health Study followed 63,469 women without known cardiovascular disease for over 8 years. Depression was associated with an increased risk of sudden death in those taking antidepressants; however there was no association between mortality and the severity of depressive symptoms.[11]

Most evidence suggests that depression is related to sudden cardiac death through an increased susceptibility to arrhythmias, and depression is a predictor of arrhythmias in patients with known coronary artery disease.[146] There is also some suggestion that the co-occurrence of anxiety with depression may have a synergistic effect, contributing more strongly to the development of ventricular arrhythmias than either of these conditions alone.[146]

■ ASSESSMENT AND DIFFERENTIAL DIAGNOSIS

Risk factors for SCD include coronary artery disease, history of prior MI, heart failure, prior sudden cardiac arrest or malignant arrhythmias, congenital heart defects, family history of heart disease, family history of SCD, high cholesterol, obesity, diabetes, tobacco use, or history of recreational drug abuse. These cardiovascular risk factors also place patients at higher risk for MDD, subclinical levels of depression, adjustment disorders, and anxiety disorders. In one study of patients at elevated risk for SCD, 24.6% had anxiety and 13.5% were depressed.[147]

Although a minority of SCD cases are due to familial cardiomyopathies or genetic conduction abnormalities, patients with family histories of SCD may have particular vulnerabilities to anxiety and depression. Assessment of these individuals should take into consideration both medical and psychosocial causes of depression. Familial cardiomyopathies and genetic conduction abnormalities may affect multiple members of a family. Individuals at risk for these conditions may have not only lost a relative from SCD, but are then faced with the decision of whether to pursue genetic testing themselves, and potentially, the emotional processing of a positive test results. A positive test result may impact personal decisions, such

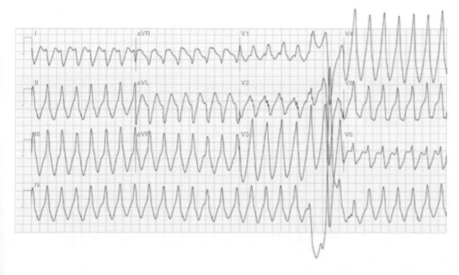

Figure 7-8 *Ventricular tachycardia. (Reproduced with permission from Longo DL, Fauci AS, Kasper DL, et al. Harrison's Principles of Internal Medicine. 18th ed. New York: McGraw-Hill, Inc; 2012.)*

as relationships and family planning. If they feel personally responsible for having passed on a genetic risk to their children, they may experience feelings of guilt. Patients at elevated risk for SCD may also develop a heightened concern about any cardiorespiratory symptoms that they may experience, attributing them to cardiac disease and believing that they presage a future catastrophic event. These individuals may be at risk not only for depression, but for grief reactions, adjustment disorders, and somatization disorders.

■ SUMMARY

Depression is associated with SCD; however it is not clear to what extent depression independently increases the risk of SCD and to what extent the elevated risk is mediated by the use of psychotropic medications. Larger scale randomized trials are needed to determine the causal relationships between depression, antidepressants, and SCD. Further study is also needed to address the role of anxiety, medication nonadherence, and substance use in the relationship between depression and SCD.

IMPLANTABLE CARDIOVERTER DEFIBRILLATORS

■ EPIDEMIOLOGY

Implantable cardioverter defibrillators (ICD) are routinely implanted in the United States and improve survival in populations at high risk for ventricular tachyarrhythmias. ICDs are placed for primary prevention in patients with left ventricular dysfunction and heart failure, and as secondary prevention in patients who have previously experienced a dangerous arrhythmia. Patients with ICDs may have heightened concern about their medical conditions, their potential for receiving shocks from their devices, and their altered body image and risk of death. A wide range of rates of depression have been reported in ICD recipients, ranging between 5% and 41% when assessed with self-report questionnaires and between 11% and 28% when using diagnostic interviews.[148]

Risk factors for depression in ICD recipients include higher NYHA functional classification,[149] younger age,[141] lower levels of education,[150] and medical comorbidities, such as angina and renal failure (**Box 7-1d**).[151] A greater length of time since ICD implantation and an increasing number of shocks received are reported as risk factors for depression in some, but not all, studies (**Box 7-7**).[149,152]

■ PATHOPHYSIOLOGY

Potential mechanisms for depression in ICD recipients relate to the pathophysiology of the underlying heart failure or arrhythmia, the psychological implications of living with an ICD, and the impact of having received shocks from the ICD (Box 7-2). Mechanisms cited to account for the development of depression in heart failure and arrhythmias include increased sympathetic nervous system activation, activation of the hypothalamic pituitary adrenal axis, systemic inflammation, nonadherence with cardiovascular medications, and

---

> ## BOX 7-7
> ## IMPORTANT DRUG–DRUG INTERACTIONS
>
> Warfarin (increased risk of bleeding with many SSRIs)
> Beta-blockers (SSRIs may interfere w/ metabolism)
> Flecainimide (antidepressants by inhibit metabolism)
> Propafenone (several SSRIs may inhibit metabolism)
> Nefazodone and Lovastatin (contraindicated)
> See Table 7-2 for more detail

alcohol use. Since depression predisposes patients to developing ventricular arrhythmias,[141] depressed patients may be at a higher risk for receiving shocks from their ICD. This may create a feedback loop with repeated shocks in turn potentiating the subsequent development of depressive symptoms. Finally, psychotropic medications, including TCAs and some SSRIs (such as citalopram at doses of greater than 40 mg), are associated with QT prolongation and ventricular arrhythmias. This may predispose patients who are taking antidepressants to arrhythmia and thus to ICD shocks.

■ CLINICAL PRESENTATION

Patients with ICDs have had a sudden cardiac arrest or dangerous arrhythmia, or are at high risk of developing such arrhythmias. Although ICDs improve survival, recipients may experience depressive symptoms not only related to their underlying cardiac disease, but due to the emotional consequences of having an ICD implanted. ICD implantation typically results in a visible scar and lump in the pectoral area which may provide patients with a physical reminder of the severity of their cardiac condition and risk of cardiac arrest. Patients may experience both fears about the possibility of being shocked by their devices, as well as doubt about whether their devices will function appropriately in response to an arrhythmia. Patients who have received shocks from their ICDs may have particular concerns about the unpredictable nature of the shocks and concerns for potential triggers of shocks. Women and younger patients may feel self-conscious about the appearance of their ICD and concerned about their physical attractiveness and the impact on social relationships. These emotional consequences of having an ICD implanted may contribute to distress and the development of depressive or anxiety symptoms in vulnerable individuals. Thus anxiety disorders, including panic disorder, agoraphobia, generalized anxiety disorder, and adjustment disorders are common, with prevalence ranging from 11% to 26% (**Box 7-8**).[148]

■ COURSE AND NATURAL HISTORY

The majority of ICD recipients experience improvement in quality of life following ICD implantation. However some patients may become depressed following implantation, and in these patients,

---

> ## BOX 7-1D
> ## IMPORTANT RISK FACTORS FOR DEPRESSION IN ICD PATIENTS
>
> **Sociodemographic**
> Younger age
> Lower level of education
> **Clinical**
> Prior history of depression
> **Medical**
> Greater time since ICD implantation
> Greater number of ICD shocks received

> ## BOX 7-8
> ## DRUGS THAT CAN CAUSE DEPRESSIVE SYMPTOMS
>
> Alpha-adrenergic blockers
> Amiodarone (due to hyper-/hypothyroidism)
> Angiotensin-converting enzyme inhibitors (rare)
> Antiarrhythmic agents (hallucinations, confusion, delirium)
> Beta-adrenergic blockers (fatigue, insomnia, lethargy, decreased libido)
> Digoxin (also visual hallucinations, delirium)
> Thiazide diuretics (fatigue, weakness, anorexia secondary to hypokalemia)

the depression is often chronic. Of patients with depression at the time of ICD implantation, 78% remain depressed after 2 years of follow-up.[149] The time elapsed since ICD implantation increases the risk of depression. One study found the highest levels of depression in patients who had their ICDs for more than 5 years.[150] There may also be an association between the number of ICD shocks and depression rates,[149] with individuals receiving multiple shocks at greatest risk for depression. However, some studies have not demonstrated differences in depression scores between patients who have and have not received shocks.[150] And although quality of life is generally better in ICD recipients than in patients receiving antiarrhythmic therapy, one large study revealed that patients who received more than five shocks did not report this improvement.[153] The relationship between depression and ICDs may be bidirectional, with depression leading to greater risk of shocks. Thus the presence of depressive symptoms in ICD recipients prospectively predicts shock treated ventricular tachyarrhythmias, with the most severe depression having the greatest association with risk of shocks.[141] Depressive symptoms have also been shown to increase all-cause mortality in ICD recipients.[151]

■ ASSESSMENT AND DIFFERENTIAL DIAGNOSIS

Differential diagnosis for depression in patients with ICDs includes adjustment disorder with depressed mood, adjustment disorder with mixed anxiety and depressed mood, and anxiety disorders (**Box 7-4**). Adjustment disorders are frequently seen immediately after ICD implantation or following an ICD shock. By definition, an adjustment disorders are time limited and resolve relatively promptly. Anxiety disorders share a number of common features with depression in patients with ICDs, including difficulty sleeping, difficulty concentrating, restlessness, and decreased enjoyment from activities. Patients who receive shocks may avoid activities or situations that they associate with them. Patients who receive multiple shocks from their devices are at risk of developing post-traumatic stress disorder-like symptoms. Features common to post-traumatic stress disorder and depression include difficulty sleeping, difficulty concentrating, and alterations in mood and cognitions, with low mood, difficulty experiencing positive emotions and feelings of guilt. Unlike depression, however, patients with post-traumatic stress disorder typically experience intrusive recollections of the ICD shocks in the form of intrusive memories, flashbacks, or nightmares.

■ SUMMARY

ICDs improve mortality rates in patients at risk for arrhythmia but may be associated with impairments in quality of life and heightened risk of depression in some vulnerable patients (Case 4). When depression associated with ICD implantation and ICD shocks does occur, the relationship may be bidirectional. As ICDs have become more advanced, with improved sensing capabilities and therapies like antitachycardia pacing, the risk of receiving shocks from ICDs has declined. However, for those patients who do receive shocks, early identification of depression and effective treatment are necessary to improve quality of life. Further studies are necessary to understand the mechanisms by which depression may lead to increased risk of arrhythmias or death.

CASE 4

IMPLANTABLE CARDIOVERTER DEFIBRILLATORS

Mr. D is a 50-year-old divorced man with a history of palpitations since childhood and the detection of a heart murmur in his 20s. After experiencing increased fatigue and shortness of breath, he was diagnosed with nonischemic cardiomyopathy in his 40s

and had an implantable cardioverter defibrillators (ICD) placed 5 years ago as primary prevention. His medical history is significant also for diabetes mellitus type 2, gout, and depression. Mr. D reports that he had received three isolated shocks for ventricular tachycardia since the implantation of his ICD. One month ago, he was admitted to the hospital after receiving 11 shocks while walking his dog in the yard. He cannot remember experiencing any physical symptoms prior to receiving the shocks. In the hospital, Mr. D's antiarrhythmic drug was changed from sotalol to amiodarone and he was discharged home. He was then readmitted 3 weeks later after receiving another 5 shocks. On interview, Mr. D reports that since his last admission, he has experienced depressed mood, has had difficulty staying asleep at night, reports that he has lost interest in his hobby of fixing old cars, and reports getting decreased enjoyment from spending time with his dogs. He also reports restlessness and significant anxiety about whether his ICD will fire again. He has been wondering how much longer he has to live.

Discussion: Mr. D is currently describing a recurrence of depressive symptoms in the setting of repeated ICD shocks. Although he had previously received single shocks from his ICD, the repeated shocks have resulted in the development of depressed mood, anhedonia, insomnia, decreased concentration, and psychomotor agitation. Mr. D also reports a component of anxiety with concerns about recurrent ICD firing and his prognosis. The feelings of helplessness and insecurity he feels are common in depression following ICD firing.

TREATMENT OF DEPRESSION IN CARDIOVASCULAR DISEASE

Treating depression in patients with cardiovascular disease can reduce the severity of depressive symptoms and improve quality of life. A range of treatment modalities are available, including antidepressants, psychotherapeutic approaches, and cardiac rehabilitation programs. This section reviews current findings on treatment of depression in patients with cardiovascular disease as well as the safety of psychotropic medications in this population and the neuropsychiatric effects of cardiac medications.

■ PHARMACOLOGIC TREATMENTS

SSRIs are first-line treatment for depression in patients with cardiovascular disease. Sertraline (dosed 50–200 mg/day) benefits patients with depression who have had recent MI or unstable angina. In the Sertraline Antidepressant Heart Attack Randomized Trial (SADHART), sertraline was effective against depression in patients with MI or unstable angina. It was safe, without any significant impact on left ventricular ejection fraction, ventricular premature complexes, or prolongation of QTc interval.[154] There was also a nonsignificant trend toward decreased mortality with sertraline.[154] However, in a follow-up study of patients with heart failure, sertraline was not shown to be superior to placebo.[155]

The Depression in Patients with Coronary Artery Disease (DECARD) study demonstrated that escitalopram prospectively prevented the development of depression following acute coronary syndromes. This suggests a possible prophylactic role for SSRI antidepressants following an acute coronary event.[156]

A large-scale trial assessed the combination of citalopram and interpersonal psychotherapy (IPT) on depressive symptoms in CHD. Patients were randomized to citalopram versus placebo and to clinical management alone versus clinical management and IPT. Citalopram (dosed 20–40 mg/day) had superior efficacy over placebo; however clinical management with IPT conferred no advantage over clinical management alone.[157]

Some SSRIs may have adverse cardiac effects. In 2011 the FDA issued a warning against doses of citalopram higher than 40 mg/day due to a risk of prolonged QT interval, in a dose-dependent manner. It also cautioned against the use of citalopram in patients with certain cardiac conditions, including congenital long QT syndrome, bradycardia, recent MI, and decompensated heart failure. In the elderly and patients with hepatic impairment, a maximum daily dose of 20 mg was recommended. Adverse cardiac effects from psychiatric drugs are reviewed in **Table 7-1**.[158]

The use of (TCAs is limited in cardiovascular disease because of their side effects. TCAs have potent anticholinergic effects, cause tachycardia, and lead to orthostatic hypotension.[159] TCAs may lead to widening of the QRS interval as a result of sodium channel blockade, which can predispose patients to developing arrhythmias.[160] TCAs are also associated with an increased risk of sudden cardiac death in a dose-dependent manner.[142]

The Myocardial Infarction and Depression-Intervention trial (MIND-IT) found that mirtazapine at doses of 30 to 45 mg/day is more effective than placebo for post-MI depression and is well tolerated with no significant adverse cardiovascular effects.[161] However, given the risk of weight gain, it is typically used as a second-line agent.

Bupropion has not been well studied for the treatment of depression in cardiovascular disease, but has been found to be safe in the treatment of smoking cessation following acute coronary syndromes and is effective in reducing short-term rates of nicotine relapse.[162]

Psychostimulants, such as methylphenidate and dextroamphetamine, can be clinically useful to address depressive apathy and anergia while waiting for the often delayed effect of antidepressants. Among young patients without cardiovascular disease, stimulant use is not associated with elevated risks of MI or SCD.[163] However, use of these agents in patients with a history of ventricular tachycardia, recent MI, CHF, uncontrolled hypertension, or tachycardia is relatively contraindicated due to their effect on blood pressure and heart rate.

In summary, SSRIs are considered safe and well tolerated in patients with CHD, unstable angina, MI, and CHF and most studies show they are effective in treating the accompanying depression. It is not known whether treatment of depression reduces cardiovascular morbidity or mortality. Although SSRIs are first-line treatment for patients with both cardiac disease and depression, they may still have adverse cardiac effects as a result of drug–drug interactions.

Sertraline appears to be a reasonable choice for depressed cardiac patients given its tolerability, relatively few drug–drug interactions, favorable side-effect profile, and lack of consistent association with QTc prolongation.[159]

■ NONPHARMACOLOGIC TREATMENTS

Several trials have shown that psychotherapeutic interventions are effective for treating depression in cardiac patients. The Enhancing Recovery in Coronary Heart Disease (ENRICHD) trial demonstrated that cognitive behavior therapy for post-MI depression improved both depressive symptoms and perceived support.[164] It did not, however, affect rates of recurrent MI or mortality.[164]

Another study found that CBT was effective for treating patients with depression post-CABG surgery. Patients were randomized to treatment with CBT, treatment with supportive stress management, or usual care. Patients receiving either CBT or supportive stress management experienced statistically significant improvement in depressive symptoms at 3 months compared to usual care. The patients receiving CBT continued to experience higher rates of remission at 9-month follow-up.[165]

Studies investigating collaborative care management of complex medical patients, usually involving a nurse or a social worker and a consulting psychiatrist who work together with a primary medical provider, have found that other psychotherapeutic interventions, such as problem-solving therapy and behavioral activation, are effective for treatment of depression symptoms in cardiac patients.[71]

The antidepressant effects of aerobic exercise have also been studied in patients with cardiovascular disease. In a large international, multicenter study, patients in an aerobic exercise group had lower mean Beck Depression Inventory II (BDI-II) scores at 3 months and at 12 months compared to usual care.[166]

In another trial of exercise training in patients with stable heart failure, depressed patients who completed an exercise training program had a statistically significant reduction in depressive symptoms, from 22% to 13%, as well as a 59% reduction in mortality, compared to those who did not complete an exercise training program.[167]

Electroconvulsive therapy (ECT) is safe and effective in patients with refractory depression and cardiovascular disease, including patients with CHD, CHF, valvular disease, atrial fibrillation, pacemakers/ICDs, after aneurysm repair, and orthotopic heart transplant.[168–170] For patients who have CHD, the degree of ischemic

TABLE 7-1 Cardiac Adverse Effects of Psychiatric Medications

Psychotropic Medication Class	Potential Cardiovascular Effects
Antipsychotics	Hypotension, orthostatic hypotension, cardiac conduction disturbances, ventricular tachycardia/fibrillation, metabolic syndrome
Bupropion	Hypertension
Monoamine oxidase inhibitors	Orthostatic hypotension
Serotonin norepinephrine reuptake inhibitors (SNRIs)	Hypertension
Selective serotonin reuptake inhibitors (SSRIs)	Reduced heart rate, occasional clinically significant sinus bradycardia or sinus arrest
Stimulants	Hypertension, tachycardia, tachyarrhythmia
Tricyclic antidepressants	Hypotension, orthostatic hypotension, Type 1A antiarrhythmic effects: slowed conduction through atrioventricular node and His bundle; heart block; QT prolongation; ventricular fibrillation
Trazodone	Orthostatic hypotension
Lithium	Sinus node dysfunction
Carbamazepine	Type 1A antiarrhythmic effects; atrioventricular block
Phosphodiesterase type 5 inhibitors	Hypotension, myocardial ischemia

TABLE 7-2 Selected Interactions Between Psychiatric Medications and Cardiac Drugs

Psychotropic	Cardiac	Warning	Mechanism	Clinical Management
Fluoxetine	Nifedipine	Concurrent use may result in increased nifedipine levels	Inhibition of CYP3A	Monitor for nifedipine toxicity, including hypotension, peripheral edema, and bradycardia. Consider dose reduction of nifedipine
	Propafenone	Concurrent use may result in increased propafenone levels and increased risk of cardiotoxicity (QT prolongation, torsades de pointes, cardiac arrest)	Inhibition of cytochrome P450 2D6. Theoretical additive effects on QT prolongation	Caution is advised
	Digoxin	Concurrent use may result in increased risk of digoxin toxicity (nausea, vomiting, arrhythmias)		Patients receiving fluoxetine and digoxin should be monitored for symptoms of digoxin toxicity. Digoxin levels should be monitored
Fluvoxamine	Quinidine	Concurrent use results in decreased clearance of quinidine which could affect cardiac conduction	Fluvoxamine inhibits quinidine metabolism	A decrease in quinidine dose may be necessary
	Warfarin	Concurrent use may result in an increased risk of bleeding	Unknown	Monitor closely for signs of increased bleeding. Check for altered anticoagulant effects with prothrombin time ratio and INR
	Propranolol	Concurrent use may result in increased propranolol levels, resulting in bradycardia and hypotension	Reduced beta-blocker metabolism	Monitor heart rate and blood pressure. Propranolol dose may need to be reduced. Alternatively, consider atenolol, a nonhepatically metabolized beta-blocker[30]
	Mexiletine	Concurrent use may result in increased mexiletine levels	Inhibition of CYP1A2	Monitor for signs and symptoms of mexiletine toxicity (nausea, dizziness, cardiac arrhythmias). Monitor liver function, complete blood count, and electrocardiogram if mexiletine toxicity is suspected, and reduce mexiletine dose as required
Nefazodone	Lovastatin	Concurrent use may result in increased lovastatin levels and increased risk of myopathy or rhabdomyolysis		Concurrent use of lovastatin and nefazodone is contraindicated. Alternatively, pravastatin is not significantly metabolized by CYP3A4, and is unaffected by nefazodone
Paroxetine	Flecainide	Concurrent use may result in an increased risk of flecainide toxicity (cardiac arrhythmia)	Inhibition CYP2D6[31]	Monitor heart rate and the EKG in patients receiving concurrent flecainide and paroxetine. Lower doses of both paroxetine and flecainide may be required. Co-administration of these agents should be approached with caution
	Warfarin	Concurrent use may increase risk of bleeding	Unknown	Monitor for signs of increased bleeding and altered anticoagulant effects
Sertraline	Metoprolol	Concurrent use may result in increased metoprolol levels	Inhibition of CYP2D6	Consider metoprolol dose reduction, and monitor heart rate and blood pressure closely
	Flecainide	Concurrent use may result in an increased risk of flecainide toxicity (cardiac arrhythmia)	Inhibition of flecainide metabolism	Co-administration of these agents should be approached with caution. Monitor the EKG. Doses of flecainide may need to be reduced
	Warfarin	Concurrent use may result in an increased risk of bleeding	Unknown	Monitor for signs of increased bleeding
	Propafenone	Concurrent use may result in an increased risk of propafenone toxicity (cardiac arrhythmias)	Inhibition of propafenone metabolism	Co-administration of these agents should be approached with caution. Monitor the EKG. Doses of propafenone may need to be reduced
	Metoprolol	Concurrent use may result in increased metoprolol levels	Inhibition of CYP2D6	Consider metoprolol dose reduction, and monitor heart rate and blood pressure closely

(continued)

TABLE 7-2 Selected Interactions Between Psychiatric Medications and Cardiac Drugs (*continued*)

Psychotropic	Cardiac	Warning	Mechanism	Clinical Management
Bupropion	Flecainide	Concurrent use may result in increased levels of flecainide	Inhibition of CYP2D6	Co-administration of bupropion and flecainide should be approached with caution. Flecainide should be initiated at the lower end of the dose range. If bupropion is added to the treatment regimen of a patient already receiving flecainide, consider decreasing the dose of flecainide
	Metoprolol	Concurrent use may result in increased metoprolol levels	Inhibition of CYP2D6	If concomitant administration is required, consider metoprolol dose reduction, and monitor heart rate and blood pressure closely
	Propafenone	Concurrent use may result in increased propafenone levels	Inhibition CYP2D6	Co-administration of bupropion and propafenone should be approached with caution. Propafenone should be initiated at the lower end of the dose range. If bupropion is added to the treatment regimen of a patient already receiving propafenone, consider decreasing the dose of propafenone

coronary artery disease is important to take into consideration when deciding whether to deliver ECT.[171] Because these patients may be at greater risk for complications arising from the increased parasympathetic and sympathetic activity during ECT. For patients with acute MI, unstable angina, or serious ventricular arrhythmias, ECT is relatively contraindicated. In any patient with cardiovascular disease and depression considering ECT, consultation between cardiology, anesthesia, and psychiatry is helpful in determining the individual's likely risks and benefits.

■ CARDIAC MEDICATIONS AND DEPRESSION

Many routinely used cardiac medications can have adverse neuropsychiatric effects, including precipitating or exacerbating depressive symptoms (Box 7-8).[158,172,173] Therefore careful review and consideration of the medications used in patients with cardiovascular disease is important in the differential diagnosis of depressive symptoms. Older alpha-adrenergic blocking agents for hypertension, including reserpine, methyldopa, and clonidine are associated with depression.[172] The antiarrhythmic agent amiodarone is associated with thyroiditis, which can result in hypothyroidism and thereby precipitate or exacerbate depression. Digoxin and digitalis can cause depression, as well as anxiety, delirium, and hallucinations. Depressed mood may be a manifestation of digitalis intoxication.[174] Thiazide diuretic use may result in hypokalemia and hyponatremia that can be manifested as weakness, fatigue, apathy, and anorexia.[172] Beta-blocking agents have long been associated with depressive symptoms, particularly lipophilic beta-blockers, such as propranolol and metoprolol, which easily cross the blood–brain barrier. However, this has not been borne out in a more recent review of randomized controlled trials, which showed no increased risk of depression with beta-blocker use.[123] It is possible that higher doses of beta-blockers or longer duration of treatment may alter risk, but further studies are needed to determine this. Several studies reported an association between low serum cholesterol levels and increased suicide risk,[175] raising concern about

the safety of the cholesterol lowering agents statins. However, multiple, large randomized clinical trials have subsequently shown that statins do not increase the risk of depression or suicide.[176] There are case reports of mood symptoms with the angiotensin-converting enzyme inhibitor (ACE-I) captopril; however in general, ACE-I, calcium channel blockers and angiotensin-II blockers have little association with depression.

■ SUMMARY

Many treatments have been evaluated in patients with depression and cardiovascular disease, including antidepressants, psychostimulants, psychotherapy, ECT, and cardiac rehabilitation. Many of these are effective treatments for depression and are well tolerated in cardiac patients. Since the effects of these treatments on cardiovascular disease progression and prognosis are still equivocal, there is a significant need for further, well-designed, adequately powered studies to determine whether treatment of depression can alter cardiac outcomes (**Box 7-9**). In the pharmacotherapy of depression in patients with cardiovascular disease, it is important to consider not only the role of individual medications, but the impact of drug–drug interactions between the cardiac and psychiatric medications (**Table 7-2**).[177–181]

**BOX 7-9
SUMMARY**

- The prevalence of depression is increased in cardiovascular diseases
- In many cardiovascular diseases, depression is associated with poorer quality of life, increased symptom burden, and increased mortality
- Treatments are effective for depression but one must be aware of the cardiac side effects of antidepressants treatments as well as potential interactions with cardiac medications

REFERENCES

1. Go AS, Mozaffarian D, Roger VL, et al. Heart disease and stroke statistics–2013 update: a report from the American Heart Association. *Circulation*. 2013;127(1):e6–e245.

2. Rudisch B, Nemeroff CB. Epidemiology of comorbid coronary artery disease and depression. *Biol Psychiatry*. 2003;54(3):227–240.

3. Kessler RC, Berglund P, Demler O, et al. The epidemiology of major depressive disorder: results from the National Comorbidity Survey Replication (NCS-R). *JAMA*. 2003;289(23):3095–3105.

4. Carney RM, Freedland KE. Depression and heart rate variability in patients with coronary heart disease. *Cleve Clin J Med*. 2009;76(Suppl 2):S13–S17.

5. Lespérance F, Frasure-Smith N. Depression in patients with cardiac disease: a practical review. *J Psychosom Res*. 2000;48(4–5):379–391.

6. Schleifer SJ, Macari-Hinson MM, Coyle DA, et al. The nature and course of depression following myocardial infarction. *Arch Intern Med*. 1989;149(8):1785–1789.

7. Connerney I, Shapiro PA, McLaughlin JS, Bagiella E, Sloan RP. Relation between depression after coronary artery bypass surgery and 12-month outcome: a prospective study. *Lancet*. 2001;358(9295):1766–1771.

8. Blumenthal JA, Lett HS, Babyak MA, et al. Depression as a risk factor for mortality after coronary artery bypass surgery. *Lancet*. 2003;362(9384):604–609.

9. Larsen KK, Agerbo E, Christensen B, Søndergaard J, Vestergaard M. Myocardial infarction and risk of suicide: a population-based case-control study. *Circulation*. 2010;122(23):2388–2393.

10. Surtees PG, Wainwright NW, Luben RN, Wareham NJ, Bingham SA, Khaw KT. Depression and ischemic heart disease mortality: evidence from the EPIC-Norfolk United Kingdom prospective cohort study. *Am J Psychiatry*. 2008;165(4):515–523.

11. Whang W, Kubzansky LD, Kawachi I, et al. Depression and risk of sudden cardiac death and coronary heart disease in women: results from the Nurses' Health Study. *J Am Coll Cardiol*. 2009;53(11):950–958.

12. Wulsin LR, Singal BM. Do depressive symptoms increase the risk for the onset of coronary disease? A systematic quantitative review. *Psychosom Med*. 2003;65(2):201–210.

13. Wassertheil-Smoller S, Shumaker S, Ockene J, et al. Depression and cardiovascular sequelae in postmenopausal women. The Women's Health Initiative (WHI). *Arch Intern Med*. 2004;164(3):289–298.

14. Lett HS, Blumenthal JA, Babyak MA, et al. Depression as a risk factor for coronary artery disease: evidence, mechanisms, and treatment. *Psychosom Med*. 2004;66(3):305–315.

15. Sullivan PF, Neale MC, Kendler KS. Genetic epidemiology of major depression: review and meta-analysis. *Am J Psychiatry*. 2000;157(10):1552–1562.

16. Sørensen C, Brandes A, Hendricks O, et al. Psychosocial predictors of depression in patients with acute coronary syndrome. *Acta Psychiatr Scand*. 2005;111(2):116–124.

17. Scherrer JF, Xian H, Bucholz KK, et al. A twin study of depression symptoms, hypertension, and heart disease in middle-aged men. *Psychosom Med*. 2003;65(4):548–557.

18. Whooley MA, de Jonge P, Vittinghoff E, et al. Depressive symptoms, health behaviors, and risk of cardiovascular events in patients with coronary heart disease. *JAMA*. 2008;300(20):2379–2388.

19. Kronish IM, Rieckmann N, Halm EA, et al. Persistent depression affects adherence to secondary prevention behaviors after acute coronary syndromes. *J Gen Intern Med*. 2006;21(11):1178–1183.

20. Grace SL, Abbey SE, Pinto R, Shnek ZM, Irvine J, Stewart DE. Longitudinal course of depressive symptomatology after a cardiac event: effects of gender and cardiac rehabilitation. *Psychosom Med*. 2005;67(1):52–58.

21. Lespérance F, Frasure-Smith N, Talajic M, Bourassa MG. Five-year risk of cardiac mortality in relation to initial severity and one-year changes in depression symptoms after myocardial infarction. *Circulation*. 2002;105(9):1049–1053.

22. Frasure-Smith N, Lespérance F, Talajic M. Depression following myocardial infarction. Impact on 6-month survival. *JAMA*. 1993;270(15):1819–1825.

23. Webb RT, Kontopantelis E, Doran T, Qin P, Creed F, Kapur N. Suicide risk in primary care patients with major physical diseases: a case-control study. *Arch Gen Psychiatry*. 2012;69(3):256–264.

24. Joynt KE, Whellan DJ, O'Connor CM. Depression and cardiovascular disease: mechanisms of interaction. *Biol Psychiatry*. 2003;54(3):248–261.

25. Dickens CM, Percival C, McGowan L, et al. The risk factors for depression in first myocardial infarction patients. *Psychol Med*. 2004;34(6):1083–1092.

26. Brummett BH, Mark DB, Siegler IC, et al. Perceived social support as a predictor of mortality in coronary patients: effects of smoking, sedentary behavior, and depressive symptoms. *Psychosom Med*. 2005;67(1):40–45.

27. Spijkerman TA, van den Brink RH, Jansen JH, Crijns HJ, Ormel J. Who is at risk of post-MI depressive symptoms? *J Psychosom Res*. 2005;58(5):425–432; discussion 433–424.

28. Doyle F, McGee HM, Conroy RM, Delaney M. What predicts depression in cardiac patients: sociodemographic factors, disease severity or theoretical vulnerabilities? *Psychol Health*. 2011;26(5):619–634.

29. Dickens C, McGowan L, Percival C, et al. Negative illness perceptions are associated with new-onset depression following myocardial infarction. *Gen Hosp Psychiatry*. 2008;30(5):414–420.

30. Martens EJ, Smith OR, Winter J, Denollet J, Pedersen SS. Cardiac history, prior depression and personality predict course of depressive symptoms after myocardial infarction. *Psychol Med*. 2008;38(2):257–264.

31. Lesperance F, Frasure-Smith N, Talajic M. Major depression before and after myocardial infarction: its nature and consequences. *Psychosom Med*. 1996;58(2):99–110.

32. Dickens C, McGowan L, Percival C, et al. New onset depression following myocardial infarction predicts cardiac mortality. *Psychosom Med*. 2008;70(4):450–455.

33. Lett H, Ali S, Whooley M. Depression and cardiac function in patients with stable coronary heart disease: findings from the Heart and Soul Study. *Psychosom Med*. 2008;70(4):444–449.

34. Frasure-Smith N, Lespérance F, Juneau M, Talajic M, Bourassa MG. Gender, depression, and one-year prognosis after myocardial infarction. *Psychosom Med*. 1999;61(1):26–37.

35. Parashar S, Rumsfeld JS, Spertus JA, et al. Time course of depression and outcome of myocardial infarction. *Arch Intern Med*. 2006;166(18):2035–2043.

36. Veith RC, Lewis N, Linares OA, et al. Sympathetic nervous system activity in major depression. Basal and desipramine-

induced alterations in plasma norepinephrine kinetics. *Arch Gen Psychiatry.* 1994;51(5):411–422.

37. Carney RM, Freedland KE, Veith RC, et al. Major depression, heart rate, and plasma norepinephrine in patients with coronary heart disease. *Biol Psychiatry.* 1999;45(4):458–463.

38. Carney RM, Freedland KE, Veith RC. Depression, the autonomic nervous system, and coronary heart disease. *Psychosom Med.* 2005;67(Suppl 1):S29–S33.

39. Kleiger RE, Miller JP, Bigger JT, Moss AJ. Decreased heart rate variability and its association with increased mortality after acute myocardial infarction. *Am J Cardiol.* 1987;59(4):256–262.

40. Otte C, Marmar CR, Pipkin SS, Moos R, Browner WS, Whooley MA. Depression and 24-hour urinary cortisol in medical outpatients with coronary heart disease: The Heart and Soul Study. *Biol Psychiatry.* 2004;56(4):241–247.

41. Vreeburg SA, Hoogendijk WJ, van Pelt J, et al. Major depressive disorder and hypothalamic-pituitary-adrenal axis activity: results from a large cohort study. *Arch Gen Psychiatry.* 2009;66(6):617–626.

42. Whooley MA, Wong JM. Depression and cardiovascular disorders. *Annu Rev Clin Psychol.* 2013;9:327–354.

43. Vaccarino V, Johnson BD, Sheps DS, et al. Depression, inflammation, and incident cardiovascular disease in women with suspected coronary ischemia: the National Heart, Lung, and Blood Institute-sponsored WISE study. *J Am Coll Cardiol.* 2007;50(21):2044–2050.

44. Kop WJ, Gottdiener JS, Tangen CM, et al. Inflammation and coagulation factors in persons > 65 years of age with symptoms of depression but without evidence of myocardial ischemia. *Am J Cardiol.* 2002;89(4):419–424.

45. Jiang W, Glassman A, Krishnan R, O'Connor CM, Califf RM. Depression and ischemic heart disease: what have we learned so far and what must we do in the future? *Am Heart J.* 2005;150(1):54–78.

46. Ziegelstein RC, Parakh K, Sakhuja A, Bhat U. Platelet function in patients with major depression. *Intern Med J.* 2009;39(1):38–43.

47. Parissis JT, Fountoulaki K, Filippatos G, Adamopoulos S, Paraskevaidis I, Kremastinos D. Depression in coronary artery disease: novel pathophysiologic mechanisms and therapeutic implications. *Int J Cardiol.* 2007;116(2):153–160.

48. Serebruany VL, Gurbel PA, O'Connor CM. Platelet inhibition by sertraline and N-desmethylsertraline: a possible missing link between depression, coronary events, and mortality benefits of selective serotonin reuptake inhibitors. *Pharmacol Res.* 2001;43(5):453–462.

49. Carneiro AM, Cook EH, Murphy DL, et al. Interactions between integrin αIIbβ3 and the serotonin transporter regulate serotonin transport and platelet aggregation in mice and humans. *J Clin Invest.* 2008;118(4):1544–1552.

50. Nakatani D, Sato H, Sakata Y, et al. Influence of serotonin transporter gene polymorphism on depressive symptoms and new cardiac events after acute myocardial infarction. *Am Heart J.* 2005;150(4):652–658.

51. McCaffery JM, Duan QL, Frasure-Smith N, et al. Genetic predictors of depressive symptoms in cardiac patients. *Am J Med Genet B Neuropsychiatr Genet.* 2009;150B(3):381–388.

52. McCaffery JM, Frasure-Smith N, Dubé MP, et al. Common genetic vulnerability to depressive symptoms and coronary artery disease: a review and development of candidate genes related to inflammation and serotonin. *Psychosom Med.* 2006;68(2):187–200.

53. Carney RM, Freedland KE. Are somatic symptoms of depression better predictors of cardiac events than cognitive symptoms in coronary heart disease? *Psychosom Med.* 2012;74(1):33–38.

54. Sanner JE, Frazier L, Udtha M. Self-reported depressive symptoms in women hospitalized for acute coronary syndrome. *J Psychiatr Ment Health Nurs.* 2013;20(10):913–920.

55. Groenewold NA, Doornbos B, Zuidersma M, et al. Comparing cognitive and somatic symptoms of depression in myocardial infarction patients and depressed patients in primary and mental health care. *PLoS One.* 2013;8(1):e53859.

56. Martens EJ, Hoen PW, Mittelhaeuser M, de Jonge P, Denollet J. Symptom dimensions of post-myocardial infarction depression, disease severity and cardiac prognosis. *Psychol Med.* 2010;40(5):807–814.

57. Simmonds RL, Tylee A, Walters P, Rose D. Patients' perceptions of depression and coronary heart disease: a qualitative UPBEAT-UK study. *BMC Fam Pract.* 2013;14:38.

58. Ladwig K, Röll G, Breithardt G, Borggrefe M. Extracardiac contributions to chest pain perception in patients 6 months after acute myocardial infarction. *Am Heart J.* 1999;137(3):528–535.

59. Spertus JA, McDonell M, Woodman CL, Fihn SD. Association between depression and worse disease-specific functional status in outpatients with coronary artery disease. *Am Heart J.* 2000;140(1):105–110.

60. Davidson KW, Kupfer DJ, Bigger JT, et al. Assessment and treatment of depression in patients with cardiovascular disease: National Heart, Lung, and Blood Institute Working Group Report. *Psychosom Med.* 2006;68(5):645–650.

61. de Jonge P, Spijkerman TA, van den Brink RH, Ormel J. Depression after myocardial infarction is a risk factor for declining health related quality of life and increased disability and cardiac complaints at 12 months. *Heart.* 2006;92(1):32–39.

62. Lauzon C, Beck CA, Huynh T, et al. Depression and prognosis following hospital admission because of acute myocardial infarction. *CMAJ.* 2003;168(5):547–552.

63. Barth J, Schumacher M, Herrmann-Lingen C. Depression as a risk factor for mortality in patients with coronary heart disease: a meta-analysis. *Psychosom Med.* 2004;66(6):802–813.

64. Bush DE, Ziegelstein RC, Tayback M, et al. Even minimal symptoms of depression increase mortality risk after acute myocardial infarction. *Am J Cardiol.* 2001;88(4):337–341.

65. Mayou RA, Gill D, Thompson DR, et al. Depression and anxiety as predictors of outcome after myocardial infarction. *Psychosom Med.* ;62(2):212–219.

66. Carney RM, Freedland KE, Steinmeyer B, et al. History of depression and survival after acute myocardial infarction. *Psychosom Med.* 2009;71(3):253–259.

67. de Jonge P, van den Brink RH, Spijkerman TA, Ormel J. Only incident depressive episodes after myocardial infarction are associated with new cardiovascular events. *J Am Coll Cardiol.* 2006;48(11):2204–2208.

68. Doyle F, Conroy R, McGee H, Delaney M. Depressive symptoms in persons with acute coronary syndrome: specific symptom scales and prognosis. *J Psychosom Res.* 2010;68(2):121–130.

69. de Jonge P, Ormel J, van den Brink RH, et al. Symptom dimensions of depression following myocardial infarction and their relationship with somatic health status and cardiovascular prognosis. *Am J Psychiatry.* 2006;163(1):138–144.

70. Davidson KW, Burg MM, Kronish IM, et al. Association of anhedonia with recurrent major adverse cardiac events and mortality 1 year after acute coronary syndrome. *Arch Gen Psychiatry.* 2010; 67(5):480–488.

71. Kronish IM, Chaplin WF, Rieckmann N, Burg MM, Davidson KW. The effect of enhanced depression care on anxiety symptoms in acute coronary syndrome patients: findings from the COPES trial. *Psychother Psychosom.* 2012;81(4):245–247.

72. Anda RF, Williamson DF, Escobedo LG, Mast EE, Giovino GA, Remington PL. Depression and the dynamics of smoking. A national perspective. *JAMA.* 1990;264(12):1541–1545.

73. Mikkelsen SS, Tolstrup JS, Flachs EM, Mortensen EL, Schnohr P, Flensborg-Madsen T. A cohort study of leisure time physical activity and depression. *Prev Med.* 2010;51(6):471–475.

74. Augestad LB, Slettemoen RP, Flanders WD. Physical activity and depressive symptoms among Norwegian adults aged 20–50. *Public Health Nurs.* 2008;25(6):536–545.

75. Glazer KM, Emery CF, Frid DJ, Banyasz RE. Psychological predictors of adherence and outcomes among patients in cardiac rehabilitation. *J Cardiopulm Rehabil.* 2002;22(1):40–46.

76. Carney RM, Freedland KE, Eisen SA, Rich MW, Jaffe AS. Major depression and medication adherence in elderly patients with coronary artery disease. *Health Psychol.* 1995;14(1):88–90.

77. Rieckmann N, Kronish IM, Haas D, et al. Persistent depressive symptoms lower aspirin adherence after acute coronary syndromes. *Am Heart J.* 2006;152(5):922–927.

78. Gehi A, Haas D, Pipkin S, Whooley MA. Depression and medication adherence in outpatients with coronary heart disease: findings from the Heart and Soul Study. *Arch Intern Med.* 2005;165(21):2508–2513.

79. Everson SA, Goldberg DE, Kaplan GA, et al. Hopelessness and risk of mortality and incidence of myocardial infarction and cancer. *Psychosom Med.* 1996;58(2):113–121.

80. Barefoot JC, Brummett BH, Williams RB, et al. Recovery expectations and long-term prognosis of patients with coronary heart disease. *Arch Intern Med.* 2011;171(10):929–935.

81. Clarke DM, Kissane DW. Demoralization: its phenomenology and importance. *Aust N Z J Psychiatry.* 2002;36(6):733–742.

82. Mangelli L, Fava GA, Grandi S, et al. Assessing demoralization and depression in the setting of medical disease. *J Clin Psychiatry.* 2005;66(3):391–394.

83. Davidson KW. Depression and coronary heart disease. *ISRN Cardiol.* 2012;2012:743813.

84. McManus D, Pipkin SS, Whooley MA. Screening for depression in patients with coronary heart disease (data from the Heart and Soul Study). *Am J Cardiol.* 2005;96(8):1076–1081.

85. Whooley MA, Avins AL, Miranda J, Browner WS. Case-finding instruments for depression. Two questions are as good as many. *J Gen Intern Med.* 1997;12(7):439–445.

86. Coventry PA, Hays R, Dickens C, et al. Talking about depression: a qualitative study of barriers to managing depression in people with long term conditions in primary care. *BMC Fam Pract.* 2011;12:10.

87. Heidenreich PA, Trogdon JG, Khavjou OA, et al. Forecasting the future of cardiovascular disease in the United States: a policy statement from the American Heart Association. *Circulation.* 2011;123(8):933–944.

88. Roger VL, Weston SA, Redfield MM, et al. Trends in heart failure incidence and survival in a community-based population. *JAMA.* 2004;292(3):344–350.

89. Rutledge T, Reis VA, Linke SE, Greenberg BH, Mills PJ. Depression in heart failure a meta-analytic review of prevalence, intervention effects, and associations with clinical outcomes. *J Am Coll Cardiol.* 2006;48(8):1527–1537.

90. Freedland KE, Rich MW, Skala JA, Carney RM, Dávila-Román VG, Jaffe AS. Prevalence of depression in hospitalized patients with congestive heart failure. *Psychosom Med.* 2003;65(1): 119–128.

91. Havranek EP, Spertus JA, Masoudi FA, Jones PG, Rumsfeld JS. Predictors of the onset of depressive symptoms in patients with heart failure. *J Am Coll Cardiol.* 2004;44(12):2333–2338.

92. Abramson J, Berger A, Krumholz HM, Vaccarino V. Depression and risk of heart failure among older persons with isolated systolic hypertension. *Arch Intern Med.* 2001;161(14):1725–1730.

93. Williams SA, Kasl SV, Heiat A, Abramson JL, Krumholz HM, Vaccarino V. Depression and risk of heart failure among the elderly: a prospective community-based study. *Psychosom Med.* 2002;64(1):6–12.

94. Francis GS, Cohn JN, Johnson G, Rector TS, Goldman S, Simon A. Plasma norepinephrine, plasma renin activity, and congestive heart failure. Relations to survival and the effects of therapy in V-HeFT II. The V-HeFT VA Cooperative Studies Group. *Circulation.* 1993;87(6 Suppl):VI40–VI48.

95. Lespérance F, Frasure-Smith N, Laliberté MA, et al. An open-label study of nefazodone treatment of major depression in patients with congestive heart failure. *Can J Psychiatry.* 2003;48(10):695–701.

96. Shores MM, Pascualy M, Lewis NL, Flatness D, Veith RC. Short-term sertraline treatment suppresses sympathetic nervous system activity in healthy human subjects. *Psychoneuroendocrinology.* 2001;26(4):433–439.

97. Güder G, Bauersachs J, Frantz S, et al. Complementary and incremental mortality risk prediction by cortisol and aldosterone in chronic heart failure. *Circulation.* 2007;115(13):1754–1761.

98. Howren MB, Lamkin DM, Suls J. Associations of depression with C-reactive protein, IL-1, and IL-6: a meta-analysis. *Psychosom Med.* 2009;71(2):171–186.

99. Dowlati Y, Herrmann N, Swardfager W, et al. A meta-analysis of cytokines in major depression. *Biol Psychiatry.* 2010;67(5): 446–457.

100. Abbate A, Van Tassell BW, Biondi-Zoccai G, et al. Effects of Interleukin-1 Blockade With Anakinra on Adverse Cardiac Remodeling and Heart Failure After Acute Myocardial Infarction [from the Virginia Commonwealth University-Anakinra Remodeling Trial (2) (VCU-ART2) Pilot Study]. *Am J Cardiol.* 2013;111(10):1394–1400.

101. Torre-Amione G, Kapadia S, Benedict C, Oral H, Young JB, Mann DL. Proinflammatory cytokine levels in patients with depressed left ventricular ejection fraction: a report from the Studies of Left Ventricular Dysfunction (SOLVD). *J Am Coll Cardiol.* 1996;27(5):1201–1206.

102. Duivis HE, Kupper N, Penninx BW, Na B, de Jonge P, Whooley MA. Depressive symptoms and white blood cell count in coronary heart disease patients: prospective findings from the Heart and Soul Study. *Psychoneuroendocrinology.* 2013;38(4):479–487.

103. DiMatteo MR, Lepper HS, Croghan TW. Depression is a risk factor for noncompliance with medical treatment: meta-analysis of the effects of anxiety and depression on patient adherence. *Arch Intern Med.* 2000;160(14):2101–2107.

104. Miura T, Kojima R, Mizutani M, Shiga Y, Takatsu F, Suzuki Y. Effect of digoxin noncompliance on hospitalization and mortality in

patients with heart failure in long-term therapy: a prospective cohort study. *Eur J Clin Pharmacol.* 2001;57(1):77–83.

105. DiMatteo MR. Social support and patient adherence to medical treatment: a meta-analysis. *Health Psychol.* 2004;23(2):207–218.

106. Pan A, Kumar R, Macey PM, Fonarow GC, Harper RM, Woo MA. Visual assessment of brain magnetic resonance imaging detects injury to cognitive regulatory sites in patients with heart failure. *J Card Fail.* 2013;19(2):94–100.

107. Lesman-Leegte I, Jaarsma T, Sanderman R, Linssen G, van Veldhuisen DJ. Depressive symptoms are prominent among elderly hospitalised heart failure patients. *Eur J Heart Fail.* 2006;8(6):634–640.

108. Watkins LL, Koch GG, Sherwood A, et al. Association of anxiety and depression with all-cause mortality in individuals with coronary heart disease. *J Am Heart Assoc.* 2013;2(2):e000068.

109. Jiang W, Kuchibhatla M, Cuffe MS, et al. Prognostic value of anxiety and depression in patients with chronic heart failure. *Circulation.* 2004;110(22):3452–3456.

110. Friedmann E, Thomas SA, Liu F, et al. Relationship of depression, anxiety, and social isolation to chronic heart failure outpatient mortality. *Am Heart J.* 2006;152(5):940.e941–948.

111. Fuster V, Gersh BJ, Giuliani ER, Tajik AJ, Brandenburg RO, Frye RL. The natural history of idiopathic dilated cardiomyopathy. *Am J Cardiol.* 1981;47(3):525–531.

112. McKenna CJ, Codd MB, McCann HA, Sugrue DD. Alcohol consumption and idiopathic dilated cardiomyopathy: a case control study. *Am Heart J.* 1998;135(5 Pt 1):833–837.

113. Hawkins LA, Kilian S, Firek A, Kashner TM, Firek CJ, Silvet H. Cognitive impairment and medication adherence in outpatients with heart failure. *Heart Lung.* 2012;41(6):572–582.

114. Frasure-Smith N, Lespérance F, Habra M, et al. Elevated depression symptoms predict long-term cardiovascular mortality in patients with atrial fibrillation and heart failure. *Circulation.* 2009;120(2):134–140, 133p following 140.

115. Jiang W, Kuchibhatla M, Clary GL, et al. Relationship between depressive symptoms and long-term mortality in patients with heart failure. *Am Heart J.* 2007;154(1):102–108.

116. Schowalter M, Gelbrich G, Störk S, et al. Generic and disease-specific health-related quality of life in patients with chronic systolic heart failure: impact of depression. *Clin Res Cardiol.* 2013;102(4):269–278.

117. Rumsfeld JS, Havranek E, Masoudi FA, et al. Depressive symptoms are the strongest predictors of short-term declines in health status in patients with heart failure. *J Am Coll Cardiol.* 2003;42(10):1811–1817.

118. Vaccarino V, Kasl SV, Abramson J, Krumholz HM. Depressive symptoms and risk of functional decline and death in patients with heart failure. *J Am Coll Cardiol.* 2001;38(1):199–205.

119. Jiang W, Alexander J, Christopher E, et al. Relationship of depression to increased risk of mortality and rehospitalization in patients with congestive heart failure. *Arch Intern Med.* 2001;161(15):1849–1856.

120. Albert NM, Fonarow GC, Abraham WT, et al. Depression and clinical outcomes in heart failure: an OPTIMIZE-HF analysis. *Am J Med.* 2009;122(4):366–373.

121. Sherwood A, Blumenthal JA, Trivedi R, et al. Relationship of depression to death or hospitalization in patients with heart failure. *Arch Intern Med.* 2007;167(4):367–373.

122. Rollman BL, Herbeck Belnap B, Mazumdar S, et al. A positive 2-item Patient Health Questionnaire depression screen among hospitalized heart failure patients is associated with elevated 12-month mortality. *J Card Fail.* 2012;18(3):238–245.

123. Ko DT, Hebert PR, Coffey CS, Sedrakyan A, Curtis JP, Krumholz HM. Beta-blocker therapy and symptoms of depression, fatigue, and sexual dysfunction. *JAMA.* 2002;288(3):351–357.

124. Israel CW, Grönefeld G, Ehrlich JR, Li YG, Hohnloser SH. Long-term risk of recurrent atrial fibrillation as documented by an implantable monitoring device: implications for optimal patient care. *J Am Coll Cardiol.* 2004;43(1):47–52.

125. Thrall G, Lip GY, Carroll D, Lane D. Depression, anxiety, and quality of life in patients with atrial fibrillation. *Chest.* 2007;132(4):1259–1264.

126. Sang CH, Chen K, Pang XF, et al. Depression, anxiety, and quality of life after catheter ablation in patients with paroxysmal atrial fibrillation. *Clin Cardiol.* 2013;36(1):40–45.

127. Goli NM, Thompson T, Sears SF, et al. Educational attainment is associated with atrial fibrillation symptom severity. *Pacing Clin Electrophysiol.* 2012;35(9):1090–1096.

128. Bettoni M, Zimmermann M. Autonomic tone variations before the onset of paroxysmal atrial fibrillation. *Circulation.* 2002;105(23):2753–2759.

129. Tsai CT, Chiang FT, Tseng CD, et al. Increased expression of mineralocorticoid receptor in human atrial fibrillation and a cellular model of atrial fibrillation. *J Am Coll Cardiol.* 2010;55(8):758–770.

130. Christiansen CF, Christensen S, Mehnert F, Cummings SR, Chapurlat RD, Sørensen HT. Glucocorticoid use and risk of atrial fibrillation or flutter: a population-based, case-control study. *Arch Intern Med.* 2009;169(18):1677–1683.

131. Guo Y, Lip GY, Apostolakis S. Inflammation in atrial fibrillation. *J Am Coll Cardiol.* 2012;60(22):2263–2270.

132. Naruse Y, Tada H, Satoh M, et al. Concomitant obstructive sleep apnea increases the recurrence of atrial fibrillation following radiofrequency catheter ablation of atrial fibrillation: clinical impact of continuous positive airway pressure therapy. *Heart Rhythm.* 2013;10(3):331–337.

133. Frasure-Smith N, Lespérance F, Talajic M, et al. Anxiety sensitivity moderates prognostic importance of rhythm-control versus rate-control strategies in patients with atrial fibrillation and congestive heart failure: insights from the Atrial Fibrillation and Congestive Heart Failure Trial. *Circ Heart Fail.* 2012;5(3):322–330.

134. Gehi AK, Sears S, Goli N, et al. Psychopathology and symptoms of atrial fibrillation: implications for therapy. *J Cardiovasc Electrophysiol.* 2012;23(5):473–478.

135. Conen D, Tedrow UB, Cook NR, Moorthy MV, Buring JE, Albert CM. Alcohol consumption and risk of incident atrial fibrillation in women. *JAMA.* 2008;300(21):2489–2496.

136. Koskinen P, Kupari M, Leinonen H, Luomanmäki K. Alcohol and new onset atrial fibrillation: a case-control study of a current series. *Br Heart J.* 1987;57(5):468–473.

137. Lange HW, Herrmann-Lingen C. Depressive Symptoms predict recurrence of atrial fibrillation after cardioversion. *J Psychosom Res.* 2007;63(5):509–13.

138. Yu SB, Hu W, Zhao QY, et al. Effect of anxiety and depression on the recurrence of persistent atrial fibrillation after circumferential pulmonary vein ablation. *Chin Med J (Engl).* 2012;125(24):4368–4372.

139. Zheng ZJ, Croft JB, Giles WH, Mensah GA. Sudden cardiac death in the United States, 1989 to 1998. *Circulation.* 2001;104(18):2158–2163.

140. Lown B, DeSilva RA. Roles of psychologic stress and autonomic nervous system changes in provocation of ventricular premature complexes. *Am J Cardiol.* 1978;41(6):979–985.

141. Whang W, Albert CM, Sears SF, et al. Depression as a predictor for appropriate shocks among patients with implantable cardioverter-defibrillators: results from the Triggers of Ventricular Arrhythmias (TOVA) study. *J Am Coll Cardiol.* 2005;45(7):1090–1095.

142. Ray WA, Meredith S, Thapa PB, Hall K, Murray KT. Cyclic antidepressants and the risk of sudden cardiac death. *Clin Pharmacol Ther.* 2004;75(3):234–241.

143. Honkola J, Hookana E, Malinen S, et al. Psychotropic medications and the risk of sudden cardiac death during an acute coronary event. *Eur Heart J.* 2012;33(6):745–751.

144. Empana JP, Jouven X, Lemaitre RN, et al. Clinical depression and risk of out-of-hospital cardiac arrest. *Arch Intern Med.* 2006;166(2):195–200.

145. Luukinen H, Laippala P, Huikuri HV. Depressive symptoms and the risk of sudden cardiac death among the elderly. *Eur Heart J.* 2003;24(22):2021–2026.

146. Watkins LL, Blumenthal JA, Davidson JR, Babyak MA, McCants CB, Sketch MH. Phobic anxiety, depression, and risk of ventricular arrhythmias in patients with coronary heart disease. *Psychosom Med.* 2006;68(5):651–656.

147. Hamang A, Eide GE, Rokne B, Nordin K, Øyen N. General anxiety, depression, and physical health in relation to symptoms of heart-focused anxiety- a cross sectional study among patients living with the risk of serious arrhythmias and sudden cardiac death. *Health Qual Life Outcomes.* 2011;9:100.

148. Magyar-Russell G, Thombs BD, Cai JX, et al. The prevalence of anxiety and depression in adults with implantable cardioverter defibrillators: a systematic review. *J Psychosom Res.* 2011;71(4):223–231.

149. Suzuki T, Shiga T, Kuwahara K, et al. Prevalence and persistence of depression in patients with implantable cardioverter defibrillator: a 2-year longitudinal study. *Pacing Clin Electrophysiol.* 2010;33(12):1455–1461.

150. Bilge AK, Ozben B, Demircan S, Cinar M, Yilmaz E, Adalet K. Depression and anxiety status of patients with implantable cardioverter defibrillator and precipitating factors. *Pacing Clin Electrophysiol.* 2006;29(6):619–626.

151. Tzeis S, Kolb C, Baumert J, et al. Effect of depression on mortality in implantable cardioverter defibrillator recipients–findings from the prospective LICAD study. *Pacing Clin Electrophysiol.* 2011;34(8):991–997.

152. Luyster FS, Hughes JW, Waechter D, Josephson R. Resource loss predicts depression and anxiety among patients treated with an implantable cardioverter defibrillator. *Psychosom Med.* 2006;68(5):794–800.

153. Irvine J, Dorian P, Baker B, et al. Quality of life in the Canadian Implantable Defibrillator Study (CIDS). *Am Heart J.* 2002;144(2):282–289.

154. Glassman AH, O'Connor CM, Califf RM, et al. Sertraline treatment of major depression in patients with acute MI or unstable angina. *JAMA.* 2002;288(6):701–709.

155. O'Connor CM, Jiang W, Kuchibhatla M, et al. Safety and efficacy of sertraline for depression in patients with heart failure: results of the SADHART-CHF (Sertraline Against Depression and Heart Disease in Chronic Heart Failure) trial. *J Am Coll Cardiol.* 2010;56(9):692–699.

156. Hansen BH, Hanash JA, Rasmussen A, et al. Effects of escitalopram in prevention of depression in patients with acute coronary syndrome (DECARD). *J Psychosom Res.* 2012;72(1):11–16.

157. Lespérance F, Frasure-Smith N, Koszycki D, et al. Effects of citalopram and interpersonal psychotherapy on depression in patients with coronary artery disease: the Canadian Cardiac Randomized Evaluation of Antidepressant and Psychotherapy Efficacy (CREATE) trial. *JAMA.* 2007;297(4):367–379.

158. Ferrando SJ, Levenson JL, Owen JA. Clinical Manual of Psychopharmacology in the Medically Ill. *American Psychiatric Publishing, Incorporated;* 2010.

159. Beach SR, Celano CM, Noseworthy PA, Januzzi JL, Huffman JC. QTc prolongation, torsades de pointes, and psychotropic medications. *Psychosomatics.* 2013;54(1):1–13.

160. Sheline YI, Freedland KE, Carney RM. How safe are serotonin reuptake inhibitors for depression in patients with coronary heart disease? *Am J Med.* 1997;102(1):54–59.

161. Honig A, Kuyper AM, Schene AH, et al. Treatment of post-myocardial infarction depressive disorder: a randomized, placebo controlled trial with mirtazapine. *Psychosom Med.* 2007;69(7):606–613.

162. Rigotti NA, Thorndike AN, Regan S, et al. Bupropion for smokers hospitalized with acute coronary disease. *Am J Med.* 2006;119(12):1080–1087.

163. Habel LA, Cooper WO, Sox CM, et al. ADHD medications and risk of serious cardiovascular events in young and middle-aged adults. *JAMA.* 2011;306(24):2673–2683.

164. Berkman LF, Blumenthal J, Burg M, et al. Effects of treating depression and low perceived social support on clinical events after myocardial infarction: the Enhancing Recovery in Coronary Heart Disease Patients (ENRICHD) Randomized Trial. *JAMA.* 2003;289(23):3106–3116.

165. Freedland KE, Skala JA, Carney RM, et al. Treatment of depression after coronary artery bypass surgery: a randomized controlled trial. *Arch Gen Psychiatry.* 2009:66(4):387–396.

166. Blumenthal JA, Babyak MA, O'Connor C, et al. Effects of exercise training on depressive symptoms in patients with chronic heart failure: the HF-ACTION randomized trial. *JAMA.* 2012;308(5):465–474.

167. Milani RV, Lavie CJ, Mehra MR, Ventura HO. Impact of exercise training and depression on survival in heart failure due to coronary heart disease. *Am J Cardiol.* 2011;107(1):64–68.

168. Task Force on Electroconvulsive Therapy. *The Practice of Electroconvulsive Therapy: Recommendations for Treatment, Training, and Privileging.* 2nd ed. Washington, DC: American Psychiatric Publishing; 2001.

169. Rasmussen KG, Rummans TA, Tsang TS, Barnes RD. Electroconvulsive therapy. *American Psychiatric Publishing Textbook of Psychosomatic Medicine. Washington, DC: American Psychiatric Publishing.* 957–978.

170. Dolenc TJ, Barnes RD, Hayes DL, Rasmussen KG. Electroconvulsive therapy in patients with cardiac pacemakers and implantable cardioverter defibrillators. *Pacing Clin Electrophysiol.* 2004;27(9):1257–1263.

171. Applegate RJ. Diagnosis and management of ischemic heart disease in the patient scheduled to undergo electroconvulsive therapy. *Convuls Ther.* 1997;13(3):128–144.

172. Levenson JL. Psychiatric issues in heart disease. *Primary psychiatry.* 2006;13(7):29–32.

173. Mechlis S, Lubin E, Laor J, Margaliot M. Amiodarone-induced thyroid gland dysfunction. *Am J Cardiol.* 1987;59(8):833–835.

174. Wamboldt FS, Jefferson JW, Wamboldt MZ. Digitalis intoxication misdiagnosed as depression by primary care physicians. *Am J Psychiatry.* 1986;143(2):219–221.

175. Neaton JD, Blackburn H, Jacobs D, et al. Serum cholesterol level and mortality findings for men screened in the Multiple Risk Factor Intervention Trial. Multiple Risk Factor Intervention Trial Research Group. *Arch Intern Med.* 1992;152(7):1490–1500.

176. Muldoon MF, Manuck SB, Mendelsohn AB, et al. Cholesterol reduction and non-illness mortality: meta-analysis of randomized clinical trials. *BMJ.* 2001;322(7277):11–15.

177. Strain JJ, Karim A, Caliendo G, Alexis JD, Lowe RS, Fuster V. Cardiac drug-psychotropic drug update. *Gen Hosp Psychiatry.* 2002;24(5):283–289.

178. *DRUG-REAX®* *System [Internet Database].* Greenwood Village, Colorado: Thomson Healthcare. Updated Periodically.

179. Kusumoto MM, Ueno KK, Oda AA, et al. Effect of fluvoxamine on the pharmacokinetics of mexiletine in healthy Japanese men. *Clin Pharmacol Ther.* 2001;69(3):104–107.

180. Wallerstedt SM, Gleerup H, Sundström A, Stigendal L, Ny L. Risk of clinically relevant bleeding in warfarin-treated patients–influence of SSRI treatment. *Pharmacoepidemiol Drug Saf.* 2009;18(5):412–416.

181. Leibovitz A, Bilchinsky T, Gil I. Elevated serum digoxin level associated with coadministered fluoxetine. *Arch Intern Med.* 1998;158(10):1152–1153.

CHAPTER 8

Depression and Gynecologic Conditions

Laura Miller, MD

Geena Athappilly, MD

Orit Avni-Barron, MD

Daniela Carusi, MD

Hadine Joffe, MD, MSc

INTRODUCTION

Depression is more common in women than in men during the reproductive years, particularly in association with reproductive transitions and several common gynecological conditions. In the first part of this chapter, we review specific evidence supporting an association of mood disturbance with puberty in girls, across the menstrual cycle, with polycystic ovary syndrome, with infertility, and during the transition to menopause. Because of the prevalence of depression in women during the reproductive years, there are some important implications for pharmacologic treatment. Some psychotropic medications can have adverse effects on the hypothalamic–pituitary–gonadal (HPG) axis, which manifest in menstrual dysfunction, as well as potentially disruptive interactions with both endogenous and exogenous reproductive hormones. In the second part of this chapter, we review what is known about the effect of psychotropic medications on the HPG axis, and discuss important interactions with reproductive hormones. Given that women of reproductive age comprise a large proportion of psychiatric patients, knowledge about these special considerations will improve treatment outcomes for a large number of women.

■ DEPRESSION AND PUBERTY IN GIRLS

Case illustration: Marta is a 13-year-old girl brought to see you by her mother, who is concerned because Marta has appeared listless, sad, and withdrawn. Marta had been a straight. A student until a couple of months ago, when she lost interest in school and had difficulty focusing on homework. Developmental history reveals that Marta's mother has had recurrent episodes of major depression, with a particularly severe, prolonged episode while pregnant with Marta. Marta was born with low birth weight. Within her first 2 years of life, she caught up and exceeded normal weight for height. Early developmental milestones were normal. Family life is characterized by frequent verbal altercations between Marta's parents. Marta tends to brood a lot after hearing these; by contrast, her older brother tends to distract himself. Marta began showing breast development by age 9, with menarche at age 11. Two months ago, Marta's best friend rejected her in favor of a more socially popular set of friends. Marta confides in you that she feels "fat and ugly," which makes her feel hopeless about ever being socially desirable. She eats for comfort even when not hungry, and then feels guilty. She has had thoughts about killing herself by overdosing on pills from the medicine cabinet, but says she would never actually do that because it would be a sin.

Epidemiology

One of the most striking aspects of the epidemiology of depression is the marked increase in prevalence in girls, but not boys, which arises in mid-puberty. In prepubertal children, studies consistently show that rates of depressive disorder are either similar in boys and girls, or slightly higher in boys.[1] Beginning at about age 13, the prevalence of depressive disorders in girls rises to about twice that in boys. In the National Comorbidity Survey – Adolescent Supplement, a nationally representative face-to-face survey of over 10,000 adolescents aged 13 to 18 years in the United States, the lifetime prevalence of major depressive disorder or dysthymia was 15.9% in girls and 7.7% in boys.[2]

Pathophysiology (Box 8-1)

The marked gender difference in vulnerability to depression that arises during puberty may be best understood from a bio-cultural framework, with gender-linked biological factors interacting with cognitive, environmental, and sociocultural contexts. Research to date has identified the following factors as especially influential:

- Low birth weight. Low birth weight is a biomarker for *in utero* stress, which may confer health risks later in life. In the prospective, longitudinal Great Smoky Mountains Study, the cumulative prevalence of depression over the 3-year period from 13 to 16 years old was 8.4% among girls with normal birth weight, but 38.1% among girls with low birth weight.[3] Low birth weight appeared to potentiate other pregnancy-linked risk factors, such as premature birth and labor complications. The effect of low birth weight on adolescent depression was considerably less marked for boys than for girls.

- Changes in gonadal hormones. A study comparing the influence of age, pubertal stage, and circulating hormone levels found that the gender difference in depression prevalence arose at a specific stage of puberty—Tanner Stage III, when breast tissue grows beyond areola and pubic hair coarsens—regardless of age. Statistical modeling showed that the link between pubertal stage and depression was largely due to estradiol and testosterone levels.[4]

- Pubertal timing. Most, but not all, studies have found that the earlier girls begin puberty, the more likely they are to develop depressive symptoms in adolescence.[5,6] The reasons for this have not yet been empirically established. One posited explanation is that girls who appear physically more developed may be treated by others as more mature than they are and they may not be developmentally ready for this. Another is that early puberty is a biomarker for early life stressors, such as family discord and/or absent father, that might confer increased risk for subsequent depression. A retrospective study suggests that only girls with certain estrogen receptor gene polymorphisms are vulnerable to experiencing early menarche in the context of family discord,[7] supporting a posited link between genetic vulnerability, early life stress, and hormonal activation of depression in adolescent girls. Other studies are exploring the role of weight in mediating links between early puberty and depression. Low-birth-weight babies who have substantial "catch up" growth early in life are vulnerable to childhood obesity. This leads to increases in leptin, a hormone manufactured in adipose tissue that plays a role in initiating the cascade of physiologic changes leading to menarche.[8] Such effects can be transgenerational; maternal antenatal depression can increase the risk of low birth weight in infants,[9] contributing to a sequence of biopsychosocial events, including childhood excessive weight gain, early puberty, and adolescent onset depression.

BOX 8-1
IMPORTANT RISK FACTORS FOR DEPRESSION IN WOMEN DURING PUBERTY

Low birth weight
Changes in gonadal hormones
Earlier puberty
Environmental stress
Cognitive styles (e.g., poor self-worth)
Gender role expectations (*e.g.*, slenderness)

- Environmental stress. Girls are substantially more likely than boys to experience sexual abuse and/or rape. Girls' exposure to these risks increases substantially at adolescence, explaining a portion of the gender difference in vulnerability to depression.[10] In addition to differential exposure, research suggests the possibility of gender differences in types of reactivity to stress. Ebstein Barr virus (EBV) titers are a biomarker for stress-linked immunocompromise. Traumatic life events have been shown to increase EBV titers in girls, but not boys, in early adolescence.[11]

- Cognitive style. Certain characteristic ways of perceiving the world and reacting to stress are correlated with increased likelihood of becoming depressed. These include rumination, expectations of abandonment, and beliefs that one is defective or unworthy. By contrast, a problem-solving approach to stressors can be protective against depression. As compared with adolescent boys, adolescent girls are more likely to endorse cognitive styles conducive to depression. There is a reciprocal relationship among cognitive styles, stress, and depressive symptoms; cognitive vulnerabilities contribute to experiencing more stress, and depressive symptoms and stress intensify cognitive vulnerabilities.[12]

- Sociocultural gender role expectations. Perceived failure to live up to gender role expectations can influence the development of depression. In social environments that value slenderness in girls, body image at puberty is a particularly salient influence on depression. At puberty, self-perception of being overweight and efforts to lose weight, regardless of actual body mass index, correlate significantly with depressive symptoms in girls but not in boys.[13]

Clinical Presentation

As compared to adolescent boys, adolescent girls with depressive disorders endorse more symptoms of guilt, body image dissatisfaction, self-blame, disappointment in themselves, fatigue, hypersomnia, and impairment in concentration. As anxiety disorders are more prevalent in adolescent girls as compared to boys, depression may present with anxiety disorder spectrum comorbidity. Girls are also substantially more likely than boys to attempt suicide; this gender difference declines in young adulthood.[14] Girls are less likely than boys to experience anhedonia and morning symptom intensification.[15]

Course and Natural History

Among adolescents who develop major depressive episodes, female sex is associated with longer episode duration and a greater likelihood of recurrent episodes in young adulthood. Among adolescent girls, but not boys, conflict with parents predicts young adult recurrence of depressive episodes.[16,17]

Assessment and Differential Diagnosis

Recognition that girls enter a high-risk time for developing depression at mid-puberty can alert clinicians to assess for depression at that time. Detection of major depression can be improved by routine screening with a validated tool. The 9-item Patient Health Questionnaire is a public domain self-report depression screening tool that is linked with Diagnostic and Statistical Manual criteria for major depression. It has been validated for use in adolescents,[18] and can be used to measure symptom severity and track outcome after treatment. In addition to evaluating pubertal girls for the presence and severity of depressive symptoms, assessing the contextual variables in **Table 8-1** can help guide treatment.

Directly asking about thoughts of suicide is important, given the especially high risk of suicide attempts in adolescent girls. If suicidal

TABLE 8-1 Assessment of Adolescent Girls with Depressive Symptoms

- Family history of depression, including perinatal depression in the patient's mother
- Pregnancy and birth complications, including low birth weight
- Pubertal stage relative to patient's emotional and cognitive maturation
- Weight, body image, and physical activity
- History of substantial early life stress, including sexual trauma, physical violence, witnessing violence, and/or other major family discord
- Recent stressors, including interpersonal rejections
- Cognitive style and coping style, including fears of abandonment, self-deprecatory beliefs, and tendencies to ruminate instead of problem-solve
- Academic and social functioning
- Sexual activity and contraception
- Common comorbidities, including eating disorders, anxiety disorders, and substance use disorders

thoughts are present, ascertain whether the patient has a specific plan, the level of her intent to act on the plan, and her access to means (e.g., firearms or medications in the home). Also assess for protective factors, such as willingness to share her thoughts with supportive others, hopefulness about the future, impulse control, and religious beliefs.

The differential diagnosis of pubertal depression (**Box 8-2**) in girls is similar to that of depression in general. However, certain conditions deserve special emphasis in this population:

- Bipolar disorder. The first episode of bipolar disorder in females is more often depressive, while the first episode in males is more often manic.[19]
- Use of addictive substances causing or contributing to depressive symptoms.
- Iron deficiency anemia. Menstruation increases a girl's risk of developing iron deficiency. Low ferritin levels are associated with increased depressive symptoms.[20]

Treatment (Box 8-3)

The treatments with the most robust evidence for efficacy in adolescents with major depression are fluoxetine and cognitive-behavioral therapy (CBT), particularly in combination.[21] Other antidepressants that can be useful for adolescent depression are sertraline, citalopram, or escitalopram. When prescribing (explaining why just these specific agents are noted) antidepressants to adolescent girls, it is helpful to discuss contraception for those who are sexually active and at risk for unintended pregnancy. It is important to monitor closely for emerging suicidal thoughts or impulses during the course of treatment of adolescents with depression.

CBT can be especially helpful for girls with trauma histories, ruminative coping styles, and self-deprecatory or perfectionist beliefs. Other types of psychotherapy can be considered as well.

BOX 8-2
KEY CONSIDERATIONS IN DIFFERENTIAL DIAGNOSIS FOR PUBERTAL DEPRESSION IN WOMEN

Bipolar disorder
Alcohol and substance use
Iron deficiency anemia

BOX 8-3
TREATMENTS FOR PUBERTAL DEPRESSION IN WOMEN

Fluoxetine
Other SSRIs (sertraline, citalopram, escitalopram)
Cognitive behavioral therapy

Interpersonal therapy (IPT) may be especially helpful for girls whose depressive symptoms seem linked to interpersonal stressors or difficulties with navigating social roles. Family-focused therapy can be effective for girls whose depressive episodes are linked with family discord and communication difficulties.

Relatively few systematic studies have been completed about the efficacy of lifestyle changes and self-management for girls with pubertal-onset depression. Preliminary data are promising for positive effects of aerobic exercise[22] and technology-enabled biofeedback.[23]

Summary

The risk of developing depressive disorders increases substantially at mid-puberty for girls. This heightened risk may be influenced by genetic vulnerability, epigenetic influences *in utero*, gonadal hormones, environmental stressors, cognitive and coping styles, and pubertal timing. As compared to adolescent boys, adolescent girls with depressive episodes may be at greater risk of suicide attempts, longer episode duration, and subsequent recurrence. There is robust evidence for the efficacy of fluoxetine and CBT for treating major depression in adolescents.

Case outcome. Marta was diagnosed with a major depressive episode. Factors contributing to her vulnerability to depression may have included genetic predisposition, epigenetic effects of her in utero environment, early puberty, family discord, cognitive style, coping style, and current social stressors. She began fluoxetine 20 mg daily and CBT. The latter began with behavioral activation, aided by a mobile phone app, which helped Marta keep track of the activity schedule she'd set up for herself. Marta then learned problem-solving and assertiveness skills, which she used to explain to her parents how their arguing affected her and to work with them on changing family communication patterns. She also worked on identifying and reframing self-deprecatory core beliefs, by logging them on her mobile phone when they occurred and testing them against evidence. She achieved full remission, but remained on fluoxetine for 6 months to prevent recurrence.

■ DEPRESSION AND THE MENSTRUAL CYCLE

Case illustration: Denise is a 23-year-old woman whose boyfriend has asked her to seek help. He has noticed that she seems unusually grouchy at times, sometimes even throwing things toward him or storming out of the room. He has also noticed that she tends to call in sick at work on those days. He thinks there might be a premenstrual pattern to these mood and behavior changes. Denise agrees, and has noticed that a few days before each menstrual period, she becomes more irritable, anxious, and overwhelmed. She eats more, especially fatty foods, feels tired and bloated, has headaches, and sleeps more. The oral contraceptive pills she takes have not had any effect on these symptoms. When her boyfriend mentioned his concerns, Denise found an online daily symptom log and charted her symptoms across two menstrual cycles. This showed that her symptoms began 5 to 6 days before menses, peaked in severity 2 days before menses, and resolved the day after menstrual bleeding began. She is worried about getting a suboptimal performance review at work, and about ruining her relationship with her boyfriend.

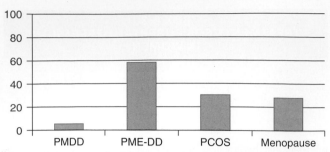

Figure 8-1 *Mean risk of depression for selected illnesses (percentage prevalence for particular disease).*

Epidemiology

There are three types of depression-related disorders linked with the menstrual cycle: premenstrual dysphoric disorder (PMDD), psychological symptoms manifesting as part of a premenstrual syndrome (PMS), and premenstrual exacerbation of depressive disorders (PME-DD) (**Fig. 8-1**). PMDD is defined as having five or more characteristic symptoms during the last week of the luteal (postovulatory) phase of all or most menstrual cycles. By definition, symptoms begin to remit within a few days after the onset of menstrual bleeding and are gone by a week after the onset of menstrual bleeding. Symptoms must be severe enough to interfere with functioning. The symptoms may include irritability, depressed mood, hopelessness, anxiety, tension, mood lability, anhedonia, change in appetite, poor concentration, fatigue, lack of energy, sleep disturbance, feeling overwhelmed, and/or physical symptoms, such as bloating or breast tenderness.[24] Using this definition, 1% to 8% of menstruating women meet criteria for PMDD in studies using prospective daily charting to confirm a premenstrual pattern.[25] PMS has no fully consensual definition; the term is often used broadly to refer to premenstrual mood and/or physical changes, regardless of distress or functional impairment. When defined as subsyndromal PMDD, for example, fewer than five symptoms, but causing distress and/or impairment, PMS has been found to affect 12% to 18% of menstruating women.[26] It is important to note that while psychological symptoms are common in PMS, diagnostic criteria for this condition can be met in the absence of any mood disturbance when physical symptoms are prominent (e.g., cramping and abdominal pain) and interfere with daily activities and/or are distressing.

The prevalence of PME-DD has not yet been rigorously studied. In a sample of 433 premenopausal depressed women from the Sequenced Treatment Alternatives to Relieve Depression (STAR*D) study, none of whom were using oral contraceptives, 64% reported that they perceived premenstrual worsening of their depressive symptoms.[27] Among 58 menstruating 13- to 53-year-old females with depressive disorders in a community sample, 58% had one or more depressive symptoms worsen before menses, based on prospective daily charting.[28] Similarly, in a cohort of 293 premenopausal women with bipolar disorder enrolled in the Systematic Treatment Enhancement Program for Bipolar Disorder (STEP-BD) study,[29] 65% reported premenstrual worsening of their underlying bipolar disorder.

Pathophysiology

Numerous studies have found alterations of neurotransmission of serotonin and gamma amino butyric acid (GABA) in women with PMDD, often specific to the luteal phase.[30,31] By contrast, most studies have found no difference in HPG axis functioning between women with and without PMDD. However, eliminating ovulation with gonadotropin releasing hormone (GnRH) analogs usually alleviates PMDD symptoms, while adding back estrogen, progesterone, or both causes symptom recurrence.[32] To explain these findings, it

is posited that women with PMDD have abnormal neurotransmitter responses to normal gonadal hormonal flux. A specific hypothesis being investigated is that women with PMDD have reduced central nervous system sensitivity to, and/or altered levels of, the progesterone metabolite allopregnanolone, which functions as a neuroactive GABA receptor modulator.[33]

Functional neuroimaging studies are being conducted to elucidate the functional neuroanatomy of PMDD. The most consistent findings to date involve increased amygdala reactivity to negative stimuli in the luteal phase, suggestive of enhanced negative emotional processing.[34,35] This is consistent with findings from studies using functional tasks, such as facial discrimination, demonstrating that in the luteal phase women with PMDD display a negative bias in the processing of nonverbal emotional stimuli.[36]

Clinical Presentation (Box 8-4)

PMDD appears to be qualitatively distinct from major depressive disorder, apart from its premenstrual temporal pattern. The most commonly endorsed mood symptoms are not depressed mood or anhedonia, but rather irritability and anger, followed by anxiety, lethargy, and mood lability.[37] Another contrast is that, although changes in appetite can be a symptom of either major depressive disorder or PMDD, the appetite change in PMDD is distinct. It is nearly always increased rather than decreased appetite, often with desires or cravings for food items that are sweet and high in fat content, happening specifically in the luteal phase.[38,39]

Although thoughts of death or suicide are not listed as a definitional symptom in PMDD, they are relatively common during symptomatic phases. In a large epidemiologic survey in the United States, women with PMDD were significantly more likely to report suicidal ideation, plans, and attempts than were women with no premenstrual symptoms.[40]

There is wide variability from woman to woman in the duration of symptoms across the menstrual cycle. Most often the most severe symptoms are reported to occur during the two days prior to menses, with milder symptoms preceding. Within individual women, symptoms tend to remain qualitatively similar from cycle to cycle, although severity may vary.[37]

In keeping with some women's experiences that they "become a different person" while premenstrual, personality scales change significantly from the follicular to the luteal phase in women with PMDD.[41] Locus of control, generally a relatively fixed characteristic, is more external in the luteal phase than in the follicular phase in women with PMDD.[42] In addition, subjective, behavioral, and neurophysiologic measures of stress reactivity are increased in the luteal phase in women with PMDD.[43] Small but significant changes in performance on attention and memory tasks are also seen in the luteal phase of women with PMDD, confirming subjective reports of reduced ability to concentrate and remember things during the symptomatic phase.[39]

Course and Natural History

Although premenstrual dysphoria is relatively common in adolescent girls,[44] PMDD does not typically begin at menarche. Once

---

BOX 8-4
IMPORTANT SYMPTOMS IN PMDD

More Common in PMDD than Depression

Irritability
Anxiety
Mood lability
Increased appetite
Cravings for sweet/fatty foods

BOX 8-5
DIAGNOSING PMS, PMDD, AND PME

Most Important Factor Is Course of Symptoms

Symptoms associated with luteal phase

Most severe symptoms begin about 2 days before menses

Symptoms remit within few days after menstrual bleeding

BOX 8-6
TREATMENTS FOR DEPRESSION IN WOMEN WITH PMDD

Serotonergic antidepressants

SSRIs (fluoxetine, sertraline, paroxetine, escitalopram using either continuous, luteal phase or symptom-onset dosing; luteal phase dosing)

Ethanyl estradiol 24/4 (drospirenone in other formulations is ineffective)

GnRH analogs

Calcium supplementation

Vitex agnus castus extract (chaste tree berry)

Cognitive behavioral therapy (mixed results)

Aerobic exercise (preliminary results)

established, the symptom pattern tends to remain stable over time but can worsen with age and childbearing.[45] To date, there are no rigorous longitudinal studies of the course of PMDD as women enter perimenopause. Case reports suggest that some women may experience symptom worsening during perimenopause, with PMDD symptoms not necessarily limited to the premenstrual phase given that cycles are irregular and ovarian steroid fluctuations are unpredictable. PMDD remits after menopause.

Assessment and Differential Diagnosis (Box 8-5)

The key to accurate diagnosis of PMS, PMDD, and PME is prospective daily symptom charting across at least two menstrual cycles. This distinguishes premenstrual mood disorders from other conditions that can present with mood shifts, such as rapid-cycling bipolar disorder and personality disorders. There are several types of daily symptom charts available in the public domain, often online and as applications for mobile devices. An instrument that is especially helpful for clinical diagnosis is the Premenstrual Tension Syndrome (PMTS) scale.[46] This has a self-rated version in the form of a visual analog scale (PMTS-VAS), which averages 68 seconds to complete, and an observer version in the form of a Likert scale (PMTS-OR). Each of these has 11 items, which correspond to the Diagnostic and Statistical Manual definitional symptoms of PMDD.

To guide interview-based diagnosis of PMDD, the Structured Clinical Interview for DSM-IV-TR-defined PMDD (SCID-PMDD) is an instrument with high sensitivity and reliability.[47] It is helpful to schedule two evaluation appointments, one in the follicular phase of the cycle and one in the late luteal phase, to observe mental status changes directly.

Treatment (Box 8-6)

In keeping with the posited role of serotonergic dysfunction in the etiology of PMDD, serotonergic antidepressants are effective in its treatment. The serotonin-selective reuptake inhibitors (SSRIs) fluoxetine, sertraline, paroxetine, and escitalopram are approved by the Food and Drug Administration (FDA) for this indication. By contrast, antidepressants that have limited to no effect on serotonergic function, such as bupropion, desipramine, and maprotiline, have not performed significantly better than placebo for PMDD.[48–50]

In addition to continuous dosing (taking the same antidepressant dose every day), numerous studies and a meta-analysis have shown that luteal phase dosing (taking antidepressants only during the 14 days prior to menses) is effective for PMDD.[51] Some studies have also found that symptom-onset dosing is effective, with a mean duration of use of 6 to 9 days during the late luteal phase of the menstrual cycle.[52,53] For PME-DD, preliminary data suggest that boosting the dose in the luteal phase is effective.[54] The rapid response and effectiveness of these dosing patterns imply that the mechanism of antidepressant action for premenstrual mood syndromes differs from that in major depressive disorder. There is some evidence to support the hypothesis that serotonergic medications alleviate premenstrual dysphoria via a rapid effect on central nervous system sensitivity to neuroactive hormonal GABA agonists.[55]

Patients who are candidates for luteal phase dosing regimens are:

- Those who prefer to minimize medication use, due to side effects and/or values.
- Those who have regular, predictable menstrual cycles that can be tracked (for luteal phase dosing and dose escalation) or who can recognize early symptoms (for symptom-onset dosing).
- Those who do not experience problematic transient side effects upon starting or discontinuing antidepressants.

Given the link between hormonal cyclicity and symptoms in PMDD, many have wondered whether hormonal interventions would be effective. Progesterone-only and combined oral contraceptive (COC) pills, at one time used relatively widely for treating PMS, have been found to be no more effective than placebo. The one exception is the COC drospirenone/ethinyl estradiol when used in a formulation that has 24 days of active agent and 4 days of placebo. Drospirenone, the progestin, is an antiandrogenic analog of spironolactone, a diuretic shown to alleviate PMS. It is not known why this particular COC is effective for treating PMDD, while others have not been shown to be effective. Factors contributing to its efficacy may include properties of its unique progestin and the shorter hormone-free interval, which maintains better suppression of the endogenous hypothalamic-pituitary-ovarian axis. This agent is FDA approved for treatment of PMDD, although the potential benefits must be weighed against a heightened risk of blood clots and other adverse effects of COCs.

Studies have begun to evaluate the efficacy of using COCs continuously, with active hormones daily and no placebo pills, therefore, no menstrual bleeding. The results of three randomized, double-blind, placebo-controlled trials of the efficacy of continuous COCs for PMDD are inconsistent. All showed a high placebo response rate; only 1 of the 3 found significantly better response to active treatment than to placebo.[56]

While COCs have not been shown to worsen PMS/PMDD, dysphoria and adverse mood symptoms have been reported as side effects. It has been difficult to definitely establish whether or not there is a relationship between COCs and depressive symptoms, in part because of the numerous varieties of COCs, but if depression is a side effect it appears to be an uncommon one.[57] One large epidemiologic study found that in 71% of women taking a COC, mood remained stable or improved, even among those with a history of depression.[58]

Other hormonal therapies are effective for PMDD, but are rarely used due to side effects. GnRH analogs, which create a temporary "chemical menopause" by suppressing estradiol and progesterone, are effective because they eliminate the hormone fluctuations, but long-term use is limited by risks associated with a hypoestrogenic menopausal state.[59] This option may be best reserved for women who are expected to reach menopause within one year, though it's use may be limited by expense and limited insurance coverage for off-label medication use. Danazol, an androgenic and anti-gonadotrophic agent, is also effective with either continuous or luteal phase dosing,[60] but is rarely used due to androgenic side effects.

Elimination of fluctuating estradiol and progesterone through bilateral oophorectomy is expected to eliminate premenstrual dysphoric symptoms, although few empiric data exist.[61] This surgical menopause should be considered as a tertiary intervention because of adverse health sequelae (hypoestrogenism, osteoporosis, sexual dysfunction, possible negative long-term health effects). Postoperative hormone replacement can cause symptom recurrence. If hysterectomy is performed with preservation of at least one ovary, symptoms are expected to persist because the hormones will continue to fluctuate despite the absence of a menstrual marker.

Among the many herbal products used in an attempt to alleviate premenstrual dysphoric symptoms, only one, vitex agnus castus extract (VACE), has demonstrated efficacy in several prospective, randomized, double-blind, placebo-controlled trials. VACE, a plant with weak estrogenic effects, is popularly known as chaste tree berry. VACE has efficacy superior to placebo and equal to fluoxetine overall, although fluoxetine is somewhat more effective for mood symptoms.[62] Optimal dosing for PMDD is 20 mg daily.[63] Side effects are similar to those of the placebo arm in controlled trials.[64]

The efficacy of psychotherapy for premenstrual mood disorders is unclear. There have been several studies of CBT with inconsistent results. This is in part due to methodologic limitations, but also due to a lack of clarity or consensus about optimal conceptual approaches to psychotherapeutic interventions for premenstrual dysphoria. For example, some therapies focus on helping women to reduce premenstrual stress by scheduling fewer activities or deadlines at that time, while other focus on maintaining normal functioning throughout the cycle. Mindfulness and acceptance-based therapies are being explored as promising interventions for premenstrual dysphoric mood states.[65]

Lifestyle interventions for PMS and PMDD are also being explored. In several studies, most relatively small and nonrandomized, aerobic exercise has led to symptom improvement.[66] The most promising nutritional intervention is calcium supplementation (1200 mg daily), which has been found to be superior to placebo in alleviating premenstrual dysphoric symptoms.[67]

Treatment studies for PME-DD are limited, with an open-label trial showing that augmentation of an antidepressant with the COC drospirenone/ethinyl estradiol alleviated premenstrual mood symptoms[68] and case reports suggesting that premenstrual dose escalation of antidepressants may be helpful.[69]

Summary

PMDD, PMS, and PME-DD are prevalent disorders that can cause substantial distress and impairment. It is posited that they arise in women who have abnormal central nervous system responses to gonadal hormonal flux, particularly in neurotransmission involving serotonin and GABA. Diagnosis is aided by prospective daily symptom charting across 2 menstrual cycles. PMDD can be treated with serotonergic antidepressants, using continuous dosing, luteal phase dosing, or symptom-onset dosing. The hormonal contraceptive drospirenone/ethinyl estradiol 24/4 is also effective for PMDD. Other promising interventions are VACE, CBT, aerobic exercise, and calcium supplementation. PME-DD may response to luteal phase escalation of antidepressant dose or augmentation with drospirenone/ethinyl estradiol 24/4, but further studies are needed.

Case outcome. Denise was diagnosed with PMDD. She was reluctant to take medication, but felt comfortable trying low-dose sertraline (50 mg daily) during the luteal phase only. This substantially reduced her irritable and anxious mood, but only somewhat alleviated her fatigue, *headaches, and bloating sensation. She began taking VACE 20 mg daily, and started using an exercise digital video disc DVD three to four times per week. Her symptoms improved. She now has only occasional mild fatigue, headaches, and irritability for 1 or 2 days before some of her menstrual cycles. She charts her cycles to predict vulnerable days, and maintains heightened awareness of her feelings and her reactions to her boyfriend and coworkers on those days.*

■ POLYCYSTIC OVARY SYNDROME (PCOS) AND DEPRESSION

Case illustration: Anne is a 32-year-old graphic designer who requests evaluation for depression. Her supervisor had become concerned after noticing that Anne, whose work had been consistently exemplary in the past, had procrastinated on several projects and had missed a couple of important deadlines over the past 3 months. Anne acknowledges that she has felt down and sluggish over that period of time, with reduced energy and difficulty getting out of bed. She has lost interest in her work, which she used to love, and has struggled to focus on it. When asked if she feels down about anything in particular, she begins to sob. She explains that she has been trying unsuccessfully to become pregnant for the past year. She is considering infertility treatment, but fears learning that something is wrong with her reproductive system, because her menses have always been irregular. She feels shaky in her marriage. She has gained weight over the past few years, especially lately, and thinks her husband finds her unattractive. He has always wanted to be a father. She fears he will leave her if evaluation reveals she is infertile. Examination is notable for hirsutism, mild acne, and central obesity.

Epidemiology

PCOS is an endocrine disorder with mutually interacting reproductive and metabolic abnormalities. Based on international consensus criteria, women are diagnosed with PCOS when at least two of three cardinal signs—hyperandrogenism (biochemical or symptomatic hirsutism, acne, male-pattern balding), anovulation or oligo-ovulation, and polycystic ovarian morphology on ultrasound—are present. These are often accompanied by insulin resistance and features of metabolic syndrome. Obesity is present in about half of women with PCOS.

Depending on diagnostic criteria used, the general population prevalence for PCOS ranges between 6% and 18% of women.[70] Women with PCOS are especially vulnerable to depressive symptoms. A meta-analysis of 26 studies found a significant increase in depressive as well as anxiety symptom scores in women with PCOS as compared to women without PCOS, with a moderate effect size.[71] Studies using Diagnostic and Statistical Manual diagnoses have found that the current prevalence of major depressive disorder is 26% to 35% of study participants with PCOS as compared to about 10% of control women.[72,73]

Pathophysiology

The relationship between PCOS and depression is likely bidirectional and multidetermined, as shown in **Figure 8-2**. Stigma and distress from some of the symptoms of PCOS, such as hirsutism, acne, male-pattern balding, and obesity, may contribute to the risk of depression. However, studies show that these factors do not fully account for the increase in depressive symptoms in women with PCOS as compared to controls.[71] Similarly, consequences of PCOS, such as subfertility, do not fully explain vulnerability to depression. When compared with women with non-PCOS infertility, women with PCOS were found to have more depressive symptoms,[74] and among women with PCOS, unfulfilled wishes to have a child have not been found to increase depressive symptoms.[75]

Studies investigating a posited link between gonadal hormone levels and depressive symptoms in women with PCOS have been

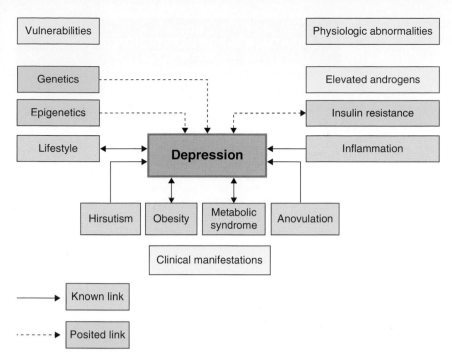

Figure 8-2 *Pathophysiology of depression in the context of PCOS.*

inconclusive. Lower circulating androgen levels have been found in some studies to correlate with more depressive symptoms in women with PCOS, but other studies have found no such link.[76,77] A more consistent finding is that women with PCOS have heightened physiologic and emotional responses to stress as compared to control women. Abnormalities include elevations in hypothalamic-pituitary-adrenal (HPA) axis response, elevated cardiovascular response, and increased psychological distress.[78] These abnormalities could contribute to depressive symptoms, although a direct link has not yet been demonstrated. Sleep apnea is more common among women with PCOS than among BMI-matched controls. Levels of pro-inflammatory cytokines have been found to be elevated in women with PCOS,[79] suggesting that PCOS includes a chronic, low-grade inflammatory state. These are other possible links with increased risk of depressive symptoms.

Clinical Presentation

PCOS comprises a cluster of reproductive and metabolic abnormalities. **Table 8-2** shows typical clinical features. The most frequent initial presenting symptoms are hirsutism and irregular menstrual cycles. Some cases are discovered due to infertility or unexplained weight gain. Although depression and anxiety are not core clinical features of PCOS,[80] some women seeking treatment for depression and anxiety may have undiagnosed comorbid PCOS.

Course and Natural History

Symptoms and signs of PCOS usually begin to be manifest in late puberty, after menarche. Since irregular menstrual cycles are relatively common in normal adolescence, often the diagnosis is not made until later. As women with PCOS become older, androgen levels and associated symptoms (e.g., hirsutism and acne) tend to decline. However, metabolic risk factors tend to worsen, with increases in blood pressure, total cholesterol, low density lipoprotein (LDL)-cholesterol, triglycerides, fasting blood sugar, insulin, and (BMI) over time.[81,82] There is no clear age link with comorbid depressive symptoms; the risk of depression appears to be elevated at all stages of the illness.

Assessment and Differential Diagnosis

For women who initially present with depression, it is important to consider a diagnosis of PCOS if they also have hirsutism, irregular menses, infertility, or other common PCOS symptoms. The key steps in assessing women for PCOS include the following:

- Assessing for the cardinal symptoms of hyperandrogenism, polycystic ovaries, and anovulation/oligo-ovulation.
- Ruling out disorders with overlapping clinical features, many of which also confer a higher risk of depressive symptoms (**Box 8-7**).
- Assessing for specific cardiovascular and other risk factors once a diagnosis of PCOS is confirmed. Consensus guidelines[83] recommend that all women with PCOS be assessed regularly for BMI, waist circumference, blood pressure, and lipid profile. Oral glucose challenge tests are recommended for those with BMI >30 kg/m², age >40 years, history of gestational diabetes mellitus, or family history of Type 2 diabetes mellitus.

TABLE 8-2 Clinical Presentation of PCOS

Reproductive-Related Abnormalities	Metabolic and Cardiovascular Abnormalities/Risks
• Elevated androgens • Irregular menstrual cycles (anovulatory or hypoovulatory) • Infertility or hypofertility • Hirsutism • Acne	• Insulin resistance • Impaired glucose tolerance • High-risk lipid profile • Impaired blood vessel function • Hypertension • Obesity (in 50% of cases)

BOX 8-7
DIFFERENTIAL DIAGNOSIS FOR DEPRESSION IN PCOS

Cushing syndrome

Congenital adrenal hyperplasia

Hyperprolactinemia

Hypothyroidism

Ovarian hyperthecosis

Given the prevalence and risks of depressive symptoms, an expert panel recommends routine assessment for depression in all women with PCOS, even when depressive symptoms are not part of the presenting complaints.[83]

Treatment

Treatment for women with PCOS is focused on alleviating current symptoms and on reducing long-term health risks. A patient's goals may include reducing signs of hyperandrogenism (e.g., hirsutism, acne), regulating menses, conceiving and maintaining a healthy pregnancy, losing weight, reducing risks of cardiovascular disease and diabetes, and treating comorbid depressive symptoms. Relevant interactions between depression and PCOS treatment are summarized below.

- Lifestyle changes. A key component of successful treatment of PCOS is to maintain a healthy diet and adequate aerobic exercise. These interventions reduce metabolic and menstrual abnormalities, improve inflammatory profiles, increase responsiveness to insulin, help maintain normal weight, and reduce cardiovascular risk. Treating comorbid depression may increase the likelihood that women with PCOS can maintain healthy eating habits and adequate physical activity. In turn, exercise and healthy eating can reduce depressive symptoms. This bidirectional improvement has not yet been studied in detail in PCOS, although preliminary results are promising. In a small open trial of eight sessions of CBT for adolescents with PCOS, obesity, and depression, participants had significant reductions in both weight and depressive symptoms.[84] Similarly, dietary and exercise interventions significantly improved depression scores in women with PCOS who had no other specific antidepressant treatment.[85]

- Insulin sensitizing agents are used in the treatment of women with PCOS in order to improve glucose tolerance and regulate menstrual cycles. The most frequently used agent is metformin. Newer agents are being studied that may have greater neuroprotective properties. A medication of particular interest in this regard is pioglitazone, a thiazolidinedione. In a 6-week double-blind trial comparing metformin to pioglitazone for women with mild to moderate major depressive episodes and PCOS, pioglitazone was superior to metformin in reducing depressive symptoms. In the absence of other treatment, 20% of study participants taking pioglitazone experienced remission of depression, as compared to none in the metformin group.[86] Further study is needed before pioglitazone could be considered for first-line use, especially studies weighing long-term benefits and risks. Pioglitazone and related agents have been implicated in increased risk of fractures and bladder cancer.

- Hormonal therapies used to treat PCOS include clomiphene to induce ovulation and improve fertility outcomes, intermittent doses of progestins to induce menses and protect the endometrium, and COCs to reduce hyperandrogenism and its associated symptoms.

- Lipid-lowering agents, particularly statins, are used to target elevated (LDL-C). Although some studies have suggested that depression may be a side effect of cholesterol-lowering medications, most data, including a recent meta-analysis, have not supported this link.[87]

- Antidepressants, when used for women (**Box 8-8**) with PCOS, can be chosen based on a side-effect profile that does not heighten preexisting risk factors. In particular, it is helpful to avoid medications with a higher likelihood of causing weight gain, such as mirtazapine. Among antidepressant augmenting agents, olanzapine is the most likely to contribute to weight gain, cholesterol elevation, and impaired glucose tolerance.[88]

BOX 8-8
TREATMENTS FOR DEPRESSION IN WOMEN WITH PCOS

Antidepressants which do not pose high risk of weight gain

Adjunctive agents (avoid weight gaining agents, such as olanzapine)

Summary

Women with PCOS are at increased risk for depressive symptoms and major depressive episodes. Untreated depressive symptoms can add to the long-term health risks associated with PCOS, and can impair ability to adhere to treatment. Exercise, healthy eating habits, and maintenance of a normal weight are first-line treatments for PCOS. Treating depression can improve adherence to these lifestyle interventions, and in turn these interventions can alleviate depressive symptoms. Choosing antidepressants that do not increase weight or worsen metabolic abnormalities is important for women with PCOS.

Case outcome. Anne was diagnosed with a major depressive episode of moderate severity. Findings of an elevated free androgen index, anovulatory bleeding patterns, and multiple ovarian cysts on ultrasound confirmed a concomitant diagnosis of polycystic ovary syndrome. Her BMI was 31, consistent with obesity. It became clear that her depressive symptoms had contributed to weight gain and psychomotor slowing, and would interfere with her ability to increase exercise and achieve healthier eating habits. Therefore, her initial treatment plan consisted of bupropion and cognitive behavioral therapy (CBT). As depressive symptoms remitted, Anne was able to establish and maintain a routine of daily aerobic exercise and strength training. She felt less of a drive toward mood-linked overeating, and was able to adhere to healthy eating guidelines recommended by a nutritionist. These focused on mindfulness about eating, and food choices based on glycemic index, rather than on calorie counting. She found this was more effective than the weight-loss diets she had tried in the past. After 9 months of treatment, she had sustained remission of depression, her BMI was 27, and her free androgen index was reduced. She had a higher percentage of ovulatory menstrual cycles. She felt more secure in her marriage, having overcome distorted negative thinking. She felt ready to resume trying to conceive. She decided to taper and discontinue bupropion, but to maintain booster CBT sessions as needed.

■ DEPRESSION AND INFERTILITY
Epidemiology

Infertility, the inability to conceive after having regular, unprotected sexual intercourse for a year, affects 6.0% of married women ages 15 to 44 years in the United States according to a National Survey of Family Growth conducted on 3,088 women.[89] Once pregnant, 10.9% of women in this age group are unable to carry a pregnancy to a live birth (impaired fecundity).[89] In a direct comparison among women with various medical conditions, psychological symptoms associated with infertility were similar to those related to cancer, hypertension, and cardiac rehabilitation.[90]

Evidence to date suggests that infertility does not increase the risk of major depression, though most studies have found an increased prevalence of subsyndromal depressive symptoms. Rates of moderate to severe depressive symptoms in women with infertility vary considerably from study to study. Nelson et al., for example, found that 19% of infertile women had moderate and 13% had severe depression.[91] Much higher rates of severe depression were found in a study by Drosdzol and Skrzypulec, with 35.4% of infertile women (in comparison to 19.47% of fertile women) scoring above the cut-off for severe symptoms of depression.[97] Methodological differences, such as varying definitions of infertility and timing of evaluation, make these findings difficult to compare. Rates of depression seem to be especially high in countries where family status and childbearing are highly valued.[93]

Women with primary infertility have never achieved a pregnancy or carried a pregnancy to term; those with secondary infertility have carried at least one child to term. Women with primary infertility are at higher risk for depressive symptoms than those with secondary infertility. The difference in levels of depression of women compared with their husbands is significantly greater for primary than for secondary infertility.[94] Additional risk factors for depression among infertile women include age over 30 years, lower level of education, lack of occupational activity, and infertility duration of 3 to 6 years relative to shorter or longer durations.[92]

Pathophysiology

Infertility is often considered a life crisis. It poses a threat to the developmental milestone of parenthood and involves multiple losses—of trust in one's body, of self-esteem, of faith and security, of expectations and hope, and of a sense of control. As such, it is associated with considerable stress, which may contribute to the development of depression in susceptible individuals.

Psychobiological characteristics may determine responsiveness to the stress of infertility. Women experience infertility as being more stressful than men, which is posited to be related to intense desire for motherhood, women's responsibilities in regard to pregnancy and childbearing, and the fact that, women are more likely to have to undergo treatment.[95] Cultural expectations and social pressure may further intensify stress. In a study conducted in Iran, 81.3% of depressed infertile women reported that the main stressor leading to their depression was relatives' comments about their infertility.[96] Infertile women who have social support, positive personal characteristics, and a satisfactory relationship with a partner show fewer signs of depression.[97]

Infertility treatment or assisted reproductive technology (ART) has also been associated with increased stress and depression. ART refers to all treatments or procedures that include in vitro handling of human oocytes, sperm, and/or embryos for the purpose of establishing a pregnancy. This encompasses in vitro fertilization (IVF) procedures, which include any transfer of fresh or cryopreserved embryos, possibly with donor eggs or sperm, and possibly with intracytoplasmic sperm injection (ICSI). Intrauterine insemination (IUI) with fresh or thawed sperm, possibly from a donor, is another form of ART. IVF typically involves hormonal treatments to stimulate ovulation or prepare the uterus for implantation, whereas IUI may or may not involve an endocrine treatment. Both forms of ART are time-consuming and cause significant emotional, physical, and financial stress, including uncertainty and potential disappointment on a monthly basis.[98] There is little a woman can do to affect the outcome of her treatment other than adherence to the treatment regimen, which does not assure success.[99] The decision whether to start infertility treatments may provoke stress and anxiety.[100] Committing to treatment, on the other hand, may be associated with decreased burden; women preparing to undergo IVF report fewer symptoms of depression than multiple comparison groups (e.g., postpartum women, primary care patients, and the general population).[101] Some attribute this finding to the healthy patient effect (women planning pregnancy tend to be physically and mentally healthy).[100] It is possible that women who choose to initiate or continue treatment have different characteristics (e.g., being able to afford ART) than those who choose to avoid or discontinue it, or that they see treatment as a way to regain control.

Hormonal medications that are used to regulate or induce ovulation may be another factor contributing to depression in infertile women undergoing ART, although this seems to be relatively rare. GnRH agonists downregulate GnRH receptors, resulting in hypogonadism.[102] Hypogonadism, in turn, has been associated with symptoms, such as depressed mood, anhedonia, fatigue, and anxiety.[103] However, findings from a prospective randomized study comparing two different controlled ovarian stimulation protocols indicate that the hypogonadal phase induced by GnRH agonists was not associated with a significant increase in depressive symptoms,[104] possibly because this phase of IVF treatment is brief. Depression is an uncommon side effect of clomiphene citrate, an oral nonsteroidal antiestrogenic agent that binds to the estrogen receptors of the hypothalamus and pituitary and stimulates ovulation. Little is known about potential effects of the more potent injectable pituitary hormone medications (e.g., FSH alone or with LH) on mood.

Just as infertility and its treatment can produce stress, substantial, prolonged stress can reduce fertility. There is variable individual sensitivity to the effects of stress on fertility.[105] It is estimated that stress is a clinically important contributor to infertility in about 5% of cases. A meta-analysis of 31 prospective studies of women undergoing infertility treatment revealed a small but significant association between stress and reduced pregnancy rates.[106] Stress may influence fertility via reciprocal interactions of the HPA axis and the HPG axis at multiple levels. Stress-induced changes in diurnal excretion patterns of cortisol mediate the downregulation of the HPG axis. The effect of cortisol on the HPG axis is dependent on the endocrine status of the ovary in its different stages within the menstrual cycle. Stress, therefore, can alter cortisol excretion patterns across the menstrual cycle, which suppress ovulation as well as disrupt the hormonal profile at critical stages of the fertilization process. Additionally, a study found that women who failed IVF showed stress-linked changes in plasma levels of adrenaline and noradrenaline.[107]

Most data show that untreated depressive symptoms do not affect fertility or response to infertility treatment. No association has been found between major depression and the likelihood of becoming pregnant.[106] Similarly, a meta-analysis of 14 prospective studies found no association between depressive symptoms and outcome of infertility treatment.[108] However, psychological burden is perhaps the most common reason to discontinue infertility treatment, affecting treatment outcome indirectly.[109]

Clinical Presentation

Infertility treatment is often described as an emotional rollercoaster involving monthly cycles of hope and hopelessness.[110] In a study focused on the emotional experience of treatment, 96% of patients described frustration, 81% experienced hopelessness, 82% endorsed depressed mood, 65% experienced anger, and nearly half to one-third had some trouble sleeping as well as some weight change.[111] Other reactions may include anxiety, cognitive impairment, and feelings of unattractiveness, as well as concerns about relationships with partners and about sexuality.[112,113] A caveat is that most research has focused on the stressful consequences of infertility and its treatment, with a selective sample of help seekers as participants.[114] Overall, as a group infertile women do not differ significantly from control or norm groups on emotional parameters.

Infertile patients face difficult decisions about treatment, taking into consideration factors, such as costs, expectations, time, and personal goals. A cycle of IVF typically requires 9 to 12 days of self-injection with medications to stimulate the production of oocytes, transvaginal retrieval of oocytes, fertilization of oocytes in a laboratory with partner or donor sperm, and transfer of the resulting embryo to the uterus. Couples then wait 2 to 3 weeks to find out whether implantation and a pregnancy have occurred. Patients have to decide how many cycles to undergo, how many embryos to transfer, whether to do reductions of multiple fetuses, and what to do with unused frozen embryos. Depressed patients, who tend to experience more decisional conflict,[110] may exhibit particular difficulty with the stresses of the ART process, potentially affecting treatment duration and outcomes. In a Danish registry study including 42,915 women treated with IVF, ICSI, frozen embryo transfer, and oocyte recipient cycles, women with a depression diagnosis prior to ART treatment initiated significantly fewer ART treatment cycles than women with no history of depression.[116]

Course and Natural History

The most common reactions to the diagnosis of infertility are shock, anger, guilt, marital distress, lowered self-esteem, sexual dysfunction, and social isolation.[117] The course thereafter is influenced by a woman's ability to adjust to ART, and ultimately to reconstruct her life if infertility treatment is unsuccessful.[118,119] After the first unsuccessful cycle, an increase in depression and anxiety has been observed.[114] Severity of depression following a failed treatment increases the duration of infertility.[120] However, this correlation between the duration of infertility and the prevalence of depression is not linear. Depression peaks between the second and third year of infertility and does not return to normal range until after 6 years of infertility.[97]

About 50% to 80% of infertile couples will eventually bear a child.[116] When ART results in a pregnancy, negative emotions tend to disappear immediately.[114] However, women with previous infertility may be at risk for developing depression during pregnancy.[112]

Assessment and Differential Diagnosis (Box 8-9)

It is important to differentiate the responses to various stressors that are associated with infertility from the diagnosis of clinical depression. Similarly, it is prudent to take potential side effects of infertility drug treatment into consideration when making the diagnosis. Anxiety is a common comorbidity, with 12% to 23% of women undergoing infertility treatment suffering from an anxiety disorder.[123–125]

Identifying women with a vulnerability to emotional problems before starting treatment enables clinicians to anticipate difficulties, offer psychosocial care, and facilitate emotional adjustment to the treatment and its outcome.[126] A comprehensive mental health assessment can uncover psychiatric disorders and functional impairment, determine the level of distress the patient is experiencing, and reveal specific fears, beliefs, goals, and coping styles.[127] Unfortunately, several studies have shown that patients' emotional cues are often missed or not responded to appropriately by providers.[128,129] One study showed that the majority of patients undergoing IVF treatment who suffered from psychiatric disorders were undiagnosed and untreated for those disorders.[125] **Table 8-3** summarizes elements of a comprehensive mental health assessment for a woman undergoing infertility treatment.

Treatment

There is an international consensus that infertility centers should address psychosocial and emotional issues, as these have been associated with premature treatment drop out, unhealthy lifestyle behaviors such as less optimal nutrition and smoking, and less

---

BOX 8-9
DIFFERENTIAL DIAGNOSIS FOR DEPRESSION IN WOMEN WITH INFERTILITY

Adjustment disorder (associated with stressor, shorter course)

Medication effects

Anxiety disorders

TABLE 8-3 Comprehensive Mental Health Assessment of Patients with Infertility

- Psychiatric disorders
- Stress and distress (about infertility and specific aspects of treatment)
- Functional impairment (social isolation, work function, reduced attention to children)
- Coping styles and abilities (avoidance, feeling overwhelmed, impaired information processing)
- Reasons for wanting a child (external pressure, way to relieve emptiness/loneliness)
- Beliefs about infertility (e.g., self-blame, guilt)
- Fantasies about the meaning of infertility
- Investment in other valued life goals

---

adaptive coping behaviors.[130–134] The debate over implementing voluntary or mandatory psychosocial counseling for infertility patients remains open. Mandatory counseling may induce suspicious or defensive behavior in some patients, while voluntary counseling can be difficult to accept for some, even in case of need. Ideally, counseling and support groups should be available at all stages of medical therapy for infertility. The goals, content, and duration of counseling should be made clear.[112]

Psychological interventions may be individual, group, or couple based, the latter focusing both on individual needs and coping styles and addressing patterns of interactions.[127,135] A treatment duration of at least six sessions results in better outcomes than shorter interventions.[136]

As shown in **Table 8-4**, CBT may include relaxation techniques, reframing of unrealistic beliefs and risk appraisals, correction of distorted thinking, gradual exposure to stress-inducing situations, and identifying other valued life goals.[127,137] CBT has been shown to attenuate autonomic and neuroendocrine responses to a stressful task in infertile women waiting for IVF.[138] In a randomized controlled clinical trial with 89 depressed infertile women participants, CBT was as effective as pharmacotherapy in decreasing mean depression scores.[139]

The efficacy of IPT was evaluated in a pilot randomized controlled study among infertile women suffering from moderate to severe depression. It produced a greater response rate than Brief Supportive Psychotherapy, with more than two-thirds of women achieving a >50% reduction in scores on the Montgomery-Åsberg Depression Rating Scale (MADRS). Gains persisted at 6-month follow-up.[140]

It is unclear whether treating psychological distress can directly improve fertility. Stress reduction has been found in several studies

---

TABLE 8-4 Cognitive Behavioral Interventions for Emotional Distress Associated with Infertility

- Relaxation techniques (in general, before and during specific interventions)
- Reframing:
  - Unrealistic beliefs about causes or meaning of infertility
  - Catastrophic thinking
  - Overgeneralization
  - Unrealistic appraisals of risks and benefits of treatment
- Gradual exposure to stress-inducing situations
- Identifying other valued life goals:
  - Maintain engagement in those goals
  - Make time for other social roles, enjoyment, and intimacy

to increase the chance of pregnancy.[138,141–143] A recent meta-analysis of 21 controlled studies of psychological interventions for patients suffering from infertility found an increased pregnancy rate in those undergoing psychological interventions, although this observation is not universal.[112] Overall, the use of antidepressants does not appear to affect pregnancy rate or live birth rate[144] directly, meta-analysis and best methodologic studies do not show this.[145] It may improve outcome indirectly, as depression can influence decisions to stop ART treatment.[126]

Summary

Infertility is a biopsychosocial condition with a multifaceted impact on patients' lives. Prior to infertility treatment, infertile women are not necessarily more depressed than fertile ones, but the treatment process may induce distress and depressive symptoms, both short- and long term. Supportive counseling, CBT, IPT, and, where indicated, antidepressant medication may decrease depressive symptoms associated with infertility and its treatment.

■ DEPRESSION AND PERIMENOPAUSE

Case illustration: Sarah is a 50-year-old married woman who has been feeling quite blue for the past 2 months. There are days in which it is difficult for her to get out of bed. Her energy and motivation are not what they used to be. Coffee chats with her friends or movie nights with her husband are no longer appealing. She cannot seem to get a good night of sleep partly because she has been experiencing night sweats. The hot flashes during the day are not as bothersome but certainly annoying. Sarah is a second-grade teacher and usually loves her job. Lately, she has been quite irritable with her students. She also finds it difficult to organize and sustain attention on tasks. This has led her to feel inadequate. Her parents live nearby; Sarah often helps care for her father, who has dementia. This has felt increasingly burdensome. Sarah's daughter is a high school senior who procrastinates on her work; Sarah often worries about her. Although her husband is generally supportive, she has become more sensitive when they argue, taking many things personally. Sarah's previous psychiatric history includes PMDD and an episode of major depression after her daughter's birth.

Epidemiology

Epidemiologic studies show no increased prevalence of major depression for women at midlife in general.[146] However, perimenopause, the several-year period of hormonal flux before and during the year after the final menstrual period, is a time of heightened risk for depressive symptoms and major depression. The Study of Women's Health Across the Nation (SWAN) prospectively tracked prevalence rates of depression across stages of menopause. According to a longitudinal analysis of data from 221 African-American and Caucasian women from the SWAN study, the risk of developing a major depressive episode during peri- or early postmenopause was found to be 2 to 4 times as likely as during premenopause.[147] The prevalence of depressive symptoms, based on high Center for Epidemiological Studies Depression Scale (CES-D) scores, was 20.9% in premenopausal women, compared to 27.8% in women during the early menopausal transition, a statistically significant difference in prevalence rates by stage.[148] The majority of women who experience a major depressive episode during the perimenopause have a prior history of depression, but major depression and, more commonly, subsyndromal depressive symptoms, may occur during the perimenopause even among those without previous depression.

Depression during perimenopause may influence the development and progression of other medical conditions. Findings from the SWAN study have linked depression during midlife to an increased risk of diabetes,[149] coronary calcifications,[150] and inflammatory and hemostatic markers.[151] Other prospective studies have correlated midlife depression with coronary heart disease,[152] headaches,[153] pain syndromes,[154] and low bone mineral density.[155]

Pathophysiology (Box 8-10)

Factors shown to influence the development of depressive symptoms during perimenopause are shown in **Figure 8-3**, and include (**Box 8-11**):

- Genetic vulnerability. The primary factor driving risk for depression during the perimenopause is a prior history of depression.[148] Family history of depression is also a risk factor for developing perimenopausal depression.[156] The existing data investigating associations between estrogen receptor genes and depression during perimenopause is largely unclear and inconclusive.[157] Nonetheless, preliminary data suggest that two polymorphisms of the estrogen alpha receptor gene may confer heightened vulnerability to depressive symptoms.[157] Fewer data are available regarding the estrogen beta receptor, but one study demonstrated an increased risk of depression with a certain polymorphism of the estrogen beta receptor gene.[158] In addition, estrogen may have a role in modulating G-proteins.[159] Polymorphisms in G-protein, in turn, may influence vulnerability to depression and lack of treatment response to antidepressants.[160]

- Hormonal flux. A history of premenstrual and postpartum mood changes predicts heightened risk for perimenopausal mood changes,[161] suggesting that a subset of women may be vulnerable to mood changes at times of hormonal flux. Estradiol (the most potent estrogen) influences the activity of serotonin, GABA, and dopamine. However, absolute differences in estradiol levels do not explain mood symptoms during the menopausal transition. Rather, the magnitude of flux of follicle stimulating hormone (FSH), luteinizing hormone, and estradiol around a woman's baseline levels is associated with a greater risk of depressive symptoms.[162] This may explain why late postmenopause, characterized by lower but more stable estradiol levels, does not confer a similar risk.

- Dehydroepiandrosterone (DHEA). DHEA is an endogenous androgen that influences mood. While some studies suggest an accelerated decline of DHEA in women during midlife,[163] more recent data from the SWAN study demonstrated a rise in adrenal DHEA during perimenopause.[164] There may be greater individual variability in circulating androgens as compared to estrogens during perimenopause.[165] DHEA's effect on perimenopausal mood warrants further investigation.

- Cascade effect of hot flashes and sleep disturbance. A leading "domino" hypothesis explaining the increased risk of depression during the perimenopause and early postmenopause is the occurrence of hot flashes and night sweats (together called vasomotor symptoms), which disrupt sleep and may therefore secondarily impair mood. Evidence to date suggests

---

BOX 8-10
POSSIBLE MEDIATORS BETWEEN MENOPAUSE AND DEPRESSION

Vulnerabilities

Genetic

Epigenetic

Life Events

Physiological Abnormalities

Fluctuations in Estrogen

Fluctuations in FSH

Fluctuations in LH

Possible influence of DHEA

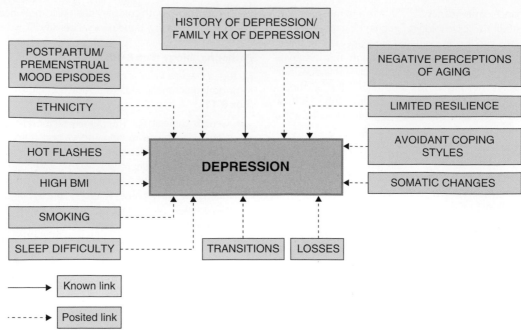

Figure 8-3 *Biopsychosocial Variables Associated with Depression during menopause.*

that this symptom cascade may be an important factor for the increased prevalence of depressive symptoms, but not major depression, during this reproductive transition. Sleep disturbance may be a key modifiable risk factor for perimenopausal major depression.[148,166,167]

- Psychosocial influences. Midlife psychosocial transitions and life events may contribute to depressive symptoms during perimenopause. Some studies have found that distressing life events are among the strongest contributory factors to perimenopausal depressive symptoms,[168] similar to depression occurring at other stages of life. These include interpersonal losses, role transitions, and mental and physical effects of aging.[169] The concept of the "empty nest"—the departure of children from the home—had been posited as a contributor to midlife depressive symptoms. However, an Australian prospective study showed that quality of life improved upon departure of children.[170] There are likely considerable individual, cultural, and generational differences in the appraisal of life events.

What may be a risk factor for one individual may be protective for another. Perceptions and coping styles may strongly influence the likelihood of becoming depressed in the face of stressors. Negative perceptions about aging,[171] limited resilience,[172] and avoidant coping styles[173] have been associated with increased risk of perimenopausal depression.

■ CLINICAL PRESENTATION

Some aspects of normal perimenopause overlap with depressive symptoms, including decreased energy and concentration, sleep disturbances, changes in sex drive, and weight gain.[174] In addition, longitudinal studies demonstrate a normative peak of irritability and mood swings in the late premenopause and early perimenopause; these mood changes decline with progression into later stages of menopause.[175] Although the aforementioned longitudinal study did not find an association of anxiety with menopausal stage, longitudinal analysis of SWAN data demonstrates a vulnerability to anxiety symptoms during the menopausal transition in individuals with low anxiety during premenopause.[148,176]

Perimenopausal depressive symptoms tend to co-occur with vasomotor symptoms and sleep disturbances.[166] Depressive symptoms also correlate with slower processing speed at perimenopause.[177] A similar pathophysiological process may underlie these symptoms. Depression may also influence appraisals of the degree of bother or impairment associated with perimenopausal changes.[178] In addition, hot flashes, night sweats, reduced sleep quality and other perimenopausal symptoms may worsen or complicate the experience of depression.[179]

Course

The average age of onset of perimenopause is about 47.5 years, with an average duration of approximately 4 years.[180] Late perimenopause seems to be the period of highest risk for depressive symptoms,[181] with risk for depression beginning to abate after about 2 years of postmenopause.[162] This appears to be the case for new onset severe depression as well as exacerbation of prior depression.[182]

Depression has been linked with an earlier age of onset of natural menopause, but not premature menopause.[183] In addition,

---

BOX 8-11
IMPORTANT RISK FACTORS FOR DEPRESSION IN WOMEN WITH MENOPAUSE

Sociodemographic

Life transitions

Personal losses

Ethnicity

Clinical

Personal history of depression

Family history of depression

Postpartum/premenstrual mood episodes

High BMI

Smoking

Negative perceptions of aging

Medical

Hot flashes

Insomnia

depressive symptoms influence several perimenopausal changes, including:

- Sexual dysfunction: Perimenopause is sometimes accompanied by increased pain during intercourse and decreased sexual interest.[184] Depression may further reduce sex drive.
- Sleep disturbance: Women in late perimenopause experience high rates of insomnia.[185] Depression may compound the sleep disturbances inherent to perimenopause.[186]
- Cardiovascular risk: Women's risk for cardiovascular disease increases at perimenopause.[187] As depression may mediate adverse cardiac outcomes independent of menopause, depression may compound cardiac risk during perimenopause.
- Psychological influences: Depressive cognitive appraisals may adversely affect reactions to transitions, life events, somatic changes and medical co-morbidities associated with midlife and perimenopause. In turn, the biological and psychosocial stressors of midlife and perimenopause may intensify negative core beliefs which had been relatively quiescent.
- Health behaviors: Depressed individuals may be less likely to adhere to medication regimens or attend necessary medical appointments,[188] and more likely to smoke.[189] This may be particularly relevant at midlife due to the increase in medical comorbidities during this life stage. Moreover, the neurovegetative symptoms of depression may contribute to a more sedentary, isolated lifestyle with less healthy eating habits.[190] Menopause may be independently associated with weight gain[191]; depression is associated with additional increases in BMI.[184]

Assessment and Differential Diagnosis

Perimenopause can be identified clinically by menstrual cycle characteristics and associated symptoms. Early perimenopause is categorized by irregularity in menstrual cycle length by at least 7 days or more, lasting for at least two menstrual cycles. During late perimenopause, FSH levels ≥25 IU/L may be present and can support the determination of perimenopause but vary widely so that an individual FSH level may be <25 IU/L, requiring that several FSH levels be obtained.[192] FSH and estradiol levels cannot be used to establish a diagnosis of depression related to the perimenopause.

The Menopause Rating Scale is a validated patient-administered tool for assessing perimenopausal symptoms, including mood changes,[193] as is the Menopause-Specific Quality of Life Scale (MENQOL), which captures psychological and somatic symptom domains comprising quality of life during the menopause transition.[194] In addition, general depression screening tools, such as the Patient Health Questionnaire-9, may be effectively used to measure depressive symptoms.

The differential diagnosis of depression during perimenopause includes the following:

- Psychological distress, defined as feeling tense or nervous, feeling blue or depressed, and feeling irritable or grouchy, has been found to be a common accompaniment of normal perimenopause.[195] Similarly, mood lability is relatively common in perimenopause.[175] A careful history of previous manic or hypomanic episodes is warranted to distinguish this from bipolar disorder.
- Adjustment disorder. Adjustment disorder develops in response to a stressor, such as midlife role transitions or new-onset health problems.
- Bereavement. Women at midlife more often experience loss of loved ones.
- Subsyndromal depression, defined as exhibiting one to four symptoms of depression causing significant distress and/or functional impairment, has a higher relative risk of occurring during perimenopause than major depression.[181]

BOX 8-12
TREATMENTS FOR DEPRESSION IN WOMEN WITH MENOPAUSE

Psychoeducation

Dietary modifications

Exercise

Relaxation techniques

Cognitive behavioral therapy

SSRIs (may also help vasomotor symptoms)

SNRIs (may help vasomotor symptoms but worsen hypertension)

Agents which improve sleep (e.g. trazodone, mirtazapine)

Bupropion (fewer sexual side effects)

Estrogen (preliminary evidence during perimenopause)

Treatment (Box 8-12)

Categorizing the nature and severity of symptoms can inform choice of interventions, as follows:

- *Mild psychological distress.* These symptoms may respond to psychoeducation, dietary, and/or exercise modifications, introduction of relaxation techniques, mobilization of supports, and reduction of perimenopausal physical symptoms.
- *Adjustment disorder.* CBT may play a role in challenging core negative beliefs that affect the appraisal of biopsychosocial changes during the menopause. IPT may be especially helpful for adjustment to midlife role transitions.
- *Bereavement.* Support strategies may include mobilizing existing resources and utilizing support groups.
- *Subsyndromal depression.* CBT and IPT are often effective treatments for milder perimenopausal depressive symptoms. CBT has also been found to be effective in alleviating distress linked with vasomotor symptoms and in reducing the frequency of stress-triggered hot flashes.[196] If estrogen is being used for other indications, such as vasomotor symptoms, osteoporosis, or urogenital atrophy, it may also be used off-label to alleviate mild depressive symptoms (does not carry an FDA approval for treatment of depressive symptoms).
- *Major depression.* Women with major depression, especially if moderate to severe, may benefit from antidepressant medication either as monotherapy or in addition to psychotherapy. The choice of antidepressant may be guided by concurrent medical comorbidities. Several trials demonstrate the efficacy of SSRI and SNRI for treatment of major depression during the perimenopause and early postmenopause.
- *Vasomotor symptoms.* Women troubled by vasomotor symptoms may benefit from an antidepressant that alleviates them. SSRI and SNRI antidepressants have been found to reduce the frequency and severity of hot flashes.[197] The effects appear not to be as robust as standard-dose hormone therapy, although head to head studies comparing the SNRI venlafaxine to the recommended low-dose estrogen therapy in the treatment of vasomotor symptoms show similar efficacy. Randomized double-blind controlled trials have demonstrated the efficacy of venlafaxine, paroxetine, fluoxetine, sertraline, citalopram, desvenlafaxine, and escitalopram in the treatment of hot flashes.[198–204] Open-label studies of duloxetine, mirtazapine, and fluvoxamine have also suggested efficacy in the treatment of hot flashes.[205–207]
- *Hypertension.* Venlafaxine and duloxetine can elevate blood pressure, particularly at higher doses. Agents less likely to have this side effect may be better choices for women with hypertension.[208]

- *Sleep.* In a multinational survey, 56.6% of midlife women were estimated to have sleep disturbances.[209] Use of antidepressants that promote sleep, such as trazodone or mirtazapine, may be beneficial for women with pronounced insomnia, provided they do not result in excessive daytime sedation. Cotherapy with hypnotic agents or behavioral therapy to target sleep may also play important roles in the treatment of depression in this population.
- *Sexual dysfunction.* Sexual dysfunction may develop from perimenopause, depression, and/or antidepressants. Decreased libido and anorgasmia as antidepressant side effects are more prominent in women than in men.[210] Bupropion has fewer sexual side effects than other antidepressants.[211] Among serotonergic agents, mirtazapine has less likelihood of sexual side effects than SSRIs.[212]
- *Cognition.* Subjective complaints of reduced cognitive capabilities are common during perimenopause. Longitudinal SWAN data show some objective validation of this. During pre- and postmenopause, cognitive processing and verbal memory improve with repeated administration of the same test, a measure of learning. By contrast, during perimenopause these cognitive measures do not improve over repeated trials, although this effect is transient and learning improves again during the postmenopause.[213] By reducing psychomotor speed, depressive symptoms could intensify subjective and/or objective cognitive slowing. Studies of the comparative effects of antidepressants on cognition have not yielded conclusive or consistent results. Paroxetine has more anticholinergic effects than most; some studies demonstrate minor adverse effects of paroxetine on visual attention processes.[214] Preliminary data demonstrate that bupropion may improve processing speed as well as visual memory in those who have lower baseline scores.[215]
- *Fracture risk.* Fracture risk can be affected by bone strength as well as propensity to fall. Some but not all epidemiologic studies in older men and women with depression have demonstrated an association between serotonergic antidepressants and low bone mineral density,[216] although it is likely that the depression itself explains this association. In addition, some antidepressants can increase fall risk by causing sedation and/or orthostatic hypotension.

Estrogen's effects on neurotransmitter activity are similar to the actions of many antidepressants. While estrogen therapy is not FDA approved for treating major depression, several well designed trials show efficacy of hormone therapy for treatment of depressive disorders occurring in perimenopausal women.[185,217,218] In contrast, hormone therapy is not effective for treatment of depressive disorders in postmenopausal women.[219] Some initial data suggest that, in perimenopausal women, estrogen therapy may augment antidepressants when there is a partial treatment response to the latter.[220]

Treatment with estrogens or estrogen–progestogen combinations involves a careful risk–benefit analysis. Adverse effects may vary depending on the age of the individual as well as timing and duration of treatment. Estrogen therapy may reduce the risk of cardiovascular disease when initiated in perimenopausal women in their early 50s.[221] By contrast, women who initiate estrogen therapy or estrogen–progestogen therapy more than 10 years after menopause have increased risk of coronary heart disease,[222] venous thromboembolic disease,[223] and stroke.[224] Estrogen-progestogen use beyond 5 years has been associated with an increased risk of breast cancer.[225] Estrogen therapy without a progestogen increases the risk of endometrial cancer.[226] While adding a progestogen may adversely affect mood in a small minority of individuals,[33] clinical trials show that progestogens have a neutral effect on mood in both depressed and nondepressed peri- and early postmenopausal women receiving estrogen therapy.[227]

Summary

Perimenopause, the period of time that begins with menstrual cycle irregularity and extends to 1 year after the final cessation of menses, is a time of heightened risk for depressive symptoms and major depressive episodes. This risk is more pronounced in women with a history of depression. Hormonal flux, Genetic vulnerability, hot flashes, sleep disturbance, and midlife stressors are additional influences. Depressive symptoms may worsen medical comorbidities as well as adversely affect the appraisal of other symptoms and stressors. Management of depression during perimenopause is multifaceted, including psychoeducation, mobilization of support, and assistance with lifestyle improvements. IPT can help women improve their interpersonal skills and relationships as they navigate midlife role changes. CBT can reduce maladaptive core beliefs and self-appraisals and improve coping skills. Antidepressant medications can be chosen based on their effects on comorbid symptoms and conditions. Although hormone replacement therapy is not FDA approved for the treatment of depression, it may be reasonable to consider adjunctive estrogen for perimenopausal women with a partial response to antidepressants, or for those with concomitant indications for estrogen.

Case outcome. Sarah was diagnosed with a major depressive episode of moderate severity. Factors that may have influenced her vulnerability to depression include previous sensitivity to mood changes at times of hormonal flux, life stressors, and the interplay of hot flashes, sleep disturbance, and mood. Her treatment included venlafaxine and interpersonal psychotherapy. Through therapy, she learned how to prioritize her goals and to delegate some aspects of caring for her father. She learned relaxation techniques and environmental changes to assist with sleep. She experienced a significant improvement in her mood and her appraisal of life events.

■ MENSTRUAL DYSFUNCTION AND REPRODUCTIVE EFFECTS OF PSYCHOTROPIC MEDICATIONS

Case illustration: Judy is a 26-year-old woman with bipolar disorder who was initially diagnosed at 22 after she presented with a manic and psychotic episode. She was treated with risperidone and lithium, which was subsequently changed to risperidone and valproate because of poor lithium tolerance. Risperidone was tapered off after her condition stabilized, and she has been maintained on valproate alone for the past 2 years. Prior to her first episode, Judy had a regular monthly menstrual cycle. After she began mood stabilizing medications, she noticed that her menstrual periods became less frequent, occurring every 40 to 60 days. She did not report this change as she assumed it was stress-related. She also gained weight, had severe acne which improved when lithium was stopped, and developed thinning of her hair after she was switched from lithium to valproate. Since her first manic episode, she has had very few menstrual periods (~1–2/year), although she had two regular menstrual periods during a 3-month period of time when she didn't take her risperidone or her lithium.

Normal menstrual cycle length (ranging from 25 to 35 days) is present in 80% to 85% of women except at the extremes of reproductive life (menarche, perimenopause).[228] The most common conditions causing irregular and skipped menses are pregnancy, lactation, PCOS, prolactinomas, and hypothalamic amenorrhea linked with stress, excessive exercise and/or being underweight. In the first 2 years after menarche, cycles are often irregular as the hypothalamic-pituitary-ovarian axis becomes entrained; in the several years leading up to the final menstrual period that comprise the perimenopause, cycles become unpredictable and less frequent.

Menstrual Cycle Dysfunction

Menstrual cycle irregularities occur more commonly in women with bipolar disorder (34.2%) than in women with unipolar mood disorders (24.5%) or in healthy women without a mental health condition (21.7%).[229] This menstrual dysfunction (cycles unpredictable within 10 days, cycles ≤25 or >35 days in length) manifests during adolescence and precedes the onset of affective symptoms, diagnosis of bipolar disorder, and the initiation of psychotropic medications. This observation suggests that some women with bipolar may have a neuroendocrine dysregulation related to their affective illness. The type of endocrinopathies that account for this increased prevalence of menstrual dysfunction are not known, and may include several different etiologies. It is notable that women with unipolar mood disorders do not appear to share this potential dysregulation. Careful documentation of the onset of menstrual dysfunction is important because several widely used psychotropic agents can independently contribute to menstrual dysfunction and ovarian suppression. It is plausible that women with preexisting cycle irregularities are more susceptible to the reproductive consequences of psychotropic medications. Regardless, this observation highlights the importance of taking a careful history of the timing of onset of menstrual cycle irregularities before attributing abnormalities to psychotropic treatment.

Valproate and PCOS

Use of the anticonvulsant valproate has been associated with the subsequent development of PCOS features in 10.5% of women with bipolar disorder participating in the Systematic Treatment Enhancement Program for Bipolar Disorder (STEP-BD) cohort study.[232] Results of a 12-month randomized trial in women with epilepsy similarly found that 7% of women assigned to valproate developed PCOS features in contrast to 1% of women receiving lamotrigine.[230] In both studies, PCOS manifested within the first year of treatment with no additional cases presenting later in the cohort study.[231] Studies of androgen-producing ovarian thecal cells demonstrate that valproate increases androgens through a direct effect on the ovary.[232] This effect of valproate has not been seen with other anticonvulsants. It is important to note that reproductive features of PCOS remit over time after valproate is discontinued and other psychotropic medications are substituted,[233] indicating reversibility of the effect of valproate on ovarian function. Therefore, this potential side effect of valproate should be weighed when treating premenopausal women, along with concern about the teratogenic effects of valproate with in-utero exposure.[234] For premenopausal women requiring maintenance treatments with valproate, close monitoring of menstrual cycle patterns and contraceptive strategies is important. Use of estrogen-containing hormonal contraceptives, has the advantage of preventing pregnancy and treating any potential PCOS features by suppressing androgens, hirsutism, and acne, although metabolic features of PCOS are not improved. Women developing PCOS features on valproate can be treated by (1) switching valproate to an alternate mood-stabilizing agent, (2) continuing valproate and initiating treatment for PCOS.

Antipsychotics and Hyperprolactinemia

Some antipsychotic agents have been associated with elevations in serum prolactin concentrations.[235] Prolactin is a peptide hormone critical for lactation that is produced in the anterior pituitary and is under tonic inhibition by dopamine. Agents that block D2 dopamine receptors release the inhibition by dopaminergic neurons to increase production of prolactin, without having an anatomic effect on the pituitary, an important distinction between the space-occupying prolactinomas and drug-induced hyperprolactinemia. High prolactin levels can subsequently suppress ovulation and induce hypoestro-

genism by suppressing secretion of GnRH. As a result, women will commonly present with oligo- or amenorrhea and possibly galactorrhea, although these symptoms are highly variable and may not be present. Fertility may be reduced in the short-term and protracted amenorrhea may contribute to risk of osteoporosis. It is because of these important health consequences that attention should be paid to the reproductive effects of prolactin-elevating antipsychotics.

The first-generation antipsychotics uniformly elevate prolactin, although typically to a lesser extent than do risperidone and amisulpride (not FDA approved), the second-generation antipsychotics that have been most clearly linked to hyperprolactinemia.[235] Hyperprolactinemia has been seen in 70% to 100% of risperidone users. Olanzapine and quetiapine have also been associated with prolactin elevation (10–40%) as has clozapine (5%), although the degree of elevation is typically mild and may be. Other newer second-generation antipsychotics (e.g., ziprasidone, asenapine, lurasidone, aripiprazole) have minimal effects on prolactin. In fact, aripiprazole reduces prolactin levels when used in combination with prolactin-elevating antipsychotics. In an 8-week randomized trial of adjunctive treatment of schizophrenia patients taking haloperidol, those assigned to aripiprazole were much more likely to have normalization of prolactin levels (88.5% vs. 3.6% on placebo) and menstrual function.[236] This observation has raised the possibility that aripiprazole may be used as the primary antipsychotic or as an adjuvant to reduce hyperprolactinemia while maintaining control of psychotic symptoms.[237]

The extent to which prolactin is elevated by an antipsychotic typically—although not universally—correlates with the likelihood and severity of the symptomatic presentation. For example, one study found symptoms of hyperprolactinemia in 44% of patients on risperidone and only 3% of those taking olanzapine,[238] consistent with a greater likelihood of much more substantial elevation on risperidone. Potential explanations for a more marked effect of specific antipsychotics on prolactin include (1) longer duration of D2 receptor antagonism, (2) reduced penetrance of the blood–brain barrier resulting in higher occupancy of D2 receptors in the pituitary relative to occupancy in the brain, and (3) relatively greater affinity for neuropeptides other than dopamine (e.g., serotonin receptors).[235]

Treatment of Antipsychotic-Induced Hyperprolactinemia

Once a pituitary adenoma, thyroid dysfunction, and renal dysfunction have been ruled-out, a decision needs to be made about whether the elevated prolactin needs to be treated or not based on age, menarchal and menopausal status of the women, and presence or absence of hyperprolactinemic symptoms. Where indicated, approaches to managing symptomatic hyperprolactinemia induced by an antipsychotic include (1) switching the antipsychotic to another that is prolactin-sparing, (2) adjunctive therapy with a dopamine agonist, (3) adjunctive therapy with an estrogenic agent (e.g., hormonal contraceptive) to prevent hypoestrogenic consequences where not contraindicated, and (4) possibly aripiprazole as a novel adjunctive therapy. Hyperprolactinemia is rapidly reversible when offending agents are withdrawn. Given the range of approaches, treatment decisions will vary with the psychiatric stability and general health of the patient as well as the risk/benefit decision about each individual treatment option.

Case outcome. Judy's mood has remained stable on valproate and she has been able to maintain a stable job and relationship over the past year. In planning for contraception, she saw a gynecologist who noted thinning of her hair, excess facial hair that she was shaving daily, and no galactorrhea. She evaluated her amenorrhea with laboratory studies revealing low/non-pregnant HCG, normal prolactin, normal TSH, normal DHEAS, elevated total testosterone (100 ng/dL), and an increased Homeostatic Model Assessment of Insulin Resistance (HOMA) ratio. Ovarian ultrasonography showed enlarged ovaries and multiple cysts

BOX 8-13
SUMMARY

- Diagnosis and treating depression in women of reproductive years requires an understanding of reproductive physiology
- Psychiatric disorders are often not associated with hormonal or menstrual factors
- In cases where they are, understand the particular diagnostic and treatment issues is central to appropriate care

around the periphery of the ovary. She was diagnosed with PCOS on the basis of her amenorrhea, hirsutism, balding, and ovarian PCO morphology. Signs of insulin resistance also raised concern. Given the timing of onset of her symptoms, she appears to have PCOS related to use of valproate. She may have previously developed hyperprolactinemia from risperidone which, although it was not investigated, is suggested by the otherwise spontaneous normalization of her menstrual pattern during the few months she was noncompliant with risperidone. Her gynecologist spoke with her psychiatrist about these endocrine symptoms. This was complicated by an emerging depressive episode. Discussions were initiated about balancing her mood stability against her PCOS reproductive and metabolic features. She was and she was switched from valproate to combination therapy with lamotrigine and quetiapine. One year later, Judy is stable on lamotrigine with small doses of quetiapine used for sleep disturbance. Her menstrual cycles normalized, as did her testosterone level. She has noticed that her hair has stopped falling out and it is thickening a bit, while she no longer needs to shave her facial hair.

■ SUMMARY (BOX 8-13)

Diagnosis and treatment of women with mental illness during the reproductive years involves special consideration of the menstrual and hormonal factors that may contribute to or complicate psychiatric illness and treatment. This chapter has reviewed several important considerations related to common gynecologic conditions and reproductive transitions. While many women with psychiatric disorders do not have any hormonal or menstrual factors underlying or complicating management of their illness, each condition discussed highlights the importance of a female-specific approach to treating mental illness when there is a particular hormonal factor at issue.

REFERENCES

1. Angold A, Costello EJ. Puberty and depression. *Child Adolesc Psychiatr Clin N Am.* 2006;15(4):919–937.

2. Merikangas KR, He J, Burstein M, et al.. Lifetime prevalence of mental disorders in US adolescents: results from the National Comorbidity Study – Adolescent Supplement (NCS-A). *J Am Acad Child Adolesc Psychiatry.* 2010;49(10):980–989.

3. Costello EJ, Worthman C, Erkanli A, Angold A. Prediction from low birth weight to female adolescent depression: a test of competing hypotheses. *Arch Gen Psychiatry.* 2007;64(3):338–344.

4. Angold A, Costello EJ, Erkanli A, Worthman CM. Pubertal changes in hormone levels and depression in girls. *Psychol Med.* 1999;29:1043–1053.

5. Mendle J, Harden KP, Brooks-Gunn J, Graber JA. Development's tortoise and hare: pubertal timing, pubertal tempo, and depressive symptoms in boys and girls. *Dev Psychol.* 2010;46(5): 1341–1353.

6. Black SR, Klein DN. Early menarcheal age and risk for later depressive symptomatology: the role of childhood depressive symptoms. *J Youth Adolesc.* 2012;41:1142–1150.

7. Manuck SB, Craig AE, Flory JD, Halder I, Ferrell RE. Reported early family environment covaries with menarcheal age as a function of polymorphic variation in estrogen receptor-α. *Devel Psychopathol.* 2011;23:69–83.

8. Dunger DB, Ahmed ML, Ong KK. Early and late weight gain and the timing of puberty. *Mol Cell Endocrinol.* 2006;254–255: 140–145.

9. Liu Y, Murphy SK, Murtha AP, et al. Depression in pregnancy, infant birth weight and DNA methylation of imprint regulatory elements. *Epigenetics.* 2012;7(7):735–746.

10. Dunn EC, Gilman SE, Willett JB, Slopen NB, Molnar BE. The impact of exposure to interpersonal violence on gender differences in adolescent-onset major depression: results from the National Comorbidity Survey Revision (NCS-R). *Depress Ann.* 2012;29:392–399.

11. Worthman CM, Costello EJ. Tracking biocultural pathways to health disparities: the value of biomarkers. *Ann Hum Biol.* 2009; 36(3):281–297.

12. Calvete E, Orue I, Hankin BL. Transactional relationships among cognitive vulnerabilities, stressors and depressive symptoms in adolescence. *Abn Child Psychol.* 213;41(3):399-410.

13. Yuan AS. Gender differences in the relationship of puberty with adolescents' depressive symptoms: do body perceptions matter? *Sex Roles.* 2007;57:69–80.

14. Lewinsohn PM, Rohde P, Seeley JR, Baldwin CL. Gender differences in suicide attempts from adolescence to young adulthood. *J Am Acad Child Adolesc Psychiatry.* 2001;40(4):427–434.

15. Bennett DS, Ambrosini PJ, Kudes D, Metz C, Rabinovich H. Gender differences in adolescent depression: do symptoms differ for boys and girls? *J Affect Disord.* 2005;89:35–44.

16. Lewinsohn PM, Rohde P, Seeley JR, Klein DN, Gotlib IH. Natural course of adolescent major depressive disorder in a community sample: predictors of recurrence in young adults. *Am J Psychiatry.* 2000;157(10):1584–1591.

17. Eaton WW, Shao H, Nestadt G, Lee HB, Bienvenu OJ, Zandi P. Population-based study of first onset and chronicity of major depressive disorder. *Arch Gen Psychiatry.* 2008;65(5):513–520.

18. Allgaier AK, Pietsch K, Frühe B, Sigl-Glöckner J, Schulte-Körne G. Screening for depression in adolescents: validity of the Patient Health Questionnaire in pediatric care. *Depress Anxiety.* 2012;29(10):906–913.

19. Kawa I, Carter JD, Joyce RR, et al. Gender differences in bipolar disorder: Age of onset, course, comorbidity, and symptom presentation. *Bipolar Disord.* 2005;7(2):119–125.

20. Vahdat Shariatpanaahi M, Vahdat Shariatpanaahi Z, Moshtaaghi M, Shahbaazi SH, Abadi A. The relationship between depression and serum ferritin level. *Eur J Clin Nutr.* 2007;61(4):532–535.

21. Reinecke MA, Curry JF, March JS. Findings from the Treatment for Adolescents with Depression Study (TADS): What have we learned? What do we need to know? *J Clin Child Adolesc Psychol.* 2009;38(6):761–767.

22. Dopp RR, Mooney AJ, Armitage R, King C. Exercise for adolescents with depressive disorders: a feasibility study. *Depress Res Treatment.* 2012;2012:257472.

23. Knox M, Lentini J, Cummings TS, McGrady A, Whearty K, Sancrant L. Game-based biofeedback for paediatric anxiety and depression. *Ment Health Fam Med.* 2011;8(3):195–203.

24. American Psychiatric Association. *Diagnostic and Statistical manual of Mental Disorders.* (4th ed., text rev.). Washington, DC: American Psychiatric Press; 2000.

25. Gehlert S, Song IH, Chang CH, Hartlage SA. The prevalence of premenstrual dysphoric disorder in a randomly selected group of urban and rural women. *Psychol Med.* 2009;39(1):129–136.

26. Potter J, Bouyer J, Trussell J, Moreau C. Premenstrual syndrome prevalence and fluctuation over time: results from a French population-based survey. *J Womens Health (Larchmt).* 2009;18(1):31–39.

27. Kornstein SG, Harvey AT, Rush AJ, et al. Self-reported premenstrual exacerbation of depressive symptoms in patients seeking treatment for major depression. *Psychol Med.* 2005;35(5): 683–692.

28. Hartlage SA, Brandenburg DL, Kravitz HM. Premenstrual exacerbation of depressive disorders in the United States. *Psychosom Med.* 2004;66(5):698–706.

29. Dias RS, Lafer B, Russo C, et al. Longitudinal follow-up of bipolar disorder in women with premenstrual exacerbation: findings from STEP-BD. *Am J Psychiatry.* 2011;168(4):386–394.

30. Inoue Y, Terao T, Iwata N, et al. Fluctuating serotonergic function in premenstrual dysphoric disorder and premenstrual syndrome: findings from neuroendocrine challenge tests. *Psychopharmacol (Berl).* 2007;190(2):213–219.

31. Sundström Poromaa I, Smith S, Gulinello M. GABA receptors, progesterone and premenstrual dysphoric disorder. *Arch Womens Ment Health.* 2003;6(1):23–41.

32. Schmidt PJ, Nieman LK, Danaceau MA, Adams LF, Rubinow DR. Differential behavioral effects of gonadal steroids in women with and in those without premenstrual syndrome. *N Engl J Med.* 1998;338(4):209–216.

33. Andrèen L, Nyberg S, Turkmen S, van Wingen G, Fernández G, Bäckström T. Sex steroid induced negative mood may be explained by the paradoxical effect mediated by GABAA modulators. *Psychoneuroendocrinol.* 2009;34(8):1121–1132.

34. Gingnell M, Morell A, Bannbers E, Wikström J, Sundström Poromaa I. Menstrual cycle effect on amygdale reactivity to emotional stimulation in premenstrual dysphoric disorder. *Horm Behav.* 2012;62(4):400–406.

35. Protopopescu X, Tuescher O, Pan H, et al. Toward a functional neuroanatomy of premenstrual dysphoric disorder. *J Affect Disord.* 2008;108(1–2):87–94.

36. Rubinow DR, Smith MJ, Schenkel LA, Schmidt PJ, Dancer K. Facial emotion discrimination across the menstrual cycle in women with premenstrual dysphoric disorder (PMDD) and controls. *J Affect Disord.* 2007;104(1–3):37–44.

37. Pearlstein T, Yonkers KA, Fayyad R, Gillespie JA. Pretreatment pattern of symptom expression in premenstrual dysphoric disorder. *J Affect Disord.* 2005;85(3):275–282.

38. Yen JY, Chang SJ, Ko CH, et al. The high sweet-fat food craving among women with premenstrual dysphoric disorder: emotional response, implicit attitude and rewards sensitivity. *Psychoneuroendocrinol.* 2010;35(8):1203–1212.

39. Reed SC, Levin FR, Evans SM. Changes in mood, cognitive performance and appetite in the late luteal and follicular phases of the menstrual cycle in women with and without PMDD (premenstrual dysphoric disorder). *Horm Behav.* 2008;54(1): 185–193.

40. Pilver CE, Libby DJ, Hoff RA. Premenstrual dysphoric disorder as a correlate of suicidal ideation, plans, and attempts among a nationally representative sample. *Soc Psychiatry Psychiatr Epidemiol.* 2013;48(3):437–446.

41. Berlin RE, Raju JD, Schmidt PJ, Adams LF, Rubinow DR. Effects of the menstrual cycle on measures of personality in women with premenstrual syndrome: a preliminary study. *J Clin Psychiatry.* 2001;62(5):337–342.

42. O'Boyle M, Severino SK, Hurt SW. Premenstrual syndrome and locus of control. *Int J Psychiatry Med.* 1988;18(1):67–74.

43. Epperson CN, Pittman B, Czarkowski KA, Stiklus S, Krystal JH, Grillon C. Luteal-phase accentuation of acoustic startle response in women with premenstrual dysphoric disorder. *Neuropsychopharmacology.* 2007;32(10):2190–2198.

44. Vichin M, Freeman EW, Lin H, Hillman J, Bui S. Premenstrual syndrome (PMS) in adolescents: severity and impairment. *J Ped Adol Gyn.* 2006;19(6):397–402.

45. Wittchen HU, Becker E, Lieb R, Krause P. Prevalence, incidence and stability of premenstrual dysphoric disorder in the community. *Psychol Med.* 2002;32(1):119–132.

46. Steiner M, Peer M, Macdougall M, Haskett R. The premenstrual tension syndrome rating scales: an updated version. *J Affect Disord.* 2011;135(1–3):82–88.

47. Accortt EE, Bismark A, Schneider TR, Allen JJ. Diagnosing premenstrual dysphoric disorder: the reliability of a structured clinical interview. *Arch Womens Mental Health.* 2011;14(3): 265–267.

48. Pearlstein TB, Stone AB, Lund SA, Scheft H, Zlotnick C, Brown WA. Comparison of fluoxetine, bupropion, and placebo in the treatment of premenstrual dysphoric disorder. *J Clin Psychopharmacol.* 1997;17(4):261–266.

49. Freeman EW, Rickels K, Sondheimer SJ, Polansky M. Differential response to antidepressants in women with premenstrual syndromepremenstrual dysphoric disorder: a randomized controlled trial. *Arch Gen Psychiatry.* 1999;56(10):932–939.

50. Eriksson E, Hedberg MA, Andersch B, Sundblad C. The serotonin reuptake inhibitor paroxetin is superior to the noradrenaline reuptake inhibitor maprotiline in the treatment of premenstrual syndrome. *Neuropsychopharmacology.* 1995;12(2):167–176.

51. Shah NR, Jones JB, Aperi J, Shemtov R, Karne A, Borenstein J. Selective serotonin reuptake inhibitors for premenstrual syndrome and premenstrual dysphoric disorder: a meta-analysis. *Obstet Gynecol.* 2008;111(5):1175–1182.

52. Freeman EW, Sondheimer SJ, Sammel MD, Ferdousi T, Lin H. A preliminary study of luteal phase versus symptom-onset dosing with escitalopram for premenstrual dysphoric disorder. *J Clin Psychiatry.* 2005;66(6):769–773.

53. Yonkers KA, Holthausen GA, Poschman K, Howell HB. Symptom-onset treatment for women with premenstrual dysphoric disorder. *J Clin Psychopharmacol.* 2006;26(2):198–120.

54. Miller MN, Newell CL, Miller BE, Frizzell PG, Kayser RA, Ferslew KE. Variable dosing of sertraline for premenstrual exacerbation of depression: a pilot study. *J Womens Health (Larchmt).* 2008;17(6):993–997.

55. Sundström I, Ashbrook D, Bäckström T. Reduced benzodiazepine sensitivity in patients with premenstrual syndrome: a pilot study. *Psychoneuroendocrinology.* 1997;22(1):25–38.

56. Freeman EW, Halbreich U, Grubb GS et al. An overview of 4 studies of a continuous oral contraceptive (levonorgestrel 90 mcgethinyl estradiol 20 mcg) on premenstrual dysphoric disorder and premenstrual syndrome. *Contraception.* 2012;85(5): 437–445.

57. Böttcher B, Radenbach K, Wildt L, Hinney B. Hormonal contraception and depression: a survey of the present state of knowledge. *Arch Gynecol Obstet*. 2012;286:231–236.

58. Fernyhough JC, Schimandle JJ, Weigel MC, Edwards CC, Levine AM. Chronic donor site pain complicating bone graft harvesting from the posterior iliac crest for spinal fusion. *Spine (Phila Pa 1976)*. 1992;17(12):1474–1480.

59. Wyatt KM, Dimmock PW, Ismail KM, Jones PW, O'Brien PM. The effectiveness of GnRHa with and without 'add-back' therapy in treating premenstrual syndrome: a meta-analysis. *BJOG*. 2004;111(6):585–593.

60. O'Brien PM, Abukhalil IE. Randomized controlled trial of the management of premenstrual syndrome and premenstrual mastalgia using luteal phase-only danazol. *Am J Obstet Gynecol*. 1999;180(1 Pt 1):18–23.

61. Cronje WH, Vashisht A, Studd JW. Hysterectomy and bilateral oophorectomy for severe premenstrual syndrome. *Hum Reprod*. 2004;19(9):2152–2155.

62. Atmaca M, Kumru S, Tezcan E. Fluoxetine versus Vitex agnus castus extract in the treatment of premenstrual dysphoric disorder. *Hum Psychopharmacol*. 2003;18(3):191–195.

63. Schellenberg R, Zimmerman C, Drewe J, Hoexter G, Zahner C. Dose-dependent efficacy of the Vitex agnus castus extract Ze 440 in patients suffering from premenstrual syndrome. *Phytomedicine*. 2012;19(14):1325–1331.

64. He Z, Chen R, Zhou Y. Treatment for premenstrual syndrome with Vitex agnus castus: a prospective, randomized, multicenter placebo controlled study in China. *Maturitas*. 2009;63(1):99–103.

65. Lustyk MK, Gerrish WG, Shaver S, Keys SL. Cognitive-behavioral therapy for premenstrual syndrome and premenstrual dysphoric disorder: a systematic review. *Arch Womens Mental Health*. 2009;12(2):85–96.

66. Daley A. Exercise and premenstrual symptomatology: a comprehensive review. *J Womens Health (Larchmt)*. 2009;18(6):895–899.

67. Thys-Jacobs S, Starkey P, Bernstein D, Tian J. Calcium carbonate and the premenstrual syndrome: effects on premenstrual and menstrual symptoms. Premenstrual Syndrome Study Group. *Am J Obstet Gynecol*. 1998;179(2):444–452.

68. Joffe H, Petrillo LF, Viguera AC, et al. Treatment of premenstrual worsening of depression with adjunctive oral contraceptive pills: a preliminary report. *J Clin Psychiatry*. 2007;68(12):1954–1962.

69. Steiner M, Pearlstein T, Cohen LS, et al. Expert guidelines for the treatment of severe PMS, PMDD, and comorbidities: the role of SSRIs. *J Womens Health (Larchmt)*. 2006;15(1):57–69.

70. March WA, Moore VM, Willson KJ, Phillips DI, Norman RJ, Davies MJ. The prevalence of polycystic ovary syndrome in a community sample assessed under contrasting diagnostic criteria. *Hum Reprod*. 2010;25(2):544–551.

71. Veltman-Verhulst SM, Boivin J, Eijkemans MJ, Faucer BJ. Emotional distress is a common risk in women with polycystic ovary syndrome: a systematic review and meta-analysis of 28 studies. *Hum Reprod Update*. 2012;18(6):638–651.

72. Hollinrake E, Abreu A, Maifeld M, Van Voorhis BJ, Dokras A. Increased risk of depressive disorders in women with polycystic ovary syndrome. *Fertil Steril*. 2007;87(6):1369–1376.

73. Rassi A, Veras AB, dos Reis M, et al. Prevalence of psychiatric disorders in patients with polycystic ovary syndrome. *Compr Psychiatry*. 2010;51(6):599–602.

74. Himelein MJ, Thatcher SS. Depression and body image among women with polycystic ovary syndrome. *J Health Psychol*. 2006;11(4):613–625.

75. Tan S, Hahn S, Benson S, et al. Psychological implications of infertility in women with polycystic ovary syndrome. *Hum Reprod*. 2008;23(9):2064–2071.

76. Pastore LM, Patrie JT, Morris WL, Dalal P, Bray MJ. Depression symptoms and body dissatisfaction associations among polycystic ovary syndrome women. *J Psychosom Res*. 2011;71(4):270–276.

77. Jedel E, Gustafson D, Waern M, et al. Sex steroids, insulin sensitivity and sympathetic nerve activity in relation to affective symptoms in women with polycystic ovary syndrome. *Psychoneuroendocrinol*. 2011;36(10):1470–1479.

78. Benson S, Arck PC, Tan S, et al. Disturbed stress responses in women with polycystic ovary syndrome. *Psychoneuroendocrinol*. 2009;34(5):727–735.

79. Escobar-Morreale HF, Botella-Carretero JI, Villuendas G, Sancho J, San Millan JI. Serum interleukin-18 concentrations are increased in the polycystic ovary syndrome: relationship to insulin resistance and to obesity. *J Clin Endocrinol Metab*. 2004;89:806–811.

80. Tasali E, Van Cauter E, Ehrmann DA. Polycystic ovary syndrome and obstructive sleep apnea. *Sleep Med Clin*. 2008;3(1):37–46.

81. Johnstone EB, Davis G, Zane LT, Cedars MI, Huddleston HG. Age-related differences in the reproductive and metabolic implications of polycystic ovary syndrome: findings in an obese, United States population. *Gynecol Endocrinol*. 2012;28(10):819–822.

82. Liang SJ, Hsu CS, Tzeng CR, Chen CH, Hsu MI. Clinical and biochemical presentation of polycystic ovary syndrome in women between the ages of 20 and 40. *Hum Reprod*. 2011;26(12):3443–3449.

83. Wild R, Carmina E, Diamanti-Kandarakis E, et al. Assessment of cardiovascular risk and prevention of cardiovascular disease in women with the polycystic ovary syndrome: A consensus statement by the Androgen Excess and Polycystic Ovary Syndrome (AE-PCOS) Society. *J Clin Endocrinol Metab*. 2010;95(5):2038–2049.

84. Rofey DL, Szigethy EM, Noll RB, Dahl RE, Lobst E, Arslanian SA. Cognitive-behavioral therapy for physical and emotional disturbances in adolescents with polycystic ovary syndrome: apilot study. *J Pediatr Psychol*. 2009;34:156–163.

85. Thompson RL, Buckley JD, Lim SS, et al. Lifestyle management improves quality of life and depression in overweight and obese women with polycystic ovary syndrome. *Fertil Steril*. 2010;94(5):1812–1816.

86. Kashani L, Omidvar T, Farzmand B, et al. Does pioglitazone improve depression through insulin-sensitization? Results of a randomized double-blind metformin-controlled trial in patients with polycystic ovarian syndrome and comorbid depression. *Psychoneuroendocrinol*. 2013;38(6):767–776.

87. O'Neil A, Sanna L, Redlich C, et al. The impact of statins on psychological wellbeing: a systematic review and meta-analysis. *BMC Medicine*. 2012;10:154–163.

88. Rummel-Kluge C, Kornossa K, Schwarz S. Head-to-head comparisons of metabolic side effects of second generation antipsychotics in the treatment of schizophrenia: a systematic review and meta-analysis. *Schiz Res*. 2010;123(2–3):225–233.

89. Chandra A, Martinez GM, Mosher WD, Abma JC, Jones J. Fertility, family planning, and reproductive health of U.S. women: data

from the 2002 National Survey of Family Growth. National Center for Health Statistics. *Vital Health Stat.* 2005;25:1–160.

90. Domar AD, Zuttermeister PC, Friedman R. The psychological impact of infertility: a comparison with patients with other medical conditions. *J Psychosom Obstet Gynaecol.* 1993;14 Suppl: 45–52.

91. Nelson CJ, Shindel AW, Naughton CK, Ohebshalom M, Mulhall JP. Prevalence and predictors of sexual problems, relationship stress, and depression in female partners of infertile couples. *J Sex Med.* 2008;5(8):1907–1914.

92. Drosdzol A, Skrzypulec V. Depression and anxiety among Polish infertile couples–an evaluative prevalence study. *J Psychosom Obstet Gynaecol.* 2009;30(1):11–20.

93. Al-Homaidan HT. Depression among women with primary infertility attending an infertility clinic in Riyadh, Kingdom of Saudi Arabia: rate, severity, and contributing factors. *Int J Health Sci (Qassim).* 2011;5(2):108–115.

94. Epstein YM, Rosenberg HS. Depression in primary versus secondary infertility egg recipients. *Fertil Steril.* 2005;83(6):1882–1884.

95. Hjelmstedt A, Andersson L, Skoog-Svanberg A, Bergh T, Boivin J, Collins A. Gender differences in psychological reactions to infertility among couples seeking IVF- and ICSI-treatment. *Acta Obstet Gynecol Scand.* 1999;78(1):42–48.

96. Noorbala AA, Ramezanzadeh F, Abedinia N, Bagheri SA, Jafarabadi M. Study of psychiatric disorders among fertile and infertile women and some predisposing factors. *J Fam Reprod Health.* 2007;1(1):6–11.

97. Domar AD, Broome A, Zuttermeister PC, Seibel M, Friedman R. The prevalence and predictability of depression in infertile women. *Fertil Steril.* 1992;58(6):1158–1163.

98. Hart VA. Infertility and the role of psychotherapy. *Issues Ment Health Nurs.* 2002;23(1):31–41.

99. Terry DJ, Hynes GJ. Adjustment to a low-control situation: Reexamining the role of coping responses. *J Pers Soc Psychol.* 1998;74(4):1078–1092.

100. Yli-Kuha AN, Gissler M, Klemetti R, Luoto R, Koivisto E, Hemminki E. Psychiatric disorders leading to hospitalization before and after infertility treatments. *Hum Reprod.* 2010;25(8):2018–2023.

101. Lewis AM, Liu D, Stuart SP, Ryan G. Less depressed or less forthcoming? Self-report of depression symptoms in women preparing for in vitro fertilization. *Arch Womens Ment Health.* 2012;16(2):87–92.

102. Shalev E, Leung PC. Gonadotropin-releasing hormone and reproductive medicine. *J Obstet Gynaecol Can.* 2003;25:98–113.

103. Warnock JK, Bundren JC, Morris DW. Depressive symptoms associated with gonadotropin-releasing hormone agonists. *Depress Anxiety.* 1998;7(4):171–177.

104. Bloch M, Azem F, Aharonov I, et al. GnRH-agonist induced depressive and anxiety symptoms during in vitro fertilization-embryo transfer cycles. *Fertil Steril.* 2011;95(1):307–309.

105. Herod SM, Dettmer AM, Novak MA, Meyer JS, Cameron JL. Sensitivity to stress-induced reproductive dysfunction is associated with a selective but not a generalized increase in activity of the adrenal axis. *Am J Physiol Endocrinol Metab.* 2011; 300(1):E28–36.

106. Matthiesen SM, Frederiksen Y, Ingerslev HJ, Zachariae R. Stress, distress and outcome of assisted reproductive technology (ART): a meta-analysis. *Hum Reprod.* 2011;26(10):2763–2776.

107. Ramezanzadeh F, Noorbala AA, Abedinia N, Forooshani AR, Naghizadeh MM. Psychiatric Intervention Improved Pregnancy Rates in Infertile Couples. *Malays J Med Sci.* 2011; 18(1):16–24.

108. Boivin J, Griffiths E, Venetis CA. Emotional distress in infertile women and failure of assisted reproductive technologies: meta-analysis of prospective psychosocial studies. *BMJ.* 2011; 342:d223.

109. van den Broeck U, Holvoet L, Enzlin P, Bakelants E, Demyttenaere K, D'Hooghe T. Reasons for dropout in infertility treatment. *Gynecol Obstet Invest.* 2009;68(1):58–64.

110. Dhaliwal LK, Gupta KR, Gopalan S, Kulhara P. Psychological aspects of infertility due to various causes-Prospective study. *Int J Fertil Womens Med.* 2004;49:44–48.

111. Mahlstedt PP, Macduff S, Bernstein J. Emotional factors and the in vitro fertilization and embryo transfer process. *J In Vitro Fert Embryo Transf.* 1987;4(4):232–236.

112. Wischmann T. Implications of psychosocial support in infertility—a critical appraisal. *J Psychosom Obstet Gynaecol.* 2008;29(2): 83–90.

113. Carter J, Applegarth L, Josephs L, Grill E, Baser RE, Rosenwaks Z. A cross-sectional cohort study of infertile women awaiting oocyte donation: the emotional, sexual, and quality-of-life impact. *Fertil Steril.* 2011;95(2):711–716.

114. Verhaak CM, Smeenk JM, van Minnen A, Kremer JA, Kraaimaat FW. A longitudinal, prospective study on emotional adjustment before, during and after consecutive fertility treatment cycles. *Hum Reprod.* 2005;20(8):2253–2260.

115. van Randenborgh A, de Jong-Meyer R, Hüffmeier J. Decision making in depression: differences in decisional conflict between healthy and depressed individuals. *Clin Psychol Psychother.* 2010;17(4):285–298.

116. Sejbaek CS, Hageman I, Pinborg A, Hougaard CO, Schmidt L. Incidence of depression and influence of depression on the number of treatment cycles and births in a national cohort of 42 880 women treated with ART. *Hum Reprod.* 2013;28(4): 1100–1109.

117. Burns LH. Psychiatric aspects of infertility and infertility treatments. *Psychiatr Clin North Am* 2007;30(4):689–716.

118. Daniluk JC. Reconstructing their lives: a longitudinal, qualitative analysis of the transition to biological childlessness for infertile couples. *J Couns Dev.* 2001;79,439–449.

119. Schmidt L, Holstein BE, Christensen U, Boivin J. Communication and coping as predictors of fertility problem stress: cohort study of 816 participants who did not achieve a delivery after 12 months of fertility treatment. *Hum Reprod.* 2005; 20(11):3248–3256.

120. Lok IH, Lee DT, Cheung LP, Chung WS, Lo WK, Haines CJ. Psychiatric morbidity amongst infertile Chinese women undergoing treatment with assisted reproductive technology and the impact of treatment failure. *Gynecol Obstet Invest.* 2002;53(4):195–199.

121. Ridenour AF, Yorgason JB, Peterson B. The Infertility Resilience Model: assessing individual, couple, and external predictive factors. *Contemporary Family Therapy.* 2009;31(1):34–51.

122. Olshansky E, Sereika S. The transition from pregnancy to postpartum in previously infertile women: a focus on depression. *Arch Psychiatr Nurs.* 2005;19(6):273–280.

123. Newton CR, Hearn MT, Yuzpe AA. Psychological assessment and follow-up after in vitro fertilization: assessing the impact of failure. *Fertil Steril.* 1990;54(5):879–886.

124. Sbaragli C, Morgante G, Goracci A, Hofkens T, De Leo V, Castrogiovanni P. Infertility and psychiatric morbidity. *Fertil Steril.* 2008;90(6):2107–2111.

125. Volgsten H, Skoog Svanberg A, Ekselius L, Lundkvist O, Sundström Poromaa I. Prevalence of psychiatric disorders in infertile women and men undergoing in vitro fertilization treatment. *Hum Reprod.* 2008;23(9):2056–2063.

126. Verhaak CM, Lintsen AM, Evers AW, Braat DD. Who is at risk of emotional problems and how do you know? Screening of women going for IVF treatment. *Hum Reprod.* 2010;25(5):1234–1240.

127. van den Broeck U, Emery M, Wischmann T, Thorn P. Counseling in infertility: individual, couple and group interventions. *Patient Educ Couns.* 2010;81(3):422–428.

128. Levinson W, Gorawara-Bhat R, Lamb J. A study of patient clues and physician responses in primary care and surgical settings. *J Am Med Assoc.* 2000;284(8):1021–1027.

129. Easter DW, Beach W. Competent patient care is dependent upon attending to empathic opportunities presented during interview sessions. *Curr Surg.* 2004;61(3):313–318.

130. Olivius C, Friden B, Borg G, Bergh C. Why do couples discontinue in vitro fertilization treatment? A cohort study. *Fertil Steril.* 2004;81(2):258–261.

131. Smeenk JM, Verhaak CM, Stolwijk AM, Kremer JA, Braat DD. Reasons for dropout in an in vitro fertilizationintracytoplasmic sperm injection program. *Fertil Steril.* 2004;81(2):262–268.

132. Verberg MF, Eijkemans MJ, Heijnen EM, et al. Why do couples drop-out from IVF treatment? A prospective cohort study. *Hum Reprod.* 2008;23(9):2050–2055.

133. Schneiderman N, Antoni MH, Saab PG, Ironson G. Health psychology: psychosocial and biobehavioral aspects of chronic disease management. *Annual Rev Psychol.* 2001;52:555–580.

134. Fekete EM, Antoni MH, Schneiderman N. Psychosocial and behavioral interventions for chronic medical conditions. *Curr Opin Psychiatry.* 2007;20(2):152–157.

135. Burnett JA. Cultural considerations in counseling couples who experience infertility. *J Multicult Couns Devel.* 2009;37(3):166–177.

136. Boivin J. A review of psychosocial interventions in infertility. *Soc Sci Med.* 2003;57(12):2325–2341.

137. Stanton AL, Dunkel-Schetter C. *Infertility: Perspectives from Stress and Coping Research.* New York, NY: Plenum; 1991:183–196.

138. Facchinetti F, Tarabusi M, Volpe A. Cognitive-behavioral treatment decrease cardiovascular and neuroendocrine reaction to stress in women waiting for assisted reproduction. *Psychoneuroendocrinology.* 2004;29(2):162–173.

139. Faramarzi M, Kheirkhah F, Esmaelzadeh S, Alipour A, Hjiahmadi M, Rahnama J. Is psychotherapy a reliable alternative to pharmacotherapy to promote the mental health of infertile women? A randomized clinical trial. *Eur J Obstet Gynecol Reprod Biol.* 2008;141(1):49–53.

140. Koszycki D, Bisserbe JC, Blier P, Bradwejn J, Markowitz J. Interpersonal psychotherapy versus brief supportive therapy for depressed infertile women: first pilot randomized controlled trial. *Arch Womens Ment Health.* 2012;15(3):193–201.

141. Tarabusi M, Facchinetti F. Psychological group support attenuates distress of waiting in couples scheduled for assisted reproduction. *J Psychosom Obstet Gynecol.* 2004;25(3–4):273–279.

142. Domar AD, Clapp D, Slawsby EA, Dusek J, Kessel B, Freizinger M. Impact of group psychological interventions on pregnancy rates in infertile women. *Fertil Steril.* 2000;73(4):805–811.

143. Terzioglu F. Investigation into effectiveness of counseling on assisted reproductive techniques in Turkey. *J Psychosom Obstet Gynaecol.* 2001;22(3):133–141.

144. Friedman BE, Rogers JL, Shahine LK, Westphal LM, Lathi RB. Effect of selective serotonin reuptake inhibitors on in vitro fertilization outcome. *Fertil Steril.* 2009;92(4):1312–1314.

145. Rahimi R, Nikfar S, Abdollahi M. Pregnancy outcomes following exposure to serotonin reuptake inhibitors: a meta-analysis of clinical trials. *Reprod Toxicol.* 2006;22(4):571–575.

146. Kessler RC, McGonagle KA, Swartz M, Blazer DG, Nelson CB. Sex and depression in the National Comorbidity Survey. I: Lifetime prevalence, chronicity and recurrence. *J Affect Disord.* 1993;29(2–3):85–96.

147. Bromberger JT, Kravitz HM, Chang YF, Cyranowski JM, Brown C, Matthews KA. Major depression during and after the menopausal transition: Study of Women's Health Across the Nation (SWAN). *Psychol Med.* 2011;41(9):1879–1888.

148. Bromberger JT, Kravitz HM. Mood and menopause: findings from the Study of Women's Health Across the Nation (SWAN) over 10 years. *Obstet Gynecol Clin North Am.* 2011;38(3):609–625.

149. Everson-Rose SA, Meyer PM, Powell LH, et al. Depressive symptoms, insulin resistance, and risk of diabetes in women at midlife. *Diabetes Care.* 2004;27(12):2856–2862.

150. Janssen I, Powell LH, Matthews KA, et al. Depressive symptoms are related to progression of coronary calcium in midlife women: the Study of Women's Health Across the Nation (SWAN) Heart Study. *Am Heart J.* 2011;161(6):1186–1191.

151. Matthews KA, Schott LL, Bromberger J, Cyranowski J, Everson-Rose SA, Sowers MF. Associations between depressive symptoms and inflammatoryhemostatic markers in women during the menopausal transition. *Psychosom Med.* 2007;69(2):124–130.

152. Schnatz PF, Nudy M, Shively CA, Powell A, O'Sullivan DM. A prospective analysis of the association between cardiovascular disease and depression in middle-aged women. *Menopause.* 2011;18(10):1096–1100.

153. Terauchi M, Hiramitsu S, Akiyoshi M, et al. Associations among depression, anxiety and somatic symptoms in peri- and postmenopausal women. *J Obstet Gynaecol Res.* 2013;39(5):1007–1013.

154. Braden JB, Young A, Sullivan MD, Walitt B, Lacroix AZ, Martin L. Predictors of change in pain and physical functioning among postmenopausal women with recurrent pain conditions in the women's health initiative observational cohort. *J Pain.* 2012;13(1):64–72.

155. Yirmiya R, Bab I. Major depression is a risk factor for low bone mineral density: a meta-analysis. *Biol Psychiatry.* 2009;66(5):423–432.

156. Woods NF, Smith-DiJulio K, Percival DB, Tao EY, Mariella A, Mitchell S. Depressed mood during the menopausal transition and early postmenopause: observations from the Seattle Midlife Women's Health Study. *Menopause.* 2008;15(2):223–232.

157. Ryan J, Ancelin ML. Polymorphisms of estrogen receptors and risk of depression: therapeutic implications. *Drugs.* 2012;72(13):1725–1738.

158. Ryan J, Scali J, Carrière I, et al. Oestrogen receptor polymorphisms and late-life depression. *Br J Psychiatry.* 2011;199(2):126–131.

159. Prossnitz ER, Oprea TI, Sklar LA, Arterburn JB. The ins and outs of GPR30: a transmembrane estrogen receptor. *J Steroid Biochem Mol Biol.* 2008;109(3–5):350–353.

160. Wilkie MJ, Smith D, Reid IC, et al. A splice site polymorphism in the G-protein beta subunit influences antidepressant efficacy in depression. *Pharmacogenet Genomics.* 2007;17(3):207–215.

161. Dennerstein L, Smith AM, Morse C, et al. Menopausal symptoms in Australian women. *Med J Australia*. 1993;159(4):232–236.

162. Freeman EW, Sammel MD, Liu L, Gracia CR, Nelson DB, Hollander L. Hormones and menopausal status as predictors of depression in women in transition to menopause. *Arch Gen Psychiatry*. 2004;61(1):62–70.

163. Laughlin GA, Barrett-Connor E. Sexual dimorphism in the influence of advanced aging on adrenal hormone levels: the Rancho Bernardo Study. *J Clin Endocrinol Metab*. 2000;85(10):3561–3568.

164. Lasley BL, Crawford S, McConnell DS. Adrenal androgens and the menopausal transition. *Obstet Gynecol Clin North Am*. 2011;38(3):467–475.

165. Crawford S, Santoro N, Laughlin GA, et al. Circulating dehydroepiandrosterone sulfate concentrations during the menopausal transition. *J Clin Endocrinol Metab*. 2009;94(8):2945–2951.

166. Joffe H, Hall JE, Soares CN, et al. Vasomotor symptoms are associated with depression in perimenopausal women seeking primary care. *Menopause*. 2002;9(6):392–398.

167. Burleson MH, Todd M, Trevathan WR. Daily vasomotor symptoms, sleep problems, and mood: using daily data to evaluate the domino hypothesis in middle-aged women. *Menopause*. 2010;17(1):87–95.

168. Bromberger JT, Schott LL, Kravitz HM, et al. Longitudinal change in reproductive hormones and depressive symptoms across the menopausal transition: results from the Study of Women's Health Across the Nation (SWAN). *Arch Gen Psychiatry*. 2010;67(6):598–607.

169. Cooke DJ, Greene JG. Types of life events in relation to symptoms at the climacterium. *J Psychosom Res*. 1981;25(1):5–11.

170. Dennerstein L, Dudley E, Guthrie J. Empty nest or revolving door? A prospective study of women's quality of life in midlife during the phase of children leaving and re-entering the home. *Psychol Med*. 2002;32(3):545–550.

171. Avis NE, McKinlay SM. A longitudinal analysis of women's attitudes toward the menopause: results from the Massachusetts Women's Health Study. *Maturitas*. 1991;13(1):65–79.

172. Morse CA, Dudley E, Guthrie J, Dennerstein L. Relationships between premenstrual complaints and perimenopausal experiences. *J Psychosom Obstet Gynaecol*. 1998;19(4):182–191.

173. Igarashi M, Saito H, Morioka Y, Oiji A, Nadaoka T, Kashiwakura M. Stress vulnerability and climacteric symptoms: life events, coping behavior, and severity of symptoms. *Gynecol Obstet Invest*. 2000;49(3):170–178.

174. Soares CN, Taylor V. Effects and management of the menopausal transition in women with depression and bipolar disorder. *J Clin Psychiatry*. 2007;68(Suppl 9):16–21.

175. Freeman EW, Sammel MD, Lin H, Gracia CR, Kapoor S. Symptoms in the menopausal transition: hormone and behavioral correlates. *Obstet Gynecol*. 2008;111(1):127–136.

176. Bromberger JT, Kravitz HM, Chang Y, et al. Does risk for anxiety increase during the menopausal transition? Study of women's health across the nation. *Menopause*. 2013;20(5):488–495.

177. Greendale GA, Wight RG, Huang MH, et al. Menopause-associated symptoms and cognitive performance: results from the study of women's health across the nation. *Am J Epidemiol*. 2010;171(11):1214–1224.

178. Seritan AL, Iosif AM, Park JH, DeatherageHand D, Sweet RL, Gold EB. Self-reported anxiety, depressive, and vasomotor symptoms: a study of perimenopausal women presenting to a specialized midlife assessment center. *Menopause*. 2010;17(2):410–414.

179. Bromberger JT, Matthews KA, Schott LL, et al. Depressive symptoms during the menopausal transition: the Study of Women's Health Across the Nation (SWAN). *J Affect Disord*. 2007;103(1–3):267–272.

180. McKinlay SM, Brambilla DJ, Posner JG. The normal menopause transition. *Maturitas*. 1992;14(2):103–115.

181. Schmidt PJ, Haq N, Rubinow DR. A longitudinal evaluation of the relationship between reproductive status and mood in perimenopausal women. *Am J Psychiatry*. 2004;161(12):2238–2244.

182. Mishra GD, Kuh D. Health symptoms during midlife in relation to menopausal transition: British prospective cohort study. *BMJ*. 2012;344:e402.

183. Harlow BW, Cramer DW, Annis KM. Association of medically treated depression and age at natural menopause. *Am J Epidemiol*. 1995;141(12):1170–1176.

184. Avis NE, Brockwell S, Randolph JF, et al. Longitudinal changes in sexual functioning as women transition through menopause: results from the Study of Women's Health Across the Nation. *Menopause*. 2009;16(3):442–452.

185. Soares CN, Almeida OP, Joffe H, Cohen LS. Efficacy of estradiol for the treatment of depressive disorders in perimenopausal women: a double-blind, randomized, placebo-controlled trial. *Arch Gen Psychiatry*. 2001;58(6):529–534.

186. Steiger A, Dresler M, Kluge M, Schüssler P. Pathology of sleep, hormones and depression. *Pharmacopsychiatry*. 2013;46(Suppl 1): S30–S35.

187. Perez-López FR, Chedraui P, Gilbert JJ, Pérez-Roncero G. Cardiovascular risk in menopausal women and prevalent related co-morbid conditions: facing the post-Women's Health Initiative era. *Fertil Steril*. 2009;92(4):1171–1186.

188. DiMatteo MR, Lepper HS, Croghan TW. Depression is a risk factor for noncompliance with medical treatment: meta-analysis of the effects of anxiety and depression on patient adherence. *Arch Intern Med*. 2000;160(14):2101–2107.

189. Harlow BL, Cohen LS, Otto MW, Spiegelman D, Cramer DW. Prevalence and predictors of depressive symptoms in older premenopausal women: the Harvard Study of Moods and Cycles. *Arch Gen Psychiatry*. 1999;56(5):418–424.

190. Roshanaei-Moghaddam B, Katon WJ, Russo J. The longitudinal effects of depression on physical activity. *Gen Hosp Psychiatry*. 2009;31(4):306–315.

191. Gambacciani M, Ciaponi M, Cappagli B, Genazzani AR. Effects of low-dose continuous combined conjugated estrogens and medroxyprogesterone acetate on menopausal symptoms, body weight, bone density, and metabolism in postmenopausal women. *Am J Obstet Gynecol*. 2001;185(5):1180–1185.

192. Harlow SD, Gass M, Hall JE, et al. Executive summary of the Stages of Reproductive Aging Workshop +10: addressing the unfinished agenda of staging reproductive aging. *Climacteric*. 2012;15(2):105–114.

193. Heinemann LA, Potthoff P, Schneider HP. International versions of the Menopause Rating Scale (MRS). *Health Qual Life Outcomes*. 2003;1:28.

194. Hilditch JR, Lewis J, Peter A, et al. A menopause-specific quality of life questionnaire: development and psychometric properties. *Maturitas*. 2008;61(1–2):107–121.

195. 5JT, Meyer PM, Kravitz HM, et al. Psychologic distress and natural menopause: a multiethnic community study. *Am J Public Health*. 2001;91(9):1435–1442.

196. Ayers B, Smith M, Hellier J, Mann E, Hunter MS. Effectiveness of group and self-help cognitive behavior therapy in reducing

problematic menopausal hot flushes and night sweats (MENOS 2): a randomized controlled trial. *Menopause*. 2012;19(7): 749–759.

197. Nelson HD, Haney E, Humphrey L, et al. Management of menopause-related symptoms. *Evid Rep Technol Assess (Summ)*. 2005;(120):1–6.

198. Suvanto-Luukkonen E, Koivunen R, Sundström H, et al. Citalopram and fluoxetine in the treatment of postmenopausal symptoms: a prospective, randomized, 9-month, placebo-controlled, double-blind study. *Menopause*. 2005;12(1):18–26.

199. Stearns V, Johnson MD, Rae JM, et al. Active tamoxifen metabolite plasma concentrations after coadministration of tamoxifen and the selective serotonin reuptake inhibitor paroxetine. *J Natl Cancer Inst*. 2003;95(23):1758–1764.

200. Loprinzi CL, Kugler JW, Sloan JA, et al. Venlafaxine in management of hot flashes in survivors of breast cancer: a randomised controlled trial. *Lancet*. 2000;356(9247):2059–2063.

201. Aedo S, Cavada G, Campodonico I, Porcile A, Irribarra C. Sertraline improves the somatic and psychological symptoms of the climacteric syndrome. *Climacteric*. 2011;14(5):590–595.

202. Barton DL, LaVasseur BI, Sloan JA, et al. Phase III, placebo-controlled trial of three doses of citalopram for the treatment of hot flashes: NCCTG trial N05C9. *J Clin Oncol*. 2010;28(20): 3278–3283.

203. Pinkerton JV, Constantine G, Hwang E, Cheng RF, Investigators S. Desvenlafaxine compared with placebo for treatment of menopausal vasomotor symptoms: a 12-week, multicenter, parallel-group, randomized, double-blind, placebo-controlled efficacy trial. *Menopause*. 2013;20(1):28–37.

204. LaCroix AZ, Freeman EW, Larson J, et al. Effects of escitalopram on menopause-specific quality of life and pain in healthy menopausal women with hot flashes: a randomized controlled trial. *Maturitas*. 2012;73(4):361–368.

205. Joffe H, Soares CN, Petrillo LF, et al. Treatment of depression and menopause-related symptoms with the serotonin-norepinephrine reuptake inhibitor duloxetine. *J Clin Psychiatry*. 2007;68(6):943–950.

206. Biglia N, Kubatzki F, Sgandurra P, et al. Mirtazapine for the treatment of hot flushes in breast cancer survivors: a prospective pilot trial. *Breast J*. 2007;13(5):490–495.

207. Oishi A, Mochizuki Y, Otsu R, Inaba N. Pilot study of fluvoxamine treatment for climacteric symptoms in Japanese women. *Biopsychosoc Med*. 2007;1:12.

208. Mbaya P, Alam F, Ashim S, Bennett D. Cardiovascular effects of high dose venlafaxine XL in patients with major depressive disorder. *Hum Psychopharmacol*. 2007;22(3):129–133.

209. Blümel JE, Cano A, Mezones-Holguín E, et al. A multinational study of sleep disorders during female mid-life. *Maturitas*. 2012;72(4):359–366.

210. Montejo AL, Llorca G, Izquierdo JA, Rico-Villademoros F. Incidence of sexual dysfunction associated with antidepressant agents: a prospective multicenter study of 1022 outpatients. Spanish Working Group for the Study of Psychotropic-Related Sexual Dysfunction. *J Clin Psychiatry*. 2001;62(Suppl 3):10–21.

211. Clayton AH, Pradko JF, Croft HA, et al. Prevalence of sexual dysfunction among newer antidepressants. *J Clin Psychiatry*. 2002;63(4):357–366.

212. Lee KU, Lee YM, Nam JM, et al. Antidepressant-induced sexual dysfunction among newer antidepressants in a naturalistic setting. *Psychiatry Investig*. 2010;7(1):55–59.

213. Greendale GA, Huang MH, Wight RG, et al. Effects of the menopause transition and hormone use on cognitive performance in midlife women. *Neurology*. 2009;72(21):1850–1857.

214. van Laar MW, Volkerts ER, Verbaten MN, Trooster S, van Megen HJ, Kenemans JL. Differential effects of amitriptyline, nefazodone and paroxetine on performance and brain indices of visual selective attention and working memory. *Psychopharmacology (Berl)*. 2002;162(4):351–363.

215. Herrera-Guzmán I, Gudayol-Ferré E, Lira-Mandujano J, et al. Cognitive predictors of treatment response to bupropion and cognitive effects of bupropion in patients with major depressive disorder. *Psychiatry Res*. 2008;160(1):72–82.

216. Shea ML, Garfield LD, Teitelbaum S, et al. Serotonin-norepinephrine reuptake inhibitor therapy in late-life depression is associated with increased marker of bone resorption. *Osteoporosis International*. 2013;24(5):1741–1749.

217. Cohen LS, Soares CN, Poitras JR, Prouty J, Alexander AB, Shifren JL. Short-term use of estradiol for depression in perimenopausal and postmenopausal women: a preliminary report. *Am J Psychiatry*. 2003;160(8):1519–1522.

218. Schmidt PJ, Nieman L, Danaceau MA, et al. Estrogen replacement in perimenopause-related depression: a preliminary report. *Am J Obstet Gynecol*. 2000;183(2):414–420.

219. Morrison MF, Kallan MJ, Ten Have T, Katz I, Tweedy K, Battistini M. Lack of efficacy of estradiol for depression in postmenopausal women: a randomized, controlled trial. *Biol Psychiatry*. 2004; 55(4):406–412.

220. Morgan ML, Cook IA, Rapkin AJ, Leuchter AF. Estrogen augmentation of antidepressants in perimenopausal depression: a pilot study. *J Clin Psychiatry*. 2005;66(6):774–780.

221. Hsia J, Langer RD, Manson JE, et al. Conjugated equine estrogens and coronary heart disease: the Women's Health Initiative. *Arch Intern Med*. 2006;166:357–365.

222. Rossouw JE, Prentice RL, Manson JE, et al. Postmenopausal hormone therapy and risk of cardiovascular disease by age and years since menopause. *JAMA*. 2007;297(13):1465–1477.

223. Curb JD, Prentice RL, Bray PF, et al. Venous thrombosis and conjugated equine estrogen in women without a uterus. *Arch Intern Med*. 2006;166(7):772–780.

224. Prentice RL, Manson JE, Langer RD, et al. Benefits and risks of postmenopausal hormone therapy when it is initiated soon after menopause. *Am J Epidemiol*. 2009;170(1):12–23.

225. Chlebowski RT, Hendrix SL, Langer RD, et al. Influence of estrogen plus progestin on breast cancer and mammography in healthy postmenopausal women: the Women's Health Initiative Randomized Trial. *JAMA*. 2003;289(24):3243–3253.

226. Grady D, Gebretsadik T, Kerlikowske K, Ernster V, Petitti D. Hormone replacement therapy and endometrial cancer risk: a meta-analysis. *Obstet Gynecol*. 1995;85(2):304–313.

227. Rogines-Velo MP, Heberle AE, Joffe H. Effect of medroxyprogesterone on depressive symptoms in depressed and nondepressed perimenopausal and postmenopausal women after discontinuation of transdermal estradiol therapy. *Menopause*. 2012;19(4):471–475.

228. Treloar AE, Boynton RE, Behn BG, Brown BW. Variation of the human menstrual cycle through reproductive life. *Int J Fertil*. 1967;12(1 Pt 2):77–126.

229. Joffe H, Kim DR, Foris JM, et al. Menstrual dysfunction prior to onset of psychiatric illness is reported more commonly by women with bipolar disorder than by women with unipolar

depression and healthy controls. *J Clin Psychiatry*. 2006;67(2): 297–304.

230. Morrell MJ, Hayes FJ, Sluss PM, et al. Hyperandrogenism, ovulatory dysfunction, and polycystic ovary syndrome with valproate versus lamotrigine. *Ann Neurol*. 2008;64(2):200–211.

231. Joffe H, Cohen LS, Suppes T, et al. Valproate is associated with new-onset oligoamenorrhea with hyperandrogenism in women withbipolar disorder. *Biol Psychiatry*. 2006;59(11):1078–1086.

232. Nelson-DeGrave VL, Wickenheisser JK, Cockrell JE, et al. Valproate potentiates androgen biosynthesis in human ovarian theca cells. *Endocrinology*. 2004;145(2):799–808.

233. Joffe H, Cohen LS, Suppes T, et al. Longitudinal follow-up of reproductive and metabolic features of valproate-associated polycystic ovarian syndrome features: A preliminary report. *Biol Psychiatry*. 2006;60(12):1378–1381.

234. Ornoy A. Valproic acid in pregnancy: how much are we endangering the embryo and fetus?*Reprod Toxicol*. 2009;28(1):1–10.

235. Ajmal A, Joffe H, Nachtigall LB. Psychotropic-induced hyperprolactinemia: a clinical review. *Psychosomatics*. 2014;55(1):29–36.

236. Shim JC, Shin JG, Kelly DL, et al. Adjunctive treatment with a dopamine partial agonist, aripiprazole, for antipsychotic-induced hyperprolactinemia: a placebo-controlled trial. *Am J Psychiatry*. 2007;164(9):1404–1410.

237. Chang S, Chen C, Lu M. Cabergoline-induced psychotic exacerbation in schizophrenic patients. *Gen Hosp Psychiatry*. 2008;30(4):378–380.

238. Melkersson K. Differences in prolactin elevation and related symptoms of atypical antipsychotics in schizophrenic patients. *J Clin Psychiatry*. 2005;66(6):761–767.

CHAPTER 9

Depression in Obstetrical Conditions

Laura Miller, MD
Leena Mittal, MD
Lindsay Merrill, MD
Audra Robertson Meadows, MD

PERINATAL DEPRESSION

Depression is a common complication of pregnancy and the post-partum period, with significant implications for a woman, her fetus, and her family. The biological, psychological, and social changes inherent in this time all contribute to the propensity toward mood disorder during this critical period. Women with mood disorders during the perinatal period are faced with challenging decisions when considering treatment. Mental health and obstetrical providers have important roles in helping women and their families weigh the impact of untreated mental health symptoms against the impact of potential treatments.

Case illustration: Shanté, a 23-year-old single woman, gave birth to her first child 6 weeks ago. Labor and delivery had been painful but uncomplicated, and her baby, a son she named Ryan, was healthy. Shanté was happy, although tired. She began to feel vulnerable and upset when she tried breastfeeding Ryan and he had difficulty latching on. Although the hospital nurse assured her this happens often, and a lactation consultant gave her tips about helping Ryan to latch, Shanté began to wonder if she would be able to parent Ryan successfully. After taking Ryan home 2 days later, she began to feel overwhelmed. She became afraid to fall asleep in case she would miss Ryan's crying or be unprepared to feed him. She felt exhausted. By 3 weeks postpartum, she felt emotionally numb and lost interest in food. She stopped showering, getting dressed or answering her phone, instead sitting leadenly in a chair near Ryan's crib as he napped. One night Ryan slept longer than usual, and Shanté became convinced he was dead. Even after seeing that he was breathing comfortably, she had the thought that unlike other mothers, she would be unable to keep her baby alive, so did not deserve to be alive herself. She had fleeting thoughts of overdosing on over-the-counter pills from the medicine cabinet, but did not act on these because she felt she could not burden anyone else with taking care of Ryan.

EPIDEMIOLOGY

Depression is one of the most common disorders in the perinatal period, with higher prevalence than gestational hypertension or diabetes mellitus (**Fig. 9-1**). The risk of depression is elevated during pregnancy and the first year postpartum, particularly during the first 3 months postpartum. Meta-analysis shows a 7.5% incidence of major depression during pregnancy and 6.5% in the first 3 months of postpartum[1] with point prevalence of major and minor depression of 11.0% in the first trimester and 8.5% later in pregnancy. In the first postpartum year, 13.9% of mothers and 3.6% of fathers develop unipolar, nonpsychotic major depression.[2] Point prevalence rises postpartum to a high of 12.9% in the 3rd month, then drops to 9.9% to 10.6% from the 4th to 12th postpartum months, declining after that to 6.5%.[1] The incidence of major depression was higher for mothers in the first year postpartum than in subsequent years.

Perinatal depression prevalence varies widely among subsets of women. Comparing women from 40 countries,[3] prevalence of postpartum major depression using DSM criteria ranged from 3.4% in a Swedish sample to 34.7% in a South African sample. Similarly, studies using Edinburgh Postnatal Depression Scale scores to measure depression show a range of 0.5% in Singapore to 57.0% in Guyana.[3] In the United States, ethnicity, socioeconomic status, age, and trauma history serve as both independent and interactive risk factors. The odds of developing perinatal depressive symptoms are higher in African American women and Hispanic women than

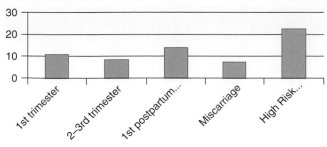

Figure 9-1 *Mean risk of depression for selected conditions (percentage prevalence for particular disease).*

in non-Hispanic Caucasian women, even after adjusting for other demographic variables.[4,5] Although the cause of these differences is unknown, possible factors include differences in levels of exposure to environmental stressors, availability of protective resources, stigma, biological vulnerabilities, interpretations and conceptualizations of distress, and communication of symptoms. In studies using structured clinical interviews rather than self-reports, prevalence of major depression is comparable among different socioeconomic groups, while the prevalence of sub-syndromal depressive symptoms is higher among women of lower socioeconomic position.[1] Adolescents have a higher risk for perinatal depression than adults, especially in the context of early life trauma.[6,7]

Women with pre-existing bipolar disorder have significantly more episodes during pregnancy and postpartum than women with unipolar depression, and significantly more episodes postpartum than during pregnancy.[8] Among untreated women with bipolar disorder, the rate of recurrence during pregnancy is doubled and tripled during the postpartum period.[9,10] Most postpartum bipolar mood episodes occur in the first month postpartum.[11] In addition, while postpartum psychotic episodes are relatively rare (1 in 1,000 women who give birth),[12] women with pre-existing bipolar disorder are at substantially higher risk of psychotic and nonpsychotic episodes.

PATHOPHYSIOLOGY

The perinatal period is a time of substantial biological and social flux. Hormonal shifts, heightened inflammatory responses, and changes in circadian rhythm occur throughout pregnancy and in the postpartum period (**Box 9-1** and **Box 9-2**). Genetic susceptibility intensifies mood changes in response to these perturbations. **Table 9-1** summarizes factors which have been shown to increase vulnerability to perinatal depression.[13–20]

BOX 9-1
IMPORTANT RISK FACTORS FOR DEPRESSION IN PERIPARTUM AND POSTPARTUM PERIOD

Sociodemographic
Ethnicity (African American, Hispanic)
Young age
Trauma history
Low socioeconomic status
Poor social support
Clinical
Personal history of depression, bipolar disorder or psychosis
Family history of depression, bipolar disorder, or psychosis
Medical
Gestational diabetes

BOX 9-2
POSSIBLE MEDIATORS BETWEEN PERINATAL FACTORS AND DEPRESSION

Genetic
Hormonal
Receptor changes
Inflammation
Stress
Social Support

Postpartum psychotic mood episodes are not associated with stress, lack of social support, or negative attitudes toward pregnancy.[12] There is a strong familial aggregation of postpartum psychotic mood episodes. In a genetic study of bipolar disorder, women with a family history of puerperal psychosis were six times more likely to have a psychotic episode within 6 weeks of giving birth.[21]

CLINICAL PRESENTATION

Major depressive episodes present differently in the antepartum, postpartum, and nonperinatal periods (**Box 9-3**).[22] When compared to women with onset of major depression postpartum, women with new episodes of major depression during pregnancy are more likely to have had unplanned pregnancies, inadequate social support, a history of physical and/or sexual abuse, and a history of major depression, as well as more complicated pregnancies and/or neonatal medical problems. In contrast, postpartum depressive episodes are more likely to include obsessive symptoms. Ego-dystonic, intrusive, violent thoughts, especially about harming the baby, are relatively common postpartum. In one study, 41% of mothers with postpartum depression and 7% of nondepressed control mothers had such thoughts.[23] The risk of women acting on such thoughts is low. By contrast, the delusional, ego-syntonic thoughts of harming

---

TABLE 9-1 Influences on Vulnerability to Perinatal Unipolar Depression

Vulnerability Factors	Evidence
Genetic susceptibility	The 5-HTTLPR-ss allele predicts postpartum depressive symptoms in the presence of negative life events.
Hormonal flux and stress reactivity	Compared to controls, women with histories of perinatal depression produce more cortisol in response to CRH after abrupt withdrawal of estrogen and progesterone.
Perinatal changes in serotonin	Serotonin (5HT-1A) receptor binding is reduced in women with postpartum depression compared to controls.
Pro-inflammatory cytokines	Pro-inflammatory cytokines increase near the end of pregnancy, and are further increased by pain, sleep deprivation, and stress. Higher levels correlate with perinatal depressive symptoms.
Stress	Consistent risk factors for perinatal depression include stressful life events, intimate partner violence, unintended pregnancy, and low socioeconomic status.
Insufficient social support	Paucity of social support strongly correlates with risk of perinatal depression. The presence of strong social and cultural support is protective.

Confounding
Fatigue
Heightened emotions (baby blues)
Appetite changes
Insomnia
More typical in depression
Thoughts of hurting child
Confusion

"Baby Blues"
Thyroid disease
Anemia
Vitamin D deficiency

babies which sometimes occur during episodes of postpartum psychosis pose substantially greater risk of being acted upon.

There are phenomenologic differences between postpartum and nonpostpartum psychotic mood episodes as well. Postpartum psychotic episodes are more often characterized by a subjective sense of confusion, disorganized thinking, lability, and homicidal ideation.[24] The waxing and waning nature of postpartum psychotic symptoms can contribute to underrecognition or underestimation of risk; patients can manifest severe symptoms at times and can appear much better hours later, with symptoms intensifying again shortly thereafter.

COURSE AND NATURAL HISTORY

Women with postpartum depressive symptoms or episodes have a high likelihood of subsequent depression, both during postpartum periods and in general, which may be as much as four times the risk for mothers without perinatal depression.[25] On the other hand, women whose first major depressive episode occurred within the first 4 weeks postpartum have a lower risk of recurrence than women those whose first episode is unrelated to pregnancy.[26] Effective treatment reduces recurrence rates.[27] Women with postpartum bipolar mood episodes have a particularly high likelihood of subsequent episodes.[28]

Perinatal depression has intergenerational effects. Thus maternal antenatal depression is associated with an increased risk of preterm birth[29] and long-term risks to offspring. These risks may stem in part from depression-linked maternal behavioral changes during pregnancy, such as reduced prenatal care, worse nutrition, reduced physical activity, and increased use of alcohol and tobacco. Some effects of maternal depression may be mediated via fetal programming, a term for epigenetic influences on fetal development that have enduring effects on emotions, behavior or cognitive abilities. Antenatal maternal depression is associated with increased methylation affecting glucocorticoid receptor gene expression, potentially influencing fetal hypothalamic pituitary adrenal (HPA) axis programming.[30] Resultant increased risks for offspring include poorer growth, increased risk of infection, and more difficult temperaments.[31–33]

Postpartum depression can adversely affect parenting capability, although it does not do so consistently. Mothers with postpartum depression may have impaired ability to read infant cues, reduced responsiveness to infant distress, constricted ability to communicate a full range of emotions, provide fewer enrichment activities for babies, and maintain less healthy feeding and sleeping practices.[34] Children and adolescents whose mothers were depressed postpartum experience poorer health-related quality of life,[35] higher rates of HPA abnormalities and depression,[36] higher rates of behavioral disturbance,[37] and lower cognitive abilities.[38]

Women with bipolar disorder are at greater risk during pregnancy for addictive substance use, being overweight, and needing instrumental delivery or Cesarean section.[39] Effects on offspring are not well studied, though there may be increased likelihood of low birth weight (OR 1.66), premature birth (OR 2.08), and being small for gestational age (OR 1.47).[40] In a controlled study of mother–infant dyadic interactions, mothers with bipolar disorder were less expressive and showed more negative communication styles.[41]

ASSESSMENT AND DIFFERENTIAL DIAGNOSIS

Normal somatic changes of pregnancy, such as increased appetite, weight gain, sleep disturbances, and reduced energy, overlap with the diagnostic criteria for depression (**Box 9-4**). The Edinburgh perinatal depression scale (EPDS) is a valid and sensitive tool that is less likely to be influenced by these potential confounds.[42,43] It is a 10-item self-report tool available in over 20 languages. The EPDS has a sensitivity of 0.88 to 1.00 and a specificity from 0.71 to 0.79 using a cutoff score ranging from 10 to 12.[43] Several general depression screening tools, including the Beck depression inventory (BDI), the Center for epidemiologic studies depression (CES-D) Scale, and the patient health questionnaire (PHQ), have also been validated for perinatal use, and compare favorably with the EPDS. The postpartum depression screening scale is specifically for postpartum use, taking into account the context of new motherhood,[44] and though less well studied, has psychometric properties that compare favorably to the EPDS.

Normal postpartum mood changes known as "baby blues" may be confused with postpartum depression. Although the term "blues" suggests a mild form of depression, normal postpartum "blues" are a qualitatively different experience in which the predominant mood is happiness[45] that is interspersed with intense reactivity of mood and heightened emotional responses to stimuli, resulting in frequent tearfulness and mood lability. For example, a woman with postpartum "blues" might be happy most of the time, but cry upon hearing a love song, feel highly anxious when reading about a train accident, and become irritable and overwhelmed from everyday stresses. These mood changes occur in approximately 50% of postpartum women, peaking from days 3 to 5 after delivery and lasting several days to weeks.[46]

Medical conditions that can present with perinatal depressive symptoms include:

- Thyroid disease: Increased thyroid synthesis is required to meet fetal needs during pregnancy, and subclinical hypothyroidism in the antenatal period may confer a higher risk of postpartum depressive symptoms.[47,48] The postpartum period also confers a heightened risk of thyroiditis.
- Anemia: Repleting iron in pregnant women with iron-deficiency anemia has been shown to reduce rates of clinically significant depression.[49]
- Vitamin D deficiency: Low vitamin D levels are associated with increased perinatal depressive symptoms,[50] however, it is unknown whether vitamin D supplementation reverses depressive symptoms in the absence of other treatment for depression.

TREATMENT

Treatments with well-established efficacy for perinatal depression include interpersonal psychotherapy (IPT), cognitive-behavioral therapy (CBT), electroconvulsive therapy (ECT), and antidepressant medication (**Box 9-5**). Estrogen therapy, phototherapy, transcranial magnetic stimulation, and omega-3 fatty acid supplementation also appear to have promising efficacy though further study of these interventions is needed.

◼ ANTIDEPRESSANTS

Many conflicting findings have emerged in studies about the risks of antidepressant medications during pregnancy. This is in part because there are no randomized, double-blind, placebo-controlled trials. Retrospective database studies track prescriptions rather than actual medication exposure and chart-recorded diagnoses rather than active symptoms. Many such studies test correlations among numerous congenital anomalies and multiple medications, often without statistical correction for multiple queries. In addition, correcting for the influence of major confounds is difficult. The most reliable data for the risks of antidepressant medications come from adequately powered, prospective, controlled studies and meta-analyses of these studies, summarized in **Table 9-2**.[51–58]

For women with moderate to severe and/or recurrent depressive episodes, decisions about the use of antidepressant medication during pregnancy must take into account the likelihood of relapse and the risks of untreated symptoms. A study of pregnant psychiatric patients suggested an increased incidence of depressive relapse following discontinuation of treatment during pregnancy,[59] whereas an obstetrical sample was not found to be at increased risk of relapse following discontinuation of antidepressant medication.[60] This conflicting evidence may relate to differences in severity of disease and/or higher dose/duration of therapy.

In the postpartum period, the decision to use antidepressants must consider effects on sleep, weight, and sexual function. Sedating agents, even if they do not cause daytime drowsiness, may interfere with a woman's ability to hear and respond safely to her baby during the night. Agents that interfere with sleep may compound postpartum sleep deprivation. Medications that cause weight gain may interfere with a woman's ability to lose pregnancy weight. Adverse effects on sexual function can add to postpartum stresses as partners attempt to maintain intimate relationships as they transition to parenthood.

For women who are breastfeeding, the effects of medications on their breastfeeding babies are also key factors in choice of agent. **Table 9-3** summarizes breastfeeding exposure (as estimated weight-adjusted percent of maternal dose received by a breastfeeding baby) and reported effects on breastfeeding babies for commonly used antidepressants.[61]

◼ LITHIUM

Treatment of bipolar depression during pregnancy can be especially challenging. Lithium fully equilibrates across the placenta,[62] and may be a weak cardiovascular teratogen, although findings are equivocal. Although individual studies have reported an increased risk of cardiovascular defects, especially right-sided defects, such as Ebstein's anomaly, prospective studies, and meta-analysis, have not.[63] In utero lithium, exposure has not been found to affect subsequent growth or neurodevelopment.[64] Lithium can cause transient fetal nephrogenic diabetes insipidus (DI) by impairing the

TABLE 9-2 Risks of Antidepressant Medications During Pregnancy

Type of Risk	Findings from High-Quality Studies In Human Pregnancy
Congenital anomalies	No increased risk in most prospective, controlled studies and meta-analyses.
Miscarriage	Meta-analysis of the highest-quality studies showed no increased risk. However, several but not all prospective controlled studies show a statistically significant increase in miscarriage rate after first trimester antidepressant exposure. In most of those studies, the miscarriage rate in the exposed group was similar to the general population rate.
Premature labor	Meta-analysis of 13 high-quality studies found a pooled OR of 1.55 ($p < 0.001$). Gestational age is reduced by 3–4 days with antidepressant exposure. Most studies could not adequately control for the influence of depression. One study comparing continuous depressive symptom exposure to continuous antidepressant exposure throughout pregnancy found they each had similar effects on premature labor.
Fetal size	Meta-analysis of 20 studies showed statistically significant birth weight reduction after in utero SSRI exposure, with a small effect size (mean reduction 74 g). Most studies could not adequately control for the influence of depression. Two studies directly compared effects of depression and antidepressants on growth. One found no significant differences for infant weight, length or head circumference among groups with SSRIs, untreated major depression, or neither. Another found that fetal growth was no different from controls with SSRI exposure, but was slower with exposure to depression.
Offspring neuro-development	Prospective studies have found no IQ reductions and no increased risk of behavior problems in children up to age 7 exposed in utero to tricyclics, SSRIs or venlafaxine. In a direct comparison study, delayed language maturation was associated with antenatal exposure to maternal depressive symptoms but not SSRIs.
Neonatal side effects	Side effects after antenatal antidepressant exposure can present in up to 30% of newborns, usually beginning within hours of birth and lasting 1–2 days. They can include respiratory distress, irritability, tremor, jitteriness, restlessness, shivering, increased or decreased muscle tone, fewer different behavioral states, eating difficulties, seizures, prolonged QT intervals, and cardiac arrhythmias.
Neonatal persistent pulmonary hypertension (PPHN)	Most, but not all studies have found increased risk of neonatal persistent pulmonary hypertension (PPHN) after SSRI exposure in late pregnancy. PPHN is rare with or without SSRI exposure; the general population prevalence is about 1.9/1,000, and the prevalence within combined reported cases after SSRI exposure is 2.0/1,000.

TABLE 9-3 Antidepressant Medications and Breastfeeding

Medication	Maternal Dose to Baby (%)	Reported Side Effects to Breastfeeding Babies[a]
Bupropion	2.0–5.1	Possible seizures
Citalopram	2.5–9.4	Uneasy sleep, drowsiness, irritability, weight loss, restlessness
Desipramine	1.0	None
Desvenlafaxine	5.5–8.1	None
Duloxetine	0.14–0.82	None
Escitalopram	3.9–7.9	Enterocolitis
Fluoxetine	1.1–12.0	Excessive crying, irritability, vomiting, watery stools, difficulty sleeping, tremor, somnolence, hypotonia, decreased weight gain, hyperglycemia, hyperactivity, reduced rooting, reduced nursing, grunting, moaning
Mirtazapine	0.6–3.5	More rapid weight gain, sleeping through the night earlier
Nortriptyline	1.3	None
Paroxetine	0.1–4.3	Agitation, difficulty feeding, irritability, sleepiness, constipation, syndrome of inappropriate antidiuretic hormone secretion (SIADH)
Sertraline	0.4–2.3	Benign sleep myoclonus, transient agitation
Venlafaxine	3.0–11.8	None

[a]Based on case reports or case series of exposure as monotherapy during breastfeeding; no causal relationship is established in most cases.

concentrating ability of the fetal kidney,[65] which can present with polyhydramnios and resultant uterine enlargement. As this progresses, it can cause maternal shortness of breath if the diaphragm has insufficient room to fully expand. DI can last a week or more after birth. Lithium is also associated with premature labor[66] and transient neonatal hypothyroidism.[67] Newborns can develop toxicity, which is greater at higher serum levels and associated with lower Apgar scores and longer infant hospital stays.[68] Signs of neonatal toxicity include flaccidity, hypotonia, hyporeflexia (decreased Moro reflex, poor suck), cyanosis, lethargy, poor feeding, abnormal breathing, cardiac arrhythmias, and poor myocardial contractility. Perinatal women are also at heightened risk of lithium toxicity under certain circumstances, summarized in **Table 9-4**.[62]

Guidelines for prescribing lithium during pregnancy include:

- Avoid lithium during the period of cardiac formation when possible. Consider ultrasound evaluation for cardiac anomalies during weeks 16 to 18 when there has been early exposure.
- Monitor for signs of fetal DI (maternal shortness of breath, uterine enlargement, and/or polyhydramnios).
- Monitor lithium serum level. Dose increases are often required as pregnancy progresses because pregnancy-linked pharmacokinetic changes, including increased glomerular filtration rate and increased total body water, may reduce serum lithium level at a given dose.

- Consider divided doses near the end of pregnancy to reduce toxic peaks for the newborn.
- Consider cutting the dose in half at labor onset to reduce the risks of maternal and neonatal toxicity, then resuming the pre-pregnancy dose postpartum.

Breastfeeding babies whose mothers are taking lithium have serum lithium levels that average about 25% of maternal levels, but can be higher. Infants are vulnerable to lithium toxicity if they become dehydrated. Elevations of TSH, BUN, and creatinine are seen in infants exposed to lithium in breast milk. Monitoring infant serum lithium level, TSH, BUN, and creatinine is warranted.[69]

■ ANTIEPILEPTIC DRUGS

Table 9-5 summarizes the rates of birth defects associated with valproate, carbamazepine, and lamotrigine.[70,71–73]

Valproic acid among antiepileptic drugs (AEDs) used as mood stabilizing agents, valproic acid confers the most risk to offspring exposed in utero, including neural tube defects and other anomalies, developmental delay, lower IQ, and possibly autism.[70,74–76] Obesity and folate deficiency, which are more prevalent in women with bipolar disorder, further increase the risk of neural tube defects.

Carbamazepine increases the risk of neural tube defects although not as much as valproic acid.[77] Whether or not carbamazepine increases the risk of IQ reduction or developmental delay is equivocal; two studies showed these risks,[74,78] however, several others and

TABLE 9-4 Risk Factors for Maternal Perinatal Lithium Toxicity

Risk Factor	Explanation
Perinatal GFR[a] changes	GFR increases during pregnancy; rapidly returns to normal postpartum
Hyperemesis gravidarum	Reduced lithium absorption if emesis happens shortly after ingestion, but increased lithium concentration due to fluid loss and hyponatremia
Preeclampsia	Increased lithium concentration from reduced GFR due to intrarenal vasospasm
Postpartum fluid loss	Blood, amniotic fluid, sweat, emesis

[a]Glomerular filtration rate.

TABLE 9-5 Comparison of Malformation Rates in Offspring Exposed to Antiepileptic Mood Stabilizing Medications during Pregnancy

Exposure During Pregnancy	Rate of Major Malformations (%)
Carbamazepine	2.2–6.3
Lamotrigine	2.0–5.4
Valproic acid	6.2–16.3
Untreated epilepsy	3.5–5.2
Nonepileptic controls	2.1

Depression in Obstetrical Conditions

a meta-analysis did not.[79] Carbamazepine also increases the risk of reduced fetal size,[80] transient neonatal hepatic dysfunction,[81] and Vitamin K depletion via enzyme induction. Low vitamin K levels can impair clotting ability, which can increase the risk of neonatal hemorrhage. Vitamin K is often administered to newborns exposed to carbamazepine in utero to mitigate this risk. Administering vitamin K supplements to pregnant women taking carbamazepine has not been found to alter the risk of neonatal bleeds.[82] Other guidelines for prescribing carbamazepine during pregnancy include administering folate before and during pregnancy to reduce the additive risk of neural tube defects, and obtaining free (not total) serum levels when needed, since carbamazepine protein binding changes somewhat during pregnancy and total serum levels are therefore less reliable estimates of biological activity.[83]

Lamotrigine is of particular importance due to its relative efficacy in treating bipolar depressive symptoms, which are more prominent in women with bipolar disorder than in men with bipolar disorder. The North American AED pregnancy registry showed that infants exposed to lamotrigine in the first trimester were more likely to have cleft palates[84]; however, several subsequent studies have not borne out this association[85,86] and a population-based case–control study surveying 3.9 million births found an odds ratio of 0.8 for developing oral clefts after first trimester lamotrigine monotherapy exposure versus no AED exposure.[87] No increases in neurodevelopmental or cognitive abnormalities have been found in children exposed to lamotrigine in utero.[74]

Because pregnancy changes the pharmacokinetics of lamotrigine, the serum blood level achieved at a given dose is lowered by 50% to 60% with considerable l variation among individuals.[88] This change begins early in pregnancy and becomes most pronounced by the third trimester, making it important to check reference blood serum levels preconception or in early pregnancy and then to monitor serum levels monthly and increase the dose by 20% to 25% as needed.[89] The pre-pregnancy dose can be resumed postpartum.

It is estimated that breastfeeding babies ingest 3.1% to 21.1% of the maternal dose of lamotrigine, with a mean of 9.2%.[90] The serum levels in breastfeeding infants whose mothers take lamotrigine are 18% to 30% of maternal serum levels; this is substantially higher than antidepressant serum levels in breastfeeding infants whose mothers take antidepressants. Lamotrigine is less protein-bound in infants, and its half-life is longer in infants. There is a case report of severe apnea and cyanosis in an exposed infant.[91]

Antipsychotic Mood Stabilizers

Prospective, controlled studies of second-generation antipsychotic (SGA) mood stabilizing agents in human pregnancy have found no increases in birth defects, gestational age, mode of delivery, Apgar scores, mean weight, or height or head circumference.[92,93] However, one study[93] did find significantly more exposed infants met criteria for low birth weight. Scores on Bailey developmental scales were lower in the exposed group at 2 months, but showed no significant differences at 12 months. This study may have been confounded by exposure to the effects of maternal schizophrenia, and higher maternal body mass index (BMI) compared to controls, which may also have influenced birth weight and neurodevelopment.

Tables 9-6 and 9-7 summarize clinical considerations for prescribing SGAs during pregnancy and breastfeeding.[61]

■ SUMMARY

There is a high prevalence of both unipolar and bipolar depressive mood episodes during pregnancy and postpartum. Depressive episodes in the postpartum period are more likely to include intrusive, ego-dystonic thoughts, particularly low-risk thoughts of harming the baby. Postpartum bipolar depressive episodes have a higher likelihood

TABLE 9-6 Second-generation Antipsychotic Agents during Pregnancy

Agent	Considerations during Pregnancy
Aripiprazole	• Not systematically studied in human pregnancy • Least likely among SGAs to cause orthostatic hypotension

Clozapine	• Increased risk of
	  • neonatal seizures
	  • agranulocytosis
	  • gestational diabetes mellitus
	• May accumulate in fetus
	• May reduce placental perfusion due to orthostatic hypotension

Olanzapine	• No increased risk of anomalies in prospective, controlled study and registry data
	• Increased risk of
	  • gestational diabetes mellitus
	  • excessive weight gain

Risperidone	• May reduce fertility due to prolactin elevation • No increased risk of anomalies in prospective, controlled study
Quetiapine	• Sedation may interfere with parenting • No increased risk of anomalies in prospective, controlled study • Less placental passage than olanzapine or risperidone
Ziprasidone	• Not systematically studied in human pregnancy • Less orthostatic hypotension than most SGAs

TABLE 9-7 Mood Stabilizing Medications during Breastfeeding

Medication	Breastfeeding (infant exposure level[a]; reported adverse effects[b])
Aripiprazole	– <0.7% of mother's dose – None, but limited data
Carbamazepine	– 0–2.6 mg/L infant serum concentration – Transient mild liver function abnormalities; poor suck; vomiting
Lamotrigine	– 3.1–21.1% of mother's dose Increased platelet counts; apneic episode, rash
Lithium	– 0.0–30.0% of mother's dose – Cyanosis, restlessness, muscle twitches, lethargy, hypothermia
Olanzapine	– 0.3–4.0% of mother's dose – Sedation, poor suck, shaking, rash, diarrhea, somnolence
Quetiapine	– 0.09–0.43% of mother's dose – None, but limited data
Risperidone	– 0.84–4.3% of mother's dose – None, but limited data
Valproate	– Infant serum concentration 0.9–40.0% of mother's – None
Ziprasidone	– Unknown – None, but limited data

[a]Reported as weight-adjusted percent of mother's dose experienced by breastfeeding baby when known, or as infant serum concentrations.
[b]Based on case reports or case series of exposure as monotherapy during breastfeeding; no causal relationship is established in most cases.

of psychotic features, and comparatively more lability and confusion. Untreated symptoms during pregnancy and/or postpartum can pose substantial risks to offspring as well as to affected women. IPT, CBT, pharmacotherapy, and ECT are effective treatments. The risks of untreated symptoms must be compared with the risks of antidepressant and mood stabilizing medication to optimize treatment.

Case Outcome: Shanté's friend Linda became increasingly worried when Shanté would not answer her phone, and persisted in ringing the doorbell until Shanté answered. Linda persuaded Shanté to see her obstetrician, who diagnosed a major depressive episode with postpartum onset. Upon hearing about treatment possibilities, Shanté initially refused medication due to worries about Ryan being exposed through breastfeeding. She also refused CBT because she did not want to leave Ryan with anyone, and also did not want to expose Ryan to germs by bringing him on the bus to sessions. Eventually, with support from Linda and empathic discussion of risks and benefits by her obstetrician, Shanté agreed to CBT with Linda caring for Ryan during sessions. After a few sessions, Shanté felt better equipped to manage stressors and parenting, but she still felt depressed and anhedonic and struggled with self-care. She then agreed to add sertraline. Within a few weeks, she achieved full remission.

PERINATAL LOSS AND DEPRESSION

Case Illustration: Sarah is a 26-year-old married woman who delivered a stillborn baby boy at 32 weeks of gestation after having developed preeclampsia. She and her husband Sam named their son Billy, and held a memorial service for him. At first they felt supported by one another, but in the weeks that followed they often clashed. Sarah did not understand Sam's way of dealing with the loss, which she described as "partying" with friends. Sam called Sarah "selfish" and "depressing to be around." Sarah was frequently tearful and wanted to talk about Billy. She felt guilty for not preventing his death, and spent hours online researching preeclampsia to see what she could have done differently. Sometimes she heard Billy cry. She did not want to kill herself, but at times wanted to be dead so she could be with her son. She became socially isolated, in part because she felt overwhelming sadness when she saw other women with babies. She identified herself as a mother, but did not actually have a live baby, so felt disconnected from other mothers. She refused Sam's requests to go out for relaxing outings, feeling she would betray Billy by enjoying herself. After nine months, Sam left and moved in with his parents. Sarah told her sister, "I hate my life; I'm just going through the motions."

EPIDEMIOLOGY

In the United States, miscarriage is defined as death of a fetus before 20 weeks of gestation and stillbirth as death of a fetus after 20 weeks of gestation. Neonatal death refers to death within the first week of life; sudden infant death syndrome (SIDS) refers to unexpected death after the first week and within the first year of life. About 15% of recognized pregnancies end in miscarriage.[94] The prevalence of stillbirth varies from 3 to 4/1,000 births in high-income countries to 30 to 40/1,000 births in low-income countries, with an overall worldwide estimate of 3.2 million stillbirths per year.[95] In the United States, the prevalence of neonatal death varies substantially by region, but overall is about 4/1,000 births.[96] SIDS affects about 0.57/1,000 babies born in the United States.[97]

It is difficult to determine the prevalence of depressive symptoms or major depression in women who have experienced perinatal loss, in part because the difficulties in distinguishing between normal grief and depression. Most studies rely on self-report symptom checklists, such as the EPDS, the BDI, the CES-D, and the Zung Self-Rating Depression Scale, which do not inquire about grief as the source of the elevated scores. Using these measures, the prevalence of depressive symptoms among women shortly after perinatal loss ranges widely, from 19% to 91%,[98–100] depending on the population studied, the type of loss, the measures used, the cut-off scores

chosen, and the time elapsed between the loss and the measurement. A study using the structured clinical interview for diagnosis (SCID) found that 7.5% of women met criteria for major depression 3 months after a miscarriage.[101] Amidst this variability, several consistent findings emerge:

- Women who have experienced a perinatal loss endorse significantly more depressive symptoms than perinatal women who have not experienced a loss.
- Women are at higher risk than men for a longer duration of depressive symptoms after a perinatal loss.
- The risk of depressive symptoms is higher after stillbirth than after miscarriage.[100]
- The risk of depressive symptoms after miscarriage is not affected by type of miscarriage—for example, surgical, medical, or spontaneous.[102] However, the number of miscarriages experienced is strongly correlated with more depressive symptoms and a greater likelihood of a diagnosis of depression.[103]
- Strong social support can reduce the risk of depressive symptoms after perinatal loss.[100] The baby's father's willingness to talk about the stillborn baby may have a particularly strong influence on the likelihood of maternal depression.[104]

PATHOPHYSIOLOGY

For some causes of perinatal loss, there may be pathophysiologic links to depression. The most common known causes of miscarriage are fetal genetic abnormalities and uterine anatomic abnormalities. Increases in inflammatory cytokines caused by depression and/or stress may be another cause of miscarriage. Examination of decidual tissue after miscarriages reveals higher levels of mast cells, tumor necrosis factor α, and cytotoxic T cells in the placentas of women with high stress scores.[105] Among women with at least two prior miscarriages, those with higher levels of depressive symptoms were significantly more likely to have another miscarriage.[106]

A direct link between maternal depression and SIDS has not been demonstrated, but indirect links have been suggested. Several factors that increase the risk of SIDS also correlate with depression, including reduced prenatal care, tobacco and alcohol use, and low birth weight.[107] It has been hypothesized that a serotonin gene transporter promoter polymorphism (5-HTTLPR) that is linked with vulnerability to depression is also linked with SIDS, but studies have not borne this out.

Probable cause for any stillbirth can be determined approximately 60% of the time via a postmortem examination.[108] The most frequent causes are placental abnormalities, fetal genetic and/or structural abnormalities, infection, umbilical cord abnormalities, and maternal medical conditions, such as hypertension. Maternal obesity and smoking, both of which correlate with depression, are predictors of stillbirth; however, these factors explain very little of the variance.[109]

CLINICAL PRESENTATION

Grief after perinatal loss varies widely, and may include intense sadness, irritability, anger, guilt, sleep, and appetite disturbances. The initial reaction may include a sense of numbness, shock, unreality, and confusion over the sudden loss of the parental role.[110] Parents may be preoccupied with the loss and attempt to find meaning in it. Qualitative studies have emphasized the influence on mood of self-blaming thoughts in women who have experienced miscarriage. Some women wonder if their diets, behaviors, stress levels, or attitudes toward the baby caused the miscarriage.[111] In a qualitative analysis of women's reactions to stillbirth,[110] participants frequently described having had premonitions of the death, such as reduced fetal movement or a sense of heaviness. Many noticed changes in the body language of clinical personnel, such as ultrasound technicians, and became especially tense if the clinicians would not talk to them. Many were frightened of having a dead baby inside, and wanted the baby to come out quickly. Some feared vaginal delivery but felt good about it later, in the sense that their bodies were functioning normally. The baby's silence at birth often came as a shock. Some were frightened by the baby's appearance, and needed guidance as to how to handle the baby. Afterward, some women experience hallucinations (e.g., hearing the baby cry, feeling fetal movement). Grieving styles may differ between partners, contributing to an increased incidence of relationship breakups if these differences are not understood or accepted.[112]

COURSE AND NATURAL HISTORY

Depressive symptoms increase after a perinatal loss,[113,114] and are notable for their long duration, particularly following stillbirth. After miscarriage, scores on depressive symptom scales remain significantly higher than those of nonpregnant controls until a year after the loss.[115] Having no subsequent pregnancy within 3 years after a stillbirth significantly increases the risk of prolonged depressive symptoms.[116] The subsequent birth of a healthy baby has been found to reduce depressive symptoms in fathers, but not mothers,[117] for whom depressive symptoms remain elevated for 3 to 8 years after the birth of a subsequent healthy baby.[113,118]

ASSESSMENT AND DIFFERENTIAL DIAGNOSIS

There is considerable overlap between normal grief reactions and depressive symptoms after perinatal loss. Several rating scales have been developed specifically[119] to distinguish perinatal grief and depression. It is important not to misconstrue normal grieving as clinical depression and to note the characteristics of either grief or depression that could lead to problematic outcomes. Excessive guilt, active suicidal thoughts, and prolonged difficulty re-engaging with life are signs of potential psychopathology. A key aspect of perinatal grief is the centrality of yearning and longing. The emphasis may vary on yearning for the lost baby, the lost pregnancy, or a lost sense of healthy womanhood. The sense of longing is linked with anticipations, hopes, and plans for the future.

TREATMENT

■ OBSTETRIC CARE AND IMMEDIATE FOLLOW-UP

Approaching perinatal loss in ways that may reduce the risk of adverse psychiatric sequelae[120] includes:

- Describing possible causes of stillbirth in clear language, accompanied by a willingness to repeat the same information several times, sometimes to significant others as well.
- Involving parents in decision making—for example, about withdrawal of life support from a critically ill infant.
- Consider possibly allowing the parents to see and hold a stillborn baby. Although some data indicate an increased risk of depressive and posttraumatic stress symptoms among women who have contact with stillborn infants,[121] optimal grieving styles vary among individuals. Most data support following maternal wishes. Subsequent depressive symptoms increase when women who wish to hold their stillborn baby are not able to do so.[116] In addition, women have fewer depressive symptoms in a subsequent pregnancy if they have seen and held their stillborn babies.[99]
- Providing mementos of a stillborn baby or neonate may facilitate grieving for some parents but not others. Hospitals may give mementos, such as photographs, ultrasound pictures, handprints, footprints, and hospital identification bracelets upon request, and it is also advisable to keep these available for several months for parents who later decide they want to have them.
- Helping the mother decide whether or not to suppress lactation is beneficial. Some women choose to do this because

lactation is too intensely evocative of their loss; others maintain lactation to foster a feeling of connection with the lost baby.

- Helping parents decide if or how to commemorate the baby and the loss—for example, whether to name the baby, have a funeral, send announcements, etc. Distress about these decisions may be intensified in cases where the parents' inclinations differ from their culture's practices—for example, parents who want to honor the baby's death but whose ethnic or religious group does not believe that a stillborn baby has a soul.
- Aiding members of a couple to articulate, understand, respect and support one another's grieving styles.
- Referring parents to a mental health provider is indicated when parents have active suicidal thoughts, prolonged and excessive guilt, or difficulty re-engaging in other aspects of life several months after a perinatal loss.

Meetings between parents and an obstetric clinician a few weeks after a loss provide opportunities for reviewing possible causes of the infant's death, reviewing autopsy reports, and articulating and countering irrational self-blame. It is also helpful to discuss future pregnancy when parents are ready to do so. Whether to recommend waiting for a specific length of time—for example, a year—before trying to conceive after a loss is controversial and the one-year recommendation is based on the notion that incomplete grieving might result in problems, such as attachment difficulties, with the subsequent child as well as the parents. Indeed, there is a significantly higher likelihood of maternal depressive symptoms during the pregnancy that follows a miscarriage when that subsequent pregnancy occurs within 6 months of the loss.[122] There is also a significantly higher rate of disorganized attachment behavior in infants born after a stillbirth.[123] These attachment problems do not correlate with maternal depressive symptoms, but do strongly correlate with maternal unresolved feelings about the loss, as measured by the Adult Attachment Interview. Based on these findings, the most relevant determinant of readiness for a subsequent pregnancy may be adequate resolution of grief, the timing of which may vary among individuals and couples.

During a subsequent pregnancy, because it is a high risk time for depressive symptoms, more frequent prenatal visits than usual may be indicated. To facilitate proactive compassionate care, patients' charts can be flagged for the time of the prior loss. All staff, including ultrasound personnel and childbirth educators, can be informed about the loss and guided about how to interact.[124]

PSYCHOTHERAPEUTIC TREATMENTS

Brief (3–6 sessions) psychoeducational and CBT-based interventions have been shown to significantly reduce depressive symptoms after miscarriage, with efficacy greater for women than men.[125] In randomized controlled trials, single-session counseling has not been proven effective in reducing depressive symptoms after miscarriage. Self-help videotapes and workbooks using coaching techniques have been developed, but have not demonstrated efficacy. Computerized interventions for psychiatric sequelae of pregnancy loss are being developed[126] but have not yet been systematically evaluated.

There is insufficient evidence about whether psychotherapy after stillbirth reduces depression. However, emerging data[127] suggest that useful aspects of psychotherapy and/or support groups include:

- Educating parents about the wide range of styles and expressions of grief.
- Addressing worries about the causes of the stillbirth, including excessive self-blame.
- Helping parents re-engage in self-care and pleasurable activities over time, and addressing guilt and/or fears that this represents a betrayal of the lost child.

- Gradually reducing avoidance of people or activities that trigger symptoms, such as pregnant women or stores that carry baby items.
- Planning for anniversaries, considering whether parents would benefit from engaging in rituals to remember the baby.

■ SUMMARY

Intense grief and depressive symptoms are highly prevalent after perinatal loss, and can be especially pronounced and prolonged after stillbirth, neonatal death or recurrent miscarriage. Strong social support can reduce depressive symptoms. By contrast, inability to talk to a partner about the loss, or living within a cultural context that does not condone expressions of grief for a fetus or newborn, can intensify depression and isolation. Depressive symptoms often increase during a subsequent pregnancy. Intense self-blame, suicidal thoughts and prolonged inability to re-engage with life are indications of the need for mental health intervention. Intervention is also helpful for couples whose individual grieving styles differ in ways that cause friction in the relationship. Initial intervention can include psychoeducation about the wide range of expressions of grieving perinatal loss. Psychotherapy includes a focus on reframing guilt-inducing thoughts, finding adaptive ways to maintain a sense of connection with the lost child, re-engaging in other activities, and gradually reducing avoidance of grief triggers.

Case Outcome: Sarah's sister persuaded her to join a support group for parents who had experienced stillbirth. There she learned that parents grieved their babies in a variety of ways. She came to see Sam's reactions in a new light, realizing that though his grief took a different form, it was as intense as hers. Other parents helped her relinquish her preoccupation with figuring out how she could have prevented the stillbirth. She began working on ways to honor Billy's memory while re-engaging with life. She created a Facebook page for Billy, with inspirational quotes and pictures of him. She also created a charity organization in his name to help other parents dealing with loss. She asked Sam to help her with this. She is not sure they will get back together, but she feels ready to give it a try.

TREATMENT OF PRE-EXISTING DEPRESSION

For a woman with a history of any mood disorder who is planning a pregnancy, the most important information to gather is her illness and treatment history, and a clarification of which treatment regimen has resulted in the most euthymic stability It is important to consider whether she has been effectively maintained on any monotherapy, and whether she has engaged in any nonpharmacologic treatments previously. For example, a patient with unipolar depression may currently be taking a medication but may also have a history of full remission of symptoms in the past while engaged in psychotherapy. If this patient is not engaged in psychotherapy while planning a pregnancy, the preconception period is an ideal time to re-enter psychotherapy.

For a woman with a history of mood disorder who is already pregnant and presenting for consultation for treatment planning, it is most important to clarify her current treatment and current symptoms. The goal is to minimize switching of agents during pregnancy to minimize the risk of additional exposures, while also limiting the exposure to untreated symptoms of depression or anxiety. If she is already on an antidepressant, the efficacy of the current regimen must be assessed. If her symptoms are well managed, the goal would be to minimize switching and maintain her euthymia. If her symptoms on a current regimen are partially treated, maximizing her dose on her current regimen is greatly favored over switching. As pregnancy progresses, patients may require dose escalation owing to physiologic changes of pregnancy. Emergence of symptoms will often respond to increase in dosage of current treatments.

GESTATIONAL DIABETES MELLITUS AND DEPRESSION

■ EPIDEMIOLOGY

Gestational diabetes mellitus (GDM) is defined as glucose intolerance with first onset, or first recognition, during pregnancy. In the United States, GDM occurs in about 3% to 8% of pregnancies and the risk of GDM varies among ethnic groups, with higher rates in African American, Asian, Latina and Native American women than in non-Latina white women. The prevalence of GDM has increased in recent years.[128]

Pregnant women with diabetes have a greater risk of being depressed than pregnant women without diabetes (Box 9-1).[129] However, this is largely accounted for by women whose diabetes preceded pregnancy. Women with GDM may be about twice as likely to have depressive symptoms,[130] but do not appear to have an increased risk of major depression, when compared to pregnant women without diabetes.[131] Depressive symptoms during pregnancy can influence course and prognosis for women with GDM, regardless of whether they preceded pregnancy or whether they meet criteria for major depression (see *Course and natural history*).

PATHOPHYSIOLOGY

During normal pregnancy, maternal insulin resistance increases. Since maternal glucose freely crosses the placenta but maternal insulin does not, this facilitates transport of glucose across the placenta. Insulin resistance returns to normal within 6 weeks postpartum. In GDM, the pancreatic islet β cells are unable to compensate for the increase in insulin resistance, leading to impaired maternal glucose tolerance and hyperglycemia. It is posited that the resultant increase in fetal insulin production promotes excessive fetal growth and adiposity, heightening the risk of fetal macrosomia. In essence, pregnancy can be viewed as a biological stressor that unmasks vulnerability to diabetes and related cardiometabolic abnormalities. Genetic, epigenetic, and environmental factors appear to play a role in this vulnerability.

Depression is not known to have a direct effect on the pathophysiology of GDM, but by influencing eating patterns and food choices, depression may have an indirect effect.

CLINICAL PRESENTATION

Due to adverse effects of hyperglycemia on pregnancy outcome, women with GDM are advised to maintain tight glycemic control. This process can be arduous, involving glucose self-monitoring several times per day, a carefully controlled diet, frequent clinic visits, and insulin when necessary. Among women with GDM, better glycemic control correlates with lower levels of depressive symptoms.[132] It is posited that women who are less depressed are better able to self-manage their diabetes, and also that women who successfully maintain good glycemic control experience greater self-efficacy and therefore better moods.

COURSE AND NATURAL HISTORY

Among women with GDM, those with excessive gestational weight gain and those who have Cesarean sections have a greater likelihood of developing postpartum depressive symptoms.[133] In the longer term, women with GDM are at high risk for subsequent metabolic, inflammatory, and cardiovascular abnormalities. Between 18% and 50% develop diabetes mellitus within 5 years postpartum. As compared to women without a history of GDM, women who have had GDM have increased glucose, triglycerides, and C-reactive protein, and decreased adiponectin, after the first postpartum year.[134] Depression can also increase the risk of subsequent metabolic and cardiovascular abnormalities; it remains to be studied whether women with both GDM and depression are at higher risk for such problems in the future.

The likelihood of developing diabetes and other cardiovascular risk factors after GDM can be influenced by postpartum exercise, diet, weight reduction, and breastfeeding. Each of these can be influenced by perinatal depressive symptoms. Depressive symptoms during pregnancy and postpartum are correlated with greater postpartum weight retention.[135] Postpartum depression is correlated with reduced intensity and maintenance of breastfeeding.[136]

ASSESSMENT AND DIFFERENTIAL DIAGNOSIS

Since untreated perinatal depressive symptoms could adversely affect glycemic control, increase postpartum weight retention, and reduce breastfeeding, screening for depressive symptoms in all women with GDM is indicated.

The American College of Obstetrics and Gynecology (ACOG), the American Diabetic Association (ADA), the United States Preventive Services Task Force, the Joslin Diabetes Center, the World Health Organization, and the International Diabetes Center have each generated guidelines for assessing GDM.[137] Most of these guidelines recommend assessing all pregnant women for their level of risk of GDM. Women in the lowest risk category are those who are less than 25 years old, Caucasian, with normal pre-pregnancy BMI and no history of adverse pregnancy outcomes. Those who are at highest risk are women with prior GDM, obesity, and a strong family history of diabetes

Diagnosis of GDM is made with by checking blood glucose levels after administration of an oral glucose load. Guidelines and practices differ regarding the amount, form, and delivery of the glucose load and recommend some leeway in interpreting results. For example, both ACOG and ADA guidelines suggest 130 mg/dL or 140 mg/dL as the cutoff for a diagnosis of GDM after a 50 g oral glucose load, depending on the desired sensitivity and/or the clinical particulars.

TREATMENT

Two large clinical trials have demonstrated that treatment of GDM reduces pregnancy complications, including macrosomia, pre-eclampsia, and excessive maternal weight gain.[138,139] It has been posited that treating comorbid depressive symptoms could further improve maternal and infant outcomes, perhaps by increasing women's ability to adhere to GDM treatment. Empirically, there are insufficient data about the effects of treating comorbid depression on outcome for women with GDM.[140] Most studies, including a randomized controlled trial, of nonpregnant patients with type 2 diabetes suggest that treating depression improves metabolic parameters.[141] Aerobic exercise alleviates maternal depressive symptoms while also reducing risks of infant macrosomia.[142]

Choice of antidepressants for women with GDM is informed by relative safety during pregnancy, effects of the antidepressant on glucose metabolism, and effects of the antidepressant on weight. Among agents that are relatively well studied and pose fewer risks during pregnancy, fluoxetine and sertraline tend to improve sensitivity to insulin and reduce hyperglycemia. By contrast, agents with more noradrenergic activity tend to worsen hyperglycemia. The tricyclics desipramine (highly noradrenergic) and nortryptiline (noradrenergic and serotonergic) have been found to improve depressive symptoms but elevate glucose levels in nonpregnant patients with diabetes.[143] Mirtazapine and paroxetine tend to lead to more weight gain than other antidepressants; bupropion is less likely to cause weight gain.[144]

■ SUMMARY

Antenatal depression can reduce the ability of women with GDM to maintain tight glycemic control, thus potentially increasing the risk of adverse pregnancy outcomes. Postpartum depression can increase the risk of subsequent metabolic, inflammatory, and cardiovascular pathology in women with GDM by reducing breastfeeding and increasing postpartum weight retention. Screening for depressive symptoms is indicated for all women with GDM. When using antidepressants for women with GDM, it is best to avoid those which have a greater likelihood of causing weight gain (such as mirtazapine and paroxetine) and those which can elevate glucose levels (such as desipramine and nortryptiline).

■ HIGH-RISK PREGNANCIES AND DEPRESSION

Case Illustration: Anne is a 26-year-old woman at 26 weeks gestational age in her third pregnancy. Anne has had two prior second trimester pregnancy losses. Earlier in her current pregnancy, she was treated with a cerclage to prevent recurrent loss, and now has symptoms of pressure and cramping. She was diagnosed with cervical insufficiency by ultrasound, and is now hospitalized due to signs of preterm labor. Anne's nurse informs her obstetrician that Anne has been tearful and withdrawn.

EPIDEMIOLOGY

High-risk pregnancy is defined as a pregnancy in which a condition in the patient or fetus places the woman, the fetus, or both at higher risk for complications during or after pregnancy and birth. Hypertension, diabetes, seizure, and clotting disorders are among the most common maternal medical high-risk conditions. Obstetric conditions, such as cervical insufficiency, multiple gestation, premature contractions, and placental problems, are also commonly considered high risk. Fetal conditions that confer higher risk include structural abnormalities, chromosomal abnormalities, genetic syndromes, congenital heart conditions, infections, and intrauterine growth problems.[145]

Studies suggest that the incidence of depression during and after a high-risk pregnancy is approximately two and half times higher than in typical pregnancy,[146] and 19% to 25% of women with high-risk pregnancies meet the criteria for major depression.[147-149] Some studies have investigated the relationship between pre-existing depression and high risk pregnancies. A meta-analysis found a significant association between antenatal maternal depression and premature labor, but not pre-eclampsia or low birth weight.[29]

PATHOPHYSIOLOGY

Factors that elevate risk for depression in pregnancy may be heightened in high-risk pregnancy. For example and as noted above, inflammation may play a role in perinatal depression (Box 9-1 and Box 9-2). High-risk conditions, including preeclampsia, preterm labor, and gestational diabetes, exacerbate immune and inflammatory disruptions.[150]

Stress is also known to increase risk of postpartum depression, and the physical and psychological impact of high-risk conditions, including perception of risk and physical discomfort, may increase stress. For example, diagnosis of incompetent cervix positively correlates with elevation in antenatal EPDS scores, whereas other obstetric diagnoses do not demonstrate any such relationship to severity of depressive symptoms.[147] Women with medical disorders during their third trimester of pregnancy compared to pregnant women without illnesses do not have any known differences in diurnal cortisol patterns, or any correlation between levels of depression or anxiety and salivary cortisol.[151]

Social and interpersonal factors influencing the risk of antenatal depression in high-risk pregnancy include relationship satisfaction and maternal fetal attachment.[147] Stressors identified among women admitted for antepartum hospitalization include separation from spouse and children, loss of control, feelings of helplessness, and concern for fetal well-being.[152]

BOX 9-6
ANXIETY DISORDERS DURING PREGNANCY AND IN THE POSTPARTUM PERIOD

Prevalence
- GAD 8.5%
- Panic 1.3–2.0%
- OCD 0.2–1.2% during pregnancy; 2.7–3.9% postpartum
- PTSD 2.3–7.7%

Presentation in the perinatal period
- Pregnancy related anxiety can be nonpathologic (e.g., concerns about health of fetus, self-appraisal of role as a parent, changing body image, discomforts of pregnancy)
- Pathologic anxiety can result in avoidance of partner, requests for termination or cesarean, avoidance of baby
- Obsessional thoughts about infant can occur, including thoughts of harm to infant

Treatment
- SSRI
- Short-term benzodiazepine
- CBT
- Exposure therapy

Data from Ross LE, Mclean LM. Anxiety disorders during pregnancy and the postpartum period: A systemic review. J Clin Psychiatry. 2006;67(8): 1285–1298.

CLINICAL PRESENTATION

Pregnant women with medical complications have higher scores on depression and anxiety scales than pregnant women without these conditions (**Box 9-6**). In addition, women with pregnancy-related medical disorders, including preeclampsia, hyperemesis gravidarum, gestational diabetes, and placenta previa, have higher depressive symptom scores than pregnant women with other medical conditions, such as hematologic conditions, diabetes mellitus, thyroid disorder, cardiac disorder, lupus, asthma, and cancer.[151]

COURSE AND NATURAL HISTORY

Many women with high-risk pregnancies are prescribed bed rest, either in a hospital or at home. Antepartum hospitalization for bed rest suggests a serious situation requiring a high level of intervention, and is often associated with uncertainty. Patients who need to be on bed rest may experience fear, boredom, loss of control, loneliness, low self-esteem, and/or feeling imprisoned. In women hospitalized for full bed rest (due to preterm labor, premature rupture of membranes, cervical incompetence, placental abruption, placenta previa, or multiple fetuses), depressive symptom scores and measures of dysphoria decrease through the course of hospitalization. However, those hospitalized for longer durations (e.g., 4 weeks) still have clinically significant depressive symptoms despite some symptom reduction from the time of hospital admission. Postpartum dysphoria negatively correlates with gestational age at birth and positively correlates with objective clinical risk.[153,154]

ASSESSMENT AND DIFFERENTIAL DIAGNOSIS

Given the prevalence of depressive disorders and symptoms in women with high-risk pregnancy and the risks associated with antenatal depression, screening for depression is indicated. The EPDS has been validated for use in a high-risk population.[148] It is important to separate the symptoms of depression from the symptoms of the high-risk conditions themselves. In addition, it is important to clarify the magnitude of risk during the pregnancy as well as the patient's subjective perception of that risk. Consider the impact of treatments, such as bed rest, cerclage, or medication, on depression

symptoms as well. Pay special attention to any history of prior high-risk pregnancy, poor pregnancy outcome or perinatal loss, as this may inform and influence the patient's perception of risk in her current pregnancy, and whether or not she may experience recurrent grief or posttraumatic symptoms.

TREATMENT

The basic principles of treatment of depressive symptoms during pregnancy apply when treating a patient with high-risk pregnancy. Use prevention strategies first and then nonpharmacologic treatments in the case of mild symptoms. Weigh the risks associated with untreated depressive symptoms against the risks of medication in deciding whether to use pharmacotherapy.

Consider potential adverse effects on maternal health and pregnancy as well. For example, if there is a risk of premature and precipitous delivery, avoid benzodiazepines in order to avoid neonatal intoxication at the time of delivery. In pregnancies in which there are known fetal conditions, consult a maternal fetal medicine specialist and/or neonatologist about the risks of medication side effects on the neonate versus the risks of untreated depression. In preeclampsia avoid medications with metabolic effects that can elevate blood pressure, such as SNRI antidepressants. In patients with hyperemesis gravidarum, mirtazapine may be helpful in treating comorbid depressive symptoms as well as ongoing nausea, insomnia, and low appetite.[155]

Focus psychotherapeutic approaches on symptom management and prevention. Brief exposure therapy may be helpful for women with intense anxiety related to delivery or anticipation of morbidity in the neonate. In patients with prior perinatal loss and current high-risk pregnancies, psychotherapy focused on bereavement or posttraumatic symptoms may be warranted. IPT can be modified to specifically address complications related to pregnancy.[156,157]

Psychosocial interventions that reduce the stress of antepartum hospitalization may also reduce risk of depression. These include providing education and support to patients and families, promoting family contact with flexible visiting hours and video chats, and reducing boredom and isolation with social interactions and daytime scheduling.[152]

■ SUMMARY

Pregnancies are considered high risk when medical, obstetric, and/or fetal conditions increase the likelihood of adverse outcomes (**Box 9-7**). There may be a higher risk of maternal depressive symptoms associated with high-risk pregnancies. Inflammation, stress, and social and interpersonal variables contribute to the risk of depressive symptoms in these high-risk pregnancies. Women who need to be on bed rest and/or hospitalized during pregnancy may experience separation from loved ones, loss of control, feelings of helplessness, and worries about fetal well-being. In addition to screening for depressive symptoms, clinical assessment includes clarifying the magnitude of risk, patients' perceptions of risk,

BOX 9-7
SUMMARY

- Depression is common in the perinatal and postpartum period. Certain factors, such as gestational diabetes and high-risk pregnancies, can worsen the risk. Psychotic symptoms represent an emergency situation.
- Diagnosis is complicated by overlapping symptoms and potential medical illnesses but can be done by using a standardized approach.
- Treatments are complicated by the concern over the possible effects on the fetus, but in some cases these have been exaggerated and a rational approach to treatment includes psychotherapy and selected medications.

patients' reactions to interventions, and prior pregnancy outcomes. CBT and IPT are effective psychotherapeutic interventions for depressive symptoms during high-risk pregnancies. When needed, antidepressant medication can be chosen based on the side-effect profile least likely to exacerbate the high-risk condition.

Case Outcome: Anne completed the EPDS and scored 13. Psychiatric consultation was obtained, which revealed that Anne had a history of a prior depressive episode at age 22 for which she was treated with antidepressants and weekly individual psychotherapy. For 2½ weeks prior to her hospitalization, Anne had been experiencing sustained sad and anxious mood, increasing impairment of focus and concentration, excessive guilt, and anhedonia. She had been isolating herself from her family and friends. She was diagnosed with major depressive disorder with recurrent episodes, and a plan was established for a course of CBT and a trial of sertraline. In addition, Anne's nurse arranged for the patient's family to bring in her laptop so she could video chat with her husband and parents. Anne's symptoms improved over the next 2 weeks while she remained hospitalized. Anne delivered prematurely at 34 weeks. Her baby required hospitalization in the neonatal intensive care unit (NICU) for 4 weeks. During that time, Anne's anxiety intensified, but she did not develop postpartum depression. She continued taking sertraline, and was able to utilize her cognitive skills and relaxation exercises to attain remission of anxiety symptoms. Upon discharge of her baby, Anne had completed her course of CBT. She was nervous, but felt supported by her husband and family. She accepted a referral for a visiting nurse and a support group of parents of former patients of the NICU.

REFERENCES

1. Gavin NI, Gaynes BN, Lohr KN, Meltzer-Brody S, Gartlehner G, Swinson T. Perinatal depression: a systematic review of prevalence and incidence. *Obstetr Gynecol.* 2005;106:1071–1083.

2. Davé S, Petersen I, Sherr L, Nazareth I. Incidence of maternal and paternal depression in primary care: a cohort study using a primary care database. *Arch Pediatr Adolesc Med.* 2010;164(11): 1038–1044.

3. Halbreich U, Karkun S. Cross-cultural and social diversity of prevalence of postpartum depression and depressive symptoms. *J Affect Disord.* 2006;91:97–111.

4. Howell EA, Mora PA, Horowitz CR, Leventhal H. Racial and ethnic differences in factors associated with early postpartum depressive symptoms. *Obstet Gynecol.* 2005;105(6):1442–1450.

5. Orr ST, Blazer DG, James SA. Racial disparities in elevated prenatal depressive symptoms among black and white women in eastern North Carolina. *Ann Epidemiol.* 2006;16(6):463–468.

6. Meltzer-Brody S, Bledsoe-Mansori SE, Johnson N et al. A prospective study of perinatal depression and trauma history in pregnant minority adolescents. *Am J Obstet Gynecol.* 2013;208(3):211.e1–7.

7. Kingston D, Heaman M, Fell D, Chalmers B. Comparison of adolescent, young adult, and adult women's maternity experiences and practices. *Pediatrics.* 2012;129(5):1228–1237.

8. Viguera AC, Tondo L, Koukopoulos AE, Reginaldi D, Lepri B, Baldessarini RJ. Episodes of mood disorders in 2,252 pregnancies and postpartum periods. *Am J Psychiatry.* 2011;168(11):1179–1185.

9. Viguera AC, Nonacs R, Cohen LS, Tondo L, Murray A, Baldessarini RJ. Risk of recurrence of bipolar disorder in pregnant and nonpregnant women after discontinuing lithium maintenance. *Am J Psychiatry.* 2000;157(2):179–184.

10. Viguera AC, Whitfield T, Baldessarini RJ, et al. Risk of recurrence in women with bipolar disorder during pregnancy: prospective study of mood stabilizer discontinuation. *Am J Psychiatry.* 2007;164(12):1817–1824.

11. Di Florio A, Forty L, Gordon-Smith K, et al. Perinatal episodes across the mood disorder spectrum. *JAMA Psychiatry.* 2013;70(2):168–175.

12. Valdimarsdóttir U, Hultman CM, Harlow B, Cnattingius S, Sparén P. Psychotic illness in first-time mothers with no previous psychiatric hospitalizations: a population-based study. *PLoS Med.* 2009;6(2):e13.

13. Mehta D, Quast C, Fasching PA, et al. The 5-HTTLPR polymorphism modulates the influence on environmental stressors on peripartum depression symptoms. *J Affect Disord.* 2012; 136(3):1192–1197.

14. Bloch M, Rubinow DR, Schmidt PJ, Lotsikas A, Chrousos GP, Cizza G. Cortisol response to ovine corticotropin releasing hormone in a model of pregnancy and parturition in euthymic women with and without a history of postpartum depression. *J Clin Endocrinol Metab.* 2005;90(2):695–699.

15. Moses-Kolko EL, Wisner KL, Price JC, et al. Serotonin 1A receptor reductions in postpartum depression: a positron emission tomography study. *Fertil Steril.* 2008;89(3):685–692.

16. Kendall-Tackett K. A new paradigm for depression in new mothers: the central role of inflammation and how breastfeeding and anti-inflammatory treatments protect maternal mental health. *Int Breastfeed J.* 2007;2:6.

17. Maes M, Lin AH, Ombelet W, et al. Immune activation in the early puerperium is related to postpartum anxiety and depressive symptoms. *Psychoneuroendocrinol.* 2000;25(2):121–137.

18. Lancaster CA, Gold KJ, Flynn HA, Yoo H, Marcus SM, Davis MM. Risk factors for depressive symptoms during pregnancy: a systematic review. *Am J Obstet Gynecol.* 2010;202(1):5–14.

19. Xie RH, He G, Koszycki D, Walker M, Wen SW. Prenatal social support, postnatal social support, and postpartum depression. *Ann Epidemiol.* 2009;19(9):637–643.

20. Eberhard-Gran M, Garthus-Niegel S, Garthus-Niegel K, Eskild A. Postnatal care: a cross-cultural and historical perspective. *Arch Womens Mental Health.* 2010;13(6):459–466.

21. Jones I, Craddock N. Familiarity of the puerperal trigger in bipolar disorder: results of a family study. *Am J Psychiatry.* 2001;158(6): 913–917.

22. Altemus M, Neeb CC, Davis A, Occhiogrosso M, Nguyen T, Bleiberg KL. Phenotypic differences between pregnancy-onset and postpartum-onset major depressive disorder. *J Clin Psychiatry.* 2012;73(12) e1485–E191.

23. Jennings KD, Ross S, Popper S, Elmore M. Thoughts of harming infants in depressed and nondepressed mothers. *J Affect Disord.* 1999;54(1–2):21–28.

24. Attia E, Downey J, Oberman M. Postpartum psychoses. In: Miller LJ, ed. *Postpartum Mood Disorders.* Washington, DC: American Psychiatric Press; 1999:99–117.

25. Josefsson A, Sydsjö G. A follow-up study of postpartum depressed women: recurrent maternal depressive symptoms and child behavior after four years. *Arch Womens Mental Health.* 2007;10(4):141–145.

26. Serretti A, Olgiati P, Colombo C. Influence of postpartum onset on the course of mood disorders. *BMC Psychiatry.* 2006;6:4.

27. Dennis CL, Dowswell T. Psychosocial and psychological interventions for preventing postpartum depression. *Cochrane Database Syst Rev.* 2013;2:CD001134.

28. Robertson E, Jones I, Hague S, Holder R, Craddock N. Risk of puerperal and non-puerperal recurrence of illness following bipolar affective puerperal (postpartum) psychosis. *Brit J Psychiatry.* 2005;186:258–259.

29. Grigoriadis S, Vonderporten EH, Mamisashvili L, et al. The impact of maternal depression during pregnancy on perinatal outcomes: a systematic review. *J Clin Psychiatry*. 2013;74(4):e321–e341.

30. Oberlander TF, Weinberg J, Papsdorf M, Grunau R, Misri S, Devlin AM. Prenatal exposure to maternal depression, neonatal methylation of human glucocorticoid receptor gene (NR3C1) and infant cortisol stress responses. *Epigenetics*. 2008;3(2):97–106.

31. Rahman A, Iqbal Z, Bunn J, Lovel H, Harrington R. Impact of maternal depression on infant nutritional status and illness: a cohort study. *Arch Gen Psychiatry*. 2004;61(9):946–952.

32. Traviss GD, West RM, House AO. Maternal mental health and its association with infant growth at 6 months in ethnic groups: results from the Born-in-Bradford birth cohort study. *PLoS One*. 2012;7(2):e30707.

33. Huot RL, Brennan PA, Stowe ZN, Plotsky PM, Walker EF. Negative affect in offspring of depressed mothers is predicted by infant cortisol levels at 6 months and maternal depression during pregnancy, but not postpartum. *Ann N Y Acad Sci*. 2004;1032:234–236.

34. Paulson JF, Dauber S, Leiferman JA. Individual and combined effects of postpartum depression in mothers and fathers on parenting behavior. *Pediatrics*. 2006;118(2):659–668.

35. Darcy JM, Grzywacz JG, Stephens RL, Leng I, Clinch CR, Arcury TA. Maternal depressive symptomatology: 16-month follow-up of infant and maternal health-related quality of life. *J Am Board Fam Med*. 2011;24(3):249–257.

36. Halligan SL, Herbert J, Goodyer I, Murray L. Disturbances in morning cortisol secretion in association with maternal postnatal depression predict subsequent depressive symptomatology in adolescents. *Biol Psychiatry*. 2007;62(1):40–46.

37. Brennan PA, Hammen C, Andersen MJ, Bor W, Najman JM, Williams GM. Chronicity, severity, and timing of maternal depressive symptoms: relationship with child outcomes at age 5. *Devel Psychol*. 2000;36(6):759–766.

38. Galler JR, Ramsey FC, Harrison RH, Taylor J, Cumberbatch G, Forde V. Postpartum maternal moods and infant size predict performance on a national high school entrance examination. *J Child Psychol Psychiatry*. 2004;45(6):1064–1075.

39. Bodén R, Lundgren M, Brandt L, Reutfors J, Andersen M, Kieler H. Risks of adverse pregnancy and birth outcomes in women treated or not treated with mood stabilizers for bipolar disorder: population based cohort study. *BMJ*. 2012;345:e7085.

40. Lee HC, Lin HC. Maternal bipolar disorder increased low birthweight and preterm births: a nationwide population-based study. *J Affect Disord*. 2010;121(1–2):100–105.

41. Vance YH, Huntley Jones S, Espie J, Bentall R, Tai S. Parental communication styles and family relationships in children of bipolar parents. *Br J Clin Psychol*. 2008;47(Pt. 3):355–359.

42. Cox J, Holden J: International and cultural issues. In *Perinatal Mental Health: A Guide to the Edinburgh Postnatal Depression Scale*. London: Gaskell; 2003:21–25.

43. Miller LJ, Gupta R, Scremin AM. The evidence for perinatal depression screening and treatment. In: Handler A, Kennelly J, Peacock N, eds. *Reducing Racial/Ethnic Disparities in Reproductive and Perinatal Outcomes: The Evidence from Population-Based Interventions*. New York, NY: Springer; 2011:301–327.

44. Beck CT, Gable RK. Comparative analysis of the performance of the postpartum depression screening scale with two other depression instruments. *Nurs Res*. 2001;50(4):242–250.

45. Kendell RE, McGuire RJ, Connor Y, Cox JL. Mood changes in the first three weeks after childbirth. *J Affect Disord*. 1981;3:317–326.

46. Miller LJ, Rukstalis M. Beyond the "blues": hypotheses about postpartum reactivity. In: Miller LJ, ed. *Postpartum Mood Disorders*. Washington, DC: American Psychiatric Press; 1999: 3–19.

47. Pederson CA, Johnson JL, Silva S, et al. Antenatal thyroid correlates of postpartum depression. *Psychoneuroendocrinol*. 2007; 32(3):235–245.

48. Sylvén SM, Elenis E, Michelakos T, et al. Thyroid function tests at delivery and risk for postpartum depressive symptoms. *Psychoneuroendocrinol*. 2012;(12);S0306—4530.00339-3.

49. Khalaffalah AA, Dennis AE, Ogden K, et al. Three-year follow up of a randomised clinical trial of intravenous versus oral iron for anaemia in pregnancy. *BMJ Open*. 2012;2(5):e000998.

50. Cassidy-Bushrow AE, Peters RM, Johnson DA, Li J, Rao DS. Vitamin D nutritional status and antenatal depressive symptoms in African American women. *J Womens Health (Larchmt)*. 2012;21(11):1189–1195.

51. Ross LE, Grigoriadis S, Mamisashvili L, et al. Selected pregnancy and delivery outcomes after exposure to antidepressant medication: a systematic review and meta-analysis. *JAMA Psychiatry*. 2013;70(4):436–443.

52. Wisner KL, Sit DK, Hanusa BH, et al. Major depression and antidepressant treatment: impact on pregnancy and neonatal outcomes. *Am J Psychiatry*. 2009;166(5):557–566.

53. Wisner KL, Bogen DL, Sit D, et al. Does fetal exposure to SSRIs or maternal depression impact infant growth? *Am J Psychiatry*. 2013;170(5):485–493.

54. El Marroun H, Jaddoe VW, Hudzick JJ, et al. Maternal use of selective serotonin reuptake inhibitors, fetal growth, and risk of adverse birth outcomes. *Arch Gen Psychiatry*. 2012;69(7): 706–714.

55. Nulman I, Koren G, Rovet J, et al. Neurodevelopment of children following prenatal exposure to venlafaxine, selective serotonin reuptake inhibitors, or untreated maternal depression. *Am J Psychiatry*. 2012;169(11):1165–1174.

56. Weikum WM, Oberlander TF, Hensch TK, Werker JF. Prenatal exposure to antidepressants and depressed maternal mood alter trajectory of infant speech perception. *Proc Natl Acad Sci USA*. 2012;109(Suppl 2):17221–17227.

57. Levinson-Castiel R, Merlob P, Linder N, Sirota L, Klinger G. Neonatal abstinence syndrome after in utero exposure to selective serotonin reuptake inhibitors in term infants. *Arch Pediatr Adolesc Med*. 2006;160(2):173–176.

58. Ochiogrosso M, Omran SS, Altemus M. Persistent pulmonary hypertension of the newborn and selective serotonin reuptake inhibitors: lessons from clinical and translational research. *Am J Psychiatry*. 2012;169(2):134–140.

59. Cohen LS, Altshuler LL, Harlow BL, et al. Relapse of major depression during pregnancy in women who maintain or discontinue antidepressant treatment. *JAMA*. 2006;295(5):499–507.

60. Yonkers KA, Gotman N, Smith MV, et al. Does antidepressant use attenuate the risk of a major depressive episode in pregnancy? *Epidemiol*. 2011;22(6):848–854.

61. United States National Library of Medicine, Toxnet Toxicology Data Network, Available at http://toxnet.nlm.nih.gov/cgi-bin/sis/htmlgen?LACT, accessed April 28, 2013.

62. Newport DJ, Viguera AC, Beach AJ, Ritchie JC, Cohen LS, Stowe ZN. Lithium placental passage and obstetrical outcome: implications for clinical management during late pregnancy. *Am J Psychiatry*. 2005;162(11):2162–2170.

63. McKnight RF, Adida M, Budge K, Stockton S, Goodwin GM, Geddes JR. Lithium toxicity profile: a systematic review and meta-analysis. *Lancet*. 2012;379(9817):721–728.

64. van der Lugt NM, van de Maat JS, van Kamp IL, Knoppert-van der Klein EA, Hovens JG, Walther FJ. Fetal, neonatal and developmental outcomes of lithium-exposed pregnancies. *Early Hum Devel*. 2012;88(6):375–378.

65. Krause S, Ebbersen F, Lange AP. Polyhydramnios with maternal lithium toxicity. *Obstet Gynecol*. 1990;75(3 Pt 2):504–506.

66. Troyer WA, Pereira GR, Lannon RA, Belik J, Yoder MC. Association of maternal lithium exposure and premature delivery. *J Perinatol*. 1993;13(2):123–127.

67. Frassetto F, Tourneur MF, Barjhoux CE, Villier C, Bot BL, Vincent F. Goiter in a newborn exposed to lithium in utero. *Ann Pharmacother*. 2002;36(11):1745–1748.

68. Kozma C. Neonatal toxicity and transient neurodevelopmental deficits following prenatal exposure to lithium: another clinical report and a review of the literature. *Am J Med Genet A*. 2005;132(4):441–444.

69. Viguera AC, Newport DJ, Ritchie J, et al. Lithium in breast milk and nursing infants: clinical implications. *Am J Psychiatry*. 2007;164(2):342–345.

70. Morrow J, Russell A, Guthrie E, et al. Malformation risks of antiepileptic drugs in pregnancy: a prospective study from the UK Epilepsy and Pregnancy Register. *J Neurol Neurosurg Psychiatry*. 2006;77(2):193–198.

71. Mawer G, Briggs M, Baker GA, et al. Pregnancy with epilepsy: obstetric and neonatal outcome of a controlled study. *Seizure*. 2010;19(2):112–119.

72. Hernández-Díaz S, Smith CR, Shen A, et al. Comparative safety of antiepileptic drugs during pregnancy. *Neurol*. 2012;78(21):1692–1699.

73. Vajda FJ, Graham J, Roten A, Lander CM, O'Brien TJ, Eadie M. Teratogenicity of the newer antiepileptic drugs—the Australian experience. *J Clin Neurosci*. 2012;19(1):57–59.

74. Cummings C, Stewart M, Stevenson M, Morrow J, Nelson J. Neurodevelopment of children exposed in utero to lamotrigine, sodium valproate and carbamazepine. *Arch Dis Child*. 2011;96(7):643–647.

75. Meador KJ, Baker GA, Browning N, et al. Fetal antiepileptic drug exposure and cognitive outcomes at age 6 years (NEAD study): a prospective observational study. *Lancet Neurol*. 2013;12(3):244–252.

76. Christensen J, Grønborg TK, Sørensen MJ, et al. Prenatal valproate exposure and risk of autism spectrum disorders and childhood autism. *JAMA*. 2013;309(16):1696–1703.

77. Jentink J, Dok H, Loane MA, et al. Intrauterine exposure to carbamazepine and specific congenital malformations: systematic review and case-control study. *BMJ*. 2010;341:c6581.

78. Jones KL, Lacro RV, Johnson KA, Adams J. Patterns of malformations in the children of women treated with carbamazepine during pregnancy. *New Eng J Med*. 1989;320(25):1661–1666.

79. Banach R, Boskovic R, Einarson T, Koren G. Long-term developmental outcome of children of women with epilepsy, unexposed or exposed prenatally to antiepileptic drugs: a meta-analysis of cohort studies. *Drug Saf*. 2010;33(1):73–79.

80. Pennell PB, Klein AM, Browning N, et al. Differential effects of antiepileptic drugs on neonatal outcomes. *Epilepsy Behav*. 2012;24:449–456.

81. Frey B, Braegger CP, Ghelfi D. Neonatal cholestatic hepatitis from carbamazepine exposure during pregnancy and breast-feeding. *Ann Pharmacother*. 2002;36(4):644–647.

82. Kaaja E, Kaaja R, Matila R, Hiilesmaa V. Enzyme-inducing antiepileptic drugs in pregnancy and the risk of bleeding in the neonate. *Neurol*. 2002;58(4):549–553.

83. Yerby MS, Friel PN, McCormick K, et al. Pharmacokinetics of anticonvulsants in pregnancy: alterations in plasma protein binding. *Epilepsy Res*. 1990;5(3):223–228.

84. Holmes LB, Baldwin EJ, Smith CR, et al. Increased frequency of isolated cleft palate in infants exposed to lamotrigine during pregnancy. *Neurol*. 2008;70(22 Pt 2):2152–2158.

85. Cunnington MC, Weil JG, Messenheimer JA, Ferber S, Yerby M, Tennis P. Final results from 18 years of the International Lamotrigine Pregnancy Registry. *Neurol*. 2011;76(21):1817–1823.

86. Mølgaard-Nielsen D, Hviid A. Newer-generation antiepileptic drugs and the risk of major birth defects. *JAMA*. 2011;305(19):1996–2002.

87. Dolk H, Jentink J, Loane M, et al. Does lamotrigine use in pregnancy increase orofacial cleft risk relative to other malformations? *Neurol*. 2008;71(10):714–722.

88. Tomson T, Landmark CJ, Battino D. Antiepileptic drug treatment in pregnancy: changes in drug disposition and their clinical implications. *Epilepsia*. 2013;54(3):405–414.

89. Sabers A. Algorithm for lamotrigine dose adjustment before, during, and after pregnancy. *Acta Neurol Scand*. 2012;126(1):e1–e4.

90. Newport DJ, Pennell PB, Calamaras MR, et al. Lamotrigine in breast milk and nursing infants: determination of exposure. *Pediatrics*. 2008;122(1):e223–e231.

91. Nordmo E, Aronsen L, Wasland K, Småbrekke L, Verren S. Severe apnea in an infant exposed to lamotrigine in breast milk. *Ann Pharmacother*. 2009;43(11):1893–1897.

92. McKenna K, Koren G, Tetelbaum M, et al. Pregnancy outcome of women using atypical antipsychotic drugs: a prospective comparative study. *J Clin Psychiatry*. 2005;66(4):444–449.

93. Peng M, Gao K, Ding Y, et al. Effects of prenatal exposure to atypical antipsychotics on postnatal development and growth of infants: a case-controlled, prospective study. *Psychopharmacol (Berl)*. 2013;228(4):577–584.

94. Lang K, Nuevo-Chiquero A. Trends in self-reported spontaneous abortions: 1970–2000. *Demography*. 2012;49:989–1009.

95. McClure EM, Pasha O, Gouder SS, et al. Epidemiology of stillbirth in low-middle income countries: a Global Network study. *Acta Obstet Gynecol Scand*. 2011;90(12):1379–1385.

96. Straney LD, Lim SS, Murray CJ. Disentangling the effects of risk factors and clinical care of subnational variation in early neonatal mortality in the United States. *PLoS One*. 2012;7(11):e49399.

97. Lisonkova S, Hutcheon JA, Joseph KS. Sudden infant death syndrome: a re-examination of temporal trends. *BMC Preg Childbirth*. 2012;12:59.

98. Boyle FM, Vance JC, Najman JM, Thearle MJ. The mental health impact of stillbirth, neonatal death or SIDS: prevalence and patterns of distress among mothers. *Soc Sci Med*. 1996;43(8):1273–1282.

99. Cacciatore J, Rådestad I, Frøen JF. Effects of contact with stillborn babies on maternal anxiety and depression. *Birth*. 2008;35(4):313–320.

100. Obi SN, Onah HE, Okafor II. Depression among Nigerian women following pregnancy loss. *Int J Gynecol Obstet*. 2009;105(1):60–62.

101. Sham A, Yiu M, Ho W. Psychiatric morbidity following miscarriage in Hong Kong. *Gen Hosp Psychiatry*. 2010;32(3):284–293.

102. Kong GW, Lok IH, Yiu AK, Hui AS, Lai BP, Chung TK. Clinical and psychological impact after surgical, medical or expectant management of first-trimester miscarriage—a randomized controlled trial. *Aust N Z J Obstet Gynecol*. 2013;53(2):170–177.

103. Toffol E, Koponen P, Partonen T. Miscarriage and mental health: results of two population-based studies. *Psychiatr Res*. 2013;205:151–158.

104. Surkan PJ, Rådestad I, Cnattingius S, Steineck G, Dickman PW. Social support after stillbirth for prevention of maternal depression. *Acta Obstet Gynecol Scand*. 2009;88(12):1358–1364.

105. Arck PC, Rose M, Hartwig K, Hagen E, Hildebrandt M, Klapp BF. Stress and immune mediators in miscarriage. *Hum Reprod*.2001;16(7):1505–1511.

106. Sugiura-Ogasawara M, Furukawa TA, Nakano Y, Hori S, Aoki K, Kitamura T. Depression as a potential causal factor in subsequent miscarriage in recurrent spontaneous abortions. *Hum Reprod*. 2002;17(10):2580–2584.

107. Athanasakis E, Karavasiliadou S, Styliadis I. The factors contributing to the risk of sudden infant death syndrome. *Hippokratia*. 2011;15(2):127–131.

108. Bukowski R, Carpenter M, Conway D, et al. Causes of death among stillbirths. *JAMA*. 2011;306(22):2459–2468.

109. Bukowski R, Carpenter M, Conway D, et al. Association between stillbirth and risk factors known at pregnancy confirmation. *JAMA*. 2011;306(22):2459–2468.

110. Trulsson O, Radestad I. The silent child–mothers' experiences before, during, and after stillbirth. *Birth*. 2004;31(3):189–195.

111. Adolfsson A, Larsson PG, Wijma B, Berterö C. Guilt and emptiness: women's experiences of miscarriage. *Health Care Women Int*. 2004;52:543–560.

112. Gold KL, Sen A, Hayward RA. Marriage and cohabitation outcomes after pregnancy loss. *Pediatrics*. 2010;125(5):1202–1207.

113. Blackmore ER, Côté-Arsenault D, Tang W, et al. Previous prenatal loss as a predictor of perinatal depression and anxiety. *Brit J Psychiatry*. 2011;198(5):373–378.

114. Couto B, Couto E, Vian B, et al. Quality of life, depression and anxiety among pregnant women with previous adverse pregnancy outcomes. *Sao Paulo Med J*. 2009;127(4):185–189.

115. Lok IH, Yip AS, Lee DT, Sahota D, Chung TK. A 1-year longitudinal study of psychological morbidity after miscarriage. *Fertil Steril*. 2010;93(6):1966–1975.

116. Surkan PJ, Rådestad I, Cnattingius S, Steineck G, Dickman PW. Events after stillbirth in relation to maternal depressive symptoms: a brief report. *Birth*. 2008;35(2):153–157.

117. Armstrong DS. Perinatal loss and parental distress after the birth of a healthy infant. *Adv Neonatal Care*. 2007;7(4):200–206.

118. Turton P, Evans C, Hughes P. Long-term psychosocial sequelae of stillbirth: phase II of a nested case-control cohort study. *Arch Womens Mental Health*. 2009;12:35–41.

119. Brier N. Grief following miscarriage: a comprehensive review of the literature. *J Womens Health (Larchmt)*. 2008;17(3):451–464.

120. Badenhorst W. Psychological aspects of perinatal loss. *Best Pract Res Clin Obstet Gynecol*. 2007;21(2):249–259.

121. Hughes P, Turton P, Hopper E, Evans CD. Assessment of guidelines for good practices in psychosocial care of mothers after stillbirth: a cohort study. *Lancet*. 2002;360(9327):114–118.

122. Gong X, Hao J, Tao F, Zhang J, Wang H, Xu R. Pregnancy loss and anxiety and depression during subsequent pregnancies: data from the C-ABC study. *Eur J Obstet Gynecol Reprod Biol*. 2013;166(1):30–36.

123. Hughes P, Turton P, Hopper E, McGauley GA, Fonagy P. Disorganised attachment behaviour among infants born subsequent to stillbirth. *J Child Psychol Psychiatry*. 2001;42(6):791–801.

124. Lamb EH. The impact of previous perinatal loss on subsequent pregnancy and parenting. *J Perinat Educ*. 2002;11(2):33–40.

125. Swanson KM, Chen HT, Graham JC, Wojnar DM, Petras A. Resolution of depression and grief during the first year after miscarriage: a randomized controlled clinical trial of couples-focused interventions. *J Womens Health (Larchmt)*. 2009;18(8):1245–1257.

126. Kersting A, Kroker K, Schlicht S, Wagner B. Internet-based treatment after pregnancy loss: concept and case study. *J Psychosom Obstet Gynecol*. 2011;32(2):72–78.

127. Cacciatore J, Schnebly S, Frøen JF. The effects of social support on maternal anxiety and depression after stillbirth. *Health Soc Care Community*. 2009;17(2):167–176.

128. Dabelea D, Snell-Bergeon JK, Hartsfield CL, Bischoff KJ, Hamman RF, McDuffie RS. Increasing prevalence of gestational diabetes mellitus (GDM) over time and by birth cohort. *Diabetes Care*. 2005;28(3):579–584.

129. Kozhimannil KB, Pereira MA, Harlow BL. Association between diabetes and perinatal depression among low-income mothers. *JAMA*. 2009;301(8):842–847.

130. Lydon K, Dunne FP, Owens L, et al. Psychological stress associated with diabetes during pregnancy: a pilot study. *Ir Med J*. 2012;105(5 Suppl):26–28.

131. Katon JG, Russo J, Gavin AR, Melville JL, Katon WJ. Diabetes and depression in pregnancy: is there an association? *J Womens Health (Larchmt)*. 2011;20(7):983–989.

132. Langer N, Langer O. Comparison of pregnancy mood profiles in gestational diabetes and preexisting diabetes. *Diab Educ*. 2000;26:667–672.

133. Nicklas JM, Miller LJ, Zera CA, Davis RB, Levkoff SE, Seely EW. Factors associated with depressive symptoms in the early postpartum period among women with recent gestational diabetes mellitus. *Matern Child Health J*. 2013;17(9):1665–1672.

134. Heitritter SM, Solomon CG, Mitchell GI, Skali-Ouris N, Seely EW. Subclinical inflammation and vascular dysfunction in women with previous gestational diabetes mellitus. *J Clin Endocrinol Metab*. 2005;90(7):3983–3988.

135. Pedersen P, Baker JL, Henriksen TB, et al. Influence of psychosocial factors on postpartum weight retention. *Obesity (Silver Spring)*. 2011;19(3):639–646.

136. Dennis CL, McQueen K. Does maternal postpartum depressive symptomatology influence infant feeding outcomes? *Acta Paediatr*. 2007;96(4):590–594.

137. Mulhoolad C, Njoroge T, Mersereau P, Williams J. Comparison of guidelines available in the United States for diagnosis and management of diabetes before, during, and after pregnancy. *J Womens Health*. 2007;16(6):790–801.

138. Crowther CA, Hiller JE, Moss JR, et al. Effect of treatment of gestational diabetes mellitus on pregnancy outcomes. *New Eng J Med*. 2005;352(24):2477–2486.

139. Landon MB, Spong CY, Thom E, et al. A multicenter, randomized trial of treatment for mild gestational diabetes. *New Eng J Med*. 2009;361(14):1339–1348.

140. Markowitz S, Gonzalez JS, Wilkinson JL, Safren SA. A review of Treating Depression in Diabetes: Emerging Findings. *Psychosomatics.* 2011;52(1):1–18.

141. Lustmann PJ, Griffiths LS, Freedland KE, Kissel SS, Clouse RE. Cognitive behavioral therapy for depression in type 2 diabetes mellitus. A randomized, controlled trial. *Ann Intern Med.* 1998;129:613–621.

142. Barakat R, Pelaez M, Lopez C, Lucia A, Ruiz JR. Exercise during pregnancy and gestational diabetes-related adverse effects: a randomised controlled trial. *Br J Sports Med.* 2013;47(10):630–636.

143. McIntyre RS, Soczynska JK, Konarski JZ, Kennedy SH. The effect of antidepressants on glucose homeostasis and insulin sensitivity: synthesis and mechanisms. *Expert Opin Drug Saf.* 2006;5(1):157–168.

144. Fava M. Weight gain and antidepressants. *J Clin Psychiatry.* 2000;61(Suppl 11):37–41.

145. Society of Maternal Fetal Medicine. *Maternal-Fetal Medicine: High-Risk Pregnancy Care, Research, and Education for Over 35 Years.* Available from https://www.smfm.org/attachedfiles/SMFMMonograph3.1.pdf. Washington, DC; 2010.

146. Thiagayson P, Krishnaswamy G, Lim ML, et al. Depression and anxiety in Singaporean high-risk pregnancies—prevalence and screening. *Gen Hosp Psychiatry.* 2013;35:112–116.

147. Brandon AR, Trivedi MH, Hynan LS, et al. Prenatal depression in women hospitalized for obstetric risk. *J Clin Psychiatry.* 2008;69(4):635–643.

148. Adouard F, Glangreaud-Freudenthal NM, Golse B. Validation of the Edinburgh postnatal depression scale in a sample of women with high-risk pregnancies in France. *Arch Womens Ment Health.* 2005;8:89–95.

149. Zadeh MA, Khajehei M, Sharif F, et al. High risk pregnancy: effects on postpartum depression and anxiety. *Brit J Midwifery.* 2012;20(2):104–113.

150. Osborne LM, Monk C. Perinatal depression—the fourth inflammatory morbidity of pregnancy? Theory and literature review. *Psychoneuroendocrinology.* 2013;38(10):1929–1952.

151. King NM, Chambers J, O'Donnell K. Anxiety, depression and saliva cortisol in women with medical disorder during pregnancy. *Arch Womens Ment Health.* 2010;13:339–345.

152. Heaman M. Psychosocial impact of high-risk pregnancy: hospital and home care. *Clin Obstet Gynecol.* 1998;41(3):629–639.

153. Maloni J, Park S, Anthony M, et al. Measurement of antepartum depressive symptoms during high risk pregnancy. *Res Nurs Health.* 2005;28:16–26.

154. Maloni JA, Kane JH, Suen L, et al. Dysphoria among high-risk pregnant hospitalized women on bed rest: a longitudinal study. *Nurs Res.* 2002;51(2):92–99.

155. Guclu S, Gol M, Dogan E, et al. Mirtazipine use in resistant hyperemesis gravidarum: report of three cases and review of the literature. *Arch Gynecol Obstet.* 2005;272:298–300.

156. Spinelli MG, Endicott J. Controlled clinical trial of interpersonal psychotherapy versus parenting education program for depressed pregnant women. *Am J Psychiatry.* 2003;160:555–562.

157. O'Hara M, Stuart S, Gorman LL, et al. Efficacy of interpersonal psychotherapy for postpartum depression. *Arch Gen Psychiatry.* 2000;57:1039–1045.

CHAPTER 10

Depression and Rheumatological and Immune Disorders

David Kroll, MD
Inder Kalra, MD
Naomi Schmelzer, MD
Charles Surber, MD
Jeffrey Katz, MD, MSc

INTRODUCTION

It is easy to think about rheumatologic illnesses, including chronic inflammatory and arthritic conditions such as rheumatoid arthritis (RA), as disorders that primarily affect the musculoskeletal and immune systems. But these rheumatologic disorders have prominent neuropsychiatric symptoms and many other confounding and complicating factors. Pain, systemic inflammation, disability, fatigue, sleep disruption, and treatment effects—all of these accompany rheumatologic conditions, and are associated with depression in and of themselves.

Although some rheumatologic illnesses—most notably systemic lupus erythematosus—directly cause neuropsychiatric symptoms, the depression occurring in most of these patients is multifactorial. This chapter reviews the diagnosis and treatment of depression when it occurs in the context of a rheumatologic disease. It includes an initial discussion of the role of two salient factors common to rheumatologic disease in general—systemic inflammation and corticosteroid treatment—and then turns to the specific diseases whose association with depression has been studied: systemic lupus, RA, scleroderma, and fibromyalgia.

SYSTEMIC INFLAMMATION AND DEPRESSION

The relationship of depression to inflammatory processes has long been a subject of investigation.[1] Significant associations were discovered between inflammation and depression, including epidemiologic observations (the high female to male ratio, and lower rates of depression in cultures with diets rich in fish) and biological associations (e.g., between symptoms of depression and pro-inflammatory cytokines). Although there is strong evidence of a link between depression and inflammation, the precise mechanisms remain elusive.

Depression is substantially more prevalent in patients with rheumatologic illnesses than in the general population,[2] and depression is highly correlated with disease-related morbidity within this population. Compared to other major medical comorbidities, patients with rheumatologic illness exhibit the strongest correlation between depression and lower quality of life measurements.[3] Depression also appears to predict work disability more strongly in this population than among patients without a rheumatic illness.[4]

The link between depression and rheumatologic illnesses likely includes both psychological and biological components. Restricted independence, higher medical burden, and patients' concerns about appearance (e.g., skin lesions or musculoskeletal deformities) have all been associated with depression in these patients.[5,6]

What is known about the biological link between depression and systemic inflammation remains limited, but some associations have been demonstrated in research studies (Chapters 1 and 2). Healthy test subjects given an endotoxin (which promotes systemic inflammation as manifested by a rise in body temperature and in pro-inflammatory cytokines) (**Table 10-1**) develop depressed mood, anxiety, and memory impairment.[7] Patients with existing major depression have higher concentrations of TNFa and IL-6 even without stimulation by an endotoxin.[8]

Furthermore, antidepressants may reduce at least some markers of systemic inflammation. A meta-analysis showed an inconsistent association between treatment with SSRIs, SNRIs, and TCAs and a reduction in TNFa and IL-6 levels and a consistent association with reduction in IL-1-beta (IL1B).[9] The association between

TABLE 10-1 Proinflammatory Cytokines Studied in Depression

Tumor necrosis factor alpha (TNF-alpha)[a,b]
Interleukin-6 (IL-6)[a,b]
Interleukin-1-beta (IL-1beta)[a]
Interferon-gamma (IFN-gamma)
Interleukin-10 (IL-10)
Interleukin-4
Interleukin-2
Interleukin-8

[a]Antidepressant therapy may affect levels.
[b]Increased levels in patients with MDD.
Data from Dowlati Y, Herrmann N, Swardfager W, et al. A meta-analysis of cytokines in major depression. Biol Psychiatry. 2010;67(5):446–457.

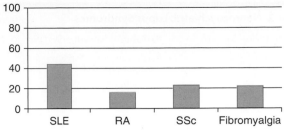

Figure 10-1 *Mean risk of depression for selected illnesses (percentage prevalence for particular disease).*

antidepressants and reduced IL-6 levels was stronger for SSRIs than for other antidepressant classes.

Nonpharmacologic treatment modalities for depression have been examined to a lesser extent in this regard. The evidence supporting these treatments for patients with specific rheumatologic disorders is discussed later in this chapter under the disorder subheadings. It is additionally worth noting that one study demonstrated that cognitive-behavioral therapy (CBT) correlated with lower IL-6 levels in women with depression who did not have a rheumatologic illness.[10] Electroconvulsive therapy (ECT), by contrast, was shown to increase proinflammatory markers, including TNFa and IL-6, after a single session, although repeat sessions did not further affect these parameters.[11] Studies examining the efficacy of repetitive transcranial magnetic stimulation (rTMS) in treating rheumatic pain have been conducted but have not consistently shown a benefit.[12]

Conversely, some immunosuppressive and anti-inflammatory agents have been associated with antidepressant effects in studies, although because these agents have an established, powerful effect in lowering disease activity (and thereby reducing pain and disability) these findings must be interpreted with caution. Etanercept was associated with a reduction in depressive symptoms when administered to patients with psoriasis.[13] Celecoxib was associated with greater reductions depressive symptoms and in IL-6 levels when provided as an adjunct to sertraline, compared to sertraline with a placebo adjunct.[14]

THE ROLE OF PRESCRIBED GLUCOCORTICOIDS (BOX 10-8)

Glucocorticoids (GCs), which are frequently prescribed in rheumatologic disorders, affect mood and other psychiatric symptoms. In addition to the systemic risks attributed to GC therapy, which include osteoporosis, cardiovascular effects, diabetes mellitus, and weight gain,[15] associated neuropsychiatric side effects include depression, mania, psychosis, delirium, cognitive impairment and memory dysfunction, suicide,[16,17] and sleep.[18] Historically, the risk of neuropsychiatric side effects from GCs has been considered to be very low at doses below 40 mg per day of prednisone (or equivalent), and higher at doses greater than 80 mg per day.[19] However, more recent evidence suggests that lower doses of prednisone (7.5 mg per day or greater) also appear to increase the risk of depression when prescribed for at least 6 months.[20]

Among affective symptoms, depression appears to be most closely associated with chronic GC therapy,[16] while short courses of treatment are more commonly associated with mania.[21,22] Paradoxically, however, some patients with preexisting depression often experience an improvement in their moods with GC administration.[21] Some authors have argued that a steroid-induced mood disorder (either depression or mania) may more closely resemble

bipolar disorder than major depression—not only in symptomatology but possibly also in its response to treatment.[16]

The evidence regarding the choice of the agent to treat steroid-induced mood symptoms is limited.[16] Studies of conventional antidepressants have demonstrated improvement in depression[16,23] in some and adverse outcomes such as agitation and psychosis in others.[24] Lithium provides effective prophylaxis against steroid-induced psychosis,[25] and lamotrigine reduces negative effects of prescribed GCs on memory function.[26] Evidence supporting the use of antipsychotics in treating steroid-induced mood symptoms is positive but remains primarily based on uncontrolled trials[27] and case reports,[16] and meanwhile use of these treatments necessitates considering their potentially unfavorable side-effect profiles. Steroid-induced mood disorders are typically reversible with discontinuation of the GC.[16]

SYSTEMIC LUPUS ERYTHEMATOSUS

Systemic lupus erythematosus (SLE) is an autoimmune disease that causes inflammation and tissue destruction in multiple organ systems. The prevalence of lupus varies between 0.03% and 0.14% worldwide[28]; it is more common among women and among nonwhite ethnic groups.[29]

■ EPIDEMIOLOGY

The reported prevalence of depressive symptoms in patients with SLE ranges between 17% and 71% (**Fig 10-1**). Despite this wide range, it is clear that major depressive disorder is more prevalent among patients with SLE than in the general population,[30,31] and suicide is more prevalent in this group as well.[32] Depression is associated with poorer quality of life in patients with SLE—perhaps even more strongly than for indicators of disease activity[33]—poorer cognitive functioning,[34] and medication nonadherence.[35]

Some studies (**Box 10-1**) have found an association with depression severity and SLE disease activity[36,37] as well; however, this finding has not shown consistency across all populations.[38] Among patients with SLE, higher depression severity has additionally been

BOX 10-1
IMPORTANT RISK FACTORS FOR DEPRESSION IN RHEUMATIC DISEASES

Sociodemographic
Clinical
Disease severity (inconsistent)
Pain
Steroid use
Insomnia
Medical
White matter hyperintensities
Vasculopathies (limited data)

TABLE 10-2 Neuropsychiatric Lupus Syndromes

Central Nervous System	Peripheral Nervous System
Aseptic meningitis	Acute inflammatory demyelinating polyradiculopathy
Cerebrovascular disease	Autonomic disorder
Demyelinating syndrome	Mononeuropathy
Headache	Myasthenia gravis
Movement disorder	Cranial neuropathy
Myelopathy	Plexopathy
Seizure disorder	Polyneuropathy
Acute confusional state	
Anxiety disorder	
Cognitive dysfunction	
Mood disorder	
Psychosis	

Adapted with permission from The American College of Rheumatology nomenclature and case definitions for neuropsychiatric lupus syndromes, Arthritis Rheum. 1999 Apr;42(4):599–608.

associated with pain, arthritis, and prednisone doses greater than 7.5 mg.[31]

■ PATHOPHYSIOLOGY

The American College of Rheumatology has formally defined 19 syndromes affecting the central and peripheral nervous systems that fall under the heading of "neuropsychiatric lupus," or NPSLE (**Box 10-2**). These are listed in **Table 10-2**. The five psychiatric NPSLE syndromes include delirium, anxiety disorder, mood disorder, cognitive dysfunction, and psychosis. Distinguishing between NPSLE (a.k.a. a psychiatric disorder "due to a general medical condition") and other depressive disorders that occur in the context of SLE has proved notoriously difficult,[39] particularly given that neuropsychiatric lupus can by definition occur at any time during the course of SLE or even predate its onset.[39] In truth, trying to make this distinction might mislead us in the same way that trying to understand depression as either a purely organic or purely psychological phenomenon misleads us. Several neurobiological mechanisms for NPSLE have been proposed; four are described below.

■ CEREBROVASCULAR DYSFUNCTION

SLE is highly associated with vascular disease,[40] and both inflammation and thrombotic phenomena contribute to its vascular manifestations.[41] It has been proposed that cerebrovascular occlusion and/or hemorrhage may underlie or contribute to NPSLE,[42] although rigorous studies to investigate this mechanism have not been conducted. Cerebrovascular pathology consistent with this

model has been demonstrated in postmortem studies of patients with SLE,[43] and a difference in cerebral perfusion between SLE patients and controls has been observed with magnetic resonance imaging (MRI).[44]

■ ANTIBODY-MEDIATED

Higher levels of circulating serum antibodies to the human N-methyl-D-aspartate (NMDA) NR2 receptor have been associated with increased depression as well as hypomania and some cognitive measures[45] in SLE patients, although in at least one study this association was found only with CSF NR2 antibodies and not with serum antibodies.[46] Anti-ribosomal P (anti-P) antibody has also been implicated in the pathogenesis of NPSLE, but the association between serum anti-P levels was not supported by a meta-analysis of the existing literature.[47] Thus the role of antibodies in NPSLE remains to be further clarified.

■ INFLAMMATORY CYTOKINES

Consistent with studies of inflammatory markers in non-SLE depression, significantly higher levels of CSF IL-6 are found in patients with NPSLE compared to other patients with SLE and to healthy controls.[48] Murine research has implicated a TNF family ligand (TWEAK) as another potential mediator between SLE, NPSLE, and depression.[49]

■ BLOOD–BRAIN BARRIER DISRUPTION

There is an absence of definitive studies on how closely blood–brain barrier (BBB) disruption and NPSLE are linked, although this association has been supported by case reports.[50] The difficulties in measuring BBB disruption probably contribute to this. The degree of BBB disruption in patients with SLE is typically measured indirectly, by the presence or quantity of proteins (e.g., albumin or immunoglobulins) or serum molecules in the CSF. These markers require lumbar puncture to obtain, are often transient, and can be reduced or reversed by treatment with corticosteroids.

■ CLINICAL PRESENTATION, COURSE, AND NATURAL HISTORY

Patients with SLE commonly present with symptoms that overlap with DSM IV criteria for major depressive disorder, including fatigue, psychomotor retardation, and sleep disturbance (**Box 10-3**).[51] Cognitive problems are commonly reported as well.[34] Therefore, the somatic and cognitive symptoms of SLE may lead to false positive symptoms of depression screening tools.[51]

■ ASSESSMENT AND DIFFERENTIAL DIAGNOSIS

When depression is identified in the context of SLE, assessment of cognitive functioning, energy, and sleep should be part of the

---

BOX 10-2
POSSIBLE MEDIATORS BETWEEN RHEUMATOLOGIC DISORDERS AND DEPRESSION

Physical disability
Autoimmune
Inflammation
Cerebrovascular dysfunction
Blood–Brain barrier disruption
Neurotransmitter dysfunction
HPA axis hyperactivity

BOX 10-3
IMPORTANT SYMPTOMS

Confounding
  Fatigue
  Psychomotor slowing
  Insomnia
  Cognitive dysfunction
  Appetite disturbances
  Preoccupation with changes in physical appearance
More typical in depression
  Anhedonia
  Suicidal ideation

BOX 10-4
DIFFERENTIAL DIAGNOSIS

Primary depressive disorder concurrent with rheumatic illness
Depressive disorder secondary to the rheumatic illness (e.g., NPSLE)
Other neuropsychiatric disorders (delirium, anxiety disorder, other mood disorder, cognitive dysfunction, psychosis)

---

initial workup (**Box 10-4** and **Box 10-5**). NPSLE is difficult to rule out, and therefore a rheumatologist should be consulted to assist in investigating other disease parameters if this is possible. Because further treatment might include use of GC, immuno-modulators, antimalarial agents, and/or anticoagulants depending upon the specific NPSLE syndrome, consideration to the effects these treatments may have on neuropsychiatric symptoms should be given as well.

■ TREATMENT

Controlled studies establishing the optimal use of antidepressants in patients with depression and SLE are lacking, although clinical experience suggests that the SSRIs are the first-line agents of choice (**Box 10-6** to **Box 10-8**). However, there are case reports of an association between bupropion[52] and sertraline[53] with cutaneous and systemic lupus symptoms, respectively. There are reports of successful treatment of NPSLE depression with ECT.[54]

There are currently no studies establishing the efficacy of psychotherapy in treating major depressive disorder when it coexists with SLE. CBT has, however, been shown to improve depressive symptoms, stress, and other quality-of-life measures in patients with SLE.[55] Negative cognitions related to physical appearance are commonly observed and are predictive of depression among SLE patients and therefore might be anticipated in psychotherapy.[6]

RHEUMATOID ARTHRITIS

Rheumatoid arthritis is an idiopathic, chronic, multisystem disease that occurs with a prevalence of approximately 0.5% to 1.0%.[56] It affects women three times more often than men. RA presents with symmetrical, peripheral, inflammatory synovitis. Patients with RA additionally have laboratory evidence of both autoantibodies and systemic inflammation.[57] Destruction and erosion of cartilage and bone from the synovitis is the hallmark of advanced disease. These destructive changes can compromise functional status and lead to loss of valued activities, including employment, recreational activities, and higher levels of independence.

BOX 10-5
COMMON COMORBIDITIES

Pain
Sexual dysfunction
Cognitive impairment
Insomnia
Anxiety
Physical appearance changes
Other medical diseases:
Gastrointestinal disorders
Pulmonary disorders
Renal disorders
CVS disorders
Diabetes

BOX 10-6
TREATMENTS FOR DEPRESSION IN PATIENTS WITH RHEUMATOLOGIC DISEASE

SSRIs
SNRIs (with comorbid pain)
TCAs (with comorbid pain)
ECT
CBT
Exercise (fibromyalgia)
Antipsychotics or mood stabilizers (with concurrent corticosteroid use)
Etanercept (psoriasis, preliminary data)
Celecoxib (adjunctive, preliminary data)

■ EPIDEMIOLOGY

The prevalence of depression ranges from 13% to 20% in patients with RA,[58–61] and RA symptom severity is correlated with the number of depressive symptoms (Fig. 10-1).[62] Although depression in RA is often attributed to chronic pain, a meta-analysis of patients with chronic pain syndromes showed that depression was more common in patients with RA compared to those with osteoarthritis when controlled for pain severity.[61] Depression has been associated with a poorer response to anti-TNF treatment in patients with RA.[63,64]

■ PATHOPHYSIOLOGY

Systemic inflammation may be a key link between RA and depression, although the body of evidence supporting this link in patients with RA remains small (Box 10-2). One study found a significant correlation between interleukin-17 and anxiety, although not depression, in RA patients.[65] Activation of the p38 mitogen-activated protein kinase (MAPK), an important factor in the pathogenesis of RA symptoms,[66] has been associated with decreased CSF levels of serotonin metabolites in animal studies.[67] The negative effects of RA on sleep may also play a direct role in the pathogenesis of depression, since inadequate sleep is associated with increased perception of pain and decreased overall sense of well-being in this patient population.[67,68]

■ CLINICAL PRESENTATION, COURSE, AND NATURAL HISTORY

Among RA patients, those who are also depressed have higher levels of inflammation, pain,[69] and of physical disability (Box 10-3).[70] Patients with RA also commonly report sexual dysfunction.[71] Cognitive impairment has been described as being more prevalent in RA patients compared to the general population,[72] but

---

BOX 10-7
IMPORTANT DRUG–DRUG INTERACTIONS BETWEEN ANTIDEPRESSANTS AND RHEUMATOLOGICAL TREATMENTS

NSAIDs: metabolism inhibited by fluoxetine

Tramadol: metabolism inhibited by fluoxetine and paroxetine; risk of serotonin syndrome with SSRIs

Codeine: therapeutic effect diminished by fluoxetine and paroxetine

Data from Cayot A, Laroche D, Disson-Dautriche A, et al: Cytochrome P450 interactions and clinical implication in rheumatology. Clin Rheumatol. 2014;33(9):1231–1238.

whether or not RA actually causes cognitive dysfunction remains controversial.[73] RA is associated with disruption of many sleep parameters, and both disease activity and depression are associated with greater sleep disruption.[74]

■ ASSESSMENT AND DIFFERENTIAL DIAGNOSIS

Because of the strong association between RA and the somatic symptoms described above, evaluation of sleep, cognition, pain, and sexual function should be assessed in all patients (Box 10-4 and Box 10-5). Whether or not patients are currently taking GC should also be noted, not only because of their potential effects on mood but also because these medications have been independently associated with cognitive impairment in patients with RA.[72] Patients with RA are more likely to smoke compared to the general population,[75] and smoking status is critical for these patients because they are also at higher risk of cardiovascular disease and stroke.[76]

■ TREATMENT

Little research on the treatment of depression in patients with RA exists (Box 10-6). One study with a small sample size randomized patients to pharmacotherapy plus CBT, pharmacotherapy plus an attention control treatment, and pharmacotherapy alone showed improvement in all three of the groups receiving pharmacotherapy compared to a nonrandomized group that opted out of treatment. There were no statistically significant differences among the three active treatment groups.[77]

SCLERODERMA

The term "scleroderma" refers to a group of autoimmune connective tissue disorders characterized by sclerosis of the skin and other organ systems. A diffuse, progressive form and a limited form (involving calcinosis, Raynaud's phenomenon, esophageal involvement, sclerodactyly, telangiectasias) of systemic sclerosis exist; localized scleroderma syndromes exist as well. Depression has been studied more rigorously in association with systemic sclerosis (SSc) than with localized scleroderma.

■ EPIDEMIOLOGY

The prevalence of SSc among adults in the United States has been estimated at 0.03%, and it is substantially more common among women and African-Americans.[78] Onset typically occurs between the fourth and sixth decade of life,[79] with a mean survival of approximately 11 years.[78] The lifetime risk of developing major depressive disorder (MDD) in SSc has been reported to be 23%,[80] and depression appears to be the strongest symptom-predictor of poor social adjustment for patients with scleroderma.[81]

■ PATHOPHYSIOLOGY

Neuropsychiatric symptoms in SSc are likely multifactorial in etiology—sleep disruption, pain, pruritus, fatigue, body image distress, and sexual dysfunction have all been shown to correlate with depression in SSc patients and may play a role in its causation on both biological and psychological fronts.[82] White matter hyperintensities appear frequently on brain MRI of patients with SSc and are also correlated with depression, as well as with headaches and the extent of peripheral vascular disease, which suggests that CNS

vasculopathy may also contribute to neuropsychiatric symptoms,[83] although research in this area remains limited.

■ CLINICAL PRESENTATION, COURSE, AND NATURAL HISTORY

SSc typically presents with symptoms in multiple organ systems. Skin changes, which can be disfiguring, occur in virtually all cases, and end-organ manifestations in many patients might include pulmonary hypertension, pulmonary fibrosis, gastrointestinal symptoms, and occasionally renal failure. Patients with SSc also typically experience constitutional symptoms, such as fatigue and sleep disruption.

Sleep disturbance carries independent associations with respiratory and gastrointestinal symptoms[84] and pain[85] as well as with depression. Among patients with depression and scleroderma, negative cognitions regarding appearance—particularly facial appearance[86]—contribute substantially to psychological distress and should be anticipated.

■ ASSESSMENT AND DIFFERENTIAL DIAGNOSIS

Somatic SSc symptoms that overlap with major depression (e.g., decreased energy, sleep changes) may complicate diagnostic efforts and measurement of depression severity. If a PHQ-9 survey is to be used, it is important to note that patients with SSc will score somatic survey items (e.g., sleep, appetite) more highly than patients without a chronic inflammatory condition, and therefore somatic items may contribute disproportionately to their total PHQ-9 scores).[87]

Depression in patients with SSc is often comorbid with anxiety, fatigue, global disability, and hand and mouth disability; therefore, the assessment should include attention to these other conditions as well.[88]

■ TREATMENT

Much remains to be understood about how the presence of scleroderma may affect depression treatment. It is likely that antidepressant medications and/or CBT can be helpful here, as they are in other inflammatory conditions, but research into this topic is lacking. Similarly, while attention to psychosocial losses associated with scleroderma may identify important treatment targets, no successful randomized controlled trials of psychosocial interventions for depression in SSc have been published.[82]

FIBROMYALGIA

Fibromyalgia is a common, complex condition characterized by widespread pain associated with nonspecific symptoms that include fatigue, sleep disturbances, cognitive dysfunction, and depressive episodes. The condition has been described under various names because it lacks objective physical or clearly defined pathological findings. The original American College of Rheumatology (ACR) diagnostic criteria required the presence of 11 of 18 specified tender points in addition to widespread pain. The ACR criteria have since been revised to incorporate other associated symptoms, including fatigue, waking unrefreshed, and cognitive symptoms, and to allow for ease of use in the primary care setting by eliminating the need for examination of tender points.[89]

■ EPIDEMIOLOGY

The prevalence of fibromyalgia in the general population is estimated between 2% and 8%.[90] A global review of prevalence studies found a mean prevalence of 2.7% to 4.1% in women and 1.4% in men—with wide variability across countries.[91] Fibromyalgia is commonly comorbid with other somatic diagnoses that are also difficult to measure with objective tests, including migraine, chronic fatigue syndrome, and irritable bowel syndrome.[92]

Fibromyalgia is associated with significant psychiatric comorbidity. In a Canadian survey, 22% of patients with fibromyalgia had concurrent major depression.[93] In this study, comorbid depression was associated with younger age, female gender, being unmarried, food insecurity, number of chronic conditions, and limitations in activity. Studies conducted in the United States suggest that the prevalence of major depression among patients with fibromyalgia may be even higher.[94] Anxiety disorders and bipolar disorder also appear common in this group; their relationship to fibromyalgia has not been studied as extensively.[95]

■ PATHOPHYSIOLOGY

The high comorbidity between fibromyalgia and depression may be related to several pathophysiological links, although the precise connections have not been established. Indeed, the pathophysiology of fibromyalgia itself remains poorly understood, although many experts believe it is a primary disorder of pain centralization,[90] a term that emphasizes the role of the central nervous system (as opposed to peripheral nociceptors) in amplifying the body's experience of pain. Heritable factors are likely, as fibromyalgia cases congregate within families.[94]

Abnormalities in neurotransmitter and neuroendocrine functioning may play a significant role in both aberrant mood regulation and pain pathway signaling. Serotonin and norepinephrine metabolite levels are decreased in the cerebrospinal fluid of patients with fibromyalgia levels compared to controls,[96] and this relative deficiency has been suggested as a possible explanatory mechanism for the abnormality in central pain processing.[97] Dysfunction of the hypothalamic-pituitary-adrenal axis may also play a role. Thus patients with fibromyalgia may have decreased baseline cortisol levels compared to controls,[98] and cortisol suppression by dexamethasone has been shown to be higher in patients with fibromyalgia.[99]

Functional brain neuroimaging of patients with comorbid fibromyalgia and depression reveals distinctly different pathways for processing the sensory and affective components of pain.[100] This suggests that despite the commonalities between depression and fibromyalgia, the mechanism linking the two may be indirect or multifactorial. In addition, depression may predispose patients to lifestyles that either exacerbate fibromyalgia or adversely impact their quality of life and occupational disability.[101]

■ CLINICAL PRESENTATION, COURSE, AND NATURAL HISTORY

Fibromyalgia and depressive disorders share considerable symptom overlap. Because fatigue, sleep difficulties, weakness, problems with attention and memory, and appetite and weight fluctuations occur in both conditions, the diagnosis of depression may be delayed or obscured in patients with fibromyalgia. Other comorbid pain disorders may also exist, and patients with fibromyalgia may exhibit sensory hyper-responsiveness—a phenomenon described in the literature as "somatosensory amplification," which is often associated with a "pan-positive review of systems" when taking a medical history, which may further complicate the clinical picture.[90,102]

Some studies have attempted to characterize the temperamental and personality traits of fibromyalgia patients[103] but have found them to be a heterogeneous group.[104] A history of abuse is common[105] and stressful life events have been reported to precipitate fibromyalgia in susceptible individuals.[106]

■ ASSESSMENT AND DIFFERENTIAL DIAGNOSIS

For a suspected diagnosis of fibromyalgia, a musculoskeletal history, complete physical examination, and basic laboratory studies, including thyroid hormone studies, should be performed. Indiscriminate testing for antinuclear and other autoantibodies should be avoided

BOX 10-9
ANXIETY SUMMARY

Anxiety is known to be more prevalent in SLE (1), RA, (2), SSc, (3), and FM (4) and is often comorbid with depression.

Benzodiazepines may have a dual role in the treatment of anxiety and pain related to rheumatic illnesses but may also exacerbate fatigue and other somatic symptoms (5); gabapentin might be considered as an alternative with a smaller evidence base supporting its use as an anxiolytic (6)

1. Meszaros ZS, Perl A, Faraone SV. Psychiatric symptoms in systemic lupus erythematosus: a systematic review. *J Clin Psychiatry*. 2012;73(7):993–1001.
2. Covic T, Cumming SR, Pallant JF, et al. Depression and anxiety in patients with rheumatoid arthritis: prevalence rates based on comparison of the depression, anxiety and stress scale (DASS) and the hospital, anxiety and depression scale (HADS). *BMC Psychiatry*. 2012;12:6.
3. Del Rosso A, Mikhaylova S, Baccini M, Lupi I, Cerinic MM, Bongi SM. In systemic sclerosis, anxiety and depression assessed by Hospital Anxiety Depression Scale are independently associated with disability and psychological factors. *BioMed Res Int*. 2013; doi:10.1155/2013/507493.
4. Arnold LM, Hudson JI, Keck PE, Auchenbach MB, Javaras KN, Hess EV. Comorbidity of fibromyalgia with psychiatric disorders. *J Clin Psychiatry*. 2006;67:1219–1225.
5. Tarpley EL. Evaluation of diazepam (Valium) in the symptomatic treatment of rheumatic disorders: a controlled comparative study. *J Chron Dis*. 19645;18:99–106.
6. Pande AC, Pollack MH, Crockatt J, et al. Placebo-controlled study of gabapentin treatment of panic disorder. *J Clin Psychiatr*. 2000;20(4): 467–471.

because these are often abnormal in healthy, otherwise asymptomatic individuals.[90] Patients should be screened for depression, bipolar disorder, and anxiety disorders (**Box 10-9**) after a diagnosis of fibromyalgia is made.

■ TREATMENT

Patients with fibromyalgia and depression require an interdisciplinary, multimodal approach that typically includes a formal exercise plan in addition to pharmacologic treatments and cognitive behavioral therapy.[90] Fortunately, there is considerable overlap between recommended psychiatric treatments for both depression and fibromyalgia, and strategies can be modified based on a patient's symptoms and coping style.

Duloxetine has been approved by the FDA for treatment of both fibromyalgia and MDD when prescribed at a dose of 60 mg/d; it appears to be less effective in reducing pain at lower doses.[107] Evidence supporting the use of venlafaxine in this group is less robust but suggests that it too may be an appropriate choice for treating co-occurring depression and pain.[108] Milnacipran, a SNRI that is used less commonly for depression, has been approved by the FDA for the treatment of fibromyalgia but not depression; however, its efficacy and tolerability as an antidepressant appears to be comparable to the efficacy and tolerability of other antidepressants.[109] Selective-serotonin reuptake inhibitors (SSRIs) are a less effective therapy for fibromyalgia pain, particularly high-selectivity SSRIs, such as citalopram.[110]

Among the TCAs, amitryptiline has been shown to reduce pain in patients with fibromyalgia.[111] However, despite the potential for TCAs to be uniquely helpful as monotherapy for these patients, a recent industry-funded study found that they are rarely used, and when they are used it is most often in combination with other agents.[112]

If a patient responds poorly to initial monotherapy, additional strategies to consider include switching to a second antidepressant or augmenting with another antidepressant. Pregabalin, which is approved by the FDA for the treatment of fibromyalgia, is associated with a reduction in pain although not with a reduction in depression per se.[113]

CHRONIC FATIGUE SYNDROME

Although the relationship between depression and myalgic encephalomyelitis/chronic fatigue syndrome (ME/CFS) also appears to be very strong, this chapter will not discuss the relationship between these two conditions in detail. ME/CFS remains poorly understood in its own right, and this diagnosis appears to represent a very heterogeneous patient population[114]; therefore, attempting to fairly and accurately describe this complex relationship based on the existing (limited) evidence is beyond the reach of this chapter. It is important to note that a debate exists on whether ME/CFS has a specific medical etiology or a primary psychiatric one.[114] Complicating this question is the publication of multiple studies attempting to demonstrate efficacy for conventional depression treatments, including cognitive behavioral therapy and antidepressants, in directly treating ME/CFS symptoms, which show mixed results.[115,116] However, emerging evidence supports the hypothesis that ME/CFS is a primary medical condition, and a number of possible biological etiologies have been described and studied.[117,118] Treatment considerations for ME/CFS relevant to patients with concurrent depression may include the incorporation of exercise and/or yoga, stabilization of insomnia, and reduction or elimination of sedating medications.[119–121] A recent Institute of Medicine report has proposed a revised set of diagnostic criteria for this condition and renaming it "systemic exertion intolerance disease," or SEID, in order to further clarify which patients should receive this diagnosis and facilitate higher-quality research.[122]

CONCLUSION

The relationship between rheumatologic illnesses and depression is complex (**Box 10-10**). It is likely that some direct pathophysiologic links exist between this group of illnesses and depression; it is certain that the chronic pain, inflammation, disability, and insomnia common to these conditions adversely affect mental and behavioral health. Much remains to be learned about this topic. However, it is safe to assert that a comprehensive approach to diagnosis and treatment that addresses both the biological and the psychosocial aspects of these diseases will yield the best outcomes for the patients who bear them.

REFERENCES

1. Smith RS. The macrophage theory of depression. *Med Hypotheses*. 1991;35:298–306.

2. Sundquist K, Li X, Hemminki K, Sundquist J. Subsequent risk of hospitalization for neuropsychiatric disorders in patients with rheumatic diseases. *Arch Gen Psychiatry*. 2008;65(5):501–507.

3. Wolfe F, Michaud K, Li T, Katz RS. Chronic conditions and health problems in rheumatic diseases: comparisons with rheumatoid arthritis, noninflammatory rheumatic disorders, systemic lupus erythematosus, and fibromyalgia. *J Rheumatol*. 2010;37: 305–315.

4. Lowe B, Willand L, Eich W, et al. Psychiatric comorbidity and work disability in patients with inflammatory rheumatic diseases. *Psychosom Med*. 2004;66:395–402.

5. Fuller-Thomson E, Shaked Y. Factors associated with depression and suicidal ideation among individuals with arthritis or rheumatism: findings from a representative community survey. *Arthritis Rheum*. 2009;61(7):944–950.

6. Monaghan SM, Sharpe L, Denton F, Levy J, Schrieber L, Sensky T. Relationship between appearance and psychological distress in rheumatic diseases. *Arthritis Rheum*. 2007;57(2):303–309.

7. Reichenberg A, Yirmiya R, Schuld A, et al. Cytokine-associated emotional and cognitive disturbances in humans. *Arch Gen Psychiatry*. 2001;58:445–452.

8. Dowlati Y, Hermann N, Swardfager W, et al. A meta-analysis of cytokines in major depression. *Biol Psychiatry*. 2010;67:446–457.

9. Hannestad J, DellaGiola N, Block M. The effect of antidepressant medication treatment on serum levels of inflammatory cytokines: a meta-analysis. *Neuropsychopharmacology*. 2011;36:2452–2459.

10. Doering LV, Cross R, Vredevoe D, Martinez-Maza O, Cown MJ. Infection, depression, and immunity in women after coronary artery bypass: a pilot study of cognitive behavioral therapy. *Altern Ther Health Med*. 2007;13(3):18–21.

11. Fluitman S, Heijnen CJ, Denys DA, Nolen WA, Balk FJ, Westenberg HG. Electroconvulsive therapy has acute immunological and neuroendocrine effects in patients with major depressive disorder. *J Affect Disord*. 2011;131:388–392.

12. Perocheau D, Laroche F, Perrot S. Relieving pain in rheumatology patients: repetitive transcranial magnetic stimulation (rTMS), a developing approach. *Joint Bone Spine* 2013;81:22–26.

13. Krishnan R, Cella D, Leonard C, et al. Effects of etanercept therapy on fatigue and symptoms of depression in subjects treated for moderate to severe plaque psoriasis for up to 96 weeks. *Br J Dermatol*. 2007;157:1275–1277.

14. Abbasi S, Hosseini F, Modabbernia A, Ashrafi M, Akhondzadeh S. Effect of celecoxib add-on treatment on symptoms and serum IL-6 concentrations in patients with major depressive disorder: randomized double-blind placebo-controlled study. *J Affect Disord*. 2012;141:308–314.

15. Duru N, van der Goes MC, Jacobs JW, et al. EULAR evidence-based and consensus-based recommendations on the management of medium to high-dose glucocorticoid therapy in rheumatic diseases. *Ann Rheum Dis*. 2013;0:1–9.

16. Brown ES. Effects of glucocorticoids on mood, memory, and the hippocampus. *Ann NY Acad Sci*. 2009;1179:41–55.

17. Lupien SJ, McEwen BS. The acute effects of corticosteroids on cognition: integration of animal and human model studies. *Brain Res Rev*. 1997;24:1–27.

18. Chrousos GA, Kattah JC, Beck RW, Cleary PA. Side effects of glucocorticoid treatment. *JAMA*. 1993;259:2110–2112.

19. The Boston Collaborative Drug Surveillance Program. Acute adverse reactions to prednisone in relation to dosage. *Clin Pharmacol Therapeut*. 1972;13(5):694–698.

20. Bolanos SH, Khan DA, Hanczyc M, Bauer MS, Dhanani N, Brown ES. Assessment of mood states in patients receiving long-term corticosteroid therapy in controls with patient-rated and clinician-rated scales. *Ann Allergy Asthma Immunol*. 2004;92:500–505.

21. Brown ES, Suppes T, Khan DA, Carmody TJ. Mood changes during prednisone bursts in outpatients with asthma. *J Clin Psychopharmacol*. 2002;22(1):55–61.

22. Naber DN, Sand P, Heigl B. Psychopathological and neuropsychological effects of 8-days' corticosteroid treatment. A prospective study. *Psychoneuroendocrinology*. 1996;21(1):25–31

23. Wada K, Yamada N, Sato T, et al. Corticosteroid-induced psychotic and mood disorders. *Psychosomatics*. 2001;42:461–466.

24. Hall RC, Popkin MK, Kirkpatrick B. Tricyclic exacerbation of steroid psychosis. *J Nerv Ment Dis*. 1978;166(10):738–742.

25. Falk WE, Mahnke MW, Poskanzer DC. Lithium prophylaxis of corticotropin-induced psychosis. *JAMA*. 1979;241:1011–1012.

26. Brown ES, Zaidel L, Allen G, McColl R, Vazquez M, Ringe WK. Effects of lamotrigine on hippocampal activation in corticosteroid-treated patients. *J Affect Disord*. 2010;126(3):415–419.

27. Brown ES, Chamberlain W, Dhanani N, Paranjpe P, Carmody TJ, Sargeant M. An open-label trial of olanzapine for corticosteroid-induced mood symptoms. *J Affect Disord*. 2004;83: 277–281.

28. Fortuna G, Brennan MT. Systemic lupus erythematosus: epidemiology, pathophysiology, manifestations, and management. *Dent Clin N Am*. 2013;57:631–655.

29. Gonzalez LA, Toloza SM, McGwin G, Alarcon GS. Ethnicity in systemic lupus erythematosus (SLE): its influence on susceptibility and outcomes. *Lupus*. 2013;22:1214–1224.

30. Bachen EA, Chessney MA, Criswell LA. Prevalence of mood and anxiety disorders in women with systemic lupus erythematosus. *Arthritis Rheum*. 2009;61(6):822–829.

31. Karol DE, Criscione-Schreiber LG, Lin M, Clowse ME. Depressive symptoms and associated factors in systemic lupus erythematosus. *Psychosomatics*. 2013;54:443–450.

32. Harris EC, Barraclough BM. Suicide as an outcome for medical disorders. *Medicine (Baltimore)*. 1994;73(6):281–96.

33. Moldovan I, Katsaros E, Carr FN, et al. The patient reported outcomes in lupus (PATROL) study: role of depression in health-related quality of life in a Southern California lupus cohort. *Lupus*. 2011;20:1285–1292.

34. Petri M, Naqibuddin M, Carson KA, et al. Depression and cognitive impairment in newly diagnosed systemic lupus erythematosus. *J Rheumatol*. 2008;37(10):2032–2038.

35. Julian LJ, Yelin E, Yazdany J, et al. Depression, medication adherence, and service utilization in systemic lupus erythematosus. *Arthritis Rheum*. 2009;61(2):240–246.

36. Nery FG, Borba EF, Hatch JP, Soares JC, Bonfa E, Neto FL. Major depressive disorder and disease activity in systemic lupus erythematosus. *Compr Psychiatry*. 2007;48:14–19.

37. Skare T, de Silva Magalhaes VD, Siqueira RE. Systemic lupus erythematosus activity and depression. *Rheumatol Int*. 2012;34(3): 445–446.

38. Jarpa E, Babul M, Calderon J, et al. Common mental disorders and psychological distress in systemic lupus erythematosus are not associated with disease activity. *Lupus*. 2011;20:58–66.

39. ACR Ad Hoc Committee on Neuropsychiatric Lupus Nomenclature. The American College of Rheumatology nomenclature and case definitions for neuropsychiatric lupus syndromes. *Arthritis Rheum*. 1999;42(4):599–608.

40. Greco CM, Li T, Sattar A, et al. Association between depression and vascular disease in systemic lupus erythematosus. *J Rheumatol*. 2012;39(2):262–268.

41. Belmont HM, Abramson SB, Lie JT. Pathology and pathogenesis of vascular injury in systemic lupus erythematosus. *Arthritis Rheum*. 1996;39(1):9–22.

42. Rhiannon JJ. Systemic lupus erythematosus involving the nervous system: presentation, pathogenesis, and management. *Clinic Rev Allerg Immunol*. 2008;34:356–360.

43. Hanly JG, Harrison MJ. Management of neuropsychiatric lupus. *Best Pract Res Clin Rheumatol*. 2005;19(5):799–782.

44. Gasparovic C, Qualls C, Greene ER, Sibbitt WL, Roldan CA. Blood pressure and vascular dysfunction underlie elevated cerebral blood flow in systemic lupus erythematosus. *J Rheumatol*. 2012;39(4):752–758.

45. Omdal R, Brokstad K, Waterloo K, Koldingsnes W, Jonsson R, Mellgren SI. Neuropsychiatric disturbances in SLE are associated with antibodies against NMDA receptors. *Eur J Neurol*. 2005;12:392–298.

46. Fragoso-Loyo H, Cabiedes J, Orozco-Narvaez A, et al. Serum and cerebrospinal fluid autoantibodies in patients with neuropsychiatric lupus erythematosus. Implications for diagnosis and pathogenesis. *PLoS One*. 2008;3(10):e3347.

47. Karassa FB, Afeltra A, Ambrozic A, et al. Accuracy of anti-ribosomal P protein antibody testing for the diagnosis of neuropsychiatric systemic lupus erythematosus. *Arthritis Rheum*. 2006;54(1):312–324.

48. Fragoso-Loyo H, Richaud-Patin Y, Orozco-Narvaez A, et al. Interleukin-6 and chemokines in the neuropsychiatric manifestations of systemic lupus erythematosus. *Arthritis Rheum*. 2007;56(4):1242–1250.

49. Wen J, Xia Y, Stock A, et al. Neuropsychiatric disease in murine lupus is dependent on the TWEAK/Fn14 pathway. *J Autoimmun*. 2013;43:44–54.

50. Abbot NJ, Mendonca LL, Dolman DE. The blood-brain barrier in systemic lupus erythematosus. *Lupus*. 2003;12:908–915.

51. Iverson GL. Screening for depression in systemic lupus erythematosus with the British Columbia major depression inventory. *Psychol Rep*. 2002;90:1091–1096.

52. Cassis TB, Callen JP. Bupropin-induced subacute cutaneous lupus erythematosus. *Australas J Dermatol*. 2005;46:266–269.

53. Hussain HM, Zakaria M. Drug-induced lupus secondary to sertraline. *Aust N Z J Psychiatry*. 2008;42:1074–1075.

54. Douglas CJ, Schwartz HI. ECT for depression caused by lupus cerebritis: a case report. *Am J Psychiatry*. 1982;139(12):1631–1632.

55. Navarrete-Navarrete N, Peralta-Ramirez MI, Sabio-Sanchez JM, et al. Efficacy of cognitive behavioural therapy for the treatment of chronic stress in patients with lupus erythematosus: a randomized controlled trial. *Psychother Psychosom*. 201;79:107–115.

56. Helmick CG, Felson DT, Lawrence RC, et al. Estimates of the prevalence of arthritis and other rheumatic conditions in the United States. Part I. *Arthritis Rheum*. 2008;58(1):15–25.

57. Aletaha D, Neogi T, Silman AJ, et al. An American College of Rheumatology/European League Against Rheumatism collaborative initiative. *Arthritis Rheum*. 2010;62(9):2569–2581.

58. Creed F. Psychological disorders in rheumatoid arthritis: a growing consensus? *Ann Rheum Dis*. 1990;49:808–812

59. Creed F, Murphy S, Jayson MV. Measurement of psychiatric disorder in rheumatoid arthtitis. *J Psychom Res*. 1990;34:79–87.

60. Murphy S, Creed FH, Jayson MI. Psychiatric disorders and illness behavior in rheumatoid arthritis. *Br J Rheumatol*. 1988;27:357–363.

61. Dickens C, McGowan L, Clark-Carter D, Creed F. Depression in Rheumatoid Arthritis: A Systematic Review of the Literature with Meta-Analysis. *Psychosom Med.* 2002;64:52–60.

62. Godha E, Shi L, Mavronicolas H. Association between tendency towards depression and severity of rheumatoid arthritis from a national representative sample: the Medical Expenditure Panel Survey. *Curr Med Res Opin.* 2010;26(7):1685–1690.

63. Hider SL, Tanveer W, Brownfield A, Mattey DL, Packham JC. Depression in RA patients treated with anti-TNF is common and under-recognized in the rheumatology clinic. *Rheumatology.* 2009;48:1152–1154.

64. Mattey DL, Dawes PT, Hassell AB, Brownfield A, Packham JC. Effect of psychological distress on continuation of anti-Tumor Necrosis Factor therapy in Patients with Rheumatoid Arthritis. *J Rheumatol.* 2010;37:2021–2024.

65. Liu Y, Ho RC, Mak A. The role of interleukin (IL)-17 in anxiety and depression of patients with rheumatoid arthritis. *Int J Rheum Dis.* 2012;15:183–187.

66. Malemud CJ, Miller AH. Pro-inflammatory cytokine-induced SAPK/MAPK and JAK/STAT in rheumatoid arthritis and the new anti-depression drugs. *Expert Opin Ther Targets.* 2008;12(2):171–183.

67. Sanchez MM, Alagbe O, Felger JC, et al. Activated p38 MAPK is associated with decreased CSF 5-HIAA and increased maternal rejection during infancy in young adult rhesus monkeys. *Mol Psychiatry.* 2007;10:895–897.

68. Nicassio PM, Ormseth SR, Kay M, Custodio M, Iwin MR, Olmstead R, Weisman MH. The contribution of pain and depression to self-reported sleep disturbance in patients with rheumatoid arthritis. *Pain.* 2011;153:107–112.

69. Kojima M, Kojima T, Suzuki S, et al. Depression, inflammation, and pain in patients with rheumatoid arthritis. *Arthritis Care Res.* 2009;61(8):1018–1024.

70. Van den Hoek J, Roorda LD, Boshuizen HC, et al. Long-term physical functioning and its associated with somatic comorbidity and comorbid depression in patients with established rheumatoid arthritis: a longitudinal study. *Arthritis Care Res.* 2013;65(7):1157–1165.

71. Coskun B, Coskun BN, Atis G, Ergenekon E, Dilek K. Evaluation of sexual function in women with rheumatoid arthritis. *Urol J.* 2013;10(4):1081–1087.

72. Shin SY, Katz P, Wallhagen M, Julian L. Cognitive impairment in persons with rheumatoid arthritis. *J Rheumatol.* 2013;40(3):236–243.

73. Meade T. Assessing cognitive function in rheumatoid arthritis: comment on the article by Shin et al. *Arthritis Care Res.* 2013;65(8):1390–1392.

74. Sariyildiz MA, Batmaz I, Bozkurt M, et al. Sleep quality in rheumatoid arthritis: relationship between the disease severity, depression, functional status and the quality of life. *J Clin Med Res.* 2014;6(1):44–52.

75. Boyer J, Gourraud P, Cantagrel A, Davignon J, Constantin A. Traditional cardiovascular risk factors in rheumatoid arthritis: a meta-analysis. *Joint Bone Spine.* 2011;78:179–183.

76. Dougados M, Soubrier M, Antunez A, et al. Prevalence of comorbidities in rheumatoid arthritis and evaluation of their monitoring: results of an international, cross-sectional study (COMORA). *Ann Rheum Dis.* 2014;73:62–68.

77. Parker JC, Smarr KL, Slaughter JR, et al. Management of depression in rheumatoid arthritis: a combined pharmacologic and cognitive-behavioral approach. *Arthritis Rheum.* 2003;49(6):766–777.

78. Mayes MD, Lacey JV, Beebe-Dimmer J, et al. Prevalence, incidence, survival, and disease characteristics of systemic sclerosis in a large US population. *Arthritis Rheum.* 2003;48(8):2246–2255.

79. Thombs BD, Van Lankveld W, Bassel M, et al. Psychological health and well-being in systemic sclerosis: state of the science and consensus research agenda. *Arthritis Care Res.* 2010;62(8):1181–1189.

80. Jewett LR, Razykov I, Husdon M, Baron M, Thombs BD. Prevalence of current, 12-month and lifetime major depressive disorder among patients with systemic sclerosis. *Rheumatology.* 2013;52:669–675.

81. Benrud-Larson LM, Haythornthwaite JA, Heinberg LJ, et al. The impact of pain and symptoms of depression in scleroderma. *Pain.* 2002;95:267–275.

82. Malcarne VL, Fox RS, Mills SD, Gholizadeh S. Psychosocial aspects of systemic sclerosis. *Curr Opin Rheumatol.* 2013;25:707–713.

83. Mohamed RH, Nassef AA. Brain magnetic resonance imaging findings in patients with systemic sclerosis. *Int J Rheum Dis.* 2010;13:61–67.

84. Frech T, Hays RD, Maranian P, Clements PJ, Furst DE, Khanna D. Prevalence and correlates of sleep disturbance in systemic sclerosis–results from the UCLA scleroderma quality of life study. *Rheumatology.* 2011;50:1280–1287.

85. Milette K, Razykov I, Pope J, et al. Clinical correlates of sleep problems in systemic sclerosis: the prominent role of pain. *Rheumatology.* 2011;50:921–925.

86. Amin K, Clarke A, Sivakumar B, et al. The psychological impact of facial changes in scleroderma. *Psychol Health Med.* 2011;16(3):304–312.

87. Leavens A, Patten SB, Hudson M, Baron M, Thombs BD. Influence of somatic symptoms on Patient Health Questionnaire-9 depression scores among patients with systemic sclerosis compared to a health general population sample. *Arthritis Care Res.* 2012;64(8):1195–1201.

88. Del Rosso A, Mikhaylova S, Baccini M, Lupi I, Cerinic MM, Bongi SM. In systemic sclerosis, anxiety and depression assessed by Hospital Anxiety Depression Scale and independently associated with disability and psychological factors. *Biomed Res Int.* 2013;2013:507493.

89. Wolfe F, Clauw DJ, Fitzcharles M, et al. The American College of Rheumatology preliminary diagnostic criteria for fibromyalgia and measurement of symptoms severity. *Arthritis Care Res.* 2010;62(5):600–610.

90. Clauw DJ. Fibromyalgia: a clinical review. *JAMA.* 2014;311(15):1547–1555.

91. Querioz LP. Worldwide epidemiology of fibromyalgia. *Curr Pain Headache Rep.* 2013;17(8):356.

92. Hudson JI, Goldenberg DL, Pope HG, Keck PE, Schlesinger L. Comorbidity of fibromyalgia with medical and psychiatric disorders. *Am J Med.* 1992;92:363–367.

93. Fuller-Thompson E, Nimigon-Young J, Brennenstuhl S. Individuals with fibromyalgia and depression: findings from a nationally representative Canadian survey. *Rheumatol Int.* 2012;32:853–862.

94. Hudson JI, Arnold LM, Keck PE, Auchenbach MB, Pope HG. Family study of fibromyalgia and affective spectrum disorder. *Biol Psychiatry.* 2004;56:884–891.

95. Arnold LM, Hudson JI, Keck PE, Auchenbach MB, Javaras KN, Hess EV. Comorbidity of fibromyalgia with psychiatric disorders. *J Clin Psychiatry.* 2006;67:1219–1225.

96. Russell IJ, Vaeroy H, Javors M, Nyberg F. Cerebrospinal fluid biogenic amine metabolites in fibromyalgia/fibrositis syndrome and rheumatoid arthritis. *Arthritis Rheum*. 1992;35(5):550–556.

97. Smith HS, Harris R, Clauw D. Fibromyalgia: an afferent processing disorder leading to a complex pain generalized syndrome. *Pain Physician*. 2011;14:E217–E245.

98. Tak LM, Cleare AJ, Ormel J, et al. Meta-analysis and meta-regression of hypothalamic-pituitary-axis activity in functional somatic disorders. *Biol Psychiatry*. 2011;87:183–194.

99. Wingenfeld K, Wagner D, Schmidt I, Meinlschmidt G, Hellhammer DH, Heim C. The low-dose dexamethasone suppression test in fibromyalgia. *J Psychosom Res*. 2007;62:85–91.

100. Giesecke T, Gracely RH, Williams DA, Geisser ME, Petzke FW, Claw DJ. The relationship between depression, clinical pain, and experimental pain in a chronic pain cohort. *Arthritis Rheum*. 2005;52(5):1577–1584.

101. Kurtze N, Gundersen KT, Svebak S. Quality of life, functional disability and lifestyle among subgroups of fibromyalgia patients: the significance of anxiety and depression. *Br J Med Psychol*. 1999;72:471–484.

102. Nakao M, Barsky AJ. Clinical application of somatosensory amplificatino in psychosomatic medicine. *Biopsychosoc Med*. 2007;1:17.

103. Gencay-Can A, Can SS. Temperament and character profile of patients with fibromyalgia. *Rheumatol Int*. 2012;32:3957–3961.

104. Salgueiro M, Aira Z, Buesa I, Bilbao J, Azkue JJ. Is psychological distress intrinsic to fibromyalgia syndrome? Cross-sectional analysis in two clinical presentations. *Rheumatol Int*. 2012;32:3463–3469.

105. Bohn D, Bernardy K, Wolfe F, et al. The association among child maltreatment, somatic symptoms intensity, depression, and somatoform dissociative symptoms in patients with fibromyalgia syndrome? A single-center cohort study. *J Trauma Dissociation*. 2013;14:342–358.

106. Lucini D, Pagani M. From stress to functional syndromes: an internist's point of view. *Eur J Intern Med*. 2012;23:295–301.

107. Arnold LM, Zhang S, Pangallo BA. Efficacy and safety of duloxetine 40mg/d in patients with fibromyalgia. *Clin J Pain*. 2012;28:775–781.

108. Sayar K, Aksu G, Ak I, Tosun M. Venlafaxine treatment of fibromyalgia. *Ann Pharmacother*. 2003;37(11):1561–1565.

109. Nakagawa A, Watanabe N, Omori IM, et al. Milnacipran versus other antidepressive agents for depression. *Cochrane Database Syst Rev*. 2009;(3):CD006529.

110. Anderberg UM, Marteinsdottir I, von Knorring L. Citalopram in patients with fibromyalgia–a randomized, double-blind, placebo-controlled study. *Eur J Pain*. 2000;4(1):27–35.

111. Hauser W, Wolfe F, Tolle T, Uceyler N, Sommer C. The role of antidepressants in the management of fibromyalgia syndrome: a systematic review and meta-analysis. *CNS Drugs*. 2012;26(4):298–307.

112. Reed C, Birnbaum HG, Ivanova JI, et al. Real-world role of tricyclic antidepressants in the treatment of fibromyalgia. *Pain Practice*. 2012;12(7):533–540.

113. Arnold LM, Leon T, Whalen E, Barrett J. Relationships among pain and depressive and anxiety symptoms in clinical trials of pregabalin in fibromyalgia. *Psychosomatics*. 2010;51(6):489–497.

114. Christley Y, Duffy I, Everall IP, Martin CR. The neuropsychiatric and neuropsychological features of chronic fatigue syndrome: revisiting the enigma. *Curr Psychiatry Rep*. 2013;15:353.

115. Arnold LM, Blom TJ, Welge JA, Mairutto E, Heller A. A randomized, placebo-controlled, double-blinded trial of duloxetine in the treatment of general fatigue in patients with chronic fatigue syndrome. *Psychosomatics*. 2015;56(3):242–253.

116. Flo E, Chalder T. Prevalence and predictors of recovery from chronic fatigue syndrome in a routine clinical practice. *Behav Res Ther*. 2014;63:1–8.

117. Maes M, Ringel K, Kubera M, et al. In myalgic encephalomyelitis/chronic fatigue syndrome, increased autoimmune activity against 5-HT is associated with immuno-inflammatory pathways and bacterial translocation. *J Affective Disord*. 2013;150:223–230.

118. Barnden LR, Crouch B, Kwiatek R, Burnet R, Del Fante P. Evidence in chronic fatigue syndrome for severity-dependent upregulation of prefrontal myelination that is independent of anxiety and depression. *NMR Biomed*. 2015;28:404–413.

119. Larun L, Brurberg KG, Odgaard-Jensen J, Price JR. Exercise therapy for chronic fatigue syndrome. *Cochrane Database Syst Rev*. 2015;2:CD003200.

120. Oka T, Tanahashi T, Chijiwa T, Lkhagvasuren B, Sudo N, Oka K. Isometric yoga improves the fatigue and pain of patients with chronic fatigue syndrome who are resistant to conventional therapy: a randomized, controlled trial. *Biopsychosocial Med* 2014;8(1):27.

121. Kallestad H, Jacobsen HB, Landro N, Borchgrevink PC, Stiles TC. The role of insomnia in the treatment of chronic fatigue. *J Psychosom Res*. 2015;78(5):427–432.

122. Committee on the Diagnostic Criteria for Myalgic Encephalomyelitis/Chronic Fatigue Syndrome; Board on the Health of Select Populations; Institute of Medicine. Beyond myalgic encephalomyelitis/chronic fatigue syndrome: redefining an illness. Washington (DC): National Academies Press (US); 2015.

CHAPTER 11

Depression and Infectious Diseases

John Grimaldi, MD

Jessica Harder, MD

Megan Oser, PhD

Paul Sax, MD

INTRODUCTION

Depression and infectious diseases are linked in multiple ways. Depression contributes to initial infection in several diseases; for example depression predisposes to both hepatitis C (HCV) and HIV acquisition. Conversely, depression may result from the stress of living with a serious infectious disease, or may stem from the effect of an infectious disease on the immune and central nervous systems (CNS). In addition, the medications used to treat infectious diseases may cause depression. The interrelationship is further complicated by the fact that depression may be more prevalent among groups at greater risk of infection, such as individuals with substance-related conditions or individuals who are homeless or living in poverty.

Early identification and treatment of depression leads to improved quality of life and may improve medical outcomes by facilitating engagement in and adherence to the medical regimen. Given shared underlying pathophysiologic mechanisms, effective treatment of depression may in some instances even influence the course of disease. This chapter will address the salient features of depression found among those infectious diseases most commonly associated with mood disturbances.

HEPATITIS C

■ EPIDEMIOLOGY (FIG. 11-1)
Prevalence and Incidence of Depressive Disorders

Patients with HCV are disproportionately affected by depression, the most common mental health concern among HCV-infected individuals.[1-4] Compared to the general population, depression is three to four times more prevalent in individuals with HCV.[5-7] Current prevalence rates for depressive disorders among individuals with HCV range from 28% to 35%,[3,7-9] and lifetime rates are reported to be between 34% and 44%.[3,7] The prevalence of particular depressive disorders varies widely depending on the study; the prevalence of major depressive disorder (MDD) is variously reported between 8% and 25%.[3,7,10] The most common depressive diagnosis is adjustment disorder with depressed mood, reported in 40% of cases, while the least prevalent is dysthymia or depressive disorder NOS (3%).[3]

One alarming result of MDD is suicidal ideation and suicide attempts. HCV patients are twice as likely to have attempted suicide as matched controls.[11] The suicide risk is greater for males and those under 45 years of age.[12]

Risk Factors and Correlates of Depression

Increasing age is associated with greater risk for depression and severity of depression in those with HCV (**Box 11-1**).[3,13] As in the general population, the prevalence is higher in women (44%) with HCV than in men (22%).[3]

One explanation of the increased prevalence of depression in HCV may be the increased rate of substance use in this population, since intravenous drug use is the leading cause of HCV infections in the United States.[14] Individuals who are depressed may be more likely to engage in intravenous or intranasal drug use, putting them at greater risk of HCV.[7] Another possible reason for the heightened depressive comorbidity is the pathophysiology of the disease itself,[3,15,16] in that depressive disorder may be the direct result of the infectious process itself.[17] Finally, the stress of living with a stigmatized, serious illness may also increase the vulnerability to

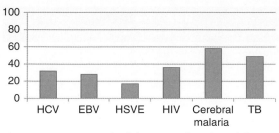

Figure 11-1 *Mean risk of depression for selected illnesses (% prevalence for particular disease).*

developing depression.[7,18] Indeed, increasing depressive symptom severity has been linked to poor acceptance of HCV and HCV-related stigma.[3]

■ PATHOPHYSIOLOGY

Depressive symptoms may result from changes in immunological functioning, in particular, interleukin-1 and tumor necrosis factor[19] and/or from changes in platelet 5-HT functioning (**Box 11-2**).[3,15,16,20]

■ CLINICAL PRESENTATION

Depression in HCV patients is often characterized by fatigue and malaise (**Box 11-3**).[21,22] However, the neurovegetative and somatic symptoms of depression are often caused by the hepatitis infection itself.[23] The Beck Depression Inventory-II has been used to distinguish depressive symptoms from HCV symptoms using a somatic factor and a cognitive-affective factor. Patients with current MDD score significantly higher on both factors than those without MDD, but the cognitive-affective factor may become a more valid measure of depression as liver disease progresses.[23]

Patients with chronic HCV experience an impaired quality of life (QoL).[21] This is not associated with age, gender, mode of acquiring the virus, alanine aminotransferase (ALT) levels, substance use or social support,[24,25] but instead is related to depressive symptoms and fatigue.[22,23] One source of this diminished QoL is the emotional distress and uncertainty that accompany HCV.[18,26,27] Illness uncertainty has been related to depressive symptoms in a cross-sectional study of HCV patients. Ambiguity about the disease is the primary component of illness uncertainty associated with depressive symptoms, diminished quality of life, and fatigue.[22]

Eighty-five percent of HCV-infected Veterans have one or more past or current psychiatric disorders.[11] The most prevalent psychiatric comorbidities with HCV, in addition to depressive disorders, are alcohol use disorder, substance use disorder, and anxiety disorders (**Box 11-4**). Lifetime prevalence rates of alcohol use disorder range from 81% to 86%[8,9] and point prevalence of substance use disorders ranging from 30% to 60%.[1,8,9,11] Approximately 71% of HCV patients have a past or current anxiety disorder,[11] and 62% have PTSD (**Box 11-5**).[8]

BOX 11-1
IMPORTANT RISK FACTORS FOR DEPRESSION IN INFECTIOUS DISEASES

Sociodemographic

Age (increased)

Stigma surrounding the infectious disease

Clinical

Substance use

Medical

Worsening infectious disease

BOX 11-2
POSSIBLE MEDIATORS BETWEEN INFECTIOUS DISEASE AND DEPRESSION

Immunological functioning:

IL-1

TNF

Changes in platelet 5-HT functioning

Altered monoamine activity

Changes in amygdala and hippocampal volumes (HSVE)

Changes in subcortical volumes (HIV)

Prefrontal hypoperfusion (HSVE)

Epigenetic changes (HSVE)

Stress of Illness uncertainty

Poor adherence

■ COURSE AND NATURAL HISTORY
Depression and Antiviral Medication

There is some evidence that quality of life with HCV improves after antiviral therapy or liver transplantation.[21] Antiviral therapy (AVT), consisting of interferon and ribavirin, was the standard treatment for HCV, but the antiviral treatment landscape is now changing rapidly. The recent addition of more effective and less toxic antiviral agents has improved treatment success rates for the most prevalent HCV genotypes.[14] The side effect profile of interferon-free HCV therapies is markedly improved, with a drastic reduction in psychiatric side effects.

Between 50% and 60% of HCV patients treated with interferon experience clinically significant depressive symptoms,[28–31] with 25% developing a major depressive episode.[32] Interestingly, interferon therapy in patients with HCV is associated with depression more frequently than when used in other patient populations (e.g., multiple sclerosis).[33] See **Box 11-6**.

Depression and Adherence to Antiviral Medication and Disease Outcome

Untreated depression negatively affects the course of HCV. It jeopardizes the receipt of HCV treatment and engagement in care.[3] During antiviral therapy, depression can lead to nonadherence, and alcohol and/or substance relapse.[34] Although two studies have found that an increase in depression during AVT was associated with lower rates of virologic response to treatment,[35,36] other studies showed that patients whose depression began during AVT had significantly higher rates of treatment completion.[34,37] In addition, the development of a depressive disorder during AVT did not negatively impact virologic response rates.[34,37,38] One possible explanation is that HCV patients who experience more depressive and neuropsychiatric side effects during AVT may also be experiencing a more robust immunological activation response, resulting in viral suppression.[34,39]

Impact of Comorbid Depression on the Course of HCV, HCV Severity, and Chronicity

Depression may have adverse effects on the amplification of physical symptoms, treatment engagement and adherence, and

---

BOX 11-3
IMPORTANT SYMPTOMS

Neurovegetative symptoms: e.g., Fatigue (may be a primary symptom of the infection)

Affective symptoms and cognitive symptoms more reliable indicators of depression

BOX 11-4
COMMON COMORBIDITIES

Alcohol and substance use disorders

Anxiety disorders

PTSD

Other infectious illnesses (e.g., HIV and HCV)

functioning and quality of life.[3,7] Several studies have found that severity of the HCV infection does not differ significantly in those with and without current depression.[7] However, depression appears to have more of an impact on fatigue and functional impairment than does HCV disease severity.[7]

■ ASSESSMENT AND DIFFERENTIAL DIAGNOSIS

All HCV patients should be systematically assessed for psychiatric disorders, particularly depression, as recommended by treatment and practice guidelines and consensus reports (**Box 11-7**).[40,41] As discussed above, assessing depressive symptoms among HCV patients is made more difficult by the overlap between the somatic symptoms of depression and those of HCV and AVT side effects. However, due to the persistent under-detection of depressive disorders among individuals with HCV,[3,8] assessing and monitoring all depressive symptoms is recommended.[42] Several self-report and clinician administered depression scales are recommended for use in this population: Self-report scales include the Patient Health Questionnaire-9 (PHQ-9), Center for Epidemiologic Studies-Depression Scale (CES-D), and the Beck Depression Inventory (BDI-II).[43] The HAM-7 is a clinician administered scale whose accuracy in detecting depression among HCV patients is comparable to that of the PHQ-9.[43]

BOX 11-6
DRUGS THAT CAN CAUSE DEPRESSIVE SYMPTOMS

HIV Medication	Adverse Effects
Efavirenz	Depression, derealization, depersonalization and sleep disturbance
HCV medication	Adverse effects
Interferon	Depression
TB medication	Adverse effects
INH	Depression and delusional ideation
Cyclosporine	Depression and anxiety
Malarial medication	Adverse effects
Mefloquine	Depression

References: 28–31, 131, 138, 139, 140, 161, 186.

■ TREATMENT OF DEPRESSION IN HCV
Pharmacotherapy

Serotonin reuptake inhibitors (SSRIs) are considered first-line treatment in this setting. General principles for treatment of depression in HCV still apply. Side effect profile and pharmacokinetic considerations should guide choice of agents. For example, SSRI treatment may be limited for some patients due to the associated risk of GI bleeding or hepatic insufficiency. ECT has also been reported to be effective.[44]

Much of the empirical evidence for the pharmacotherapy of depression in HCV comes from trials of antiviral therapy with interferon.[45–49] In light of the recent development of interferon-free HCV therapies, these data may be of limited relevance. In the largest randomized controlled trial of interferon-based therapy, escitalopram

BOX 11-5
ANXIETY AND INFECTIOUS DISEASES

- The prevalence of generalized anxiety disorder and panic disorder was 15.8% and 10.5%, respectively in a nationally representative estimate of persons in HIV care, greatly exceeding that found in the general population (1).

- Similarly, the rate of anxiety disorders was 32% in a Veterans Administration Hospital sample of persons with chronic hepatitis C (HCV) compared with 17% of veterans without HCV (2). Generalized anxiety disorder and panic disorder were overrepresented (3).

- PTSD and social anxiety may predispose to acquisition of HIV, HCV, and syphilis (4, 5).

- Comorbid anxiety is not a contraindication to initiation of therapy for HIV, HCV, and/or TB. Successful completion of therapy is possible with adequate management of anxiety symptoms. SSRIs, benzodiazepines and cognitive–behavioral therapy, alone or in combination, are preferred treatments for anxiety (6–8).

- The following medications used to treat HIV, HCV, TB, and malaria, respectively may be associated with anxiety: efavirenz, interferon, INH/cyclosporine, and mefloquine (8–11).

Bing EG, Burnam MA, Longshore D, Fleishman JA, et al. Psychiatric disorders and drug use among human immunodeficiency virus-infected adults in the United States. *Arch Gen Psychiatry*. 2001;58(8):721–728.

Rifai MA, Gleason OC, Sabouni D. Psychiatric care of the patient with hepatitis C: a review of the literature. *Prim Care Companion J Clin Psychiatry*. 2010;12(6). pii: PCC .09r00877.

Adinolfi LE, Nevola R, Lus G, Restivo L, et al. Chronic hepatitis C virus infection and neurological and psychiatric disorders: an overview. *World J Gastroenterol*. 2015;21(8):2269–2280.

Shoptaw S, Peck J, Reback CJ, Rotheram-Fuller E. Psychiatric and substance dependence comorbidities, sexually transmitted diseases, and risk behaviors among methamphetamine-dependent gay and bisexual men seeking outpatient drug abuse treatment. *J Psychoactive Drugs*. 2003;35 Suppl 1:161–168.

Pantalone DW, Hessler DM, Bankoff SM, Shah BJ. Psychosocial correlates of HIV-monoinfection and HIV/HCV-coinfection among men who have sex with men. *J Behav Med*. 2012;35(5):520–528.

Willie TC, Overstreet NM, Sullivan TP, Sikkema KJ, Hansen NB. Barriers to HIV medication adherence: examining distinct anxiety and depression symptoms among women living with HIV who experienced childhood sexual abuse. *Behav Med*. 2016; 42(2):120–127.

Martín-Santos R, Díez-Quevedo C, Castellví P, Navinés R, et al. De novo depression and anxiety disorders and influence on adherence during peginterferon-alpha-2a and ribavirin treatment in patients with hepatitis C. *Aliment Pharmacol Ther*. 2008;27(3):257–265.

Vega P, Sweetland A, Acha J, Castillo H, Guerra D, et al. Psychiatric issues in the management of patients with multi-drug-resistant tuberculosis. *Int J Tuberc Lung Dis*. 2004;8(6):749–759.

Dieperink E, Willenbring M, Ho S. Neuropsychiatric symptoms associated with hepatitis C and interferon alpha: A review. *Am J of Psychiatry*. 2000;157(6):867–876.

Rihs TA, Begley K, Smith DE, Sarangapany J, et al. Efavirenz and chronic neuropsychiatric symptoms: a cross-sectional case control study. *HIV Med*. 2006;7(8):544–548.

Schneider C, Adamcova M, Jick SS, Schlagenhauf P, Miller MK, Rhein HG, Meier CR. Antimalarial chemoprophylaxis and the risk of neuropsychiatric disorders. *Travel Med Infect Dis*. 2013;11(2):71–80.

BOX 11-7
DIFFERENTIAL DIAGNOSIS

Infectious disease itself

Complications of infectious disease (e.g., hypogonadism)

Recommend erring on side against under detection of depression

Self-report scales may help

outperformed placebo in both preventing incident depression and in treating depressive symptoms.[50]

Psychosocial Interventions

Guidelines for assessing and monitoring depression before and during HCV treatment were developed prior to the introduction of interferon-free HCV therapies. The relevance of these recommendations in the absence of interferon is limited. For patients receiving interferon-based therapy, regular monitoring of depressive symptoms during the course of antiviral therapy is recommended (approximately every 4 weeks), even among those patients not exhibiting depression before starting the treatment. Those with moderate to severe depression should be followed closely (i.e., at least 2 weeks) by a mental health professional, and also considered for antidepressants.[38] In this setting, the depression accompanying HCV is characterized by pronounced somatic and neurovegetative symptoms, as opposed to cognitive-affective symptoms, which may require modification of the standard psychotherapies for depression. Cognitive and behavioral interventions may therefore target the somatic side effects first.[51] There is currently insufficient data to recommend similar guidelines for patients undergoing HCV treatment with novel antiviral agents.

Studies evaluating psychological interventions for depression are lacking. It has been recommended that CBT be initiated before interferon-based antiviral therapy is begun in patients with premorbid mood symptoms in order to build coping skills.[51] One RCT of CBT for depression prophylaxis in patients undergoing interferon-based antiviral therapy for HCV reported a trend favoring the CBT arm although overall the results were inconclusive.[52] The therapy consisted of mood monitoring, pleasant activity scheduling, constructive thinking, and social skills and assertiveness training.[52]

Several empirically supported psychological treatment approaches can be adapted for treating comorbid depression in HCV. These include the Cognitive–Behavioral Treatment for Depression and Adherence (CBT-AD) model that combines CBT with problem-solving skills targeting medication adherence and motivational interviewing.[53] Another model is the Cognitive–Behavioral Stress Management (CBSM) intervention, a group-based intervention focused on stress management and relaxation skills, assertiveness and communication training, and anger management.[53,54] Finally, an acceptance-based behavioral therapy, such as Acceptance and Commitment Therapy, has potential to treat depression in the HCV population.[52]

■ SUMMARY

Individuals living with HCV are at substantially increased risk for depression and experience more neurovegetative and somatic depressive features due to the overlap with HCV symptoms themselves. In line with national practice guidelines, we recommend assessing all HCV patients for depression and providing information to HCV patients about treatment options. A sound evidence base exists for pharmacological treatment, structured skills-based psychotherapies, and for the integrated behavioral healthcare delivery of both.

HERPES VIRUSES

The herpes viruses, including herpes simplex viruses (HSV) 1 and 2, varicella zoster virus, Epstein–Barr virus, and cytomegalovirus, are some of the most widespread worldwide, and there is some evidence that immune responses to all of them are associated with depression and anxiety.[55]

EPSTEIN–BARR VIRUS

■ EPIDEMIOLOGY (FIG. 11-1)

Epstein–Barr virus infection is ubiquitous in human populations throughout the world, often acquired in early childhood with subclinical primary infection or in adolescence with an infectious mononucleosis syndrome (glandular fever).[56] There is some evidence to suggest that active EBV infection or reactivation of the virus is associated with depressive disease. One study evaluated depressive symptoms after "glandular fever" and found that MDD was the most common new diagnosis in patients with EBV (28% of subjects) and non-EBV glandular fever (14% of subjects), and was significantly more common in those populations than in patients with recent upper respiratory infection (URI). The relative risk of a new MDD with EBV was 2.5 that with an ordinary URI. Interestingly, all depressive disorders occurring after glandular fever resolved fairly quickly, at a median of 3 weeks.[57] The association with depression appears strongest for highly symptomatic EBV primary infection—mononucleosis syndrome.

■ PATHOPHYSIOLOGY, CLINICAL PRESENTATION, COURSE, AND NATURAL HISTORY

An association has been reported between severity of depressive symptoms and seropositivity for EBV antibodies in patients with seasonal affective disorder (SAD).[58] The fact that this relationship was still present in the summer months, when SAD sufferers were unaffected by depressive symptoms, and that chronic fatigue syndrome (CFS) sufferers showed a similar relationship between severity of symptoms and seropositivity for EBV antibodies, led the authors to suggest that EBV seropositivity could indicate susceptibility to fatiguing illness.[58] However, the relationship between EBV antibodies and CFS remains controversial. Many infectious disease specialists consider this association unproven since the same antibody patterns are found in nonfatigued controls.

Pregnant depressed women are more likely to have EBV reactivation than nondepressed pregnant women (48% vs. 30%) after controlling for confounders.[59] This suggests that depression and stress lead to EBV reactivation rather than EBV reactivation itself leading to depression. However, there has been no work thus far to definitively disentangle cause and effect.

Several case reports indicate that delusional depression can be associated with elevated titers to Epstein–Barr virus.[60] The psychiatric consequences of Epstein–Barr infection may not be limited to depressive disorders however; evaluation of the relationship between early-life exposure to EBV and psychotic experiences in early adolescence found that EBV exposure increased the risk of psychotic experiences five-fold.[61,62]

■ ASSESSMENT AND DIFFERENTIAL DIAGNOSIS

Although the assessment of depression in the patient with Epstein–Barr infection has not been studied, one diagnostic consideration is worth mentioning. CFS, the much-debated entity theorized to be associated with certain viral infections and potentially other immunologic triggers, may present with many of the same symptoms (fatigue, low mood, somatic symptoms) as depression and is an important differential diagnostic consideration.

■ TREATMENT

To the extent that antibodies may be associated with depressive symptoms after Epstein–Barr infection, immune-modulatory therapies may be a treatment consideration in addition to the usual array of antidepressants. One small open label study suggested that in a subgroup of patients with depressive symptoms and elevated EBV antibodies and CFS, antiviral therapy may reduce CNS symptoms by suppressing viral activity.[63]

■ SUMMARY

Although evidence suggests that primary infection and reactivation of Epstein–Barr virus may be associated with both depressive disorders and other psychiatric symptoms as well, not enough data exist to clarify the pathophysiology of depressive disorders in this context or to comment on the unique considerations for treatment in these populations.

HERPES SIMPLEX

■ EPIDEMIOLOGY

HSV infection is common, with prevalence estimates of infection with either HSV-1, HSV-2, or both around 90% in the general population.[64] Labial or peri-oral lesions are caused by HSV-1 whereas anogenital herpes usually results from infection with HSV-2. In both types symptoms are typically mild. While treatment can speed healing and reduce risk of active lesions, the infection establishes chronic latency and is not cleared. Among seropositive patients, there is wide variation in the frequency of symptomatic reactivation.[65]

In contrast, herpes simplex virus encephalitis (HSVE) is a rare but serious necrotizing brain infection with a high mortality rate and high rate of permanent neuropsychiatric sequelae among those who survive. It is the most common sporadic encephalitis in the West, with incidence between 1 in 250,000 and 1 in 1,000,000 persons per year.[66] Over 90% of HSVE cases are attributable to HSV-1, with the remainder caused by HSV-2.[66] HSVE occurs sporadically, without preceding systemic illness or localized case clustering or epidemics.[66]

In cross-sectional studies, HSV infection is associated with depressive symptoms. In patients with acute coronary syndrome, chronic latent HSV infection was found in 100% of patients with the worst depressive symptoms, significantly more than the 43% infection rate in the lowest symptom group.[67] A greater overall pathogen burden, as measured by antibodies to HSV, cytomegalovirus, and Epstein–Barr virus, was also significantly associated with more severe depressive symptoms.[67]

In the one longitudinal study of HSV and depression, more than 95% of patients were seropositive for HSV-1 at inception, and no relationship was found between this infection and incident depression.[65] Although there is limited support in the literature, individuals with HSV-2—anogenital herpes—may be at increased risk for depression due to feelings of stigma, shame, or anxiety related to having a chronic, incurable, sexually transmitted infection. This could be relevant even when latent, as the virus still could be transmitted to others.

The prevalence of depression following HSVE is a different phenomenon. Neurologic deficits are common in patients after this severe infection. One study of (HSVE) survivors found that 45% had changes in behavior and personality, with 17% of them experiencing depression despite a negative prior psychiatric history.[68] Other studies have found somewhat lower numbers: Among 13 HSVE survivors, two had severe behavioral disturbance and two others had depression.[69] Psychiatric symptoms including depression may precede the diagnosis of HSVE, and may also emerge sometime after the acute illness has been treated.[64]

■ PATHOPHYSIOLOGY

The effects of HSVE on neurotransmitter levels in animal models suggest several possible mechanisms for the neuropsychiatric features of the disease (Box 11-2). Rabbits with HSVE have substantially decreased levels of serotonin and a serotonin metabolite in their raphe nuclei, as well as decreased hemispheric serotonin.[70] Dopamine level alterations have also been implicated: rabbits with HSVE have decreased dopamine receptor (D2) density in the substantia nigra and ventral tegmental area on the side contralateral to inoculation, with associated movement disturbances.[71] There may be involvement of acetylcholine as well. The expression of certain viral genes appears to be associated with diminished acetylcholinesterase activity, at least in vitro.[72]

Behavioral changes have been associated with left prefrontal hypoperfusion and left amygdala damage. Patients with HSVE have reduced amygdala and hippocampal volumes, and prefrontal hypoperfusion. The latter may result from diminished inputs from damaged amygdalar efferents to the frontal lobes.[69] It was thought that the psychiatric disturbances common after HSVE may be related to the dysfunction of the amygdalar-prefrontal circuits.

At the genetic level, HSV-1 binds to a number of proteins and modifies the expression of multiple genes, producing a host/ pathogen "interactome" involving well over 1000 host genes, including genes thought to increase susceptibility to depression and other neuropsychiatric disorders.[73]

■ CLINICAL PRESENTATION

As noted above, HSVE is an acute illness—patients are usually febrile, confused, and agitated. Psychiatric disturbance may also occur and typically includes depression as well as aggression, anxiety, apathy, irritability, mania, and panic. As mentioned previously, these symptoms can precede the onset of neurological symptoms and occur well after encephalitis has been treated and the patient discharged from the hospital.[64] Persistent problems with social and occupational functioning are most closely tied to behavioral changes rather than to the memory deficits that are also common in HSVE survivors.[69] This is an important consideration is the rehabilitation of postencephalitis patients.

The psychiatric presentations, if any, associated with latent HSV infection are less clear. The psychological impact of anogenital herpes and associated shame and stigma of living with an incurable sexually transmitted disease are discussed above.

■ COURSE AND NATURAL HISTORY

Psychiatric symptoms associated with HSVE have been reported to occur prior to, during, and after the acute illness.[64] Acute and subacute changes in psychiatric status initially thought to be due to functional disorders can in fact be early manifestations of HSVE and respond to acyclovir treatment.[74] Acute encephalitis should be considered in the differential diagnosis of any patient with acute changes in mental status until laboratory or imaging investigations suggest otherwise.

Although many patients with HSVE demonstrate psychiatric symptoms early in the course of their illness, a delayed presentation is possible. The onset of behavioral and emotional disturbance (including insomnia, hostility, and agitation) has been reported as long as 6 months after resolution of HSVE.[75] In this case, there were no EEG abnormalities or other medical findings to explain the presentation, but encephalomalacia and gliosis were noted in temporal and frontal lobes, suggesting a possible etiology of the delayed presentation.[75] On the other hand, there is also evidence that many patients continue to improve after the acute injury and that depression is not a major cause of ongoing morbidity in most HSVE survivors.[76]

■ ASSESSMENT AND DIFFERENTIAL DIAGNOSIS

Little is known about the assessment of depression specifically in HSV infection or HSVE. Differential diagnostic considerations should include the possibility of relapse; in one study a significant minority of patients with HSVE experienced a relapse.[68] Thus, acute worsening in mental status, even in patients treated successfully with acyclovir, should raise concern for HSVE recurrence rather than simply secondary psychiatric manifestations.

■ TREATMENT

There are no large-scale studies of depression treatment after HSVE. Research to evaluate whether some agents are more beneficial than others will be extremely valuable. In the absence of such evidence, treatment of depression and other accompanying disorders should proceed with attention to medication side effects and comorbidities that may inform treatment. For example, patients with a history of HSVE are at high risk for seizures, which may preclude bupropion as a therapeutic choice even in patients with prominent amotivational symptoms. Conversely, treatment of comorbid seizure disorder should take into account psychiatric symptoms that may be aggravated by selection of seizure medication. A few case reports suggest that carbamazepine may provide some benefit in management of residual psychiatric disturbance after HSVE.[75,77] Ropinorole has also been suggested to have some benefit.[78]

■ SUMMARY

Chronic HSV infection, which is common in the general population, has not been clearly demonstrated to be associated with an increased risk for depression, though some studies are suggestive. HSVE, however, is associated with serious psychiatric presentations and sequelae, including depression. Treatment of the infection with acyclovir is an important step in resolution of all manifestations of the disease, but depressive and other debilitating psychiatric symptoms may persist as a result of damage to medial temporal and frontal brain regions and may require independent treatment.

HIV/AIDS

■ EPIDEMIOLOGY
Prevalence and Incidence of Depressive Disorders

Recent CDC surveillance data estimate that there are 1,148,200 people living with HIV in the United States, 18.1% of whom are unaware they are infected.[79,80] Despite widespread knowledge about effective prevention methods, the HIV incidence rate has remained constant over the past decade with roughly 50,000 new infections annually.[81]

In numerous studies, the prevalence of lifetime and current depressive disorders exceeded expected rates both in those at risk for HIV as well as in HIV seropositive individuals. Data from the HIV Cost and Services Utilization Study of HIV-infected individuals estimated a 12 month prevalence of MDD of 36%, nearly five times higher than 7.6% found in the National Household Survey on Drug Abuse (NHSDA).[82] 26.5% of the sample screened positive for dysthymia (not assessed by the NHSDA) and 21% screened positive for both major depression and dysthymia.[82] More recent nationally representative data of HIV-infected individuals receiving medical care in the United States in 2009 found a prevalence of current major depression of 12.4%, or 3.1 times that found in the general population.[83] In early studies, suicide rates among individuals with HIV/AIDS were as high as 36 times that of the general population.[84,85] More recent studies have found lower rates corresponding to the introduction of antiretroviral therapies in the mid-1990s.[86]

See **Table 11-1**: Comparison of Epidemiologic Studies of Depression in HIV.[82,87,88–90]

■ PATHOPHYSIOLOGY

HIV has a predilection for subcortical structures including the putamen and globus pallidus as well as the hippocampus (Box 11-2).[91] Although attempts to correlate results of neuropsychological assessments with neuroimaging findings have been problematic, neurocognitive impairment appears to be associated with loss of synapses and dendrites as well as neuronal loss and atrophy in deep subcortical structures.[91–93] These findings suggest that each individual's neuroinflammatory response is partially under genetic control and determines the degree of cognitive and psychiatric morbidity observed clinically.[91]

Several endogenous and exogenous molecular targets have been studied as possible links between psychiatric and neurological processes in HIV. Genes regulating opioid-related neurotransmitter and receptor functioning have been one area of study. Delta-opioid agonists may possess antidepressant properties[91,94] and opioid ligands may be involved in cellular resistance to HIV.[91,95] Evidence for this hypothesis comes from studies demonstrating that morphine upregulates CCR5 expression, thereby increasing HIV infectivity of target cells.[91,96]

■ CLINICAL PRESENTATION

Accurate identification of clinical depression in HIV may be complicated by the presence of HIV-related somatic symptoms that are difficult to distinguish from the somatic symptoms produced by depression. In addition, psychomotor and neurocognitive impairments such as diminished concentration, and mental and motor slowing, may be a direct consequence of HIV CNS involvement and can be difficult to distinguish from similar symptoms found in uncomplicated depression. Untangling these clinical phenomena may be even more challenging since combination antiretroviral therapies may have CNS adverse effects that mimic somatic depressive symptoms. They have also prolonged survival, which in turn has been associated with an increased prevalence of milder forms of HIV-associated neurocognitive disorders.

Some studies suggest a subtype of depression secondary to the effect of HIV on subcortical brain structures.[97] For example, data from The Multicenter AIDS Cohort Study found an increase in depressive symptoms beginning 18 months before a diagnosis of AIDS. This finding suggested that depressive symptoms were a harbinger of clinical progression of disease and a proxy for HIV CNS activity. However, other studies have not supported these findings.[98]

■ COURSE AND NATURAL HISTORY
Depression and Progression of HIV Disease, Morbidity, and Mortality

Several large, longitudinal cohort studies, both before and after the introduction of effective combination therapies, have attempted to characterize the impact of depression on the course and variability in outcomes of HIV disease.[98,99,100,101–103] The San Francisco Men's Health Study followed a cohort of HIV-infected gay men over a 9-year period and found that at the 7-year mark, those men with significant depressive symptoms at every visit were at 67% greater risk of dying compared to men without depressive symptoms, after adjusting for antiretroviral use.[104,105]

In the era following the introduction of highly active antiretroviral therapy (HAART), the HIV Epidemiologic Research Study (HERS) followed a cohort of HIV-positive women for a maximum of 7 years and measured HIV-related mortality and decline in cd4 cell count.[98] Chronic depressive symptoms were associated with HIV progression, patient death and greater cd4 cell count decline. These findings persisted after adjusting for substance use, clinical characteristics, antiretroviral medication use, viral load, and baseline cd4 cell count.[98] Similar studies found that women with chronic

TABLE 11-1 Comparison of Epidemiologic Studies of Depression in HIV

Study	Type	Measures	Comment
Dew 1997	Prospective, 12-month 113 HIV-positive, 57 HIV-negative controls Allegheny County, PA	Lifetime prevalence at baseline, 12-month incidence of major depressive disorder DSM-IV diagnosis (SCID)	Incidence HIV-positive: 36.5% HIV-negative controls 15.1% Lifetime prevalence HIV-positive: 47.8% HIV-negative controls: 36.8% No significant difference
Ciesla, Roberts (1988–98)	Meta-analysis of 10 studies using HIV-positive and HIV-negative controls $n = 2596$	Prevalence of current (1–6 months) major depressive disorder DSM criteria	HIV-positive: 9.4% HIV-negative controls 5.2%
Bing (2001)	Nationally representative study using probability sampling method (data from HIV CSUS)[a] $n = 2864$	12-month prevalence of psychiatric and drug use disorders UM-CIDI[b] brief screener	Major depressive disorder 36% Dysthymia 26.5% Comorbid major depressive disorder and dysthymia 21%
Ikovics (2001)	Prospective 7-year exclusively HIV-positive female cohort (HERS)[c] $n = 765$	Chronic depression Intermittent depressive symptoms CES-D[d]	Chronic depression 42% Intermittent depressive symptoms 35%
Lopes (2012)	Nationally representative sample from NESARC[e] Wave 2 HIV-positive and HIV-negative adults stratified by sex (2004–2005)	12-month rates of psychiatric disorders AUDADIS-IV[f]	12.5% of HIV-infected men had major depressive disorder compared to 3.6% of HIV-uninfected men Among women, rates of major depressive disorder did not differ significantly between HIV-positive and HIV-negative groups, 5.9% vs. 8.1%

[a]HIV CSUS: HIV Cost and Services Utilization Study.
[b]UM-CIDI: University of Michigan Composite International Diagnostic Interview.
[c]HERS: HIV Epidemiologic Research Study.
[d]CES-D: Center for Epidemiologic Studies Depression Scale: chronic depression = score ≥ 16 for 75% of study visits (9 out of 12); intermittent depression = score >16 for 26–74% of study visits.
[e]NESARC: National Epidemiologic Survey on Alcohol and Related Conditions.
[f]AUDADIS-IV: Alcohol Use Disorders and Associated Disabilities Interview Schedule DSM-IV Version.

depressive symptoms were more likely to die than women without depression after controlling for clinical and sociodemographic variables and substance use.[102] Over 50% of women in the terminal phase of their HIV disease suffered from significant depressive symptoms.[102] However, Rabkin's longitudinal study of HIV-infected homosexual man over a period of 4 years found no change in depressive symptoms despite significant disease progression and mortality.[106]

Depression and Adherence to Antiretroviral medications

Depression has emerged as the psychiatric disorder with the strongest association with medication nonadherence.[104,105] A meta-analysis of 95 studies comprising 35,000 patients found an association between depression and HIV treatment nonadherence with an effect size similar to that found between depression and treatment nonadherence in other chronic diseases such as diabetes.[104,107]

Importantly, depressed patients treated with antidepressant medications are more likely to be adherent to the antiretroviral medication regimen than untreated depressed patients.[99,108–110]

■ ASSESSMENT AND DIFFERENTIAL DIAGNOSIS

As noted previously, there is considerable overlap between the symptoms of HIV and those of depression: four out of the nine symptoms listed in the DSM criteria for MDD may also be caused by HIV: (1) change in appetite and weight, (2) sleep disturbance, (3) fatigue

or loss of energy and (4) diminished ability to think or concentrate or indecisiveness (Box 11-7). Many clinician-investigators in the field recommend taking an inclusive view of major depression by counting these symptoms. The degree to which other cognitive and affective symptoms are also present will increase confidence in the diagnosis.

Individuals with HIV CNS involvement may present with symptoms that clinically resemble depressive symptoms including blunted affect, apathy, and lethargy and psychomotor slowing. They may also exhibit mild to moderate cognitive impairment and complain of problems with reading comprehension and speed and fine motor dexterity. In addition, depression may coexist with HIV-associated neurocognitive impairment and both may require therapeutic intervention.

Opportunistic conditions affecting the CNS that may present with an acute change in mental status with depressive symptoms include toxoplasmosis, cryptococcal meningitis, cytomegalovirus, neurosyphilis, TB, progressive multifocal leukoencephalopathy, and lymphoma. In any patient with significant immunosuppression, usually reflected in a cd4 cell count of less than 200, a thorough medical and neurological exam is indicated for new onset psychiatric symptoms, including depression, to rule out CNS HIV-related infections and cancers.

Due to shared transmission risk factors, between 15% and 30% of HIV-infected individuals are coinfected with HCV.[111] HCV can be associated with fatigue and dysphoria that can mimic depressive

TABLE 11-2 Medical Differential Diagnosis of Change in Mental Status with Depressed Mood

CNS Opportunistic Conditions

Toxoplasmosis

Cryptococcal meningitis

CMV encephalitis

Progressive multifocal leukoencephalopathy

Lymphoma

Tuberculosis

Neurosyphilis

HIV-associated neurocognitive disorder

Malnourishment

B12 deficiency

Folate deficiency

Hypogonadism

Chronic hepatitis C infection

Addison disease

Anemia

Immune reconstitution syndrome

HIV medications

Efavirenz, raltegravir

symptoms and therefore should also be considered in the differential diagnosis.[112] Hypogonadism may also mimic depression and should be considered in both men and women who present with depression, weight loss, fatigue, and sexual dysfunction.[113,114]

See **Table 11-2**, Medical differential diagnosis of change in mental status with depressed mood.

■ TREATMENT OF DEPRESSION IN HIV
Pharmacotherapy

Psychopharmacologic trials have concentrated mostly on tricyclic antidepressants and SSRIs, although other nonconventional agents such as testosterone and modafinil have also been studied (**Box 11-8**). In general, these studies concluded that the use of antidepressant medications in HIV is safe, effective, does not negatively impact immune functioning, and that no single drug(s) is superior to others. A meta-analysis of seven randomized controlled trials of tricyclic and selective serotonin inhibitors antidepressants concluded that antidepressant medications were effective in treating depression in HIV and were as effective as antidepressants in depressed non-HIV-infected outpatients.[115]

A prominent review of both double blind and open label studies of antidepressant medications as well as psychotherapy studies of depression offered useful guidance. Although fluoxetine is the most frequently studied SSRI, citalopram may be a better choice. It is less likely to interact with HIV medications via cytochrome P450 pathways and preliminary evidence points to its comparability to fluoxetine in effectiveness.[116,117] However, in light of a recent FDA and manufacturer warning about elevated risk for cardiac adverse events at doses of citalopram greater than 40 mg daily, and 20 mg daily in the elderly population, this agent may have lost some of its appeal as a first-line treatment among clinicians.[118]

Due to drug interactions between psychiatric medications and HIV-related drugs a cautious approach similar to that in geriatric populations is advised, with low initial dosing and slower drug titration.[119]

For additional studies not included in above text, see Box 11-8.

Psychosocial Interventions

Among intervention studies of psychological and psychosocial therapies, there was evidence for the effectiveness of cognitive–behavioral stress management, both individual and group cognitive–behavioral therapy (CBT) and other therapies that incorporated a cognitive–behavioral component.[120] One randomized controlled trial found CBT effective for both depression and medication adherence.[120,121] Markowitz et al. compared four treatment groups consisting of interpersonal therapy, CBT, supportive therapy and imipramine combined, and supportive therapy alone. He found that interpersonal therapy and imipramine combined with supportive therapy were more effective than either cognitive–behavioral or supportive therapy alone.[122]

Drug–Drug Interactions

Among the antiretroviral medication classes used to treat HIV, the protease inhibitors, especially ritonavir, and the nonnucleoside reverse transcriptase inhibitors such as efavirenz and nevirapine have been most widely studied in relation to interactions with psychiatric medications. Interactions involving these drugs may be bidirectional, involving inhibition and/or induction of CYP450 2D6 and 3A4 pathways affecting metabolism of psychiatric medications (**Box 11-9**).

Although ritonavir likely has no clinically significant effect on citalopram,[123] efavirenz may potentially either increase or decrease blood levels.[123] For further information about specific drug interactions between antiretroviral and other HIV-related medications and

BOX 11-8
TREATMENTS FOR DEPRESSION IN PATIENTS WITH HIV

Medication	Study	Comparison Group	Comment
Fluoxetine	Zisook et al. (1998)[124]	Fluoxetine and group therapy vs. group therapy alone	Difference in outcome between groups significant only in severe depression
Fluoxetine	Rabkin et al. (1999)[125]	Fluoxetine vs. placebo	Fluoxetine superior to placebo
Fluoxetine	Schwartz and McDaniel (1999)[126]	Fluoxetine vs. desipramine	Both groups showed significant response to treatment
Paroxetine	Elliot et al. (1998)[127]	Paroxetine vs. imipramine vs. placebo	Both paroxetine and imipramine superior to placebo
Fluoxetine	Rabkin et al. (2004)[128]	Fluoxetine vs. testosterone vs. placebo, male patients	Testosterone noninferior to fluoxetine
Imipramine	Rabkin et al. (1994)[129]	Imipramine vs. placebo	Imipramine superior to placebo
Fluoxetine	Targ et al. (1994)[130]	Fluoxetine and group therapy vs. placebo and group therapy	No difference in outcome between groups

BOX 11-9
IMPORTANT DRUG–DRUG INTERACTIONS BETWEEN ANTIDEPRESSANTS AND HIV/TB TREATMENTS

HIV Medication	Antidepressant Medication	Suggested Alternatives
Ritonavir	Fluoxetine associated with serotonin syndrome	Citalopram, escitalopram
	Quetiapine toxicity	
	Buproprion levels may be either decreased or increased	
	Trazodone levels increased	
	Tricyclic antidepressant levels increased	
	Methadone level decreased	
	Sildenafil, tadalafil, vardenafil levels increased	
	Carbamazepine level increased	
	Alprazolam and triazolam increased	Lorazepam, oxazepam
	Methyphenidate and dextroamphetamine levels increased	
	Lamotrigine level decreased	
Efavirenz	Fluoxetine associated with serotonin syndrome	
	Buproprion levels decreased	
	Carbamazepine and methadone levels decreased	
Anti-TB Medication	Antidepressant Medication	Suggested Alternatives
Linezolid	SSRI and SNRIs associated with serotonin syndrome	

psychiatric medications, two websites are recommended: http://hivinsite.ucsf.edu and http://hiv-druginteractions.org.

See Box 11-9. Important drug–drug interactions between HIV/TB and antidepressant medications.[115,118,119,123,131–133,134,135,136,137]

Neuropsychiatric Adverse Effects of Antiretroviral Medications

The antiretroviral medication efavirenz is associated with neuropsychiatric side effects in about 50% of patients, with depression, derealization, depersonalization, and prominent sleep disturbances including vivid or unusual dreams being most common (Box 11-6).[131,138,139] In most cases, these effects occur within the first week and resolve after about 4 weeks. In a subgroup of patients these adverse effects may persist longer and include irritability and anxiety as well as depression.[138,139] There are case reports of patients with pre-existing depression whose mood symptoms worsened after starting raltegravir.[140]

■ SUMMARY

Depression is the most common psychiatric disorder found in people living with HIV. It often predates HIV acquisition, may contribute to risk for transmission, and frequently occurs with other behavioral health comorbidities such as alcohol and substance abuse as well as PTSD and other mood and anxiety disorders. Despite substantial

research documenting its high prevalence and adverse impact on quality of life, engagement in care, and medical outcomes, depression is under-diagnosed and untreated in a significant proportion of patients. Aggressive efforts to identify and treat depression in HIV patients should be a public health priority, especially in light of strong evidence that depression responds well to both pharmacologic and psychotherapeutic intervention, and that improvement is associated with better adherence to HIV medical therapies.

LYME DISEASE

■ EPIDEMIOLOGY

Lyme disease is a spirochetal infection caused by the organism *Borrelia burgdorferi*. It is transmitted to humans via the bites of Ixodes ticks. It takes a minimum 1 to 2 days of feeding for the spirochete to multiply in the tick's gut and then migrate through its salivary glands into the human host. Treatment with a single dose of doxycycline at this stage nearly always prevents the infection.[141]

If enough bacteria are injected, they may multiply and gradually migrate centrifugally from the site of the bite, often but not invariably leading to an enlarging round to oval rash with concentric rings of inflammation and recovery known as erythema migrans (EM). Lyme disease affects the heart, the joints, and the nervous system, with 10% to 15% of patients developing symptomatic nervous system involvement. Importantly, a positive screening test for Lyme disease, typically ELISA (measuring antibody levels) depends on an immune response that persists long after successful eradication of the disease.[141] This suggests that simply correlating psychiatric symptoms with antibody levels could have little relevance, if the active infection was eradicated long ago.

There has been extensive debate over the possible effects of Lyme disease on the nervous system, and over what psychiatric and systemic symptoms could result. In that context, and with the profusion of "post-Lyme," "Lyme-associated," and "chronic Lyme" syndromes, it becomes exceedingly difficult to establish accurate prevalence data for depression.

■ PATHOPHYSIOLOGY

It is not entirely clear how Lyme disease induces the broad range of CNS abnormalities described in the literature. In direct spirochete invasion of the CNS, monocytes produce a B-cell-attracting chemokine in response to *B. burgdorferi* outer surface proteins. The B-cell proliferation that results leads to pleocytosis in the CSF and local production of specific antibody. It is less clear how generalized inflammation can result, or how neurologic damage can persist, despite treatment of the bacterial infection. Inflammatory cytokines may be in part responsible.

Psychological factors may also be involved, especially in the chronic, post-Lyme, syndromes whose biological basis is unclear. A cross sectional study of persistent symptoms including depression attributed to Lyme disease found that catastrophizing, low positive affect and high negative affect were significantly associated with these ongoing symptoms.[142]

■ CLINICAL PRESENTATION

Neurologic involvement in Lyme disease can involve cranial nerve palsies, mononeuropathy, lymphocytic meningitis, encephalopathy, or encephalitis.[141] Some data support an illness syndrome, sometimes called Lyme encephalopathy, characterized by poor performance on memory tests[143,144] and other cognitive deficits.[143] In addition to Lyme encephalopathy, which should be used to describe the symptoms of active, ongoing systemic disease, there may be an entity known as post treatment Lyme disease syndrome, referring to ongoing symptoms in patients already treated for the inciting organism.[145] "Chronic Lyme disease," a vague entity incorporating a number of nonspecific symptoms, is of even less clear status.[145] In addition, there have been reports of a wide variety of neuropsychiatric symptoms attributed to Lyme disease,[146] including depression as well as anxiety, paranoia, and hallucinations. This section will focus on the presence of depression in later stages of infection, rather than in acute encephalitis.

Depression is not a prominent symptom of Lyme disease. Patients with late, disseminated Lyme disease (with, e.g., cardiac conduction anomalies or arthritis) have been studied extensively before and after antibiotic treatment. Some have clinical signs of encephalopathy (e.g., disordered cognition) without the typical peripheral nervous system manifestations (e.g., neuropathy, radiculopathy) of Lyme disease. The cognitive deficits, present across multiple modalities, improve with treatment. Beck Depression Inventory scores, while below the clinical threshold for treatment, nonetheless decrease with treatment of the Lyme disease, which may reflect improved overall health.[147] The literature suggests that while subtle CNS disturbance like fatigue, memory difficulties, and impairments in executive functioning may indeed accompany Lyme disease, depression is not a central component of this syndrome.

If depression does occur after Lyme infection, its severity is generally below the threshold for a clinical diagnosis. A meta-analysis of the literature on the presence of a distinct and definable post-Lyme borreliosis syndrome confirmed the presence of a triad of fatigue, musculoskeletal pain, and neurocognitive difficulties that can persist for up to several years following Lyme infection.[143] Depressive symptom scores are below those of clinically depressed patients, and the depressive symptoms do not appear to influence impaired cognitive performance.[148] A large retrospective cohort study found no association between depression and IgG antibodies to Borrelia.[149]

However, some studies suggest that Lyme disease patients have more depressive symptoms than controls. Patients with past Lyme disease or post Lyme symptoms have more neuropsychological deficits and higher depression scores than normal controls.[140] In one study, 30% of patients with a history of documented severe neuroborrelliosis had Beck Depression Inventory scores in the depressed range.[150]

Instead of examining the rates of depression in patients with Lyme disease, some studies have assessed the prevalence of Lyme infection in psychiatric populations. A prospective study of psychiatric inpatients in an area endemic for *B. burgdorferi* found only one false positive result.[151] suggesting that such screening is low yield and that Lyme infection is not more likely in psychiatric patients.

Overall, the evidence is mixed, but does not indicate a prominent or unique role for depression in Lyme disease or post-Lyme infection syndromes.

■ COURSE AND NATURAL HISTORY

With so much debate over the course of Lyme-associated symptoms, including neuropsychiatric manifestations such as depression, it is not possible to accurately describe the course and natural history of comorbid depression in this illness. The following link provides an excellent summary of Lyme related controversies: http://www.thelancet.com/journals/laninf/article/ePIIS1473–3099(11)70034–2/abstract

■ ASSESSMENT AND DIFFERENTIAL DIAGNOSIS

The Beck Depression Inventory (BDI) is the most commonly used instrument for assessing depression in Lyme disease, with the Minnesota Multiphasic Personality Inventory (MMPI), scale 2, also a popular choice. Differential diagnostic considerations include the proposed post-Lyme syndromes, fibromyalgia, and CFS, among others. Assessment of personality structure and coping style may also help to determine whether the depression present is a physiologic response to neurologic or systemic inflammation, or a psychological response to chronic illness.

■ TREATMENT

The controversy and confusion over the existence of the syndrome known variously as Lyme encephalopathy, neuroborreliosis, or chronic Lyme, have made it very difficult to assess treatment efficacy. Currently, a large randomized controlled trial (RCT) for persistent Lyme symptoms, as well as systematic and Cochrane reviews are underway, but not yet completed.[152] In a small series of patients with Lyme encephalopathy, 50% of whom reported minor depression on the BDI, treatment with ceftriaxone 2 g IV for 30 days resulted in both subjective global improvement and objective memory and CSF protein improvement at 6- and 12 to 24 months.[153] However, neuropsychiatric outcomes were not well characterized, and the study lacked a placebo arm. Another study evaluated the efficacy of ceftriaxone 2 g IV daily for 30 days followed by oral doxycycline 200 mg daily for 60 days in patients with a history of Lyme disease and ongoing symptoms despite previous treatment. Initial mean scores on the BDI and MMPI scale 2 were consistent with mild depression. Although scores on depression inventories improved significantly after treatment, this improvement did not separate from placebo.[154] Overall, there is not compelling evidence to support the use of antibiotics to treat post Lyme depression.

It is not known whether standard antidepressant regimens are effective treatment for post Lyme depression or whether any special considerations are needed for use of antidepressants in this population. However, it seems self-evident that effective treatment of depression may hasten recovery. Low-dose tricyclic antidepressant medications may be useful in patients with sleep disturbance or neuropathic pain[155]

■ SUMMARY

In summary, the relationship between depression and Lyme disease remains incompletely characterized, with conflicting data on prevalence and presentation. At most, it is possible to say that depression at times accompanies or follows infection with B. burgdorferi, with plausible mechanisms including both immune-mediated and psychological. Treatment of primary Lyme infection may help to resolve depression for a number of reasons, but repeated courses of antibiotics are unlikely to be beneficial.

MALARIA

■ EPIDEMIOLOGY

Malaria, caused by the protozoan *Plasmodium* and transmitted by a mosquito vector, is one of the greatest burdens of disease worldwide. There were an estimated 400 million cases in 2012, with over 600,000 estimated deaths.[156] Despite its high incidence, the literature on depression or other neuropsychiatric disturbances in malaria is sparse. One study of community-dwelling adults in Ghana found that a history of falciparum malaria (infection with *Plasmodium falciparum*) was associated with significant elevations in self-report items relating to depression and anxiety.[157] Although these symptoms were subclinical, it is notable that they persisted at least one year beyond the most recent malarial illness.[157]

■ PATHOPHYSIOLOGY

The cerebral pathophysiology of malarial infection is complex, but all processes are secondary to the infection; the parasite itself does not actually enter brain parenchyma. Sequestration, locally released cytokines, changes in blood–brain barrier (BBB) permeability, and metabolic abnormalities all probably play a role. Sequestration refers to the parasitized red blood cells lodging in small vessels and further impeding blood flow by adhering to uninfected red blood cells. Inflammatory mediators are also thought to play a role; one proposed mediator of cytokine effect on neural function is nitric oxide, which can easily diffuse across the BBB. However, evidence for this has been mixed. It is not clear what alters BBB permeability in malaria, and changes in pH, sequestration, cytokine activity, microhemorrhages, and increased cerebral blood flow from heightened local metabolic demands have all been proposed to contribute. All of the above may contribute to psychiatric disturbance associated with malaria, but more research will be needed to clarify the interactions between these multiple pathological processes.[158]

■ CLINICAL PRESENTATION, COURSE, AND NATURAL HISTORY

Malaria-associated behavioral and cognitive changes may persist for a long time after resolution of the acute illness. As noted above, subclinical depression and anxiety symptoms can persist for at least one year after infection.[157] Vietnam era war veterans who had had cerebral malaria were more likely to suffer from major depression than wounded veterans who had not contracted malaria many years after infection (58% vs. 30%). In addition, the survivors of cerebral malaria were more likely to have problems with emotional lability, subjective distress, personality change, and memory impairment, and were more likely to engage in domestic violence.[159] These findings of emotional and behavioral disturbance more than 20 years after malaria infection suggests that even a single episode of infection can have an enduring neuropsychiatric impact.

Children exposed to malaria may fare even worse. Kenyan children who had contracted cerebral malaria were at increased risk of behavioral problems as well as a range of neurocognitive developmental impairments (in attention, memory, speech and language, and motor skills) years after infection.[160]

■ ASSESSMENT AND DIFFERENTIAL DIAGNOSIS

Although *Plasmodium* infection increases the risk of developing depression and other neuropsychiatric symptoms, treatment and prevention of the infection itself bring similar risks. A number of case reports have suggested that mefloquine in particular may be responsible for acute depressive symptoms,[161] psychosis,[162] or both,[163] and for this reason it is contraindicated in patients with a recent history of depression, generalized anxiety disorder, or psychosis.[66,164] In clinical practice in the United States, mefloquine is generally not prescribed for anyone with a history of psychiatric disease.

Some research has sought to clarify the relative risk of psychiatric symptoms associated with mefloquine versus other major prophylactic/treatment drugs such as chloroquine or atovaquone/proguanil. One study surprisingly found relatively little increased risk for neuropsychiatric disturbance amongst the prophylactic agents.[165] An RCT of malarial prophylaxis similarly found no significant difference in mood profiles across four different treatment regimens, although women taking mefloquine reported more fatigue and confusion than did men[166] and it appears to be better tolerated in younger patients rather than older.[164]

■ TREATMENT

There are not specific data available to guide the treatment of depression in malaria. Clinicians should therefore follow the guidelines for the use of antidepressants in general in the medically ill.

■ SUMMARY

Malaria is common and carries significant morbidity in those who survive acute infection. There is evidence to suggest that prior malaria infection is associated with increased risk for a wide range of behavioral and cognitive disorders, including depression. In addition, prophylaxis and treatment, in particular with mefloquine, may carry their own risks for emotional and behavioral disturbance. At this time there is a paucity of data on the association between malaria and neuropsychiatric disorders, but more research is clearly indicated given the global burden of this disease.

NEUROCYSTICERCOSIS

■ EPIDEMIOLOGY AND PATHOPHYSIOLOGY

Neurocysticercosis (NCC) results when humans ingest the eggs of a pork tapeworm Taenia solium from contaminated food or water, and the larval cysticerci lodge in the brain. Epilepsy frequently results. Although the global prevalence of NCC is unknown, the prevalence in persons with epilepsy across Latin American, sub-Saharan Africa, and Southeast Asia has been estimated to be 29%.[167] The point prevalence of NCC lesions in rural Mexico was 9.15.[167] One recent study of the prevalence of depression in NCC patients found a rate of 85%.[168]

■ CLINICAL PRESENTATION

NCC can present in myriad ways; focal seizures or elevated intracranial pressure from hydrocephalus are most typical. However, the disease can also present as a sudden change (e.g., a cerebral infarct), more gradually as in dementia, or as psychosis, mania, catatonia, or depression.[169]

■ COURSE AND NATURAL HISTORY

A Brazilian study found that active NCC disease was associated with depression.[170] However, another study found no difference in depression rates among NCC patients with cysts and those with calcifications. Interestingly, in this study, measures of active disease, such as elevated total protein in the cerebrospinal fluid (CSF), were associated with milder or no depression.[171]

■ ASSESSMENT AND DIFFERENTIAL DIAGNOSIS

Diagnosis of NCC is usually made by correlating signs of the illness, such as seizure, with observation of cystic lesions on brain imaging. Confirmatory serum antibodies can be obtained as well. Assessing for depression can proceed as in patients unaffected by neurocysticerci; there is no evidence to support the use of a particular scale or approach in this population.

■ TREATMENT

It seems self-evident that addressing the underlying disorder disease process with antihelminthic agents would help to treat secondary psychiatric disturbance as well, but as yet these data do not exist. In addition, many of the clinical manifestations of NCC arise from the host's inflammatory response to the dying organisms; hence antimicrobial therapy can paradoxically worsen symptoms in some patients. Antidepressant treatment can be pursued, with attention paid to the elevated risk for seizures in this population, which may guide antidepressant selection away from those agents that lower seizure threshold, like bupropion and clomipramine, and toward those that do not destabilize neuronal membranes at therapeutic levels, such as selective SSRIs.

An additional treatment complication in this population results from the need to administer steroids during the course of malaria treatment. The associated risks attending steroid use of exacerbating or provoking psychiatric disturbances may suggest the need for additional monitoring.

■ SUMMARY

Limited existing data suggest that depression is quite common in patients with NCC; more research is needed to clarify prevalence, natural disease history, and best practices for treatment.

SYPHILIS

Syphilis is a sexually transmitted disease caused by infection with treponema pallidum, a spirochete bacterium. Its clinical course is characterized by four stages. Primary syphilis is manifested by skin lesions or "chancre" commonly seen in the anogenital region or oral mucosa, that occur soon after initial exposure. Secondary syphilis follows within four to ten weeks and is accompanied by a rash usually involving the trunk and extremities. An asymptomatic latent period typically lasting years precedes tertiary syphilis that in turn is known for many different clinical presentations. A more acute form of CNS involvement can occur during primary or secondary syphilis, and be associated with meningitis or stroke.

Psychiatric symptoms result from CNS involvement with treponema pallidum. Invasion of the CNS occurs early in the course of infection and may lead to a range of neuropsychiatric symptoms encompassed by the term neurosyphilis that may be seen at any point along the entire course of disease. However, psychiatric manifestations are most commonly seen in late stage disease and are believed to be related to brain parenchymal involvement.

■ EPIDEMIOLOGY

By 2000, primary and secondary syphilis had reached their lowest-ever incidence rates of 2.1 cases per 100,000 population in the United States. From near eradication, rates have subsequently more than doubled with the large majority of cases now occurring in men who have sex with men (MSM).[172] Although the prevalence and incidence of depression in primary or secondary syphilis have not been well investigated, elevated rates similar to those seen in HIV would seem likely.[173] It has been postulated that persons coinfected with HIV and syphilis may be less likely to clear treponema pallidum after early entry into the CNS. Coinfected MSM might therefore be at greater risk for developing late stage neurosyphilis and associated neuropsychiatric complications.

■ PATHOPHYSIOLOGY

The mechanisms underlying the psychiatric manifestations of neurosyphilis are not fully understood. In symptomatic late stage disease, neurosyphilis may involve either CNS vasculature and meninges or brain parenchyma or have clinical features of both.[174] Psychiatric symptoms result from injury to parenchymal structures and neuronal loss.[175] One study assessed the relationship between depression and magnetic resonance imaging (MRI) neuroradiologic findings.[176] Twenty HIV-negative patients newly diagnosed with neurosyphilis were compared to 20 healthy subjects. Compared to the healthy subjects, the group with active disease had significantly more focal lesions in cortical gray and white matter in multiple arterial distributions likely reflecting areas of ischemia. There was also a significant association between frontal lesions and more severe depressive symptoms. However, the one patient with MDD had no significant neuroradiologic findings.[177] Another study using single photon emission computed tomography (SPECT) and positron emission tomography (PET) found a correlation between psychiatric symptoms and diminished cerebral blood flow.[178]

■ CLINICAL PRESENTATION

Much of our knowledge of the clinical presentation of neuropsychiatric complications of syphilis comes from retrospective studies of psychiatric populations and case reports. Though rigorous descriptions of clinical affective features are generally lacking in many cases, the initial presentation consisted of depressive or manic symptoms. In one study, 27% of patients with neurosyphilis presented with what was termed simple depression. Most also exhibited neurological signs such as abnormal reflexes, tremors, slurred speech, ataxia, and pupillary abnormalities.[179] This contrasted with another study in which only 5% of patients demonstrated signs of depression and 3.3% exhibited manic symptoms.[180] In a review, depressed patients with neurosyphilis were described as "typically slowed, quiet, often suicidal, and may manifest melancholia, nihilistic delusions and all other neurovegetative symptoms".[181,182] As mentioned previously, many cases of neurosyphilis occur when there is coexisting HIV infection. However, in one study, approximately one-third of patients with neurosyphilis were HIV negative. This group presented with mental status abnormalities consisting of bizarre behavior or hallucinations.[183]

■ COURSE AND NATURAL HISTORY

Neuropsychiatric complications of neurosyphilis may not improve despite adequate treatment of the underlying infection if there has been significant neuronal injury.[175] The prognostic significance of mood disturbance associated with neurosyphilis is not known. However, patients with mood symptoms in the absence of initial presenting neurological symptoms would seem to follow the same course as infected patients without neuropsychiatric involvement. If left untreated, significant cognitive impairment usually follows with progression to dementia and death.[175]

Syphilis is associated with stigma and shame that may impact mood, especially in individuals already predisposed to depression. In addition, the majority of incident syphilis now occurs in MSM who are already members of a psychiatrically vulnerable and stigmatized group. Drug abuse also poses a risk for infection as well as psychiatric comorbidity.

■ ASSESSMENT AND DIFFERENTIAL DIAGNOSIS

A discussion of the diagnosis of neurosyphilis is beyond the scope of this chapter. Most investigators interested in psychiatric aspects of this area have focused on establishing screening guidelines for syphilis in psychiatric populations. Screening serves the dual purpose of preventing progression in patients with early disease and identifying those whose psychiatric symptoms are attributable to previously undetected syphilis.[175] There are no established guidelines to assist in the identification of mood disorders in this setting and therefore evaluation should proceed in the same manner as in patients who do not have syphilis.

■ TREATMENT

The treatment literature on depression in neurosyphilis is limited, although case reports offer some guidance. Common sense suggests that the principles that apply to the pharmacotherapy of depression in HIV and other CNS conditions would also apply to syphilis. In a report of five cases of neurosyphilis, antidepressant medications included bupropion extended release 150 mg daily for anhedonia and anergia, and mirtazapine 30 mg daily for anhedonia, anergia and insomnia.[178] Haloperidol, risperidone, and quetiapine were used to control agitation, aggressive behavior, and psychosis while divalproex sodium was used for mood lability.[178]

■ SUMMARY

There has been an upsurge in the incidence of syphilis over the past decade, predominantly in MSM, that has been closely linked to the HIV epidemic. Both diseases are transmitted through sexual contact and organisms responsible for both conditions enter the CNS early in the course of illness. Persistent CNS involvement throughout the latent phase of disease in both diseases may manifest years after initial infection with neuropsychiatric symptoms. Early identification and effective treatment of both psychiatric symptoms as well as the underlying infection can greatly impact morbidity and mortality, enhance compliance with medical treatment and improve quality of life.

TUBERCULOSIS

Tuberculosis (TB) is an infectious disease caused by the bacterium mycobacterium tuberculosis. Only a small proportion of infected persons develop active TB. TB most commonly affects the lung although other organ systems including the CNS may also be involved.

Risk factors for TB include HIV, poor nutrition, diabetes mellitus, overcrowded living conditions, homelessness, and drug and alcohol abuse. Increasing attention has focused on comorbid depression due to its impact on morbidity and mortality, medication adherence, development of antibiotic drug resistance and transmission.[135]

■ EPIDEMIOLOGY

Mood disorders occur more commonly with TB than with other medical illnesses, though there is a wide variability in the reported prevalence of comorbid depression (Fig. 11-1).[184] A prominent literature review of individuals receiving TB treatment reported a current prevalence of depression between 11.3% and 80.2%, with a mean weighted prevalence of 48.9%. Another review reported rates of current depression and anxiety ranging from 46% to 72% in patients with TB.[185] Sixty-eight percent of hospitalized TB patients have been found to have mild to severe depression.[184] The prevalence of depression was reported to be three to six times higher among outpatients with TB than in a healthy control group.[135] A retrospective study reported that 52% of patients starting multidrug-resistant TB therapy (MDR-TB) were depressed at inception and 12% developed depression during treatment.[186]

Conversely, having a mood disorder appears to confer added risk for having latent TB compared to being diagnosed with other psychiatric disorders.[184]

■ PATHOPHYSIOLOGY

Pathophysiologic mechanisms mediating the relationship between TB and depression are not well understood. Neuroendocrine and psychoneuroimmunologic processes similar to those seen with other chronic infectious diseases apparently play a role.[185] So does the psychological stress associated with risk factors such as diminished social support and stigma.

The emergence of drug-resistant TB threatens global public health and has drawn attention to the adverse psychiatric effects of anti-TB medications. Understanding the mechanisms underlying the side effects that too often result in treatment interruption and noncompliance may offer clues to pathways linking TB and depression. Cycloserine (CS), a second line anti-TB drug, may cause psychiatric symptoms including depression and anxiety. Isoniazid (INH), a powerful first-line anti-TB drug, is also associated with psychiatric side effects including depression and delusional ideation (Box 11-6). INH-induced neurotoxicity may result from its inhibition of monoamine oxidase or through INH-induced pyridoxine deficiency that may lead to diminished production of norepinephrine, dopamine, serotonin and GABA.[186]

■ CLINICAL PRESENTATION

Depression is both the result of neuroimmunologic processes on the one hand, and of TB-associated social, interpersonal, psycho-logical and financial factors on the other. For example, individuals may experience guilt or fear of infecting others. In addition, loss of occupational functioning and physical limitations may occur, leading to depression.

In populations with high TB prevalence, tuberculous meningitis occurs more commonly in young children, whereas in low prevalence areas adults are more likely to be affected. HIV greatly increases the risk of coinfection with TB in general and more specifically of TB CNS infection. However, comorbid HIV does not appear to alter the clinical manifestations of tuberculous meningitis.[187] The literature on neuropsychiatric complications of tuberculous meningitis is limited. In one retrospective review of 194 children treated for tuberculous meningitis, 43% were either mildly or severely psychiatrically impaired.[188] In another study, 10% of 74 children who survived tuberculous meningitis suffered long-term psychiatric complications.[189]

■ COURSE AND NATURAL HISTORY

Two thirds of patients receiving treatment for MDR-TB who presented with depression prior to anti-TB therapy had depressive symptoms that were mild or remitted spontaneously. In those patients who developed depression after initiation of therapy, the large majority required antidepressant medications, which were effective. The investigators were unable to identify any social or medical variable associated with depression.[186]

There is an association between depression and the severity and duration of TB and the response to anti-TB therapy.[185,190] Evidence also suggests that active intervention with psychotherapy is associated with improved TB therapy and clinical outcome.[135,136] As already mentioned, depression, both before and after diagnosis with TB, diminishes treatment adherence.

■ ASSESSMENT AND DIFFERENTIAL DIAGNOSIS

Assessment and differential diagnosis should follow the same principles used in evaluating depression co-occurring with any disease with overlapping somatic symptoms. Fatigue, anorexia and weight loss and psychomotor slowing should be considered, while suicidal ideation, hopelessness, social withdrawal and anhedonia strengthen confidence in the diagnosis. The Beck Depression Inventory is the most frequently used screening tool.[135]

■ TREATMENT

There are no controlled studies or consensus guidelines to assist medication choice in the treatment of depression in TB. Selective SSRI are generally recommended as first-line agents due to their more benign side effect profile when compared to tricyclic antidepressants and MAOIs. The most controversial issue involves potential interactions between SSRIs and INH due to its MAOI activity. In general, combining SSRIs with an MAOI is contraindicated because their interaction may lead to serotonin syndrome. However, according to some sources there is insufficient evidence to recommend against this combination.[137,191] Trenton et al. suggest that among the SSRIs, paroxetine may be the safest choice due to its use primarily of the CYP 2D6 isoenzyme which has limited activity in INH metabolism.[184] Linezolid which is used in the treatment of MDR-TB and has weak MAOI activity, has been associated with serotonin syndrome when used in combination with SSRIs and serotonin norepinephrine reuptake inhibitors (SNRIs). Case reports exist for this adverse interaction between linezolid and citalopram, escitalopram, sertraline, fluoxetine, paroxetine, venlafaxine, and duloxetine.[191] The combination of linezolid with an MAO inhibitor should be done with caution, and only when absolutely necessary.

Cycloserine, a second line anti-TB drug may be associated with depression that in most cases responds well to antidepressant medication without interruption of anti-TB therapy.[186] (See Box 11-9: Important Drug–Drug Interactions between antidepressants and HIV/TB treatments[115,118,119,123,131–133,134,137,184,191].)

As with pharmacotherapy, there are no specific guidelines regarding psychotherapy of comorbid depression in TB. Individual psychotherapy for depression has a beneficial effect on TB treatment adherence and outcome.[136] Psychosocial support groups are effective in addressing stigma, grief, and hopelessness.[186]

■ SUMMARY

Depression commonly co-occurs with TB and may occur with more frequency in TB than in other medical disorders. CNS involvement is frequent and depression and TB share multiple risk factors that may partially explain their coexistence. In addition, depression may result from anti-TB therapy, especially INH and cyclosporine. Depression is associated with poor compliance with the TB medication regimen, which has contributed to the appearance of MDR-TB. Evidence suggests that effective treatment of depression can improve adherence to TB therapy and lead to improved outcomes. Together these findings suggest that early identification and treatment of depression in these patients is effective.

BACTERIAL, VIRAL, AND FUNGAL MENINGITIS

■ EPIDEMIOLOGY AND PATHOPHYSIOLOGY

The most common causes of bacterial meningitis are *Neisseria meningitides, Streptococcus pneumonia* and *Staphylococcus aureus* while viral meningitis is often due to seasonal enteroviruses and arboviruses.[192] *Cryptococcus neoformans* is the most common cause of fungal meningitis. Prevalence studies examining rates of depression following recovery from meningitis have produced conflicting results. One study compared 17 HIV-seronegative patients who had been successfully treated for Cryptoccocal meningitis (CM) with 26 healthy controls. 35% of the patient group had mild-to-severe depression. They were significantly more likely than controls to have CM-related positive findings on brain MRI and impairment in executive and visuo-constructive functioning. Depressed patients also exhibited poorer performance on tests of executive functioning and visuo-constructive functions, thus linking depression to frontal-subcortical circuits. In addition, CM-related structural damage in the thalamus, basal ganglion and cerebral cortex may be linked to depressive symptoms.[193] In contrast, another study of 118 patients fully recovered from either bacterial (BM) or viral meningitis (VM) were compared to 30 healthy controls. Although the BM group demonstrated greater neuropsychological impairment compared to the VM group, there was no significant difference between any of the groups in depression.[194] Childhood hydrocephalus secondary to meningitis may also be associated with higher than expected rates of depression.[195]

■ CLINICAL PRESENTATION

Depression may be the presenting manifestation of meningitis or may occur as a sequela in patients fully recovered from it. Case reports describe patients with CM who presented with depression accompanied by worsening cognitive functioning. These patients were treated with antidepressant medication before the underlying fungal infection was discovered.[196] Hesueh and Lin describe a patient treated for 10 months for depression without a therapeutic response. After he demonstrated worsening cognitive impairment, MRI revealed bilateral ventricular enlargement and *Cryptoccocus neoformans* was cultured from his CSF.[197]

■ CLINICAL COURSE AND NATURAL HISTORY

There are limited data regarding the clinical course and history of depression either as a symptom accompanying acute onset of meningitis or as a sequela. Case reports suggest that medical intervention for the underlying infectious disease may result in resolution of depressive symptoms without direct pharmacologic treatment of mood.[196]

■ ASSESSMENT AND DIFFERENTIAL DIAGNOSIS

Given the association between depression and positive neuropsychological and neuroimaging findings, careful neurocognitive assessment is warranted in patients presenting with depressive symptoms following successful treatment of meningitis. There is no evidence to suggest that any particular approach to diagnosis is preferable, and no published guidelines to follow in assessing depressive symptoms in this setting.

■ TREATMENT

There is no evidence to support the use of any particular antidepressant agent in patients with meningitis. It seems self-evident that treatment of the underlying infectious disease should precede or accompany treatment of depressive symptoms, but there is no data to support one approach over another. In patients at elevated risk for seizures, bupropion and clomipramine should be avoided since they may lower the seizure threshold to a greater extent than do other agents.

■ SUMMARY

Current evidence suggests that depression may either be a presenting symptom of meningitis, especially CM, or may follow effective treatment of meningitis as sequelae. The association between depression and neurocognitive and neuroimaging studies suggests a common pathophysiologic mechanism related to underlying neuroinflammatory or structural abnormalities. Future research is needed to elucidate this relationship.

CONCLUSION

Clinicians should screen for depression in infectious diseases (**Box 11-10**). The rationale for early detection and intervention of depression rests on several observations. Prevalence rates of depression appear to exceed those found in the general population and to be at least comparable to rates found in other medical illnesses. Pharmacologic and psychosocial therapies are as safe and effective treatments as in nonmedically ill depressed patients. And alleviation of depressive symptoms may be associated with improved quality of life and medical outcomes either through improved adherence to medical treatment or by more directly affecting the course of the underlying infection. Further research is needed to clarify the bidirectional relationship between depression and the neuroimmunologic processes involved in infectious diseases which may in turn deepen our understanding of the pathophysiology of mood disorders.

**BOX 11-10
SUMMARY**

Individuals with infectious disease are at a substantially increased risk for depression

It can be difficult to distinguish depression given the overlapping (neurovegetative symptoms)

There is a good evidence base for standard depression treatments, both pharmacological and structured psychotherapies

---

REFERENCES

1. Yates W, Gleason O. Hepatitis C and depression. *Depress Anxiety*. 1998;7(4):188–193.

2. Bayliss MS, Gandeck KM, Bungay KM, Sugano D, Hsu MA, Ware JE. A questionnaire to assess the generic and disease-specific health outcomes of patients with chronic hepatitis C. *Qual Life Res*. 1997;7(1):39–55.

3. Golden J, O'Dwyer A, Conroy R. Depression and anxiety in patients with hepatitis C: prevalence, detection rates and risk factors. *Gen Hosp Psych*. 2005;27(6):431–438.

4. Fontana RJ, Hussain K B, Schwartz SM, Moyer CA, Su GL, Lok AS. Emotional distress in chronic hepatitis C patients not receiving antiviral therapy. *J Hepatology*. 2002;36(3):401–407.

5. Nelligan JA, Loftis JM, Matthews AM, Zucker BL, Linke AM, Hauser P. Depression comorbidity and antidepressant use in veterans with chronic hepatitis C: results from a retrospective chart review. *J Clin Psych*. 2008;69:810–816.

6. Basseri B, Yamini D, Chee G, Enayati P, Tran T, Poordad F. Comorbidities associated with the increasing burden of hepatitis C infection. *Liver Int*. 2010;30:1012–1018.

7. Dwight M, Kowdley K, Russo J, Ciechanowski P, Larson A, Katon W. Depression, fatigue, and functional disability in patients with chronic hepatitis C. *J Psychosomatic Research*. 2000;49(5):311–317.

8. Lehman C, Cheung R. Depression, anxiety, post-traumatic stress, and alcohol-related problems among veterans with chronic hepatitis C. *Am J Gasteroenterol*. 2002;97:2640–2646.

9. Fireman M, Indest DW, Blackwell A, Whitehead AJ, Hauser P,. Addressing tri-morbidity (hepatitis C, psychiatric disorders, and substance use): The importance of routine mental health screening as a component of a comanagement model of care. *Clin Infectious Dis*. 2005;40(S5):S286–S291.

10. Yovtcheva S, Aly Rifai M, Moles J, Van Der Linden B. Psychiatric comorbidity among hepatitis C-positive patients. *Psychosomatics*. 2001;42(5):411–415.

11. El-Serag H, Kunik M, Richardson P, Rabeneck L. Psychiatric disorders among veterans with hepatitis C infection. *Gastroenterol*. 2002;123:476–482.

12. Kristiansen MG, Lochen ML, Gutteberg TJ, Mortensen L, Eriksen BO, Florholmen J. Total and cause specific mortality rates in a prospective study of community-acquired hepatitis C virus infection in northern Norway. *J Viral Hepat*. 2011;18(4):237–244.

13. Kraus MR, Schäfer A, Schöttker K, et al. Therapy of interferon-induced depression in chronic hepatitis C with citalopram: a randomised, double-blind, placebo-controlled study. *Gut*. 2008;57(4):531–536.

14. Centers for Disease Control and Prevention. Hepatitis C information for professionals. Available at http://www.cdc.gov/hepatitis/HCV/index.htm. Accessed June 15, 2013.

15. McDonald E, Mann A, Thomas H. Interferons as mediators of psychiatric morbidity: an investigation in a trial of recombinant α-interferon in hepatitis-B carriers. *Lancet*. 1987;330(8569):1175–1178.

16. Denicoff KD, Rubinow DR, Papa MZ, Simpson C, Seipp CA, Lotze MT, Rosenberg SA. The neuropsychiatric effects of treatment with interleukin-2 and lymphokine-activated killer cells. *Ann intern med*. 1987;107(3):293–300.

17. Carta M, Hardoy M, Garofalo A, et al. Association of chronic hepatitis C with major depressive disorders: irrespective of interferon-alpha therapy. *Clin Pract Epidemiol Ment Health*. 2007;3(1):22.

18. Glacken M, Kernohan G, Coates V. Diagnosed with hepatitis C: a descriptive exploratory study. *Int J Nurs Stud*. 2001 ;38(1):107–116.

19. Loftis J, Huckans M, Ruimy S, Hinrichs D, Hauser P. Depressive symptoms in patients with chronic hepatitis C are correlated with elevated plasma levels of interleukin-1beta and tumor necrosis factor-alpha. *Neurosci Lett*. 2008;430:264–268.

20. Schwaiger M, Pich M, Franke L, et al. Chronic hepatitis C infection, interferon-alpha treatment and peripheral serotenergic dysfunction. Poster presented at: 54th Annual Meeting of the American Association for the Study of Liver Diseases; October 24–28, 2004; Boston, Mass.

21. Lim JK, Cronkite R, Goldstein MK, Cheung RC. The impact of chronic hepatitis C and comorbid psychiatric illnesses on health-related quality of life. *J Clin Gastroenterol*. 2006;40(6):528.

22. Bailey D Jr, Landerman L, Barroso J, et al. Uncertainty, symptoms, and quality of life in persons with chronic hepatitis C. *Psychosomatics*. 2009;50(2):138–146.

23. Patterson A, Morasco B, Fuller B, Indest D, Loftis J, Hauser P. Screening for depression in patients with hepatitis C using the Beck Depression Inventory-II: do somatic symptoms compromise validity? *Gen Hospital Psychiatry*. 2011;33(4):354–362.

24. Miller ER, Hiller JE, Shaw DR. Quality of life in HCV infection: lack of association with ALT levels. *Aust NZ J Public Health*. 2001;25:355–361.

25. Hussain KB, Fontana R J, Moyer CA, Su GL, Sneed-Pee N, Lok AS. Comorbid illness is an important determinant of health-related quality of life in patients with chronic hepatitis C. *Am J Gastroenterol*. 2001;96(9):2737–2744.

26. Grassi L, Satriano J, Serra A, et al. Emotional stress, psychosocial variables and coping associated with hepatitis C virus and human immunodeficiency virus infections in intravenous drug users. *Psychother Psychosom*. 2002;71:342–349.

27. Sgorbini M, O'Brien L, Jackson D. Living with hepatitis C and treatment: The personal experiences of patients. *J Clin Nursing*. 2009;18:2282–2291.

28. Dieperink E, Wiilenbring M, Ho S. Neuropsychiatric symptoms associated with hepatitis C and interferon alpha: A review. *Am J Psychiatry*. 2000;157(6):867–876.

29. Loftis J, Socherman R, Howell C, Whitehead A, Hill J, Dominitz J, Hauser P. Association of interferon-alpha-induced depression and improved treatment response in patients with hepatitis C. *Neurosci Lett*. 2004;365(2): 87–91.

30. Dieperink E, Ho S, Thuras P, Willenbring M. A prospective study of neuropsychiatric symptoms associated with interferon-a-2b and ribavirin therapy for patients with chronic hepatitis C. *Psychosomatics*. 2003;44(2):104–112.

31. Smith KJ, Norris S, O'Farrelly C, O'Mara SM. Risk factors for the development of depression in patients with hepatitis C taking interferon-α. *Neuropsychiatr Dis Treat*. 2011;7:275.

32. Udina M, Castellví P, Moreno-España J, et al. Interferon-induced depression in chronic hepatitis C: a systematic review and meta-analysis. *J Clin Psych*. 2012;73(8):1128–1138.

33. Pavlovic Z, Jasovic-Gasic M, Delic D, Maric N, Vukovic O, Pejovic S. Prevalence, severity and course of depressive symptomatology in chronic hepatitis c patients on pegylated interferon alpha: a 72-week prospective study. *Eur Psychiatry*. 2013;28:1680–1681.

34. Evon D, Ramcharran D, Belle S, Terrault N, Fontana R, Fried M; Virahep-C study group. Prospective analysis of depression during peginterferon and ribavirin therapy of chronic hepatitis C: Results of the Virahep-C study. *Am J Gastroenterol.* 2009;104:2949–2958.

35. Raison C L, Broadwell SD, Borisov AS, et al. Depressive symptoms and viral clearance in patients receiving interferon-α and ribavirin for hepatitis C. *Brain Behav Immun.* 2005;19(1):23–27.

36. Maddock C, Landau S, Barry K, et al. Psychopathological symptoms during interferon-alpha and ribavirin treatment: effects on virologic response. *Mol Psychiatry.* 2005;10:332–333.

37. Chapman J, Oser M, Hockemeyer J, Weitlauf J, Jones S, Cheung R. Changes in depressive symptoms and impact on treatment course among Hepatitis C patients undergoing Interferon-α and Ribavirin therapy: A prospective evaluation. *Am J Gastroenterol.* 2011;106:2123–2132.

38. Loftis J, Hauser P. Hepatitis C in patients with psychiatric disease and substance abuse: screening strategies and co-management models of care. *Curr Hepat Rep.* 2003;2:93–100.

39. Loftis JM, Hauser P. The phenomenology and treatment of interferon-induced depression. *J Affective Disorders.* 2004;82(2):175–190.

40. Yee H, Chang M, Pocha C, et al. Update on the management and treatment of hepatitis C virus infection: recommendations from the Department of Veterans Affairs Hepatitis C Resource Center Program and the National Hepatitis C Program Office. *Am J Gastroenterol.* 2012;107(5):669–689.

41. Management of hepatitis C: 2002. *NIH Consens State Sci Statements.* 2002;19(3) 1–46.

42. Ramasubbu R, Taylor VH, Samaan Z. The Canadian Network for Mood and Anxiety Treatments (CANMAT) task force recommendations for the management of patients with mood disorders and select comorbid medical conditions. *Ann Clin Psychiatry.* 2012;24:91–109.

43. Sockalingam S, Links P, Abbey S. Suicide risk in hepatitis C and during interferon alpha therapy: a review and clinical update. *J viral hepatitis.* 2011;18(3):153–160.

44. Lotrich FE. Psychiatric clearance for patients started on interferon-alpha-based therapies. *Am J Psych.* 2013;170(6):592–597.

45. Batki SL, Canfield KM, Ploutz Snyder R. Psychiatric and substance use disorders among methadone maintenance patients with chronic hepatitis C infection: effects on eligibility for hepatitis C treatment. *Am J Addictions.* 2011;20(4):312–318.

46. Morasco BJ, Rifai MA, Loftis JM, Indest DW, Moles JK, Hauser P. A randomized trial of paroxetine to prevent interferon-α-induced depression in patients with hepatitis C. *J Affective Disorders.* 2007;103(1):83–90.

47. Morasco BJ, Loftis JM, Indest DW, et al. Prophylactic antidepressant treatment in patients with hepatitis C on antiviral therapy: a double-blind, placebo-controlled trial. *Psychosomatics.* 2010;51:401–408.

48. Diez-Quevedo C, Masnou H, Planas R, et al. Prophylactic treatment with escitalopram of pegylated interferon alfa-2a-induced depression in hepatitis C: a 12-week, randomized, double-blind, placebo-controlled trial. *J Clin Psych.* 2011;72:522–528.

49. De Knegt RJ, Bezemer G, Van Gool AR, et al. A Randomised clinical trial: escitalopram for the prevention of psychiatric adverse events during treatment with peginterferon-alfa-2a and ribavirin for chronic hepatitis C. *Aliment Pharmacol Ther.* 2011;34:1306–1317.

50. Schaefer M, Sarkar R, Knop V, et al. Escitalopram for the prevention of peginterferon-α2a–associated depression in hepatitis C virus–infected patients without previous psychiatric disease: a randomized trial. *Ann Intern Med.* 2012;157:94–103.

51. Evon DM, Golin CE, Fried MW, Keefe FJ. Chronic hepatitis C and antiviral treatment regimens: Where can psychology contribute? *J Consul Clin Psychol.* 2013;81(2):361–374.

52. Ramsey SE, Engler PA, Stein MD, et al. Effect of CBT on depressive symptoms in methadone maintenance patients undergoing treatment for hepatitis C. *J Addict Res Ther.* 2011;2(2):2–10.

53. Safren SA, O'Cleirigh C, Tan JY, et al. A randomized controlled trial of cognitive behavioral therapy for adherence and depression (CBT-AD) in HIV-infected individuals. *Health Psychology.* 2009;28:1–10.

54. Antoni M, Ironson G, Schneiderman N. *Cognitive-Behavioral Stress Management: Treatments that Work.* New York, NY: Oxford University Press: 2007.

55. Coughlin S. Anxiety and depression: linkages with viral disease. *Public Health Rev.* 2012;34(2):92.

56. Hjalgrim H, Friborg J, Melbye M. The epidemiology of EBV and its association with malignant disease. In: Arvin A, Campadelli-Fiume G, Mocarski E, et al. eds. *Human Herpesviruses: Biology, Therapy, and Immunoprophylaxis.* Cambridge: Cambridge University Press; 2007.

57. White PD, Thomas JM, Amess J, et al. Incidence, risk and prognosis of acute and chronic fatigue syndromes and psychiatric disorders after glandular fever. *Br J Psychiatry.* 1998;173:475–481.

58. Natelson B, Ye N, Moul D, et al. High titers of anti-Epstein–Barr virus DNA polymerase are found in patients with severe fatiguing illness. *J Med Virol.* 1994 42:42–46.

59. Haeri S, Johnson N, Baker AM, et al. Maternal depression and Epstein-Barr virus reactivation in early pregnancy. *Obstet Gynecol.* 2011;117(4):862–866.

60. White PD, Lewis SW. Delusional depression after infectious mononucleosis. *Br Med J.* 1987;295:97–98.

61. Khandaker G, Stochl J, Zammit S, Lewis G, Jones P. Childhood Epstein–Barr virus infection and subsequent risk of psychotic experiences in adolescence: A population-based prospective serological study. *Schizophr Res.* 2014;158:19–24.

62. Khandaker GM, Zimbron J, Dalman C, Lewis G, Jones PB. Childhood infection and adult schizophrenia: A meta-analysis of population-based studies. *Schizophr Res.* 2012;139(1–3):161–168.

63. Kogelnik AM, Loomis K, Hoegh-Petersen M, Rosso F, Hischier C, Montoya J. Use of valganciclovir in patients with elevated antibody titers against human herpesvirus-6 (HHV-6) and Epstein–Barr virus (EBV) who were experiencing central nervous system dysfunction including long-standing fatigue. *J Clin Virology.* 2006;37(Suppl 1):S33–S38.

64. Hokkanen L, Launes J. Neuropsychological sequelae of acute-onset sporadic viral encephalitis. *Neuropsychol Rehabil.* 2007;17(4–5):450–477.

65. Simanek A, Cheng C, Yolken R, Uddin M, Galea S, Aiello A. Herpesviruses, inflammatory markers and incident depression in a longitudinal study of Detroit residents. *Psychoneuroendocrinology.* 2014;50:139–148.

66. Granerod J, Crowcroft NS. The epidemiology of acute encephalitis. *Neuropsychol Rehabil.* 2007;17(4–5):406–428.

67. Miller GE, Freedland KE, Duntley S, Carney RM. Relation of depressive symptoms to C-reactive protein and pathogen burden (cytomegalovirus, herpes simplex virus, Epstein-Barr virus) in patients with earlier acute coronary syndromes. *Am J Cardiol.* 2005;95(3):317–321.

68. McGrath N, Anderson NE, Croxson MC, Powell KF. Herpes simplex encephalitis treated with acyclovir: diagnosis and long term outcome. *J Neurol Neurosurg Psychiatry.* 1997;63(3):321–326.

69. Caparros-Lefebvre D, Girard-Buttaz I, Reboul S, et al. Cognitive and psychiatric impairment in herpes simplex virus encephalitis suggest involvement of the amygdalo-frontal pathways. *J Neurol.* 1996;243(3):248–256.

70. Päivärinta MA, Marttila RJ, Lönnberg P, Rinne UK. Decreased raphe serotonin in rabbits with experimental herpes simplex encephalitis. *Neurosci Lett.* 1993;156(1–2):1–4.

71. Päivärinta MA, Marttila RJ, Rinne JO, Rinne UK. Decrease in mesencephalic dopamine autoreceptors in experimental herpes simplex encephalitis. *J Neural Transm Gen Sect.* 1992;89 (1–2):71–80.

72. Päivärinta MA, Röyttä M, Hukkanen V, Marttila RJ, Rinne UK. Nervous system inflammatory lesions and viral nucleic acids in rabbits with herpes simplex virus encephalitis-induced rotational behaviour. *Acta Neuropathol.* 1994;87(3): 259–268.

73. Carter CJ. Susceptibility genes are enriched in those of the herpes simplex virus 1/ host interactome in psychiatric and neurological disorders. *Pathog Dis.* 2013;69:240–261.

74. Boyapati R, Papadopoulos G, Olver J, Geluk M, Johnson PD. An unusual presentation of herpes simplex virus encephalitis. *Case Rep Med.* 2012;2012:241710.

75. Gaber TA, Eshiett M. Resolution of psychiatric symptoms secondary to herpes simplex encephalitis. *J Neurol Neurosurg Psychiatry.* 2003;74(8):1164; author reply 1164.

76. Hokkanen L, Launes J. Cognitive recovery instead of decline after acute encephalitis: a prospective follow up study. *J Neurol Neurosurg Psychiatry.* 1997;63:222–227.

77. Vallini AD, Burns RL. Carbamazepine as therapy for psychiatric sequelae of herpes simplex encephalitis. *South Med J.* 1987;80(12):1590–1592.

78. Kohno N, Nabika Y, Toyoda G, Bokura H, Nagata T, Yamaguchi S. The effect of ropinirole on apathy and depression after herpes encephalitis. *Cogn Behav Neurol.* 2012;25(2):98–102.

79. Centers for Disease Control and Prevention. HIV/AIDS Available at http://www.cdc.gov/hiv/pdf/statistics_2010_HIV_Surveillance_Report_vol_17_no_3. Accessed May 11, 2013.

80. Centers for Disease Control and Prevention. Vital signs: HIV prevention through care and treatment–United States. *Morb Mortal Wkly Rep.* 2011;60(47):1618–1623.

81. Centers for Disease Control and Prevention. HIV/AIDS Available at http://www.cdc.gov/hiv/surveillance/resources/reports/2010supp_vol17no4/. Accessed May 11, 2013.

82. Bing EG, Burnam MA, Longshore D, et al. Psychiatric disorders and drug use among human immunodeficiency virus-infected adults in the United States. *Arch Gen Psychiatry.* 2001;58(8): 721–728.

83. Do AN, Rosenberg ES, Sullivan PS, et al. Excess burden of depression among HIV-infected persons receiving medical care in the United States: Data from the Medical Monitoring Project and the Behavioral Risk Factor Surveillance System. *PLoS ONE.* 2014;9(3):e92842.

84. Komiti A, Judd F, Grech P, et al. Suicidal behaviour in people with HIV/AIDS: a review. *Aust N Z J Psychiatry.* 2001;35(6): 747–757.

85. Marzuk PM, Tierney H, Tardiff K, et al. Increased risk of suicide in persons with AIDS. *JAMA.* 1988;259(9):1333–1337.

86. Jia CX, Mehlum L, Qin P. AIDS/HIV infection, comorbid psychiatric illness, and risk for subsequent suicide: a nationwide register linkage study. *J Clin Psychiatry.* 2012;73(10):1315–1321.

87. Dew MA, Becker JT, Sanchez J, et al. Prevalence and predictors of depressive, anxiety and substance use disorders in HIV-infected and uninfected men: a longitudinal evaluation. *Psychol Med.* 1997;27(2):395–409.

88. Ciesla JA, Roberts JE. Meta-analysis of the relationship between HIV infection and risk for depressive disorders. *Am J Psychiatry.* 2001;158(5):725–730.

89. Ickovics JR, Hamburger ME, Vlahov D, et al. HIV Epidemiology Research Study Group Mortality, CD4 cell count decline, and depressive symptoms among HIV-seropositive women: longitudinal analysis from the HIV Epidemiology Research Study. *JAMA.* 2001;285(11):1466–1474.

90. Lopes M, Olfson M, Rabkin J, et al. Gender, HIV status, and psychiatric disorders: results from the National Epidemiologic Survey on Alcohol and Related Conditions. *J Clin Psychiatry.* 2012;73(3):384–391.

91. Kopnisky KL, Bao J, Lin YW. Neurobiology of HIV, psychiatric and substance abuse comorbidity research: workshop report. *Brain Behav Immun.* 2007;21(4):428–441.

92. Woods SP, Moore DJ, Weber E, Grant I. Cognitive neuropsychology of HIV-associated neurocognitive disorders. *Neuropsychol Rev.* 2009;19(2):152–168.

93. Masliah E, Heaton RK, Marcotte TD, et al. Dendritic injury is a pathological substrate for human immunodeficiency virus-related cognitive disorders. HNRC Group. The HIV Neurobehavioral Research Center. *Ann Neurol.* 1997;42(6):963–972.

94. Jutkiewicz EM. The antidepressant -like effects of delta-opioid receptor agonists. *Mol Interv.* 2006;6(3):162–169.

95. McCarthy L, Wetzel M, Sliker JK, Eisenstein TK, Rogers TJ. Opioids, opioid receptors, and the immune response. *Drug Alcohol Depend.* 2001;62(2):111–123.

96. Wang GJ, Chang L, Volkow ND, et al. Decreased brain dopaminergic transporters in HIV-associated dementia patients. *Brain.* 2004;127(Pt 11):2452–2458.

97. Treisman G, Fishman M, Schwartz J, Hutton H, Lyketsos C. Mood disorders in HIV infection. *Depress Anxiety.* 1998;7(4):178–187.

98. Ickovics JR, Hamburger ME, Vlahov D, et al. HIV Epidemiology Research Study Group. Mortality, CD4 cell count decline, and depressive symptoms among HIV-seropositive women: longitudinal analysis from the HIV Epidemiology Research Study. *JAMA.* 2001;285(11):1466–1474.

99. Rabkin JG. HIV and depression: 2008 review and update. *Curr HIV/AIDS Rep.* 2008 ;5(4):163–171.

100. Leserman J. HIV disease progression: depression, stress, and possible mechanisms. *Biol Psychiatry.* 2003;54(3):295–306.

101. Farinpour R, Miller EN, Satz P, et al. Psychosocial risk factors of HIV morbidity and mortality: findings from the Multicenter AIDS Cohort Study (MACS). *J Clin Exp Neuropsychol.* 2003;25(5):654–670.

102. Cook JA, Grey D, Burke J, Cohen MH, et al. Depressive symptoms and AIDS-related mortality among a multisite cohort of HIV-positive women. *Am J Public Health.* 2004;94(7):1133–1140.

103. Rabkin J. Depression and HIV. *Focus*. 2004;19(10):1–5.

104. Gonzalez JS, Batchelder AW, Psaros C, Safren SA. Depression and HIV/AIDS treatment nonadherence: a review and meta-analysis. *J Acquir Immune Defic Syndr*. 2011;58(2):181–187.

105. Starace F, Ammassari A, Trotta MP, et al. AdICoNA Study Group. NeuroICoNA Study Group. Depression is a risk factor for suboptimal adherence to highly active antiretroviral therapy. *J Acquir Immune Defic Syndr*. 2002;31(Suppl 3):S136–S139.

106. Rabkin JG, Goetz RR, Remien RH, Williams JB, Todak G, Gorman JM. Stability of mood despite HIV illness progression in a group of homosexual men. *Am J Psychiatry*. 1997;154(2):231–238.

107. Bottonari KA, Tripathi SP, Fortney JC, et al. Correlates of antiretroviral and antidepressant adherence among depressed HIV-infected patients. *AIDS Patient Care STDS*. 2012;26(5):265–273.

108. Horberg MA, Silverberg MJ, Hurley LB, et al. Effects of depression and selective serotonin reuptake inhibitor use on adherence to highly active antiretroviral therapy and on clinical outcomes in HIV-infected patients. *J Acquir Immune Defic Syndr*. 2008;47(3):384–390.

109. Yun LW, Maravi M, Kobayashi JS, Barton PL, Davidson AJ. Antidepressant treatment improves adherence to antiretroviral therapy among depressed HIV-infected patients. *J Acquir Immune Defic Syndr*. 2005;38(4):432–438.

110. Cruess DG, Kalichman SC, Amaral C, et al. Benefits of adherence to psychotropic medications on depressive symptoms and antiretroviral medication adherence among men and women living with HIV/AIDS. *Ann Behav Med*. 2012;43(2):189–197.

111. Hughes CA, Shafran SD. Treatment of hepatitis C in HIV-coinfected patients. *Ann Pharmacother*. 2006;40(3):479–489; quiz 582–583.

112. Martin KA, Krahn LE, Balan V, Rosati MJ. Selective serotonin reuptake inhibitors in the context of hepatitis C infection: reexamining the risks of bleeding. *J Clin Psychiatry*. 2007;68(7):1024–1026.

113. Rietschel P, Corcoran C, Stanley T, et al. Prevalence of hypogonadism among men with weight loss related to human immunodeficiency virus infection who were receiving highly active antiretroviral therapy. *Clin Infect Dis*. 2000;31(5):1240–1244.

114. Grinspoon S, Corcoran C, Stanley T, Rabe J, Wilkie S. Mechanisms of androgen deficiency in human immunodeficiency virus-infected women with the wasting syndrome. *J Clin Endocrinol Metab*. 2001;86(9):4120–4126.

115. Himelhoch S, Medoff DR. Efficacy of antidepressant medication among HIV-positive individuals with depression: a systematic review and meta-analysis. *AIDS Patient Care STDS*. 2005;19(12):813–822.

116. Ferrando SJ, Freyberg Z. Treatment of depression in HIV positive individuals: a critical review. *Int Rev Psychiatry*. 2008;20(1):61–71.

117. Rabkin JG, McElhiney MC, Rabkin R, McGrath PJ, Ferrando SJ. Placebo-controlled trial of dehydroepiandrosterone (DHEA) for treatment of nonmajor depression in patients with HIV/AIDS. *Am J Psychiatry*. 2006;163(1):59–66.

118. Freudenreich O, Goforth HW, Cozza KL, et al. Psychiatric treatment of persons with HIV/AIDS: an HIV-psychiatry consensus survey of current practices. *Psychosomatics*. 2010;51(6):480–488.

119. Repetto MJ, Petitto JM. Psychopharmacology in HIV-infected patients. *Psychosom Med*. 2008;70(5):585–592.

120. Sherr L, Clucas C, Harding R, Sibley E, Catalan J. HIV and depression-a systematic review of interventions. *Psychol Health Med*. 2011;16(5):493–527.

121. Safren SA, O'Cleirigh C, Tan JY, et al. A randomized controlled trial of cognitive behavioral therapy for adherence and depression (CBT-AD) in HIV-infected individuals. *Health Psychol*. 2009;28(1):1–10.

122. Markowitz JC, Spielman LA, Sullivan M, Fishman B. An exploratory study of ethnicity and psychotherapy outcome among HIV-positive patients with depressive symptoms. *J Psychother Pract Res*. 2000;9(4):226–231.

123. Hill L, Lee KC. Pharmacotherapy considerations in patients with HIV and psychiatric disorders: focus on antidepressants and antipsychotics. *Ann Pharmacother*. 2013;47(1):75–89.

124. Zisook S, Peterkin J, Goggin KJ, et al. Treatment of major depression in HIV-seropositive men. HIV Neurobehavioral Research Center Group. *J Clin Psychiatry*. 1998;59(5):217–224.

125. Rabkin JG, Wagner GJ, Rabkin R. Fluoxetine treatment for depression in patients with HIV and AIDS: A randomized placebo-controlled trial. *Am J Psychiatry*. 1999;156:101–107.

126. Schwartz JA, McDaniel JS. Double-blind comparison of fluoxetine and desipramine in the treatment of depressed women with advanced HIV disease: A pilot study. *Depress Anxiety*. 1999;9:70–74.

127. Elliott AJ, Uldall KK, Bergam K, et al. Randomized, placebo-controlled trial of paroxetine versus imipramine in depressed HIV-positive outpatients. *Am J Psychiatry*. 1998;155(3):367–372.

128. Rabkin JG, Wagner GJ, McElhiney MC, et al. Testosterone versus fluoxetine for depression and fatigue in HIV/AIDS: a placebo controlled trial. *J Clin Psychopharmacol*. 2004;24:379–385.

129. Rabkin JG, Rabkin R, Harrison W, Wagner G. Effect of imipramine and enumerative measures of immune status in depressed patients with HIV illness. *Am J Psychiatry*. 1994;151:516–523.

130. Targ EF, Karasic DH, Diefenbach PN, et al. Structured group therapy and fluoxetine to treat depression in HIV-positive persons. *Psychosomatics*. 1994;35:132–137.

131. Watkins CC, Pieper AA, Treisman GJ. Safety considerations in drug treatment of depression in HIV-positive patients: an updated review. *Drug Saf*. 2011;34(8):623–639.

132. DeSilva KE, Le Flore DB, Marston BJ, Rimland D. Serotonin syndrome in HIV-infected individuals receiving antiretroviral therapy and fluoxetine. *AIDS*. 2001;15(10):1281–1285.

133. Greenblatt DJ, von Moltke LL, Harmatz JS, et al. Short-term exposure to low-dose ritonavir impairs clearance and enhances adverse effects of trazodone. *J Clin Pharmacol*. 2003;43(4):414–422.

134. Thompson A, Silverman B, Dzeng L, Treisman G. Psychotropic medications and HIV. *Clin Infect Dis*. 2006;42:1305–1310.

135. Sweetland A, Oquendo M, Wickramaratne P, Weissman M, Wainberg M. Depression: a silent driver of the global tuberculosis epidemic. *World Psychiatry*. 2014;13:325–326.

136. Janmeja AK, Das SK, Bhargava R, et al. Psychotherapy improves compliance with tuberculosis treatment. *Respiration*. 2005;72:375–380.

137. Malek-Ahmadi P, Chavez M, Contreras SA. Coadministration of isoniazid and antidepressant drugs. *J Clin Psychiatry*. 1996;57(11):550.

138. Rihs TA, Begley K, Smith DE, et al. Efavirenz and chronic neuropsychiatric symptoms: a cross-sectional case control study. *HIV Med*. 2006;7(8):544–548.

139. Mollan KR, Smurzynski M, Eron JJ, et al. Association between efavirenz as initial therapy for HIV-1 infection and increased risk for suicidal ideation or attempted or completed suicide: an analysis of trial data. *Ann Intern Med*. 2014;161(1):1–10.

140. Harris M, Larsen G, Montaner JS. Exacerbation of depression associated with starting raltegravir: a report of four cases. *AIDS.* 2008;22(14):1890–1892.

141. Halperin J. Nervous system Lyme disease. *J R Coll Physicians Edinb.* 2010;40:248–255.

142. Hassett AL, Radvanski DC, Buyske S, Savage SV, Sigal LH. Psychiatric comorbidity and other psychological factors in patients with "chronic Lyme disease". *Am J Med.* 2009;122(9):843–850.

143. Cairns V, Godwin J. Post-Lyme borreliosis syndrome: a meta-analysis of reported symptoms. *Int J Epidemiol.* 2005;34(6):1340–1345.

144. Kaplan RF, Jones-Woodward L, Workman K, Steere AC, Logigian EL, Meadows ME. Neuropsychological deficits in Lyme disease patients with and without other evidence of central nervous system pathology. *Appl Neuropsychol.* 1999;6(1):3–11.

145. Halperin JJ. Lyme disease: neurology, neurobiology, and behavior. *Clin Infect Dis.* 2014;58(9):1267–1272.

146. Fallon BA, Nields JA. Lyme disease: a neuropsychiatric illness. *Am J Psychiatry.* 1994;151(11):1571–1583.

147. Halperin JJ, Pass HL, Anand AK, Luft BJ, Volkman DJ, Dattwyler RJ. Nervous system abnormalities in Lyme disease. *Ann N Y Acad Sci.* 1988;539:24–34.

148. Kaplan RF, Meadows ME, Vincent LC, Logigian EL, Steere AC. Memory impairment and depression in patients with Lyme encephalopathy: comparison with fibromyalgia and nonpsychotically depressed patients. *Neurology.* 1992;42(7):1263–1267.

149. Grabe HJ, Spitzer C, Lüdemann J, et al. No association of seropositivity for anti-Borrelia IgG antibody with mental and physical complaints. *Nord J Psychiatry.* 2008;62(5):386–391.

150. Gustaw K, Beltowska K, Studzińska MM. Neurological and psychological symptoms after the severe acute neuroborreliosis. *Ann Agric Environ Med.* 2001;8(1):91–94.

151. Nadelman RB, Herman E, Wormser GP. Screening for Lyme disease in hospitalized psychiatric patients: prospective serosurvey in an endemic area. *Mt Sinai J Med.* 1997;64(6):409–412.

152. Berende A, Ter Hofstede H, Donders A, et al. Persistent Lyme Empiric Antibiotic Study Europe (PLEASE)—design of a randomized controlled trial of prolonged antibiotic treatment in patients with persistent symptoms attributed to Lyme borreliosis. *BMC Infect Dis.* 2014;14(1):543.

153. Logigian E, Kaplan R, Steere A. Successful treatment of Lyme encephalopathy with intravenous ceftriaxone. *J Infect Dis.* 1999;180:377–383.

154. Kaplan RF, Trevino RP, Johnson GM, et al. Cognitive function in post-treatment Lyme disease: do additional antibiotics help? *Neurology.* 2003;60:1916–1922.

155. Nields JA, Grimaldi JA. Infectious Diseases. In: Schein LA, Bernard HS, Spitz HI, Muskin PR, eds. *Psychosocial Treatment for Medical Conditions, Principles and Techniques.* New York, NY: Hove; 2003:305.

156. http://www.who.int/mediacentre/factsheets/fs094/en/

157. Dugbartey AT, Dugbartey MT, Apedo MY. Delayed neuropsychiatric effects of malaria in Ghana. *J Nerv Ment Dis.* 1998;186(3):183–186.

158. Postels DG, Birbeck GL. Cerebral malaria. *Handb Clin Neurol.* 2013;114:91–102.

159. Varney NR, Roberts RJ, Springer JA, Connell SK, Wood PS. Neuropsychiatric sequelae of cerebral malaria in Vietnam veterans. *J Nerv Ment Dis.* 1997;185(11):695–703.

160. Carter JA, Ross AJ, Neville BG, et al. Developmental impairments following severe falciparum malaria in children. *Trop Med Int Health.* 2005;10:3–10.

161. Caillon E, Schmitt L, Moron P. Acute depressive symptoms after mefloquine treatment. *Am J Psychiatry.* 1992;149(5):712.

162. Tran TM, Browning J, Dell ML. Psychosis with paranoid delusions after a therapeutic dose of mefloquine: a case report. *Malar J.* 2006;5:74.

163. Peterson AL, Seegmiller RA, Schindler LS. Severe neuropsychiatric reaction in a deployed military member after prophylactic mefloquine. *Case Rep Psychiatry.* 2011;2011:350417.

164. Wooltorton E. Mefloquine: contraindicated in patients with mood, psychotic or seizure disorders. *CMAJ.* 2002;167(10):1147.

165. Schneider C, Adamcova M, Jick SS, et al. Antimalarial chemoprophylaxis and the risk of neuropsychiatric disorders. *Travel Med Infect Dis.* 2013;11(2):71–80.

166. Schlagenhauf P, Johnson R, Schwartz E, Nothdurft HD, Steffen R. Evaluation of mood profiles during malaria chemoprophylaxis: a randomized, double-blind, four-arm study. *J Travel Med.* 2009;16(1):42—45.

167. Ndimubanzi PC, Carabin H, Budke CM, et al. A systematic review of the frequency of neurocyticercosis with a focus on people with epilepsy. *PLoS Negl Trop Dis.* 2010;4:e870.

168. de Almeida SM, Gurjão SA. Frequency of depression among patients with neurocysticercosis. *Arq Neuropsiquiatr.* 2010;68(1):76–80.

169. Srivastava S, Chadda RK, Bala K, Majumdar P. A study of neuropsychiatric manifestations in patients of neurocysticercosis. *Indian J Psychiatry.* 2013;55(3):264–267.

170. Forlenza OV, Filho AH, Nobrega JP, et al. Psychiatric manifestations of neurocysticercosis: a study of 38 patients from a neurology clinic in Brazil. *J Neurol Neurosurg Psychiatry.* 1997;62(6):612–616.

171. de Almeida SM, Gurjão SA. Is the presence of depression independent from signs of disease activity in patients with neurocysticercosis? *J Community Health.* 2011;36(5):693–697.

172. Patton ME, Su JR, Nelson R, Weinstock H. Primary and secondary syphilis, United States, 2005–2013. *Morb Mortal Wkly Rep.* 2014;63(18):402–406.

173. Su JR, Weinstock H. Epidemiology of co-infection with HIV and syphilis in 34 states, United States–2009. In: proceedings of the 2011 National HIV Prevention Conference, August 13–17, 2011, Atlanta, GA.

174. Tramont EC. Treponema pallidum (Syphilis). In: *Principles and Practice of Infectious Disease.* 7th ed. Philadelphia, PA: Elsevier Churchill Livingston; 2010.

175. Hutto B. Syphilis in clinical psychiatry: A review. *Psychosomatics.* 2001;42(6):453–460.

176. Overall JE, Gorham DR. The brief psychiatric rating scale. *Psychol Rep.* 1962;10:799–812.

177. Russouw HG, Roberts MC, Emsley RA, Truter R. Psychiatric manifestations and magnetic resonance imaging in HIV-negative neurosyphilis. *Biol Psychiatry.* 1997;41:467–473.

178. Sanchez FM, Zisselman MH. Treatment of psychiatric symptoms associated with neurosyphilis. *Psychosomatics.* 2007;48(5):440–445.

179. Dewhurst K. The neurosyphilitic psychoses today: A survey of 91 cases. *Br J Psych.* 1969;115:31–38.

180. Hooshmand H, Escobar MR, Kopf SW. Neurosyphilis, A study of 241 patients. *JAMA*. 1972;219(6):726–729.

181. Rundell JR, Wise MG. Neurosyphilis: A psychiatric perspective. *Psychosomatics*. 1985;26(4):287–295.

182. Lishman WA. Organic psychiatry – the psychological consequences of cerebral disorder. Oxford, Alden Press, 1983:388–406.

183. Lair L, Naidech AM. Modern neuropsychiatric presentation of neurosyphilis. *Neurology*. 2004;63:1331–1333.

184. Trenton AJ, Currier GW. Treatment of comorbid tuberculosis and depression. *Prim Care Companion J Clin Psychiatry*. 2001;3(6):236–243.

185. Pachi A, Bratis D, Mousses G, Tselebis A. Psychiatric morbidity and other factors affecting treatment adherence in pulmonary tuberculosis patients. *Tuberc Res Treat*. 2013;2013:1–37.

186. Vega P, Sweetland A, Acha J, et al. Psychiatric issues in the management of patients with multi-drug-resistant tuberculosis. *Int J Tuberc Lung Dis*. 2004;8(6):749–759.

187. Thwaites G, Chau TT, Mai NT, et al. Tuberculous meningitis. *J Neurol Neurosurg Psychiatry*. 2000;68:289–299.

188. Todd RM, Neville JG. The sequelae of tuberculous meningitis. *Arch Dis Childh*. 1964;39:213–225.

189. Wait JW, Schoeman JF. Behavioral profiles after tuberculous meningitis. *J Trop Pediatrics*. 2010;56(3):166–171.

190. Natani GD, Jain NK, Sharma TN. Depression in tuberculosis patients: correlation with duration of disease and response to anti-tuberculous chemotherapy. *Ind J Tuberc*. 1985;32(4):195–198.

191. Doherty AM, Kelly J, McDonald C, et al. A review of the interplay between tuberculosis and mental health. *Gen Hosp Psych*. 2013;35:398–406.

192. Rajnik M, Ottolini MG. Serious infections of the central nervous system: encephalitis, meningitis and brain abscess. *Adolesc Med*. 2000;11(2):401–425.

193. Chen CH, Chang CC, Chang WN, Tsai NW. Neuropsychological sequelae in HIV-negative cryptococcal meningitis after complete anti-fungal treatment. *Acta Neurologica Taiwanica*. 2012;21(1):8–17.

194. Schmidt H, Heiman B, Djukic M, et al. Neuropsychological sequelae of bacterial and viral meningitis. *Brain*. 2006;129(2):3333–3345.

195. Gupta N, Park J, Solomon C, Kranz DA, Wrensch M, Wu YW. Long-term outcomes in patients with treated childhood hydrocephalus. *J Neurosurg*. 2007;106(5 Suppl):334–339.

196. Holikatti PC, Kar N. Psychiatric manifestations in a patient with HIV-associated neurocognitive symptoms and cryptococcal meningitis. *Indian J Psychol Med*. 2012;34(4):381–382.

197. Hsueh KL, Lin PY. Treatment-resistant depression prior to the diagnosis of cryptococcal meninitis: a case report. *Gen Hosp Psych*. 2010;32:560.e9–560.e10.

CHAPTER 12

Dermatologic Disease

Sejal Shah, MD
Naomi Schmelzer, MD, MPH
Vivian Ecker, MD
Arturo Saavedra, MD, PhD, MBA

INTRODUCTION

The skin is the largest organ of the body, and skin disease is unique in often being immediately visible to others. This is one reason why dermatologic disease is accompanied by significant psychological distress and psychiatric morbidity.[1,2]

Many dermatologic disorders are associated with negative quality of life, and psychiatric disturbances are reported in at least 30% of these patients.[2,3] There are many reasons for the elevated frequency of psychiatric disturbance in dermatologic patients, including disfigurement, perceived social stigma, and unforeseen changes in lifestyle. Although less common, the dermatologist may also encounter primary psychiatric disorders, including obsessive-compulsive disorder, trichotillomania, dysmorphophobia, delusions of parasitosis, and factitious disorder. Skin conditions and psychiatric symptoms may be present concomitantly in some illnesses, such as systemic lupus erythematosus or porphyria. And medications utilized in dermatologic practice, such as corticosteroids, may precipitate psychiatric symptoms.

The connection between brain and skin begins in the embryo, when the nervous system and epidermis originate from the same tissue layer (ectoderm). They then maintain close neural, endocrine, and immunologic connections throughout life, including being targets of the same immunologic processes, neurotransmitters, neuropeptides, and second messengers.[4,5] It is hypothesized that chemical messengers released by epidermal keratinocytes influence the brain, and this may account for an association between the severity of certain skin diseases (e.g., atopic dermatitis, psoriasis) and depression or anxiety.[5] When a large area of skin is involved, cytokine levels may be of sufficient concentration to affect mental state.[6]

This chapter focuses on the most common dermatologic illnesses associated with depression: acne vulgaris, herpes zoster (HZ) (shingles), psoriasis, vitiligo, and atopic dermatitis (**Fig. 12-1**).

ACNE VULGARIS

■ INTRODUCTION

Acne is very common in adolescence and is strongly associated with depressive symptoms. Acne has an adverse effect on quality of life comparable to that of epilepsy, asthma, diabetes, and arthritis. Although the disorder is self-limited for many, even patients with mild to moderate acne may have significant psychosocial difficulties. Acne can also be severe and disfiguring, with profound and lifelong consequences for a significant number of patients. Sequelae include hypertrophic or pitted scarring, poor body image, interpersonal problems, social withdrawal, higher unemployment rates, lower self-esteem, depression, anxiety, suicidal ideation, and suicide. Further complicating care, acne is exacerbated by emotional and psychosocial stress and associated with major depression.[7,8]

■ EPIDEMIOLOGY

Facial acne has an overall prevalence of 54%, though most is mild, and clinically significant facial acne is present in 3% of men and 12% of women (**Box 12-1**).[9] It typically begins early in puberty, triggered by hormonal changes. It may precede menarche in girls by one or more years.[10] Acne may become chronic and persist into adulthood and a small percentage of cases develop after age 25. Acne is found in 85% of the population between 12 and 24 years

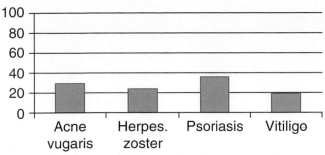

Figure 12-1 *Mean risk of depression for selected illnesses (percentage prevalence for particular disease).*

of age and is moderate to severe in 15% to 20% of those affected. Fifty percent of boys aged 10 and 11 and 78% of girls between ages 8 and 12 have some degree of acne. Visible acne is present in up to 64% of people ages 20 to 29, 43% in ages 30 to 39 years, and 24.3% in ages 40 to 49.[11]

■ PATHOPHYSIOLOGY

Acne is a disorder of the pilosebaceous unit that involves obstructive desquamation of keratinocytes lining the hair follicle, excess sebum production, development of noninflammatory lesions (open and closed comedones), inflammatory lesions (papules, pustules, nodules), and the presence of *Propionibacterium acnes* (**Box 12-2**).[10] Acne has a significant genetic component, occurring in up to 78% of first-degree relatives and 75% of second-degree relatives.[12] In patients with positive family history, acne begins at a younger age and tends to be more severe.[13,14]

Epidermal cells have androgen and interleukin (IL)-1 receptors. In acne IL-1 is upregulated, triggering an immune response of IL-1.[15] Before microcomedone formation, there is follicular inflammatory infiltration with memory and effector T-cells of the immune system, thought to be a response to an antigen produced by the bacteria *P. acnes*.

P. acnes binds to receptors on sebocytes, dendritic cells, and keratinocytes. That receptor in turn triggers multiple chemokines, including tumor necrosis factor (TNF)-α, IL-8, and IL-6, which causes infiltration of lymphocytes, monocytes, neutrophils, and macrophages that also produce these cytokines. The keratinocytes lining the follicle infundibulum thus proliferate, delay desquamation, and obstruct the outflow of sebum resulting in comedone formation (**Fig. 12-2**).[15]

Sebaceous glands also contain multiple receptors for hormones, cytokines, and neurotransmitters and increase production of sebum in response to these. Substance P is released during stress

and potentiates sebaceous gland response to cytokines and TNF-α. Progression of this process can lead to follicular membrane disruption and fatty acid egress into the dermis with dissolution of extracellular matrix. This results in papules, pustules, and nodules.

Androgens must be present for sebum production in both normal and acne-affected skin. Hyperkeratinized sebaceous gland development and production of adult sebum is mediated by androgen receptors on sebocytes and keratinocytes. Skin cells themselves also manufacture androgen hormones from cholesterol.

Sebaceous glands have numerous receptors for androgen and estrogen hormones, TSH, histamine, prostaglandins, corticotropin-releasing hormone, neurotransmitters, neuropeptides, and other chemical messengers. There are changes in the quantity and composition of sebum produced at the onset of puberty, which is thought to support increased proliferation of *P. acnes*. Although the mechanism of the coordination of onset between puberty and acne is unclear, it is hypothesized that this is due to the hypothalamic–pituitary–adrenal axis.[15]

■ CLINICAL PRESENTATION AND ASSESSMENT OF DEPRESSION IN ACNE

The relationships among depression, psychological stress, and acne are complex. Acne occurs predominantly in adolescence, and adolescents are at high risk for suicidal behavior (**Box 12-3**). The prevalence of suicidal ideation is greater in adolescents with subthreshold anxiety or subthreshold depression and greater still in patients who meet criteria for depression or anxiety disorder.[16]

Most studies that consider the psychological effects of acne find decreased quality of life and increased psychiatric comorbidity. Most are uncontrolled and collect data with self-report questionnaires to measure the severity of acne and psychiatric symptoms. A summary of 16 studies published between 1981 and 2007[17] demonstrated an increased risk of psychiatric comorbidity in patients with acne, though methods and populations in the studies varied and two of the studies do not show increased risk of depression or anxiety.[18,19] In the most significant of these studies[20] patients with acne were at higher risk than a non-acne comparison group for depression (29.5% vs. 0%) and anxiety (26.2% vs. 0%); there was no significant difference in age or gender between the groups. No correlations were found between acne severity and depression or anxiety, or quality of life.

The effect of acne on emotional status has been examined and compared to a random sample of the general population and to patients with other chronic medical illnesses. Although quality of life measures do not correlate with acne severity, self-esteem scores in acne patients are significantly lower, particularly for women. Acne patients are at higher risk for nonpsychotic psychiatric disorders (41% vs. 31%).[21] When compared to patients with asthma, epilepsy, diabetes, arthritis, and coronary heart disease, those with acne had significant impairments in mental health, social functioning,

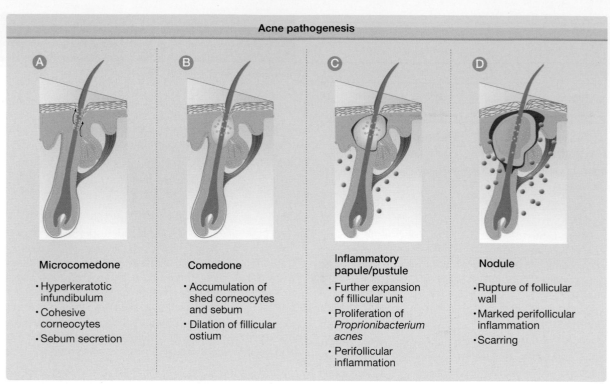

Acne pathogenesis

A **Microcomedone**
- Hyperkeratotic infundibulum
- Cohesive corneocytes
- Sebum secretion

B **Comedone**
- Accumulation of shed corneocytes and sebum
- Dilation of fillicular ostium

C **Inflammatory papule/pustule**
- Further expansion of fillicular unit
- Proliferation of *Proprionibacterium acnes*
- Perifollicular inflammation

D **Nodule**
- Rupture of follicular wall
- Marked perifollicular inflammation
- Scarring

Figure 12-2 *A-D: Acne pathogenesis. (Reproduced with permission from Goldsmith LA, Katz SI, Gilchrest BA, et al. Fitzpatrick's Dermatology in General Medicine. 8th ed. New York: McGraw-Hill, Inc; 2012.)*

energy/vitality, and role limitations due to emotional problems.[21] Although acne patients did not view themselves as ill on the perceived health dimension (community subjects with these chronic illnesses did), the mental health scores for acne patients were worse than for these other chronic illnesses. Role limitations for emotional reasons were worse for the other medical conditions, except for diabetes and coronary heart disease.[21]

The risk of suicidality is elevated in acne patients.[22] A large study of patients with chronic and potentially disfiguring dermatologic disorders, specifically noncystic facial acne, alopecia areata, atopic dermatitis, and psoriasis,[23] found that acne patients had significantly higher risk of depression and of active suicidal ideation than all other groups except for inpatients with psoriasis. Patients with acne were younger, and this may have contributed to the higher rate of active suicidality.

Community-based studies show variable associations between acne, psychological distress, psychiatric disorders, and suicidality.[22] A large New Zealand survey of adolescents revealed an association between greater subjective acne severity ("having really bad or terrible problem with acne") and severity of depressive and anxiety symptoms, and an increased risk of suicide attempts.[24] The association between acne and suicide attempts persisted after controlling for depressive and anxiety.[24]

Patients with depression and anxiety may perceive their acne as more severe due to the cognitive-emotional effects of their

mood symptoms.[24] It is also possible that depression and/or anxiety physiologically affect the actual severity of acne. Alternatively, hormonal changes of puberty may independently affect both the rates of acne and of mood/anxiety disorders. In addition, acne may contribute to depression and anxiety via negative cutaneous body image, lower self-esteem, and impaired social functioning.

In sum, although study findings are inconsistent, undiagnosed mood and anxiety disorders clearly carry significant risk in this population. These include developmental, psychosocial, and functional impairment and increased rates of suicidality in patients with acne. These risks are not clearly associated with the objective severity of acne. Suicidal thoughts and behaviors may not correlate with the presence of psychiatric syndromes. It is strongly recommended that clinicians treating patients with acne assess mood and anxiety symptoms and specifically inquire about suicidal ideation and behaviors.

■ TREATMENT
Acne Medications and Depression

Important issues to consider when treating comorbid depression and acne are the effects of acne medications on mood, the dermatological side effects of psychotropics, and drug–drug interactions.

There are numerous topical acne treatments, prescription and over-the-counter.[10] These do not have known adverse psychiatric effects, with the possible exception of dapsone,[25] and there are no known drug–drug interactions between psychiatric medications and these topical agents (**Table 12-1**).

Systemic acne therapies include antibiotics, hormone therapy, glucocorticoids, gonadotropin-releasing hormone agonists, antiandrogens, and isotretinoin (**Box 12-4**).[10] Isotretinoin has a controversial association with depression and suicidality, and from its release in 1982 until 2000 the FDA received reports of depression, suicidal ideation, suicide attempts, and completed suicide. Sixty-two percent of these patients had past psychiatric history or other risk

---

BOX 12-3
IMPORTANT CONFOUNDING SYMPTOMS

Poor energy

Suicidality

Insomnia

Anger and hostility

TABLE 12-1 Commonly Available Topical Prescription Acne Preparations

Retinoids	Tretinoin	Adapalene	Tazarotene	
Retinoid Combinations	Tretinoin/clindamycin	Adapalene-benzoyl peroxide		
Antimicrobials	Benzoyl peroxide	Clindamycin	Erythromycin	Dapsone
	Benzoyl peroxide-hydrocortisone	Benzoyl peroxide-clindamycin		
Miscellaneous	Sodium sulfacetamide	Sodium sulfacetamide with sulfur	Azelaic acid	

Data from Goldsmith LA, Katz SI, Gilchrest BA, et al: Fitzpatrick's Dermatology in General Medicine. 8th ed. New York: McGraw-Hill, Inc; 2012.

factors for suicidality.[26] One-hundred ten patients with a median age of 17 years were hospitalized for depression, suicidal ideation, and suicide attempts while using or after stopping isotretinoin. Sixty-nine percent had a previous psychiatric history or other potentially contributing factors.

However, determining the role that isotretinoin may play in suicidality is challenging. As noted above, since adolescents and individuals with acne have increased prevalence of mood symptoms and suicidal ideation. A review of 12 controlled studies[26] found no increased risk for depression, anxiety, or suicide attempts, and on the contrary suggested that isotretinoin improved depression in comparison to the control population or the baseline patient's status. This improvement in depressive symptoms was associated with improvement of severe acne in these studies. Although other studies show no increased risk of depression or suicide in patients taking isotretinoin, a retrospective cohort study and a case–control study both showed a slight increase in the relative risk of suicide attempts in patients taking isotretinoin.[27,28] There may be a small subpopulation of patients who are at increased risk for depression or suicide attempts when exposed to isotretinoin[26] and depression in these patients apparently improved after drug cessation.

Clinicians should consider patients' past psychiatric histories, assess for depressive symptomatology and suicidal ideation, and maximize communication with patients who experience depression on isotretinoin. Discussing likely outcomes of isotretinoin treatment may help patients to have more realistic expectations of therapy, which may reduce the occurrence of "lost hope." In some cases, it may be beneficial to obtain a psychiatric consultation before initiating this agent.

Psychotropic Medications and Acne

Dermatologic adverse drug reactions often occur with psychotropic medications; 2% to 5% of patients taking psychiatric medications experience adverse skin reactions (**Box 12-5**).[29] Acne-type adverse skin reactions are common with lithium.[30] The literature reveals no established increased incidence of specifically acne with all classes of antidepressants (TCA, SSRI, SNRI, MAOI, bupropion).[31] With the exception of isolated case reports, there is no known association of increased frequency of acne with

anticonvulsants commonly prescribed for psychiatric disorders (valproic acid/divalproex, lamotrigine, gabapentin, oxcarbazepine, carbamazepine) or antipsychotic medications. However, acne may occur secondarily as part of psychotropic-associated endocrine syndromes, such as hyperprolactinemia or polycystic ovarian syndrome.[32,33]

Other dermatologic reactions, both mild (e.g., rash, pruritus) and serious (erythema multiforme, Steven Johnson syndrome, toxic epidermal necrolysis), may occur with many psychotropics.

Drug–Drug Interactions

There are numerous potential drug–drug interactions between systemic treatments for acne and psychotropic medications, especially as many different classes of medication are prescribed for acne (**Box 12-6** and **Table 12-2**). Potential effects include cytochrome P450–mediated interactions, additive QT prolongation, cumulative lowering of seizure threshold, electrolyte imbalances increasing risk of QT prolongation, decreased renal clearance of lithium or unpredictable effects on lithium levels, synergistic hyperprolactinemia, increased risks of hyponatremia and SIADH, and increased risk of orthostatic hypotension.[34] Specific interactions of selected medications are summarized in Table 12-2.

■ SUMMARY

There appears to be a synergistic, bidirectional relationship between acne vulgaris and depression. Clinical research has shown increased risks of depression and suicidality in patients with acne, although confounding factors (e.g., developmental stage of onset of acne) are difficult to exclude. Laboratory research has elucidated pathophysiologic relationships between depression and acne, potentially linking cutaneous disease with neuroendocrine, neurotransmitter, and neuroimmunologic processes of depression. In view of the high prevalence of acne and its association with depressive symptoms, including suicidality, increased awareness of this comorbidity, and

---

BOX 12-4
DRUGS THAT CAN CAUSE DEPRESSIVE SYMPTOMS

Dapsone (possible)

Isotretinoin (controversial)

Corticosteroids

Opioids

Gabapentin, pregabalin (including suicide: controversial)

BOX 12-5
TREATMENTS FOR DEPRESSION IN PATIENTS WITH DERMATOLOGICAL DISORDERS

SSRIs: usually safe with acne, may trigger psoriasis

Bupropion: studies have been inconsistent: may improve or worsen psoriasis

Moclobemide: may improve psoriasis

Some antidepressants, such as doxepin and mirtazapine, may also reduce dermatological symptoms (e.g., pruritus)

Photochemotherapy

Cognitive behavioral therapy

Behavioral therapies and relaxation therapies (e.g., to reduce scratching behaviors in atopic dermatitis)

TABLE 12-2 Selected Interactions of Psychotropic and Acne Medications

	Sulfamethoxazole-Trimethoprim: may prolong QTc	Erythromycin: may prolong QTc, inhibits CYP3A4	Azithromycin: may prolong QTc	Dexamethasone	Prednisone	OCP: Ortho Tri-Cyclen; Estrostep; Yaz Ortho Tri-Cyclen	Spironolactone	Isotretinoin
Antidepressants								
Amitriptyline	↑QTc, TdP.	↑QTc, TdP; rarely problematic	↑QTc, TdP.					
Clomipramine	↑QTc, TdP.	↑QTc, TdP; rarely problematic	↑QTc, TdP.					
Desipramine	↑QTc, TdP.	↑QTc, TdP; rarely problematic	↑QTc, TdP.					
Imipramine	↑QTc, TdP.	↑QTc, TdP; rarely problematic	↑QTc, TdP.					
Nortriptyline	↑QTc, TdP.	↑QTc, TdP; rarely problematic	↑QTc, TdP.					
Bupropion				sz risk increased	sz risk increased			
Desvenlafaxine							Hyponatremia	
Citalopram	↑QTc, TdP.	↑QTc, TdP.	↑QTc, TdP.			inhibit CYP; increased citalo, increased QTc	QTc, TdP if e-lyte abnl	
Duloxetine							Hyponatremia, Hypotension	
Escitalopram	↑QTc, TdP.	↑QTc, TdP.	↑QTc, TdP.				Hyponatremia	
Fluoxetine		↑QTc, TdP.	↑QTc, TdP.				Hyponatremia	
Fluvoxamine							Hyponatremia	
Mirtazapine		inhib CYP3A4 →↑mirtaz level					Hyponatremia	
Paroxetine							Hyponatremia	
Sertraline							Hyponatremia	
Trazodone	↑QTc, TdP.	inhib CYP3A4 →↑traz level	↑QTc, TdP.					
Venlafaxine	↑QTc, TdP.	↑QTc, TdP.	↑QTc, TdP.				Hyponatremia	

Antianxiety							
Alprazolam		inhib CYP3A4 →↑alpraz level					
Buspirone		inhib CYP3A4 →↑busp level up to 6x		induces CYP; decreased busp			
Diazepam		inhib CYP3A4 →↑diaz level					
Lorazepam							
Mood Stabilizers/AEDs							
Carbamazepine		inhib CYP3A4; ↑carbam level				induces CYP; decreased hormonal effect	
Gabapentin							
Lithium							Li toxicity
Oxcarbazepine						induces CYP; decreased hormonal effect	
Valproic Acid							
Antipsychotics							
Aripiprazole	↑QTc, TdP.	↑QTc, TdP. Inhib CYP3A4 →↑arip level	↑QTc, TdP.	induces CYP; decreased aripip			
Chlorpromazine	↑QTc, TdP.	↑QTc, TdP.	↑QTc, TdP.				
Clozapine	↑QTc, TdP.	↑QTc, TdP. Inhib CYP3A4 →↑cloz level	↑QTc, TdP.	induces CYP; decreased cloz			Hypotension
Fluphenazine	↑QTc, TdP.	↑QTc, TdP.	↑QTc, TdP.				
Haloperidol	↑QTc, TdP.	↑QTc, TdP.	↑QTc, TdP.	QTc, TdP if e-lyte abnl	QTc, TdP if e-lyte abnl		Hypotension
Iloperidone	↑QTc, TdP.	↑QTc, TdP.	↑QTc, TdP.				Hypotension (alpha blockade)
Lurasidone		inhib CYP3A4; ↑ luras level		induces CYP; decrease luras			Hypotension (alpha blockade)
Olanzapine	↑QTc, TdP.	↑QTc, TdP.	↑QTc, TdP.				Hypotension
Perphenazine	↑QTc, TdP.	↑QTc, TdP.	↑QTc, TdP.				
Quetiapine	↑QTc, TdP.	↑QTc, TdP. Inhib CYP3A4 →↑quet level	↑QTc, TdP.	↑QTc, TdP.	↑QTc, TdP.		
Risperidone	↑QTc, TdP.	↑QTc, TdP.	↑QTc, TdP.				Hypotension
Ziprasidone	↑QTc, TdP; contraind	↑QTc, TdP; contraind					Additive photosensitization

recognition and active treatment of both these conditions, could have enduring beneficial effects.

HERPES ZOSTER (SHINGLES)

■ INTRODUCTION

HZ ("shingles") is a neurocutaneous infection caused by reactivation of endogenous varicella zoster virus (VZV) in the dorsal sensory ganglia after initial infection with varicella ("chickenpox"). Upon initial infection, VZV passes from cutaneous and mucosal lesions into sensory nerve endings and is transported up the sensory nerves to the sensory ganglia.[35] Infected T-cells may also transport VZV via sensory ganglia. There the virus becomes dormant and resides until reactivation.

Reactivation most often occurs in the context of declining cellular immunity with aging, immunosuppression, immunocompromise due to illness (e.g., HIV/AIDS), emotional stress, tumor involvement of the spinal cord, dorsal root ganglia and nearby structures, spinal irradiation, trauma, or spinal surgery, and frontal sinusitis (for ophthalmic zoster). Reactivation spreads the virus from within the ganglion to the innervated dermatome. Neural pathology includes neural necrosis and inflammation causing severe pain, termed postherpetic neuralgia (PHN).[36]

■ EPIDEMIOLOGY

The incidence of HZ is approximately 4 cases per 1000 in the U.S. general population and 10 cases per 1,000 in those aged 60 and older (Fig. 12-2).[37] There are an estimated 1,000,000+ new cases of HZ in the United States every year. More than half of these cases occur in patients aged ≥60 years. Approximately one out of three people in the United States develops shingles during his or her lifetime.

Depression is among the risk factors for the development of HZ. A case–control study found that an HADS depression score ≥8 (OR 4.15, 95% CI 1.88–9.16), a recent negative life event (OR 3.40, 95% CI 1.67–6.93), and a family history of HZ (OR 3.69, 95% CI 1.81–7.51) were significantly associated with HZ.[38] Another case–control study[39] found that depression increased the risk of HZ by over 10% (adjusted OR [99% CI] 1.15 [1.10–1.20]). And a longitudinal study[40] showed that patients with no past history of any depressive disorder at the time of HZ onset had an elevated risk of subsequently developing depressive disorder compared with the control group, after adjusting for demographics and comorbid medical diseases. Interestingly in this study there was a decreased risk of developing major depression and any depressive order among older patients newly diagnosed with HZ.

PHN is a serious complication of HZ. The overall incidence of PHN is 10% although the risk of PHN increases significantly with age.[41] It is the second most common neuropathic pain condition, second to painful diabetic neuropathy. Although there are no currently available studies of the relationship between depression and PHN, chronic pain is known to be associated with increased risk of depression.

■ PATHOPHYSIOLOGY

A pathophysiologic relationship between HZ and depression has been suggested by case–control studies of cell-mediated immunity to VZV in depressed patients, and as previously noted, depression may affect VZV cell–mediated immunity. Cellular immunity, in turn, has been implicated in the pathogenesis of depression (Box 12-2).

■ CLINICAL PRESENTATION

HZ presents with characteristic dermatomal pain and vesicular rash (**Box 12-3**). It occurs most often in the dermatomes that are most heavily affected during the initial varicella outbreak: the first ophthalmic division of the trigeminal nerve and spinal sensory ganglia from T1 to L2. The infection may spread centrally to the meninges, spinal cord, and CNS causing leptomeningitis, CSF pleocytosis, myelitis, and meningoencephalitis. Anterior horn motor neurons may also become infected and cause local palsies in the area of the skin eruption. Acute and severe pain is a central feature of VZV and may persist after resolution of the VZV episode resulting in PHN. PHN is defined as persistent pain for more than 90 days after rash onset.[42]

HZ and PHN are associated with significant adverse effects on quality of life,[43] including neurovegetative symptoms and general activities. Patients with PHN are more likely to have mood problems, anxiety or depression, impaired ability to enjoy life, and sleep difficulties. Although no published studies have examined whether depression is a precipitating factor for HZ depression may affect VZV cell–mediated immunity as measured by VZV-specific responder cell frequency (RCF)[44] and may increase the risk of HZ (**Fig. 12-3**). To date there are no published studies that examine the semiology of depression co-occurring with HZ.

■ TREATMENT

The treatment of HZ aims to reduce severity and duration of the eruptive phase and to reduce pain in the acute phase.[45] Pain reduction is important because it affects quality of life and because severe acute pain is a risk factor for PHN. Systemic antivirals, acyclovir, valacyclovir, and famciclovir are used to treat the eruptive phase.

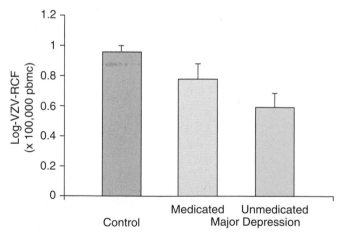

Figure 12-3 *Varicella-zoster virus specific responder cell frequency (VZV-RCF) at baseline in elderly subjects with major depressive disorder stratified on the basis of current use of antidepressant medication (n = 29) or not (n = 23) versus controls. VZV-RCF differed across the three groups (F = 7.6; df = 2, 103; p < 0.001) with depressed subjects not on antidepressants having lower levels as compared to controls (t = 4.0, p <0.001), and the depressed subjects who were taking antidepressant medications (t = 2.0, p = 0.06). Mean ± SEM. (Reproduced with permission from Irwin MR, Levin MJ, Carrillo C, et al. Major depressive disorder and immunity to varicella-zoster virus in the elderly, Brain Behav Immun. 2011;25(4):759–766.)*

A variety of analgesics are used in the acute phase of HZ and in PHN. Acetaminophen, NSAIDs, or tramadol is often used for mild to moderate pain. Gabapentin, pregabalin, tricyclic antidepressants, corticosteroids, and opiate analgesics may be used for moderate to severe pain. Neural blockade is considered for severe cases that are unresponsive to systemic medications. In addition topical lidocaine and topical capsaicin may provide some relief for PHN pain.

Herpes Zoster/PHN Medications and Depression

No association between acyclovir, valacyclovir, or famciclovir and depression has been reported in HZ patients. Manufacturer's prescribing information for valacyclovir[46] cites an elevated rate of depression in the treatment for genital herpes (herpes simplex) but not in the treatment of HZ. Depression is a possible adverse effect of corticosteroids and opiates. The risk of depression in patients using gabapentin[47] and pregabalin[48] is estimated to be 2%. Both of these antiepileptic medications carry specific FDA warnings regarding increased risk of suicidal behavior and ideation. The rate of suicidal behavior and ideation in AED-treated patients was 0.43%, compared to 0.24% among placebo-treated patients in pooled analyses of antiepileptic drugs given for several medical and psychiatric conditions.[49] However, the association of suicidal behavior and ideation with anticonvulsants remains controversial.[50-52]

Psychotropic Medications and Herpes Zoster/PHN

Depression may affect VZV cell–mediated immunity. A 2013 study demonstrated diminished cell-mediated immunity response to HZ vaccine in depressed patients and treatment with antidepressant medication was associated with normalization of the CMI in response to the vaccine.[53]

Drug–Drug Interactions

There are numerous drug–drug interactions among systemic treatments for the pain of HZ and PHN and antidepressant medication (Box 12-6 and **Table 12-3**). These interactions may be pharmacodynamic, for example, risk of serotonin syndrome, lowering of seizure threshold, or additive sedative effects, or pharmacokinetic, for example, P450-mediated interactions. No drug–drug interactions have been found between these psychotropic medications and acyclovir, valacyclovir, and famciclovir.[34] Specific interactions of selected medications are summarized in Table 12-3.

■ SUMMARY

HZ is common, particularly in older adults, and significantly impairs quality of life. Depression increases the risk and morbidity of HZ. Further research may help identify the ways in which the pathophysiology of depression affects cell-mediated immunity in HZ.

PSORIASIS

Psoriasis is a chronic systemic inflammatory disease that most commonly affects the skin.

■ PATHOPHYSIOLOGY

Psoriasis involves an autoimmune inflammatory response among infiltrating T-lymphocytes, resident skin cells, and a range of pro-inflammatory cytokines, chemokines, and chemical mediators. The exact mechanisms, however, are still under investigation.[54] The release of cytokines, such as TNF-α, interferon (IFN)-γ, IL-6, IL-8, IL-12, IL-12, and IL-22, lead to systemic inflammation. In psoriasis, these cytokines are thought to induce hyperplasia of the epidermis as well as growth and dilation of superficial blood vessels leading to the characteristic red, raised, and scaly skin lesions.[55]

In addition to the psychological impact of disfiguring psoriatic lesions, shared mechanisms of pathophysiology between psoriasis and psychiatric disorders are implicated in the comorbidity of these conditions. Increased concentrations of inflammatory cytokines are associated with the pathogenesis of both psoriasis and major depression, and reducing the effects of these mediators may improve symptoms in both conditions.[56,57]

■ EPIDEMIOLOGY

Psoriasis occurs in 1.5% to 2% of the population and affects both genders equally (Fig. 12-2).[58] Although it can occur at any age, onset is typically during early adulthood with mean age of 33 years.[54,59] Patients with psoriasis are more likely to suffer psychiatric illness than patients with other skin diseases.[56] A wide range of psychopathology is seen in this population, including elevated rates of depression, anxiety, alcoholism, poor self-esteem, sexual dysfunction, and suicidal ideation (**Box 12-7** and **Box 12-8**).[58,60] The effect of psoriasis on psychosocial disability is often not correlated with the dermatologic severity of the disease.[56,61]

The prevalence of depression in patients with psoriasis ranges from 10% to 62%. The wide variability in estimates is due to differences in study methods, as depression is often assessed with screening instruments rather than diagnostic interviews.[56,62] The prevalence of suicidal ideation in outpatients and inpatients with psoriasis is 2.5% and 7.2%, respectively.[23] A retrospective study found that patients with psoriasis recalled significantly more moderate and severe depression prior to the onset of the illness.[63]

■ CLINICAL PRESENTATION

Skin manifestations are characterized by focal, inflamed red plaques. In addition to cosmetic disfigurement, psoriasis is associated with significant psychosocial morbidity[23] and with cardiovascular, metabolic, gastrointestinal, and ocular manifestations.[56] A review of the literature does not reveal any specific factors unique to depression when it co-occurs with psoriasis.

■ TREATMENT

The treatment of co-occurring depression in psoriasis encompasses several modalities, including pharmacotherapy, photochemotherapy, psychotherapy, and support groups (Box 12-5).[60] New biologic therapies targeting inflammatory cytokines and other immune-modifying agents may be used to treat moderate to severe psoriasis. In addition to reducing clinical severity of lesions, these agents may also improve depressive symptoms.[57,64] In contrast, photochemotherapy with psoralen plus ultraviolet A (PUVA) therapy, while significantly reducing psoriasis-related disability, does not improve depression, anxiety, or worry.[65]

Use of antidepressants in patients with psoriasis requires careful consideration. There are few rigorous studies evaluating the efficacy of antidepressants in this specific population, and case reports suggest that specific medications may trigger psoriasis symptoms. In one small study of patients with psoriasis who were treated with anti–TNF-α therapy, patients who were also using escitalopram regimen had reduced depression, anxiety, and pruritus.[66] However, there are also case reports that implicate SSRIs in induction of psoriasis several months after starting treatment.[67,68] Conversely, there is a case report of bupropion-induced exacerbation of preexisting psoriasis.[69] However, in another small study, nondepressed patients started on bupropion showed improvement in psoriasis symptoms that returned to baseline after stopping bupropion.[70] A study of the monoamine oxidase inhibitor moclobemide (not available in the United States) showed improvement both in severity of psoriasis

TABLE 12-3 Specific Interactions of Selected Antidepressant and VZV-PHN Medications

	Tramadol	Oxycodone	Morphine	Gabapentin; Pregabalin	NSAIDs	Prednisone
Antidepressants	↑ seizure risk; ↑ risk of serot. syn.					
Amitriptyline	↑ seizure risk; ↑ risk of serot. syn.			↑ CNS depression; ↑ seizure risk		
Clomipramine	↑ seizure risk; ↑ risk of serot. syn.			↑ CNS depression; ↑ seizure risk		
Desipramine	↑ seizure risk; ↑ risk of serot. syn.			↑ CNS depression; ↑ seizure risk		
Imipramine	↑ seizure risk; ↑ risk of serot. syn.			↑ CNS depression; ↑ seizure risk		
Nortriptyline	↑ seizure risk; ↑ risk of serot. syn.			↑ CNS depression; ↑ seizure risk		
Bupropion	↑ seizure risk					↑seizure risk
Desvenlafaxine	↑ seizure risk; ↑ risk of serot. syn.					
Citalopram	↑ seizure risk; ↑ risk of serot. syn.		↑ risk of serot. syn.		↓ platelet agg, ↑ bleeding	↑QTc, TdP if e-lyte abnl
Duloxetine	↑ seizure risk; ↑ risk of serot. syn.				↓ platelet agg, ↑ bleeding	
Escitalopram	↑ seizure risk; ↑ risk of serot. syn.				↓ platelet agg, ↑ bleeding	
Fluoxetine	↑ seizure risk; ↑ risk of serot. syn.		↑ risk of serot. syn.		↓ platelet agg, ↑ bleeding	
Fluvoxamine	↑ seizure risk; ↑ risk of serot. syn.	inhib CYP3A4 →↑ oxycod level; ↑risk of serot. syn.			↓ platelet agg, ↑ bleeding	
Mirtazapine	↑ seizure risk; ↑ risk of serot. syn.				↓ platelet agg, ↑ bleeding	
Paroxetine	↑ seizure risk; ↑ risk of serot. syn.				↓ platelet agg, ↑ bleeding	
Sertraline	↑ seizure risk; ↑ risk of serot. syn.		↑ risk of serot. syn.		↓ platelet agg, ↑ bleeding	
Trazodone	↑ seizure risk; ↑ risk of serot. syn.		↑ CNS depression; ↑ risk serot. syn.			
Venlafaxine	↑ seizure risk; ↑ risk of serot. syn.				↓ platelet agg, ↑ bleeding	
Lithium	↑ risk of serot. syn.				↑ risk of Li toxicity	

symptoms and Beck Depression Inventory (BDI) scores at the end of 6 weeks.[71]

■ SUMMARY

Further research is needed into the pathophysiology and treatment of depression in patients with psoriasis. New biological therapies show promise in reducing both clinical severity of psoriasis and depressive symptoms. The effect of antidepressant and antipsychotic medications on psoriasis is unclear. When deciding on a treatment strategy, a collaboration between the psychiatrist, the dermatologist, and patient should take into account the severity of both depression and psoriasis and develop a tailored approach, including both pharmacologic and nonpharmacologic options. Antidepressants should be used cautiously and providers should closely monitor for exacerbation of psoriatic symptoms when prescribing these medications.

BOX 12-7
COMMON COMORBIDITIES

Suicidality
Anxiety
Alcoholism
Sexual dysfunction

VITILIGO

■ INTRODUCTION

Vitiligo is a skin disorder of depigmentation resulting from selective destruction of melanocytes.

BOX 12-8
ANXIETY IN DERMATOLOGIC DISEASE

- Anxiety is quite prevalent in the dermatologic population, with up to 8% to 52% in worldwide studies of both inpatients and outpatients (1,2).
- Of various anxiety disorders, mild GAD (25%), severe GAD (8.7%), social phobia (4%), and obsessive compulsive disorder (1.4%) are the most common (2).
- The highest prevalence of anxiety is found in psoriasis patients and lowest in nonmelanoma skin cancer (3).
- In dermatologic patients, anxiety is associated with higher unemployment rate, female gender, higher joint count involvement and patient-reported factors, such as disability, pain, and fatigue, are associated with both depression and anxiety (4).
- Patients with early-onset psoriasis are more anxious than patients with late-onset psoriasis (5).
- Patient with acne vulgaris are at significantly increased risk for anxiety and depression but the odds of anxiety appear to be greater than for depression in some studies (6–8).

References:

1. AlShahwan MA. The prevalence of anxiety and depression in Arab dermatology patients. *J Cutaneous Med Surg.* 2014;(18):1–7.
2. Woodruff PWR, Higgins EM, Du Vivier AWP, et al. Psychiatric illness in patients referred to a dermatology-psychiatry clinic. *Gen Hosp Psychiatr.* 1997;19(1):29–35.
3. Dalgard F, Gieler U, Tomas-Aragones L, et al. The psychological burden of skin diseases: a cross-sectional multicenter study among dermatological out-patients in 13 European countries. *J Invest Dermatol.* 2015; 135(4):984–991.
4. McDonough E, Ayearst R, Eder L, et al. Depression and anxiety in psoriatic disease: prevalence and associated factors. *J Rheumatol.* 2014; 41(5):887–896.
5. Remrod C, Sjostrom K, Svensson A. Psychological differences between early- and late-onset psoriasis: a study of personality traits, anxiety and depression in psoriasis. *Brit J Dermatol.* 2013;169(2):344–350.
6. Gul AI, Colgecen E. Personality traits and common psychiatric conditions in adult patients with acne vulgaris. *Ann Dermatol.* 2015;27: 48–52.
7. Silverberg JI, Silverberg NB. Epidemiology and extracutaneous comorbidities of severe acne in adolescence: a U.S. population-based study. *Brit J Dermatol.* 2014;170:1136–1142.
8. Niemeier V, Kupfer J, Gieler U. Acne Vulgaris – Psychosomatic Aspects. *Journal der Deutschen Dermatologischen Gesellschaft* 2006; 4:1027–1036.

■ EPIDEMIOLOGY

The prevalence in the U.S. population is 1%, with worldwide prevalence ranging from 0.1% to 8%. Although men and women are equally affected, women may be overrepresented in practice as they are more likely to seek treatment for the condition.[72,73]

■ PATHOPHYSIOLOGY

The disease is categorized by the extent of involvement and distribution of depigmentation, with generalized vitiligo being the most common presentation. The etiology is unknown; hypotheses suggest that it is autoimmune, autocytotoxic, or neurally mediated.

■ CLINICAL PRESENTATION

Vitiligo is clinically manifested by hypopigmented macules or patches of variable progression. The disorder commonly begins before age 20. Later age of onset is more often associated with autoimmune diseases, such as thyroid dysfunction, rheumatoid arthritis, diabetes mellitus, anemia, or alopecia areata.

The disfiguring appearance of depigmentation can be psychologically devastating, but the impact on perceived quality of life and psychological well-being is variable. Patients with generalized vitiligo may have emotional problems of comparable severity to those of patients with psoriasis, eczema, chronic hand dermatitis, and acne.[74] Patients report feelings of increased anxiety, embarrassment, discrimination, low self-esteem, poor self-image, lack of confidence, inferiority, stigmatization, and interference with sexual relationships. The social stigma of the disease and misperceptions about underlying etiology (e.g., believing that it is caused by leprosy or sexually transmitted infections) may complicate marriage and employment opportunities in some areas. Patients may feel uncomfortable around strangers, whom they perceive to stare, make rude remarks, or discriminate.[72–73,75]

■ ASSESSMENT AND DIFFERENTIAL DIAGNOSIS

Psychiatric comorbidities include major depression, persistent depressive disorder (dysthymia), adjustment disorder, anxiety, and sleep disturbance (Boxes 12-6 and **12-9**).[72] International studies report prevalence rates of 16% to 22% for depressive disorders, 7% to 9% for persistent depressive disorder (dysthymia), 10% for suicidal ideation, 3.3% for suicide attempts, and 56% to 75% for adjustment disorder.[75] A Turkish study comparing youths with vitiligo to age-matched controls found that vitiligo was related to depression in children but the same effect was not seen in the adolescent group.[76]

■ TREATMENT

Because of the psychological distress, treatment for vitiligo should address both recovery of pigmentation and relief of the psychosocial burden.[77] Clinical interventions that successfully reduce visibility of depigmentation are believed to ease psychiatric symptoms. Few studies have evaluated the efficacy of this or other interventions on the psychological aspects of the disease.[75] It is recommended that patients, regardless of disease severity, be screened for psychiatric comorbidities such as depression and adjustment disorders with depressed mood, given their high prevalence rates. To date, little is known about specialized treatment strategies for depression in patients with comorbid vitiligo.

ATOPIC DERMATITIS

■ INTRODUCTION

Atopic dermatitis, also referred to as atopic eczema, is a chronically relapsing skin disease that is most often diagnosed in early infancy and childhood. It can be thought of as the cutaneous expression of the atopic state, characterized by a family history of asthma, allergic rhinitis, or eczema. There is no distinguishing feature of atopic dermatitis, and rather, it is diagnosed based upon a constellation of clinical findings that include intense pruritus, xerosis, inflammatory lesions, and lichenification in flexural areas. The strongest link to depression and anxiety has been noted with nodular lesions, termed prurigo nodularis. Whereas chronic "rubbers" may show clinical features consistent with lichenification, chronic "pickers"

BOX 12-9
DIFFERENTIAL DIAGNOSIS

Other psychiatric disorders:

Anxiety

Substance use disorders

Adjustments disorders

will instead create hyperpigmented, nodular lesions and excoriations limited to sites that the patient can reach. Of note, prurigo nodularis may be seen in patients with or without other features of atopic dermatitis.

■ EPIDEMIOLOGY

The prevalence of atopic dermatitis is 10% to 20% in children[78] and 1% to 3% in adults.[1] There has been a more than threefold increase in the prevalence of atopic dermatitis since the 1960s.[1] This increase has been attributed to a change in environmental allergens, deficient antigen exposure in early life (hygiene hypothesis), climate, environmental pollution, and tobacco smoke exposure.

No specific data exist on the prevalence of depression in atopic dermatitis. However, hospital-treated atopic disorders increase the risk of developing a severe depression up to threefold.[79] Health-related quality of life is more closely associated with psychiatric morbidity than is physician-rated disease severity,[3] suggesting that the impact on the patients' daily activities is the driving factor for psychological issues rather than the disease itself.[80]

Although gender data are sparse, it is known that women respond differently from men to skin illness, particularly if it is disfiguring.[81] Women report more subjective stress and worry in dermatologic illness,[82] and it has been speculated that the incidence of depressive illness is, therefore, higher in women. Clinically manifest atopic disorders increase the risk of diagnosable depression up to 2.7-fold in women, but not in men,[83] and 31-year prospective follow-up indicates that atopy increases the risk of depression up to 4.7-fold in women. However, it should be noted that a gender difference in disease-related quality of life is not been found in all studies.[84]

Age is inversely related to psychological symptoms and disease-related quality of life,[85] which may be explained by older adults having fewer emotional reactions to living with skin disease or having developed coping mechanisms to deal more adaptively with chronic illness.

■ PATHOPHYSIOLOGY
Genetics

A large proportion (64%) of the association between atopy and depression is due to additive genetic effects[86] suggesting there is some shared genetic covariance between atopic disorders and depressive symptoms.

Stress and Psychosocial Effects

Psychiatric assessments and self-report inventories in various studies have revealed increased levels of comorbid depression and anxiety in atopic dermatitis patients,[87,88] but what remains unclear to what extent psychological symptoms precede the skin disease and to what extent the disease leads to increased psychological symptoms. A one-way relationship is often assumed when considering psychological distress and atopic dermatitis in which the skin illness is presumed to lower quality of life and psychological dysfunction. However, it is now thought that the relationship between the psychological symptoms and the skin disorder is bidirectional.

Psychosocial factors negatively impact the development and prognosis of atopic disorders, and the effect of atopic disease on future mental health is stronger than that of psychosocial factors on atopic disease development and progression.[89] The onset or exacerbation of atopic dermatitis, however, often follows stressful life events, and an increase in perceived psychological stress has been linked to a decline in cutaneous permeability barrier function.[90] The reciprocal relationship between psychosocial factors and atopic disorders may also be mediated by behavioral

and socioeconomic factors. For example, psychosocial stress may exacerbate atopy via behaviors, such as poor diet, lack of exercise, sleep disturbance, frequent smoking, substance abuse, unhygienic living environment, and poor medical adherence. Conversely, atopic diseases could have an adverse impact on mental health via distressing somatic symptoms, consistent unsuccessful treatment and cumulative medical cost, and social functioning impairment at home, school, or workplace.[91] Individual variation in vulnerability to stress-related disease among people with similar life experiences is determined largely by the way stressors are perceived and by the quality of social support.[93]

Common Biologic Pathways
Immunologic and Serotonergic Pathways

There appears to be a biologic link between allergic conditions and depression, as adults with depression have higher than normal IgE-mediated allergies.[93,94] Cytokines play a key role in pathogenesis of allergic disorders and serve as chemical mediators between the immune system and the brain.[95] In atopic states, there is a shift from T-helper (Th) 1 to Th2 responses from Th lymphocyte precursors. Th2 cells produce IL-4, which has an effect on serotonin (5-HT) metabolism and regulatory effects on serotonin transporter genotypes (5-HTT).[96] 5-HT is an important mediator of bidirectional interactions between the nervous and immune systems, and genetic polymorphism of the serotonin transporter is associated with depression.[97] Thus the link between atopic dermatitis and depression may be explained by altered 5-HT metabolism in the brain.

In addition, two major pathways, the hypothalamic–pituitary–adrenal (HPA) axis and the sympathetic nervous system (SNS), are involved in the bidirectional interaction between the brain and immune system. Proinflammatory cytokines are released by the IgE-stimulation of tissue mast cells and basophils during allergic hypersensitivity reactions, which subsequently activate both the HPA axis and SNS. This, in turn, can lead to depressed mood states.

Histamine

Not all studies indicate a link between IgE-mediated immune reaction and depression,[98] and the comorbidity of depression and atopy might be related to chronic pruritic dermatosis, which leads to depression, anxiety, and sleep disturbances. This may involve metabolism of histamine, which is released from activated mast cells during hypersensitivity reactions. Histamine mediates suppression of some ILs and stimulates the secretion of others.[99] Furthermore, histamine acts as a neurotransmitter in the brain; histamine turnover in the diencephalon may be related to the pathology of the depressive state[100] and histamine H3 receptor antagonists have antidepressive effects.[101] Antihistamines, or H1 receptor antagonists, also have immunological effects as they inhibit the wheal and flare response to allergens and psychological effects, including decreasing anxiety.

■ CLINICAL PRESENTATION

The stigmatization, social isolation, frequent medical visits, and the need to constantly apply topical remedies all add to the burden of disease, and result in a variety of psychiatric symptoms that are seen in atopic dermatitis.[102] Depression and anxiety are the most common, and patients with atopic dermatitis are more likely to report depressive symptoms and medically unexplained somatic symptoms.[103] They have significantly lower quality of life and higher state and trait anxiety as compared with healthy controls,[104] as well as difficulties dealing with anger and hostility.[105] Atopic dermatitis also affects interpersonal relationships. For example, a large study revealed that more than half of eczema patients and a third of their spouses reported that the illness had a negative impact on their sex lives.[106]

These patients' mood disorder may become so severe that concerns about suicide arise. Suicidal ideation has been reported in 2.1% of mild to moderately affected adult atopic dermatitis patients.[107] A study of completed suicides among patients with eczema revealed that 72% of them occurred in the first half of the year.[108] This seasonal distribution in suicide was not found in the non-atopic patients.[108] The seasonality of suicide in atopic patients parallels that of depression[109] and suggests a possible common etiological basis.

■ COURSE AND NATURAL HISTORY

The course of depression in atopic dermatitis parallels that of the skin disorder itself and follows a relapsing-remitting course. There is a direct correlation between pruritus and depression ratings, suggesting that the depressed clinical state may lower the threshold for pruritus.[110]

Depression leads to reduced treatment adherence for chronic illnesses in general,[111,112] and this is particularly true for atopic dermatitis,[113] though empirical evidence linking depression and medication nonadherence in this population is lacking. However, it is likely that such a relationship does exist and it would help to explain the relationship between psychological distress and poor disease outcomes.[114]

■ ASSESSMENT AND DIFFERENTIAL DIAGNOSIS

There are no specific instruments for assessing depressive symptoms in patients with atopic dermatitis. Please refer to the "Assessment" Chapter 3 for an overview of screening for depression Elevated symptom scores for depression and anxiety in atopic dermatitis patients do not necessarily indicate the presence of diagnosable disorder. Indeed, subthreshold symptoms that do not quite reach the level of diagnosable disorder characterize many such patients.[115,116]

There are several assessment tools to measure the quality of life of dermatologic patients such as the Dermatology Quality of Life Index[117] and Skindex.[118] There is also an instrument to evaluate the psychosomatic and psychosocial issues for adult patients with atopic dermatitis.[119] The Psychosomatic Scale for Atopic Dermatitis (PSS-AD) is a simple and reliable measure of stress-induced exacerbations, quality of life, and emotions, such as anger, associated with the disorder. It is also important to screen for anxiety, particularly since this symptom may be a clue to an underlying depressive disorder.

Given the elevated prevalence of depression in atopic dermatitis patients, dermatologists should be urged to screen for it in order to identify affected patients.

■ TREATMENT

There are several behavioral techniques to reduce the scratching behaviors that tend to perpetuate the itch–scratch cycle in this illness. These include biofeedback,[120] cognitive behavioral approaches,[121] specific management of scratching behaviors,[122] and relaxation training (Box 12-5).[121] Relaxation therapy, cognitive behavioral treatment, and combined relaxation and cognitive behavioral treatment have been shown to lead to significant additional treatment benefit in skin conditions beyond those of standard dermatological care.[123] Thus standard dermatological treatments combined with progressive relaxation and hypnosis are associated with greater improvement of the atopy at 14-month follow-up than standard treatment alone.[124] Relaxation training ameliorates stress-induced exacerbation of atopic dermatitis[125] and may improve psychological functioning, particularly in relation to avoidance.[126]

There are no specific guidelines regarding the pharmacotherapy of depression in atopic dermatitis and some of the above-mentioned

BOX 12-10
SUMMARY

Owing largely to disfigurement, perceived social stigma, and unforeseen changes in lifestyle, psychiatric illness is reported in at least 30% of patients with dermatologic disorders.

Dermatologic and psychiatric disorders possess shared mechanisms of pathophysiology, including inflammatory, immune-mediated, hormonal, neurally mediated, and genetic.

Pharmacologic interventions for dermatologic disorders should be carefully considered given drug–drug interactions with psychotropic agents, dermatologic side effects of psychotropic agents, as well as psychiatric side effects of dermatologic agents.

cognitive and behavioral techniques may reduce or avoid reliance on antidepressant pharmacotherapy.[125] The pharmacotherapy of atopic dermatitis should aim to interrupt the itch–scratch cycle and optimize night-time sleep, which is frequently a problem.[127] Several studies suggest using antidepressants with sedating properties to specifically address the insomnia secondary to pruritus.[70] Antidepressants are also used to specifically treat pruritus: bupropion reduces affected body surface area in patients with atopic dermatitis who are not depressed.[128] Mirtazapine reduced pruritus in a case report[129] and a pilot study.[130] Thus, antidepressant medications may be helpful in treating these dermatologic disorders even in the absence of comorbid depression.[107] It is postulated that this is related to antihistaminic, anticholinergic, and centrally mediated analgesic effects, independent of antidepressant effects.[123]

■ SUMMARY

The importance of collaboration between dermatologists and psychiatrists is made apparent by the clear association between atopic dermatitis and depression (**Box 12-10**). Addressing both conditions simultaneously appears prudent, particularly given the bidirectional relationship between psychological symptoms and skin illness.

REFERENCES

1. Hughes JE, Barraclough BM, Hamblin LG, White JE. Psychiatric symptoms in dermatology patients. *Br J Psychiatry*. 1983;143: 51–54.

2. Fried RG, Gupta MA, Gupta AK. Depression and skin disease. *Dermatol Clin*. 2005;23:657–664.

3. Picardi A, Abeni D, Melchi C, Puddu P, Pasquini P. Psychiatric morbidity in dermatological outpatients: an issue to be recognized. *Br J Dermatol*. 2000;143:983–991.

4. Arck PC, Slominski A, Theoharides TC, Peters EM, Paus R. Neuroimmunology of stress: skin takes center stage. *J Invest Dermatol*. 2006;126(8):1697–1704.

5. Denda M, Takei K, Denda S. How does epidermal pathology interact with mental state? *Med Hypotheses*. 2013;80(2): 194–196.

6. Miller AH, Maletic V, Raison CL. Inflammation and its discontents: the role of cytokines in the pathophysiology of major depression. *Biol Psychiatry*. 2009;65:732–741.

7. Chiu A, Chon SY, Kimball AB. The response of skin disease to stress: changes in the severity of acne vulgaris as affected by examination stress. *Arch Dermatol*. 2003;139(7):897–900.

8. Gupta MA, Gupta AK. Psychiatric and psychological co-morbidity in patients with dermatologic disorders: epidemiology and management. *Am J Clin Dermatol*. 2003;4(12):833–842.

9. Goulden V, Stables GI, Cunliffe WJ. Prevalence of facial acne in adults. *J Am Acad Dermatol.* 1999;41(4):577–580.

10. Zaenglein AL, Graber EM, Thiboutot DM. Chapter 80. Acne Vulgaris and Acneiform Eruptions. In: Goldsmith LA, Katz SI, Gilchrest BA, Paller AS, Leffell DJ, Dallas NA, eds. *Fitzpatrick's Dermatology in General Medicine.* 8th ed. New York, NY: McGraw-Hill; 2012. http://www.accessmedicine.com.ezp-prod1.hul.harvard.edu/content.aspx?aID = 56046904.

11. Burke BM, Cunliffe WJ. The assessment of acne vulgaris–the Leeds technique. *Br J Dermatol.* 1984;111(1):83–92.

12. Wei B, Pang Y, Qu L, et al. The epidemiology of adolescent acne in North East China. *J Eur Acad Dermatol Venereol.* 2010;24: 953–957.

13. Ghodsi SZ, Orawa H, Zouboulis CC. Prevalence, severity, and severity risk factors of acne in high school pupils: a community based study. *J Invest Dermatol.* 2009;129:2136–2141.

14. Schäfer T, Nienhaus A, Vieluf D, Berger J, Ring J. Epidemiology of acne in the general population: the risk of smoking. *Br J Dermatol.* 2001;145(1):100–104.

15. Taylor M, Gonzalez M, Porter R. Pathways to inflammation: acne pathophysiology. *Eur J Dermatol.* 2011;21(3):323–333.

16. Balazs J, Miklosi M, Kereszteny A, et al. Adolescent subthreshold-depression and anxiety: psychopathology, functional impairment and increased suicide risk. *J Child Psychol Psychiatry.* 2013;54(6):670–677.

17. Saitta P, Keehan P, Yousif J, Way BV, Grekin S, Brancaccio R. An update on the presence of psychiatric comorbidities in acne patients, part 1: overview of prevalence. *Cutis.* 2011;88(1):33–40.

18. Aktan S, Ozmen E, Sanli B. Anxiety, depression, and nature of acne vulgaris in adolescents. *Int J Dermatol.* 2000;39:354–357.

19. Niemeier V, Kupfer J, Demmelbauer-Ebner M, Stangier U, Effendy I, Gieler U. Coping with acne vulgaris. Evaluation of the chronic skin disorder questionnaire in patients with acne. *Dermatology.* 1998;196(1):108–115.

20. Yazici K, Baz K, Yazici AE, et al. Disease-specific quality of life is associated with anxiety and depression in patients with acne. *J Eur Acad Dermatol Venereol.* 2004;18:435–439.

21. Mallon E, Newton JN, Klassen A, Stewart-Brown SL, Ryan TJ, Finlay AY. The quality of life in acne:comparison with general medical conditions using generic questionnaires. *Br J Dermatol.* 1999;140(4):672–676.

22. Picardi A, Lega I, Tarolla E. Suicide risk in skin disorders. *Clin Dermatol.* 2013;31(1):47–56.

23. Gupta MA, Gupta AK. Depression and suicidal ideation in dermatology patients with acne, alopecia areata, atopic dermatitis, and psoriasis. *Br J Dermatol.* 1998;139(5):846–850.

24. Purvis D, Robinson E, Merry S, et al. Acne, anxiety, depression and suicide in teenagers: a cross-sectional survey of New Zealand secondary school students. *J Paed Child Health.* 2006;42:793–796.

25. Highlights of Prescribing Information ACZONE (dapsone) Gel 5%, 2013. Allergan, Inc. http://www.allergan.com/assets/pdf/aczone_pi.pdf. Accessed April 30, 2013.

26. Wolverton SE, Harper JC. Important controversies associated with isotretinoin therapy for acne. *Am J Clin Dermatol.* 2013; 14(2):71–76.

27. Sundstrom A, Alfredsson L, Sjolin-Forsberg G, Gerdén B, Bergman U, Jokinen J. Association of suicide attempts with acne and treatment with isotretinoin: retrospective Swedish cohort study. *BMJ.* 2010;341:c5812.

28. Azoulay L, Blais L, Koren G, LeLorier J, Bérard A. Isotretinoin and the risk of depression in patients with acne vulgaris: a case-crossover study. *J Clin Psych.* 2008;69(4):526–532.

29. Bliss SA, Warnock JK. Psychiatric medications: Adverse cutaneous drug reactions. *Clin Dermatol.* 2013;31:101–109.

30. Yeung CK, Chan HH. Cutaneous adverse effects of lithium: epidemiology and management. *Am J Clin Dermatol.* 2004;5(1):3–8.

31. Du-Thanh A, Kluger N, Bensalleh H, Guillot B. Drug-Induced Acneiform Eruption. *Am J Clin Dermatol.* 2011;12(4):233–245.

32. Carvalho MM, Góis C. Hyperprolactinemia in mentally ill patients. *Acta Med Port.* 2011;24(6):1005–1012.

33. Ajmal A, Joffe H, Nachtigall LB. Psychotropic-induced hyperprolactinemia: a clinical review. *Psychosomatics.* 2014;55:29–36.

34. http://www.clinicalpharmacology-ip.com.ezp-prod1.hul.harvard.edu/Forms/Reports/intereport.aspx Drug Interaction Reporting. Accessed April 30, 2014.

35. Schmader KE, Oxman MN. Chapter 194. Varicella and herpes zoster. In: Goldsmith LA, Katz SI, Gilchrest BA, Paller AS, Leffell DJ, Dallas NA, eds. *Fitzpatrick's Dermatology in General Medicine.* 8th ed. New York, NY: McGraw-Hill; 2012. http://www.accessmedicine.com.ezp-prod1.hul.harvard.edu/content.aspx?aID=56046904.

36. Gharibo C, Kim C. Neuropathic Pain of Postherpetic Neuralgia. *Pain Medicine News.* 2011;9:84–92

37. http://www.cdc.gov/shingles/hcp/clinical-overview.html#reference. Accessed May 8, 2014.

38. Lasserrea A, Blaizeaua F, Gorwood P, et al. Herpes zoster: Family history and psychological stress—Case–control study. *J Clin Virol.* 2012;55:153–157.

39. Forbes HJ, Bhaskaran K, Thomas SL, Smeeth L, Clayton T, Langan SM. Quantification of risk factors for herpes zoster: population based case-control study. *BMJ.* 2014;348:g2911.

40. Chen MH, MD, Wei HT, MD, Su TP, MD, et al. Risk of depressive disorder among patients with herpes zoster: A Nationwide Population-Based Prospective Study. *Psychosom Med.* 2014;76: 285–291.

41. Watson CP. Herpes zoster and postherpetic neuralgia. *CMAJ.* 2010;182(16):1713–1714.

42. Coplan PM, Schmader K, Nikas A, et al. Development of a measure of the burden of pain due to herpes zoster and postherpetic neuralgia for prevention trials: adaptation of the Brief Pain Inventory. *J Pain.* 2004;5:344–356.

43. Drolet M, Brisson M, Schmader KE, et al. The impact of herpes zoster and postherpetic neuralgia on health-related quality of life: a prospective study. *CMAJ.* 2010;182:1731–1736.

44. Irwin MR, Levin MJ, Carrillo C, et al. Major depressive disorder and immunity to varicella- zoster virus and the elderly. *Brain Behav Immun.* 2011;25(4):759–766.

45. Gan EY, Tian EA, Tey HL. Management of herpes zoster and postherpetic neuralgia", *Am J Clin Dermatol.* 2013;14(2): 77–85.

46. *Valtrex (Valacyclovir) Package Insert.* Research Triangle Park, NC: GlaxoSmithKline; 2013.

47. *Neurontin (gabapentin) package insert.* New York, NY: Parke Davis; 2013.

48. *Lyrica (pregabalin) package insert.* New York, NY: Pfizer; 2012.

49. US Food and Drug Administration. Guidance for industry: suicidal ideation and behavior: prospective assessment of

occurrence in clinical trials. Available at http://www.fda.gov/downloads/drugs/guidancecomplianceregulatoryinformation/guidances/ucm225130.pdf; 2012.

50. Pugh MJ, Hesdorffer D, Wang CP, et al. Temporal trends in new exposure to antiepileptic drug monotherapy and suicide-related behavior. *Neurology* 2013;81:1900–1906.

51. Harden CL, Meador KJ. Do antiepileptic drugs cause suicidal behavior?*Neurology*. 2013;81(22):1889–1890.

52. Pereira A, Gitlin MJ, Gross RA, Posner K, Dworkin RH. Suicidality associated with antiepileptic drugs: implications for the treatment of neuropathic pain and fibromyalgia. *Pain*. 2013;154(3):345–349.

53. Irwin MR, Levin MJ, Laudenslager ML, et al. Varicella zoster virus-specific immune responses to a herpes zoster vaccine in elderly recipients with major depression and the impact of antidepressant medications. *Clin Infect Dis*. 2013;56(8):1085–1093.

54. Krueger JG, Bowcock A. Psoriasis pathophysiology: current concepts of pathogenesis. *Ann Rheum Dis*. 2005;64(suppl II): ii30–ii35.

55. Mattozzi C, Salvi M, D'Epiro S, et al. Importance of regulatory T cells in the pathogenesis of psoriasis: review of the literature. *Dermatology*. 2013;227:134–145.

56. Rieder E, Tausk F. Psoriasis, a model of dermatologic psychosomatic disease: psychiatric implications and treatments. *Int J Dermatol*. 2012;51:12–26.

57. Tyring S, Gottlieb A, Papp K, et al. Etanercept and clinical outcomes, fatigue, and depression in psoriasis: double-blind placebo-controlled randomized phase III trial. *Lancet*. 2006;367:29–35.

58. Russo PA, Ilchef R, Cooper AJ. Psychiatric morbidity in psoriasis: A review. *Aust J Dermatol*. 2004;45:155–161.

59. Nevitt GJ, Hutchinson PE. Psoriasis in the community: prevalence, severity and patient's beliefs and attitudes towards the disease. *Br J Dermatol*. 1996;135:533–537.

60. Gupta MA, Gupta AK. Psychodermatology: An update. *J Am Acad Derm*. 2006;34:1030–1046.

61. Remrod C, Sjostrom K, Svensson A. Psychological differences between early and late onset psoriasis: A study of personality traits, anxiety and depression. *Br J Dermatol*. 2013;169(2):344–350.

62. Esposito M, Saraceno R, Giunta A, Maccarone M, Chimenti S. An Italian study on psoriasis and depression. *Dermatology*. 2006;212:123–127.

63. Devrimci-Ozguven H, Kundakci N, Kumbasar H, Boyvat A. The depression, anxiety, life satisfaction and affective expression levels in psoriasis patients. *JEADV*. 2000;14:267–271.

64. Langley RG, Feldman SR, Han C, et al. Ustekinumab significantly improves symptoms of anxiety, depression, and skin-related quality of life in patients with moderate-to-severe psoriasis: Results from a randomized, double-blind, placebo-controlled phase III trial. *J Am Acad Derm*. 2010;63:457–465.

65. Fortune DG, Richards HL, Kirby B, McElhone K, Main CJ, Griffiths CE. Successful treatment of psoriasis improves psoriasis-specific but not more general aspects of patients' well-being. *Br J Dermatol*. 2004;151:1219–1226.

66. D'Erme AM, Zanieri F, Campolmi E, et al. Therapeutic implications of adding the psychotropic drug escitalopram in the treatment of patients suffering from moderate-severe psoriasis and psychiatric comorbidity: a retrospective study. *JEADV*. 2012;28(2):246–249.

67. Hemlock C, Rosenthal JS, Winston A. Fuoxetine-induced psoriasis. *Ann Pharmacother*. 1992;26(2):211–212

68. Osborne SF, Stafford L, David G. Paroxetine-Associated Psoriasis. *Am J Psychiatry*. 2002;159:2113–2113.

69. Cox NH, Gordon PM, Dodd H. Generalized Pustular and erythodermic psoriasis associated with bupropion treatment. *Br J Dermatol*. 2002;146:1061–1063.

70. Modell JG, Boyce S, Taylor E, Katholi C. Treatment of atopic dermatitis and psoriasis vulgaris with bupropion-SR: a pilot study. *Psychosom Med*. 2002;64:835–840.

71. Alpsoy E, Ozcan E, Cetin L, et al. Is the efficacy of topical corticosteroid therapy for psoriasis vulgaris enhanced by concurrent moclobemide therapy? *J Am Acad Derm*. 1997;38:197–200.

72. Alikhan A, Felsten LM, Daly M, Petronic-Rosic V. Vitiligo: A comprehensive overview. *J Am Acad Derm*. 2011;65:473–491.

73. Kovacs SO. Vitiligo. *J Am Acad Derm*. 1998;38:647–664.

74. Linthorst Homan MW, Spuls PI, de Korte J, Bos JD, Sprangers MA, Wietze van der Veen JP. The burden of vitiligo: Patient characteristics associated with quality of life. *J Am Acad Derm*. 2009;61:411–419.

75. Ongenae K, Beelart L, van Geel N, Naeyaert JM. Psychosocial effects of vitiligo. *JEADV*. 2006;20:1–8.

76. Bilgic O, Bilgic A, Akis HK, Eskioglut F, Kilic EZ. Depression, anxiety and health-related quality of life in children and adolescents with vitiligo. *Clin Exp Dermatol*. 2011;36:360–365.

77. Chan MF, Chua TL, Goh BK, Derrick CW, Thng TG, Lee SM. Investigating factors associated with depression of vitiligo patients in Singapore. *J Clin Nurs*. 2011;21:1614–1621.

78. Odhiambo JA, Williams HC, Clayton TO, Robertson CF, Asher MI; ISAAC Phase Three Study Group. Global variations in prevalence of eczema symptoms in children from ISAAC Phase Three. *J Allergy Clin Immunol*. 2009;124:1251–1258.

79. Gupta MA. Psychiatric comorbidity in dermatologic disorders. In: Walker C, Papadopoulos L, eds. *Psychodermatology: The Psychological Impact of Skin Disorders*. New York, NY: Cambridge University Press; 2005:30–34.

80. Schulz-Larsen F, Hanifin JM: Epidemiology of atopic dermatitis. *Immunol Allergy Clin N Am*. 2002;22:1.

81. Alexander F. *Psychosomatic Medicine*. New York, NY: Norton; 1950.

82. Wittkowski A, Richards HL, Griffiths CE, Main CJ. The impact of psychological and clinical factors on quality of life in individuals with atopic dermatitis. *J Psychosom Res*. 2004;57:195–200.

83. Timonen M, Hakko H, Miettunen J, et al. Association between atopic disorders and depression: findings from the Northern Finland 1966 birth cohort study. *Am J Med Genet*. 2001;105: 216–217.

84. Roenigk RK, Roenigk HH Jr. Sex differences in the psychological effects of psoriasis. *Cutis*. 1978;21:529–533.

85. Ginsburg IH. The psychosocial impact of skin disease. *Dermatol Clin*. 1996;14:473–484.

86. Timonen M, Jokelainen J, Silvennoinen-Kassinen S, et al. Association between skin-test diagnosed atopy and professionally diagnosed depression: a Northern Finland 1966 birth cohort study. *Biol Psychiatry*. 2002;52:349–355.

87. Zachariae R, Zachariae C, Ibsen HH, Mortensen JT, Wulf HC. Psychological symptoms and quality of life of dermatology outpatient and hospitalized dermatology patients. *Acta Derm Venereol*. 2004;84:205–212.

88. Wamboldt M, Hewitt J, Schmitz S, et al. Familial association between allergic disorders and depression in adult Finnish twins. *Am J Med Genet*. 2000;6:146–153.

89. Ginsburg IH, Pystowsky JH, Kornfield DS, Wolland H. Role of emotional factors in adults with atopic dermatitis. *Int J Dermatol*. 1993;32:656–660.

90. Buske-Kirschbaum A, Geiben A, Hellhammer D. Psychobiological aspects of atopic dermatitis: an overview. *Psychchother Psychosom*. 2001;70:6–16.

91. Seiffert K, Hilbert E, Schaechinger H, Zouboulis CC, Deter H. Psychophysiological reactivity under mental stress in atopic dermatitis. *Dermatology*. 2005;210:286–293.

92. Garg A, Chren M, Sands LP, et al. Psychological stress perturbs epidermal permeability barrier homeostasis: Implications for the pathogenesis of stress-associated skin disorders. *Arch Dermatol*. 2001;137:53–59.

93. Chida Y, Hamer M, Steptoe A. A birdrectional relationship between psychosocial factors and atopic disorders: a systematic review and meta-analysis. *Psychosom Med*. 2008;70:102–116.

94. Marshall GD, Roy SR. Stress and allergic diseases. In: Ader R, ed. *Psychoneuroimmunology*. Amersterdam: Academic Press; 2007;799–824.

95. McEwen BS. Protective and damaging effects of stress mediators. *N Engl J Med*. 1998;338:171–179.

96. Bell I, Jasnoski M, Kagan J, Kin D. Depression and allergies: survey of a nonclinical population. *Psychother Psychosom*. 1991;55:24–31.

97. Kennedy B, Morris R, Schwab J. Responsivity of allergic depressed subjects to antidepressant medications: a preliminary study. *Depression*. 1996;3:286–289.

98. Kronfol Z, Remick DG. Cytokines and the brain: implications for clinical psychiatry. *Am J Psychiatry*. 2000;157:683–694.

99. Mossner R, Daniel S, Schmitt A, Albert D, Lesch KP. Modulation of serotonin transporter function by interleukin-4. *Life Sci*. 2001;68:873–880.

100. Lesch KP. Serotonergic gene expression and depression: implications for developing novel antidepressants. *J Affect Disord*. 2001;62:57–76.

101. Yang YW, Tseng KC, Chen YH, Yang JY. Associations among eczema, asthma, serum immunoglobulin E and depression in adults: a population-based study. *Allergy*. 2010;65:801–802.

102. Lundberg L, Johannesson M, Silverdahl M, Hermansson C, Lindberg M. Health-related quality of life in patients with psoriasis and atopic dermatitis measured with SF-36, DLQI and a subjective measure of disease activity. *Acta Derm Venereol*. 2000;80:430–434.

103. Elenkov IJ, Wilder RL, Chrousos GP, Vizi ES. The sympathetic nerve—an integrative interface between two supersystems: the brain and the immune system. *Phamacol Rev*. 2000;52:595–638.

104. Ito C, Shen H, Toyota H, et al. Effects of the acute and chronic restraint stresses on the central histaminergic neuron system of Fischer rat. *Neurosci Lett*. 1999;262:143–145.

105. Ito C. The role of brain histamine in acute and chronic stresses. *Biomed Pharmacother*. 2000;54:263–267.

106. Hashiro M, Okumura M. Anxiety, depression and psychosomatic symptoms in patients with atopic dermatitis: comparison with normal controls and among groups of different degrees of severity. *J Dermatol Sci*. 1997;14:63–67.

107. Linnet J, Jemec GB. An assessment of anxiety and dermatology life quality in patients with atopic dermatitis. *Br J Dermatol*. 1999;140:268–272.

108. White A, Horne DJ, Varigos GA: Psychological profile of the atopic eczema patient. *Australas J Dermatol*. 1990;31:13–16.

109. Misery L, Finlay AY, Martin N, et al. Atopic dermatitis: impact on the quality of life of patients and their partners. *Dermatology*. 2007;215:123–129.

110. Gupta MA, Gupta AK, Ellis CN. Antidepressant drugs in dermatology: an update. *Arch Dermatol*. 1987;123:647–652.

111. Timonen M, Viilo K, Helina H, Särkioja T, Meyer-Rochow VB, Räsänen PK. Is seasonality of suicides stronger in victims with hospital-treated atopic disorders? *Psych Res*. 2004;126:167–175.

112. Maes M, Meltzer HY, Suy E, De Meyer F. Seasonality in severity of depression: relationships to suicide or homicide. *Acta Psychiatrica Scandinavica*. 1998;43:313–314.

113. Gupta MA, Gupta AK, Schork MA, Ellis CN. Depression modulates pruritus perception: A study of pruritus in psoriasis, atopic dermatitis, and chronic idiopathic urticaria. *Psychom Med*. 1994;56:36–40.

114. Dimatteo R, Lepper H, Croghan T. Depression is a risk factor for noncompliance with medical treatment: meta-analysis of the effects of anxiety and depression on patient adherence. *Arch Intern Med*. 2000;160:2101–2107.

115. Krejci-Manwaring J, Tusa M, Carroll C, et al. Stealth monitoring of adherence to topical medication: adherence is very poor in children with atopic dermatitis. *J Am Acad Dermatol*. 2007;56:1–9.

116. Kelsay K, Klinnert M, Bender B. Addressing psychosocial aspects of atopic dermatitis. *Immunol Allergy Clin N Am*. 2010;30:385–396.

117. Leung DY, Bieber T. Atopic dermatitis. *Lancet*. 2003;361:151–160.

118. Misery L, Thomas L, Jullien D, et al. Comparative study of stress and quality of life in outpatients consulting for different dermatoses in 5 academic departments of dermatology. *Eur J Dermatol*. 2008;18:412–415.

119. Magin P, Pond C, Smith W, Watson AB, Goode SM. A cross-sectional study of psychological morbidity in patients with acne, psoriasis, and atopic dermatitis in specialist dermatology and general practices. *J Eur Acad Dermatol Venereol*. 2008;22:1435–1444.

120. Finlay AY, Khan GK. Dermatology life quality index (DLQI)-A simple practical measure for routine clinical use. *Clin Exp Dermatol*. 1994;19:210–216.

121. Chren MM, Lasek RJ, Flocke SA, Zyzanski SJ. Improved discriminative and evaluative capability of a refined version of Skindex, a quality-of-life instrument for patients with skin disease. *Arch Dermatol*. 1997;133:1433–1440.

122. Ando T, Hashiro M, Noda K, et al. Development and validation of the psychosomatic scale for atopic dermatitis in adults. *J of Dermatol*. 2006;33:439–450.

123. Brown D, Bettley F. Psychiatric treatment of eczema: a controlled trial. *Br Med J*. 1971;2:729–734.

124. Haynes SN, Wilson CC, Jaffe PG, Britton BT. Biofeedback treatment of atopic dermatitis: controlled case studies of eight cases. *Biofeedback Self Regul*. 1979;4:195–209.

125. Horne DJ, White AE, Varigos GA. A preliminary study of psychological therapy in the management of atopic eczema. *Br J Med Psychol*. 1989;62:241–248.

126. Cole WC, Roth HL, Saches LB. Group psychotherapy as an aid in the medical treatment of eczema. *J Am Acad Dermatol*. 1988;18:286–291.

127. Chida Y, Steptoe A, Hirakawa N, Sudo N, Kubo C. The effects of psychological intervention on atopic dermatitis. *Int Arch Allergy Immunol*. 2007;144:1–9.

128. Wittkowski A, Richards H. How beneficial is cognitive behaviour therapy in the treatment of atopic dermatitiss? A single-case study. *Psychol Health Med*. 2007;12:445–449.

129. Ehlers A, Stangier U, Gieler U. Treatment of atopic dermatitis: a comparison of psychological and dermatological approaches to relapse prevention. *J Consult Clin Psychol*. 1995;63:624–635.

130. Bender B, Ballard R, Canono B, Murphy JR, Leung DY. Disease severity, scratching, and sleep quality in patients with atopic dermatitis. *J Am Acad Dermatol*. 2008;58:415–420.

CHAPTER 13

Depression and Gastrointestinal Disease

Robert Boland, MD

Florina Haimovici, MD

Megan Oser, PhD

Pamela Mirsky, MD

Joshua Korzinek, MD

Psychiatry has enjoyed a particularly interesting relationship with the gastrointestinal (GI) illnesses since the brain–gut relationship was considered one of the core examples of how psychological stress could influence autonomic processes,[1] until increasing understanding regarding the pathophysiology underlying stomach and duodenal disorders diminished interest in this relationship. Still, it remains a fact that the brain and digestive tract are intimately connected and more recent—and more modest—research reveals strong evidence for direct and indirect influences of one on the other. Considering that depression can be a consequence of both physiological and psychological stress, it should be no surprise that depressive disorders very commonly co-occur with GI disorders. This chapter will consider several examples of the complex relationship between depressive disorders and GI disorders, including peptic ulcer disease, irritable bowel syndrome (IBS), inflammatory bowel disease (IBD), and various diseases of the liver.

PEPTIC ULCERS

■ INTRODUCTION

Peptic ulcers are erosions of the GI lining that extend through the mucosa of the GI lumen. Ulcers can occur anywhere along the alimentary tract; however, they are most likely to occur in the stomach or in the proximal bulb of the duodenum: the "peptic" regions, so called because these are the areas that have the most contact with the corrosive digestive juices gastric acid and pepsin. This is why gastric and duodenal ulcers are collectively referred to as "peptic ulcers," and as they are pathologically similar, they are usually considered together. The peptic lumen has adapted to protect against the effects of constant contact with acids and proteolytic enzymes through adaptations of the mucosal lining and its protective mucus layer; ulcers only occur when some pathological process disrupts this normal protection. Considered a disorder of the modern age,[2] the incidence of peptic ulcer disease rose dramatically in the 19th century, peaked in the first half of the 20th century, and then began to decline after the 1950s with advances in diagnosis and treatment. Despite these advances, they remain common, with an estimated prevalence of about 8% in the United States and an estimated cost of more than 3 billion dollars per year. The relationship of peptic ulcers to psychiatry is particularly interesting: thought to be a classic "psychosomatic" disease for much of the 20th century, research on the psychological aspect of ulcers was largely abandoned after it was discovered that the great majority were infectious in etiology. However, this understanding is incomplete and there is some renewed interest in the role of psychological stress and psychiatric disease, both as risk factors, perpetuating factors, and as possible complications of this disease.

■ EPIDEMIOLOGY

Epidemiological studies support an association between depression and peptic ulcer disease (**Fig. 13-1, Box 13-1**). A large epidemiological study in the United States demonstrated the association between mood and anxiety disorders and peptic ulcer disease: for the mood disorders, this association was strongest for chronic depressive disorder and persistent depressive disorder (dysthymia) (OR = 3.59).[3] Alcohol and nicotine use explained some, but not all of this association. A large international epidemiological survey also found depression to be independently associated with peptic ulcer onset (OR = 1.3 for major depression or persistent depressive

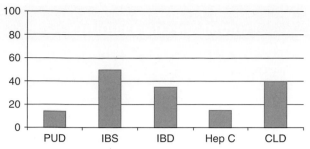

Figure 13-1 *Mean risk of depression for selected illnesses (percentage prevalence for particular disease).*

Neuroendocrine responses

HPA dysregulation

Immune systems

Autonomic dysfunction

Inflammation

disorder [dysthymia]).[4] This study had the advantage of only including episodes of depression that preceded ulcer onset.

Studies of patients with recurrent depression also show a high incidence of ulcers. For example, one large case–control study of patients with two or more episodes of major depression found that these patients were more likely to have peptic ulcers (OR = 4.31).[5] However, another survey[6] did not find an increased rate of peptic ulcers in persons who had had major depressive episodes in the past year. The discrepancy may be one of chronicity, as the second study did not select for recurrent depression.

■ PATHOPHYSIOLOGY

The majority of ulcers result from infection with *Helicobacter pylori*, which causes inflammation and disrupts the normal defensive and reparative processes of the mucosa. Nonsteroidal anti-inflammatory medications (NSAIDs), which impede the normal protective effects of prostaglandin, are the next most common cause. Much less common are ulcers due to other GI diseases (e.g., Crohn disease [CD]), other infections, medications, tumors, mechanical damage to the mucosa because of radiation or hiatal hernias, and hypersecretory states (e.g., Zollinger–Ellison syndrome). Ulcers can also be the result of severe insults to the body, such as a severe systemic illness, major surgery, severe head injury, or burns—such ulcers are referred to as "stress ulcers"—a term which occasionally causes confusion given the multiple meanings of the word "stress," in this case referring to severe physical stress. The etiology of stress ulcers is not entirely understood, but thought to be due to splanchnic hypoperfusion: in life-threatening situations, the circulatory system typically shunts blood away from the GI system to muscles and other organs where the need is more pressing.

Up to 20% of peptic ulcers have no clear cause. It is assumed that in many of these cases the patients have undiagnosed *H. pylori* or are unaware that some medication they take has nonsteroidal anti-inflammatory properties. However, in some of these cases, emotional stress is thought to play a role.

Sociodemographic

Clinical

Alcohol use

Nicotine use

Insomnia

Poor diet

NSAID use

Physical or sexual abuse

Medical

Psychological Factors and Peptic Ulcers

Psychological explanations for peptic ulcers have had a long and interesting history. After it became apparent that the 19th century model of acid hypersecretion could only explain a small fraction of occurrences and as no other cause was evident many looked for psychological explanations. These explanations were derived from psychoanalytic theory, invoking concepts of various conflicts and frustrated drives. Support for these theories mainly came from anecdotal cases and uncontrolled, correlative studies. This remained the dominant explanation for peptic ulcers throughout the 20th century until the 1970s when *H. pylori* bacilli were identified and cultured from the gastric epithelium around areas of inflammation.[7] Subsequent studies demonstrated dramatic improvements following eradication of the bacteria and emergence of the disease after one of the investigators ingested the bacilli. These spelled the end of the psychosomatic theory of ulcer formation.[8]

Subsequently, some researchers studying the effects of stress on disease suggested that it was a mistake to entirely abandon psychological investigations, opining that, as with most chronic diseases, peptic ulcer disease would benefit from a biopsychosocial perspective. It was noted, for example, that a lack of central nervous influences on this and other GI diseases would be surprising, given the multiple intimate connections between the two organ systems, which include multiple points of contact between the autonomic nervous system and the hypothalamic–pituitary–adrenal (HPA) axis. Instances were noted in which the risk of peptic ulcers increased dramatically following stressful mass events.[9] Better controlled prospective studies then demonstrated a link between psychosocial factors and peptic ulcers.[10] A good deal of this association likely reflects incorrect diagnoses and recall biases and much of this association may be accounted for by behaviors that are associated with both stress and ulcers, including smoking, sleeplessness, poor diet, alcohol use, and medication use (particularly NSAIDs). However, it appears that even when all these factors are accounted for, there remains a small but significant relationship between psychosocial stress and the incidence of peptic ulcers. Thus, studies controlling for these health risk behaviors still found an elevated risk of peptic ulcer in individuals experiencing high levels of stress (OR = 1.7–2.9).[11–13] As a whole, although each of these studies had methodological problems and none accounted for all possible confounders, the weight of evidence suggests some direct relationship between stress and peptic ulcer risk. These epidemiological data were also supported, in part, by animal models in which the induction of psychological stress increased the risk for ulcers, as well as the persistence and extent of ulceration in affected animals.[14]

The exact mechanism by which stress can contribute to ulcer formation is not known but remains a ripe area for speculation: as already noted, the GI system and the central nervous system are closely linked (**Box 13-2**). Most frequently implicated are neuroendocrine responses to stress mediated by the HPA axis as well as through the autonomic system.[15,16] For example, autonomic hyperactivity can decrease gastric emptying and perfusion,[17] both of which can predispose to ulcer formation, and stress-related hypercortisolemia

BOX 13-3
IMPORTANT SYMPTOMS

Confounding

Psychological distress

Poor appetite

Weakness

Sexual dysfunction

More typical of depression

Anhedonia

Guilty or other depressive ruminations

Suicidality

BOX 13-4
COMMON COMORBIDITIES

Alcohol use disorders

Nicotine use disorders

Anxiety disorders

can delay wound healing.[18] Various other mechanisms, such as decreased resistance to *H. pylori* due to glucocorticoid-mediated inhibition of the immune response, are possible as well.

This said, it must be appreciated that correlation is not causation, and the fact that there is a relationship between stress and ulcer formation says little about the nature of that relationship. For example, one study showed a significant decrease in anxiety following definitive peptic ulcer treatment by eradication of *H. pylori*,[19] supporting the idea that psychological stress can be the result of peptic ulcers rather than the cause. Although this remains to be worked out, it seems reasonable to assume a complex and bidirectional relationship.

Depression and Peptic Ulcers

Given the above discussion on the relationship between stress and ulcers, one should expect there to be a high rate of depression in individuals with peptic ulcers, in that depression can be considered a disorder of chronic stress. Indeed, most animal models of depression are actually models of chronic mild stress.[20] Thus, the same strategies used for animal stress studies (e.g., forced swimming tests, chronic aversive stimuli) can also support a relationship between depression and peptic ulcer disease.[21] Similar mechanisms of action have been suggested as well, including, most commonly, disruptions of the HPA axis.[21]

As noted above, epidemiological studies also support a relationship between depression and peptic ulcer disease, with national and world survey data showing increased risks of depression in patients suffering from peptic ulcer disease. However, the directionality of the relationship remains unclear and is, again, most likely bidirectional.

■ CLINICAL PRESENTATION, ASSESSMENT, AND DIFFERENTIAL DIAGNOSIS

Diagnosing major depression in patients with peptic ulcers presents the same dilemma encountered when diagnosing depression with other medical disorders (**Box 13-3** to **Box 13-4**). Many of the symptoms associated with the ulcers, including the psychological distress caused by pain, loss of appetite, and occasional weakness can overlap with depression. That said, patients with peptic ulcers do not usually develop systemic symptoms and we would recommend an inclusive approach, in which patients who exhibit the full spectrum of symptoms associated with a major depressive disorder be treated as having such, even when alternative explanations for individual symptoms are possible.

In addition to diagnosing depression in this population, it is important to look for other common comorbid psychiatric disorders that can worsen the course of both diseases. Of most concern are alcohol and nicotine use disorders, as both are also risk factors for

peptic ulcer disease. In addition, anxiety disorders, particularly panic disorder, may be comorbid as well.

■ COURSE AND NATURAL HISTORY

Typically, ulcers can be eradicated with appropriate pharmacotherapy (antimicrobial therapy for *H. pylori* infection and proton pump inhibitors), and refractory ulcers are rare; in such cases nonadherence or some other underlying pathology (such as hypersecretory states) should be suspected. In the case of NSAID-related ulcers, cessation of the NSAID should obviously be added to the standard anti-ulcer regimen.

There is some evidence to suggest that depression can worsen the course of peptic ulcer disease and one study of 75 patients with duodenal ulcers found that those who were depressed spent more time than psychologically well ulcer patients experiencing ulcer-related symptoms over an approximately 3-year follow-up period.[22] Some of that difference may have been mediated by having greater life or socioeconomic stress.

Although not studied sufficiently in this particular disorder, we know that comorbid medical illnesses invariably worsen the course of major depressive episodes,[23] arguing for early and aggressive treatment of depressive symptoms.

■ TREATMENT

Given the data that depression is frequently associated with peptic ulcers, and that the presence of depression might worsen the course of the disease, it is reasonable to hope that treatment of depression would improve the course of peptic ulcer disease (**Box 13-5**). However, investigations of that proposition have been disappointing. Studies of psychotherapy, including cognitive therapy and stress management approaches, have generally not shown any effect on the course of peptic ulcer disease. Similarly, antidepressant pharmacotherapy has little role in ulcer treatment per se. It has been occasionally noted that some antidepressants, particularly tricyclic antidepressants (TCAs), have some effect as anti-ulcer agents, largely owing to their potency as antihistamines. In addition, fluoxetine may have anti-ulcer effects although the mechanism is not as clear.[24] At any rate, both agents are inferior to current ulcer treatments and in practice are rarely used for that purpose.

For patients with comorbid peptic ulcer disease and depression, it remains important to treat their depression as well as their ulcers. Although improvement of psychiatric symptoms following primary treatment of peptic ulcers has been reported, both disorders should

BOX 13-5
TREATMENTS FOR DEPRESSION IN PATIENTS WITH GI DISEASE

SSRIs, SNRIs (need to monitor for gastric bleeding and other gastrointestinal side effect, particularly in patients with peptic ulcers and other risk factors for bleeding)

TCAs (may help when pain or diarrhea is present)

Cognitive behavioral therapy

Exercise

be treated independently. Studies examining the treatment of depression with comorbid peptic ulcer disease are largely lacking but it makes sense to assume that the standard treatments for depression, both in terms of psychotherapy and pharmacology, are indicated here as well. This approach is somewhat tempered by the concern that selective serotonin reuptake inhibitors (SSRIs) may cause GI bleeding through inhibition of platelet function,[25] particularly in the elderly.[26] Some have questioned the prevalence of this adverse effect, and at least one endoscopic study of patients with a variety of upper GI diseases found no adverse effects in individuals who were taking SSRIs for at least a month.[27] That said, in patients with active peptic ulcer disease, particularly elderly patients, non-SSRI antidepressants should be considered. In such patients for whom SSRIs are preferred (e.g., because of a good response in the past), careful monitoring for GI bleeding is indicated and adjunctive acid-suppressing agents should be considered.

■ SUMMARY

Peptic ulcer disease has had a particularly dramatic relationship with psychiatry. Considered to be a psychosomatic disorder for most of the 20th century, research on the psychological aspects of peptic ulcer disease virtually ceased after the discovery that most cases of the disease were infectious in origin. The last decade and a half, however, has seen some modest but meaningful recrudescence of interest in the role that psychosocial factors, particularly psychological stress, could play in the onset and course of the disease. The weight of evidence supports a direct relationship between stress and ulcers, perhaps mediated by the HPA axis or autonomic regulation of the gut. It therefore follows that psychiatric disorders associated with chronic stress, including depression, are associated with peptic ulcer disease and may represent independent risk factors for it. Further research is needed to better elucidate the mechanisms connecting the disorders, and, perhaps, improve treatments for both.

IRRITABLE BOWEL SYNDROME

■ INTRODUCTION

IBS is the most common of the "functional bowel disorders," so named because they are defined by their effect on bowel functioning rather than any consistent pathological finding. IBS's primary feature is chronic abdominal bowel pain that is relieved by defecation. Other features include changes in the appearance and frequently of stool as well as feelings of bloating, urgency, incomplete evacuation, and flatulence. IBS is usually divided into two types depending on whether it is associated with diarrhea or constipation. These symptoms are found in many GI disorders and the diagnosis often rests more on the lack of systemic symptoms (fever, weight loss) or other symptoms that would imply a specific underlying condition (e.g., GI bleeding). Multiple studies have failed to elucidate a consistent underlying pathology or pathophysiological mechanism for this disorder, and it is commonly associated with other non-GI functional disorders, such as chronic headaches, fibromyalgia, and other forms of chronic pain. It is also frequently associated with a number of psychiatric disorders.

■ EPIDEMIOLOGY

The majority of people with IBS do not seek medical attention,[28] making epidemiological studies difficult to interpret, but it is thought to be very common and affects perhaps 10% to 15% of the general population (Fig. 13-1).[29] Interestingly, whereas the disorder is more often seen in women in the United States and other western countries, in Asian countries it is more commonly found in men.

As noted above, psychiatric comorbidity is common, although exact reports vary widely, with estimates ranging from approxi-

---

BOX 13-6
ANXIETY DISORDERS AND GI DISEASE

Look for Comorbid Anxiety. Along with mood disorders, anxiety disorders (including panic disorder and generalized anxiety) are strongly associated with peptic ulcers, IBS, IBD, HCV, and other GI disorders

Look for Subclinical Anxiety. Some symptoms of anxiety are very common in GI disorder, even if they don't reach the level of a discrete disorder

Consider the Possibility that Anxiety Is Secondary to the Medical Cause. Proinflammatory cytokines, such as those seen in IBD, can cause a sickness syndrome that includes symptoms of anxiety.

Treat the Primary Cause. At least one study suggested that anxiety improves with eradication of H. pylori independent of primary anxiety treatments

Treat the Symptoms. Anxiety symptoms can worsen the course of GI disease and negatively affect quality of life. Standard treatment for anxiety appears to be effective in these settings as well

---

mately half of patients with IBS to nearly all.[30] Among psychiatric disorders, depressive disorders are the most common, followed by anxiety disorders (**Box 13-6**). Patients with IBS are two to five times more likely to suffer depression or anxiety (odds ratio 2.7–4.6)[31–38] than those without. Directionality of the relationship between depression and IBS is understandably hard to establish–frequently the depressive symptoms precede the GI symptoms; however, the opposite is reported as well.[29]

Despite the reports that depression is very frequently associated with IBS, this may be population-specific and apply mainly to those patients seeking medical care, particularly in tertiary medical centers. Most community samples suggest that the rates of comorbid psychopathology are much lower in persons with IBS who do not regularly seek medical attention.

Certain risk factors shared by IBS and depression may help explain the relationship; of particular note is the observation that patients with IBS often have a history of physical or sexual abuse or other early life traumas.[39–42]

■ PATHOPHYSIOLOGY

There is a great deal of speculation regarding the underlying pathology behind IBS; however, the disorder has defied simple explanations; this likely reflects the heterogeneous nature of this disorder (Box 13-2). Theories include altered stress responses (similar to those described above for peptic ulcer disease), autonomic hypersensitivity, inflammatory processes, and abnormal serotonin signaling. Altered stress responses have been noted in some studies, for example, increased corticotropin response to corticotropin-releasing factor, as well as changes in the HPA axis.[43] Similarly, abnormal sympathetic and parasympathetic activity has been reported in some IBS patients.[44] In addition, hypersensitivity to pain likely plays a role. For example, distention of the rectum or gut, even within a normal range, is felt more intensely and perceived to be painful at a lower threshold by patients with IBS.[45] A role of inflammatory processes seems likely for at least some forms of the disorder; this is supported by the fact that patients with IBS often previously had some sort of GI infection, and biopsies have shown increases in inflammatory cell types (e.g., T-cells, mast cells).[46] These observations have led to the characterization of a "post infectious" subtype of IBS. A role for serotonin has been suggested as well. From a psychiatric perspective, it is notable that 90% of all serotonin in the body is located in the enterochromaffin cells of the GI tract, where it acts as a hormone regulating gastric motility, and the normal functioning of serotonin in this system has been reported to be disrupted.[47,48]

It should be stressed, however, that all these theories lack empirical support and no consistent pathology underlying IBS has been demonstrated. They are, of course, not mutually exclusive and it is likely that IBS is a heterogeneous disorder that results from multiple physiological disturbances.

Given this lack of a clear pathology, the many speculations about the role of depression in IBS are equally preliminary. Nonetheless, numerous pathophysiologic links between depression and IBS have been suggested. Depression can affect the perception of pain, and make individuals overly sensitive to normal stimuli, and depression's effect on the pain threshold may be the mediating factor between depression and IBS.[34] However, there may be more direct links. As noted above, dysregulation of the autonomic nervous system, serotonin, and the HPA axis have all been speculated to underlie IBS and these are also thought to be important in the pathophysiology of mood disorders as well. Many connections between the brain and GI system have led some investigators to refer to a "brain–gut" axis.[49] Theories range from those that suggest that depression and IBS are distinct disorders sharing underlying mechanisms to some who propose that IBS is a *forme fruste* of depression. More confident statements regarding the many possible relationships await a better understanding of the pathophysiology of the depressive disorders

■ CLINICAL PRESENTATION

The main features of IBS are distinct from the primary symptoms of depression as the disorder is defined by recurrent abdominal pain or discomfort and changes in the frequency or appearance of stool (Box 13-2 and **Table 13-1**). However, a number of systemic symptoms can be associated with IBS, particularly in its more severe forms, including fatigue, insomnia, and sexual dysfunction and these overlap with symptoms of depression. As with the discussion of peptic ulcers, in cases of possible overlap it is usually best to take an inclusive approach, diagnosing both IBS and depression in cases in which patients meet both criteria.

■ ASSESSMENT AND DIFFERENTIAL DIAGNOSIS

Definitive diagnosis is complicated by the heterogeneity of the functional disorders. There has been, however, some effort to identify more homogeneous subgroups based on tighter diagnostic criteria for IBS (e.g., the Rome Criteria III; Table 13-1) and on clinical features, including IBS diarrhea predominant, IBS constipation predominant, and postinfectious IBS. Much of the diagnostic workup for IBS involves ruling out other potential causes for abdominal

TABLE 13-1 Rome III Diagnostic Criteria* for Irritable Bowel Syndrome

Recurrent abdominal pain or discomfort** at least 3 days/month in the last 3 months associated with two or more of the following:
1. Improvement with defecation
2. 2.Onset associated with a change in frequency of stool
3. Onset associated with a change in form (appearance) of stool

*Criterion fulfilled for the last 3 months with symptom onset at least 6 months prior to diagnosis

**"Discomfort" means an uncomfortable sensation not described as pain.
In pathophysiology research and clinical trials, a pain/discomfort frequency of at least 2 days a week during screening evaluation is recommended for subject eligibility.
Copyright 2014 by Rome Foundation, Inc.
(Data from Rome III Diagnostic Criteria for Functional Gastrointestinal Disorders. Appendix A. Rome Foundation, Inc., 2014.)

pain, for which the list is long, but usually suggested by such "alarm" symptoms as fever, weight loss, or GI bleeding.[29]

When depression is comorbid, it is likely similar to that seen in depressed patients without IBS, with the addition of some amplification of the IBS symptoms. As noted above, it is a common comorbid condition, but not invariably associated. Thus, although one should investigate for mood disorders in IBS patients, we cannot assume their presence. A comprehensive diagnostic workup for depression and psychopathology is always indicated; as noted above it is usually best to take an inclusive approach toward symptoms consistent with a major depressive episode when considering such a diagnosis.

■ TREATMENT

Primary treatment of IBS usually involves symptomatic treatment of the diarrhea or constipation. A recent review comparing various approaches found no benefit with bulking agents (i.e., fiber supplements) but did see some with antispasmodics (such as cimetropium/dicyclomine, peppermint oil, pinaverium, and trimebutine).[50] Education is a critical component of care for these illnesses to reinforce reassurance about the nature of the disease as well as good dietary and hygiene practices.

Many patients with IBS receive anxiolytics and antidepressants.[31] Even absent comorbid depression, antidepressants can be helpful for IBS patients: SSRIs have been shown to improve overall symptoms and TCAs may be preferentially effective for abdominal pain.[50] The use of TCAs is limited by their many side effects, particularly anticholinergic side effects. In patients without comorbid depression, lower doses can be used to take advantage of the anticholinergic effects without their becoming intolerable. In depressed patients, SSRIs may be the initial drug of choice. Among the SSRIs, paroxetine is particularly anticholinergic; although often a downside of this drug, it may be an advantage for patients with diarrhea-predominant IBS.[51,52] Non-SSRIs, such as the SNRI duloxetine, are likely to be helpful as well although to date their support is mainly through open-label studies.[53] Indeed, although data are lacking, it is reasonable to assume that the standard antidepressants that show efficacy for depression in other situations will be useful in this context.

A variety of psychotherapies have been used for IBS—both for the disorder itself and for the comorbid depression, including CBT, psychodynamic psychotherapy, various relaxation therapies, and hypnosis. All have at least some positive clinical trials[29]; however when taken as a whole the effects of such therapies, particularly for IBS absent depression, have been equivocal.[54] Some of these disappointing results can be attributed to methodological problems with many of the studies, and more rigorous studies have shown significant improvement of IBS symptoms with CBT,[55,56] including self-administered CBT.[57] The CBT used emphasizes such techniques as self-monitoring, cognitive reappraisal, worry control, and problem-solving training.

CBT is, of course, an effective treatment for depression, including depression that is comorbid with IBS. Whether the improvement in IBS symptoms from psychotherapeutic treatments is related to treatment of underlying depression is unclear, but the mechanism of effect is thought to relate to more nonspecific factors, such as general stress reduction.[58] However, there may be more specific effects—one interesting study examined response to CBT in IBS patients using positron emission tomography (PET) and found that improvement was related to areas of the brain associated with attention to fear stimuli, danger orientation, and vigilance (e.g., anterior cingulated cortex and amygdale).[59]

INFLAMMATORY BOWEL DISEASE

■ EPIDEMIOLOGY

Patients with IBD have a high incidence of psychiatric comorbidity, predominantly depressive and anxiety symptoms, as well as major depressive disorder. Compared with the general population, IBD patients are twice as likely to have a depressive disorder (Fig. 13-1).[60] However, persistent depressive disorder (dysthymia) does not appear to be more prevalent in individuals with IBD than the general population.[60] The prevalence of depression and/or anxiety in IBD is estimated at 15% to 35% during remission and up to 60% for depression and 80% for anxiety during relapse.[61] Symptoms of IBD, which include abdominal pain, diarrhea, fatigue, malnutrition, weight loss, anemia, joint pain, anemia, hematochezia, and skin lesions,[62] can cause considerable psychiatric distress and lead to a significant decrement in quality of life.[63]

■ PATHOPHYSIOLOGY

IBD is a chronic, relapsing, and remitting bowel disorder involving inflammation of the intestinal mucosa (Box 13-2). There are two main subtypes: CD and ulcerative colitis (UC), which differ in the extent of GI tract involvement and mucosal injury. The exact etiology of IBD is unknown, but immunological, genetic, and environmental factors have been implicated as contributing causes.[64]

Inflammation may play a part in the pathogenesis of depression[65,66] as well. Individuals with depression have higher levels of proinflammatory cytokines,[67,68] which influence metabolism of monoamines such as serotonin, dopamine, and norepinephrine, all targets of currently used antidepressants.[69] Cytokines also induce changes in the HPA axis function, which in turn also induces mood changes.[70,71]

■ CLINICAL PRESENTATIONS

CD and UC may have overlapping clinical presentations and may be difficult to differentiate at initial onset (Box 13-3). Common symptoms of IBD include diarrhea, fever, abdominal pain, GI bleeding, weight loss, and fatigue. A hallmark of UC is bloody diarrhea whereas CD, particularly involving the ileum or right colon, is less likely to produce bleeding. As many as 10% of CD patients have flares without diarrhea and some children may present solely with poor growth. The systemic manifestations of fatigue or low-grade fevers as well as abdominal pain are more commonly associated with CD than UC, though they can be seen in both diseases. Complications more specific to CD include bowel obstruction or perforation, abdominal abscess, and fistulas. Symptoms may vary depending on the involvement of the GI tract.

The influence of depression in altering the clinical presentation of these diseases has not been well investigated and may not alter symptomatology. There also does not appear to be evidence indicating that the presentation of depression in patients with IBD is different than in that of the general population. However, since symptoms associated with inflammation, such as fatigue and sleep disturbances, can also be symptoms of depression, it is important to do a thorough assessment of the clinical picture.

■ COURSE AND NATURAL HISTORY

The cause and effect relationships between depression and IBD remain controversial.[63] Most studies examining the relationship between depression and the course of IBD suggest that depressive symptoms are more likely to be elevated around periods of active disease. It does appear that individuals are particularly vulnerable to depression around the time of diagnosis of IBD, as well as during disease flares.[72–74]

Depression prior to diagnosis may be a predisposing factor for the development of CD (RR, 2.39; CI, 1.40–3.98) though not for UC.[75] Depression appears to lead to more frequent and earlier relapses[60,72,74]; however, this remains somewhat controversial[61,73] and there is no conclusive evidence that depression contributes to or exacerbates IBD flares. Depression also negatively impacts quality of life[76] and treatment outcomes in individuals[77] with IBD.

Corticosteroids are the treatment for active IBD symptoms yet are also known to cause depressive symptoms in some individuals.[78] These generally occur later rather than early in the course of treatment and are dose-related.[79] In outpatient management, preferred dosages of prednisone are 40 mg daily or less, though higher doses are frequently used. Duration of treatment is generally limited to less than 3 months; however, in clinical practice, corticosteroid administration is often extended, which likely contributes to the burden of depression. Because corticosteroids are not effective in maintaining remission and long-term treatment carries many risks, they are used episodically in most patients. On the other hand, the successful treatment of IBD reduces the risk of depression in patients with IBD.[73]

■ ASSESSMENT AND DIFFERENTIAL DIAGNOSIS

The clinical history remains the most important tool in the diagnosis of IBD, but it is supplemented with laboratory tests (C-reactive protein and sedimentation rates), radiologic tests (particularly CT scans or MR imaging), and endoscopy to evaluate the nature and extent of inflammation.

As depression often co-occurs with IBD, clinicians need to remain alert to the possibility of comorbid psychiatric illness. The depression that accompanies IBD does not have a characteristic or distinctive clinical presentation that differentiates it from depression occurring in other medical illnesses. But given its frequency in IBD and its impact on both disease course and quality of life, routine screening is recommended.[61] There is no consensus on the best screening tool to use, but the Patient Health Questionnaire-9 (PHQ-9) is frequently used in primary care and specialty settings.

Proinflammatory cytokines, seen in inflammatory states, such as IBD, are known to produce a "sickness syndrome," which resembles depression in that it includes sleep disturbances, anorexia, cognitive dysfunction, fatigue, anxiety/irritability, and anhedonia.[80] Since these symptoms overlap with the symptoms of depression, it is important to use screening tools to aid in the diagnosis of depression in patients with IBD.

Elevated rates of anxiety are also found in IBD. There is an increased lifetime prevalence of panic disorder, generalized anxiety disorder, and obsessive-compulsive disorder in these patients.[60]

■ TREATMENT

Medications used in the treatment of IBD include aminosalicylates (in UC), corticosteroids, immunomodulators, biologics, and antibiotics (in CD). Some of these medications carry the risk of adverse effects on mood. As noted above, corticosteroids can often cause depression, and have also been known to cause symptoms of mania or hypomania, anxiety and/or irritability, and even psychosis.[79]

Reliable data to guide treatment of depression in patients with IBD are not currently available. Thus, the clinician should use general guidelines for treatment of depression until further evidence is available (**Box 13-5**), keeping in mind that SSRIs and serotonin-norepinephrine reuptake inhibitors (SNRIs) have GI side effects, including nausea, vomiting, and diarrhea. These are generally dose-related and tend to decrease over the first week or two of treatment. Sertraline seems to cause more diarrhea than other SSRIs. The risk of upper GI bleeding must also be considered and can be increased with SSRIs and venlafaxine.[26]

Choosing a form of psychotherapy also follows the more general guidelines for treating depression in general as there is currently no evidence favoring one particular form of psychotherapy for patients with both depression and IBD. Psychotherapy, particularly cognitive behavioral therapy (CBT), may be effective in treating depression in patients with IBD,[81] and may also improve global functioning and decrease IBD disease severity.[81,82] Improvement in psychiatric symptoms with the use of CBT lasts up to 1 year after treatment.[83]

■ SUMMARY

Depressive disorders are common in individuals with IBD, and screening for depression in these patients should be done regularly. Treatment of depression can lead to improved quality of life, and possibly to improvements in IBD activity.

LIVER DISEASE

■ INTRODUCTION

A large proportion of gastroenterology patients have chronic liver disease (CLD). CLD is usually caused by long-term injury to the liver from hepatotropic viruses, fatty liver, alcohol, and autoimmune hepatitis.[84] The vast majority of the research on depressive disorders among those living with CLD has focused on hepatitis C virus (HCV). This section on liver disease is divided into two parts. The first section is devoted exclusively to HCV and the latter section covers other liver diseases.

HEPATITIS C

■ EPIDEMIOLOGY[1]

Individuals living with HCV are disproportionately affected by depression, which is three to four times more prevalent in them than in the general US population (Fig. 13-1).[85–87] Individuals with HCV have a lifetime prevalence rate of depression between 34% and 44%[87,88] and current prevalence rates range from 28% to 81%.[85,87–91] Within samples of both veterans and civilians, rates for major depressive disorder ranged from 8% to 23%.[87,88,92] The most prevalent current diagnosis was adjustment disorder with depressed mood (40%) and the least prevalent was persistent depressive disorder (dysthymia) or depressive disorder not otherwise specified.[88]

Suicide is an important consideration in this population. Among HCV patients, the risk is higher in men and in those under the age of 45.[93] Compared to matched controls, HCV patients are twice as likely to have documented suicide attempts.[94] Rates of suicidal ideation range between 3.5% and 26% during antiviral treatment,[95,96] and suicidal ideation is a reason for early termination of antiviral therapy.[94] However, actual suicide attempts and completed suicides during antiviral therapy are rare (0.02%).[97]

In addition to depression, the most prevalent psychiatric disorders among individuals with HCV include alcohol and substance use disorders and anxiety disorders. The current prevalence of alcohol use disorder is 21% and the prevalence of a lifetime alcohol use disorder reaches 86%.[89–91] Current substance use disorders range from 30% to 60%,[90,91] and current posttraumatic stress disorder is found in 19% to 62%. The current lifetime prevalence of anxiety disorders can reach 71%.[89–91,95,98]

Increasing age is also associated with greater risk for depression,[88,99] and women with HCV are about twice as likely to have depression as men.[88] Methadone maintenance is an alarming risk factor for depression in HCV, with a fivefold increased risk of depression in HCV patients who are currently treated with methadone.[88]

■ PATHOPHYSIOLOGY

The HCV population in the United States has a high prevalence of intravenous (IV) and intranasal (IN) drug use, and current and former IV or IN drug users have an increased risk of psychiatric disorder, independent of HCV status (Box 13-1).[100] This has been posited as an explanation for the elevated depression prevalence in HCV, that is, the high prevalence of depression among HCV patients may be linked to the increased prevalence of IV/INDU, rather than to HCV per se. Another contributing factor for depression may be the stigma of living with

HCV.[87,101] Thus, increasing depressive symptom severity is associated with HCV-related stigma and poor acceptance of HCV.[88] The emotional consequences of living with HCV may account for impairments in quality of life and contribute to depressive disorders.[101,102] Finally, the specific pathophysiology activity of the HCV is also thought to contribute to the higher prevalence of depression,[88,103,104] since even those without a history of substance use disorders were found to have elevated rates of major depressive disorders.[105]

Both central and peripheral nervous system pathologies are implicated in HCV-associated depression.[106] Depressive symptoms may result from immunological changes, specifically interleukin-1 and tumor necrosis factor (TNF)[107] and/or from platelet serotonin (5-HT) changes.[88,103,104,108] Interferon-induced depression in patients undergoing interferon-based antiviral therapy may involve a decrease in 5-HT, HPA axis and cytokine activation, increased nitric oxide levels and intercellular adhesion molecule-1, and decreased peptidase levels.[109] Higher TNF–α levels and lower 5-HT prior to starting interferon-based antiviral therapy is associated with worsening somatic depressive symptoms during initial weeks of antiviral therapy.[110]

■ CLINICAL PRESENTATION AND COURSE

No significant differences have been found in HCV disease severity between those with current depressive disorders and those without.[87] However, depression seems to contribute significantly to fatigue and functional impairment, even more than HCV disease severity does,[87] and may adversely affect HCV by amplifying physical symptoms and by impairing treatment adherence and engagement and quality of life.[87,88] Those living with chronic HCV tend to experience an impaired quality of life.[111] Interestingly, these impairments in quality of life are associated with depressive symptoms and fatigue but not with age, gender, mode of acquiring the virus, alanine aminotransferase test (ALT) levels (a proxy for liver disease severity and injury), substance use, or social support.[112,113]

Among men infected with HCV who receive a liver transplant, recurrence of HCV is associated with depression.[114] Similarly, a 2011 study evaluated three distinct trajectories of depression following liver transplantation for alcoholic liver disease: low depression, increasing depression, high depression. A larger percentage of HCV patients were in the high depression group than in the low and increasing depression groups. Depressive symptom severity, the strongest predictor of survival following liver transplant for patients with alcoholic liver disease, predicted poorer survival rates independent of HCV status.[115]

The neurovegetative and somatic symptoms of depression are also common symptoms of chronic HCV.[102,111] Fatigue and malaise are the most common symptoms in patients with co-occurring HCV and depressive disorders. Due to this overlap in symptoms, it is important to differentiate depression from HCV. The cognitive-affective subscales of the Beck Depression Inventory-Second Edition (BDI-II) appear to be a more valid measure of depression in these patients than is the somatic subscale.[116] The overlap between the BDI somatic subscale and the side effects of antiviral therapy provides an additional reason for relying on the cognitive-affective subscale of the BDI-II to differentiate depression from HCV.

There is little evidence regarding the natural course of depression in patients with untreated HCV, but there are abundant data on depression during the course of interferon-based antiviral treatment. Interferon-based antiviral therapy was the gold standard for treating HCV until 2013 and is well known to be associated with onset or exacerbation of depressive symptoms.[95,107,117–119] Twenty to sixty percent of HCV patients treated with interferon-based antiviral therapy may develop depression.[120]

Depression can profoundly impact interferon-based antiviral treatment through both behavioral and biological pathways. First,

---

[1]This is an abbreviated review of depression and hepatitis C. For a thorough review please see Chapter 11, Depression and Infectious Diseases.

regarding the behavioral pathways, depressive disorders jeopardize engagement and adherence in HCV treatment.[85] Thus, during HCV treatment, depressive disorders can lead to noncompliance and relapse on alcohol or substances.[121] In addition, emergent depression is a major reason both for withholding and discontinuing interferon-based antiviral treatment.[122] However, some data suggest that experiencing depression during antiviral therapy may be associated with *lower* rates of discontinuing treatment, thought to occur because these patients may be better connected to mental health treatment and access to resources for HCV treatment assistance.[121,123] In terms of biological pathways, there are mixed findings regarding the impact of depression on the viral response to HCV therapy. Some studies suggest that depressive symptoms may be associated with lower rates of viral response to treatment,[124,125] while other studies suggest that the onset of depressive symptoms does not negatively impact viral response.[121,123,124]

■ ASSESSMENT AND DIFFERENTIAL DIAGNOSIS

HCV practice guidelines and consensus reports recommend that all HCV patients be systematically assessed for psychiatric disorders.[126,127] Because of the persistent underdiagnosis of depressive disorders among individuals with HCV,[88,89] and because of the overlap between depressive and HCV symptoms, repeated assessment of depressive symptoms is highly recommended.[128] Self-report scales recommended for use in this population include the Patient Health Questionnaire-9 (PHQ-9), Center for Epidemiologic Studies-Depression Scale (CES-D), and the BDI-II.[129,130] The HAM-7 is a clinician-administered scale that has comparable accuracy as the PHQ-9 in detecting depression in this population.[130]

■ TREATMENT
Pharmacotherapy

Much of the empirical evidence for pharmacologic treatment of depression in HCV comes from studies of patients experiencing emergent or worsening depressive symptoms when undergoing interferon-based antiviral therapy (Box 13-5 and **Box 13-7**). Many clinical trials specifically exclude patients with pre-existing depressive disorders prior to starting interferon-based antiviral treatment. The few randomized placebo-controlled trials that exist use small samples and study either prophylactic use of antidepressant medication or treatment of depressive symptoms emerging after the initiation of antiviral therapy.[131] When compared to placebo, prophylactic treatment of depression with paroxetine or citalopram did not result in benefits,[132,133] but, when treating incident depression, citalopram resulted in decreased depressive symptoms.[134] Among HCV patients with no prior psychiatric history undergoing antiviral therapy, escitalopram outperformed placebo in preventing incident depression and in treating depressive symptoms.[135] SSRIs are considered first-line treatment, and the choice of agents should be guided by consideration of side effects and potential drug–drug interactions, especially if patients are also using combination antiviral therapies that include certain protease inhibitors, which may interfere with cytochrome 3A4 hepatic metabolism. ECT has also been reported to be effective.[136]

As the current landscape of antiviral therapies for HCV is rapidly changing, the following website is useful to obtain up-to-date information about drug interactions: www.hep-druginteractions.org

---

BOX 13-7
DRUGS THAT CAN CAUSE DEPRESSIVE SYMPTOMS

Corticosteroids

Interferon-based antivirals

Psychological Treatment

Evon et al.[137] outline empirically supported depression treatments for patients undergoing treatment of HCV. The Cognitive Behavioral Treatment for Depression and Adherence (CBT-AD) model developed by Safren et al. for HIV-infected individuals with depression combines CBT with problem-solving skills targeting medication adherence and motivational interviewing.[138] This treatment holds promise for successful treatment of depression among HCV patients. Another model for treating depression is group-based Cognitive Behavioral Stress Management (CBSM).[137,139] Exercise helps to alleviate depressive symptoms and can also decrease fatigue during antiviral therapy.[140,141] SAMSHA and the Department of Veterans Affairs HCV treatment guidelines recommend low-impact exercise, if approved by one's medical provider.

OTHER LIVER DISEASES

In this section, we discuss depression among liver diseases broadly. The term CLD encompasses several different diagnostic entities with differing etiologies: viral (hepatitis), toxic (alcohol), and metabolic (nonalcoholic fatty liver disease [NAFLD]). Cirrhosis is scarring of the liver and can occur in many types of liver disease but the most common causes of cirrhosis are chronic heavy alcohol use and hepatitis.

■ EPIDEMIOLOGY

Among patients with CLD, 14% to 24% have a diagnosis of depression, and up to 53% of patients with CLD have subclinical depressive symptoms (Fig. 13-1).[142] Women and patients who overuse alcohol are most likely to have depression.[142]

From 1988 to 2008, the prevalence of CLD in the United States has steadily increased. NAFLD contributes most to this increase.[143] Among those living with NAFLD, the presence of hypertension, smoking, history of lung disease, being female, and being non-African American increases the risk for depression.[142] Depression is significantly related to more severe hepatocyte ballooning (i.e., degeneration) among patients with NAFLD.[142]

Between 24% and 57% of patients with liver cirrhosis have moderate to severe depression, as measured by the BDI[144] or the HAM-D.[145] In patients with cirrhosis, as the number of GI symptoms increase, so does depression severity and impairment in quality of life.[146] CLD may result in liver transplantation. The prevalence of depressive disorders is elevated following liver transplantation, and occurs in 20% to 30% of liver transplant recipients.[147] Among patients undergoing liver transplantation, younger age, being unmarried, being infected with HCV, and having a history of substance use and depression are associated with increased likelihood of depression following transplantation.[115] Those with more depressive symptoms and greater symptom severity have significantly poorer survival rates following transplant. The proximity of depression following the transplantation seems to matter, but depression prior to transplant apparently does not predict posttransplant survival.[114] However, after adjusting for liver disease severity, transplant candidates who are depressed are more likely to die awaiting transplantation than nondepressed candidates.[114]

Rates of depressive disorders may be higher among patients with hepatitis B virus (HBV) than the general population, though this may be related to excessive alcohol use.[3] Patients with NAFLD have a higher prevalence of depression than patients with HBV (27% NAFLD vs. 4% HBV)[84] though this may reflect an underestimate of the prevalence of depression.[148] There is evidence that increasing severity of HBV is inversely related to quality of life; however, those with HBV generally have better quality of life, and less severe and less prevalent depressive disorders than patients with HCV.[148]

Other psychiatric disorders in addition to depression are prevalent in CLD patients. Among patients with NAFLD, 25% meet the clinical cut-off for an anxiety disorder and another 45% have subclinical anxiety.[142] Among patients with cirrhosis, sleep disorders are highly prevalent (69%), and are significantly associated with depression and psychological distress.[144]

■ PATHOPHYSIOLOGY

Depression is accompanied by an immune response among patients with cirrhosis. Increased CD8 levels in T-lymphocyte subsets is positively related to depression after controlling for age and liver disease prognosis.[145]

■ CLINICAL PRESENTATION

There are no data bearing on the differences or similarities of depression phenomenology in patients with various types of CLD. In general, patients with CLD have heightened somatic symptoms of depression as compared to the general population with depression.[144] Among those with CLD, depression may be a reactive depression due to declining health status, and there is a strong association between depressive symptom severity and liver function.[144]

■ DIAGNOSIS AND DIFFERENTIAL DIAGNOSIS

As noted above, validated self-report and clinician administered measures of depression are recommended for all patients with CLD. Once the diagnostic assessment is completed, the next step involves a search for etiological and maintaining factors to guide the choice of treatment modality. For example, if the depression assessment reveals the CLD patient's perception of declining health and functional limitations perpetuates depressive cognitions, rumination, and decreased activity, then CBT is indicated to interrupt the ruminative cycle and institute behavioral activation. In addition, a stimulant medication or antidepressant with stimulant properties may also be used to increase activation if CLD patient is suffering from pronounced fatigue.

■ TREATMENT

There are few data regarding treatment of depression in non-HCV liver disease, probably because depression is most prevalent and impactful in that group. Extrapolating from the depression treatment literature in HCV, we recommend use of evidence-based psychotherapies for treating depression among CLD patients, with a focus on psychoeducation and careful attention to the overlap between somatic symptoms due to liver disease and somatic symptoms due to depression. Antidepressant pharmacotherapy is also crucial when indicated. However, antidepressant medications can cause drug-induced liver damage. The antidepressants with the least potential for hepatotoxicity are citalopram, escitalopram, paroxetine, and fluvoxamine. Those with greater hepatotoxic risks are MAO inhibitors, tricyclic/tetracyclics, nefazadone, duloxetine, and bupropion.[149] For patients with cirrhosis, duloxetine and MAOIs should not be prescribed. Escitalopram dosages should not exceed 10 mg/day, and buproprion should be prescribed with caution, in doses not to exceed 75 mg/day. Venlafaxine dosage should be reduced by 50%, and mirtazapine dosage should be decreased as clearance is reduced by 30%.[150]

CONCLUSION

Although the early ambition of psychosomatic theorists to find examples of direct causation and associated cures now seems naive, the basic notion that our emotions can influence internal autonomic processes has become an accepted tenet in medicine (**Box 13-8**). It is clear that depression and other psychiatric disorders can worsen the course of GI disorders, and that interventions to alleviate emotional disorders can aid recovery from both disorders as well. Future research, emphasizing a holistic approach toward these disorders, holds the promise of helping to alleviate the considerable suffering caused by these often chronic diseases.

BOX 13-8
SUMMARY

- The brain and the gut are intimately connected so it should be no surprise that they had a bidirectional relationship of mutual influence
- Explanatory models relying on cause and effect relationship are usually too simplistic; it is more useful to think of how GI diseases and mental diseases can influence each other
- Although standard antidepressant treatments, including pharmacological and psychotherapeutic, remain useful for patients with comorbid GI diseases, there are some specific side effects that need to be considered

REFERENCES

1. Alexander F. The influence of psychological factors upon gastro-intestinal disturbances: a symposium. *Psychoanal Quarter*. 1934;3:501–588.

2. Malfertheiner P, Chan FK, McColl KE. Peptic ulcer disease. *Lancet*. 2009;374:1449–1461.

3. Goodwin RD, Keyes KM, Stein MB, Talley NJ. Peptic ulcer and mental disorders among adults in the community: the role of nicotine and alcohol use disorders. *Psychosom Med*. 2009;71:463–468.

4. Scott KM, Alonso J, de Jonge P, et al. Associations between DSM-IV mental disorders and onset of self-reported peptic ulcer in the World Mental Health Surveys. *J Psychosom Res*. 2013;75:121–127.

5. Farmer A, Korszun A, Owen MJ, et al. Medical disorders in people with recurrent depression. *Br J Psychiatry*. 2008;192:351–355.

6. Patten SB, Beck CA, Kassam A, Williams JV, Barbui C, Metz LM. Long-term medical conditions and major depression: strength of association for specific conditions in the general population. *Can J Psychiatry*. 2005;50:195–202.

7. Yeomans ND. The ulcer sleuths: The search for the cause of peptic ulcers. *J Gastroenterol Hepatol*. 2011;26(Suppl 1):35–41.

8. Hyman SE. Another one bites the dust: an infectious origin for peptic ulcers. *Harv Rev Psychiatry*. 1994;1:294–295.

9. Matsushima Y, Aoyama N, Fukuda H, et al. Gastric ulcer formation after the Hanshin-Awaji earthquake: a case study of Helicobacter pylori infection and stress-induced gastric ulcers. *Helicobacter*. 1999;4:94–99.

10. Levenstein S. The very model of a modern etiology: a biopsychosocial view of peptic ulcer. *Psychosom Med*. 2000;62:176–185.

11. Levenstein S, Kaplan GA, Smith MW. Psychological predictors of peptic ulcer incidence in the Alameda County Study. *J Clin Gastroenterol*. 1997;24:140–146.

12. Anda RF, Williamson DF, Escobedo LG, Remington PL, Mast EE, Madans JH. Self-perceived stress and the risk of peptic ulcer disease. A longitudinal study of US adults. *Arch Intern Med*. 1992;152:829–833.

13. Levenstein S, Kaplan GA, Smith M. Sociodemographic characteristics, life stressors, and peptic ulcer. A prospective study. *J Clin Gastroenterol*. 1995;21:185–192.

14. Overmier JB, Murison R. Restoring psychology's role in peptic ulcer. *Appl Psychol Health Well Being*. 2013;5:5–27.

15. Fink G. Stress controversies: post-traumatic stress disorder, hippocampal volume, gastroduodenal ulceration*. *J Neuroendocrinol*. 2011;23:107–117.

16. Ulrich-Lai YM, Herman JP. Neural regulation of endocrine and autonomic stress responses. *Nat Rev Neurosci*. 2009;10:397–409.

17. Yano S, Fujiwara A, Ozaki Y, Harada M. Gastric blood flow responses to autonomic nerve stimulation and related pharmacological studies in rats. *J Pharm Pharmacol*. 1983;35:641–646.

18. Ebrecht M, Hextall J, Kirtley LG, Taylor A, Dyson M, Weinman J. Perceived stress and cortisol levels predict speed of wound healing in healthy male adults. *Psychoneuroendocrinology*. 2004;29:798–809.

19. Wilhelmsen I, Berstad A. Reduced relapse rate in duodenal ulcer disease leads to normalization of psychological distress: twelve-year follow-up. *Scand J Gastroenterol*. 2004;39:717–721.

20. Levinstein MR, Samuels BA. Mechanisms underlying the antidepressant response and treatment resistance. *Front Behav Neurosci*. 2014;8:208.

21. Zhang S, Xu Z, Gao Y, et al. Bidirectional crosstalk between stress-induced gastric ulcer and depression under chronic stress. *PloS One*. 2012;7:e51148.

22. Levenstein S, Prantera C, Varvo V, et al. Long-term symptom patterns in duodenal ulcer: psychosocial factors. *J Psychosom Res*. 1996;41:465–472.

23. Boland RJ. Depression in medical illness. In: Stein MD, Kupfer D, Schatzberg AF, eds. *The American Psychiatric Press Textbook of Mood Disorders*. Washington, DC: American Psychiatric Press; 2006.

24. Abdel-Sater KA, Abdel-Daiem WM, Sayyed Bakheet M. The gender difference of selective serotonin reuptake inhibitor, fluoxetine in adult rats with stress-induced gastric ulcer. *Eur J Pharmacol*. 2012;688:42–48.

25. Andrade C, Sandarsh S, Chethan KB, Nagesh KS. Serotonin reuptake inhibitor antidepressants and abnormal bleeding: a review for clinicians and a reconsideration of mechanisms. *J Clin Psychiatry*. 2010;71:1565–1575.

26. de Abajo FJ. Effects of selective serotonin reuptake inhibitors on platelet function: mechanisms, clinical outcomes and implications for use in elderly patients. *Drugs Aging*. 2011;28:345–367.

27. Itatsu T, Nagahara A, Hojo M, et al. Use of selective serotonin reuptake inhibitors and upper gastrointestinal disease. *Intern Med*. 2011;50:713–717.

28. Talley NJ, Boyce PM, Jones M. Predictors of health care seeking for irritable bowel syndrome: a population based study. *Gut*. 1997;41:394–398.

29. Crone CC, Dobbelstein CR. Gastrointestinal disorders. In: Levenson JL, ed. *The American Psychiatric Publishing Textbook of Psychosomatic Medicine*, 2nd ed. Washington, DC: American Psychiatric Press; 2011.

30. Palsson OS, Drossman DA. Psychiatric and psychological dysfunction in irritable bowel syndrome and the role of psychological treatments. *Gastroenterol Clin N Am*. 2005;34:281–303.

31. Ladabaum U, Boyd E, Zhao WK, et al. Diagnosis, comorbidities, and management of irritable bowel syndrome in patients in a large health maintenance organization. *Clin Gastroenterol Hepatol*. 2012;10:37–45.

32. Okami Y, Kato T, Nin G, et al. Lifestyle and psychological factors related to irritable bowel syndrome in nursing and medical school students. *J Gastroenterol*. 2011;46:1403–1410.

33. Tosic-Golubovic S, Miljkovic S, Nagorni A, Lazarevic D, Nikolic G. Irritable bowel syndrome, anxiety, depression and personality characteristics. *Psychiatr Danub*. 2010;22:418–424.

34. Thijssen AY, Jonkers DM, Leue C, et al. Dysfunctional cognitions, anxiety and depression in irritable bowel syndrome. *J Clin Gastroenterol*. 2010;44:e236–e241.

35. Mykletun A, Jacka F, Williams L, et al. Prevalence of mood and anxiety disorder in self reported irritable bowel syndrome (IBS). An epidemiological population based study of women. *BMC Gastroenterol*. 2010;10:88.

36. Ladep NG, Okeke EN, Samaila AA, et al. Irritable bowel syndrome among patients attending General Outpatients' clinics in Jos, Nigeria. *Eur J Gastroenterol Hepatol*. 2007;19:795–799.

37. Son YJ, Jun EY, Park JH. Prevalence and risk factors of irritable bowel syndrome in Korean adolescent girls: a school-based study. *Int J Nurs Stud*. 2009;46:76–84.

38. Dong YY, Zuo XL, Li CQ, Yu YB, Zhao QJ, Li YQ. Prevalence of irritable bowel syndrome in Chinese college and university students assessed using Rome III criteria. *World J Gastroenterol*. 2010;16:4221–4226.

39. Beesley H, Rhodes J, Salmon P. Anger and childhood sexual abuse are independently associated with irritable bowel syndrome. *Br J Health Psychol*. 2010;15:389–399.

40. Lessa LM, Chein MB, da Silva DS, et al. Irritable bowel syndrome in women with chronic pelvic pain in a Northeast Brazilian city. *Rev Bras Ginecol Obstet*. 2013;35:84–89.

41. Bradford K, Shih W, Videlock EJ, et al. Association between early adverse life events and irritable bowel syndrome. *Clin Gastroenterol Hepatol*. 2012;10:385–390.e1–3.

42. Heitkemper MM, Cain KC, Burr RL, Jun SE, Jarrett ME. Is childhood abuse or neglect associated with symptom reports and physiological measures in women with irritable bowel syndrome? *Biol Res Nurs*. 2011;13:399–408.

43. Grover M, Herfarth H, Drossman DA. The functional-organic dichotomy: postinfectious irritable bowel syndrome and inflammatory bowel disease-irritable bowel syndrome. *Clin Gastroenterol Hepatol*. 2009;7:48–53.

44. Furgala A, Mazur M, Jablonski K, et al. Myoelectric and autonomic nervous system activity in patients with irritable bowel syndrome. *Folia Med Cracov*. 2008;49:49–58.

45. Ringel Y, Drossman DA, Leserman JL, et al. Effect of abuse history on pain reports and brain responses to aversive visceral stimulation: an FMRI study. *Gastroenterology*. 2008;134:396–404.

46. Long MD, Drossman DA. Inflammatory bowel disease, irritable bowel syndrome, or what?: A challenge to the functional-organic dichotomy. *Am J Gastroenterol*. 2010;105:1796–1798.

47. Keszthelyi D, Troost FJ, Jonkers DM, et al. Serotonergic reinforcement of intestinal barrier function is impaired in irritable bowel syndrome. *Aliment Pharmacol Ther*. 2014;40:392–402.

48. Spiller R. Recent advances in understanding the role of serotonin in gastrointestinal motility in functional bowel disorders: alterations in 5-HT signalling and metabolism in human disease. *Neurogastroenterol Motil*. 2007;19(Suppl 2):25–31.

49. Bellini M, Gambaccini D, Stasi C, Urbano MT, Marchi S, Usai-Satta P. Irritable bowel syndrome: A disease still searching for pathogenesis, diagnosis and therapy. *World J Gastroenterol*. 2014;20:8807–8820.

50. Ruepert L, Quartero AO, de Wit NJ, et al. Bulking agents, antispasmodics and antidepressants for the treatment of irritable bowel syndrome. *Cochrane Database Syst Rev*. 2011;(8):Cd003460.

51. Trinkley KE, Nahata MC. Medication management of irritable bowel syndrome. *Digestion*. 2014;89:253–267.

52. Masand PS, Pae CU, Krulewicz S, et al. A double-blind, randomized, placebo-controlled trial of paroxetine controlled-release in irritable bowel syndrome. *Psychosomatics*. 2009;50:78–86.

53. Kaplan A, Franzen MD, Nickell PV, Ransom D, Lebovitz PJ. An open-label trial of duloxetine in patients with irritable bowel syndrome and comorbid generalized anxiety disorder. *Int J Psychiatry Clin Pract*. 2014;18:11–15.

54. Zijdenbos IL, de Wit NJ, van der Heijden GJ, Rubin G, Quartero AO. Psychological treatments for the management of irritable bowel syndrome. *Cochrane Database Syst Rev*. 2009;(1):CD006442.

55. Li L, Xiong L, Zhang S, Yu Q, Chen M. Cognitive-behavioral therapy for irritable bowel syndrome: a meta-analysis. *J Psychosom Res*. 2014;77:1–12.

56. Kennedy TM, Chalder T, McCrone P, et al. Cognitive behavioural therapy in addition to antispasmodic therapy for irritable bowel syndrome in primary care: randomised controlled trial. *Health Technol Assess*. 2006;10:iii-iv, ix-x, 1–67.

57. Lackner JM, Jaccard J, Krasner SS, Katz LA, Gudleski GD, Holroyd K. Self-administered cognitive behavior therapy for moderate to severe irritable bowel syndrome: clinical efficacy, tolerability, feasibility. *Clin Gastroenterol Hepatol*. 2008;6:899–906.

58. Lackner JM, Jaccard J, Krasner SS, Katz LA, Gudleski GD, Blanchard EB. How does cognitive behavior therapy for irritable bowel syndrome work? A mediational analysis of a randomized clinical trial. *Gastroenterology*. 2007;133:433–444.

59. Lackner JM, Lou Coad M, Mertz HR, et al. Cognitive therapy for irritable bowel syndrome is associated with reduced limbic activity, GI symptoms, and anxiety. *Behav Res Therapy*. 2006;44:621–638.

60. Walker JR, Ediger JP, Graff LA, et al. The Manitoba IBD cohort study: a population-based study of the prevalence of lifetime and 12-month anxiety and mood disorders. *Am J Gastroenterol*. 2008;103:1989–1997.

61. Mikocka-Walus AA, Turnbull DA, Moulding NT, Wilson IG, Andrews JM, Holtmann GJ. Controversies surrounding the comorbidity of depression and anxiety in inflammatory bowel disease patients: a literature review. *Inflamm Bowel Dis*. 2007;13:225–234.

62. Szigethy E, McLafferty L, Goyal A. Inflammatory bowel disease. *Child Adolesc Psychiatr Clin N Am*. 2010;19:301–318, ix.

63. Lesage AC, Hagege H, Tucat G, Gendre JP. Results of a national survey on quality of life in inflammatory bowel diseases. *Clin Res Hepatol Gastroenterol*. 2011;35:117–124.

64. Actis GC, Pellicano R, Rosina F. Inflammatory bowel diseases: Current problems and future tasks. *World J Gastrointest Pharmacol Ther*. 2014;5:169–174.

65. Maes M. Major depression and activation of the inflammatory response system. *Adv Exp Med Biol*. 1999;461:25–46.

66. Haroon E, Raison CL, Miller AH. Psychoneuroimmunology meets neuropsychopharmacology: translational implications of the impact of inflammation on behavior. *Neuropsychopharmacology*. 2012;37:137–162.

67. Howren MB, Lamkin DM, Suls J. Associations of depression with C-reactive protein, IL-1, and IL-6: a meta-analysis. *Psychosom Med*. 2009;71:171–186.

68. Dowlati Y, Herrmann N, Swardfager W, et al. A meta-analysis of cytokines in major depression. *Biol Psychiatry*. 2010;67:446–457.

69. Dunn AJ, Wang J, Ando T. Effects of cytokines on cerebral neurotransmission. Comparison with the effects of stress. *Adv Exp Med Biol*. 1999;461:117–127.

70. Raison CL, Capuron L, Miller AH. Cytokines sing the blues: inflammation and the pathogenesis of depression. *Trends Immunol*. 2006;27:24–31.

71. Raison CL, Borisov AS, Woolwine BJ, Massung B, Vogt G, Miller AH. Interferon-alpha effects on diurnal hypothalamic-pituitary-adrenal axis activity: relationship with proinflammatory cytokines and behavior. *Mol Psychiatry*. 2010;15:535–547.

72. Kurina LM, Goldacre MJ, Yeates D, Gill LE. Depression and anxiety in people with inflammatory bowel disease. *J Epidemiol Community Health*. 2001;55:716–720.

73. Nahon S, Lahmek P, Durance C, et al. Risk factors of anxiety and depression in inflammatory bowel disease. *Inflamm Bowel Dis*. 2012;18:2086–2091.

74. Mittermaier C, Dejaco C, Waldhoer T, et al. Impact of depressive mood on relapse in patients with inflammatory bowel disease: a prospective 18-month follow-up study. *Psychosom Med*. 2004;66:79–84.

75. Ananthakrishnan AN, Khalili H, Pan A, et al. Association between depressive symptoms and incidence of Crohn's disease and ulcerative colitis: results from the Nurses' Health Study. *Clin Gastroenterol Hepatol*. 2013;11:57–62.

76. Nigro G, Angelini G, Grosso SB, Caula G, Sategna-Guidetti C. Psychiatric predictors of noncompliance in inflammatory bowel disease: psychiatry and compliance. *J Clin Gastroenterol*. 2001;32:66–68.

77. Persoons P, Vermeire S, Demyttenaere K, et al. The impact of major depressive disorder on the short- and long-term outcome of Crohn's disease treatment with infliximab. *Aliment Pharmacol Ther*. 2005;22:101–110.

78. Yang YX, Lichtenstein GR. Corticosteroids in Crohn's disease. *Am J Gastroenterol*. 2002;97:803–823.

79. Warrington TP, Bostwick JM. Psychiatric adverse effects of corticosteroids. *Mayo Clin Proc*. 2006;81:1361–1367.

80. Graff LA, Walker JR, Bernstein CN. Depression and anxiety in inflammatory bowel disease: a review of comorbidity and management. *Inflamm Bowel Dis*. 2009;15:1105–1118.

81. Szigethy E, Carpenter J, Baum E, et al. Case study: longitudinal treatment of adolescents with depression and inflammatory bowel disease. *J Am Acad Child Adolesc Psychiatry*. 2006;45:396–400.

82. Mackner LM, Greenley RN, Szigethy E, Herzer M, Deer K, Hommel KA. Psychosocial issues in pediatric inflammatory bowel disease: report of the North American Society for Pediatric Gastroenterology, Hepatology, and Nutrition. *J Pediatr Gastroenterol Nutr*. 2013;56:449–458.

83. Szigethy E, Hardy D, Craig AE, Low C, Kukic S. Girls connect: effects of a support group for teenage girls with inflammatory bowel disease and their mothers. *Inflamm Bowel Dis*. 2009;15:1127–1128.

84. Weinstein AA, Kallman Price J, Stepanova M, et al. Depression in patients with nonalcoholic fatty liver disease and chronic viral hepatitis B and C. *Psychosomatics*. 2011;52:127–132.

85. Nelligan JA, Loftis JM, Matthews AM, Zucker BL, Linke AM, Hauser P. Depression comorbidity and antidepressant use in veterans with chronic hepatitis C: results from a retrospective chart review. *J Clin Psychiatry*. 2008;69:810–816.

86. Basseri B, Yamini D, Chee G, Enayati PD, Tran T, Poordad F. Comorbidities associated with the increasing burden of hepatitis C infection. *Liver Int*. 2010;30:1012–1018.

87. Dwight MM, Kowdley KV, Russo JE, Ciechanowski PS, Larson AM, Katon WJ. Depression, fatigue, and functional disability in patients with chronic hepatitis C. *J Psychosom Res*. 2000;49:311–317.

88. Golden J, O'Dwyer AM, Conroy RM. Depression and anxiety in patients with hepatitis C: prevalence, detection rates and risk factors. *Gen Hosp Psychiatry*. 2005;27:431–438.

89. Lehman CL, Cheung RC. Depression, anxiety, post-traumatic stress, and alcohol-related problems among veterans with chronic hepatitis C. *Am J Gastroenterol*. 2002;97:2640–2646.

90. Fireman M, Indest DW, Blackwell A, Whitehead AJ, Hauser P. Addressing tri-morbidity (hepatitis C, psychiatric disorders, and substance use): the importance of routine mental health screening as a component of a comanagement model of care. *Clin Infect Dis*. 2005;40(Suppl 5):S286–S291.

91. El-Serag HB, Kunik M, Richardson P, Rabeneck L. Psychiatric disorders among veterans with hepatitis C infection. *Gastroenterology*. 2002;123:476–482.

92. Yovtcheva SP, Rifai MA, Moles JK, Van der Linden BJ. Psychiatric comorbidity among hepatitis C-positive patients. *Psychosomatics*. 2001;42:411–415.

93. Kristiansen MG, Løchen ML, Gutteberg TJ, Mortensen L, Eriksen BO, Florholmen J. Total and cause-specific mortality rates in a prospective study of community-acquired hepatitis C virus infection in northern Norway. *J Viral Hepat*. 2011;18:237–244.

94. Rifflet H, Vuillemin E, Oberti F, et al. [Suicidal impulses in patients with chronic viral hepatitis C during or after therapy with interferon alpha]. *Gastroenterol Clin Biol*. 1998;22:353–357.

95. Dieperink E, Ho SB, Tetrick L, Thuras P, Dua K, Willenbring ML. Suicidal ideation during interferon-alpha2b and ribavirin treatment of patients with chronic hepatitis C. *Gen Hosp Psychiatry*. 2004;26:237–240.

96. Papafragkakis H, Rao MS, Moehlen M, et al. Depression and pegylated interferon-based hepatitis C treatment. *Int J Infereron Cytokine Mediator Res*. 2012;4:25–35.

97. Sockalingam S, Links PS, Abbey SE. Suicide risk in hepatitis C and during interferon-alpha therapy: a review and clinical update. *J Viral Hepat*. 2011;18:153–160.

98. Yates WR, Gleason O. Hepatitis C and depression. *Depress Anxiety*. 1998;7:188–193.

99. Kraus MR, Schafer A, Csef H, Scheurlen M, Faller H. Emotional state, coping styles, and somatic variables in patients with chronic hepatitis C. *Psychosomatics*. 2000;41:377–384.

100. Prevention. CfDCa. Hepatitis C Information for Professionals [6/15/2013]. Available at http://www.cdc.gov/hepatitis/HCV/index.htm.

101. Glacken M, Kernohan G, Coates V. Diagnosed with Hepatitis C: a descriptive exploratory study. *Int J Nurs Stud*. 2001;38:107–116.

102. Bailey DE Jr, Landerman L, Barroso J, et al. Uncertainty, symptoms, and quality of life in persons with chronic hepatitis C. *Psychosomatics*. 2009;50:138–146.

103. McDonald EM, Mann AH, Thomas HC. Interferons as mediators of psychiatric morbidity. An investigation in a trial of recombinant alpha-interferon in hepatitis-B carriers. *Lancet*. 1987;2:1175–1178.

104. Denicoff KD, Rubinow DR, Papa MZ, et al. The neuropsychiatric effects of treatment with interleukin-2 and lymphokine-activated killer cells. *Ann Intern Med*. 1987;107:293–300.

105. Carta MG, Hardoy MC, Garofalo A, et al. Association of chronic hepatitis C with major depressive disorders: irrespective of interferon-alpha therapy. *Clin Pract Epidemiol Ment Health*. 2007;3:22.

106. Giunta B, Somboonwit C, Nikolic WV, et al. Psychiatric implications of hepatitis-C infection. *Crit Rev Neurobiol*. 2007;19:79–118.

107. Loftis JM, Huckans M, Ruimy S, Hinrichs DJ, Hauser P. Depressive symptoms in patients with chronic hepatitis C are correlated with elevated plasma levels of interleukin-1beta and tumor necrosis factor-alpha. *Neuroscie Lett*. 2008;430:264–268.

108. Schaefer M, Schwaiger M, Pich M, Lieb K, Heinz A. Neurotransmitter changes by interferon-alpha and therapeutic implications. *Pharmacopsychiatry*. 2003;36(Suppl 3):S203–S206.

109. Asnis GM, De La Garza R 2nd. Interferon-induced depression in chronic hepatitis C: a review of its prevalence, risk factors, biology, and treatment approaches. *J Clin Gastroenterol*. 2006;40:322–335.

110. Loftis JM, Patterson AL, Wilhelm CJ, et al. Vulnerability to somatic symptoms of depression during interferon-alpha therapy for hepatitis C: a 16-week prospective study. *J Psychosom Res*. 2013;74:57–63.

111. Lim JK, Cronkite R, Goldstein MK, Cheung RC. The impact of chronic hepatitis C and comorbid psychiatric illnesses on health-related quality of life. *J Clin Gastroenterol*. 2006;40:528–534.

112. Miller ER, Hiller JE, Shaw DR. Quality of life in HCV-infection: lack of association with ALT levels. *Aust N Z J Public Health*. 2001;25:355–361.

113. Hussain KB, Fontana RJ, Moyer CA, Su GL, Sneed-Pee N, Lok AS. Comorbid illness is an important determinant of health-related quality of life in patients with chronic hepatitis C. *Am J Gastroenterol*. 2001;96:2737–2744.

114. Singh N, Gayowski T, Wagener MM, Marino IR. Depression in patients with cirrhosis. Impact on outcome. *Dig Dis Sci*. 1997;42:1421–1427.

115. DiMartini A, Dew MA, Chaiffetz D, Fitzgerald MG, Devera ME, Fontes P. Early trajectories of depressive symptoms after liver transplantation for alcoholic liver disease predicts long-term survival. *Am J Transplant*. 2011;11:1287–1295.

116. Patterson AL, Morasco BJ, Fuller BE, Indest DW, Loftis JM, Hauser P. Screening for depression in patients with hepatitis C using the Beck Depression Inventory-II: do somatic symptoms compromise validity? *Gen Hosp Psychiatry*. 2011;33:354–362.

117. Dieperink E, Ho SB, Thuras P, Willenbring ML. A prospective study of neuropsychiatric symptoms associated with interferon-alpha-2b and ribavirin therapy for patients with chronic hepatitis C. *Psychosomatics*. 2003;44:104–112.

118. Udina M, Castellvi P, Moreno-Espana J, et al. Interferon-induced depression in chronic hepatitis C: a systematic review and meta-analysis. *J Clin Psychiatry*. 2012;73:1128–1138.

119. Pavlovic Z, Delic D, Maric NP, Vuković O, Jašović-Gašić M. Depressive symptoms in patients with hepatitis C treated with pegylated interferon alpha therapy: a 24-week prospective study. *Psychiatr Danub*. 2011;23:370–377.

120. Smith KJ, Norris S, O'Farrelly C, O'Mara SM. Risk factors for the development of depression in patients with hepatitis C taking interferon-alpha. *Neuropsychiatr Dis Treat*. 2011;7:275–292.

121. Evon DM, Ramcharran D, Belle SH, Terrault NA, Fontana RJ, Fried MW; Virahep-C Study Group. Prospective analysis of depression during peginterferon and ribavirin therapy of chronic hepatitis C: results of the Virahep-C study. *Am J Gastroenterol*. 2009;104:2949–2958.

122. Ho SB, Groessl E, Dollarhide A, Robinson S, Kravetz D, Dieperink E. Management of chronic hepatitis C in veterans: the potential of integrated care models. *Am J Gastroenterol*. 2008;103:1810–1823.

123. Chapman J, Oser M, Hockemeyer J, Weitlauf J, Jones S, Cheung R. Changes in depressive symptoms and impact on treatment course among hepatitis C patients undergoing interferon-alpha and ribavirin therapy: a prospective evaluation. *Am J Gastroenterol*. 2011;106:2123–2132.

124. Raison CL, Broadwell SD, Borisov AS, et al. Depressive symptoms and viral clearance in patients receiving interferon-alpha and ribavirin for hepatitis C. *Brain Behav Immun*. 2005;19:23–27.

125. Maddock C, Landau S, Barry K, et al. Psychopathological symptoms during interferon-alpha and ribavirin treatment: effects on virologic response. *Mol Psychiatry*. 2005;10:332–333.

126. Yee HS, Chang MF, Pocha C, et al. Update on the management and treatment of hepatitis C virus infection: recommendations from the Department of Veterans Affairs Hepatitis C Resource Center Program and the National Hepatitis C Program Office. *Am J Gastroenterol*. 2012;107:669–689; quiz 90.

127. Seeff LB, Hoofnagle JH. National Institutes of Health Consensus Development Conference: management of hepatitis C: 2002. *Hepatol (Baltimore, Md)*. 2002;36:S1–S2.

128. Ramasubbu R, Patten SB. Effect of depression on stroke morbidity and mortality. *Canad J Psychiatry*. 2003;48:250–257.

129. Navines R, Castellvi P, Moreno-Espana J, et al. Depressive and anxiety disorders in chronic hepatitis C patients: reliability and validity of the Patient Health Questionnaire. *J Affect Disord*. 2012;138:343–351.

130. Sockalingam S, Blank D, Al Jarad A, Alosaimi F, Hirschfield G, Abbey SE. A comparison of depression screening instruments in hepatitis C and the impact of depression on somatic symptoms. *Psychosomatics*. 2011;52:433–440.

131. Morasco BJ, Rifai MA, Loftis JM, Indest DW, Moles JK, Hauser P. A randomized trial of paroxetine to prevent interferon-alpha-induced depression in patients with hepatitis C. *J Affect Disord*. 2007;103:83–90.

132. Morasco BJ, Loftis JM, Indest DW, et al. Prophylactic antidepressant treatment in patients with hepatitis C on antiviral therapy: a double-blind, placebo-controlled trial. *Psychosomatics*. 2010; 51:401–408.

133. Diez-Quevedo C, Masnou H, Planas R, et al. Prophylactic treatment with escitalopram of pegylated interferon alfa-2a-induced depression in hepatitis C: a 12-week, randomized, double-blind, placebo-controlled trial. *J Clin Psychiatry*. 2011;72:522–528.

134. Kraus MR, Schafer A, Schottker K, et al. Therapy of interferon-induced depression in chronic hepatitis C with citalopram: a randomised, double-blind, placebo-controlled study. *Gut*. 2008; 57:531–536.

135. Schaefer M, Sarkar R, Knop V, et al. Escitalopram for the prevention of peginterferon-alpha2a-associated depression in hepatitis C virus-infected patients without previous psychiatric disease: a randomized trial. *Ann Intern Med*. 2012;157:94–103.

136. Lotrich FE. Psychiatric clearance for patients started on interferon-alpha-based therapies. *Am J Psychiatry*. 2013;170:592–597.

137. Evon DM, Golin CE, Fried MW, Keefe FJ. Chronic hepatitis C and antiviral treatment regimens: where can psychology contribute? *J Consult Clin Psychology*. 2013;81:361–374.

138. Safren SA, O'Cleirigh C, Tan JY, et al. A randomized controlled trial of cognitive behavioral therapy for adherence and depression (CBT-AD) in HIV-infected individuals. *Health Psychol*. 2009; 28:1–10.

139. Antoni MH, Ironson GH, Scheiderman N. *Cognitive-Behavioral Stress Management*. New York; Oxford: Oxford University Press; 2007:vi, 125.

140. USDVA. Viral Hepatitis. Available at http://www.hepatitis.va.gov/patient/hcv/treat/single-page.asp.

141. SAMHSA. Addressing Viral Hepatitis in People with Substance Disorders. Available at http://store.samhsa.gov/product/Addressing-Viral-Hepatitis-in-People-With-Substance-Use-Disorders/SMA13–4791.

142. Youssef NA, Abdelmalek MF, Binks M, et al. Associations of depression, anxiety and antidepressants with histological severity of nonalcoholic fatty liver disease. *Liver Int*. 2013;33: 1062–1070.

143. Younossi ZM, Stepanova M, Afendy M, et al. Changes in the prevalence of the most common causes of chronic liver diseases in the United States from 1988 to 2008. *Clin Gastroenterol Hepatol*. 2011;9:524–530.e1; quiz e60.

144. Bianchi G, Marchesini G, Nicolino F, et al. Psychological status and depression in patients with liver cirrhosis. *Dig Liver Dis*. 2005;37:593–600.

145. Ko FY, Tsai SJ, Yang AC, Zhou Y, Xu LM. Association of CD8 T cells with depression and anxiety in patients with liver cirrhosis. *Int J Psychiatry Med*. 2013;45:15–29.

146. Fritz E, Hammer J. Gastrointestinal symptoms in patients with liver cirrhosis are linked to impaired quality of life and psychological distress. *Eur J Gastroenterol Hepatol*. 2009;21:460–465.

147. DiMartini A, Dew MA, Trzepacz PT. Organ transplantation. In: Levenson JL, ed. *Textbook of Psychosomatic Medicine*. Washington, DC: American Psychiatric Press; 2004:775–803.

148. Modabbernia A, Ashrafi M, Malekzadeh R, Poustchi H. A review of psychosocial issues in patients with chronic hepatitis B. *Arch Iran Med*. 2013;16:114–122.

149. Voican CS, Corruble E, Naveau S, Perlemuter G. Antidepressant-induced liver injury: a review for clinicians. *Am J Psychiatry*. 2014;171:404–415.

150. Lewis JH, Stine JG. Review article: prescribing medications in patients with cirrhosis - a practical guide. *Aliment Pharmacol Ther*. 2013;37:1132–1156.

CHAPTER 14

Depression and Endocrine Disease

John Fromson, MD
Charles Surber, MD
Matthew Kim, MD

Endocrine disorders often cause or co-occur with depression. Thyroid, parathyroid, and adrenal disease, as well as diabetes and abnormalities in the hypothalamic–pituitary–thyroid (HPT) and hypothalamic–pituitary–adrenal (HPA) axes, can all result in depression. Treatment of these endocrine conditions often ameliorates the depressive symptoms, but If persistent, they can be addressed with somatic, behavioral, and psycho therapies.

DIABETES MELLITUS

■ DESCRIPTION

Diabetes mellitus is a group of metabolic diseases characterized by hyperglycemia that develops as a result of decreased secretion of insulin and/or impaired tissue response to insulin.[1] Type 1 diabetes is caused by autoimmune destruction of pancreatic beta cells, which leads to decreased insulin secretion. Type 2 diabetes—the most common form—is due to an impaired tissue response to insulin and decreased secretion of insulin. Untreated diabetes can lead to cardiovascular, renal, neurologic, and ophthalmologic damage. Diabetes is strongly associated with depression, as evidenced by the increased prevalence of depression in individuals with diabetes compared to the general adult population.[2] Untreated depression in those with diabetes can have a profound impact upon glycemic control and self-care behaviors, resulting in a greater risk of end-organ complications, disability, diminished quality of life, and increased mortality.

■ EPIDEMIOLOGY

In the United States, 29.1 million people (9.3% of the population) have diabetes. However, more than a quarter of them remain undiagnosed (**Fig. 14-1**).[3] Type 1 diabetes accounts for 5% of all diagnosed cases,[3] and type 2 diabetes accounts for 90% to 95% of all diabetes cases in the United States.[3] It is being diagnosed more often in children and adolescents due to increasing rates of childhood obesity.[3] Gestational diabetes affects 3% to 5% of pregnant women.[4] Postpartum, women with gestational diabetes have a 17% to 63% risk of being diagnosed with type 2 diabetes within 5 to 16 years.[5]

In the United States, there are significant racial and ethnic differences in those who are 20 years or older and diagnosed with diabetes (**Table 14-1**).

Compared with the general population, the prevalence of depression is three times greater in individuals with type 1 diabetes and almost twice as high in those with type 2.[6] Specifically, the point prevalence of depression is about 11%[6] compared to 3% to 4% in the general population.[2] The point prevalence increases to 28.5% in those diabetics with a past history of depression.[6] Women with diabetes have a higher prevalence of depression than men with diabetes.[7]

■ PATHOPHYSIOLOGY

Both types of diabetes cause impaired carbohydrate, fat, and protein metabolism. Gestational diabetes is characterized by glucose intolerance that is commonly diagnosed during the second or third trimester of pregnancy (**Box 14-1**).[3]

Other forms of diabetes include maturity onset of youth and latent autoimmune of adults. Patients with *maturity-onset diabetes of youth* have symptoms manifest before age 25 and have only

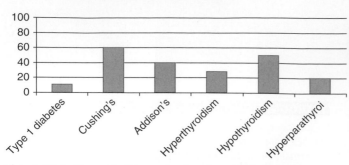

Figure 14-1 *Mean risk of depression for selected illnesses (percentage prevalence for particular disease).*

Hyperglycemia (diabetes)

Antidepressant-induced metabolic syndrome (diabetes)

Weight gain and dietary changes (diabetes)

Physical inactivity (diabetes)

Insulin sensitivity (diabetes)

Hypercortisolemia (Cushing's)

Effect of glucocorticoid and receptors (Cushing's, Addison's)

Electrolyte, metabolic imbalances

HPA and HPT axis dysregulation

Reduction of central 5-HT activity (Hypothyroidism)

impaired insulin secretion due to a monogenetic defect of beta cells with an autosomal dominant inheritance pattern.[8] *Latent autoimmune diabetes in adults* is characterized by a late diagnosis and the presence of pancreatic autoantibodies.[9] Additional causes of diabetes include pancreatic disease, infections, medication side effects, and surgery.[8] The risk for both type 1 and type 2 diabetes is increased in close relatives, suggesting a genetic predisposition, although no direct genetic link has been identified.[1]

Although studies endorse a relationship between diabetes and depressive symptoms, the relationship is bidirectional and the pathophysiological mechanisms linking them remain uncertain.[7] Lustman and Clouse have suggested that depression can induce hyperglycemia, especially in diabetic patients.[10] Findings by Eaton et al.[11] and Kawakami et al.[12] support this, finding both major depressive disorder and depressive symptoms precede and may increase the risk of type 2 diabetes.

Conversely, hyperglycemia may induce dysphoria.[11,12] In addition, antidepressant medications, such as SSRIs, influence metabolic function through weight loss or gain, and hydrazine monoamine oxidase inhibitors increase insulin sensitivity. Lustman and Clouse point out that antidepressants may also ameliorate hyperglycemia by virtue of improved antidiabetic medication adherence and dietary compliance.[10]

■ CLINICAL PRESENTATION

Typical presenting symptoms of diabetes include polyuria, polydipsia, weight loss, polyphagia, and blurred vision (**Box 14-2**).[13] Chronic hyperglycemia during childhood and adolescence may cause growth retardation and decreased resistance to infections.[13] Glucose control is essential, as uncontrolled diabetes may result in life-threatening hyperglycemia with ketoacidosis or the nonketotic hyperosmolar syndrome.[13]

There are no studies to suggest that the clinical presentation of depression differs in those with or without diabetes. However, depression in patients with type 1 and 2 diabetes is significantly

associated with hyperglycemia and may interfere with glycemic control.[14] In type 1 diabetes a direct relationship has been found between depressive symptoms and mortality risk.[15] In type 2 diabetes, depressive symptoms may not necessarily be indicative of a DSM disorder, but may instead reflect a depressive reaction to this stressful disease that requires demanding and extensive self-management. The stress of living with, adjusting to, and managing diabetes has been referred to as "diabetes distress."[15]

■ COURSE AND NATURAL HISTORY

Control of blood glucose is essential to reduce the risk of cardiovascular disease and stroke, renal dysfunction, lower limb amputations, peripheral neuropathy, nonalcoholic liver disease, periodontal disease, hearing loss, erectile dysfunction, and diabetic retinopathy and blindness.[3] Patients with diabetes and comorbid major depression who have poor glycemic control are at increased risk for retinopathy,[16] microvascular complications, and mortality.[17,18] Conversely, hypoglycemia can lead to seizures, loss of consciousness, and death. In 2010, diabetes was the seventh leading cause of death in the United States, and may be vastly underreported.[3] After adjusting for population age differences, all-cause mortality is approximately 1.5 times higher among adults with diabetes than among those without the disease.[3]

As in the general population, depression is a remitting and relapsing disorder for those with diabetes.[10] Even though most individuals will recover from the first episode of depression, there is a high likelihood of relapse[10] and its course has been described as "chronic and severe."[10] Maintenance of antidepressant medication appears to be effective in reducing recurrence rates.[10] In cross-sectional studies, glycemic control is significantly worse in those with depression than in those without.[19]

The depressive diagnosis more often follows rather than precedes the diagnosis of type 1 diabetes.[10] Longitudinal studies suggest that

TABLE 14-1 Age-Adjusted[a] Percentage of People Aged 20 Years or Older with Diagnosed Diabetes, by Race/Ethnicity, United States, 2010–2012[3]

Race	Percentage
American Indians/Alaska Natives	15.9
Non-Hispanic blacks	13.2
Hispanics	12.8
Asian Americans	9.0
Non-Hispanic whites	7.6

[a]Based on the 2000 US standard population.
Data from 2010–2012 National Health Interview Survey and 2012 Indian Health Service's National Patient Information Reporting System.

Symptoms associated with hyperglycemia (including neurovegetative)

Psychomotor retardation

Severe fatigue

Irritability

Mood lability

Anxiety

Cognitive abnormalities

Psychosis

BOX 14-3
DIFFERENTIAL DIAGNOSIS

Direct effects of the endocrine disorder

Side effects of endocrine treatments

Other psychiatric disorders (anxiety, substance use)

Sleep disorders

Chronic fatigue syndrome

Fibromyalgia

Obesity

Somatoform disorders

BOX 14-5
IMPORTANT RISK FACTORS FOR DEPRESSION IN ENDOCRINE DISORDERS

Sociodemographic
 Female gender
 Family history of depression or other psychiatric disorder (e.g., anxiety, psychoactive substance use)
 Age >60

Clinical
 "Diabetes distress"
 Sexual dysfunction
 Chronic pain

Medical
 Diabetic complications (e.g., cardiovascular, neuropathies)

major depression may increase the probability of developing type 2 diabetes.[20] This may be due to several different mechanisms, including the "…hyperglycemic effects of antidepressant medications, changes in diet and weight, and physical inactivity associated with chronic depression."[11] It is also possible that due to increased release of counter-regulatory hormones, depression may impair the disposition of carbohydrate loads and increase the chances of developing of type 2 diabetes. In addition, hyperglycemia may cause arousal states with greater risk to environmental stress and depression.

◼ ASSESSMENT AND DIFFERENTIAL DIAGNOSIS

Patients presenting with diabetes are often over 45 years old, overweight, and have unexplained weight loss, polydipsia, and polyuria. The diagnosis is confirmed by a fasting plasma glucose level >126 mg/dL, a random plasma glucose level >200 mg/dL with characteristic symptoms, a hemoglobin A_{1C} level > 6.5%, or a 2-hour plasma glucose level >200 mg/dL following an oral glucose challenge (**Boxes 14-3** and **14-4**).[21] Patients presenting with hypertension or hyperlipidemia should be screened for diabetes. During pregnancy, women are at increased risk of developing diabetes and those with gestational diabetes are at increased lifelong risk for type 2 diabetes.

Although depression in diabetes is similar to major depression in general, certain risk factors may point to a diagnosis of depression, as outlined in **Box 14-5**.

The use of screening tools to identify and monitor depression in diabetes is also highly recommended.[10] These include self-report questionnaires such as the Beck Depression Inventory, the 9-Item Patient Health Questionnaire (PHQ-9), and the Depressive Cognition Scale, as well as interviewer-administered scales, such as the Hamilton Rating Scale for Depression, the Diagnostic Interview Schedule, and the Structured Clinical Interview—DSM IV.

◼ TREATMENT

Treatment of diabetes begins with patient/family education, glucose-lowering medication, and the self-care practices of salutary dietary intake, regular physical activity, and weight control. Other crucial lifestyle changes include reducing the cardiovascular risk factors by controlling hypertension and hyperlipidemia, and curtailing nicotine use. Individuals with type 1 diabetes require life-sustaining insulin administered as multiple daily injections or as a continuous infusion supplied by a pump. Type 2 glucose levels can be controlled with similar behavioral interventions and the use of insulin and oral medications.[3]

Two-thirds of depressed diabetics do not receive treatment of their mood disorder (**Box 14-6**).[22] Yet, simply implementing glycemic control by diet, insulin, or oral hypoglycemic agents is beneficial.[23] When diagnostic criteria for major depressive disorder are met, evidence-based somatic therapy with or without cognitive behavioral therapy (CBT) is recommended.[10] CBT is effective in treating depression in type 2 diabetes patients with major depression, and results in moderate improvements in glycemic control as well.[24] Fluoxetine decreased depressive symptoms in an RCT of patients with major depression and either type 1 or type 2 diabetes.[23] In this study glycemic control improved, and this was associated more with fluoxetine's hypoglycemic affects than with remission of depressive symptoms suggesting a possible insulin sensitizing effect of fluoxetine.[23] Selective serotonin reuptake inhibitors may exacerbate hypoglycemia in diabetic patients by impairing hormonal counter-regulatory responses.[25]

Oral medications for type 2 diabetes have different interactions with commonly prescribed SSRIs (**Box 14-7**). Metformin has no interaction, but sulfonylurea drugs such as glimepiride, glyburide, glipizide, the meglitinides including repaglinide, and ᴅ-phenylalanine derivatives, such as nateglinide, may interact in a clinically significant manner requiring monitoring and dosage adjustments.

Interventions to improve diabetes self-management are also important. These include online diabetes self-management programs, assistance in problem solving, personalized health risk information, and educational material.[16]

◼ SUMMARY

Most cases of diabetes mellitus are classified as type 1 or type 2. Diabetes can also be the result of pancreatic disease, infections, medication side effects, or surgery. The diagnosis is based on measurement of hemoglobin A_{1C} level, fasting or random plasma glucose level, or the results of oral glucose tolerance testing. Depression is common in both type 1 and type 2 diabetes, and due to its chronic and severe nature has significant effects on the course and outcome of diabetes. Untreated depression can result in decreased adherence to treatment, poor metabolic control, higher complication rates, decreased quality of life, increased health-care use and costs, increased disability and lost productivity, and

BOX 14-4
COMMON COMORBIDITIES

Anxiety disorders

Substance use disorders

Delirium

BOX 14-6
TREATMENTS FOR DEPRESSION IN PATIENTS WITH DEPRESSIVE DISORDERS

Fluoxetine

Other SSRIs (although as a class may exacerbate hypoglycemia)

CBT

ECT

BOX 14-7
IMPORTANT DRUG–DRUG INTERACTIONS BETWEEN ANTIDEPRESSANTS AND PHARMACOLOGIC TREATMENTS OF TYPE 2 DIABETES

Sulfonylurea drugs (w/ SSRIs)

Meglitinides (w/ SSRIs)

D-phenylalanine derivatives (w/ SSRIs)

---

increased risk of death. SSRIs, particularly fluoxetine, and/or CBT are effective treatments. Glycemic control and the use of insulin may also improve depressed mood and sense of well-being. Depression in type 2 diabetes may often be a form of "diabetes distress" rather than a major depression. As such, it responds to self-management, assisted problem solving, and education.

HYPERCORTISOLISM

■ DESCRIPTION

Hypercortisolism (Cushing syndrome) is caused by endogenous chronic overproduction of cortisol or by prolonged exposure to exogenous glucocorticoids used in the treatment of other medical conditions. Laboratory tests confirm the diagnosis, and a variety of treatment modalities target the specific cause of Cushing syndrome. Depression is the most common psychiatric disorder affecting patients with Cushing syndrome.[26] Cushing disease is the pituitary ACTH-dependent form of Cushing syndrome.

■ EPIDEMIOLOGY

Endogenous Cushing syndrome is a rare disorder. Its precise incidence is difficult to determine because large numbers of patients are prescribed glucocorticoids and many others have subclinical features. In one Danish study the estimated annual incidence was 2–3 per million, of which benign adrenal adenomas accounted for 0.6 per million.[27] The female-to-male ratio was 3:1, and the median age for first hospitalization was 41.[27] Preliminary data suggest that patients with type 2 diabetes or osteoporosis may account for a large number of cases of subclinical Cushing syndrome.[28] The incidence of Cushing disease (pituitary ACTH-dependent Cushing syndrome) is five to six times more common than ACTH-independent adrenal Cushing syndrome caused by the secretion of excessive cortisol from benign or malignant adrenal tumors.[29]

The prevalence of depression in Cushing syndrome is high, and 50% to 70% of these patients experience a major depressive syndrome.[26]

■ PATHOPHYSIOLOGY

The production of cortisol is mediated by the HPA axis. The hypothalamus, located in the ventral diencephalon, sends corticotropin-releasing hormone (CRH) to the pituitary gland (Box 14-1). CRH then causes the pituitary to secrete adrenocorticotropin hormone (ACTH), which stimulates the adrenal glands that in turn release cortisol into the bloodstream.

Cortisol is an essential factor in the human stress response. Stress leads to rapid (seconds to minutes) activation of the sympathetic nervous system with the release of noradrenaline and adrenaline from the adrenal medulla.[30] These trigger increased vigilance, alertness, arousal, and attention. Slower (minutes to hours) stimulation of the mineralocorticoid and glucocorticoid receptors also takes place.[31]

Chronic stress results in a cumulative burden of behavioral adaptations, or "allostatic load," which interferes with homeostasis and ultimately results in neurodegenerative changes and cognitive impairment. Thus, persistently elevated circulating glucocorticoids

due to maladaptive coping can lead to depression, as well as increased abdominal obesity, osteoporosis, and cardiovascular disease.[32] The hypercortisolemia of Cushing disease and Cushing syndrome results in depression and a concomitant reduction in hippocampal volume.[33] Depression is associated with increased glucocorticoid signaling via the glucocorticoid receptors.[34] In the glucocorticoid signaling insufficiency hypothesis, hypercortisolemia is the result of primary glucocorticoid receptor resistance. This is in contrast to the glucocorticoid signaling overactivity hypothesis that suggests up-regulation at glucocorticoid receptors.[35]

■ CLINICAL PRESENTATION

The presentation of Cushing syndrome (**Table 14-2**) depends upon the duration and level of hypercortisolism and its cause, for example, adrenal adenomas that slowly secrete increasing amounts of cortisol that lead to gradual development of manifestations versus adrenal carcinomas that secrete markedly excessive amounts of cortisol over shorter intervals, often in combination with masculinizing androgens (Box 14-2). Gender and age also play a role in the clinical manifestations of hypercortisolism. Females commonly have dysmenorrhea or amenorrhea as well as facial, neck, chest, abdominal, and thigh hirsutism. Males may experience decreased or absent libido, erectile dysfunction, and infertility. Children of either sex experience impaired growth rates and obesity.[36]

The depression accompanying hypercortisolemia does not differ in clinical presentation from the depression co-occurring with other medical disorder.

■ COURSE AND NATURAL HISTORY

The course of hypercortisolism is variable and depends on its etiology as well as the patient's age at time of presentation. Excluding

---

TABLE 14-2 Most Common Features of Hypercortisolism

Cardiovascular
- Hypertension

Centripetal obesity
- Dorsocervical fat pad or "buffalo hump"
- Rounded or "moon-like" facies
- Supraclavicular adipose deposition

CNS
- Anxiety
- Cognitive abnormalities[37]
- Depression
- Insomnia
- Irritability
- Severe fatigue

Dermatologic
- Cutaneous fungal infections
- Easy bruisability
- Hyperpigmentation
- Impaired healing
- Prominent purple or pink striae
- Skin fragility

Diabetes
- Hyperglycemia

Orthopedic
- Osteoporosis
- Pathological fractures
- Proximal muscle weakness and wasting[38]

Renal
- Polydipsia
- Polyuria

cases caused by exogenous glucocorticoids, 70% of Cushing syndrome cases are due to benign, single pituitary adenomas that secrete ACTH.[39] Cortisol-producing adrenal tumors are rare and usually take the form of nonmalignant adrenal adenomas that are more likely found in women with an age of onset of about 40. Cushing disease occurs most frequently in women of reproductive age. Primary pigmented micronodular adrenal disease with tumors that produce cortisol is a condition that is usually diagnosed in children and young adults. In familial or inherited Cushing syndrome, cortisol-secreting tumors are found in the pituitary and adrenal glands as well as ectopically.[40] The least common cause of hypercortisolism is adrenocortical carcinomas, which also secrete androgens and account for rapid development of debilitating symptoms.

■ ASSESSMENT AND DIFFERENTIAL DIAGNOSIS

Diagnosis involves history, physical examination, and laboratory tests including imaging studies to locate pituitary or adrenal tumors. Tests to diagnose Cushing syndrome include 24-hour urinary free cortisol levels and/or lack of cortisol suppression after low-dose dexamethasone induction, as well as late-night salivary cortisol measurements. Dexamethasone-CRH testing is used to rule out elevated cortisol levels associated with morbid obesity, uncontrolled diabetes, and alcoholism, depression, and anxiety disorders. To distinguish between pituitary, adrenal, or ectopic sources of hypercortisolemia, ACTH levels, CRH stimulation testing, high-dose dexamethasone testing, and imaging studies are conducted.[37] The differential diagnosis for these patients should include metabolic syndrome and polycystic ovary syndrome, which can also cause aberrant menses, obesity, hirsutism, and insulin resistance.

Elevated cortisol levels are also seen in individuals with depression. Subsequent cortisol nonsuppression with the dexamethasone suppression test (DST) is found in both unipolar depression and bipolar disorders. In a meta-analysis of 144 studies, baseline DST status did not predict response to antidepressant treatment or outcome after hospital discharge. Persistent nonsuppression after treatment was associated with high risk of early relapse and poor outcome after discharge. The test lacks sufficient specificity and sensitivity to be useful.[41] Cushing syndrome should be part of the differential diagnosis when a medical etiology is considered in the presence of new or persistent psychopathology (Box 14-3).[34] Depression, anxiety, mood instability, and less commonly hypomania, psychosis, and mania[42,43] require careful assessment to rule out primary psychiatric disorders. If they are refractory to psychopharmacological interventions, then hypercortisolism should be considered as a possible etiology.[34] When atypical depression is associated with hypercortisolism, it often remits with treatment of the hypercortisolism.

■ TREATMENT

Treatment of hypercortisolism depends upon its etiology. If the cause is exogenous glucocorticoids, titration downward to the lowest effective dose doubled on alternate days may ameliorate symptoms. Another strategy is to switch to noncorticosteroid therapy. If an ACTH-secreting pituitary adenoma is the cause, trans-sphenoidal resection can be curative. Focused radiation therapy, or stereotactic radiosurgery, may be used to treat refractory cases. For ectopic ACTH syndrome, surgery, radiation, chemotherapy, immunotherapy, or combination therapy may be indicated. Cortisol-inhibiting medication or bilateral adrenalectomy is reserved for intractable cases. Cortisol-secreting adrenal tumors can usually be surgically removed.

In some depressed patients, cortisol level reductions result in significant symptom reduction.[44] In one study of Cushing syndrome, 67% of patients had a psychiatric diagnosis (52% atypical depression and 12% major depressive disorder [MDD]) prior to treatment; after successful treatment, only 24% manifested depression.[45] However,

even with aggressive treatment directed toward reducing hypercortisolism, psychiatric and cognitive problems may persist.[37] Data are not yet available to guide the treatment of refractory MDD associated with hypercortisolism that does not remit upon treatment of the hypercortisolism. Dorn et al. suggest psychiatric and endocrinologic collaborative follow-up of such patients with treatment tailored to each individual patient.[45] Hippocampal volume loss occurs in Cushing syndrome.[46] Rodent studies indicate that tianeptine, an SSRI, or electroconvulsive therapy (ECT) have effects on the hippocampus that should counter those reported in major depression, increasing adult hippocampal neurogenesis.[47,48]

■ SUMMARY

Hypercortisolism is the result of overproduction of cortisol due to benign pituitary adenomas (70%) that secrete ACTH, benign or malignant "ectopic" tumors that produce ACTH, or mostly benign adrenal tumors that secrete cortisol. Depression, which is the most common comorbid psychiatric disorder, as well as mood dysregulation, anxiety, and irritability are important presenting symptoms.

Data are not yet available to guide the treatment of MDD associated with hypercortisolism that does not remit upon treatment of the hypercortisolism.

ADRENAL INSUFFICIENCY

■ DESCRIPTION

Adrenal insufficiency can be primary (Addison disease) or secondary, representing diminished ACTH secretion due to disruption of pituitary corticotroph function, and tertiary adrenal insufficiency to represent diminished ACTH secretion due to hypothalamic suppression of CRH secretion due to exposure to exogenous glucocorticoids. Although the diagnosis of adrenal insufficiency, which has the potential to be life-threatening, is primarily made through laboratory testing, it may initially present with psychiatric symptoms.

■ EPIDEMIOLOGY

Addison disease affects 110 to 144 of every 1 million people in developed countries[49] and has an incidence of 4.7 to 6.2 per million per year in Caucasians with the age of diagnosis peaking during the fourth decade.[2] However, secondary adrenal insufficiency is much more common than Addison disease with a prevalence estimated at 150 to 280 per million, with the incidence peaking in the sixth decade.[50] Women account for the majority of cases of primary and secondary adrenal insufficiency. There is a paucity of recent literature describing the epidemiology of psychiatric symptoms in Addison disease. However, mid-century reports found their prevalence to be between 64% and 84%.[51-54] Anglin et al.[55] reviewed these studies and concluded that the primary presenting psychiatric symptoms of Addison disease are mild disturbances in mood, motivation, and behavior. Severe Addison disease and the presenting symptoms of an addisonian crisis can be psychosis, cognitive impairment, and delirium.[55]

■ PATHOPHYSIOLOGY

Addison disease results primarily from autoimmune adrenalitis, either adrenal gland specific or part of a polyglandular autoimmune syndrome (Box 14-1).[56] In developing countries tuberculosis remains the most common cause, as it did in 1855 when Thomas Addison first arrived at the diagnosis. Other causes include inborn errors of adrenal steroid biosynthesis enzymes from congenital adrenal hyperplasia, coagulation disorders or infection, leading to bilateral adrenal hemorrhage, opportunistic infections, metastatic malignancies, and iatrogenic causes. The latter include medications that inhibit cortisol biosynthesis (ketoconazole, aminoglutethimide, etomidate, and suramin) or those that enhance cortisol catabolism through hepatic microsomal-enzyme induction (rifampicin, phenytoin, and troglitazone).[57]

Secondary adrenal insufficiency is due primarily to abruptly stopping exogenous glucocorticoid therapy given for other medical conditions that causes HPA axis suppression. Megestrol acetate, prescribed for anorexia, cachexia or an unexplained, significant weight loss in patients with acquired immunodeficiency syndrome can also cause HPA suppression. Pituitary disease due to masses, surgery, or radiation may cause panhypopituitarism in addition to autoimmune, infectious, ischemic, hemorrhagic, or traumatic causes.

While the precise neuropathophysiology of psychiatric symptoms in adrenal insufficiency is not known, Anglin et al. present six possibilities.[55] The first describes electrophysiologic abnormalities, since patients with Addison disease and neuropsychiatric symptoms often have abnormal EEGs. In a small series of cases, diffuse slowing and bursts of sharp and slow wave discharges were observed. The second possible mechanism is electrolyte and metabolic abnormalities. These include commonly occurring hyponatremia that may lead to cognitive changes from an encephalopathy, as well as (less common) hypoglycemia and hypoxia due to severe hypotension. The third possibility is glucocorticoid deficiency resulting from the demise of granule cells in the hippocampal dentate gyrus, leading to memory impairment and cognitive changes.[58] Henkin[59] postulates that decreased glucocorticoids can increase conduction velocity in peripheral axons and prolong synaptic conduction, resulting in impaired perceptual ability and integration of sensory inputs. This could result in a lower threshold for developing psychosis.[59-62] The fourth possible pathophysiologic mechanism is increased endorphin secretion that may result from the anterior pituitary synthesis of proopiomelanocortin (POMC). The latter is cleaved, releasing ACTH and beta-endorphin, leading to psychosis.[63] The fifth possible mechanism involves adrenoleukodystrophy (ALD), an X-linked paroxysmal disorder due to the accumulation of very long chain fatty acids from defective beta-oxidation.[64,65] ALD usually presents in males during childhood with psychiatric symptoms of attention deficit disorder, followed by intellectual, behavioral, and neurological deterioration.[55] There are adolescent and adult forms of ALD, the latter with symptoms of adrenal insufficiency, abnormalities of gait, evidence of upper motor neuron involvement, mania, and psychosis.[55] Ten percent of all cases of adrenal insufficiency cases may be due to ALD.[66] Sixth is associated Hashimoto encephalopathy, a controversial diagnosis, with highly elevated antithyroid peroxidase antibodies in a patient with a history of treated hypothyroidism who also had Addison disease with neuropsychiatric symptoms.[55]

■ CLINICAL PRESENTATION

Sixty percent to 90% of patients with Addison disease present with apathy, social withdrawal, fatigue, anhedonia, poverty of thought, and negativism.[67] Depressive disorders are diagnosed in 30% to 50% of patients.[68] Severe cases, especially during an addisonian crisis, are associated with psychosis, impaired cognition, and delirium.[7] Rarely, catatonia, and self-mutilation may be present. However, up to 60 percent of young men with ADL may present with adrenal insufficiency before neurological problems develop.[69]

Skin and mucosal hyperpigmentation due to increased melanocyte-stimulating hormone are the most consistent findings in Addison disease.[55] Other signs and symptoms and laboratory features are in **Table 14-3**.

■ COURSE AND NATURAL HISTORY

Although the majority of patients with adrenal insufficiency come to medical attention for the symptoms described above, others may present during acute adrenal insufficiency that occurs with stressors, such as injury, infection, surgery, or pregnancy. These patients can present with dehydration resulting from vomiting and diarrhea, severe

TABLE 14-3 Signs and Symptoms of Addison Disease

Signs
Hyperpigmentation
Hypotension
Thinning of axillary and pubic hair
Vitiligo
Weight loss
Symptoms
Abdominal pain
Amenorrhea
Anorexia
Arthralgias
Constipation
Diarrhea
Fatigue
Myalgias
Postural Hypotension
Weakness and Vomiting
Laboratory Findings
Anemia
BUN and Creatinine Elevation
Eosinophilia
Hypercalcemia
Hyperchloremia
Hyperkalemia
Hyponatremia
Lymphocytosis
Metabolic Acidosis

pain in the lower back, abdomen, or legs, hypotension, and even loss of consciousness. Untreated adrenal insufficiency can lead to death.

■ ASSESSMENT AND DIFFERENTIAL DIAGNOSIS

Assessment consists of a history, physical examination, and laboratory testing. Diagnosis is confirmed with a low-dose cosyntropin stimulation test that uses 1 mcg dose to distinguish between primary and secondary adrenal insufficiency (Boxes 14-2 and 14-3). At the time of an adrenal crisis, ACTH and cortisol levels can help in determining the diagnosis. Additional laboratory findings include hyperkalemia, hyponatremia, and hypoglycemia. Ultrasound of the adrenals, tuberculin skin testing, and antibody testing for autoimmune adrenalitis are used to determine the precise etiology of adrenal insufficiency. Surgical removal of ACTH-producing pituitary or hypothalamic tumors can cause secondary adrenal insufficiency. Low or absent ACTH levels can also result from pituitary pathology in the form of diminished blood supply, infectious diseases, tumors, and radiation treatment sequelae. Computerized tomography and magnetic resonance imaging are used for diagnostic confirmation. Secondary adrenal insufficiency may be misdiagnosed as MDD in patients treated with high doses of corticosteroids for other medical problems. This is because symptoms can include severe fatigue, loss of appetite, weight loss, GI disturbances, muscle weakness, irritability, and depression. *If these are ruled out and depressive symptoms persist, then depression should be treated empirically.*

■ TREATMENT

Adrenal insufficiency is treated with oral corticosteroid replacement therapy, usually in the form of dexamethasone, hydrocortisone, or prednisone. Aldosterone deficiency that is present in primary adrenal insufficiency is treated with the mineralocorticoid fludrocortisone acetate. Emergent adrenal crisis intervention with rapid symptom reversal includes immediate intravenous administration of corticosteroids. In a review of several case series of Addison disease, 80% of cases had developed psychiatric symptoms before the diagnosis was made, suggesting that the psychiatric symptoms are attributable to Addison disease and not to corticosteroid treatment.[55] The depressive symptoms generally resolved in 1 week following corticosteroid treatment. However, in some instances the symptoms persisted for months and relapsed during an addisonian crisis.[55] There are no clear study recommendations for a particular course of treatment for persistent depression after amelioration of adrenal insufficiency.

■ SUMMARY

Primary adrenal insufficiency, Addison disease, is the result of reduced adrenal cortisol and in some patients, aldosterone production. Secondary adrenal insufficiency is caused by inadequate pituitary production of ACTH, which in turn is the basis for diminished circulating adrenal cortisol. Women account for the majority of cases of primary and secondary adrenal insufficiency. The course of adrenal insufficiency is usually slow and progressive. Common physical symptoms include fatigue, muscle weakness, loss of appetite, weight loss, and abdominal pain. The majority of patients with Addison disease present with the psychiatric symptoms of apathy, social withdrawal, fatigue, anhedonia, poverty of thought, and negativism. Depressive disorders are diagnosed in 30% to 50% of these patients. Severe cases, especially during an addisonian crisis, are associated with psychosis, impaired cognition, and delirium. These symptoms remit with aggressive glucocorticoid replacement. The precise neuropathophysiology of psychiatric symptoms in adrenal insufficiency is not known; however, the advances in neuroendocrinology may shed light in this area.

HYPERTHYROIDISM

■ DESCRIPTION

Hyperthyroidism is the result of overproduction of thyroid hormone by the thyroid gland. Nonhyperthyroid thyrotoxicosis can be caused by ingestion of toxic amounts of exogenous thyroid hormone. The most common cause of hyperthyroidism is diffuse toxic goiter (Graves disease), an autoimmune disease. Other causes include excessive production of thyroid hormone due to growth of autonomous thyroid nodules, release of preformed thyroid hormone caused by thyroiditis, excess dietary or supplemental iodine, and over dosage with prescribed synthetic or natural thyroid hormone replacement. Special populations, particularly the elderly and women during and after pregnancy, are at greater risk of developing hyperthyroidism. Mood lability, including depression and anxiety, are commonly present.[70]

■ EPIDEMIOLOGY

Hyperthyroidism occurs in approximately 1% of the US population. Women are 2 to 10 times more likely to become hyperthyroid, primarily from Graves disease or toxic diffuse goiter. Men and women older than 60 years are also more susceptible, primarily due to the growth of autonomous thyroid nodules.[71] Benign thyroid nodules or adenomas that produce excessive hormone occur in 3% to 7% of the population.[72] One in 500 pregnant women has Graves disease[73] and postpartum thyroiditis occurs during the first post partum year in 4% to 10% of birthing mothers, usually lasting for 1 to 2 months.[74] Other risk factors include a previous history or family history of thyroid disease, consuming excessive quantities of food or medication, such as amiodarone, that contain iodine, or medical conditions, including type 1 diabetes, vitamin B12 deficiency with pernicious anemia, or primary adrenal insufficiency.

Depression occurs in up to 28% of cases of hyperthyroidism.[75] Symptoms include psychomotor retardation, guilt, muscle pain, energy loss, and fatigue.[76]

■ PATHOPHYSIOLOGY

Graves disease is an autoimmune disease in which thyroid-stimulating immunoglobulins (TSI) bind to and simulate TSH receptors, resulting in overproduction of thyroid hormone. Thyroiditis can be subacute, silent, or postpartum. Subacute thyroiditis presents as painful inflammation of the thyroid gland that lasts a number of months and is usually self-limiting. Silent thyroiditis likely has an autoimmune etiology, is painless with an enlarged gland, and can lead to hypothyroidism.

Although the HPT axis is associated with major depression,[77] the precise pathophysiological mechanism linking depression with hyperthyroidism is not clear. However, studies have demonstrated that minute changes in thyroid hormone levels may have a direct effect on CNS functioning and can result in depression.[78] In addition, depressed patients without thyroid disease nonetheless have derangement of a various thyroid hormones.[77,79–83]

■ CLINICAL PRESENTATION

Since thyroid hormone affects virtually every organ system and because its clinical manifestations vary greatly, the presenting symptoms can be wide-ranging. They include irritability, mood lability (including depression), anxiety, pressured speech, upper extremity tremulousness, anergia, sleep disturbances, muscle weakness, hyperreflexia, and hyperphagia with or without weight loss, diarrhea, tachycardia, atrial fibrillation, and heat intolerance. The goiter associated with Graves disease or toxic multinodular goiter can reach massive proportions, leading to airway and esophageal obstruction in young and middle-aged adults. Older adults with Graves disease may have a nonpalpable thyroid. A minimally enlarged or nonpalpable goiter can also occur in painless or lymphocytic thyroiditis as well as in hyperthyroidism due to exogenous hormonal sources. If a solitary nodule is present, an autonomously functioning thyroid adenoma must be ruled out. Ophthalmologic lid retraction and lag, and for those with Graves disease, exophthalmos, periorbital and conjunctival edema, and dermatological pretibial myxedema, may be present.

The clinical presentation of comorbid depression in patients with Graves disease is seen when patients are returned to a euthyroid state, but still manifest depressed mood, lethargy, poor appetite, and sleep disturbances.

■ COURSE AND NATURAL HISTORY

Iodine requirements increase during pregnancy. Autoimmune Graves disease is the most common form of hyperthyroidism occurring in this period. If untreated, the possible sequelae include preeclampsia, miscarriage, and preterm delivery. Since a healthy thyroid enlarges during pregnancy and many women experience fatigue, particularly in the last trimester, thyroid dysfunction can be easily missed. Postpartum thyroiditis, also an autoimmune condition, is painless, and lasts from 1 to 2 months.

In the elderly, subclinical hyperthyroidism can cause atrial fibrillation with heart failure and stroke, and osteoporosis in women. Overtreatment of hypothyroidism with thyroid preparations can result in symptoms of hyperthyroidism. Over-consuming iodine-rich food (e.g., kelp) can also lead to hyperthyroidism.

There are no published reports addressing the precise course of comorbid depression, how often it precedes or follows thyroid disease, how often depression remits when thyroid disease remits, and the likelihood of recurrent depressive episodes.

■ ASSESSMENT AND DIFFERENTIAL DIAGNOSIS

Since the presenting symptoms of hyperthyroidism resemble a host of other medical diagnoses, in addition to careful history and physical examination, laboratory results are essential to confirm the diagnosis (Boxes 14-2 and 14-3). Thyroid function tests include blood TSH, T_3, T_4, thyroid-stimulating immunoglobulin (TSI), radioactive iodine uptake, and thyroid scan studies. The TSH level is usually <0.05 mU/L in overt hyperthyroidism. In these patients free T_4, total T_4, or total T_3 levels may be elevated. The precise etiology of hyperthyroidism is determined with these assays. TSI measures thyroid-stimulating antibody, indicative of Graves disease. The radioactive iodine uptake test measures the amount of iodine the thyroid collects from the bloodstream.[84] Low levels of iodine uptake may indicate thyroiditis while high levels may reflect underlying Graves disease or hyperthyroidism due to autonomously functioning nodules.[85] A thyroid scan indicates thyroid iodine distribution and the presence of nodules that may be hot or cold.

Depressive and anxiety disorders each have similar features to the mood changes that are seen in the acute phase of hyperthyroidism (**Box 14-8**). After the etiology of hyperthyroidism has been estab-lished and appropriate therapy instituted, if there is a continuation of psychomotor retardation, guilt, muscle pain, energy loss, and fatigue, a psychiatric evaluation for comorbid mood and anxiety disorders should be instituted.[86]

■ TREATMENT

The primary goal of treatment is the restoration of thyroid hormone levels to normal. Treatment can take the form of decreasing excessive dietary iodine intake, antithyroid medications, radioactive iodine therapy, and surgery. Beta blockers are an effective in quelling anxiety, tremors, and elevated pulse, but do not alter thyroid hormone production. Antithyroid treatment can then be achieved using thionamides, for example, carbimazole, methimazole (MMI), or propylthiouracil (PTU). Once the patient has become euthyroid, definitive treatment may involve administration of radioactive iodine therapy or surgery for large goiters and the excision of nodules. Radioactive iodine therapy is contraindicated in women who are pregnant or breastfeeding women. These treatments may result in hypothyroidism requiring synthetic thyroid replacement therapy.

Those who have comorbid depression tend to have more severe symptoms of both depression and hyperthyroidism, more difficulty adapting to their medical condition, and higher medical costs than those who do not have coexisting depression. Depression treatment can improve the outcome of hyperthyroidism treatment. Treatments for comorbid depression include antidepressant medications, focused short-term psychotherapy, or a combination. Electroconvulsive therapy (ECT) may also be considered. Treating hyperthyroidism reduces depressive symptoms and thyroxine level reduction from antidepressants can yield an enhanced therapeutic effect.[87] Lithium treatment may also cause low thyroid levels.[88] Patients receiving lithium and tricyclic antidepressants should be monitored for the development of thyroid function abnormalities. Lithium prescribed for the treatment of bipolar mood disorders has a high incidence of goiter, hypothyroidism, thyroid autoimmunity, and hyperthyroidism.[89] NB: even in the presence of thyroid dysfunction with ongoing lithium treatment, lithium can still be prescribed as long as the thyroid disease is treated.

Only those who are at risk for developing thyroid function abnormalities should be monitored when prescribed nontricyclic antidepressants.[88]

■ SUMMARY

Hyperthyroidism, when symptomatic, frequently presents with anxiety, mood lability with depression, tremors, and elevated pulse. Most of these symptoms can be treated initially with beta blockers. However, further treatment with thionamides, radioactive iodine therapy, or surgery may be required to definitively control overproduction of thyroid hormone. These treatments may ultimately cause hypothyroidism and the need for synthetic thyroid hormone to restore a euthyroid state. Data are not yet available to guide the treatment of comorbid depression when it does not remit upon treatment of the hyperthyroidism. Since there is a paucity of empirical evidence to guide depression treatment, the standard treatments for depression without thyroid disease should be employed.

HYPOTHYROIDISM

■ DESCRIPTION

Hypothyroidism is a disorder in which the thyroid gland secretes inadequate amounts of thyroid hormone. Its most common cause in the United States is chronic lymphocytic thyroiditis (Hashimoto disease).[71] It also results from surgery, radiation, and medications taken for other conditions, such as hyperthyroidism, bipolar and cardiac disorders, and cancers. Consideration must also be given to its presence in special populations, particularly women who are

---

BOX 14-8
MANAGING ANXIETY IN THE PATIENT WITH ENDOCRINE DISORDERS: PEARLS TO CONSIDER

- Anxiety symptoms are often associated with endocrine disorders, especially hyperthyroidism, diabetes mellitus, pheochromocytoma, and hyperadrenalism (1)
  - Other endocrine causes of anxiety include hypothyroidism, Addison disease, hyper- and hypoparathyroidism, and less common, virilizing tumors and hypo- and hyperpituitarism (2).
- Once an endocrine disorder has been diagnosed, the presence of a primary anxiety disorder is determined by a careful history noting onset, temporal relationship with the endocrine disorder, family history, the presence of psychoactive substance use, and if the anxiety is associated with having a medical illness.
  - Primary anxiety disorders are usually associated with a clear psychosocial stressor, manifest acutely, and usually have been present for at least two years (2).
- Anxiety signs and symptoms from endocrine disorders can include diaphoresis, hyperventilation, elevated pulse, sleep disturbance, weight and libido change, fatigue, myalgias, chronic pain, and have panic and obsessional features (3).
- Treatment should be targeted to the underlying endocrine disorder.
- For co-occurring primary anxiety in the presence of an endocrine disorder, behavioral and somatic therapies should be selected based on the type of anxiety disorder.
  - Acute anxiety—benzodiazepines, relaxation techniques, and social support.
  - NB: Use benzodiazepines with caution in patients with substance use disorders, only for acute management of withdrawal or agitation.
- Generalized anxiety disorder, panic disorder—SSRIs, short-term benzodiazepines, alpha-2 antagonist, cognitive behavioral therapy (CBT) or psychotherapy, alone or combined (4).

1. Jefferson JW, Marshall JR, eds. Neuropsychiatric Features of Medical Disorders. New York: Plenum;1981:6–7.
2. Hall RCW. Anxiety. In: Hall RCW, ed. Psychiatric Presentations of Medical Illness. New York: Spectrum;1980:13–35.
3. Available at http://www.drrichardhall.com/Articles/anxiety.pdf; Accessed August 31, 2015.
4. Hunot V, Churchill R, Silva de Lima M, Teixeira V. Psychological therapies for generalised anxiety disorder. *Cochrane Database Syst Rev.* 2007.

pregnant or postpartum. Depression is commonly associated with hypothyroidism.[90]

■ EPIDEMIOLOGY

The prevalence of hypothyroidism in the United States in those over the age of 12 is approximately 4.6% (Fig. 14-1).[71] It is five to eight times more common in women, especially those who are small at birth and during childhood.[91,92] Depressive symptoms are present in nearly 50% of those with hypothyroidism.[75]

■ PATHOPHYSIOLOGY

The HPT axis is involved in the pathophysiology of major depression.[78] However, the direct pathophysiological mechanism linking depression and hypothyroidism is not clear. Minute changes in thyroid hormone levels may have a direct effect on CNS functioning and result in depression.[79] When patients with depression are compared to healthy controls, a number of complicated findings have been reported.[93] Depressed patients without thyroid disease have evidence of derangement of a various thyroid hormones.[77,80–83] Cleare et al. explored whether central 5-HT activity is reduced in hypothyroidism, since this might lower the threshold for developing depression.[93] Depressed patients had higher TSH levels than nondepressed patients, and TSH levels were positively correlated with HAM-D and BDI scores. Higher TSH levels predicted lower 5-HT–mediated endocrine responses, as well as the presence of clinical depression. These results suggest that hypothyroidism reduces central 5-HT activity.[94]

■ CLINICAL PRESENTATION

Hypothyroidism is usually slow to develop, so patients may not be aware of the symptoms (**Table 14-4**) that result from generalized metabolic slowing.[95] Metabolic abnormalities can include hyponatremia, elevated serum creatinine,[96] hypercholesterolemia, and hyperlipidemia. The metabolism of medications such as mood stabilizers, benzodiazepines, opioids, and anticoagulants may be impaired, resulting in elevated levels of circulating medications. Hematological changes include a normochromic, normocytic hypoproliferative anemia, and decreased hematocrit.[97]

■ COURSE AND NATURAL HISTORY

Hypothyroidism is most commonly caused by an autoimmune chronic lymphocytic thyroiditis or Hashimoto disease. It occurs primarily in middle-aged women and progresses insidiously so that it may be years before it is detected. It may also be part of type 2 polyglandular autoimmune syndrome (PGA II) co-occurring with adrenal insufficiency and type 1 diabetes or type 1 polyglandular

TABLE 14-4 Symptoms of Hypothyroidism

- Anergia
- Cold intolerance
- Constipation
- Decreased heart rate
- Depression
- Dry skin
- Goiter
- Infertility
- Irregular or heavy menses
- Joint and muscle pain
- Loss of the lateral one third of eyebrow hair eyebrow hair
- Orbital and facial edem
- Thinning hair
- Weight gain

autoimmune syndrome (PGA I) with adrenal insufficiency, hypoparathyroidism, and cutaneous fungal infections.

Hypothyroidism may also result from other forms of thyroiditis that initially cause thyrotoxicosis but subsequently result in hypothyroidism. These include painful subacute thyroiditis; Hashimoto disease during pregnancy; autoimmune and painless postpartum thyroiditis that can be mistaken for postpartum blues; and painless or "silent" autoimmune thyroiditis that can lead to permanent hypothyroidism.

Hypothyroidism may also be iatrogenic, following surgical removal of the thyroid for hyperthyroidism, or due to obstructive goiter or benign or malignant nodules. Treatment with radioactive iodine for hyperthyroidism, or treatment with external beam radiation for Hodgkin disease or head and neck cancers can also cause hypothyroidism. Medications prescribed for other medical conditions that can cause hypothyroidism include lithium, amiodarone, interferon alpha, and interleukin-2. In the setting of bipolar disorder, if there is a minor elevation of TSH supplementation with T_4 may ameliorate the breakthrough mood symptoms. With frank hypothyroidism, thyroid hormone replacement therapy is necessary, but there is usually no need to actually stop lithium therapy. Alternative mood stabilizers may be used, but if the patient has responded to lithium and thyroid supplementing works, this intervention is not necessary.

There is no clear empirical evidence about the precise course of depression when it occurs in hypothyroidism, its frequency prior to or following thyroid disease, or its rate of recurrence.

■ ASSESSMENT AND DIFFERENTIAL DIAGNOSIS

Individuals older than 60 years, women, particularly women who are pregnant or have had a child within the past 6 months, are all at increased risk of developing hypothyroidism. A careful history is required to search for predisposing conditions. These include an individual or family history of thyroid disease, surgery, or goiter, radiation to the thyroid, neck, or chest, and other autoimmune diseases including systemic lupus erythematosis, Sjögren syndrome, type 1 diabetes, or rheumatoid arthritis. Physical examination may reveal a goiter or the presence of nodules.

Patients presenting with first episode or atypical depression should have thyroid function testing (serum TSH and free T_4) to rule out the presence of hypothyroidism. Even depressed patients without overt clinical hypothyroid signs and symptoms require thyroid function testing, since thyroid dysfunction may be present without symptoms (subclinical) and is quite common.[98]

In addition to the many forms of thyroid pathology, since hypothyroidism often presents with a multiplicity of nonspecific symptoms, the differential diagnosis (Box 14-3) is extensive. However, with respect to depressive symptoms, other diagnoses to consider include sleep disorders, chronic fatigue syndrome, fibromyalgia, obesity,[99] and hypochondriasis.[100]

■ TREATMENT

The primary goals of treatment are to ameliorate symptoms, halt disease progression, and correct aberrant metabolic abnormalities. For primary hypothyroidism, replacement therapy with levothyroxine (LT$_4$) is facilitated by close monitoring and reversal of elevated TSH and low free T_4.[101] Free T_4 levels are used to monitor and calibrate treatment for patients with central pituitary or hypothalamic mediated hypothyroidism. In pregnant patients, TSH and free T_4 levels are used to titrate LT$_4$ dosing.[90]

Patients with comorbid depression tend to have more severe symptoms of both depression and hypothyroidism, more difficulty adapting to their medical condition, and more medical costs than those without comorbid depression. Treating the depression may improve the course of treatment for hypothyroidism. Treatment for those whose depression does not respond to thyroid replacement therapy includes antidepressant medications, focused short-term psychotherapy, or a combination of both. ECT may also be considered. Treating hypothyroidism will also reduce depressive symptoms. Lithium treatment may also cause low thyroid levels.[87] Patients receiving lithium and tricyclic antidepressants should be monitored for the development of thyroid function abnormalities. Only those who are at risk for developing thyroid function abnormalities should be monitored when prescribed nontricyclic antidepressants.[102]

■ SUMMARY

Hypothyroidism commonly occurs in women, during pregnancy, and in those older than 60 years. Causes include Hashimoto disease, thyroiditis, and the overtreatment of hyperthyroidism. The mainstay of treatment for primary hypothyroidism is synthetic LT_4 with monitoring of TSH and free T_4. Studies suggest that hypothyroidism reduces central 5-HT activity. Higher TSH levels may predict both lower 5-HT–mediated endocrine responses and the presence of clinical depression. Treating hypothyroidism with replacement T_4 or in combination with T_3 will reduce depressive symptoms. For nonresponders to thyroid hormone replacement, antidepressant medications, focused short-term psychotherapy, or combination therapy can return the patient to euthymia.

HYPERPARATHYROIDISM

■ INTRODUCTION

There are primary and secondary forms of hyperparathyroidism. Primary hyperparathyroidism is caused by the increased production of parathyroid hormone, usually from one or more of the four parathyroid glands, which results in hypercalcemia and hypophosphatemia. Primary hyperparathyroidism is typically the result of growth of a single adenoma. Secondary hyperparathyroidism is caused by disorders that lower blood calcium levels or increase phosphate levels. These include a paucity of vitamin D due to dietary deficiency, diminished exposure to sunlight, malabsorption syndromes, and renal failure.

■ EPIDEMIOLOGY

Primary hyperparathyroidism (pHPT) occurs in 22 per 100,000 person-years and is associated with significant cognitive and mood symptoms (Fig. 14-1).[103] The peak incidence of hyperparathyroidism is in the third and fifth decades, but can occur in all stages of life. Depression is highly prevalent in patients with pHPT, with about 10% to 30% of patients meeting criteria for MDD.[104–106]

■ PATHOPHYSIOLOGY

The direct pathophysiological mechanism of depression associated with hyperparathyroidism remains unclear. Some studies have found that neuropsychiatric symptoms correlate with elevated calcium and parathyroid hormone (PTH) levels, but others have failed to replicate these findings. There are reports of changes in brain physiology and neurotransmitters in patients before and following parathyroidectomy.[107] Improvements in mood and quality of life have been correlated with cerebral blood flow measurements,[107] cerebrospinal fluid levels of 5-hydroxyindole-acetic acid (serotonin metabolite), and homovanillic acid (metabolite of norepinephrine and dopamine),[108] and medial prefrontal cortex activity.[109]

■ CLINICAL PRESENTATION

Most patients are diagnosed while asymptomatic due to relatively frequent routine screening of serum calcium. For those with unusually rapid progression of the disease or who have not had routine medical examinations, initial presenting findings and symptoms may include nephrolithiasis, anorexia, nausea, vomiting, constipation, bone pain, depression, anxiety, fatigue, lethargy, and memory complaints.

■ COURSE AND NATURAL HISTORY

The course of hyperparathyroidism is variable and depends upon whether it is primary or secondary, as well as on the patient's age at time of presentation. Those with mild to moderate elevations of calcium may be closely monitored and many never progress to symptomatic illness. Others have a rapid course resulting in dangerously high levels of calcium with risk of cardiac arrhythmias and significant morbidity from symptoms of hypercalcemia and hypophosphatemia.

■ ASSESSMENT AND DIFFERENTIAL DIAGNOSIS

In an asymptomatic patient, laboratory findings of hypercalcemia and elevated PTH or normal PTH in the face of high calcium levels are usually the first indications of primary hyperparathyroidism (Boxes 14-2 and 14-3). The symptomatic patient with primary hyperparathyroidism may present with polydipsia, polyuria, constipation, nausea, and decreased appetite precipitated by hypercalcemia. Elevated PTH levels can cause bone pain from osteitis fibrosa cystica, nephrolithiasis, and neuromuscular symptoms of weakness and fatigue. Other conditions to consider with abnormally elevated calcium levels include secondary hyperparathyroidism, familial hypocalciuric hypercalcemia (FHH), and malignancy.

Neuropsychiatric symptoms include depression, anergia, decreased psychomotor activity, cognitive deficits, and even psychosis.[110] There is currently no empiric evidence to distinguish the comorbid depression with hyperparathyroidism from that seen in other medical illnesses.

■ TREATMENT

Surgical excision of overactive parathyroid gland(s) is the treatment of choice. Although this typically results in cure of the hyperparathyroid state, there is the future possibility of overactivity in the remaining parathyroid gland(s) and the subsequent need for additional surgery. However, removal of all or most of the parathyroid gland tissue can result in a hypoparathyroid state.

Depression as a comorbid symptom and possible reason for parathyroidectomy was explored by Espiritu et al.[104] who compared the depression scores of patients with primary hyperparathyroidism who were observed without intervention, those with primary hyperparathyroidism who underwent parathyroidectomy, and a control group undergoing thyroid surgery. All three groups experienced a reduction in depressive symptoms, but the group undergoing parathyroidectomy had the greatest reduction. A limitation of the study was that patients in the surgery arm had significantly higher depression scores at baseline, and likely had more severe hyperparathyroidism.

Studies are needed to guide the treatment of depression co-occurring with hyperparathyroidism that persists after treatment of hyperparathyroidism. Therefore, the general guidelines for depression treatment in Chapter 4 should be followed.

■ SUMMARY

Hyperparathyroidism, when symptomatic, can frequently present with depression. When the depression is associated with the hyperparathyroid state, it often remits with treatment of the hyperparathyroidism. Data are not yet available to guide the treatment of comorbid depression that does not remit with treatment of the hyperparathyroidism. Therefore, the general principles outlined earlier apply.

HYPOPARATHYROIDISM

■ INTRODUCTION

Hypoparathyroidism is a disorder in which the parathyroid glands secrete inadequate amounts of PTH resulting in hypocalcemia and hyperphosphatemia.

■ EPIDEMIOLOGY

Primary hypoparathyroidism is rare. There is a paucity of literature elucidating the epidemiology of depression that co-occurs with hypoparathyroidism. There are reports of mood and behavior problems in the congenital absence of the parathyroid glands (DiGeorge syndrome), 22q11 chromosome abnormalities, and velocardiofacial syndrome, but depression in these cases is likely due to the other manifestations of these disorders rather than a direct effect of hypoparathyroidism or hypocalcemia. The incidence of depression in patients with hypoparathyroidism is unknown.

■ PATHOPHYSIOLOGY

Parathyroid hormone's primary function is to maintain a normal range of calcium in the extracellular fluid. Hypoparathyroidism results in decreased calcium levels and can be both congenital and idiopathic; however, most cases are secondary to gland removal or devitalization during neck surgeries.[111]

■ CLINICAL PRESENTATION

Hypoparathyroidism presents with low calcium and low or absent parathyroid hormone. The presentation is characterized by muscle spasms and tetany, and by nerve function abnormalities, including perioral numbness, paresthesias, and in severe cases seizures.[111]

■ COURSE AND NATURAL HISTORY

Primary hypoparathyroidism presents with symptoms mentioned above that are the direct effects of low calcium. Most cases of hypoparathyroidism are the result of iatrogenic injury to the glands during surgery. Less commonly, it results from the treatment for hyperthyroidism with radioactive iodine, treatment with external radiation, or from metabolic alkalosis, hypomagnesemia, DiGeorge syndrome, adrenal insufficiency, or type I polyglandular autoimmune syndrome (PGA I). There is no empiric evidence about the precise nature of comorbid depression, its prevalence, incidence, symptoms, and course.

■ ASSESSMENT AND DIFFERENTIAL DIAGNOSIS

Assessment primarily consists of history and physical examination, especially when the patient presents following neck surgery. Subsequent laboratory evaluation demonstrating low calcium levels and low parathyroid hormone confirm the diagnosis. Low calcium with normal or high parathyroid hormone would indicate insufficient vitamin D levels, diminished absorption of calcium in the intestines, or renal wasting of calcium. Since there are no well-established guidelines for the assessment of comorbid depression in those with hypoparathyroidism, the differential diagnosis should include those outlined in Chapter 4.

■ TREATMENT

The treatment of hypoparathyroidism is replacement of calcium and vitamin D with supplements. Studies are needed to guide the treatment of comorbid depression. Therefore, the general guidelines for depression treatment in Chapter 4 should be followed.

■ SUMMARY

Hypoparathyroidism is a rare condition that in most cases is iatrogenic. There is no literature demonstrating a link between hypoparathyroidism and depression.

CONCLUSIONS

Depression can be caused by endocrine disorders or can co-occur with them. Often the presentation of endocrine-induced depression is identical to depression arising from other causes (**Box 14-9**). This necessitates careful diagnostic assessment, including laboratory testing. When endocrine abnormalities are found, treatment of the underlying condition is usually indicated. If depression remains unabated, co-occurring depression will usually respond to standard treatment protocols.

BOX 14-9 SUMMARY

- Depression is common in endocrine disorders, but underrecognized
- Untreated depression can worsen the course of endocrine disorders
- Standard antidepressant treatments remain effective in these cases

---

REFERENCES

1. Tuomi T. Type 1 and type 2 diabetes: what do they have in common? *Diabetes*. 2005;54(suppl 2):S40–S45.

2. Gavard JA, Lustman PJ, Clouse RE. Prevalence of depression in adults with diabetes: An epidemiological evaluation. *Diabetes Care*. 1993;16:1167–1178.

3. Centers for Disease Control and Prevention. *National Diabetes Statistics Report*. 2014. Available at http://www.cdc.gov/diabetes/pubs/statsreport14.htm. Accessed August 23, 2014.

4. Ben-Haroush A, Yogev Y, Hod M. Epidemiology of gestational diabetes mellitus and its association with Type 2 diabetes. *Diabet Med*. 2004;21:103–113.

5. Hanna FW, Peters JR. Screening for gestational diabetes; past, present and future. *Diabet Med*. 2002;19:351–358.

6. Anderson RJ, Freedland KE, Clouse RE, Lustman PJ. The prevalence of comorbid depression in adults with diabetes: a meta-analysis. *Diabetes Care*. 2001;24:1069–1078.

7. Roy T, Lloyd CE. Epidemiology of depression and diabetes: a systematic review. *J Affect Disord*. 2012;142Suppl:S8–S21.

8. American Diabetes Association. Diagnosis and classification of diabetes mellitus. *Diabetes Care*. 2010;33(suppl 1):S62–S69.

9. Unger J. Latent autoimmune diabetes in adults. *Am Fam Physician*. 2010;81(7):843–847.

10. Lustman PJ, Clouse RE. Depression in diabetic patients, the relationship between mood and glycemic control. *J Diabetes and Its Complications*. 2005;19:)113–122.

11. Eaton WW, Armenian H, Gallo J, Pratt L, Ford DE. Depression and risk for onset of type II diabetes. A prospective population-based study. *Diabetes Care*. 1996;19:1097–1102.

12. Kawakami N, Takatsuka N, Shimizu H, Ishibashi H. Depressive symptoms and occurrence of type 2 diabetes among Japanese men. *Diabetes Care*. 1999;22:1071–1076.

13. American Diabetes Association. Diagnosis and classification of diabetes mellitus. *Diabetes Care*. 2009;32(Suppl 1):62–67.

14. Lustman PJ, Anderson RJ, Freedland KE, de Groot M, Carney RM, Clouse RE. Depression and poor glycemic control: a meta-analytic review of the literature. *Diabetes Care*. 2000;23:934–942.

15. *American Diabetes Association's 74th Scientific Sessions*. Available at http://www.diabetes.org/newsroom/press-releases/2014/diabetes-distress-vs-depression.html#sthash.X2Dem0u1.dpuf. Accessed August 24, 2014.

16. Kovacs M, Mukerji P, Drash A, Iyengar S. Biomedical and psychiatric risk factors for retinopathy among children with IDDM. *Diabetes Care*. 1995;18:1592–1599.

17. Lloyd CE, Matthews KA, Wing RR, Orchard TJ. Psychosocial factors and complications of IDDM. The Pittsburgh Epidemiology of Diabetes Complications Study. VIII. *Diabetes Care*. 1992;15, 166–172.

18. Katon WJ, Rutter C, Simon G, et al. The association of comorbid depression with mortality in patients with type 2 diabetes. *Diabetes Care*. 2005;28(11):2668–2672.

19. Lustman PJ, Griffith LS, Freedland KE, Clouse RE. The course of major depression in diabetes. *General Hospital Psychiatry*. 1997;19:138–143.

20. Talbot F, Nouwen A. A review of the relationship between depression and diabetes in adults: is there a link? *Diabetes Care*. 2000;23:1556–1562.

21. Patel P, Macerollo A. Diabetes mellitus: diagnosis and screening. *Am Fam Physician*. 2010;81(7):863–870.

22. Kovacs M, Obrosky DS, Goldston D, Drash A. Major depressive disorder in youths with IDDM: a controlled prospective study of course and outcome. *Diabetes Care*. 1997;20:45–51.

23. Lustman PJ, Freedland KE, Griffith LS, Clouse RE. Fluoxetine for depression in diabetes: a randomized double-blind placebo-controlled trial. *Diabetes Care*. 2000;23:618–623.

24. Lustman PJ, Griffith LS, Freedland KE, Kissel SS, Clouse RE. Cognitive behavior therapy for depression in type 2 diabetes mellitus. A randomized, controlled trial. *Annals of Internal Medicine*. 1998;129:613–621.

25. Sanders NM, Wilkinson CW, Taborsky Jr GJ, et al. The selective serotonin reuptake inhibitor sertraline enhances counter-regulatory responses to hypoglycemia. *Am J Physiol Endocrinol Metab*. 2008;294(5):E853–E860.

26. Sonino N, Fava GA. Psychosomatic aspects of Cushing's disease. *Psychother Psychosom*. 1998;67:140–146.

27. Lindholm J, Juul S, Jorgensen JO, et al. Incidence and late prognosis of Cushing's syndrome: a population-based study. *J Clin Endocrinol Metab*. 2001;86:117–123.

28. Steffensen C, Bak AM, Rubeck KZ, Jørgensen JO. Epidemiology of Cushing's syndrome. *Neuroendocrinology*. 2010;92 Suppl 1:1–5.

29. Carpenter PC. Diagnostic evaluation of Cushing's syndrome. *Endocrinol Metab Clin North Am*. 1988;17:445–472.

30. de Kloet ER, Joëls M, Holsboer F: Stress and the brain: from adaptation to disease. *Nat Rev Neurosci*. 2005;6:463–475.

31. Pereira AM, Tiemensma J, Romijn JA. Neuropsychiatric disorders in Cushing's syndrome. *Neuroendocrinology*. 2010;92(suppl 1):65–70

32. Brown ES, Varghese FP, McEwen BS. Association of depression with medical illness: does cortisol play a role? *Biol. Psychiatry*. 2004;55:1–9.

33. Sheline YI, Sanghavi M, Mintun MA, Gado MH. Depression duration but not age predicts hippocampal volume loss in medically healthy women with recurrent major depression. *J Neurosci*. 1999;19:5034–5043.

34. Tang A, O'Sullivan AJ, Diamond T, Gerard A, Campbell P. Psychiatric symptoms as a clinical presentation of Cushing's syndrome. *Ann Gen Psychiatry*. 2013;12:23.

35. Wolkowitz OM, Burke H, Epel ES, Reus VI. Glucocorticoids: mood, memory and mechanisms. Glucocorticoids and mood. *Ann N Y Acad Sci*. 2009, 1179:19–40.

36. Chan LF, Storr HL, Grossman AB, Savage MO. Pediatric Cushing's syndrome: clinical features, diagnosis, and treatment. *Arq Bras Endocrinol Metab*. 2007;51(8):1261–1271.

37. Arnaldi G, Angeli A, Atkinson B, et al. Diagnosis and complications of Cushing's syndrome: a consensus statement. *J Clin Endocrinol Metab*. 2003;88(12):5593–5602.

38. Ross EJ, Linch DC. Cushing's syndrome–killing disease: discriminatory value of signs and symptoms aiding early diagnosis. *Lancet*. 1982;2:646–649.

39. Nieman LK, Ilias I. Evaluation and treatment of Cushing's syndrome. *The Journal of American Medicine*. 2005;118(12):1340–1346.

40. NIH Conference. Multiple endocrine neoplasia type 1: Clinical and genetic topics. *Ann Int Med*. 1998;29(6):484–494.

41. Ribeiro SC, Tandon R, Grunhaus L, Greden JF. The DST as a predictor of outcome in depression: A meta-analysis. *Am J Psychiatry*. :1993;150(11):1618–1629.

42. Kathol RG, Delahunt JW, Hannah L. Transition from bipolar affective disorder to intermittent Cushing's syndrome: case report. *J Clin Psychiatry*. 1985;46:194–196.

43. Hirsh D, Orr G, Kantarovich V, Hermesh H, Stern E, Blum I. Cushing's syndrome presenting as a schizophrenia-like psychotic state. *Isr J Psyuchiatry Relat Sci*. 2000;37:46–50.

44. Kelly WF, Kelly MJ, Faragher B. A prospective study of psychiatric and psychological aspects of Cushing's syndrome. *Clin Endocrinol*. 1996;45:715–720.

45. Dorn LD, Burgess ES, Friedman TC, Dubbert B, Gold PW, Chrousos GP. The longitudinal course of psychopathology in Cushing's syndrome after correction of hypercortisolism. *J Clin Endocrinol Metab*. 1997;82:912–919.

46. Starkman M, Gebarski S, Berent S, Schteingart D. Hippocampal formation volume, memory dysfunction, and cortisol levels in patients with Cushing's syndrome. *Biol Psychiatry*. 1992;32: 756–764.

47. Malberg J, Eisch A, Nestler E, Duman R. Chronic antidepressant treatment increases neurogenesis in adult rat hippocampus. *J Neurosci*. 2000;20:9104–9110.

48. Scott B, Wojtowicz J, Burnham W. Neurogenesis in the dentate gyrus of the rat following electroconvulsive shock seizures. *Exp Neurol*. 2000;165:2231–2237.

49. Betterle C, Morlin L. Autoimmune Addison's disease. In: Ghizzoni L, Cappa M, Chrousos G, eds. *Pediatric Adrenal Diseases. Endocrine Development*. Vol. 20. Padova, Italy: Karger Publishers; 2011:161–172.

50. Arlt W, Allolio B. Adrenal insufficiency. *Lancet*. 2003;361(9372): 1881–1893.

51. Engel GI, Margolin SG. Neuropsychiatric disturbances in internal disease. *Arch Int Med*. 1942;70:236–259.

52. Sorkin SZ. Addison's disease. *Medicine*. 1949; 28:371–425.

53. Cleghorn RA. Adrenal cortical insufficiency: psychological and neurological observations. *Can Med Assoc J*. 1951;65:449–454.

54. Smith CK, Barish J, Correa J, et al. Psychiatric disturbance in endocrinologic disease. *Psychosom Med*. 1972;34:69–86.

55. Anglin RE, Rosenbush PI, Mazurek MF. The neuropsychiatric profile of Addison's disease: revisiting a forgotten phenomenon. *J Neuropsychiatry Clin Neurosci*. Fall 2006;18(4):450–459.

56. Betterle C, Dal Pra C, Mantero F, et al. Autoimmune adrenal insufficiency and autoimmune polyendocrine syndromes: Autoantibodies, autoantigens, and their applicability in diagnosis and disease prediction. *Endocr Rev*. 2002;23(3):327–364.

57. Edwards OM, Courtenay-Evans RJ, Galley JM, Hunter J, Tait AD. Changes in cortisol metabolism following rifampicin therapy. *Lancet*. 1974;304(7880):549–551.

58. Squire LR, Zola-Morgan S. Memory: brain systems and behavior. *Trends Neurosci*. 1988;11:170–175.

59. Henkin RI. The effects of corticosteroids and ACTH on sensory systems. *Prog Brain Res*. 1970;32:270–294.

60. Henkin RU, Gill JR, Warmolts JR, et al. Steroid-dependent increase of nerve conduction velocity in adrenal insufficiency. *J Clin Invest*. 1963;42:941.

61. Henkin RI, Gill JR, Bartter FC. Studies on taste thresholds in normal man and in patients with adrenal cortical insufficiency: the role of adrenal cortical steroids and of serum sodium concentration. *J Clin Invest*. 1973;42:727–735.

62. Henkin FI, Daly RL. Auditory detection and perception in normal man and in patients with adrenal cortical insufficiency: effect of adrenal cortical steroids. *J Clin Invest*. 1968;47:1269–1280.

63. Johnstone PA, Rundell JR, Esposito M. Mental status changes of Addison's disease. *Psychosomatics*. 1990;31:103–107.

64. Garside S, Rosebush PI, Levinson AJ, et al. Late-onset adrenoleukodystrophy associated with long-standing psychiatric symptoms. *J Clin Psychiatry*. 1999;60:460–468.

65. Rosebush PI, Garside S, Levinson AJ, et al. The neuropsychiatry of adult-onset adrenoleukodystrophy. *J Neuropsychiatry Clin Neurosci*. 1999;11:315–327.

66. Laureti S, Aubourg P, Calcinaro F, et al. Etiological diagnosis of primary adrenal insufficiency using an original flow chart of immune and biochemical markers. *J Clin Endocrinol Metab*. 1998;83:3163–3168.

67. Popkin MK, MacKenzie TB. Psychiatric presentations of endocrine dysfunction. In: Hall RC, eds. *Psychiatric Presentations of Medical Illness*. New York, NY: Spectrum Publications; 1980:139–156.

68. Kornstein SG, Sholar EF, Gardner DG. Endocrine disorders. In: Stoudemire A, Fogel BS, Greenberg D, eds. *Psychiatric Care of the Medical Patient*. 2 nd ed. New York, NY: Oxford Univ Press; 2000:801–819.

69. Sadeghi-Dejad A, Senior B. Adrenomyeloneuropathy presenting as Addison's disease in childhood. *N Engl J Med* 1990; 322:13–16.

70. Trzepacz PT, Klein I, Roberts M, et al. Graves' disease: an analysis of thyroid hormone levels and hyperthyroid signs and symptoms. *Am J Med*. 1989;87:558–561.

71. Golden SH, Robinson KA, Saldanha I, et al. Prevalence and incidence of endocrine and metabolic disorders in the United States: a comprehensive review. *J Clin Endocrinol Metabolism*. 2009;94(6):1853–1878.

72. Gharib H, Papini E, Paschke R, et al. American Association of Clinical Endocrinologists, Associazione Medici Endocrinologi, and European Thyroid Association medical guidelines for clinical practice for the diagnosis and management of thyroid nodules. *Endocr Pract*. 2010;16(s1)1–43.

73. Komal PS, Mestman JH. Graves hyperthyroidism and pregnancy: a clinical update. *Endocr Pract*. 2010;16(1):118–129.

74. . Ogunyemi DA. Autoimmune thyroid disease and pregnancy. Available at http://emedicine.medscape.com/article/261913-overview. Updated March 12, 2012. Accessed August 8, 2014.

75. Boswell EB, Anfinson TH, Nemeroff CB. Depression associated with endocrine disorders. In: Robertson MM, Katona CL, eds. *Depression and Physical Illness*. England: Wiley, Chichester; 1997:256–292.

76. Demet MM, Ozmen B, Deveci A, Boyvada S, Adigüzel H, Aydemir O. Depression and anxiety in hyperthyroidism. *Arch Med Res*. 2002;33(6):552–556.

77. Stipcevic T, Pivac N, Kozaric-Kovacic D, Mück-Seler D. Thyroid Hormones in Depression, Coll. *Antropol*. 2008;32:973–976

78. Bahls SC, Carvalho GA. Relation between thyroid function and depression. *Rev Bras Psiquiatr*. 2004;26(1):40–48

79. Berlin I, Payan C, Corruble E, Puech AJ. Serum thyroid-stimulating-hormone concentration as an index of severity of major depression. *Int J Neuropsychopharmacol*. 1999;2:105.

80. Rao ML, Ruhrmann S, Retey B, Liappis N, Fuger J, Kraemer M. Low plasma thyroid indices of depressed patients are attenuated by antidepressant drugs and influence treatment outcome. *Pharmacopsychiat*. 29(5):180–186.

81. Sagud M, Pivac N, Muck Seler D, Jakovljevic M, Mihaljevic-Peles A, Korsic M. Effects of sertraline treatment on plasma cortisol, prolactin and thyroid hormones in female depressed patients. *Neuropsychobiol*. 45(3):139–143.

82. Rupprecht R, Rupprecht C, Rupprecht M, Noder M, Mahlstedt J. Triiodothyronine, thyroxine, and TSH response to dexamethasone in depressed patients and normal controls. *Biol Psychiat*. 25(1):22–32.

83. Kirkegaard C, Korner A, Faber J. Increased production of thyroxine and inappropriately elevated serum thyrotropin in levels in endogenous depression. *Biol Psychiat*. 27(5):472–476.

84. Davey RX, Clarke MI, Webster AR. Thyroid function testing based on assay of thyroid-stimulating hormone: assessing an algorithm's reliability. *Med J Aust*. 1996;164:329–331.

85. *National Endocrine and Metabolic Diseases Information Service (NEMDIS) fact sheet Thyroid Function Tests*. Available at http://www.endocrine.niddk.nih.gov/. Accessed August 11, 2014.

86. Sauvage MF, Marquet P, Rousseau A, Raby C, Buxeraud J, Lachâtre G. Relationship between psychotropic drugs and thyroid function: a review. *Toxicol Appl Pharmacol*. 1998;149(2):127–135.

87. Kupka RW, Nolen WA, Post RM, et al. High rate of autoimmune thyroiditis in bipolar disorder: lack of association with lithium exposure. *Biol Psychiatry*. 2002;51(4):305–311.

88. Barbesino G. Drugs affecting thyroid function. *Thyroid*. 2010;20(7): 763–770.

89. Bou Khalil R, Richa S. Thyroid adverse effects of psychotropic drugs: a review. *Clin Neuropharmacol*. 2011;34(6):248–255.

90. Rack SK, Makela EH. Hypothyroidism and depression: a therapeutic challenge. *Ann Pharmacother*. 2000;34(10):1142–1145.

91. Aoki Y, Belin RM, Clickner R, et al. Serum TSH and total T4 in the United States population and their association with participant characteristics: National Health and Nutrition Examination Survey (NHANES 1999–2002). *Thyroid*. 2007;17:1211–1223.

92. Kajantie E, Phillips DI, Osmond C, et al. Spontaneous hypothyroidism in adult women is predicted by small body size at birth and during childhood. *J Clin Endocrinol Metab*. 2006;91:4953–4956.

93. Cleare AJ, McGregor A, O'Keane V. Neuroendocrine evidence for an association between hypothyroidism, reduced central 5-HT activity and depression. *Clin Endocrinol*. 1995;43(6):713–719

94. Smith TJ, Bahn RS, Gorman CA. Connective tissue, glycosaminoglycans, and diseases of the thyroid. *Endocr Rev*. 1989;10:366–391.

95. Kreisman SH, Hennessey JV. Consistent reversible elevations of serum creatinine levels in severe hypothyroidism. *Arch Intern Med*. 1999;159:79–82.

96. Green ST, Ng JP. Hypothyroidism and anaemia. *Biomed Pharmacother*. 1986;40:326–331.

97. Hollowell JG, Staehling NW, Flanders WD, et al. Serum TSH, T(4), and thyroid antibodies in the United States population (1988

to 1994): National Health and Nutrition Examination Survey (NHANES III). *J Clin Endocrinol Metab*. 2002;87:489–499.

98. Luppino FS, de Wit LM, Bouvy PF, et al. Overweight, obesity, and depression: A systematic review and meta-analysis of longitudinal studies. *Arch Gen Psychiatry*. 2010;67(3):220–229.

99. Kreitman N, Sainsbury P, Pearce K, Costain WR. Hypochondriasis and depression in out-patients at a General Hospital. *Br J Psychiatry*. 1965;111:607–615.

100. Grozinsky-Glasberg S, Fraser A, Nahshoni E, Weizman A, Leibovici L. Thyroxine-triiodothyronine combination therapy versus thyroxine monotherapy for clinical hypothyroidism: meta-analysis of randomized controlled trials. *J Clin Endocrinol Metab*. 2006;91(7):2592–2599.

101. LeBeau SO, Mandel SJ. Thyroid disorders during pregnancy. *Endocrinol Metab Clin North Am*. 2006;35(1):117–136, vii.

102. Bou Khalil R, Richa S. Thyroid adverse effects of psychotropic drugs: a review. *Clin Neuropharmacol*. 2011;34(6):248–255.

103. Wermers RA, Khosla S, Atkinson EJ, et al. Incidence of primary hyperparathyroidism in Rohester, Minnesota, 1993–2001: an update on the changing epidemiology of the disease. *J Bone Miner Res*. 2006;21:171–177.

104. Espiritu RP, Kearns AE, Vickers KS, Grant C, Ryu E, Wermers RA. Depression in Primary Hyperparathyroidism: Prevalence and Benefit of Surgery. *J Clin Endocrinol Metab*. 2011;96(11):E1737–E1745.

105. Weber T, Keller M, Hense I, et al. Effect of parathyroidectomy on quality of life and neuropsychological symptoms in primary hyperparathyroidism. *Wrold J Surg*. 2007;31:1202–1209.

106. Wilhelm SM, Lee J, Prinz RA. Major depression due to primary hyperparathyroidism: a frequent and correctable disorder. *Am Surg*. 2004;70:175–179; discussion 179–180.

107. Mjaland O, Normann E, Halvorsen E, Rynning S, Egeland T. Regional cerebral blood flow in patients with primary hyperparathyroidism before and after successful parathyroidectomy. *B J Surg*. 2003;90:732–737.

108. Joborn C, Hetta J, Rastad J, Agren H, Akerstrom G, Ljunghall S. Psychiatric symptoms and cerebrospinal fluid monoamine metabolites in primary hyperparathyroidism. *Biol Psychiatry*. 1988;23:149–158.

109. Perrier ND, Coker LH, Rorie KD, et al. Preliminary report: Functional MRI of the brain may be the ideal tool for evaluating neuropsychologic and sleep complaints of patients with primary hyperparathyroidism. *World J Surg*. 2006;30:686–696.

110. Coker LH, Rorie K, Cantley L, et al. Primary hyperparathyroidism, cognition, and health-related quality of life. *Ann Surg*. 2005;242:642–650.

111. Cusano NE, Rubin MR, Sliney J Jr, Bilezikian JP. Mini-Review: new therapeutic options in hypoparathyroidism. *Endocrine*. 2012;41:410–414.

CHAPTER 15

Depression in Chronic Kidney Disease, Hypertension, and Nutritional Deficiencies

Katy LaLone, MD
Elizabeth Alfson, MD
David Gitlin, MD

INTRODUCTION

One in five patients with chronic kidney disease (CKD) will experience at least one major depressive episode, which is likely to be detrimental to the course of their kidney disease and significantly limit their quality of life. Most patients with major depressive disorder (MDD) in the setting of CKD are undiagnosed and untreated, which suggests a significant opportunity for psychiatrists to work collaboratively to optimize the treatment of depression in this high-risk population and provide guidance for both patients and their families around complex issues like dialysis withdrawal.

There is clearly a direct association between depression and hypertension as both have been identified as risk factors in precipitating the occurrence of the other. Psychiatrists should be vigilant about the appropriate management of hypertension and be familiar with medications that can exacerbate hypertension.

As many as four out of five adults in the United States report inadequate intake of fruits and vegetables according to national dietary standards and there are direct relationships between vitamin deficiencies and depressive symptoms. Psychiatrists have the opportunity to educate patients about appropriate nutrition and should be especially careful to recognize and appropriately treat nutritional deficiencies.

CHRONIC KIDNEY DISEASE AND DEPRESSION

■ EPIDEMIOLOGY

Chronic kidney disease (CKD) is defined as the presence of kidney damage or decreased kidney function (glomerular filtration rate [GFR] <60 mL/min/1.73m^2) for 3 or more months. It is a highly prevalent condition affecting over 8 million Americans each year.[1] Common etiologies include diabetes mellitus, hypertension, generalized arteriosclerosis, lupus, AIDS, and primary renal diseases, such as chronic glomerulonephritis, polycystic kidney disease, and other congenital and hereditary renal disorders. Around 80,000 Americans will progress to end-stage renal disease (ESRD) each year joining the more than 500,000 who are being treated for ESRD. Seventy-five percent of those with ESRD are on maintenance dialysis. The majority of these are treated with hemodialysis (HD), with less than 10% by home peritoneal dialysis (PD). The remaining 25% have a functioning kidney transplant, which is the treatment of choice for patients as it increases survival and quality of life.[2]

Depression is the most common psychiatric disorder in the CKD and ESRD population, with prevalence rates as high as 20% to 25% in recent studies, although many of these studies have used non-standard measures for assessing depression.[3,4] In one study, 27.4% of CKD patients had evidence of depressive symptoms,[5] while in others, 20% to 22% of patients with CKD have major depressive disorder.[6,7] The prevalence does not appear to vary widely with the stage of renal disease.[8] Variables associated with a major depressive episode were diabetes mellitus, comorbid psychiatric illness, and history of drug or alcohol abuse. Taken together, the current data suggest that one in five patients with CKD will have at least one major depressive episode.[8]

Early studies on suicide in ESRD patients reported very high rates (100- to 400-fold greater risk than the general population), but these studies did not distinguish suicide from dialysis withdrawal, now considered to be distinct entities.[9] In addition, early data were drawn from a highly select population undergoing a much more rudimentary and arduous dialysis procedure.[9] Since 1990, the ESRD

Death Notification Form has listed dialysis withdrawal and suicide as separate causes of death, allowing for more accurate data collection.[9] What is unique about suicide consideration in this population is the ease of access to lethal methods that dialysis allows, either by noncompliance with medications or dialysis therapy, dietary excess, or by manipulating one's shunt. Despite this, more recent data from the US Renal Data System (USRDS) indicate that suicide occurs at a modestly increased rate compared to the general population.[9,10] Data from the USRDS indicated that patients with ESRD had an 84% higher rate of suicide compared to the general population, but this rate is comparable to that of other chronic or debilitating illnesses, such as HIV, chronic lung disease, and stroke.[9]

ESRD appears to exacerbate a pre-existing vulnerability or tendency toward suicidal behavior among certain high-risks groups, particularly individuals with a history of alcohol dependence and previous hospitalizations for substance abuse and/or mental illness.[10] The increased risk for suicide is associated with age >75, male gender, white or Asian race, ischemic heart disease, peripheral vascular disease, cancer, COPD, alcohol or drug dependence, low serum albumin, and hospitalization within the preceding 12 months.[9] For example, prior psychiatric hospitalization is associated with a fivefold increase in suicide risk. The risk for suicide is highest in the first 3 months of dialysis initiation but then diminishes steadily over time, and it has been suggested that suicide may be driven by a failure to cope with the stress of adjusting to the lifestyle demands of dialysis.[9] Clearly, the ESRD population deserves thoughtful assessment of suicide risk, especially those with a history of mental illness in addition to a high global burden of disease.[9]

The incidence of ESRD is disproportionately higher in African Americans and Hispanic Americans (compared with Caucasian Americans) and is thought to be related to both genetic and socioeconomic factors.[11] African-American patients comprise approximately one-third of ESRD patients in the United States and have an incidence of disease about threefold that of Caucasian patients.[10] There is an increased prevalence of the APOL1 gene among those of West African ancestry, which appears to contribute to the higher frequency of certain common etiologies of CKD (e.g., focal segmental glomerulosclerosis) observed among African and Hispanic Americans.[11]

Patients with CKD and depression are also more likely to be of lower socioeconomic status (**Box 15-1**). Patients with moderate to severe depressive symptoms were found more likely to lack a high school diploma, have an annual income of $20,000 or less, and receive public aid for health insurance.[5] Indeed, socioeconomic

factors such as low income, poor education, residence in low-income areas, and poor access to healthcare are strong predictors of the development of ESRD.[12] Minority populations in the ESRD program were at twice the risk of low socioeconomic status. This may contribute to the increased prevalence of depression among minority patients with CKD, who are also much less likely to seek mental health treatment and be prescribed antidepressants.[5,12] Other risk factors for depression in patients with CKD are being old, female, single, and unemployed. Among individuals with chronic HD, those who were female, unemployed, and had less education were over-represented in the subgroup with comorbid depression. Sixty percent of those who screened positive for depression were either single or widowed.[6,11,13]

Finally, some data suggest that depression itself may be a risk factor for the development of CKD. Depressed patients have a higher prevalence of CKD at baseline compared with nondepressed participants in one multivariable analysis. Depression has been prospectively associated with incident ESRD, a rapid decline in estimated GFR, and acute kidney injury (AKI).[14] The authors also found that elevated depressive symptoms are associated with subsequent adverse renal disease outcomes.[14] Depression has been shown to precede a decrease in serum albumin concentration in dialysis patients, implying that the depression may result in malnutrition.[12]

Depressive symptoms also substantially increase the risk of adverse renal outcomes in adults with CKD. A major depressive episode is associated with nearly doubling the risk of death, dialysis therapy initiation, or hospitalization in male veterans with CKD.[4] Patients with comorbid CKD and MDD were twice as likely to be admitted to the hospital and more than 3 times as likely to progress to ESRD and maintenance dialysis initiation as CKD patients without depression, even after adjusting for other medical comorbidity.[7] In a prospective cohort of diabetic patients with stage 5 CKD, those with comorbid major depression had an almost threefold greater risk of mortality compared to those without major depression.[6] What's more, depression has been shown to be a risk factor for subsequent peritonitis rates and to independently correlate with mortality in PD patients.[15]

Additional risk factors that can affect the development of CKD include hypertension, diabetes mellitus, autoimmune disease, family history of renal disease, a previous episode of AKI, presence of proteinuria, abnormal urinary sediment, or structural abnormalities of the urinary tract.[11] In the United States, the leading cause of ESRD is diabetes mellitus, currently accounting for nearly 55% of newly diagnosed cases of ESRD and associated with a 15% to 25% greater mortality risk among ESRD patients compared to those without diabetes.[6,16] Depression has been found to be commonly comorbid with both diabetes and hypertension. Symptoms of chronic pain and insomnia in addition to a past history of depression are also associated with increased risk of depression in patients with CKD.[10,12]

■ PATHOPHYSIOLOGY

While most of the risk factors for CKD are relatively fixed, depression remains an important modifiable risk factor in patients with ESRD (**Box 15-2**).[3] Several behavioral and physiologic factors have been proposed as mechanisms through which depression can influence outcomes in patients with renal diseases.

Depression has been shown to negatively influence adherence with all the components of ESRD treatment, including medical appointments, the dialysis procedure itself, dietary control, fluid restriction, and the medication regimen.[5] High rates of nonadherence to antihypertensives (85.2%) and oral phosphate binders (72.9%) have been found in depressed dialysis patients, and depression, anxiety, and stress have been negatively correlated with adherence.[17] In addition, depression has been found to be negatively correlated with adherence to the dialysis regimen.[10] Finally, depressed patients are more likely to engage in unhealthy

---

BOX 15-1
IMPORTANT RISK FACTORS FOR DEPRESSION IN RENAL DISEASE AND HYPERTENSION

Sociodemographic

Lower SES

Minority status

Age (elderly)

Gender (female)

Marital status (single)

Clinical

Hypertension

Chronic pain

Insomnia

Medical

Diabetes mellitus

Other psychiatric disorders

Substance use disorders

BOX 15-2
POSSIBLE MEDIATORS BETWEEN RENAL DISEASE, HYPERTENSION, AND DEPRESSION

Non adherence

Sedentary and unhealthy lifestyles

Cytokines and other inflammatory processes

Stress reactions, including sympathetic, parasympathetic, and circadian dysregulation

Insomnia

Obesity

behaviors, including a sedentary lifestyle, cigarette smoking, and alcohol overuse.[6,14]

There is increasing evidence to support a direct physiologic effect of depression and stress on the immune system and internal cytokine milieu.[3,12] Depression has been shown to increase inflammation, alter platelet reactivity, lead to dysregulation of the autonomic nervous system and the hypothalamic–pituitary–adrenal (HPA) axis, and contribute to endothelial dysfunction.[5] Kimmel et al. showed elevations in proinflammatory cytokines such as IL-1 and β-endorphin correlated with increasing levels of depression and marital discord, and was associated with increased mortality.[3,10] C-reactive protein (CRP), another inflammatory biomarker, has been linked to depression in patients without CKD. This is of particular importance as elevations of CRP in ESRD has been associated with increased mortality.[18] Research has revealed alterations in tumor necrosis factor (TNF-α) and IL-6 in setting of uremia, and evidence suggests that increased levels of TNF-α may drive the cachexia that occurs in CKD patients.[12] Since peptide and steroid hormones (e.g., cortisol) undergo metabolism by the kidney, they often circulate at much higher levels in patients with renal disease as than in patients without renal disease, and thus create an internal biochemical milieu similar to that of a chronic stress response.[12] This chronic proinflammatory state intrinsic to ESRD, and exacerbated by the presence of depression, likely contributes to the higher than expected rates of cardiovascular disease and other medical comorbidity, leading to increased mortality in this population.[12]

■ CLINICAL PRESENTATION

Assessment of clinical depression in the setting of CKD can be challenging and major depression should be distinguished from subthreshold depression and dysthymia (**Box 15-3**). Exploring the cognitive rather than somatic symptoms of depression may be useful in differentiating between an appropriate adaptive reaction to the physiologic effects of CKD and a maladaptive cognitive schema that would suggest a depressive disorder.[19] Hallmark symptoms suggesting major depression in ESRD patients include worthlessness, guilt, thoughts of death, and suicidal ideation.[10] It is also important to consider the time course of depressive symptoms in making the diagnosis. For example, the transition to dialysis can be an exceptionally stressful time. In this context, it has been suggested that a diagnosis of major depression should not be made until 3 to 6 months after

BOX 15-3
IMPORTANT SYMPTOMS

Symptoms in common

Somatic/neurovegetative symptoms

Symptoms suggestive of depression

worthlessness, guilt, thoughts of death, and suicidal ideation

beginning dialysis, as there seems to be a normal "settling in period" following which depressive symptoms tend to decrease. Depressive symptoms that improve following adaptation to an acute stressor would suggest an adjustment disorder whereas those that continue to persist would indicate a more severe clinical depression.[10]

One of the shortcomings of the literature is the use of widely differing instruments for assessing depression in CKD.[15] Earlier studies have mostly relied on screening tools such as the Hamilton Rating Scale for Depression (HRSD) or the Beck Depression Inventory© (BDI) to quantify depressive symptoms rather than on making a clinical diagnosis of depressive disorder.[3] The BDI has been used extensively in the ESRD populations and many authors suggest higher cutoffs (i.e., BDI >15) than are used in the general population (BDI >10) because of the higher prevalence of somatic symptoms in patients with ESRD, including fatigue, loss of energy, decreased appetite, sleep disturbance, and difficulty concentrating.[4] Wuerth et al. demonstrated a BDI cutoff of 11 has 84% sensitivity in predicting a diagnosis of depression.[18] More recent studies have used the BDI to screen patients for referral to psychiatric providers who then confirm the diagnosis with a clinical evaluation utilizing DSM criteria.[4] Scales assessing quality of life in CKD are often inversely related to dimensional measures of depression, as both chronic pain and insomnia frequently complicate depression in patients with renal disease.[3]

Negative affect due to depression can be difficult to distinguish from the known uremic symptoms of irritability, cognitive dysfunction, and encephalopathy.[19] While the early stages of CKD are usually not associated with somatic symptoms, patients in the later stages may develop the uremic syndrome, whose clinical features include anorexia, dysquesia, nausea, vomiting, constipation, lassitude, pruritus, disturbances in memory and concentration, and sleep changes. Neuromuscular effects include muscle twitching, muscle cramps, restless leg syndrome, and peripheral neuropathy.[8,11,12]

The initiation of dialysis in the setting of ESRD is often associated with significant psychological and biological stress, lifestyle changes, and decreased quality of life.[6] Several factors contributing to emotional distress include impairments in physical and cognitive functioning, decreased mobility, decreased role function within the family, loss of occupation, and loss of independence.[8,20] Decreased marital satisfaction, disturbances in family dynamics, and lower socioeconomic status have been associated with poorer health outcomes. These factors may also effect patients' perception of social support and increase depression.[12] ESRD and dialysis can also impact the patient's family. Over 40% of spouses of patients on dialysis experience moderate to severe degrees of distress resulting from role changes, loss of employment or income, increasing household responsibilities, and reduced recreational and social activity.[21] PD, which is often preferred because it can be done at home and allows for more autonomy, still places many demands on the patient and his/her support system. PD requires a substantial time commitment, can cause disruption of the home environment, requires a large bedroom machine (which can affect the bed partner), and a surgically implanted catheter (which can affect self-esteem, body image, and sexual functioning).[21] Moreover, dialysis patients have significant sexual dysfunction in part due to hormone dysregulation.[15] Sexual dysfunction is related to quality of life, and improvement in sexual function results in improvement in quality of life.[21] Finally, the perception of disability and the discomfort associated with the peritoneal procedure can also drive symptoms of depression and hopelessness.[15]

Depressed patients with CKD may also suffer from comorbid symptoms of anxiety (**Box 15-4**). Various stresses appear to drive anxiety in this population, most notably impaired functioning, time constraints, fear of disability and death, loss of supportive relationships, loss of employment, and financial stressors.[21] Rates of anxiety

BOX 15-4
RENAL DISORDERS AND ANXIETY

Anxiety is very common in the ESRD population and may be particularly intense during or in anticipation of dialysis sessions. Fluid overload can exacerbate hypoxia, shortness of breath, tachycardia leading to symptoms of panic. Post-dialysis, electrolyte and fluid shifts can often cause nausea, emesis, hypotension, and muscle cramps, all of which can exacerbate anxiety.

Up to a third of patients with CKD suffer from anxiety and commonly worry about the impact of their illness on their daily routines, dietary changes, functional limitations, fears of disability and death, relationship stress and marital discord, sexual dysfunction, loss of employment, and financial difficulties.

There is a negative correlation between anxiety and adherence to the dialysis regimen. Helping to identify the primary sources of anxiety may be useful for clinicians so they can target these concerns directly.

For further details regarding medications commonly used to treat anxiety disorders, see Table 15-2.

Sources: Refs. 4, 12, 17, 21, and 97.

BOX 15-6
DIFFERENTIAL DIAGNOSIS

Other mood disorders

Anxiety disorders

Substance use disorders

Sleep disorders

Dementia

Cognitive disorder

Delirium

Depressed individuals have a higher expectation that their needs for security, safety, acceptance, and respect will not be met. Patients with depression also demonstrate impaired autonomy that interferes with their perceived ability to survive, function independently, or perform successfully.[19] These findings are consistent with the psychodynamic literature, which discusses themes of "aloneness" and "ineffectiveness" as hallmarks of the depressogenic changes associated with ESRD treatment.[19]

Withdrawal from Dialysis

Despite major technological advances over past 30 years, the short- and long-term adjustments to dialysis still exact a heavy toll on ESRD patients. Withdrawal from dialysis is common; approximately 20% of patients withdraw voluntarily, leading to about 10,000 deaths in the United States each year.[10,22] Although there has long been controversy around patient decision-making capacity to discontinue dialysis, cessation of dialysis is now recognized as an appropriate treatment option. Clinical practice guidelines[23] on dialysis withdrawal recommend a shared decision-making process, which takes into account prognostic information along with individual treatment preferences, ideally through an advanced directive. Less than one-third of ESRD patients complete advanced directives. At the time of dialysis withdrawal, nearly half of patients will lack the capacity to participate in this complex decision and, consequently, the burden will fall to their surrogates.[23] Reassurance can be offered that dialysis withdrawal generally results in a peaceful and pain-free death, and the average duration from the last day of cessation until death is 8 days.[23] (Practice guidelines from the American Society of Nephrology and Renal Physicians Association are available at http://www.renalmd.org).[23]

Age, medical complications, dementia, and failure to thrive are common important reasons associated with the decision to withdraw ESRD therapy.[10] In a retrospective review of over 460, 000 patients in the USRDS those withdrawing from dialysis had mean age of 71, were predominately white, more likely to be on HD (rather than PD), and had a higher burden of illness, malnutrition, physical impairment, dementia, malignancy, and other comorbid chronic diseases. African-American patients are half as likely to withdraw as white or Asian patients and the likelihood of dialysis withdrawal is the highest within the first year after initiating dialysis.[9,22]

Depression is also an important factor affecting the decision to withdraw from dialysis. Patients with depression are more likely to eventually withdraw from dialysis compared to those without depression.[22,23] While concern has been raised that depression may lead to a premature decision to withdraw, it is not known whether this would decrease with improved recognition and treatment of depression. Despite this, it is prudent to consider psychiatric evaluation for depression when ESRD patients make an unexpected decision to discontinue dialysis. A low threshold for treatment, either psychotherapy, pharmacotherapy, or both, is indicated when patients meet criteria for major depression.

in CKD have been estimated as high as 27% but rates of comorbid depression and anxiety are substantially lower, and it appears that anxiety exists independently of depression in this population.[19] In a study of urban HD patients, 29% had a current depressive disorder, 27% had a current anxiety disorder, up to 19% had a substance use disorder, and 10% had a current psychotic disorder (**Box 15-5**).[19]

■ COURSE AND NATURAL HISTORY

Depression results in substantial functional impairment and decreased quality of life in ESRD patients, and symptoms of depression do not appear to remit spontaneously in untreated patients.[4] Untreated depression is likely to adversely affect progression of kidney disease. Kop et al. showed that depressive symptoms pose an increased risk for the development of poor kidney function and clinical progression to ESRD and AKI.[14] It is hypothesized that effective treatment of depression will improve adverse ESRD outcomes, including poor nutritional status and treatment adherence, which will in turn affect survival.[12] However, this remains unproven given the existing low rates of adequate treatment. While nearly one in four patients with stage 5 CKD qualify for a DSM diagnosis of MDD, estimates suggest that only 16% to 20% of these patients are being treated with antidepressants.[4,15,19] More research is needed to demonstrate the benefit of effective treatment, but it is likely that adequate therapy would ameliorate depressive symptoms, which in turn would improve quality of life and functioning.[18]

As CKD progresses, the presence of depressive symptoms has been shown to increase. Fischer et al. demonstrated that for every 10 mL/min/1.73m² decrease in GFR, there was a 9% increased odds of elevated depressive symptoms. These authors also found a significantly greater frequency of BDI scores >11 (positive screen for depression) in patients with GFR <30 mL.[5]

Finally, progressive renal dysfunction leads to poorer health status. In the setting of comorbid depression, this CKD progression is significantly associated with a perception of lower quality of life.[19]

BOX 15-5
COMMON COMORBIDITIES

Anxiety disorders

Substance use disorders

Psychotic disorders

BOX 15-7
TREATMENTS FOR DEPRESSION IN PATIENTS WITH RENAL DISEASE

Antidepressants: limited data

SSRIs: usually first line (watch for bleeding, falls)

TCAs and MAOIs usually avoided due to cardiovascular effects

SNRIs, bupropion: may increase blood pressure

Atypical antipsychotics (watch for metabolic side effects)

CBT

Marital and family counseling

More frequent dialysis

Exercise

■ ASSESSMENT AND DIFFERENTIAL DIAGNOSIS

The assessment and differential diagnosis of depression in patients with CKD is similar to that for all medically ill patients (see chapter on Assessment of Depression) (**Box 15-6**). Prior history of depression, family history, and other comorbid medical illnesses associated with depression should not be overlooked. Differential diagnoses that should always be considered include other mood disorders, particularly bipolar affective disorder, anxiety disorders, and substance use disorders. In patients with chronic or ESRD, additional consideration should include sleep disorders, dementia or other cognitive disorder, and delirium.

■ TREATMENT

Chronic kidney disease may affect antidepressant (AD) pharmacokinetics unpredictably (**Box 15-7**). Most importantly, decreases in GFR may result in impaired drug excretion. Unless more than 70% of a drug excretion is by a nonrenal route, such as hepatic elimination, the maintenance doses of many drugs will likely need to be adjusted.[11] Antidepressants are highly protein bound and not significantly cleared by the dialysis procedure and as such do not require substitution dosing following dialysis. They commonly undergo hepatic metabolism, but many have active metabolites that are excreted renally, leading to accumulation of potentially toxic metabolites in patients with decreased GFR (**Table 15-1**).[4] Specific agents with reduced clearance in advanced CKD include selegiline, amitriptyline, venlafaxine, desvenlafaxine, and bupropion. Dose reduction is recommended with these agents. Mirtazapine has a reduced plasma clearance after oral intake but not a prolonged elimination half-life so dose adjustment may not be needed (**Table 15-2**).[24]

TABLE 15-1 Pharmacokinetic Changes in ESRD

Elevated urea can cause alkalinization of gastric fluid à reduce enteral absorption of drugs
Changes in body fat/lean body mass composition à altered volume of distribution
Polypharmacy, elevated levels of urea and other toxins, loss of serum albumin à increased competition for binding sites on albumin à higher free fractions of drugs
Decline in chemical reduction and hydrolysis (while preserved rates of glucuronidation, microsomal oxidation, and sulfate conjugation) à may lead to accumulation of drugs and metabolites
Decline in GFR leads to reduced renal clearance of drugs and their metabolites à may lead to toxic accumulation

Source: Refs. 4, 11, and 97.

There is a paucity of data describing the safety and efficacy of AD medications in patients with advanced CKD and ESRD as these patients have generally been excluded from large AD trials because of concern for adverse effects. In addition, there are insufficient data to clearly suggest that the treatment of MDD is either effective in CKD or that treatment of depression changes outcomes in advanced CKD or ESRD.[4] Most of the known studies are small, lack placebo control, and fail to utilize DSM-based criteria for diagnosing depression.[4]

Although there is limited evidence suggesting that ADs are more effective than placebo in treating patients with CKD, they are still recommended as first-line treatment of depression.[24] A recent review of AD drug therapy in CKD patients showed that ADs were more effective that placebo, with NNT = 6.[24] A systematic review of RCTs and observational studies of AD use in patients with CKD stages 3 to 5 found only 28 studies, and the data in these studies were so sparse and heterogeneous that they precluded a meta-analysis.[24] Nine nonrandomized trials all suggested benefit for the AD under investigation but the response was not significantly greater than placebo, with up to one-third of patients responding to placebo. Even though side effects were considered mild in most patients, an average of 21% discontinued treatment making it even more difficult to accurately assess outcomes.[24] The authors concluded that current evidence was insufficient, but still advised active treatment for depression given its negative influence on survival and quality of life. When choosing an agent, SSRIs are preferred and the authors recommend an 8–12-week trial and a reduction in starting dosage by one-third.[12,24] Once medication is initiated, response to treatment, need for dose adjustment, and the development of side effects should be monitored closely. Dose escalation should not be done sooner than 1 to 2 weeks and only as tolerated, with special attention to drug interactions and to assessment of suicidal ideation (**Box 15-8**).[4]

Many barriers prevent patients who do get diagnosed with depression from obtaining the appropriate treatment. These include patient refusal of psychiatric referral, reluctance to accept AD therapy in the context of an already complex pharmacologic regimen, and medication side effects.[15] In a study of the efficacy of several different ADs over 12 weeks, improvement in depressive symptoms was observed in all groups. However, only 50% of patients who screened positive for depression agreed to referral, and nearly 25% of that group refused to initiate pharmacotherapy. Of those who did take medication, only 50% successfully completed a 12-week trial.[25]

Depression treatment seems to vary with sociodemographic factors and comorbid psychiatric disorders. Female patients with depression are more likely to be on medication than males. Minority populations, who have up to 1.5-fold increased prevalence of depressive symptoms, are much less likely to be on medication.[5] Patients with depression who use tobacco or illicit drugs are more likely to receive AD treatment. It is reassuring that those with more severe depressive symptoms are more likely to be on an antidepressant medication.[5] Patients with comorbid substance abuse and with axis II personality disorders are much more likely to prematurely discontinue antidepressant therapy.[18]

There are limited data to suggest a direct effect of renal medications on symptoms of depression, except for the antihypertensives (which are reviewed elsewhere in this chapter). However, there is an increased risk of drug–drug interactions in patients with CKD as they

---

BOX 15-8
IMPORTANT DRUG–DRUG INTERACTIONS BETWEEN ANTIDEPRESSANTS AND RENAL TREATMENTS

Affected by dialysis:

selegiline, amitriptyline, venlafaxine, desvenlafaxine, and bupropion.

TABLE 15-2 Pharmacotherapy in CKD and ESRD

Medications by Class	Comments
Selective Serotonin Reuptake Inhibitors	
Monitor for bleeding risks	Considered first line for treatment of depression in CKD/ESRD
GI symptoms: nausea, diarrhea	No more than 2/3 max dose
CNS effects: agitation, anxiety	Reduce paroxetine dose: max 20 mg/day
Sexual dysfunction, hyponatremia	Monitor for CYP1A2 inhibition: fluvoxamine
	Monitor for CYP2D6 inhibition: fluoxetine, paroxetine, sertraline
Serotonin Norepinephrine Reuptake Inhibitors	
Monitor for bleeding risks	May consider as alternative to TCAs for neuropathic pain, due to better tolerability
GI symptoms: nausea, diarrhea	No more than 2/3 max dose
CNS effects: agitation, anxiety	Reduce dose of venlafaxine: max 112.5 mg/day
Sexual dysfunction, hyponatremia	Monitor for CYP2D6 inhibition: duloxetine
Monitor for hypertension	
Atypical Antidepressants	
Mirtazapine	
May have enhanced CNS effects, somnolence, weight gain, hypotension	Use more cautiously in CKD/ESRD patients
Bupropion	Dose reduce by 30–50%
Active metabolite accumulation could increase risk of seizures, cardiac dysrhythmia, widen QRS, GI effects of nausea, insomnia, appetite suppression	Use more cautiously in CKD/ESRD patients
	No more than 2/3 max dose
	Monitor for CYP2D6 inhibition
Trazodone/Nefazodone	Use more cautiously in CKD/ESRD patients
May have enhanced CNS effects, somnolence, hypotension, priapism, QT prolongation	No more than 2/3 max dose
Hepatotoxicity (nefazodone)	
Tricyclic Antidepressants	
Anticholinergic effects: urinary retention, constipation, tachycardia	Generally not recommended
Monitor for hypotension, QRS prolongation, increased risk of cardiac arrhythmias, CNS effects: sedation, falls	Serum levels and EKGs should be monitored
Monoamine Oxidase Inhibitors	
Significant risk of drug–drug interactions	Generally not recommended
Risk of hypertensive crisis with tyramine-rich foods	
Monitor for orthostatic hypotension	
Anxiolytics/Sedatives	
Benzodiazepines	Most are hepatically metabolized, well-tolerated, with wide therapeutic index
Monitor for enhanced CNS effects: somnolence, ataxia, falls, respiratory suppression	Most are highly protein bound which can have higher potency in CKD/ESRD
Increased risk of delirium	Dosing should be cautiously titrated
Buspirone	May have additive effects with other sedatives
Monitor for enhanced CNS effects: somnolence, dizziness, falls	Considerable variability in metabolism in ESRD of both parent compound and active metabolites
Zolpidem	Use more cautiously in CKD/ESRD patients
Monitor for enhanced CNS effects: somnolence, dizziness, falls	Dose reduce by 25–50%
	Use more cautiously in CKD/ESRD patients
	Dose reduce by 50%

Source: Refs. 4, 24, and 97.

are commonly on multiple medications, frequently have other medical comorbidity, and have increased risk of metabolic derangements.

Several antidepressant classes, such as serotonin modulators, tricyclics antidepressants (TCAs), and tetracyclics, can have cardiac effects, such as QTc prolongation, arrhythmias, and orthostatic hypotension. This can be especially concerning in the large proportion of CKD and ESRD patients who also suffer from cardiovascular diseases.[4] TCAs, monoamine oxidase inhibitors (MAOIs), and herbal treatments such as St. John wort should be avoided in ESRD patients due to the risks of arrhythmias, other cardiac events, and orthostatic hypotension.[12,18] In addition, some observational data suggest that both TCAs and selective serotonin reuptake inhibitors (SSRIs) antidepressants may increase the risk of falls in elderly patients. SSRIs have been associated with an increased risk of bleeding. This could become problematic in advanced CKD as uremia also leads to platelet dysfunction, potentially compounding the risk. Adverse gastrointestinal side effects of SSRIs can exacerbate symptoms of nausea and vomiting in patients with CKD and ESRD.[4] Given these interactions, nephrologists are often timid about adding any additional medications to patients who are already on complicated regimens.[4]

Lithium and Chronic Kidney Disease

Since the 1970s, lithium has been used as an important augmentation agent in treatment-refractory major depression and has been associated with reduction in self-harm, suicide, and all-cause mortality.[26,27] More recently, research into the unique neuroprotective properties of lithium has demonstrated potential benefits for healing after acute brain injury and stabilization of chronic neurodegenerative diseases, and it is likely to continue as a key therapeutic agent for psychiatric illness in the years to come.[26,28] Lithium can affect the kidney in three major ways: (1) AKI often associated with acute lithium toxicity; (2) impaired urinary concentrating ability or nephrogenic diabetes insipidus (NDI); and (3) lithium-induced nephropathy with decline in GFR, and progression to CKD.[29]

Lithium has a narrow therapeutic index (0.8–1.2 mEq/L) and requires regular serum monitoring and assessment of renal function.[30] Lithium toxicity may develop at levels >1.5 mEq/L and may become life-threatening above 2 mEq/L and may require emergent HD. Symptoms of lithium toxicity include nausea, diarrhea, blurred vision, tremor, confusion, lethargy, and, if untreated, convulsions and death.[31,32] Risk factors for AKI include older age, past AKI, past episodes of lithium toxicity, use of certain antihypertensives, diuretics, and anti-inflammatory agents (**Table 15-3**).[33] To minimize risks of acute lithium toxicity, adequate hydration is imperative. Other considerations include cessation or reduction of lithium during acute illness, more frequent monitoring of serum lithium levels and renal function (every 3–6 months) in patients older than 60 and in any patient with history of renal disease.[33]

It is estimated that up to 40% of patients treated with lithium have evidence of impaired urinary concentrating ability (UOsm <300 mOsm/kg) due to direct effects of lithium on renal collecting ducts. Symptoms of NDI include increased thirst, polydipsia, or polyuria defined as >3 L urine output per day.[34] Most patients can manage increased urine output by compensating with increased fluid intake. However, in elderly patients or those unable to access adequate hydration, NDI can lead to dehydration, hypernatremia, and acute lithium toxicity.[35] Risk factors for NDI include advanced age, concurrent use of antipsychotics, use of slow release lithium formulations, higher lithium-serum concentration, and longer duration of lithium use.[33] In addition, several studies have shown that lithium dosed once daily can reduce adverse effects, enhance compliance, and minimize polyuria.[32] There are no standard recommendations for screening for NDI and the collection of a 24-hour urine sample can be cumbersome. There is some evidence that urine-specific gravity (USG) as part of a standard urinalysis may have some utility as a screening tool for NDI. Rej et al. demonstrated that USG <1.010 (performed after 10 hours of water restriction) strongly correlated

TABLE 15-3 Medications Which May Impair Excretion of Lithium

COX-2 inhibitors
NSAIDs
ACEIs
ARBs
Thiazides
Loop diuretics

Source: Ref. 31.

with UOsm <300 mOsm/kg with sensitivity of 0.78 and specificity of 0.93.[34] Fortunately, the presence of NDI does not appear to predict loss of GFR[27]; however, if severe, it can predispose to lithium toxicity and AKI, and thereby enhance long-term progression to CKD.

The most feared renal complication of lithium use is progression to ESRD, which fortunately is considered a rare event and associated with long-term use. Pathological changes consistently demonstrated in patients on chronic lithium therapy for 10 years or more include evidence of tubular atrophy, interstitial fibrosis, and 1- to 2-mm microcysts, found in the zones of atrophy and fibrosis, and appear to originate from both cortical and medullary collecting ducts.[29,36] Although it is not clear how these anatomical changes directly affect glomerular function, as many as 15% to 30% of patients treated with lithium for more than 10 years show evidence of reduced GFR compared to controls, which can further complicate the changes in renal function that are due to age. After the 4th decade, renal function begins to decline by 10% per decade.[31] As many as 40% of all community dwelling Americans >70 years have moderate to severe CKD (GFR <60 mL/min/1.73m²). Similarly, up to 50% of patients treated with lithium for longer than 20 years will have evidence of CKD and thus necessitate referral to a nephrologist and consideration of lithium discontinuation, which may help to slow rates of progression to ESRD.[31,37] Other risk factors for CKD include repeated episodes of AKI, high maintenance plasma lithium levels, concurrent medications, and comorbid illnesses (e.g., hypertension, diabetes, ischemic heart disease).[30] Strategies to minimize risk of CKD include use of the lowest effective lithium dose, regular monitoring of renal function, optimizing treatment of blood pressure, diabetes, obesity, and other modifiable risk factors.[32]

■ NONPHARMACOLOGIC TREATMENT OF DEPRESSION IN CKD

Several nonpharmacologic therapies have demonstrated efficacy in depression treatment, including more frequent dialysis, exercise regimens, and cognitive behavioral therapy. In one study, 85 HD patients with MDD were assigned to standard care or cognitive–behavioral group therapy. BDI scores decreased significantly in the study group versus the control group over the follow-up period.[4,38] In another study, a 6-month exercise rehabilitation program for HD patients produced a statistically significant decrease in BDI scores.[18] Other psychosocial interventions to consider in the ESRD population include marital and family counseling, referral to appropriate treatment facilities (e.g., addiction centers), and eliciting involvement of other support services, for example, church groups, extended family, community agencies, or groups to support treatment compliance and overall functioning.[18,21] Social support has been associated with decreased depressive affect in ESRD patients.[39] Religious beliefs have been shown to enhance coping and thus decrease depressive affect in patients being treated for ESRD. Greater spirituality and religious involvement has been associated with decreased BDI and cognitive depression scores.[10]

■ SUMMARY

As many as one in five patients with CKD will experience a major depressive episode, and depression is associated with poorer outcomes in patients with ESRD and in those receiving dialysis. Given this high prevalence, patients with CKD should be routinely screened for depression. Additional vigilance is indicated for female, minority, or lower socioeconomic status patients. Patients with more severe CKD and/or a previous history of psychiatric illness or substance abuse are also at higher risk of depression.[5] Further attention should also be paid to improving education about depression and its effects on renal disease in order to decrease stigmatization and encourage patients to consider treatment.[24]

More evidence-based data are needed in order to develop best practices for the pharmacologic treatments of depression in patients with CKD and ESRD. One would hope that further research would demonstrate that adequate depression treatment not only improves depressive symptoms and quality of life but also improves medical outcomes.[3] Nonpharmacologic treatments may provide equal benefit without potential harms and can represent valuable alternatives to antidepressant drug therapy.[24] Another area that requires more investigation is the effect of renal transplantation on depression.[3] Finally, supporting patients through dialysis withdrawal, a natural consequence of severe renal disease, is an important way in which physicians can help to reduce suffering and maximize the autonomy of our patients.[22]

HYPERTENSION AND DEPRESSION

■ EPIDEMIOLOGY

Approximately 30% of adults (65 million individuals) in the United States have hypertension, defined as having one of the following: systolic blood pressure ≥140 mm Hg, diastolic blood pressure ≥90 mm Hg, or taking antihypertensive medications.[40] High blood pressure is considered one of the most important preventable causes of premature morbidity and mortality and doubles the risk of developing renal failure, cardiovascular diseases, stroke, and peripheral arterial disease.[41] Although antihypertensive therapy clearly reduces the risks of cardiovascular and renal disease, up to 50% of those with hypertension are either untreated or inadequately treated.[40]

The incidence of hypertension increases with age, with prevalence rates as high as 65% in individuals older than 60 years.[40] Male gender is a risk factor for development of hypertension, related in part to male sex-hormones.[42] In addition, men are more likely to have unhealthy behaviors and less likely to perceive themselves at risk for health problems. Premenopausal women have relatively lower rates related to protective effects of estrogen, but postmenopausal women have increased prevalence of hypertension as they age.[42] The increasing prevalence of hypertension in the United States is thought to be related to increasing rates of obesity. Obesity and weight gain are known to be strong independent risk factors for hypertension with an estimated 60% of hypertensive patients being more than 20% above their ideal body weight. The prevalence of hypertension is also associated with high dietary intake of sodium chloride.[40]

Family studies show a significant heritability of blood pressure levels and hypertension, in the range 15% to 35%. The onset of hypertension before age 55 occurs 3.8 times more often among those with a positive family history of hypertension.[40] It has been suggested that hypertension and depression may share common genetic susceptibility.[43] In African Americans, hypertension appears to present at an earlier age, is generally more severe, and results in higher rates of ESRD, general medical morbidity, and mortality than in white Americans.[40] Lower socioeconomic status has also been associated with an elevated prevalence of hypertension, which may suggest that this population has less knowledge about hypertension risks and fewer opportunities for treatment.[42]

The rate of hypertension in patients with MDD is somewhat higher than in nondepressed patients, especially with advancing age.[42] Depression is associated with both the cross-sectional prevalence and the longitudinal incidence of hypertension.[43,44] Several large cohort studies have reported up to a twofold increase in odds of incident hypertension among adults with baseline depressive symptoms.[45] A recent meta-analysis concluded that there was a 42% increased risk for hypertension in depressed cohorts and that depression was likely an independent risk factor for hypertension.[43] A prospective cohort study found an increased risk of hypertension in subjects with recurrent depressive episodes over time that becomes evident in later adulthood. Even after controlling for increasing age and other covariates, those with more severe and recurrent depression developed hypertension more frequently (about 7% increased incidence), with men showing increased incidence at an earlier age than women.[46] Another study showed that middle-aged subjects with depression were 65% more likely to be diagnosed with hypertension in the follow-up period when compared to age-matched controls without depression.[44] In contrast, however, one study found that subjects with major depression had a significantly lower mean systolic blood pressure and were less likely to have isolated systolic hypertension.[47]

■ PATHOPHYSIOLOGY

The relationship between depression and hypertension is complex and bidirectional. Depression is associated with alterations in catecholamine secretion as well as dysregulation of circadian rhythm. Both these systems are important in neuroregulatory feedback mechanisms of blood pressure, and impairment in these systems may be associated with the development of hypertension. Chronic hypertension may then lead to further impact on catecholamine homeostasis, which can affect the ability to respond to chronic stress and thus further precipitate depressive illness.[45]

Insomnia and decreased sleep duration are common symptoms of depression that are thought to mediate the relationship with hypertension.[45] In normal individuals, blood pressures during sleep are generally 10% to 20% lower than those during the daytime.[40] It is thought that depression may influence this physiologic nocturnal decrease in blood pressure, and one study has demonstrated an association between depressive symptoms and blunted nocturnal fall in systolic blood pressure.[45] In a prospective study, Gangwisch et al. found that depressed participants reporting chronic short sleep duration (<5 hours/night) were 50% more likely to develop hypertension than those with 7 to 8 hours sleep/night. The authors proposed that chronic sleep deprivation could condition the cardiovascular system to adapt to a higher pressure equilibrium.[44] Moreover, insomnia can increase activation of HPA axis with subsequent elevations in cortisol,[44,48] and elevated cortisol levels and lack of suppression on dexamethasone suppression tests (DST) have been significantly correlated with elevated blood pressure.[46]

Depression is associated with autonomic dysfunction, including increased sympathetic and decreased parasympathetic activity, which could also contribute to an elevation of blood pressure. Autonomic dysregulation may result from diminished vagal function, as evidenced by reduced heart rate variability.[43,49] Even subtle changes in autonomic regulation can cause increased blood pressure reactivity when stress is encountered, and this has been suggested as the mechanism whereby psychological traits and stress may lead to hypertension.[50,51] Depression (and anxiety) can alter neuropeptide Y, which modulates norepinephrine signaling by suppressing sympathetic activity and therefore decreases blood pressure, which might explain why systolic blood pressure has also been shown to be lower in some depressed patients.[41,52]

Growing evidence suggests that patients with depression can manifest immune dysfunction and increased release of inflammatory cytokines, and hypertensive patients show increases in circulating inflammatory markers, for example, CRP, which can predict the onset of hypertension.[49]

Depression commonly cooccurs with anxiety disorders, which themselves have been implicated in the development of hypertension. Cross-sectional studies of depressed persons provide evidence of increased sympathetic activity, for example, autonomic arousal and increased blood pressure reactivity. This suggests that taken together, anxiety and depression may have a pressor effect on the cardiovascular system that could lead to the development of hypertensions.[48]

Finally, persons with MDDs might be more frequently exposed to psychotropic drugs that may contribute to weight gain and the consequent development of hypertension.[42]

■ CLINICAL PRESENTATION

Hypertension is relatively asymptomatic and therefore unlikely to have symptoms that overlap with those of depression. Thus, the diagnosis of depressive disorder in patients with hypertension does not differ significantly from that discussed in Chapter 3.

■ COURSE AND NATURAL HISTORY

Depression and hypertension share several common risk factors, including behaviors such as diminished self-care, a sedentary lifestyle, drinking, smoking, and obesity (Box 15-1). The lack of physical activity, smoking, alcohol abuse, metabolic syndrome, and obesity account for a significant portion of the relative risk of incident hypertension in depressed patients, suggesting that these behaviors might be mediators of the relationship between depression and hypertension.[43]

These unhealthy lifestyle behaviors can affect the management and prognosis of hypertension, as can medication nonadherence.[42] Poor adherence to antihypertensive pharmacotherapy is a major contributor to poor blood pressure control and subsequent adverse clinical outcomes. A large sample of community dwelling elderly adults revealed poorer adherence in those with a depressive disorder, with women more adherent than men. Adherence to medication decreased significantly over time with rates falling to 59% after 2 years in the depressed cohort.[53] A meta-analysis also demonstrated a statistically significant relationship between depression and poor adherence to antihypertensive medications.[54]

The course of untreated hypertension can also contribute to the development of depression in late life. Thus, elderly men with depressive symptoms have a higher frequency of hypertension early in life.[49] Hypertension in early life can lead to cerebrovascular changes, with white matter lesions and cortical atrophy involving frontolimbic and frontostriatal pathways, leading to subsequent mood changes.

■ ASSESSMENT AND DIFFERENTIAL DIAGNOSIS

The assessment of depression in patients with hypertension is not significantly different from the depression evaluation discussed in Chapter 3 (Box 15-6). Differential diagnoses include bipolar disorder, anxiety disorders, comorbid substance use disorder, sleep disorder, dementia or cognitive disorder, or in an acute medical setting, delirium. In the patient with hypertension, the assessment should consider the temporal relationship between the onset of hypertension and development of depression. If a strong relationship exists, greater emphasis may be placed on the aggressive management of the hypertension. In addition, symptoms that suggest cerebrovascular disease related to the hypertension should lead to more complete neuropsychiatric evaluation, with potential addition of neuroimaging that may help guide depression treatment.

■ TREATMENT

Pharmacotherapy is the mainstay in the treatment of hypertension, in addition to the management of dietary habits, low salt diet, weight loss, and regular exercise (Box 15-7).[53] In addition, attention to smoking cessation, alcohol, and drug use is important. The association between short sleep duration and hypertension suggests that improving sleep hygiene practices are particularly important in patients with hypertension and comorbid depression.[44]

Psychiatric Side Effects of Antihypertensive Agents

Reserpine, clonidine, methyldopa, β-blockers, calcium channel blockers, and agents targeting angiotensin, for example, angiotensin-converting

---

BOX 15-9
DRUGS THAT CAN CAUSE DEPRESSIVE SYMPTOMS

Classically described: reserpine, clonidine, methyldopa, β-blockers, calcium channel blockers, angiotensin converting enzyme (ACE) inhibitors, angiotensin II-receptor blockers (ARBs).

Note that modern studies have found the associations and depression to be much weaker than originally described.

---

enzyme (ACE) inhibitors, angiotensin II-receptor blockers (ARBs), have been associated with depression, but these associations are probably much weaker than originally believed (**Box 15-9**).[55,56]

Reserpine leads to the depletion of cathecholamine neruotransmitters by monoamine oxidase. Early studies reported an incidence of subsyndromal depressive symptoms (including fatigue, malaise, and sedation) of up to 15% with reserpine. But more recent studies have found low rates of depression with reserpine.[55] The centrally acting α-agonist clonidine has been associated with sedation and fatigue in up to a third of patients, but rarely (1–2%) leading to mood disturbance. Older studies of methyldopa, a central α_2-agonist (now rarely used except in pregnancy-induced hypertension), revealed side effects of fatigue, sedation, and depression (thought to be related to reduced norepinephrine levels) in up to a third of patients, particularly in patients with a history of depression. However, more recent reviews have not shown a significant association between methyldopa and depression.[55]

β-Blockers have been the most extensively studied of the antihypertensive agents.[56] Although lipophilic β-blockers (e.g., propranolol, metoprolol) cross the blood–brain barrier much more easily than nonlipophilic β-blockers, there is no clear evidence to suggest they have higher rates of neuropsychiatric sequelae. A large metaanalysis did not find a significant association between β-blockers and depressive symptoms, and there was no difference between lipophilic and nonlipophilic agents in this regard.[55] Furthermore, pindolol, which has effects at 5-HT1A receptors, has been actively studied as a potential augmenting agent in treatment of depression, and has been found to increase the speed of response to SSRIs.[55] Finally, Celano et al. found that β-blockers were not associated with cognitive symptoms of depression but did increase some somatic symptoms (fatigue and sleep problems), and as such may be misinterpreted as evidence of depression.[55]

Studies of calcium-channel blockers suggest an increase in fatigue but no association with depression. Nimodipine has been shown superior to placebo in augmenting antidepressant treatment in patients with vascular depression. A study of patients with coronary artery disease (CAD) and hypertension treated with verapamil SR found a significant improvement in depressive symptoms at 1-year follow-up, suggesting that verapamil may be preferred over other β-blockers in patients with CAD and depression.[57]

Other antihypertensive agents, including diuretics, ACE inhibitors, and ARBs, are generally not associated with neuropsychiatric effects or depression.[55] Some case reports have implicated ACE inhibitors and ARBs in the onset of depressive symptoms but controlled study data are lacking. Nonetheless, it is certainly possible that all antihypertensive agents may cause some symptoms of depression, most commonly fatigue, and could be implicated in exacerbating a subsyndromal depression into a more clinically significant depressive episode. As such, it appears prudent to monitor patients prescribed these agents for evolving symptoms of depression.[56]

Effects of Antidepressants on Blood Pressure

Antidepressant use is associated with a higher prevalence of elevated blood pressure in patients with MDD.[42] MAOIs and TCAs, in addition to the serotonin-norepinephrine reuptake inhibitor

(SNRI) venlafaxine, appear to have direct effects on blood pressure and could contribute to the development and/or exacerbation of hypertension.[58] This effect on blood pressure may be mediated by potentiation of noradrenergic transmission and by anticholinergic effects on heart rate.[58] Other agents that may also affect blood pressure include bupropion and the antipsychotics, which are commonly used as adjunctive agents in the treatment of depression.[56,58]

TCAs can produce orthostatic hypotension via blockade of α_1 receptors, as well as increasing systolic blood pressure via their anticholinergic effects on cardiac vagal control.[52] In a study of 2,600 adults with hypertension and comorbid depression, those taking TCAs had higher systolic and diastolic blood compared to those on other antidepressant agents.[52] Post-hoc analysis of a study by Delaney et al. revealed a strong association between TCAs and hypertension.[47] A more recent meta-analysis of the blood pressure effects of venlafaxine and imipramine revealed blood pressure changes with imipramine therapy that were relatively benign, and 75% of the cases with elevated systolic and diastolic blood pressure remitted spontaneously during the continuation phase.[58] Many of the studies of TCAs and blood pressure have focused on older patients, often with serious medical comorbidity, and these patients may be more prone to the development of orthostatic hypotension, a potentially serious side effect for which all patients on TCAs should be monitored.[58]

Similar to the TCAs, the nonselective MAOIs can cause relatively high rates of orthostatic hypotension, which also deserves close clinical monitoring.[58] MAOIs exhibit their antidepressant effect by inhibition of monoamine oxidase, which enhances synaptic levels of dopamine, serotonin, and norepinephrine. These agents have been associated with hypertension and a very serious risk of hypertensive crisis. It may be prudent to avoid MAOIs in patients with chronic hypertension. Most importantly, patients on MAOIs must be appropriately educated about their dietary intake of tyramine, a vasoactive amine that occurs naturally in aged meats, alcoholic beverages, and aged cheeses. Dietary tyramine is converted to norepinephrine (NE). When NE degradation is inhibited by an MAOI, even moderate consumption of tyramine can lead to a rapid increase in blood pressure and possibly hypertensive crisis. Dangerous elevations in blood pressure and toxic levels of serotonin (e.g., serotonin syndrome) can also occur when MAOIs are combined with other drugs that enhance catecholamine or serotonin levels.[59] All patients taking MAOIs must be closely monitored with use of other pharmacologic agents, including over-the-counter agents, to avoid these dangerous drug interactions (**Table 15-4**).[41,58,59]

SNRIs have been found to increase diastolic blood pressure less than either TCAs or MAOIs. This may be partially due to effects on vagal control, but the complete mechanism remains unknown. In a large review of depressed patients on venlafaxine, those on >300 mg/day of venlafaxine had a small but statistically significant increase in the incidence of blood pressure elevation. This effect persisted during continuation therapy, and there was a small but significant incidence of new cases of elevated blood pressure during longer term therapy. Blood pressure effects were observed in up to 11% of patients on venlafaxine. Of note, venlafaxine did not negatively affect the control of blood pressure in patients who were on antihypertensive therapy. It is, therefore, recommended that venlafaxine be tried at lower doses before advancing to 300 mg or higher, with serial monitoring of blood pressure in patients on >300 mg/day.[58]

Bupropion has been shown to increase blood pressure, likely through dopaminergic pathways, although neither a dose–response relationship nor the exact incidence of sustained blood pressure elevation has been examined in detail.[58]

Atypical antipsychotics are increasingly being used as augmentation agents for the treatment of MDD.[42] Both first- and second-generation antipsychotic agents have been associated with elevated blood pressure in patients with MDD. A recent review suggests that

TABLE 15-4 Drugs Contraindicated with MAOIs

Sympathomimetics
    Amphetamines
    Phenylephrine
    Cocaine
    Vasoconstrictive agents
Opiates/Analgesics
    Dextromethorphan
    Methadone
    Meperidine
    Tramadol
Anesthetic agents
Antibiotics
    Linezolid
Antidepressants/Anxiolytics
    SSRIs, SNRIs, TCAs, other MAOIs
    Bupropion, Buspirone
Antiepileptic Agents
    Carbamazepine
    Oxcarbazepine
Dibenzazepine-related agents
    Cyclobenzaprine
    Perphenazine
St. John's Wort

Source: Ref. 59.

although these agents do appear to be effective in treating depression when compared to placebo, they may be associated with serious and relatively common long-term side effects, such as weight gain, hypercholesterolemia, and metabolic syndrome and as such should be used cautiously with continued monitoring of blood pressure.[42]

■ SUMMARY

Hypertension is one of the most preventable causes of premature morbidity and mortality, and there is some evidence of an association with depression. The bidirectional mechanisms by which depression and hypertension affect each other are not well understood. Multiple pathways have been suggested, including sleep disruption, alteration of catecholamine secretion, and autonomic regulation, in addition to the effects of cortisol and inflammation. There are limited data on the effect that early recognition and treatment of depression might have on decreasing the risk of developing hypertension and to what extent long-term morbidity and mortality related to hypertension might be decreased. Further complicating the picture, several antidepressants can directly contribute to elevated blood pressure. However, given the high prevalence of both conditions, evaluation of possible depression in patients with hypertension and for hypertension in patients with depression, and ensuring adequate treatment of both conditions, seems likely to improve their outcomes.

NUTRITIONAL DEFICIENCIES

■ INTRODUCTION

Vitamin and nutritional deficiencies may occur as a result of medical illness or as part of a dietary pattern contributing to medical illness, as in diabetes or cardiovascular disease. A number of nutritional deficiencies have been linked to depression (see **Table 15-5**). Nutritional factors can impact depression pathophysiology by

TABLE 15-5 Nutritional Deficiencies and Depression[1]

Nutrient	Conditions Associated with Deficiency	Medications Causing Deficiency	Signs and Symptoms	Mechanism in Depression	Dietary Sources
Folate	Heavy alcohol use, dietary insufficiency, pregnancy and lactation, cancer, hemolytic anemia, hemodialysis, liver disease, malabsorption, tobacco	Oral contraceptives Sulfasalazine Phenytoin Primidone Methotrexate Triamterene Pyrimethamine Trimethoprim	↑Homocysteine, hypersegmented neutrophils Macrocytic anemia ± fatigue, shortness of breath, weakness	Required for synthesis of monoamine neurotransmitters in one-carbon cycle	Green leafy vegetables, legumes, orange juice
Magnesium	Malabsorption, Crohn's disease, Celiac disease, prolonged diarrhea, resection of parts of intestine, intestinal inflammation caused by radiation, renal disease, diabetes, heavy alcohol use, older age	Long-term diuretic use	Hypomagnesemia, hypocalcemia in spite of adequate dietary calcium, hypokalemia, sodium retention, ↓PTH, tremor, tetany, muscle spasms, anorexia, nausea and vomiting, personality changes	Required for ion transport across membranes as part of neuronal transmission and for synthesis of glutathione	Oat bran, 100% bran cereal, brown rice, spinach, almonds, Swiss chard, lima beans, molasses
Selenium	Dietary insufficiency, resection of part of small intestine, Crohn's disease. metabolic disorders requiring specialized diets	None	No clinical manifestations unless severe deficiency Impaired immunity, cardiomyopathy, muscle weakness and wasting	Required for thyroid hormone activation; component of glutathione peroxidase; supports antioxidant effects of vitamin E	Brazil nuts, organ meats, seafood, meats, some whole grains
Vitamin B2 (riboflavin)	Dietary insufficiency, heavy alcohol use, anorexia nervosa, lactose intolerance, adrenal insufficiency, hypothyroidism	None	Sore throat, swelling and redness of mucous membranes, cheilosis, angular stomatitis, redness and inflammation of tongue, seborrheic dermatitis, corneal vascularization	Required for folate activation, regeneration of glutathione, and generation of uric acid, an antioxidant	Milk, eggs, almonds, spinach, chicken, beef, asparagus, salmon, broccoli
Vitamin B6 (pyridoxine)	Hemodialysis,[3] heavy alcohol use	Oral contraceptives[4]	Seizures and EEG changes, irritability, depression, confusion, inflammation of tongue, mouth ulcers, angular cheilitis	Cofactor in neurotransmitter synthesis	Potato, chicken, salmon, banana, turkey, spinach, vegetable juice, hazelnuts
Vitamin B12	Pernicious anemia, atrophic gastritis, resection of parts of stomach or ileum, malabsorption, pancreatic insufficiency, heavy alcohol use, AIDS, strict vegan/vegetarian diet	Proton pump inhibitors (≥3 years of use) Metformin Nitrous oxide Colchicine Neomycin Chloramphenicol Cholestyramine	↑Homocysteine, ↑methylmalonic acid, signs/symptoms of folate deficiency, peripheral neuropathy, ataxia, memory loss, disorientation, dementia ± mood disturbance	Required for synthesis of monoamine neurotransmitters in one-carbon cycle; cofactor for production of SAMe; required for folate metabolism	Meat, poultry, fish, shellfish, milk

(continued)

TABLE 15-5 Nutritional Deficiencies and Depression (*continued*)

Nutrient	Conditions Associated with Deficiency	Medications Causing Deficiency	Signs and Symptoms	Mechanism in Depression	Dietary Sources
Vitamin C	Dietary insufficiency	Estrogen-containing oral contraceptives Aspirin (frequent use)	Fatigue, joint pain and swelling, easy bruising and bleeding, loss of hair and teeth	Required for production of BH4, a coactivator for enzymes that produce monoamine neurotransmitters; antioxidant; involved in methylation cycle	Fruits Vegetables
Vitamin D	Older age, low sunlight exposure, dark skin, skin covering when outside, cystic fibrosis, cholestatic liver disease, inflammatory bowel disease, small bowel resection, obesity	None	Rickets, osteomalacia, muscle weakness and pain	May impact nerve growth factor production, neurotransmitter synthesis, brain calcium homeostasis, inflammation[2]	Canned salmon, sardines, mackerel, fortified foods
Vitamin E	Severe malnutrition, fat malabsorption, cystic fibrosis, cholestatic liver disease	Cholestyramine Colestipol Isoniazid Orlistat Sucralfate Carbamazepine Phenytoin Phenobarbitol	Symptoms may be delayed up to 10–20 years in adulthood Ataxia, peripheral neuropathy, myopathy, pigmented neuropathy	Antioxidant; enhances vasodilation	Vegetable oils, nuts, whole grains, green leafy vegetables
Zinc	Infants and children, age 65 and older, severe burns, prolonged diarrhea, pregnancy and lactation, acrodermatitis enteropathica, TPN, malnutrition, anorexia nervosa, malabsorption, inflammatory bowel disease, sickle cell anemia, alcoholic liver disease	Iron supplements	Growth/development retardation, delayed puberty, skin changes, diarrhea, immune Deficiency, impaired wound healing, anorexia, impaired taste, night blindness, corneal swelling and clouding, behavioral disturbance	Involved in synaptic neurotransmittion,[5] deficiency may disrupt HPA axis[6]; cofactor for enzyme that increases bioavailability of dietary folate	Shellfish, beef, other red meats, nuts, legumes

1. Unless otherwise cited, information from Higdon and Drake (2012).

2. Harrisons (2012).

3. Stahl (2008).

4. Bjelland et al. (2003).

5. Papakostas et al. (2004).

6. Descombes et al. (1993).

acting on neurotransmitter formation or directly on neuronal receptors. Nutritional factors also effect the protection of neuronal membranes from damage by reactive oxygen species, either as antioxidants themselves or as cofactors in antioxidant systems, such as the glutathione cycle.

Psychiatrists can identify nutritional deficiencies by screening for signs and symptoms of deficiency, for medical or surgical conditions placing patients at risk, and for medications that interfere with nutrient absorption or utilization. They should also counsel patients, particularly those with comorbid chronic medical illness, on the importance of a healthy diet. In 2009, only 14% of American adults reported meeting government recommendations of two or more servings of fruit and three or more servings of vegetables per day.[60] Based on the link between poor diet and chronic disease, this number is likely lower in those with medical illness. Psychiatrists may choose to recommend a Mediterranean diet pattern, which, in addition to reducing risk in cardiovascular disease and improving GFR in kidney disease,[61] decreases risk of depression,[62] and when combined with nut consumption, increases BDNF levels in patients with depression.[63]

■ FOLATE AND VITAMIN B12

Epidemiology

Folate is of particular relevance for patients with depression since studies have demonstrated that folate levels are lower in patients with major depression than in healthy controls.[64,65] Both worsening depression severity and increasing episode length are associated with low serum or RBC folate.[66,67] Folate deficiency may result from insufficient dietary folate, hemolytic anemias, long-term HD, liver disease, congestive heart failure, chronic inflammatory disorders, chronic infections, and malabsorption.[68] Heavy alcohol use decreases both folate intake and folate absorption. Folate demands increase with higher rates of cell division, as in pregnancy and cancer.[69] Some medications, in particular anticonvulsants and methotrexate, can interfere with folate uptake or utilization (see Table 15-5).

Deficiency of vitamin B12 is seen in 10% to 15% of those over age 60[69] and in one study, in 30% of patients hospitalized for depression.[70] However, unlike low folate, low B12 does not impair antidepressant efficacy.[71] Conditions predisposing to B12 deficiency include strict vegan or vegetarian diets; AIDS; pernicious anemia; malabsorption caused by atrophic gastritis, Celiac disease, or tropical sprue; resection of portions of the stomach or small intestine; heavy alcohol use; and pancreatic insufficiency. Three or more years of continuous use of proton-pump inhibitors can also interfere with B12 absorption.[69]

Pathophysiology

Both folate and B12 are required for methylation pathways of the one-carbon cycle, a crucial step in monoamine neurotransmitter synthesis. Both folate, in the form of 5-methyltetrahydrofolate (5MTHF) and B12, interact with the enzyme methionine synthase, which converts homocysteine to methionine. Deficiency of folate or B12 leads to elevated homocysteine, which is more common in patients with depression.[72] Homocysteine is then converted to S-adenosylmethionine (SAMe), an endogenous antidepressant and building block for monoamine neurotransmitters.[69,72] In this manner, folate deficiency leads to disruption of serotonin, norepinephrine, and dopamine metabolism, which is implicated in the pathophysiology of depression.

Folate cannot cross the blood–brain barrier in its dietary form, but must first be converted to 5-methyltetrahydrofolate by methylenetetrahydrofolate reductase (MTHFR). Patients with depression are more likely to have a point mutation in this MTHFR gene,[73] resulting in higher folate needs than those without the mutation.[74] 5MTHF is required for synthesis of tetrahydrobiopterin, a rate-limiting cofactor for tyrosine hydroxylase and tryptophan hydroxylase in monoamine synthesis[75];

this represents another mechanism by which folate deficiency can disrupt neurotransmitter balance.

Clinical Presentation

The presentation of depression resulting from nutritional deficiencies does not differ significantly from depression related to other causes. Detection of possible nutritional deficiencies requires clinicians to inquire about nonpsychiatric symptoms. In addition to depressive symptoms, patients with folate or B12 deficiency may also have symptoms of anemia, such as shortness of breath, weakness, and fatigue.[68,69] Anorexia, diarrhea, or constipation, angular cheilosis, glossitis, jaundice, and skin hyperpigmentation may also result from folate or B12 deficiency.[68] B12 deficiency impacts the nervous system directly and may result in peripheral neuropathy, ataxia, memory loss, disorientation, and dementia with or without mood disturbance.[68,69] Because B12 deficiency traps folate in an unusable form, symptoms of folate deficiency, including msegaloblastic anemia, can develop as a result of B12 deficiency.

Course and Natural History

Early folate and B12 deficiency may be asymptomatic, with only depressed serum levels or elevated homocysteine and/or MMA present. Megaloblastic anemia, seen in more severe cases of folate and B12 deficiency, may take up to 4 months to manifest, as red blood cells live for 4 months in circulation.[69] Once megaloblastic anemia is present, two-thirds of patients will also have an associated neuropsychiatric manifestation.[76] Affective disturbances, such as depression, were the most common neuropsychiatric disturbance in folate deficiency, while peripheral neuropathy was most common in B12 deficiency. When anemia is severe, patients may develop a mild fever.[68]

Assessment and Differential Diagnosis

Vitamin B12 and folate deficiencies are diagnosed by laboratory testing. Serum folate reflects recent diet, while RBC folate tests total body folate and is impacted less by recent diet. RBC folate levels may be low in severe cobalamin deficiency. Normal serum cobalamin levels range from 118–148 pmol/L (160–200 ng/L) to 738 pmol/L (1000 ng/L), with levels 74 to 148 pmol/L (100–200 ng/L) considered borderline.[68] Some authors have suggested that 300 ng/L be regarded as the lower limit of normal in the elderly, due to their higher risk for cobalamin deficiency.[77]

Elevated serum homocysteine and MMA are more sensitive markers for functional or subclinical folate and B12 deficiency.[69,78] Elevated homocysteine may be the only marker of early folate deficiency[69] but is also elevated in B12 deficiency. A normal methylmalonic acid effectively rules out B12 deficiency.[78] Testing for methylmalonic acid, which is elevated in B12 deficiency but in not folate deficiency, can assist the clinician in differentiating between these deficiency states.

Macrocytic anemia and hypersegmented neutrophils may also be seen on laboratory examinations. The anemias of folate deficiency and B12 deficiency are indistinguishable, so a finding of macrocytic anemia warrants further investigation.

Psychiatrists should consider referring patients to their primary care doctor for workup of the cause of B12 deficiency.

Treatment

Oral folate supplements of 5 to 15 mg daily are usually adequate even in cases of severe malabsorption. Therapy should be continued for at least 4 months, until a new population of folate-rich RBCs has replaced folate-deficient RBCs. Because large doses of folate can mask B12 deficiency, patients should be tested for B12 deficiency before treatment with supplemental folate is initiated. Patients taking methotrexate may require folinic acid, a stable form of fully reduced folate. Deplin provides a metabolically active form of folate (L-methylfolate) that does not require metabolism by 5MTHFR, and theoretically may benefit those with mutations in the folate activation pathway.

Patients with B12 deficiency typically require intramuscular repletion. Therapy may be lifelong if the cause of the deficiency cannot be corrected. When IM repletion is not possible, oral and sublingual preparations are also available.[68]

■ ZINC

Epidemiology

Numerous studies have documented lower zinc levels in patients with depression,[79,80] as well as an association between low zinc and both treatment-resistance and depression severity.[81] Zinc deficiency is more common in the elderly and in infants and children. Conditions associated with zinc deficiency include severe burns, prolonged diarrhea, pregnancy and lactation, acrodermatitis enteropathica, malnutrition, anorexia nervosa, malabsorption, inflammatory bowel disease, sickle cell anemia, and alcoholic liver disease.[69] Penicillamine, ethambutol, and iron supplements can cause zinc deficiency.[68]

Pathophysiology

Zinc is the second most abundant transition metal in the brain, after iron.[82] It appears to both impact neurotransmission and function as a neurotransmitter.[82]

Zinc is active in brain regions and neurotransmitter systems involved in the pathophysiology of depression. It blocks NMDA receptors[83] and protects against glutamatergic excitotoxicity.[84,85] Zinc also modulates AMPA and GABA receptors.[86,87] Zinc-specific synaptic vesicles contain the majority of zinc in the brain.[88] It is concentrated in the amygdala and hippocampus.[89] The hippocampus seems particularly sensitive to chronic zinc deficiency.[90] Zinc deficiency activates the HPA axis,[91,92] which is felt to mediate increased depression-like behavior in zinc-deprived rats.[93]

Clinical Presentation

Mild zinc deficiency impairs growth in children and causes hypogeusia.[68] Impaired humoral immunity results from alterations in glucocorticoid secretion,[92] resulting in higher rates of pneumonia in zinc-deficiency elderly nursing home residents.[94]

Course and Natural History

More severe chronic zinc deficiency is a cause of hypogonadism and dwarfism in the Middle East.[68] Other symptoms of zinc deficiency include diarrhea, impaired wound healing, anorexia, night blindness, and corneal clouding and swelling.[69] Zinc absorption is altered in acrodermatitis enteropathica, an autosomal recessive disorder, resulting in a characteristic rash accompanied by hair loss, muscle wasting, diarrhea, depression, and irritability.[68]

Assessment and Differential Diagnosis

Blood zinc level less than 12 μmol/L is diagnostic of zinc deficiency. Zinc levels can be depressed in pregnancy and with oral contraceptive use. Hypoalbuminemia and acute illness also lower zinc levels.[68]

Treatment

Sixty milligrams twice a day of elemental zinc effectively treats zinc deficiency.[68] Zinc supplementation of 25 mg daily is an effective adjunct to traditional antidepressant treatment, resulting in significant improvements in depression scores at 6 and 12 weeks compared to antidepressant treatment alone.[95] Augmentation with 25 mg daily of zinc improved response to imipramine in patients with treatment-resistant depression.[96]

BOX 15-10
SUMMARY

One in five patients with CKD will experience at least one Major Depressive Episode

Depression is likely to be detrimental to the course of kidney disease and quality of life

Most patients with MDD in the setting of CKD are undiagnosed and untreated

Psychiatrists have a unique opportunity to work collaboratively with medical providers to maximize the treatment of depression in this high-risk population and provide guidance for both patients and their families around complex issues like dialysis withdrawal

There is clearly a direct association between depression and hypertension as both have been identified as a risk factor in precipitating the occurrence of the other

Psychiatrists should closely collaborate with medical providers to ensure appropriate management of hypertension and be cautious with use of psychotropics, which can further exacerbate hypertension

As many as 4 out of 5 adults in the United States have reported inadequate intake of fruits and vegetables according to national dietary standards

There are direct relationships between vitamin deficiencies and depressive symptoms

Psychiatrists have the unique opportunity to educate patients about appropriate nutrition and should be especially careful to recognize and appropriately treat nutritional deficiencies in their patients

■ CONCLUSION

Numerous vitamin and mineral deficiencies have been implicated in depression (see **Table 15-5**). Psychiatrists can identify dietary contributions to depression by taking a dietary history, by screening for conditions that are risk factors for nutrient deficiencies, or for some deficiencies, by obtaining a blood level. When repletion is needed, liaison with primary care providers may be appropriate depending on the comfort level of the treating psychiatrist (**Box 15-10**).

REFERENCES

1. KDIGO. 2012 Clinical practice guidelines for the evaluation and management of chronic kidney disease. *Kidney Int Suppl.* 2013;3:5.

2. Levenson JL. *Textbook of Psychosomatic Medicine: Psychiatric Care of the Medically Ill.* IInd ed. Arlington, VA: American Psychiatric Publishing; 2010.

3. Kimmel PL, Cukor D, Cohen S, Peterson RA. Depression in end-stage renal disease patients: A critical review. *Adv Chronic Kidney Dis.* 2007;14(4):328–334.

4. Hedayati SS, Yalamanchili V, Finkelstein FO. A practical approach to the treatment of depression in patients with chronic kidney disease and end-stage renal disease. *Kidney Int.* 2012;81(3):247–255.

5. Fischer MJ, Xie D, Jordan N, et al. Factors associated with depressive symptoms and use of antidepressant medications among participants in the Chronic Insufficiency Cohort (CRIC) and Hispanic-CRIC Studies. *Am J Kidney Dis.* 2012;60(1):27–38.

6. Young BA, Von Kroff M, Heckbert SR, et al. Association of major depression and mortality in Stage 5 diabetic chronic kidney disease. *Gen Hosp Psychiatry.* 2010;32(2):119–124.

7. Hedayati SS, Minhajuddin AT, Afshar M, Toto RD, Trivedi MH, Rush AJ. Association between major depressive episodes in patients with chronic kidney disease and initiation of dialysis, hospitalization, or death. *JAMA*. 2010;303(19):1946–1953.

8. Hedayati SS, Minhajuddin AT, Toto RD, Morris DW, Rush AJ. Prevalence of major depressive episode in CKD. *Am J Kidney Dis*. 2009;54(3):424–432.

9. Kurella M, Kimmel P, Young B, Chertow GM. Suicide in the United States End-Stage Renal Disease Program. *J Am Soc Nephrol*. 2005;16(3):774–781.

10. Kimmel PL, Peterson RA. Depression in end-stage renal disease patients treated with hemodialysis: tools, correlates, outcomes, and needs. *Semin Dial*. 2005;18(2):91–97.

11. Bargman JM, Skorecki K. Chronic kidney disease. In: Longo DL, Fauci AS, Kasper DL, et al. *Harrison's Principles of Internal Medicine*. 18th ed. New York, NY: McGraw-Hill Inc.; 2012.

12. Cukor D, Cohen SD, Peterson RA, Kimmel PL. Psychosocial aspects of chronic disease: ESRD as a paradigmatic illness. *J Am Soc Nephrol*. 2007;18(12):3042–3055.

13. Ibrahim S, El Salamony O. Depression, quality of life and malnutrition-inflammation scores in hemodialysis patients. *Am J Nephrol*. 2008;28(5):784–791.

14. Kop WJ, Seliger SL, Fink JC, et al. Longitudinal association of depressive symptoms with rapid kidney function decline and adverse clinical renal disease outcomes. *Clin J Am Soc Nephrol*. 2011;6(4):834–844.

15. Lew SQ, Piraino B. Quality of life and psychological issues in peritoneal dialysis patients. *Semin Dial*. 2005;18(2):119–123.

16. Liu KD, Chertow GM. Dialysis in the Treatment of Renal Failure. In: Longo DL, Fauci AS, Kasper DL, et al. *Harrison's Principles of Internal Medicine*. 18th ed. New York, NY: McGraw-Hill Inc.; 2012.

17. Garcia-Llana H, Remor E, Selgas R. Adherence to treatment, emotional state and quality of life in patients with end-stage renal disease undergoing dialysis. *Psicothema*. 2013;25(1):79–86.

18. Wuerth D, Finkelstein SH, Finkelstein FO. The Identification and Treatment of Depression in Patients Maintained on Dialysis. *Semin Dial*. 2005;18(2):142–146.

19. Cukor D, Coplan J, Brown C, et al. Depression and anxiety in urban hemodialysis patients. *Clin J Am Soc Nephrol*. 2007;2(3):484–490.

20. Turk S, Atalay H, Altintepe L, et al. Treatment with antidepressant drugs improved quality of life in chronic hemodialysis patients. *Clin Nephrol*. 2006;65(2):113–118.

21. Wuerth D, Finkelstein SH, Finklestein FO. Psychosocial assessment of the patient on chronic peritoneal dialysis: An overview. *Adv Chronic Kidney Dis*. 2007;14(4):353–357.

22. Tamura MK, Goldstein MK, Perez-Stable EJ. Preferences for dialysis withdrawal and engagement in advance care planning within a diverse sample of dialysis patients. *Nephrol Dial Transplant*. 2010;25(1):237–242.

23. Cohen LM, Germain MJ, Poppel DM. Practical considerations in dialysis withdrawal: "To Have That Option Is a Blessing," *JAMA*. 2003;289(16):2113–2119.

24. Nagler EV, Webster AC, Vanholder R, Zoccali C. Antidepressants for depression in stage 3–5 chronic kidney disease: a systematic review of pharmacokinetics, efficacy and safety with recommendations by European Renal Best Practice (ERBP). *Nephrol Dial Transplant*. 2012;27(10):3736–3745.

25. Wuerth D, Finkelstein SH, Kilger AS, Finkelstein FO. Chronic peritoneal dialysis patients diagnosed with clinical depression: Results of pharmacologic therapy. *Semin Dial*. 2003;16(6):424–427.

26. Kishore BK, Ecelbarger CM. Lithium: a versatile tool for understanding renal physiology. *Am J Physiol Renal Physiol*. 2013;304(9):F1139–F1149.

27. Adam WR, Sshweitzer I, Walker R. Editorial. Trade-off between the benefits of lithium treatment and the risk of chronic kidney disease. *Nephrology*. 2012;17:772–779.

28. Aprahamian I, Santos FS, dos Santos B, et al. Long-term, low-dose lithium treatment does not impair renal function in the elderly: A 2-year randomized, placebo-controlled trial followed by single-blind extension. *J Clin Psychiatry*. 2014;75(70):e672–e678.

29. Karaosmanoğlu AD, Butros SR, Arellano R. Imaging findings of renal toxicity in patients on chronic lithium therapy. *Diagn Interv Radiol*. 2013;19:299–303.

30. Minay J, Paul R, McGarvey D, et al. Lithium usage and renal function testing in a large UK community population: A case-control study. *Gen Hosp Psychiatry*. 2013;35:631–635.

31. Rej S, Herrmann N, Shulman K. The effects of lithium on renal function in older adults—a systematic review. *J Geriatric Psychiatr Neurol*. 2012;25(1):51–61.

32. Carter L, Zolezzi M, Lewczyk A. An updated review of the optimal lithium dosage regimen for renal protection. *Can J Psychiatry*. 2013;58(10):595–600.

33. Rej S, Elie D, Mucsi I, et al. Chronic kidney disease in lithium-treated older adults: A review of the epidemiology, mechanisms, and implications for the treatment of late-life mood disorders. *Drugs Aging*. 2015;32:31–42.

34. Rej S, Segal M, Low NC, et al. The McGill Geriatrics Lithium-Induced Diabetes Insipidus Clinical Study (McGLIDICS). *Can J Psychiatry*. 2014;59(6):327–334.

35. Lam SS, Kjellstrand C. Emergency treatment of lithium-induced diabetes insipidus with nonsteroidal anti-inflammatory drugs. *Ren Fail*. 1997;19(1):183–188.

36. Wu JY, Wadhwa N. Case 192: Lithium-induced nephropathy. *Radiology*. 2013;267(1):308–312.

37. Boccheta A, Ardau R, Fanni T, et al. Renal function during long-term lithium treatment: A cross-sectional and longitudinal study. *BMC Med*. 2015;13(12):1–7.

38. Duarte PS, Miyazaki MC, Blay SL, Sesso R. Cognitive-behavioral group therapy is an effective treatment for major depression in hemodialysis patients. *Kidney Int*. 2009;76(4):414–421.

39. Stenvinkel P, Ketteler M, Johnson R, et al. Interleukin-10, IL-6, and TNF-alpha: Central factors in the altered cytokine network of uremia-the good, bad, and the ugly. *Kidney Int*. 2005;67:1216–1233.

40. Kotchen T. Hypertensive vascular diseases. In: Longo DL, Fauci AS, Kasper DL, et al. *Harrison's Principles of Internal Medicine*. 18th ed. New York, NY: McGraw-Hill Inc.; 2012.

41. Michal M, Wiltink J, Lackner K, et al. Association of hypertension with depression in the community: results from the Gutenberg Health Study. *J Hypertens*. May;31(55):893–899.

42. Wu EL, Chen IC, Lin CH, Chou YJ, Chou P. Increased risk of hypertension in patients with major depressive disorder: A population-based study. *J Psychosomatic Res*. 2012;73:169–174.

43. Meng L, Chen D, Yang Y, Zheng Y, Hui R. Depression increases the risk of hypertension incidence: a meta-analysis of prospective cohort studies. *J Hypertens*. 2012;30(55):842–851.

44. Gangwisch J, Malaspina D, Posner K, et al. Insomnia and sleep duration as mediators of the relationship between depression and hypertension incidence. *Am J Hypertens*. 2010; 23(1): 62–69.

45. Hamer M, Fraser-Smith N, Lespérance F, Harvey BH, Malan NT, Malan L. Depressive symptoms and 24-hour ambulatory blood pressure in Africans: The SABPA Study. *Int J Hypertens.* 2012;2012:426803.

46. Nabi H, Chastang JF, Lefèvre T, et al. Trajectories of depressive episodes and hypertension over 24 years: The Whitehall II Prospective Cohort Study. *Hypertension.* 2011;57(4):710–716.

47. Delaney J, Oddson B, Kramer H, Shea S, Psaty BM, McClelland RL. baseline depressive symptoms are not associated with clinically important levels of incident hypertension during two years of follow-up: The multi-ethnic study of atherosclerosis. *Hypertension.* 2010;55:408–414.

48. Jonas B, Franks P, Ingram D. are symptoms of anxiety and depression risk factors for hypertension?: Longitudinal Evidence from the National Health and Nutrition Examination Survey I Epidemiologic Follow-Up Study. *Arch Fam Med.* 1997;6:43–49.

49. Siennicki-Lantz A, Andre-Peterson L, Elmstahl S. Decreasing blood pressure over time is the strongest predictor of depressive symptoms in octogenarian men. *Am J Geriatr Psychiatry.* 2013;21(9):863–871.

50. Rutledge T, Hogan B. A quantitative review of prospective evidence linking psychological factors with hypertension development. *Psychosom Med.* 2002;64:758–766.

51. Yan L, Liu K, Matthews K, et al. Psychosocial factors and the risk of hypertension: the coronary artery risk development in young adults (CARDIA) study. *JAMA.* 2003;290(7):2138–2148.

52. Licht C, de Geus E, Seldenrijk A, et al. Depression is associated with decreased blood pressure, but antidepressant use increases the risk for hypertension. *Hypertension.* 2009;53:631–638.

53. Gentil L, Vasiliadis HM, Preville M, Bossé C, Berbiche D. Association between depressive and anxiety disorders and adherence to antihypertensive medication in community-living elderly adults. *J Am Geriatr Soc.* 2012;60(12):2297–2301.

54. Eze-Nilam C, Thombs B, Lima B, Smith C, Ziegelstein RC. The association of depression with adherence to antihypertensive medications: a systematic review. *J Hypertens.* 2010;28(9):1785–1795.

55. Celano C, Freudenreich O, Fernandez-Robles C, Stern TA, Caro MA, Huffman JC. Depressogenic effects of medications: A review. *Dialogues Clin Neurosci.* 2011;13:109–125.

56. Kotlyar M, Dysken M, Adson D. Update on drug-induced depression in the elderly, *Am J Geriatr Psychopharmacol.* 2005;3(4):29–300.

57. Reid ID, Tueth M, Handberg E, Kupfer S, Pepine CJ; INVEST Study Group. A Study of antihypertensive drugs and depressive symptoms (SADD-Sx) in patients treated with a calcium antagonist versus an atenolol hypertension treatment strategy in the International Verapamil SR-Trandaloprol Study (INVEST). *Psychosom Med.* 2005;67:398–406.

58. Thase M. Effects of venlafaxine on blood pressure: A meta-analysis of original data from 3744 depressed patients. *J Clin Psychiatry.* 1998;59:502–508.

59. Flockhart DA. Dietary restriction and drug interactions with monoamine oxidase inhibitors: an update. *J Clin Psychiatry.* 2012;73(I):17–24.

60. Center for Disease Control and Prevention. "State Indicator Report on Fruits and Vegetables. 2009. " Available at http://www.cdc.gov/nutrition/downloads/StateIndicatorReport2009.pdf Accessed on March 30, 2013.

61. Diaz-Lopez A, Bullo M, Martinez-Gonzales MA, et al.; PREDIMED Reus Study Investigators. Effects of Mediterranean diets on

kidney function: a report from the PREDIMED trial. *Am J Kidney Dis.* 2012;60(3):380–389.

62. Sánchez-Villegas A, Delgado-Rodríguez M, Alonso A, et al. Association of the Mediterranean dietary pattern with the incidence of depression: the Seguimiento Universidad de Navarra/University of Navarra follow-up (SUN) cohort. *Arch Gen Psychiatry.* 2009;66:1090–1098.

63. Sanchez-Villegas A, Galbete C, Martinez-Gonzales MA, et al. The effect of the Mediterranean diet on plasma brain-derived neurotrophic factor (BDNF) levels: The PREDIMED-NAVARRA randomized trial. *Nutr Neurosci.* 2011;14(5):195–201.

64. Ghadhiran AM, Anath J, Engelsmann F. Folic acid deficiency in depression. *Psychosomatics.* 1980;21:926–929.

65. Bottiglieri T, Hyland K, Laundy M, et al. Folate deficiency, biopterin and monoamine metabolism in depression. *Psychol Med.* 1992;22:871–876.

66. Abou-Saleh MT, Coppen A. Serum and red blood cell folate in depression. *Ata Psychiatr Scand.* 1989;80:78–82.

67. Wesson VA, Levitt AJ, Joffe RT. Change in folate status with antidepressant treatment. *Psychiatry Res.* 1994;53:313–322.

68. Longo DL, Fauci AS, Kasper DL, et al. *Harrison's Principles of Internal Medicine.* 18th edi. New York, NY: McGraw-Hill Medical; 2012

69. Higdon J, Drake VJ. *An Evidence-based Approach to Vitamins and Merinals: Health Benefits and Intake Recommendations.* New York, NY: Thieme; 2012.

70. Carney MW, Sheffield BF. Serum folic acid and B12 in 272 psychiatric in-patients. *Psychol Med.* 1978;8:139–144.

71. Papakostas GI, Petersen T, Mischoulon D, et al. Serum folate, vitamin B12, and homocysteine in major depressive disorder, Part 1: predictors of clinical response in fluoxetine-resistant depression. *J Clin Psychiatry.* 2004;65:1090–1095.

72. Bottiglieri T, Laundy M, Crellin R, Toone BK, Carney MW, Reynolds EH. Homocysteine, folate, methylation, and monoamine metabolism in depression. *J Neurol Neurosurg Psychiatry.* 2000;69:228–232.

73. Bjelland I, Tell GS, Vollset SE, Refsum H, Ueland PM. Folate, vitamin B12, homocysteine, and the NTHFR 677C->T polymorphism in anxiety and depression: the Hordaland Homocysteine Study. *Arch Gen Psychiatry.* 2003;60:618–626.

74. deBree A, Verschuren WM, Bjorke-Monsen AL, et al. Effect of the methylenetetrahydrofolate reductase 677C->T mutation on the relations among folate intake and plasma folate and homocysteine concentrations in a general population sample. *Am J Clin Nutr.* 2003;77:687–693.

75. Stahl SM. L-methylfolate: a vitamin for your monoamines. *J Clin Psychiatry.* 2008;69:1352–1353.

76. Shorvon SD, Carney MW, Chanarin I, Reynolds EH. The neuropsychiatry of megaloblastic anaemia. *Br Med J.* 1980;281(6247):1036–1038.

77. Yao Y, Yao SL, Yao SS, Yao G, Lou W. Prevalence of vitamin B12 deficiency among geriatric outpatients. *J Fam Pract.* 1992;35:524–528.

78. Carmel R. Biomarkers of cobalamin (vitamin B-12) status in the epidemiological setting: a critical overview of content, applications, and performance characteristics of cobalamin, methylmalonic acid, and holotranscobalamin II. *Am J Clin Nutr.* 2011;94:348S–358S.

79. Maes M, D'Haese PC, Scharpe S, D'Hondt P, Cosyns P, De Broe ME. Hypozincemia in depression. *J Affect Disord.* 1994;42:349–358.

80. Maes M, De Vos N, Demedts P, Wauters A, Neels H. Lower serum zinc in major depression in relation to changes in serum acute phase proteins. *J Affect Disord*. 1999;56:189–194.

81. Maes M, Vandoolaeghe E, Neels H, et al. Lower serum zinc in major depression is a sensitive marker of treatment resistance and of the immune/inflammatory response in that illness. *Biol Psychiatry*. 1997;42:349–358.

82. Huang EP. Metal ions and synaptic transmission: Think zinc. *Proc Natl Acad Sci U S A*. 1997;94:13386–13387.

83. Vogt K, Mellor J, Tong G, Nicoll R. The actions of synaptically released zinc at hippocampal mossy fiber synapses. *Neuron*. 2000;26:187–196.

84. Bancila V, Nikonenko I, Dunant Y, Bloc A. Zinc inhibits glutamate release via activation of pre-synaptic KATP channels and reduces ischaemic damage in rat hippocampus. *J Neurochem*. 2004;90:1243–1250.

85. Cohen-Kfir E, Lee W, Eskandari S, Nelson N. Zinc inhibition of gamma-aminobutyric acid transporter 4 (GAT4) reveals a link between excitatory and inhibitory neurotransmission. *Proc Natl Acad Sci U S A*. 2005;102:6154–6159.

86. Smart TG, Xie X, Krishek BJ. Modulation of inhibitory and excitatory amino acid receptor ion channels by zinc. *Prog Neurobiol*. 1994;42:393–441.

87. Nakashima AS, Dyck RH. Zinc and Cortical Plasticity. *Brain Res Rev*. 2009;59:347–373.

88. Frederickson CJ. Neurobiology of zinc and zinc-containing neurons. *Int Rev Neurobiol*. 1989;31:145–238.

89. Takeda A, Sawashita J, Okada S. Biological half-lives of zinc and manganese in rat brain. *Brain Res*. 1995;695:53–58.

90. Takeda A, Minami A, Takefuta S, Tochigi M, Oku N. Zinc homeostasis in the brain of adult rats fed zinc-deficient diet. *J Neurosci Res*. 2001;63:447–452.

91. Fraker PJ, Osati-Ashtiani F, Wagner MA, King LE. Possible roles for glucocorticoids and apoptosis in the suppression of lymphopoiesis during zinc deficiency: a review. *J Am Coll Nutr*. 1995;14:11–17.

92. King LE, Osati-Ashtiani F, Fraker PJ. Apoptosis plays a distinct role in the loss of precursor lymphocytes during zinc deficiency in mice. *J Nutr*. 2002;132:974–979.

93. Takeda A, Tamano H, Ogawa T, et al. Significance of serum glucocorticoid and chelatable zinc in depression and cognition in zinc deficiency. *Behav Brian Res*. 2012;226(1):259–264.

94. Meynadi SN, Barnett JB, Dallal GE, et al. Serum zinc and pneumonia in nursing home elderly. *Am J Clin Nutrition*. 2007;86:1167–1173.

95. Nowak G, Siwek M, Dudek D, Zieba A, Pilc A. Effect of zinc supplementation on antidepressant therapy in unipolar depression: a preliminary placebo-controlled study. *Pol J Pharmacol*. 2003;55:1143–1147.

96. Siwek M, Dudek D, Paul IA, et al. Zinc supplementation augments efficacy of imipramine in treatment resistant patients: a double blind, placebo-controlled study. *J Affect Disord*. 2009;118(1–3):187–195.

97. Cohen LM, Tessier EG, Germain MJ, Levy NB, et al. Update on medication use in renal disease. *Psychosomatics*. 2004;45:34–48.

CHAPTER 16

Depression in Pulmonary Disease

David Wolfe, MD, MPH
Hilary Goldberg, MD, MPH

Diseases of the lung are diverse in pathophysiology, course, and treatment, creating several challenges for the assessment and treatment of comorbid depression. The anxiety associated with shortness of breath—at times nearly indistinguishable from that of a panic—may be the most prominent psychiatric symptom in individuals with lung disease. However, depression of various degrees is also common (**Fig. 16-1**) and associated with significant morbidity and mortality. This chapter will first review the major classes of pulmonary diseases and the known epidemiology of depression in these groups. Subsequent sections will discuss over-arching pathophysiologic mechanisms, as well as the novel features of depression onset, progression, and treatment in this population.

Asthma, the chronic inflammation of airways characterized by smooth muscle hyper-reactivity, is common, and likely results from a combination of environmental and genetic factors. Worldwide, the prevalence of asthma has risen dramatically in recent years, especially among children and adolescents. In the United States, asthma prevalence increased from 7.3% in 2001 to 8.4% in 2010, making it one of the most common chronic diseases.[1] Exercise, infection, allergens, and other airborne irritants can all be associated with the onset of an asthma attack, which is typically marked by wheezing, dyspnea, chest discomfort, and coughing. Although there is no cure, there is effective treatment to prevent and treat acute asthmatic attacks. Depression has been reported in 15% to 50% of individuals with asthma.[2–4] Asthma has also been linked to suicidal thoughts, behaviors, and attempts, though the causal mechanisms remain poorly understood.[5]

Chronic obstructive pulmonary disease (COPD) involves the gradual, progressive narrowing of airways over time, but unlike asthma, these changes are not reversible. The associated tissue pathology may arise from cigarette smoke, other environmental exposures, and/or genetic disposition, such as in alpha-1 antitrypsin deficiency. Progression of COPD may slow sufficiently to allow psychological and social adjustment to the illness, though depression still arises in approximately 20% to 25% of cases, a rate higher than found in the general population.[6,7] One study of elderly patients with COPD found rates of clinical depression above 40%.[8] Mood may also be acutely worsened by episodic complications of the disease, including infections, hospitalizations, and the need for supplemental oxygen. While depression does not directly correlate with pulmonary function (e.g., percent expected FEV_1), there is evidence that mood tends to worsen with advancing stages of disease.[9]

Cystic fibrosis (CF) arises from one of many autosomal recessive mutations in the CF transmembrane conductance regulator (CFTR) gene. As a consequence, sodium and chloride balance is disturbed across epithelial membranes, most critically in the lungs but also in the liver and pancreas. Diabetes, infertility, and gastrointestinal malabsorption with subsequent malnutrition are all typical complications of CF, though respiratory complications, arising from inflammation and infection, remain the most common cause of mortality. Depression prevalence ranges from approximately 11% to 17%, and is associated with poorer quality of life.[10,11] One center reported PHQ-9 scores in the clinically depressed range in 33% of CF patients, with 10% endorsing suicidal thoughts.[12]

Interstitial lung disease (ILD) can arise from environmental insults, autoimmune processes, or idiopathic mechanisms. Silicosis, systemic lupus erythematosis, rheumatoid arthritis, and drug adverse reactions are all examples of this group. Since the etiology varies, the

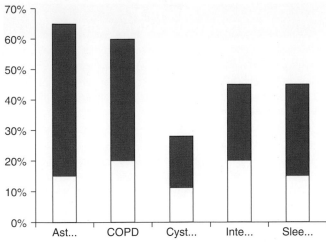

Figure 16-1 *Ranges of depression prevalence observed in pulmonary diseases.*

course, severity, and prognosis in this group of diseases are variable and unpredictable, and when serious, may progress to pulmonary fibrosis. Sarcoidosis is a systemic inflammatory disease in which the lungs are the most commonly affected organ. Approximately half of patients develop permanent disease, with less than 15% progressing to pulmonary fibrosis. In idiopathic pulmonary fibrosis (IPF), the onset typically occurs after age 50, and the symptoms may progress suddenly and unpredictably. Transplantation may become an urgent consideration in severe cases of ILD, especially in those with IPF. Similar to COPD, depression prevalence in individuals with ILD is approximately 20% to 25%, and is significantly correlated with level of dyspnea and functional status.[13–15] Compared to matched controls, significant elevations in depression scores have been described in individuals with occupational silicosis.[16]

Sleep apnea (SA), marked by decreased or abnormal breathing during sleep, can arise from central or obstructive causes (OSA), with the latter accounting for the vast majority of cases. Surprisingly, many patients are unaware of their breathing difficulties and sleep disturbance. As a consequence, SA can occur for long periods without detection or treatment, gradually leading to cognitive impairment and changes in mood. The prevalence of depression in this population is estimated at 15% to 30%, with the severity of SA increasing the longitudinal risk of developing depression in multivariate models.[17] Preliminary evidence also suggests that the combination of insomnia and major depression appears to increase the risk of having OSA compared to having either condition alone.[18] Daytime fatigue is the symptom that is most predictive of depression, and may serve as a mediating factor in the relationship between sleep disorder and depressed mood in this population.[19] It is important to note that disrupted sleep is common in pulmonary disease in general, even in the absence of OSA; a "negative" sleep study should not preclude further assessment and treatment of dyssomnia.

Pulmonary hypertension is characterized by elevation of blood pressure in the vasculature of the lung. It can represent a primary disease process, or arise as a complication of cardiac, vascular, or pulmonary dysfunction. Idiopathic and familial variants are relatively rare compared to pulmonary hypertension arising from scleroderma, rheumatoid arthritis, or systemic lupus erythematosus. Pulmonary causes include COPD, ILD, and SA, though the latter tends to have a relatively minimal effect. Among patients with pulmonary arterial hypertension (PAH), depressive symptoms as measured by PHQ-8 have been suggestive of major depressive disorder in 15% of cases, with 40% of individuals reporting symptoms in the mild to moderate range.[20]

BOX 16-1
POSSIBLE MEDIATORS BETWEEN PULMONARY DISEASE AND DEPRESSION

Cytokines

Vitamin D deficiency

Sleep disruption

Low testosterone

Oxidative stress

Environmental stress

PATHOPHYSIOLOGY

The possibility that pulmonary disease and depression share an underlying pathophysiology remains intriguing, though relatively unexplored (**Box 16-1**). There is increasing recognition of an "inflammatory type" of depression, marked by elevations in pro-inflammatory cytokines, such as interleukin-1 (IL-1), IL-6, and tumor necrosis factor (TNF)-α, ultimately leading to oxidative and nitrosative stress as well as disrupted serotonin metabolism in the brain.

Although cytokines and these other stressors can produce a depressed phenotype, inflammation is not necessarily observed in all cases of depression. This discrepancy may in part depend on the timing of the measurement of inflammatory markers in relation to the onset of mood symptoms. Interestingly, COPD is also associated with systemic, as well as localized, inflammation in many but not all cases.[21] There is increasing focus on understanding these inflammatory factors as they are somewhat distinct among lung diseases, and can guide more effective treatment.[22]

Depression may represent a cause or effect of the variation in inflammatory factors. One of the few studies to link these phenomena revealed that asthmatics with moderate-to-severe depression had significantly higher levels of serum and sputum TNF-α, as well as lower levels of the anti-inflammatory cytokine IFN-γ, when compared to matched nondepressed asthmatics as well as healthy controls.[23] In a study of patients with COPD, elevated serum levels of TNF-α were correlated with more severe depressive symptoms.[24] In a larger COPD cohort, however, physiologic measures of inflammation were not associated with the incidence of depression.[25] Inflammation also plays a prominent role in the pathophysiology of CF and ILDs, but specific links with mood disorders have not been elucidated.

Other shared mechanisms may exist. Vitamin D deficiency represents a common complication of CF, and is a theoretical risk factor for developing depression. Although studies examining the relationship between vitamin D level and mood have been generally mixed, one cross-sectional study of children with CF did find an association between lower serum vitamin D levels and higher depression scores.[26] Larger, longitudinal studies are necessary to confirm this finding, though proactive monitoring of vitamin D levels and supplementation are nonetheless reasonable recommendations in this population. While the precise mechanism linking vitamin D to depression is not well understood, high-dose supplementation in CF patients does appear to reduce levels of IL-6 and TNF-α, though other factors, including IL-1, are not changed significantly.[27]

Although sleep dysfunction is observed in SA as well as depression, the precise physiologic relationship linking the diseases remains unknown. One study of middle-aged men found lower serum testosterone levels, and significantly higher depression scores, in patients with OSA when compared to matched controls.[28] Another growing theory suggests that oxidative stress may mediate the relationship. Increased production of superoxide radicals, along with decreased serum nitrate and nitrite levels, represents an indicator of systemic oxidative stress. The overall level of oxidative stress appears to be positively correlated with the degree of sleep fragmentation, nocturnal hypoxemia, daytime fatigue, and depressive symptoms.[29] Oxidative stress also activates inflammatory pathways, providing a theoretical explanation for why SA can lead to cardiac and metabolic diseases, as well as mood and cognitive disorders.

Notably, environmental stress and associated exposures can lead to comorbid pulmonary disease and mood disorders. The most dramatic instances of this phenomenon include experienced acts of war and terrorism, such as the attacks on the World Trade Center in 2001. In the years following September 11, upper and lower respiratory conditions arising from exposure to dust and smoke, primarily asthma, occurred in approximately 20% to 30% of police and civilian responders.[30] While epidemiologic studies have found a PTSD prevalence of approximately 10% in this population, probable depression was also found in a significant 9% to 10% of individuals near the attacks.[31,32] As a consequence, screening for depression, as well as PTSD symptoms, is critical in patients presenting with pulmonary sequelae from occupational or traumatic exposures.

CLINICAL PRESENTATION

In pulmonary illness, the clinical presentation of depression potentially has several distinctive features (**Fig. 16-2**). Comorbid anxiety, especially around dyspnea or hypoxia, is relatively prevalent, with panic attacks closely resembling acute exacerbations of asthma or COPD (**Box 16-2**).[33] Because anxiety is such a prominent and dramatic symptom, it may mask underlying depression and other psychiatric comorbidities. Fatigue is a common symptom in both chronic lung disease and depression, though is certainly not specific to either. Thus, careful screening for negative or depressive thoughts (hopelessness, helplessness, and self-blaming) can be more informative than relying on neurovegetative or somatic indicators of depression.

For patients with chronic lung disease, especially COPD or ILD, any history of smoking, regardless of duration or known causality, can lead to specific feelings of guilt. Similarly, the inability to quit smoking as the disease progresses can engender self-blame and hopelessness. Encouragement, reassurance, and aggressive interventions to promote smoking cessation may address these concerns. It is important to note that the presence of depression predicts a lower rate of success at quitting smoking, underscoring the need for proactive screening and treatment of mood symptoms.[34]

BOX 16-2
ANXIETY AND PULMONARY DISEASE

Anxiety is common in pulmonary disease and may be severe to enough to overshadow other symptoms of depression.

The acute anxiety associated with dyspnea can present similarly to panic attacks, requiring a thorough assessment of the triggers, quality, and duration of symptoms.

Some pulmonary medications, such as inhaled beta agonists, can precipitate acute anxiety.

Given the overlap in symptoms between asthma and panic attacks, a methacholine or histamine challenge may be beneficial in guiding diagnosis and treatment in unclear cases.

Patients dependent on supplemental oxygen often develop some early anxiety about their appearance, or about running out of oxygen outside of the home. In some cases these fears can lead to social anxiety or agoraphobia.

Given the extensive overlap of mood, sleep, and lung function, insomnia may serve as a heralding symptom of depression. Patients with subjective sleep disturbance and daytime fatigue should be evaluated for depression, keeping in mind that the primary pulmonary illness coexists. Sleep studies should be considered in patients with any refractory sleep disturbance, especially if they experience daytime fatigue.

COURSE AND NATURAL HISTORY

Since many studies of depression in these populations are cross-sectional or involve relatively few points of measurement, the question of how mood specifically interacts with the course of pulmonary disease remains largely unknown. In addition, the course of pulmonary disease itself varies widely, ranging from self-limited, mild asthma symptoms to rapidly progressing forms of ILD, or systemic diseases, such as scleroderma. That said, depression has been associated with an overall increased mortality risk in COPD and asthma.[35–37] Depressed mood has also been associated with medication nonadherence in patients with COPD and CF, though these relationships appear to be complex and multifactorial.[38,39]

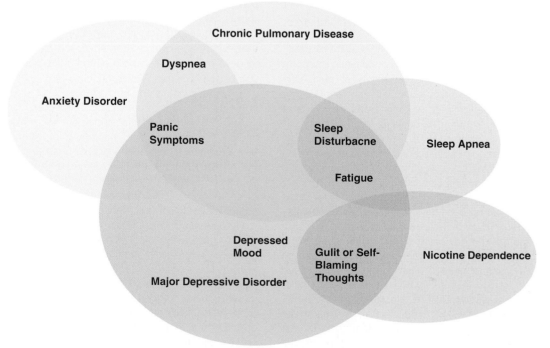

Figure 16-2 *Overlap of common symptoms in pulmonary and psychiatric disorders.*

Milestone events in pulmonary illness can lead to acute mood symptoms, resembling adjustment disorders or exacerbations of major depression (**Box 16-3**). In cases of ILD, the onset of pulmonary symptoms can be innocuous, sudden, and relatively late in life, creating a risk of significant adjustment disorder symptoms. Hospital admissions for COPD flares or CF cleanouts can lead to discouragement and hopelessness. The point at which individuals first require supplemental oxygen can be a particularly stressful time; this outward manifestation of their illness that can curtail mobility and lead to feelings of embarrassment or, in severe cases, guilt. Assessing mood longitudinally, especially at these stressful points, can be useful.

For patients with advanced, progressive disease, lung transplantation may arise as a consideration. While the specific screening procedures vary somewhat among transplant centers, psychological and social assessments are typically required as part of the evaluation for candidacy. These assessments provide a critical opportunity for depression screening as they often arise in the stressful context of end-stage disease, impaired quality of life, and the risky prospect of transplantation. In severe cases, such as with untreated major depression, further psychiatric treatment may be necessary prior to determining candidacy for transplant. Patients who are listed for a lung transplant face an unpredictable wait, and generally report increased depression and anxiety as well as lower quality of life when compared to norms.[40] Even 2 years following successful lung transplant, the prevalence of major depression and depressed-type adjustment disorder has been observed to be 30% and 10%, respectively.[41]

ASSESSMENT AND DIFFERENTIAL DIAGNOSIS

A depressed mood can arise from several causes, and keeping a broad differential in mind is important (**Box 16-4**). Although detailed epidemiological data are lacking, adjustment disorders are common in this population, especially in the context of complications, hospitalizations, supplemental oxygen use, and transplantation (**Box 16-5**). Dysthymia, major depression, and comorbid anxiety disorder, such as panic disorder, may also be present.

In the patient with advanced pulmonary disease, or with acute exacerbations, delirium should be excluded at the outset. The more common hypoactive type of delirium is marked by affective blunting and social withdrawal, resembling depression though typically without actual dysphoria. Similarly, cognitive impairment

arising from chronic hypoxia or SA can be manifest by psychomotor retardation, fatigue, and decreased volition.[42] Sleep disturbance can arise in many pulmonary diseases, however, and not solely OSA. Some pulmonary medications such as steroids, discussed below in more detail, can directly influence mood symptoms, making careful accounts of the timing and dosing of these agents critical elements in the history. Neuropsychological testing or a sleep study may help guide treatment in complex cases.

TREATMENT

■ MEDICATIONS

Selective serotonin reuptake inhibitors (SSRIs) remain the first-line treatment for depression arising in the context of pulmonary disease (**Box 16-6**). Pilot trials of citalopram, escitalopram, and bupropion in depressed asthma patients have all shown promise in decreasing depression as well as asthma severity, although larger studies are needed.[43–45] While SSRIs are typically well tolerated and have minimal potential for interactions with routine pulmonary medications, there is some theoretical basis linking these drugs with PAH. Depression and PAH share a serotonin hypothesis, with receptor and transporter variants linked with the pathogenesis of both disorders. Consequently, SSRIs could have an impact on the course of PAD, though the clinical significance of this relationship remains unknown. In various observational studies, SSRIs have been associated with increased as well as decreased mortality, and it remains unclear if this is attributable to the drug itself or to the underlying depression (and related factors).[46,47]

Bupropion, an atypical antidepressant that inhibits reuptake of norepinephrine and dopamine, has demonstrated efficacy in promoting smoking cessation as well as in treating depression. In patients with comorbid smoking and depression, bupropion may prove especially beneficial as a first-line agent, though its relatively activating clinical effects may exacerbate anxiety symptoms in some patients. Its dopaminergic activity can also precipitate confusion in patients at risk for delirium, limiting its routine use in the acute hospital setting.[48]

Cachexia frequently accompanies advanced COPD and is associated with decreased survival. While the exact mechanisms for this decrease in body mass remain under investigation, inflammation, malnutrition, and disuse atrophy are all possible contributors. For patients with significant weight loss or low appetite, the norepinephrine and serotonin antagonist mirtazapine can be specifically useful in targeting these symptoms, as well as depression and sleep disturbance. While not specifically tested for this indication in COPD, mirtazapine has shown promise in slowing anorexia and cachexia arising from cancer.[49]

Drug–drug interactions among pulmonary and antidepressant medications are relatively few, with the notable exception of fluvoxamine which, due to its inhibitory effect on cytochrome P4501A2, can lead in increased theophylline levels and related toxicity (**Box 16-7**).[50] One additional, though relatively uncommon, exception is in patients requiring the antibiotic linezolid. Often an agent of last resort employed in CF-related infections, linezolid can lead to serotonin syndrome and hypertensive crisis when administered with SSRIs.[51] As a consequence, it is generally recommended that patients who may need linezolid in the future be given antidepressants with a relatively short half-life (e.g., not fluoxetine) to facilitate a rapid taper.

Although the risk appears to be somewhat idiosyncratic, pulmonary medications can lead to depression in some individuals (**Box 16-8**). Corticosteroids, primarily oral prednisone, can elicit depressive and psychotic, as well as (hypo-)manic symptoms, generally in a dose-related fashion.[52] Cases of theophylline-induced depression have also been reported, and a cohort study of 664 patients found an association between theophylline use and suicidal ideation.[53,54] The leukotriene-modifying agents, such as montelukast, zafirlukast, and zileuton, have been associated with cases of suicide, prompting FDA warnings, though large cohort studies have not been conducted to explore this risk.[55]

Roflumilast, a phosphodiesterase inhibitor recently approved for reducing COPD exacerbations, has also been associated with suicidal behaviors.[56] While this incidence is relatively low, on the order of 1:10,000, there is still no clear understanding of this phenomenon or if there are any modifying risk factors. As a consequence, frequent monitoring of mood and screening for suicidal thoughts are recommended in patients taking roflumilast.

■ BEHAVIORAL AND PSYCHOLOGICAL THERAPIES

Among the psychotherapies, variations of cognitive behavioral psychotherapy (CBT) have been the most formally studied in pulmonary disease, primarily COPD. A systematic review of CBT in COPD does reveal some positive effects on depression, though the

evidence remains limited.[57,58] A randomized clinical trial of CBT in a group setting showed significant improvements in quality of life and depression scores among individuals with COPD.[59]

One somewhat unique resource available to patients with advanced lung disease is pulmonary rehabilitation. These programs provide patients with education, support, socialization, and encouragement. Studies of individuals undergoing pulmonary rehabilitation generally find improvements in functional capacity as well as depression scores.[60] Preliminary evidence suggests that such programs can actually improve coping with the illness.[61] Small sample sizes and relatively low baseline mood symptoms have likely masked the potential positive effect of this intervention, though fortunately larger trials have been proposed.[62,63]

■ SUMMARY

Depression, as well as anxiety, is common in lung disease (**Box 16-9**). Inflammation and abnormalities in serotonin metabolism may represent direct pathophysiologic links between many pulmonary diseases and depression, although further study is needed to elucidate these correlations and to identify the direction of any potential causality. Nonetheless, the presence of depression with most lung diseases is associated with increased mortality, reduced quality of life, and related poor outcomes, such as lower success at quitting smoking. As a result, concerted, repeated screening for depression is essential throughout the disease process, especially around vulnerable time points such as hospitalizations, onset of supplemental oxygen, and transplant evaluation. A sleep study may be indicated in patients with daytime fatigue to discern depression from OSA or other causes of dyssomnia. As steroids and other pulmonary agents can lead to mood symptoms with some frequency, the potential for drug-induced depression should be considered when medications are changed or increased. For identified cases of depression, first-line depression treatments are generally recommended and well tolerated, though relatively unique treatments, such as pulmonary rehabilitation and group therapies, may offer additional options in this population.

REFERENCES

1. Akinbami LJ, Moorman JE, Bailey C, et al. Trends in asthma prevalence, health care use, and mortality in the United States, 2001–2010. *NCHS data brief*. 2012(94):1–8.

2. Zielinski TA, Brown ES, Nejtek VA, Khan DA, Moore JJ, Rush AJ. Depression in Asthma: Prevalence and Clinical Implications. *Prim Care Companion J Clin Psychiatry*. 2000;2(5):153–158.

3. Lavoie KL, Joseph M, Favreau H, et al. Prevalence of Psychiatric Disorders among Patients Investigated for Occupational Asthma. *Am J Respir Crit Care Med*. 2013;187(9):926–932.

4. Katz PP, Morris A, Julian L, et al. Onset of depressive symptoms among adults with asthma: results from a longitudinal observational cohort. *Prim Care Respir J*. 2010;19(3):223–230.

5. Goodwin RD, Demmer RT, Galea S, Lemeshow AR, Ortega AN, Beautrais A. Asthma and suicide behaviors: results from the Third National Health and Nutrition Examination Survey (NHANES III). *J Psychiatr Res*. 2012;46(8):1002–1007.

6. Schnell K, Weiss CO, Lee T, et al. The prevalence of clinically-relevant comorbid conditions in patients with physician-diagnosed COPD: a cross-sectional study using data from NHANES 1999–2008. *BMC Pulm Med*. 2012;12:26.

7. Zhang MW, Ho RC, Cheung MW, Fu E, Mak A. Prevalence of depressive symptoms in patients with chronic obstructive pulmonary disease: a systematic review, meta-analysis and meta-regression. *Gen Hosp Psychiatry*. 2011;33(3):217–223.

8. Yohannes AM, Baldwin RC, Connolly MJ. Depression and anxiety in elderly outpatients with chronic obstructive pulmonary disease: prevalence, and validation of the BASDEC screening questionnaire. *Int J Geriatr Psychiatry*. 2000;15(12):1090–1096.

9. Iguchi A, Senjyu H, Hayashi Y, et al. Relationship Between Depression in Patients With COPD and the Percent of Predicted FEV1, BODE Index, and Health-Related Quality of Life. *Respir Care*. 2013;58(2):334–339.

10. Burke P, Meyer V, Kocoshis S, et al. Depression and anxiety in pediatric inflammatory bowel disease and cystic fibrosis. *J Am Acad Child Adolescent Psychiatry*. 1989;28(6):948–951.

11. Yohannes AM, Willgoss TG, Fatoye FA, Dip MD, Webb K. Relationship between anxiety, depression, and quality of life in adult patients with cystic fibrosis. *Respir Care*. 2012;57(4):550–556.

12. Latchford G, Duff AJ. Screening for depression in a single CF centre. *J Cyst Fibros*. 2013;12(6):794–796.

13. Ryerson CJ, Arean PA, Berkeley J, et al. Depression is a common and chronic comorbidity in patients with interstitial lung disease. *Respirology*. 2012;17(3):525–532.

14. Ryerson CJ, Berkeley J, Carrieri-Kohlman VL, Pantilat SZ, Landefeld CS, Collard HR. Depression and functional status are strongly associated with dyspnea in interstitial lung disease. *Chest*. 2011;139(3):609–616.

15. Goracci A, Fagiolini A, Martinucci M, et al. Quality of life, anxiety and depression in sarcoidosis. *Gen Hosp Psychiatry*. 2008;30(5):441–445.

16. Wang C, Yang LS, Shi XH, Yang YF, Liu K, Liu RY. Depressive symptoms in aged Chinese patients with silicosis. *Aging Ment health*. 2008;12(3):343–348.

17. Peppard PE, Szklo-Coxe M, Hla KM, Young T. Longitudinal association of sleep-related breathing disorder and depression. *Arch Intern Med*. 2006;166(16):1709–1715.

18. Ong JC, Gress JL, San Pedro-Salcedo MG, Manber R. Frequency and predictors of obstructive sleep apnea among individuals with major depressive disorder and insomnia. *J Psychosom Res*. 2009;67(2):135–141.

19. Jackson ML, Stough C, Howard ME, Spong J, Downey LA, Thompson B. The contribution of fatigue and sleepiness to depression in patients attending the sleep laboratory for evaluation of obstructive sleep apnea. *Sleep Breath*. 2011;15(3):439–445.

20. McCollister DH, Beutz M, McLaughlin V, et al. Depressive symptoms in pulmonary arterial hypertension: prevalence and association with functional status. *Psychosomatics*. 2010;51(4):339–339 e338.

21. Burgel PR, Mannino D. Systemic inflammation in patients with chronic obstructive pulmonary disease: one size no longer fits all! *Am J Respir Crit Care Med*. 2012;186(10):936–937.

22. Sethi S, Mahler DA, Marcus P, Owen CA, Yawn B, Rennard S. Inflammation in COPD: implications for management. *Am J Med*. 2012;125(12):1162–1170.

23. Du YJ, Li B, Zhang HY, et al. Airway inflammation and hypothalamic-pituitary-adrenal axis activity in asthmatic adults with depression. *J Asthma*. 2013;50(3):274–281.

24. Al-shair K, Kolsum U, Dockry R, Morris J, Singh D, Vestbo J. Biomarkers of systemic inflammation and depression and fatigue in moderate clinically stable COPD. *Respir Res*. 2011;12:3.

25. Hanania NA, Mullerova H, Locantore NW, et al. Determinants of depression in the ECLIPSE chronic obstructive pulmonary disease cohort. *Am J Respir Crit Care Med*. 2011;183(5):604–611.

26. Smith BA, Cogswell A, Garcia G. Vitamin D and Depressive Symptoms in Children with Cystic Fibrosis. *Psychosomatics*. 2013;55(1):76–81.

27. Grossmann RE, Zughaier SM, Liu S, Lyles RH, Tangpricha V. Impact of vitamin D supplementation on markers of inflammation in adults with cystic fibrosis hospitalized for a pulmonary exacerbation. *Eur J Clin Nutr*. 2012;66(9):1072–1074.

28. Bercea RM, Patacchioli FR, Ghiciuc CM, Cojocaru E, Mihaescu T. Serum testosterone and depressive symptoms in severe OSA patients. *Andrologia*. 2012;45(5):345–350.

29. Franco CM, Lima AM, Ataide L Jr, et al. Obstructive sleep apnea severity correlates with cellular and plasma oxidative stress parameters and affective symptoms. *J Mol Neurosci*. 2012;47(2):300–310.

30. Luft BJ, Schechter C, Kotov R, et al. Exposure, probable PTSD and lower respiratory illness among World Trade Center rescue, recovery and clean-up workers. *Psychol Med*. 2012;42(5):1069–1079.

31. Stellman JM, Smith RP, Katz CL, et al. Enduring mental health morbidity and social function impairment in world trade center rescue, recovery, and cleanup workers: the psychological dimension of an environmental health disaster. *Environ Health Perspect*. 2008;116(9):1248–1253.

32. Galea S, Ahern J, Resnick H, et al. Psychological sequelae of the September 11 terrorist attacks in New York City. *N Eng J Med*. 2002;346(13):982–987.

33. Livermore N, Butler JE, Sharpe L, McBain RA, Gandevia SC, McKenzie DK. Panic attacks and perception of inspiratory resistive loads in chronic obstructive pulmonary disease. *Am J Respir Crit Care Med*. 2008;178(1):7–12.

34. Berlin I, Covey LS. Pre-cessation depressive mood predicts failure to quit smoking: the role of coping and personality traits. *Addiction*. 2006;101(12):1814–1821.

35. Atlantis E, Fahey P, Cochrane B, Smith S. Bidirectional associations between clinically relevant depression or anxiety and chronic obstructive pulmonary disease (COPD): a systematic review and meta-analysis. *Chest*. 2013;144(3):766–777.

36. Walters P, Schofield P, Howard L, Ashworth M, Tylee A. The relationship between asthma and depression in primary care patients: a historical cohort and nested case control study. *PloS One*. 2011;6(6):e20750.

37. Abrams TE, Vaughan-Sarrazin M, Van der Weg MW. Acute exacerbations of chronic obstructive pulmonary disease and the effect of existing psychiatric comorbidity on subsequent mortality. *Psychosomatics*. 2011;52(5):441–449.

38. Khdour MR, Hawwa AF, Kidney JC, Smyth BM, McElnay JC. Potential risk factors for medication non-adherence in patients with chronic obstructive pulmonary disease (COPD). *Eur J Clin Pharmacol*. 2012;68(10):1365–1373.

39. Smith BA, Modi AC, Quittner AL, Wood BL. Depressive symptoms in children with cystic fibrosis and parents and its effects on adherence to airway clearance. *Pediatr Pulmonol.* 2010; 45(8):756–763.

40. Chen L, Huang D, Mou X, Chen Y, Gong Y, He J. Investigation of quality of life and relevant influence factors in patients awaiting lung transplantation. *J Thorac Dis.* 2011;3(4):244–248.

41. Dew MA, DiMartini AF, DeVito Dabbs AJ, et al. Onset and risk factors for anxiety and depression during the first 2 years after lung transplantation. *Gen Hosp Psychiatry.* 2012;34(2):127–138.

42. Grant I, Prigatano GP, Heaton RK, McSweeny AJ, Wright EC, Adams KM. Progressive neuropsychologic impairment and hypoxemia. Relationship in chronic obstructive pulmonary disease. *Arch Gen Psychiatry.* 1987;44(11):999–1006.

43. Brown ES, Vigil L, Khan DA, Liggin JD, Carmody TJ, Rush AJ. A randomized trial of citalopram versus placebo in outpatients with asthma and major depressive disorder: a proof of concept study. *Biol Psychiatry.* 2005;58(11):865–870.

44. Brown ES, Howard C, Khan DA, Carmody TJ. Escitalopram for severe asthma and major depressive disorder: a randomized, double-blind, placebo-controlled proof-of-concept study. *Psychosomatics.* 2012;53(1):75–80.

45. Brown ES, Vornik LA, Khan DA, Rush AJ. Bupropion in the treatment of outpatients with asthma and major depressive disorder. *Int J Psychiatry Med.* 2007;37(1):23–28.

46. Shah SJ, Gomberg-Maitland M, Thenappan T, Rich S. Selective serotonin reuptake inhibitors and the incidence and outcome of pulmonary hypertension. *Chest.* 2009;136(3):694–700.

47. Sadoughi A, Roberts KE, Preston IR, et al. Use of Selective Serotonin Reuptake Inhibitors and Outcomes in Pulmonary Arterial Hypertension. *Chest.* 2013;144(2):531–541.

48. Mack DR, Barbarello-Andrews L, Liu MT. Agitated delirium associated with therapeutic doses of sustained-release bupropion. *Int J Clin Pharm.* 2012;34(1):9–12.

49. Riechelmann RP, Burman D, Tannock IF, Rodin G, Zimmermann C. Phase II trial of mirtazapine for cancer-related cachexia and anorexia. *Am J Hosp Palliat Care.* 2010;27(2):106–110.

50. Sperber AD. Toxic interaction between fluvoxamine and sustained release theophylline in an 11-year-old boy. *Drug Saf.* 1991;6(6):460–462.

51. Go AC, Golightly LK, Barber GR, Barron MA. Linezolid interaction with serotonin reuptake inhibitors: report of two cases and incidence assessment. *Drug Metabol Drug Interact.* 2010; 25(1–4):41–47.

52. Brown ES, Vera E, Frol AB, Woolston DJ, Johnson B. Effects of chronic prednisone therapy on mood and memory. *J Affect Disord.* 2007;99(1–3):279–283.

53. Murphy MB, Dillon A, Fitzgerald MX. Theophylline and depression. *Br Med J.* 1980;281(6251):1322.

54. Favreau H, Bacon SL, Joseph M, Labrecque M, Lavoie KL. Association between asthma medications and suicidal ideation in adult asthmatics. *Respir Med.* 2012;106(7):933–941.

55. Schumock GT, Lee TA, Joo MJ, Valuck RJ, Stayner LT, Gibbons RD. Association between leukotriene-modifying agents and suicide: what is the evidence?. *Drug Safety.* 2011;34(7):533–544.

56. Pinner NA, Hamilton LA, Hughes A. Roflumilast: a phosphodiesterase-4 inhibitor for the treatment of severe chronic obstructive pulmonary disease. *Clin Ther.* 2012;34(1):56–66.

57. Coventry PA, Gellatly JL. Improving outcomes for COPD patients with mild-to-moderate anxiety and depression: a systematic review of cognitive behavioural therapy. *Br J Health Psychol.* 2008;13(Pt 3):381–400.

58. Hynninen MJ, Bjerke N, Pallesen S, Bakke PS, Nordhus IH. A randomized controlled trial of cognitive behavioral therapy for anxiety and depression in COPD. *Respir Med.* 2010;104(7): 986–994.

59. Kunik ME, Veazey C, Cully JA, et al. COPD education and cognitive behavioral therapy group treatment for clinically significant symptoms of depression and anxiety in COPD patients: a randomized controlled trial. *Psychol Med.* 2008;38(3):385–396.

60. Bhandari NJ, Jain T, Marolda C, ZuWallack RL. Comprehensive pulmonary rehabilitation results in clinically meaningful improvements in anxiety and depression in patients with chronic obstructive pulmonary disease. *J Cardiopulm Rehabil Prev.* 2013;33(2):123–127.

61. Stoilkova A, Janssen DJ, Franssen FM, Spruit MA, Wouters EF. Coping styles in patients with COPD before and after pulmonary rehabilitation. *Respir Med.* 2013;107(6):825–833.

62. Swigris JJ, Fairclough DL, Morrison M, et al. Benefits of pulmonary rehabilitation in idiopathic pulmonary fibrosis. *Respir Care.* 2011;56(6):783–789.

63. Dowman L, McDonald CF, Hill C, et al. The benefits of exercise training in interstitial lung disease: protocol for a multicentre randomised controlled trial. *BMC Pulm Med.* 2013;13:8.

CHAPTER 17

Depression in the Patient with Chronic Pain

Robert Jamison, PhD
Ajay Wasan, MD, MSc

INTRODUCTION

There are many challenging issues presented to a clinician when dealing with persons who have a primary report of chronic pain but who also present with depression and other comorbidities (see **Table 17-1**; **Box 17-1**). In this chapter we present an overview of epidemiology of pain and depression, discuss the biological basis for depression and pain, review commonly used assessment measures for depression in persons with chronic pain, and present treatment strategies for depression and chronic pain, including psychopharmacology and psychotherapy. We also include a brief discussion of somatization and suicidal ideation associated with pain and depression. Finally, we discuss future issues related to this topic.

EPIDEMIOLOGY

Complaints of pain are the most common reason for seeing a physician in the United States, and pain is now regarded as the fifth vital sign in medically hospitalized patients (see **Table 17-2** and **Fig. 17-1**). According to the International Association for the Study of Pain, pain is defined as "an unpleasant sensory and emotional experience associated with actual or potential tissue damage or described in terms of such damage."[1] This definition describes pain as both an emotional and sensory phenomenon. Chronic pain is often classified into two broad categories of cancer pain (which includes cancer-related pain from chemotherapy, etc.) and noncancer pain (e.g., chronic low back pain). Chronic noncancer pain is an immense problem worldwide[2,3]: Approximately one out of every three individuals will experience chronic pain at some point in their lifetimes.[4] Chronic pain accounts for 21% of emergency department visits and 25% of annual missed workdays in the United States. In fact, chronic pain imposes the greatest economic burden of any health condition.[5,6] Persistent back pain in particular is one of the principal drivers of these costs, both in the United States[7] and internationally,[8] with indirect costs (e.g., lost or reduced work productivity) accounting for more than half of this economic burden.[9] In addition, the presence of a long-lasting pain syndrome is a leading risk factor for suicide, and psychosocial variables are important risk factors for suicidality in patients with pain.[10]

Chronic pain, generally defined as pain persisting for more than 6 months, or past the normal healing time, influences every aspect of a person's quality of life. It frequently interferes with sleep, employment, social functioning, and activities of daily living. Patients with persistent pain often report depression, anxiety, irritability, sexual dysfunction, and decreased energy.[11,12] Family roles are altered and worries about financial limitations and the consequences of a restricted lifestyle are common.[13,14,15,16,17] Studies suggest that most patients with chronic pain present with some psychiatric symptoms. Close to 50% of these patients have a comorbid psychiatric condition, and 35% of patients with chronic back and neck pain have a comorbid depressive or anxiety disorder (**Box 17-2**).[18,19,20] In surveys of chronic pain clinic populations, between 50% and 70% of patients have significant psychopathology, and psychiatric comorbidity is the most prevalent comorbidity in patients with chronic noncancer pain.[21,22,23] Many chronic pain patients have a history of physical or sexual abuse, or a past history of a mood disorder.[24]

Patients with chronic pain and a comorbid psychiatric disorder are more likely to report greater pain intensity, more pain-related disability, and a larger affective component to their pain than those without psychiatric comorbidity.[25,26] Patients with chronic

TABLE 17-1 Issues Associated with Chronic Pain and Depression

- Medical comorbidities (e.g., diabetes, asthma, hypertension)
- Family history of mood disorder and substance abuse
- Personal history of mood disorder and substance abuse
- History of criminal activity and/or legal problems, including DUI arrests
- Prior drug and/or alcohol rehabilitation
- Regular contact with high risk people or high-risk environments
- Problems with past employers, family members, and friends (mental disorder)
- Risk-taking or thrill-seeking behavior
- Heavy reliance on dependent substances (e.g., tobacco)
- History of suicide attempts and psychiatric hospitalization
- Psychosocial stressors

TABLE 17-2 Prevalence and Impact of Chronic Pain on Society

- Chronic pain is one of the most common conditions for which people seek medical treatment.
- Thirty five percent of Americans will suffer from chronic pain.
- Greater than 50 million Americans are partially or totally disabled by chronic pain.
- Fifty million workdays are lost per year.
- Pain is the leading cause of long-term work disability.
- Annual cost in lost productivity, medical costs, and lost income estimated at $100 billion
- Chronic pain is associated with higher medical costs than cancer, diabetes, and heart disease combined.
- Mood and anxiety disorders are two to three times higher in chronic pain patients.
- Chronic pain significantly increases the risk of major depression.
- Psychiatric disorders increase the disability associated with chronic pain.

pain and psychopathology, especially those with chronic low back pain, also typically have poorer pain and disability outcomes with treatment.[27,28,29,30] There is a significantly poorer return-to-work rate 1 year after injury among patients with both chronic pain and anxiety and/or depression compared to those without any psychopathology.[31,32] Physicians are more likely to prescribe opioids for noncancer pain on the basis of increased affective distress and pain behavior, rather than the patient's pain severity or objective physical pathology.[33] Moreover, there is some evidence that opioids may be less effective in patients with both chronic pain and psychiatric comorbidity. In one study, patients with chronic low back pain and high negative affective symptoms had 40% less analgesia with IV morphine than those in a low negative affect group.[34] In sum, psychiatric comorbidity, primarily major depression and anxiety disorders, is associated with greater levels of chronic pain, more disability, a worse response to treatment, and a greater likelihood of receiving prescription opioids.

Many pain patients with affective disorders also have co-occurring substance use disorders. Treating the affective disorder may result in decreased substance abuse behaviors, although these patients remain at risk of relapse.[35,36,37,38,39] Hasin et al. found some patients abuse opioid pain medication in an attempt to alleviate their psychiatric symptoms.[40] Thus comorbid depression and/or anxiety disorders are associated with greater opioid misuse, even in those with no history of a substance use disorder. Wasan et al. also found that increased craving for prescription opioids was associated with a greater urge to self-medicate the anxiety and depression that precede the sensations of craving.[41] These individuals with a mood disorder who self-medicate negative affective symptoms are at increased risk for substance abuse.[42] Since many patients with chronic pain frequently report mood swings and prominent anxiety and depressive symptoms, it remains important to carefully monitor all patients for psychiatric comorbidity. Individuals self-medicating their dysphoria with analgesics will then have a greater chance of receiving appropriate antidepressant and behavioral treatment instead of ineffective and potentially dangerous opioid analgesics.

BOX 17-1
CASE HISTORY

Mr. Jones is a 49-year-old disabled construction worker with a 4-year history of chronic back and left lower extremity pain. He was involved in an incident at work when he fell from a ladder and injured his back. He was seen by a number of providers and, despite receiving nerve blocks, physical therapy and many medications, still reported significant back and leg pain. He had evidence of a herniated disk in his lumbar spine and had back surgery. The surgery was unsuccessful and his symptoms worsened following the surgery. Over time his back and leg pain increased and he was prescribed oxycodone by his primary care physician. He became less inclined to leave his house and spent most of his days sitting on the couch watching television. He often became tearful when discussing his situation with others and was increasingly irritable with those around him. He preferred being by himself and became more socially isolated. He was angry that his coworkers no longer contacted him and he felt abandoned by his employer and friends. He had recurrent thoughts that life would not be worth living if he had to continue suffering in pain.

Eventually he was referred to a psychiatrist for an evaluation after reporting to his wife that he no longer wanted to live because of his pain. During the initial interview he described his back pain as very intense (8 to 10 on a 0–10 scale) and stated that the pain was burning, aching, pulling and sharp in nature and became much worse with any activity such as standing, walking, lifting, bending, or sitting for long periods. He had problems with his sleep since he could not get comfortable at night. He often felt fatigued and had problems with short-term memory and concentration. He had recurrent thoughts of suicide and of overdosing on his medication, although never acted on this plan.

During his initial evaluation it was learned that he had had a difficult childhood. He never knew his biological father and did not get along with his stepfather. He lived with his aunt and uncle during part of his adolescence and felt that they were abusive toward him. He proceeded to get into legal trouble with episodes of drug and alcohol abuse. His first marriage ended in divorce and he had a 16-year-old son from that marriage, who he rarely was able to see. His current wife had 2 children from her first marriage and there was considerable stress in their home. Mr. Jones stated that he had been sober for 3 years after a history of daily alcohol use and two DUIs. He continued to smoke a pack of cigarettes a day. He had a history of psychiatric hospitalization after attempting to overdose on prescription medication when he was 17. He has been treated for hypertension and borderline diabetes and had minimal perceived support from family members.

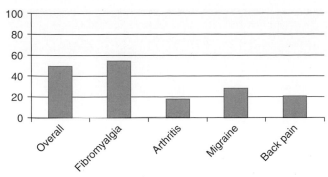

Figure 17-1 *Mean risk of depression for selected illnesses (percentage prevalence for particular disease).*

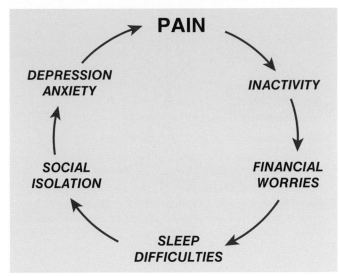

Figure 17-2 *The vicious cycle of pain.*

PATHOPHYSIOLOGY

The rate of depression among patients in pain centers has varied widely from 10% to 100% depending on the method of assessment.[43] Most studies report depression in more than 50% of chronic pain patients[24,44] and there is a direct relationship between the duration of pain and the incidence of major depression. Persons with fibromyalgia, chronic daily headache, and chronic pelvic pain have the highest rates of depression compared to patients with other chronic pain conditions.[45,46,47] Patients with two or more pain complaints are more likely to be depressed than those with a single pain complaint, and the number of pain conditions is a better predictor of major depression than pain severity or pain duration.[48] In a study of back pain patients within primary care, those whose back pain improved over time also showed significant improvement in depression and overall mood.[49] Taken together these studies provide solid support for the association between chronic pain and depression.

Prospective studies of patients with chronic noncancer pain have suggested that chronic pain can cause depression,[50] that depression can increase chronic pain,[51] and that they exist in a mutually negative reinforcing relationship in a vicious cycle[52,53] (see **Fig. 17-2**). In the majority of cases, the depressive episode began after the onset of the pain problem,[54] although many patients with chronic pain

---

BOX 17-2
ANXIETY AND PAIN

Anxiety and pain

- Patients with chronic pain frequently present with anxiety and recurrent worried thoughts (1, 2)
- Anxiety disorders are 2 to 3 times higher in chronic pain patients than comparable patients without pain (2, 3).
- Fear of pain, anxiety, and negative affect contribute to higher pain intensity ratings (4, 5)
- Anxiety and mood disorders increase the disability associated with chronic pain (6)
- Highly anxious patients with pain have: (1) a greater number of repeat surgeries, (2) higher medical expenses, and (3) higher compensation expenses compared with those with pain and lower levels of anxiety (7)
- Negative beliefs about the inevitability of pain, fear of hurting, and perceived disability are significantly associated with absenteeism and lower successful rates of return to work (6,8)
- Presurgical anxiety and depression are the best predictors of poor response from surgery (9,10)
- Anxiety and catastrophic thinking predict lower benefit from opioids and higher risk for prescription opioid misuse among chronic pain patients (11–13)

References
1. Jamison RN, Craig KD . "Psychological assessment of persons with chronic pain." In ME Lynch, KD Craig, PWH Peng, Eds., *Clinical Pain Management: A Practice Guide,* Wiley-Blackwell Publishing, Oxford, pp. 81–91.
2. Jamison RN, Edward RR. "Integrating pain management into clinical practice." *J Clin Psych Med Settings* 19:49–64.
3. Burke AL, Mathias JL., et al. "Psychological functioning of people living with chronic pain: A meta-analytic review." *Br J Clin Psychol.* 2015 54(3):345–360.
4. Vlaeyen JW, Linton SJ. Fear-avoidance and its consequences in chronic musculoskeletal pain: A state of the art. *Pain.* 2000;85:317–322.
5. Jamison RN, Edwards RR, Liu X, et al. Effect of negative affect on outcome of an opioid therapy trial among low back pain patients. *Pain Pract.* 2013;13:173–181.
6. Main CJ, Spanswick CC. *Pain Management: An Interdisciplinary Approach.* New York, NY: Churchill Livingstone; 2000.
7. DeBerard MS, Masters KS, Colledge AL, Holmes EB. Presurgical biopsychosocial variables predict medical and compensation costs of lumbar fusion in Utah workers' compensation patients. *Spine J.* 2003;3(6):420–429.
8. Boersma K, Linton SJ. Screening to identify patients at risk: Profiles of psychological risk factors for early intervention. *Clin J Pain.* 2005;21:38–43.
9. Celestin J, Edwards RR, Jamison RN. Pretreatment psychosocial variables as predictors of outcomes following lumbar surgery and spinal cord stimulation: a systematic review. *Pain Med.* 2009;10:639–653.
10. Sparkes E, Duarte RV, Mann S, Lawrence TR, Raphael JH. Analysis of psychological characteristics impacting spinal cord stimulation treatment outcomes: a prospective assessment. *Pain Physician.* 2015;18(3):369–377.
11. Quello S, Brady K, Sonne S. Mood disorders and substance use disorder: A complex comorbidity. *Sci Pract Perspect.* 2005;3:13–24.
12. Wasan AD, Gudarz D, Jamison RN. The association between negative affect and opioid analgesia in patients with discogenic low back pain. *Pain.* 2005;117:450–461.
13. Martel MO, Dolman AJ, Edwards RR, Jamison RN, Wasan AD. The association between negative affect and prescription opioid misuse in patients with chronic pain: the mediating role of opioid craving. *J Pain.* 2014;15:90–100.

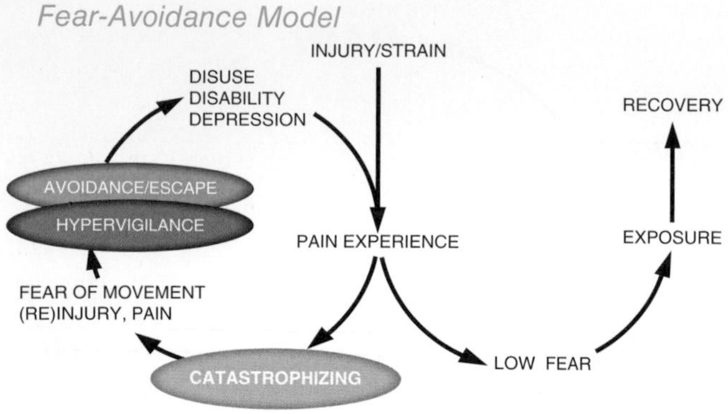

Fear-Avoidance Model

Figure 17-3 *Fear–avoidance model of pain. (Modified with permission from Vlaeyen JW, Linton SJ: Fear-avoidance and its consequences in chronic musculoskeletal pain: a state of the art, Pain. 2000;85(3): 317–332.)*

have had early childhood trauma and depressive episodes that predated their pain problem.[55] It may be useful when initiating depression treatment to embrace the notion that the pain contributed to depression rather than the other way around. This formulation avoids concerns by the patient that the pain is perceived to be "all in my head" and there is considerable empirical support for the directionality of this relationship based on epidemiologic evidence.[56]

Regardless of the directionality of the relationship, psychological symptoms and ineffective coping styles are prognostic indicators of poor outcomes (**Box 17-3**). Patients who present with poor coping skills often remain bed-bound and inactive because they mistakenly assume that chronic pain is indicative of ongoing tissue damage. Patients with poor coping skills tend not to use active self-management strategies. Pain catastrophizing, which is a cognitive distortion centered around pain and low self-efficacy, has been linked to higher levels of pain and disability and worse quality of life (**Fig. 17-3**).[57,58] Psychiatric comorbidity and pain duration are each independent predictors of pain intensity and disability.[10] High levels of anger also explains a significant portion of the variance in pain severity.[59,60]

Three core symptoms of major depression in patients with pain are low mood, impaired self-attitude, and neurovegetative signs.[61,62] For many of these patients, poor sleep, poor concentration, and lack of enjoyment are attributed to pain rather than depression. Patients with major depression have more prominent pain complaints than those without depression. Thirty percent to 60% of depressed patients complain of pain.[63] Depressed patients may in fact have a greater sensitivity to noxious stimuli and reduced pain tolerance.[64,65] Thus, patients with temporamandibular (TMJ) disorder and depression symptoms have lower pain thresholds and greater sensitivity to noxious stimuli than those with TMJ pain alone.[66,67]

BOX 17-3
IMPORTANT RISK FACTORS FOR DEPRESSION IN PAIN DISORDERS

Pain chronicity and heightened pain sensitivity

Pre-existing personality traits including high negative affect

Poor coping and pain catastrophizing

Neurovegetative symptoms and somatic preoccupation

Low self-image

Early childhood trauma, abuse history, and chaotic family background

Substance use disorder and opioid craving

BOX 17-4
POSSIBLE MEDIATORS BETWEEN PAIN AND DEPRESSION

Monoamines

Cytokines

Cortical modulation

Descending pain pathways

Studies of the brain help in understanding the relationship between pain and depression. The descending pain inhibitory system is modulated by serotonin and norepinephrine, which have a role in modulating mood (**Box 17-4**). Dysfunction of the descending\modulatory pain system, in such regions as fronto-limbic areas (e.g., prefrontal cortex and amygdala) and the periaqueductal grey, is thought to be a mechanism by which negative affective disorders amplify pain complaints.[68,69] Selective serotonin norepinephrine reuptake inhibitors (SNRIs) have a positive effect in reducing depression and pain. These medications enhance serotonergic and noradrenergic neurotransmission in descending inhibitory tracts in the brain. Other studies suggest that opioid analgesia is enhanced in the presence of concurrent antidepressant treatment[70] and decreased when serotonin and norepinephrine are depleted.[71] It has also been shown that those with major depression alone have a diminished endogenous opioid response compared with healthy normals.[72] Thus, it appears that certain biogenic amines play a role in endogenous pain modulation, and the increased pain experienced by those with major depression may be related to depletion or impaired function of amines such as serotonin and norepinephrine.

Cytokine responses can affect the initiation and maintenance of chronic pain,[73] and these responses may also affect the development of depression.[74] Depressed patients in the general population tend to have higher levels of proinflammatory cytokines and acute phase proteins, and administration of the cytokine interferon-alpha can lead to depression in 50% of patients. Proinflammatory cytokines also appear to affect neurotransmitter metabolism, neuroendocrine function, and synaptic plasticity.

Recent brain imaging studies shed light on the processing of pain and mood.[75] Cortical areas such as the anterior cingulate cortex (ACC), the insula, amygdala, and the dorsolateral prefrontal cortex (DLPFC) form functional units that can amplify pain and disability. These areas also contain opioid receptors.[76] There is evidence that the ACC, insula, and DLPFC are less responsive to endogenous opioids in persons who have high depression, anxiety and irritability (negative affect) but no pain.[77] Thus, individuals with high negative affect may experience a diminished effect of endogenous and exogenous opioids due to direct effects on supraspinal opioid binding. The multiple interactions of pain perception and psychiatric illness are still unknown, but it appears that the spinolimbic pathway (involved in descending pain inhibition) is negatively affected by psychopathology, which could in turn lead to heightened pain perception. It has also been shown that differences in pain sensitivity between patients can be related to differences in activation patterns in the ACC, the insula, and the DLPFC.[78] Anxiety has also been implicated as a mechanism to amplify pain perception. Studies have shown that anticipation for an acute painful stimulus in healthy volunteers is marked by brain activation patterns throughout the medial pain system.[79]

CLINICAL PRESENTATION AND DIAGNOSIS

There is debate about the best way to assess depressive symptoms and negative mood in chronic pain patients, but the domains to be

TABLE 17-3 Domains to be Addressed During a Patient Interview

1. Pain description
2. Aggravating and minimizing factors
3. Past and current treatments, including medications
4. Daily activities: content and level
5. Relevant medical history
6. Development, education, and employment history
7. Compensation status, engagement in litigation
8. History of drug or alcohol abuse
9. History of psychiatric disturbance
10. Current emotional status
11. Financial and social support
12. Perceived directions for treatment

considered appear in **Table 17-3**. The measures most commonly used to evaluate personality and emotional distress among persons with chronic pain include the Minnesota Multiphasic Personality Inventory—MMPI-2,[80,81,82] the Symptom Checklist 90—SCL-90-R,[83] the Millon Behavior Health Inventory—MBHI,[84] the Illness Behavior Questionnaire—IBQ,[85] the Beck Depression Inventory—BDI-II,[86] the Center for Epidemiologic Studies Depression Scale—CES-D,[87] and the Hospital Anxiety and Depression Scale—HADS (**Box 17-5**).[88] A broader consideration of the self-report measures of depressive symptoms is found in Chapter 3.

The MMPI[82] consists of 567 true-false items and yields a distinct psychological profile. These profiles can predict return-to-work in males as well as response to surgical treatment.[89] A shortened MMPI is also available.[90] Unfortunately, the profiles obtained can be misinterpreted because of the physical symptoms frequently reported by these patients,[91] and patients with chronic pain tend to dislike the test's emphasis on psychopathology. As a result it is less frequently used in pain patient populations.

The SCL-90 is a 90-item checklist with a 5-point scale that offers a global index score as well as nine subscale scores as a general assessment of emotional distress. Disadvantages include a high correlation among subscales and an absence of validity scales to detect subtle inconsistencies.[92] It is not validated in patients with medical illness and tends to attribute physical complaints to somatization. It is therefore a poor choice for psychological assessment in patients with pain.

The MBHI, includes 150 true-false items and offers 20 subscales that measure (1) styles of relating to providers, (2) psychosocial stressors, and (3) response to illness. The advantage of the MBHI is that the scales are not subject to misinterpretation due to physical symptoms. Rather, unlike other measures, the MBHI emphasizes medical rather than emotional concerns.

The IBQ is commonly used self-report measure to assess emotionality and illness behavior in chronic pain patients. This questionnaire includes 62 true-false items that yield 7 subscales measuring symptoms and abnormal illness behavior. Patients whose organic pathology does not account for their pain tend to have higher IBQ scores and these scores tend to be correlated with anxiety measures.

The BDI-II[86] is a popular measure of depressive symptoms in chronic pain patients. This 21-item self-report questionnaire is commonly used to evaluate treatment outcome. A limitation is the potential for misinterpretation of an elevated depression score as a result of the endorsement of somatic items by chronic pain patients. When a high cutoff score (e.g., >20) is used, it has a high positive predictive value for identifying major depression in patients with pain.[93]

The CES-D is an additional tool for assessment of depressive symptoms in pain patients.[87] The CES-D is a self-report measure of depressive symptoms consisting of 20 items. It is useful in patients with chronic illnesses because it contains fewer somatic items. The CES-D has good sensitivity and specificity in discriminating chronic pain patients with and without major depression,[94] provided that a higher cutoff score is used.[93] A short 10-item version of the CES-D is also available.[95]

The HADS[88] is a 14-item scale assessing anxious and depressive symptoms. It has been translated into many languages and is widely used. Scores on the depression scale >11 in patients with cancer-related pain and >9 in low back pain patients are highly correlated with the presence of comorbid major depression or anxiety disorder.[96] The HADS best functions as a uni-dimensional measure of negative affect, while retaining excellent case-finding ability.[97,98]

Of these measures, the BDI-II, CES-D, and the HADS have enjoyed the most popular use among clinicians who manage chronic pain patients.

TREATMENT

■ PSYCHOPHARMACOLOGY

Chronic pain patients often present with multiple comorbidities, physical deconditioning, vocational and marital problems, sleep disturbances, social isolation, and substance abuse (**Box 17-6**). A treatment plan that takes them all into account increases the likelihood of success. Depression subsides (but may not be resolved) when the chronic pain is relieved and pain coping improves with improvement in depressive symptoms.[99] Patients whose depression improves report that they may still have pain but that it doesn't bother them as much and is not as unpleasant, that is, diminished affective components of the pain experience (**Box 17-7**).

In a large RCT of several different antidepressants and pain education for chronic low back or knee pain and depression,[100] after 6 months of treatment, 47% of subjects achieved either a 30% or greater improvement in average daily pain and function[101] or a 50% or greater improvement in depression symptoms. Twenty nine percent improved on both outcomes. The vast majority of responders reached these benchmarks after 4 months and maintained the gains at 1-year follow-up. Venlafaxine, citalopram, mirtazapine, or buproprion did not differ in efficacy. Several of the study medications (citalopram, sertraline, mirtazapine, and buproprion) were ineffective against pain in those patients who did not have major

BOX 17-5
IMPORTANT SYMPTOMS COMMON TO PAIN AND DEPRESSION

Dysphoria
Poor self-esteem
Neurovegetative signs
Suicidality

BOX 17-6
COMMON COMORBIDITIES

Substance use disorders
Somatoform disorders
Anxiety disorders
Sleep disorders
Medical disorders

depression.[102,103] Another large RCT of antidepressants in patients with osteoarthritis pain and major depression reported similar findings.[104] As a whole, these findings strengthen the case that treating depression improves co-occurring pain.

Antidepressants are effective in significantly improving mood and pain in patients with noncancer pain and psychiatric comorbidity. The two classes of antidepressants that have analgesic properties, that is, improving pain independent of any effects on mood, are the tricyclic antidepressants (TCAs) and the selective SNRIs. There is some evidence that agents affecting both serotonin and norepinephrine are associated with a faster rate of improvement and lower relapse rates.[105] The monoamine oxidase inhibitors (MAOIs) are rarely used due to their side effect profile and medication interactions. They do, however, have analgesic properties, particularly in chronic daily headache (**Box 17-8**).

Establishing a therapeutic alliance with patients with chronic pain and depression is important. This helps in finding a satisfactory medication regimen with a side-effect profile that the patients can tolerate. Care must be taken in educating the patients with chronic

pain about the side effects of antidepressants, since they may be hypervigilant about new symptoms and prone to worry about side effects. Starting medication at lower doses may to allow habituation to adverse effects.

Although TCAs are considered first-line treatments, their side effect profile and the slower rate of titration can limit their usefulness compared to SNRIs. TCAs often are associated with a wide range of adverse effects, including weight gain, sedation, sexual dysfunction, restlessness, anticholinergic effects, and orthostatic hypotension. Amitriptyline and nortripyline have comparable rates of analgesia. Nortripyline is a preferred TCA, however, because of its lower incidence of side effects than other TCAs; however nortripyline and amitriptyline can be more sedating than desipramine.

The selective serotonin reuptake inhibitors (SSRIs) are popular because of their favorable side-effect profiles. However, they are not known for their analgesic properties. Bupropion can be useful in chronic pain because of its energetic properties, since many of these patients report fatigue and poor concentration. One study has shown that buproprion has analgesic properties in neuropathic pain,[106] but other studies failed to confirm this.[107] Among those patients with chronic pain who have treatment-resistant depression, there is some evidence that electroconvulsive therapy can be helpful for both depression and pain.[108,109]

Persons with chronic pain often report insomnia and anxiety. As a result, many of these patients are treated with benzodiazepines or other muscle relaxants. Unfortunately patients may be maintained on these medications for many years and eventually become dependent. Benzodiazepines are not adequate treatments for depression and pain and over time can worsen symptoms (**Box 17-9**). Few conditions exist for which chronic benzodiazepines are the treatment of choice and most patients should be tapered off after prolonged use.[110] The antidepressants are the medication treatment of choice for chronic anxiety and depressive symptoms.[111,112]

■ PSYCHOTHERAPY

The optimal treatment of depression in patients with chronic pain combines both psychotherapy and medication.[113,114] One of the most popular and effective psychotherapeutic approaches for chronic pain is cognitive-behavioral therapy (CBT). CBT posits that chronic pain patients become depressed in part from their inability to control their symptoms and because of their interpretations of the meaning of their symptoms. Many depressed patients are preoccupied with their pain and have an excessive fear of pain, movement, and reinjury.[115] These lead them to feel helpless and overwhelmed by the disruption in their lives that is caused by the pain.[116] The therapeutic goal is to change their view of their situation from hopeless, helpless, and out of control to feeling more resourceful and able to exert some control over their situation. The goal is to change their interpretation of information about themselves and their future condition and to change some of the behavior associated with these interpretations (Table 17-4).[117,118]

TABLE 17-4 Objectives and Components of Cognitive Behavioral Therapy

- Change patient's views of their problems from overwhelming to manageable.
- Reconceptualize personal views from passive to competent and resourceful.
- Teach patients to monitor maladaptive thoughts.
- Demonstrate how to use and when to employ these skills.
- Break problems down to "bite size" pieces.
- Identify negative thoughts and actions
- Learn positive self-statements
- Acquire distraction techniques
- Employ relaxation strategies
- Rehearse coping strategies
- Maintain gains and prevent relapse

The cognitive-behavioral therapist uses coping and communication-skills training and problem-solving strategies, and directs patients to recognize and challenge their maladaptive appraisals, interpretations, and beliefs associated with their pain. These are outlined in **Table 17-4**. Techniques include graded practice, use of homework, coping skills training, problem solving, relaxation training, and relapse prevention.[119] The therapist also prescribes a progressive, graduated, resumption of healthy activities.

In a large, well-designed, controlled intervention trial for patients with chronic low back pain, those undergoing CBT reported greater satisfaction, lower disability scores, and less cost in overall healthcare utilization than those in the control group.[120] In a careful and rigorous meta-analysis of CBT for back pain, Hoffman et al.[121] concluded that cognitive-behavioral and self-regulatory treatments were efficacious. Multidisciplinary approaches that included a psychological component, when compared with active control conditions, were also noted to have positive short-term effects on pain interference and positive long-term effects on return to work.

Acceptance and commitment therapy (ACT) for persons with chronic pain has recently received empirical support.[122] ACT uses acceptance and mindfulness strategies, combined with commitment and behavior-change strategies, to increase psychological flexibility.[123] It aims to reduce the disabling consequences of pain by developing control strategies and encouraging the tolerance of unpleasant emotions, sensations, and thoughts. ACT differs from traditional CBT in that rather than teaching patients to control their thoughts, feelings, sensations, and memories, ACT teaches them to "just notice," accept, and embrace these private events, especially previously unwanted ones. ACT facilitates the changing of associations and thought processes that are tied to unhealthy behaviors that increase pain and decrease quality of life).

SOMATIZATION AND DEPRESSION

Estimated rates of chronic pain patients with somatization and depression vary between 1% and 12%. The classical concept of somatization, which implies that there is no pathophysiological basis for physical complaints, is problematic in patients with chronic pain. This is because the majority of these patients have some underlying physical condition that is at least partially responsible for their pain.[124] The pain symptoms due to a physical or somatic cause (such as degenerative disc disease in the lumbar spine) may then be amplified by psychiatric factors such as depression, anxiety, pain-catastrophizing, fear of movement, and/or poor coping. Areas in the brain that process pain and mood together (such as the prefrontal and anterior cingulate cortices and insula, commonly termed, *the medial pain system*) may be the underlying brain substrates by which pain signals coming from the spinal cord are amplified and

perceived as heightened pain. Hence, it is more appropriate to think of somatization as a neural amplification of viscerosomatic stimuli. There may or may not be a demonstrable medical basis for the abnormal physical sensations.[125,126]

By the time chronic pain patients are referred to mental health providers, they tend not to respond to unimodal treatments and an interdisciplinary team approach with staff members who have experience dealing with chronic pain and can offer multimodal interventions have the best chance of making any improvement. It is also important that providers communicate with each other, since chronic pain patients tend to seek out multiple specialists, have many tests and procedures, and are prescribed multiple medications. For patients with a strong component of negative affect, the evidence is strong that repeated invasive procedures and implanted devices almost uniformly are unsuccessful.[127,128] Education about the nature of the problem and helping patients understand the risk associated with repeated treatments is also important.

Providers should resist a dualistic model that postulates that pain is either all physical or all mental in origin. This model alienates patients who may feel blamed for their pain and is not consistent with modern models of pain causation. Multiple lines of evidence suggest that pain is a product of efferent as well as afferent activity in the nervous system. We know that tissue damage and nociception are not necessary or sufficient for pain and the relationship between pain and nociception is highly complex. We are only beginning to understand the complexities of the relationship between pain and suffering.[118]

SUICIDALITY

Suicide is a very serious risk in patients with pain and depression, and it is often heightened by the presence of personality disorder, substance use disorder, and/or multiple medical comorbidities.[129,130] Patients with chronic pain are at greater risk for suicide attempts and completed suicide[123] compared to those without pain. The incidence of completed suicide in patients with chronic pain is two to three times that in the general population.[129] The lifetime prevalence of suicide attempts in patients with chronic pain is estimated between 5% and 14%, which is double that found in the general population. However, the pathways from suicidal ideation to suicide attempt to suicide completion are difficult to predict. Although a number of methods are used by patients with chronic pain to commit suicide, overdoses with medications are the most common.[118]

Depression and chronic illness are the most consistent predictors of suicidal ideation among pain patients.[132,133] Hopelessness, catastrophizing, low levels of activity, perceptions of poor social support, and alcohol dependence also predict suicidal ideation in patients with chronic pain.[134] The strongest predictors of *completed suicide* are family history of suicide, previous suicide attempts, and presence of comorbid depression.[52] The risk factors for *suicide attempts* include pain characteristics (intensity, location, type, duration), female gender, comorbid insomnia, catastrophizing and avoidance, desire for escape, helplessness and hopelessness, and problem-solving deficits (**Box 17-10**).[10,135,136]

■ SUMMARY

There is substantial evidence of a strong, bidirectional relationship between pain and low mood. Dualistic thinking about pain and depression as either purely psychological or medical should be avoided. It is not true that these patients cannot be adequately treated for depression until their pain is treated. Both conditions should be treated simultaneously. Persons with chronic pain and depression also often present with other medical comorbidities and heightened risk for suicidal ideation and substance use disorders. Careful monitoring to avoid prescription abuse and to identify suicidal intent should be encouraged (**Box 17-11**).

BOX 17-10
FOLLOW-UP CASE EXAMPLE

Follow-Up with Case Report

Mr. Jones was assessed to be a very high risk for suicide. He scored a 24 on the BDI-II, which suggested significant depression. He had recurrent negative thoughts, was frequently tearful, and was hopeless about the future. Mr. Jones was referred to a multidisciplinary pain management program to help manage his pain and his mood disorder. He was evaluated by both a psychiatrist and psychologist and was started on gabapentin and duloxetine for his pain and mood. He was seen for individual CBT and came to accept that he may have persistent pain for some time to come. He was introduced to coping strategies for his pain and he agreed to monitor his pain, mood, activity, medication use and side effects between visits. He learned ways to challenge recurrent worrisome thoughts and to pace his activities. His wife attended the sessions and provided support. Mr. Jones came to understand that self-management of his pain would be important and that he would need to re-think the way he remained active throughout the day. He participated in physical therapy and was able to increase his endurance and strength while using proper body mechanics. He acknowledged that he would be unable to resume his former employment and that re-training would be important. Gradually he was able to increase his function and confidence and to reduce his fear of reinjury.

A retest of the BDI-II 6 months later showed that his mood had improved and the major depression had resolved. He was gradually tapered off narcotic analgesia and continued with duloxetine and gabapentin during the day and baclofen and trazadone at night. He also took advantage of comfort measures and periodic nerve block therapy. Over time his mood improved and he made a point of going out every day to walk and to socialize with others. He eventually was re-trained as a building codes inspector and continued to work part-time through his local city council while being maintained on stable doses of nonopioid medication.

The management of chronic pain and depression will likely change dramatically over the next decade. As the U.S. population ages, greater attention will be directed to these related conditions, with evolving assessment strategies and interventions. New and promising areas of study will emerge. First, genetic testing holds promise for the identification of sensitive biological markers for pain and pain treatment. And there will likely be greater understanding of the role of inherited predispositions for chronic pain based on genomic research. Second, sophisticated imaging techniques will enable more objective assessment of pain with the use of high-resolution fMRI and computerized pain-mapping techniques. Third, nanotechnology will allow for more targeted drug development that will help

to advance personalized treatment among individuals with pain and mood disorders. Fourth, remote data entry and electronic assessment programs will offer better ways to track changes in pain and mood of the individual in his or her natural environment. Information will be summarized remotely and sent to providers. Finally, breakthroughs in pharmacology will lead to the discovery of medications for pain and depression that have low risk for abuse and adverse effects. Although the management of persons with chronic pain and depression will always be a challenge and require interdisciplinary input, the future will likely hold answers for improved treatment for those who suffer with these conditions.

REFERENCES

1. Merskey H, Bogduk N. *Classification of Chronic Pain: Description of Chronic Pain Syndromes and Definitions of Pain Terms*. Seattle, WA; IASP Press: 1994.

2. Ehrlich GE. Back pain. *J Rheumatol Suppl*. 2003;67:26–31.

3. Fordyce WE. *Back Pain in the Workplace: Management of Disability in Nonspecific Conditions*. Seattle, WA; IASP Press: 1995.

4. Institute of Medicine (US) Committee on Advancing Pain Research, Care and Education. *Relieving Pain in America: A Blueprint for Transforming Prevention, Care, Education, and Research*. Washington, DC; National Academic Press: 2011

5. Ferrari R, Russell AS. Regional Musculoskeletal Conditions: Neck Pain. *Best Pract Res Clin Rheumato*. 2003;17(1):57–70.

6. Stewart WF, Ricci JA, Chee E, Morganstein D, Lipton R. Lost productive time and cost due to common pain conditions in the US workforce. *JAMA*. 2003;290:2443–2454.

7. Becker A, Held H, Redaelli M et al. Low back pain in primary care: costs of care and prediction of future health care utilization. *Spine (Phila Pa 1976)*. 2010;35(18):1714–1720.

8. Hoy D, March L, Brooks P, et al. Measuring the global burden of low back pain. *Best Pract Res Clin Rheumatol*. 2010;24(2):155–165.

9. Phillips CJ, Harper C. The economics associated with persistent pain. *Curr Opin Support Palliat Care*. 2011;5(2):127–130.

10. Edwards RR, Smith MT, Kudel I, Haythornthwaite J. Pain-related catastrophizing as a risk factor for suicidal ideation in chronic pain. *Pain*. 2006;126:272–279.

11. Alschuler KN, Ehde DM, Jensen MP. The co-occurrence of pain and depression in adults with multiple sclerosis. *Rehabil Psychol*. 2013;58(2):217–221.

12. Jamison RN. Comprehensive pretreatment and outcome assessment for chronic opioid therapy in nonmalignant pain. *J Pain Symptom Manage*. 1996;11(4):231–241.

13. Chapman SL, Jamison RN, Sanders SH. Treatment helpfulness questionnaire: a measure of patient satisfaction with treatment modalities provided in chronic pain management programs. *Pain*. 1996;68:349–361.

14. Linton S. The socioeconomic impact of chronic back pain: is anyone benefiting. *Pain*. 1998;75:163–168.

15. Ohman M, Soderberg S, Lundman B. Hovering between suffering and enduring: the meaning of living with serious chronic illness. *Qual Health Res*. 2003;13(4):528–542.

16. Otis JD, Cardella LA, Kerns RD. The influence of family and culture on pain. In: Dworkin RH, Breitbart WS. *Psychosocial Aspects of Pain: A Handbook for Health Care Providers*. Seattle, WA; IASP Press: 29–45.

BOX 17-11
SUMMARY

- Most patients with chronic pain meet criteria for major depression.
- There are a number of associated neurobiological factors contributing to depression, chronic pain, and risk of substance use disorder.
- Interdisciplinary care is most effective in managing patients with chronic pain and depression including pharmacology, psychotherapy, and rehabilitation approaches.

17. Soderberg S, Strand M, Haapala M, Lundman B. Living with a woman with fibromyalgia from the perspective of the husband. *J Adv Nurs*. 2003;42:143–150.

18. Katz JN, Lipson SJ, Lew RA, et al. Lumbar laminectomy alone or with instrumented or noninstrumented arthrodesis in degenerative lumbar spinal stenosis. Patient selection, costs, and surgical outcomes. *Spine (Phila Pa 1976)*. 1997;22(10):1123–1131.

19. Katz JN, Stucki G, Lipson SJ, Fossel AH, Grobler LJ, Weinstein JN. Predictors of surgical outcome in degenerative lumbar spinal stenosis. *Spine (Phila Pa 1976)*. 1999;24(21):2229–2233.

20. Peloso PM, Bellamy N, Bensen W, et al. Double blind randomized placebo control trial of controlled release codeine in the treatment of osteoarthritis of the hip or knee. *J Rheumatol Suppl*. 2000;27(3):764–771.

21. Caldwell J, Hale M, Boyd RE, et al. Treatment of osteoarthritis pain with controlled release oxycodone or fixed combination oxycodone plus acetaminophen added to nonsteroidal anti-inflammatory drugs: a double blind, randomized, multicenter, placebo controlled trial. *J Rheum*. 1999;26(4):862–869.

22. Maier C, Hildebrandt J, Klinger R, Henrich-Eberl C, Lindena G; MONTAS Study Group. Morphine responsiveness, efficacy and tolerability in patients with chronic non-tumor pain–results of a double-blind placebo-controlled trial (MONTAS). *Pain*. 2002; 97(3):223–233.

23. Von Korff M, Deyo RA. Potent opioids for chronic musculoskeletal pain: flying blind? *Pain*. 2004;109(3):207–209.

24. Bair M, Robinson R, Katon W, Kroenke K. Depression and Pain Comorbidity: a literature review. *Arch Int Med*. 2003;163: 2433–2445.

25. Ang DC, Bair MJ, Damush TM, Wu J, Tu W, Kroenke K. Predictors of pain outcomes in patients with chronic musculoskeletal pain co-morbid with depression: results from a randomized controlled trial. *Pain Med*. 2010;11(4):482–491.

26. Moulin DE, Iezzi A, Amireh R, Sharpe WK, Boyd D, Merskey H. Randomised trial of oral morphine for chronic non-cancer pain. *Lancet*. 1996;347:143–147.

27. Rakvag TT, Klepstad V, Baar C, et al. The Val 158Met polymorphism of the human catechol-O-methyltransferase (COMT) gene may influence morphine requirements in cancer pain patients. *Pain*. 2005;116:73–78.

28. Rivest C, Katz JN, Ferrante FM, Jamison RN. Effects of epidural steroid injection on pain due to lumbar spinal stenosis or herniated disks: a prospective study. *Arthritis Care Res*. 1998;11(4): 291–297.

29. Rooks DS, Huang J, Bierbaum BE, et al. Effect of preoperative exercise on measures of functional status in men and women undergoing total hip and knee arthroplasty. *Arthritis Care Res*. 2006;55(5):700–708.

30. Wasan AD, Kaptchuk TJ, Davar G, Jamison RN. The association between psychopathology and placebo analgesia in patients with discogenic low back pain. *Pain Med*. 2006;7(3):217–228.

31. Fishbain D. Approaches to treatment decisions for psychiatric comorbidity in the management of the chronic pain patient. *Med Clin North Amer*. 1999;83(3):737–759.

32. Boersma K, Linton S. Screening to identify patients at risk: profiles of psychological risk factors for early intervention. *Clin J Pain*. 2005;21:38–43.

33. Breckenridge J, Clark J. Patient characteristics associated with opioid vs. nonsteroidal anti-inflammatory drug management of chronic low back pain. *J Pain*. 2003;4(6):344–350.

34. Wasan AD, Davar G, Jamison R. The association between negative affect and opioid analgesia in patients with discogenic low back pain. *Pain*. 2005;117(3):450–461.

35. Brady K, Myrick H, Sonne S. eds. *Comorbid addiction and affective disorders. Principles of Addiction Medicine*. Arlington, VA; American Society of Addiction Medicine; 1998.

36. Cornelius J, Salloum I, Salloum IM, Ehler JG, et al. Fluoxetine in depressed alcoholics: a double-blind, placebo-controlled trial. *Arch Gen Psychiatry*. 1997;54:700–705.

37. Kessler R, McGonagle K, Zhao S, et al. Lifetime and 12-month prevalence of DSM-III-R psychiatric disorders in the Unites States: results from the National Comorbidity Survey. *Arch Gen Psychiatry*. 1994;51:8–19.

38. Pribor EF, Yutzy SH, Dean JT, Wetzel RD. Briquet's syndrome, dissociation, and abuse. *Am J Psychiatry*. 1993;150:1507–1511.

39. Sonne S, Brady K. Substance abuse and bipolar comorbidty. *Psychiatry Clin North America*. 1999;22:609–627.

40. Hasin D, Liu X, Nunes E, McCloud S, Samet S, Endicott J. Effects of major depression on remission and relapse of substance dependence. *Arch Gen Psychiatry*. 2002;59:375–380.

41. Wasan AD, Ross EL, Michna E, et al. Craving of prescription opioids in patients with chronic pain: a longitudinal outcomes trial. *J Pain*. 2012;13(2):146–154.

42. Quello S, Brady K, Sonne SC. Mood disorders and substance use disorder: a complex comorbidity. *Sci Pract Prespect*. 2005;3: 13–24.

43. Romano JM, Turner JA. Chronic pain and depression: does the evidence support a relationship?. *Psychol Bull*. 1985;97(1):18–34.

44. Fishbain D, Goldberg M, Meagher BR, Steele R, Rosomoff H. Male and female chronic pain patients characterized by DSM-III psychiatric diagnostic criteria. *Pain*. 1986;26:181–197.

45. White KP, Nielson WR, Harth M, Ostbye T, Speechley M. Chronic widespread musculoskeletal pain with or without fibromyalgia: psychological distress in a representative community adult sample. *J Rheum*. 2002;29:588–594.

46. McWilliams L, Goodwin R, Cox BJ. Depression and anxiety associated with three pain conditions: results from a nationally representative sample. *Pain*. 2004;111:77–83.

47. Ligthart L, Gerrits MM, Boomsma DI, Penninx BW. Anxiety and depression are associated with migraine and pain in general: an investigation of the interrelationships. *J Pain*. 2013;14(4): 363–370.

48. Dworkin SF, Von Korff M, LeResche L. Multiple pains and psychiatric disturbance. An epidemiologic investigation. *Arch Gen Psychiatry*. 1990;47(3):239–244.

49. Von Korff M, Deyo RA, Cherkin D, Barlow W. Back pain in primary care. Outcomes at 1 year. *Spine (Phila Pa 1976)*. 1993;18: 855–862.

50. Atkinson JH, Slater MA, Patterson TL, Grant I, Garfin SR. Prevalence, onset, and risk of psychiatric disorders in men with chronic low back pain: a controlled study. *Pain*. 1991;45(2):111–121.

51. Magni G, Moreschi C, Rigatti-Luchini S, Merskey H. Prospective study on the relationship between depressive symptoms and chronic musculoskeletal pain. *Pain*. 1994;56(3):289–297.

52. Karp JF, Scott J, Houck P, Reynolds CF 3rd, Kupfer DJ, Frank E. Pain predicts longer time to remission during treatment of recurrent depression. *J Clin Psychiatry*. 2005;66(5):591–597.

53. Polatin PB, Kinney RK, Gatchel RJ, Lillo E, Mayer TG. Psychiatric illness and chronic low back pain. *Spine (Phila Pa 1976)*. 1993;18:66–71.

54. Brown GK. A causal analysis of chronic pain and depression. *J Abn Psychol.* 1990;99(2):127–137.

55. Katon W, Egan K, Miller D. Chronic pain: lifetime psychiatric diagnosis and family history. *Am J Psychiatry* 1985;142(10):1156–1160.

56. Dersh J, Mayer T, Theodore BR, Polatin P, Gatchel RJ. Do psychiatric disorders first appear preinjury or postinjury in chronic disabling occupational spinal disorders? *Spine (Phila Pa 1976).* 2007;32:1045–1051.

57. Edwards RR, Bingham CO, Bathon J, Haythornthwaite JA. Catastrophizing and pain in arthritis, fibromyalgia, and other rheumatic diseases. *Arthritis Rheum.* 2006;55:325–332.

58. Keefe FJ, Rumble ME, Scipio CD, Giordano LA, Perri LM. Psychological aspects of persistent pain: current state of the science. *J Pain.* 2004;5(4):195–211.

59. Bruehl S, Chung OY, Burns JW, Biridepalli S. The association between anger expression and chronic pain intensity: evidence for partial mediation by endogenous opioid dysfunction. *Pain.* 2003;106:317–324.

60. Bruehl S, Liu X, Burns JW, Chont M, Jamison RN. Associations between daily chronic pain intensity, daily anger expression, and trait anger expressiveness; an ecological momentary assessment study. *Pain.* 2012;153:2352–2358.

61. Jamison RN, Edwards RR, Edwards RR, Liu X, et al. Effect of negative affect on outcome of an opioid therapy trial among low back pain patients. *Pain Practice.* 2013;13:173–181.

62. Novy DM, Nelson DV, Berry LA, Averill PM. What does the Beck depression Inventory measure in chronic pain?: a reappraisal. *Pain.* 1995;61:261–270.

63. Kroenke K, Price RK. Symptoms in the community. Prevalence, classification, and psychiatric comorbidity. *Arch Intern Med.* 1993;153(21):2474–2480.

64. Adler G, Gattaz WF. Pain perception threshold in major depression. *Biol Psychiatry.* 1993;34(10):687–689.

65. Dworkin RH, Clark WC, Lipsitz JD. Pain responsivity in major depression and bipolar disorder. *Psychiatry Res.* 1995;56(2):173–181.

66. Widerstrom EG, Aslund PG, Gustafsson LE, Mannheimer C, Carlsson SG, Andersson SA. Relations between experimentally induced tooth pain threshold changes, psychometrics and clinical pain relief following TENS. A retrospective study in patients with long-lasting pain. *Pain.* 1992;51(3):281–287.

67. Widerstrom-Noga E, Dyrehag LE, Börglum-Jensen L, Aslund PG, Wenneberg B, Andersson SA. Pain threshold responses to two different modes of sensory stimulation in patients with orofacial muscular pain: psychologic considerations. *J Orofac Pain.* 1998;12(1):27–34.

68. Schweinhardt P, Kalk N, Wartolowska K, Chessell I, Wordsworth P, Tracey I. Investigation into the neural correlates of emotional augmentation of clinical pain. *Neuroimage.* 2008;40(2):759–766.

69. Apkarian AV, Hashmi JA, Baliki MN. Pain and the brain: specificity and plasticity of the brain in clinical chronic pain. *Pain.* 2011;152(3 Suppl):S49–S64.

70. Gordon NC, Heller PH, Gear RW, Levine JD. Temporal factors in the enhancement of morphine analgesia by desipramine. *Pain.* 1993;53(3):273–276.

71. Carruba MO, Nisoli E, Garosi V, Sacerdote P, Panerai AE, Da Prada M. Catecholamine and serotonin depletion from rat spinal cord: effects on morphine and footshock induced analgesia. *Pharmacol Res.* 1992;25(2):187–194.

72. Kennedy SE, Koeppe RA, Young EA, Zubieta JK. Dysregulation of endogenous opioid emotion regulation circuitry in major depression in women. *Arch Gen Psychiatry.* 2006;63(11):1199–1208.

73. Woolf CJ. Pain: moving from symptom control toward mechanism-specific pharmacologic management. *Ann Intern Med.* 2004;140:441–451.

74. Raison CL, Capuron L, Miller AH. Cytokines sing the blues: inflammation and the pathogenesis of depression. *Trends Immunol.* 2006;27(1):24–31.

75. Sprenger T, Valet M, Boecker H, et al. Opioidergic activation in the medial pain system after heat pain. *Pain.* 2006;122:63–67.

76. Peyron R, Laurent B, García-Larrea L. Functional imaging of brain responses to pain. a review and meta-analysis. *Neurophysiol Clin.* 2000;30:263–288.

77. Zubieta JK, Ketter TA, Ketter TA, et al. Regulation of human affective responses by anterior cingulate and limbic mu-opioid neurotransmission. *Arch Gen Psych.* 2003;60(11):1145–1153.

78. Coghill RC, McHaffie JG, Yen YF. Neural correlates of interindividual differences in the subjective experience of pain. *Proc Natl Acad Sci U S A.* 2003;100(14):8538–8542.

79. Ploghaus A, Tracey I, Gati JS, et al. Dissociating pain from its anticipation in the human brain. *Science.* 1999;284(5422):1979–1981.

80. Ben-Porth Y, Tellegen A. *Minnesota Multiphasic Personality Inventory - 2 Restructured Form: Technical Manual.* Minneapolis; University of Minnesota Press: 2008.

81. Block AR, Ohnmeiss DD, Guyer RD, Rashbaum RF, Hochschuler SH. The use of presurgical psychological screening to predict the outcome of spine surgery. *Spine J.* 2001;1:274–282.

82. Hathaway SR, McKinley JC, Butcher JN, et al. *Minnesota Multiphasic Personality Inventory-2: Manual for Administration.* Minneapolis, MN; University of Minnesota Press: 1989.

83. Derogatis LR, Melisaratos N. The Brief Symptom Inventory: an introductory report. *Psychol Med.* 1983;13:595–605.

84. Millon T, Green CJ, Meagher RB Jr. The MBHI: a new inventory for the psychodiagnostician in medical settings. *Prof Psychol.* 1979;10:529–539.

85. Pilowsky I, Spence ND. Patterns of illness behavior in patients with intractable pain. *J Psychosom Res.* 1975;19:279–287.

86. Beck AT, Steer RA. *Beck Depression Inventory.* San Antonio, TX; Psychological Corporation: 1993.

87. Radloff LS. The CES-D scale: a self-report depression scale for research in the general population. *Appl Psychol Measure.* 1977;1:385–401.

88. Zigmond AS, Snaith RP. The hospital anxiety and depression scale. *Acta Psychiatrica Scandinavica.* 1983;37:361–370.

89. McCreary C. Empirically derived MMPI profile clusters and characteristics of low back pain patients. *Clin Psychol.* 1985;53(4):558–560.

90. Gass CS, Luis CA. MMPI-2 short form: psychometric characteristics in a neuropsychological setting. *Assessment.* 2001;2:213–219.

91. Moore JE, McFall ME, Kivlahan DR, Capestany F. Risk of misinterpretation of MMPI Schizophrenia scale elevations in chronic pain patients. *Pain.* 1988;32:207–213.

92. Jamison RN, Rock DL, Parris WC. Empirically derived Symptom Checklist 90 subgroups of chronic pain patients: a cluster analysis. *J Behav Med.* 1988;11(2):147–158.

93. Geisser ME, Roth RS. Assessing depression among persons with chronic pain using the center for epidemiological studies

depression scale and the beck depression inventory: a comparative analysis. *Clin J Pain*. 1997;13:163–170.

94. Santor DA, Zuroff DC, Ramsay JO, Cervantes P, Palacios J Examining scale descriminability in the BDI and CES-D as a function of depressive severity. *Psychol Assess*. 1995;7:131–139.

95. Andresen EM, Malmgren JA, Carter WB, Patrick DL. Screening for depression in well older adults: evaluation of a short form of the CES-D. *Amer J Prevent Med*. 1994;10:77–84.

96. Bjelland I, Dahl AA, Haug TT, Neckelmann D. The validity of the Hospital Anxiety and Depression Scale. An updated literature review. *J Psychosom Res*. 2002;52(2):69–77.

97. Cosco TD, Doyle F, Ward M, McGee H. Latent structure of the Hospital Anxiety And Depression Scale: a 10-year systematic review. *J Psychosom Res*. 2012;72(3):180–184.

98. Doyle F, Cosco T, Conroy R. Why the HADS is still important: Reply to Coyne & van Sonderen. *J Psychosom Res*. 2012;73(1):74.

99. Salerno SM, Browning R, Jackson JL. The effect of antidepressant treatment on chronic back pain: a meta-analysis. *Arch Int Med*. 2002;162(1):19–24.

100. Kroenke K, Bair MJ, Damush TM, et al. Optimized antidepressant therapy and pain self-management in primary care patients with depression and musculoskeletal pain. *JAMA*. 2009;301:2099–2110.

101. Farrar JT, Young JP, LaMoreaux L, Werth JL, Poole RM. Clinical importance of changes in chronic pain intensity measured on an 11-point numerical pain rating scale. *Pain*. 2001;94:149–158.

102. Watson CP, Gilron I, Sawynok J, Lynch ME. Nontricyclic antidepressant analgesics and pain: are serotonin norepinephrine reuptake inhibitors (SNRIs) any better? *Pain*. 2011;152(10):2206–2210.

103. Dharmshaktu P, Tayal V, Kalra BS. Efficacy of antidepressants as analgesics: a review. *J Clin Pharmacol*. 2012;52(1):6–17.

104. Lin EH, Katon W, Von Korff M, et al.; IMPACT Investigators. Effect of improving depression care on pain and functional outcomes among older adults with arthritis: a randomized controlled trial. *JAMA*. 2003;290(18):2428–2429.

105. Rosenzweig-Lipson S, Beyer CE, Hughes ZA, et al. Differentiating antidepressants of the future: efficacy and safety. *Pharmacol Therapeutics*. 2007;113:134–153.

106. Semenchuk MR, Sherman S, Davis B. Double-blind, randomized trial of bupropion SR for the treatment of neuropathic pain. *Neurol*. 2001;57(9)1583–1589.

107. Katz J, Pennella-Vaughan J, Hetzel RD, Kanazi GE, Dworkin RH. A randomized, placebo-controlled trial of bupropion sustained release in chronic low back pain. *J Pain*. 2005;6(10):656–661.

108. Bloomstein JR, Rummans TA, Maruta T, Lin SC, Pileggi TS. The use of electroconvulsive therapy in pain patients. *Psychosomatics*. 1996;37:374–749.

109. Wasan AD, Artin K, Clark MR. A case-matching study of the analgesic properties of electroconvulsive therapy. *Pain Med*. 2004; 5(1):50–58.

110. Salzman C. The APA task force report on benzodiazepine dependence, toxicity, and abuse. *Am J Psychiatry*. 1991;148(2): 151–152.

111. Jann MW, Slade JH. Antidepressant agents for the treatment of chronic pain and depression. *Pharmacotherapy*. 2007;27(11): 1571–1587.

112. Rickels K, Schweizer E. The spectrum of generalized anxiety in clinical practice: the role of short-term, intermittent treatment. *Br J Psychiatry Suppl*. 1998;1:49–54.

113. Gilbody S, Bower P, Fletcher J, Richards D, Sutton AJ. Collaborative care for depression: a cumulative meta-analysis and review of longer-term outcomes. *Arch Int Med*. 2006;166(21):2314–2321.

114. Wasan AD, Alpay M. Chapter 78: Pain and the psychiatric comorbidities of pain. Comprehensive Clinical Psychiatry. In: Stern T, Rosenbaum JF, Fava M, Biederman J, Rauch SL. Philadelphia, PA; Elsevier: 2008:1067–1080.

115. Brox JI, Reikerås O, Nygaard Ø, Sørensen R, Indahl A, Holm I, Keller A, Ingebrigtsen T, Grundnes O, Lange JE, Friis A. Lumbar instrumented fusion compared with cognitive intervention and exercises in patients with chronic back pain after previous surgery for disc herniation: a prospective randomized controlled study. *Pain*. 2006;122(1-2):145–155.

116. Jamison RN. *Learning to Master Your Chronic Pain*. Sarasota, FL; Professional Resource Press: 1996.

117. Elliott RL. Depression in primary care. *Ethn Dis*. 2007;17(2 Suppl 2): S2–28–33.

118. Manning JS, Jackson WC. Depression, pain, and comorbid medical conditions. *J Clin Psychiatry*. 2013;74(2):e03.

119. Jamison RN. Psychological evaluation and treatment of chronic pain. In: Vacanti CA, Sikka PK, Urman RD, Dershwitz M, Segal BS. *Essential Clinical Anesthesia*. New York, NY; Cambridge University Press: 2011:901–907.

120. Lamb SE, Hansen Z, Lall R, et al.; Back Skills Training Trial investigators. Group cognitive behavioural treatment for low-back pain in primary care: a randomised controlled trial and cost-effectiveness analysis. *Lancet*. 2010;375(9718):916–923.

121. Hoffman BM, Papas RK, Chatkoff DK, Kerns RD. Meta-analysis of psychological interventions for chronic low back pain. *Health Psychol*. 2007;26(1):1–9.

122. Veehof MM, Oskam MJ, Schreurs KM, Bohlmeijer ET. Acceptance-based interventions for the treatment of chronic pain: a systematic review and meta-analysis. *Pain*. 2010;152:533–542.

123. Johnston M, Foster M, Shennan J, Starkey NJ, Johnson A. The effectiveness of an Acceptance and Commitment Therapy self-help intervention for chronic pain. *Clin J Pain*. 2010;26:393–402.

124. Kroenke K, Spitzer RL, deGruy FV 3rd, et al. Multisomatoform disorder. An alternative to undifferentiated somatoform disorder for the somatizing patient in primary care. *Arch Gen Psychiatry*. 1997;54(4):352–358.

125. Barsky AJ 3rd. Patients who amplify bodily sensations. *Ann Intern Med*. 1979;91(1):63–70.

126. Barsky AJ, Wyshak G, Klerman GL, Latham KS. (1990). The prevalence of hypochondriasis in medical outpatients. *Soc Psychiatry Psychiatr Epidemiol*. 1990;25:89–94.

127. Campbell C, Jamison RN, Edwards RR. Psychological screening/phenotyping as predictors for spinal cord stimulation. *Curr Pain Headache Rep*. 2013;17:307–314.

128. Celestin J, Edwards RR, Jamison RN. Pretreatment psychosocial variables as predictors of outcomes following lumbar surgery and spinal cord stimulation: a systematic review and literature synthesis. *Pain Med*. 2009;10(4):639–653.

129. Tang NK, Crane C. Suicidality in chronic pain: a review of the prevalence, risk factors and psychological links. *Psychol Med*. 2006;36:575–586.

130. Bernal M, Haro JM, Bernert S, et al. Risk factors for suicidality in Europe: results from the ESEMED study. *J Affect Disord*. 2007; 101:27–34.

131. Theodoulou M, Harriss L, Hawton K, Bass C. Pain and deliberate self-harm: an important association. *J Psychosom Res*. 2005;28:317–320.

132. Moller HJ. Suicide, suicidality and suicide prevention in affective disorders. *Acta Psychiatr Scand Suppl*. 2003;(418): 73–80.

133. Sokero TP, Melartin TK, Rytsälä HJ, Leskelä US, Lestelä-Mielonen PS, Isometsä ET. Suicidal ideation and attempts among psychiatric patients with major depressive disorder. *J Clin Psychiatry*. 2003;64(9):1094–1100.

134. Juurlink DN, Herrmann N, Szalai JP, Kopp A, Redelmeier DA. Medical illness and the risk of suicide in the elderly. *Arch Intern Med*. 2004;164:1179–1184.

135. Smith MT, Edwards RR, Robinson RC, Dworkin RH. Suicidal ideation, plans, attempts in chronic pain patients: factors associated with increased risk. *Pain*. 2004;111:201–208.

136. Smith MT, Perlis ML, Haythornthwaite JA. Suicidal ideation in outpatients with chronic musculoskeletal pain: an exploratory study of the role of sleep onset insomnia and pain intensity. *Clin J Pain*. 2004;20:111–118.

CHAPTER 18

Depression in Sleep Disorders

Susan Mackie, MD
John Winkelman, MD, PhD

The study of human sleep is a remarkably young field. Until the 1930s, sleep was viewed as a passive state during which the brain was "turned off." As such, there was little interest in further characterization of normal sleep or exploration of sleep disorders. In 1937, A. L. Loomis first described the characteristic electroencephalographic patterns of the stages of NREM sleep, challenging the notion of sleep as a homogeneous and passive state.[1] This was followed in 1951 by the discovery of REM sleep and its correlation with dreaming.[2] A schema of sleep architecture consisting of repeated cycles of NREM and REM sleep was formulated shortly thereafter, a concept that has persisted largely unchanged into the modern era of sleep medicine.

Discovery of the electroencephalographic substrate of sleep prompted increasing curiosity about sleep physiology. Overnight polysomnography—a technique of simultaneous recording of sleep EEG, respiratory parameters, and muscle activity—was developed and employed to describe normal and abnormal sleep patterns (**Fig. 18-1**). During the second half of the twentieth century, polysomnographic characterization of obstructive sleep apnea (OSA), insomnia, periodic leg movements of sleep (PLMS), REM behavior disorder (RBD), and narcolepsy facilitated improved understanding of the pathophysiology of these disorders and expanded treatment options.

In addition to its utility in primary sleep disorders, polysomnography was also applied to the study of a variety of neurological and psychiatric conditions. In patients with depression, consistent abnormalities of sleep architecture were identified.[3] These included shortened REM latency (time from sleep onset to the first episode of REM), prolongation of the first REM period, and increased density of eye movements during REM. These observations led to the hypothesis that "disinhibition" of REM sleep may play a role in the pathophysiology of depression. Furthermore, REM abnormalities may constitute a biomarker that predicts the onset of new depression and increased vulnerability to relapse in remitted patients.[4] Thus, the abnormalities in sleep seen in depressed patients may not be merely incidental but may be closely tied to the precipitation and perpetuation of the illness.

In light of these significant sleep abnormalities in depressed patients, primary sleep disorders may also be expected to affect mood. Indeed, a markedly increased risk for depression has been identified in a variety of sleep disorders, including insomnia, OSA, and restless legs syndrome (RLS), among others. Recognition of these epidemiologic links has spawned further research into the pathophysiologic and prognostic implications of sleep disorders in depressed patients, investigations that have improved understanding of both conditions. In this chapter, we discuss the bidirectional and complex relationships between sleep disorders and depression. Although much is known about the depression–sleep disorder relationship, much less is known about the additional influence of concurrent medical illness on this relationship. We first address epidemiologic associations between the various sleep disorders and depression. This is followed by an exploration of shared pathophysiology among these disorders. We then consider aspects of the presentation and management of depression that are particular to patients with sleep disorders. When applicable, the impact of depression and its treatment on sleep are also considered.

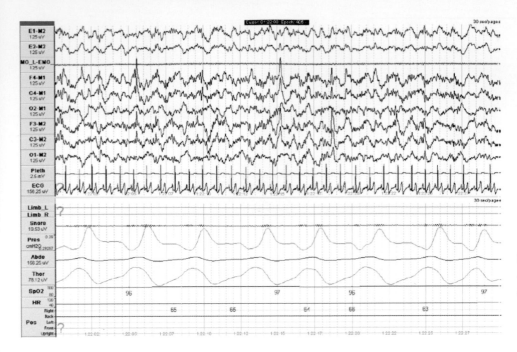

Figure 18-1 *Polysomnography. A 30-second epoch of sleep recorded by polysomnography. Eye movements, muscle tone in the chin and legs, 6 EEG channels, EKG, nasal airflow, and respiratory effort are depicted here.*

EPIDEMIOLOGY

■ INSOMNIA

Insomnia encompasses difficulty initiating sleep, difficulty maintaining sleep, and/or unrefreshing sleep, coupled with daytime impairment. Although in the past insomnia was often viewed as a symptom of depression likely to resolve with treatment of the mood disorder, recent research has focused on insomnia and depression as two independent diagnostic entities with distinct (but interrelated) characteristics and courses.[5]

Insomnia is likely both a cause and a consequence of depression, so understanding their epidemiologic relationship requires longitudinal descriptions of comorbidity. Many studies have examined insomnia symptoms as a predictor of major depression disorder (MDD). In a recent meta-analysis, the overall odds ratio of new-onset depression in individuals with insomnia compared to those without insomnia was 2.60 (CI: 1.98–3.42).[6] The incidence of new-onset depression during the follow-up period was 13.1% in the insomniacs compared to 4.0% in the group without sleep complaints.

Although the data are fewer, depression also appears to be a risk factor for new-onset insomnia. In one large survey, participants with depression but without insomnia at baseline had an OR of 6.7 of developing insomnia at 10-year follow-up.[7]

Several studies have attempted to tease out the directionality of causation between insomnia and depression. Ohayon and Roth surveyed nearly 15,000 people from the general population about sleep and psychiatric symptoms. In a large survey of the general population, insomnia symptoms preceded a first episode of a mood disorder 41% of the time, while they occurred concurrently in 29% of cases, and followed the onset of the mood disorder in another 29% of cases.[8] This study was limited by its cross-sectional nature and its reliance on subjects to recount the order of symptom appearance. Still, these findings highlight the strongly bidirectional relationship between the two disorders.

Although most patients with MDD report difficulty sleeping, a substantial minority report "hypersomnia," and this descriptor is included in the DSM 5 as a symptom of MDD. Rates of hypersomnia in MDD vary widely across studies, likely due in part to variable definitions of the term.[9] As with insomnia, hypersomnia predicts both new-onset

MDD and relapse of MDD.[10] Despite considerable literature about the prevalence of hypersomnia in MDD, few studies have established whether this subjective complaint corresponds to an objectively assessed increased propensity to sleep. Patients may have difficulty distinguishing between fatigue, avolition, and psychomotor retardation that compel them to spend excessive amounts of time in bed and true increased sleep pressure or excessive total sleep time.[11] It is incumbent on the clinician to do so, however, since true sleepiness should prompt investigation for a primary sleep disorder.

■ OBSTRUCTIVE SLEEP APNEA

Obstructive sleep apnea (OSA) is a syndrome of repetitive partial or complete airway collapse during sleep. The consequent airflow obstruction may cause oxygen desaturation and/or sleep disruption. OSA is commonly comorbid with MDD. Estimates of the prevalence of depression among OSA patients vary widely from 7% to 63%. In the National Health and Nutrition Examination Survey, snorting/stopping breathing ≥5 nights/week compared to never was strongly associated with probable major depression in men (OR = 3.1; CI: 1.8–5.2) and women (OR = 3.0; CI: 1.6–5.4).[12] Conversely, in one cross-sectional telephone survey, 18% of individuals with a diagnosis of MDD also reported symptoms consistent with probable OSA.[13] After controlling for known shared risk factors, the odds of sleep-disordered breathing was 5.26 (CI: 4.29–6.47) for those with MDD compared to those without MDD.

■ RESTLESS LEGS SYNDROME

Restless legs syndrome is another common sleep disorder frequently associated with depression. RLS is characterized by a strong urge to move the legs that is provoked by rest, relieved with movement, and worst in the evening or at night. The lifetime prevalence of MDD or dysthymia has been reported to be 36.9% in RLS patients compared to 15.2% in a control group drawn from the general population.[14] The majority (77%) reported that RLS symptoms preceded depression. Another cross-sectional analysis described increasing risk for RLS as the PHQ-9 score increased.[15] The issue has also been examined longitudinally using data from a large, long-term, prospective study. Women with RLS but no depression at baseline were more likely to develop subsequent depression at 6-year follow-up (RR = 1.5; CI: 1.1–2.1).[16] Conversely, depressive symptoms at baseline were a risk factor for incident RLS.[17] As in the case of insomnia, RLS and depression appear to have a bidirectional relationship.

The majority of RLS patients experience periodic limb movements of sleep (PLMS). PLMS are repetitive (usually every 20–40 sec) episodes of stereotyped limb movements during sleep that are often associated with EEG arousals. Both nighttime RLS symptoms and PLMS may compromise sleep quality and quantity and account for a proportion of the association between RLS and depression.[18] However, sleep disruption does not seem to be entirely explanatory. In a large cohort of patients with chronic kidney disease (CKD), Szentkiralyi and colleagues found that those with probable RLS had a higher prevalence of depressive symptoms than those without RLS (56% vs. 22%, p<0.001), and this relationship remained significant after accounting for insomnia, indicating that mechanisms independent of sleep disruption may also contribute to the association between RLS and depression.[19]

■ OTHER SLEEP DISORDERS

Shift-work sleep disorder (SWSD) occurs in patients who complain of insomnia or excessive sleepiness that is temporally related to work hours scheduled during the usual sleep period. Although such a schedule universally produces circadian misalignment, a minority of shift workers (8–15%) have extreme difficulty adapting, that is, SWSD.[20] In one cross-sectional analysis, nearly one-third of patients with SWSD also carried a diagnosis of MDD.[20] Notably, the increased risk for depression in this analysis was specific to those with symptoms of SWSD (insomnia and/or excessive sleepiness) and did not appear to be a consequence of shift work itself.

Nightmare disorder is another sleep disorder that is commonly comorbid with MDD. In one study, three-quarters of individuals with MDD reported having nightmares at least twice per week.[21]

Narcolepsy is a disorder of excessive daytime sleepiness with frequent psychiatric comorbidity, including increased rates of depressive symptoms.[22] Prevalence using self-report scales in various studies ranges from 15% to 30%.[23] Using formal psychiatric interview, Fortuyn and colleagues did not find an over-representation of MDD but did find high rates of depressive mood (30%), pathological guilt (22%), crying (25%), and anhedonia (27%), suggesting that narcoleptic patients may experience a subsyndromal form of depression.[22,24]

A complicating factor when quantifying the association between depression and sleep disorders is their myriad shared risk factors. Obesity, lack of physical activity, and low socioeconomic status are a few of the more obvious confounders. Many of the multivariate models described above have attempted to account for these. However, in consideration of the likelihood of residual confounding, these data should be interpreted with caution.

■ PATHOPHYSIOLOGY

Several lines of evidence suggest common pathophysiological mechanisms underlying sleep disorders and depression (**Box 18-1**).

BOX 18-1
POSSIBLE MEDIATORS BETWEEN INSOMNIA AND DEPRESSION

Hyperarousal
Somatic arousal
Stress
Decreased hippocampal volume
Decreased GABA in occipital and prefrontal cortices
Neurotrophins (BDNF)

NE, norepinephrine; IL—6, interleukin 6; MSLT, multiple sleep latency test
Figure 18-2 *Evidence of hyperarousal in insomnia.*

Although the link has been most thoroughly explored in insomnia, some abnormalities are shared across a range of sleep disorders. These may reflect causal relationships and/or consequences of sleep disruption itself rather than markers of a specific illness. For the most part, the directionality of these relationships remains an open question.

■ AROUSAL AND STRESS

Hyperarousal is a crucial element in the development and perpetuation of insomnia. It is evident as autonomic activation (increased heart rate, decreased heart rate variability), elevated stress hormones (e.g., cortisol and norepinephrine), higher metabolic rate (increased VO_2 and brain metabolism), electroencephalographic arousal (increased high-frequency beta activity), and behavioral evidence of decreased sleep propensity (increased latency to sleep on the MSLT) (**Fig. 18-2**).[25–27] Although the data are fewer, recent research also points toward a pattern of hyperarousal in RLS.[28]

Somatic arousal has also been classically postulated as a component of the tripartite model of depression.[29] Recently, novel EEG analysis techniques have demonstrated hyperstable vigilance in MDD, suggestive of tonic CNS arousal.[30,31] As further evidence of physiologic arousal, autonomic activation is evidenced by decreased heart rate variability, an abnormality that correlates with the severity of depression.[32] Plasma norepinephrine levels are also increased in untreated MDD patients and normalize with treatment.[33] Dysfunctional HPA axis regulation is manifest as diminished amplitude of diurnal cortisol rhythms and impaired cortisol suppression following dexamethasone challenge.[34]

Although other sleep disorders are more often marked by sleepiness rather than hyperarousal, the profile of prolonged stress response (sympathetic nervous system activation and HPA axis dysregulation) is also common to other sleep disorders. Both autonomic abnormalities and hormonal markers of stress have been examined in OSA. Abnormally decreased heart rate variability[35] and elevated cortisol levels[36] are both consistent features of OSA that improve with continuous positive airway pressure (CPAP) treatment. Muscle sympathetic nerve activity (MSNA) is another measure of sympathetic activation. OSA patients demonstrate elevation in MSNA that correlates with the degree of sleepiness and improves in parallel with reduction in sleepiness during treatment.[37,38] Similarly in MDD, elevated MSNA correlates with the severity of depression and improves with antidepressant treatment.[39] Finally, inflammatory cytokines, including IL-6 and TNF, are elevated in both MDD and OSA—an abnormality closely tied to the increased cardiovascular risk seen with both disorders.[40,41]

■ IMAGING DATA

Brain imaging provides further evidence of shared pathophysiology between depression and sleep disorders. Using structural MRI, the hippocampus is consistently smaller in patients with MDD compared to normal controls.[42] Abnormalities in hippocampal volume have also been shown in several sleep disorders, including narcolepsy and insomnia.[43,44,45] Proton magnetic resonance spectroscopy (1 H-MRS) is a type of MRI developed to measure levels of neurotransmitters *in vivo*. Using this technique, decreased gamma aminobutyric acid (GABA) in the occipital and prefrontal cortices has been a consistent finding in MDD. Similar reductions in whole brain and regional GABA have been demonstrated in insomnia patients in some[46] but not all investigations[47] and may reflect common neurochemistry between insomnia and depression.[46]

Obstructive sleep apnea patients also exhibit abnormalities by both structural and functional imaging. Changes in the cingulate, frontal cortex, hippocampus, insular cortex, cerebellum, and amygdala overlap with findings in MDD.[48–50] The hippocampus is of particular interest because there are data suggesting that hypoxia due to OSA plays a causative role in damaging this area.[48,51] These findings highlight the potential detrimental interactions between depression and OSA.

■ NEUROTROPHINS

The neurotrophic model of depression postulates that dysfunctional neuroplasticity and remodeling contribute to the pathophysiology of depression. Brain-derived neurotrophic factor (BDNF) has been the most extensively studied neurotrophin. BDNF levels measured in the serum are decreased in depressed subjects relative to controls,[52] and a functional polymorphism in the pro-BDNF gene is associated with increased risk of MDD and may mediate hippocampal atrophy.[53,54] BDNF during sleep has been shown to play a role in the generation of slow wave oscillations that mediate neuronal plasticity.[55,56] Deficits in slow wave sleep have been reported in insomnia,[57,58] and a recent study demonstrated decreased serum BDNF in insomnia patients.[59] This deficit was proportional to the severity of sleep disturbance. It is possible that decreased BDNF reflects common pathophysiology underlying the disorders, or insomnia may mediate the abnormalities seen in depression. As the authors suggest, sleep abnormalities could explain inconsistency in reports of BDNF changes during depression treatment. These relationships illustrate the subtlety and complexity of the pathophysiologic links between depression and insomnia.

■ PRESENTATION OF COMORBID DEPRESSION AND INSOMNIA

Patients with insomnia may experience distress due to fears of sleeplessness, preoccupation with the daytime consequences of poor sleep, guilt about the use of hypnotics. People with chronic insomnia report lower SF-36 scores in each of eight domains compared with good sleepers ($p < 0.001$).[60] Compared to those without insomnia, insomniacs report greater impairment in all areas (energy, mood, concentration, relationships, work, and ability to stay awake).[61]

Major depressive disorder occurring in insomniacs tends to be more severe compared to depression in those without sleep complaints. In a study by O'Brien et al., 1,057 patients with a principal diagnosis of MDD were evaluated using the Structured Clinical Interview for DSM-IV Disorders (SCID), Schedule for Affective Disorders (SADS), and self-report measures of mood and psychosocial functioning.[62] One quarter of patients with MDD have been found to have severe insomnia. These severe insomniacs, in comparison to those without severe insomnia, were older at the time of presentation, less likely to be married, less educated, had poorer social functioning, and had more severe depressive symptoms.

The presentation of insomnia is also influenced by depression. Insomnia symptoms can be divided into difficulty initiating sleep, middle-of-the-night insomnia, early morning waking, and/or nonrestorative sleep. Although it is commonly held that MDD is characterized particularly by early morning awakenings, this has not been the case in research samples. In a large study of patients with MDD, the most common presentation was the simultaneous presence of sleep onset, middle-of-the-night, and early morning insomnia symptoms (27.1%). Of these three types of insomnia symptoms, mid-nocturnal insomnia symptoms were the most commonly found alone (13.5%) and in combination with one or more other types (82.3%) (**Fig. 18-3**).[63] Another study found shorter sleep duration in depressed compared to nondepressed insomniacs.[64] These findings indicate that depression is associated with increased severity of insomnia.

■ PRESENTATION OF COMORBID DEPRESSION AND OSA

As in insomnia, patients with sleep apnea frequently experience distressing emotional consequences and reduced quality of life.

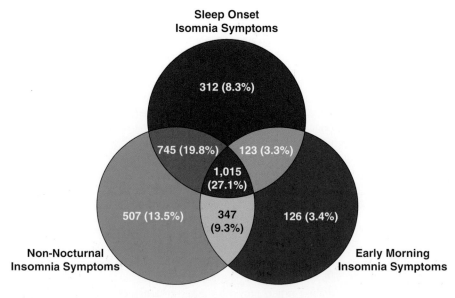

Sleep Onset Isomnia Symptoms

312 (8.3%)

745 (19.8%)   123 (3.3%)

1,015 (27.1%)

507 (13.5%)   347 (9.3%)   126 (3.4%)

Non-Nocturnal Insomnia Symptoms

Early Morning Insomnia Symptoms

Note: patients with no insomnia symptoms = 571 (15.3%).

Figure 18-3 *Insomnia symptoms in depressed patients. (Reproduced with permission from Sunderajan P, Gaynes BN, Wisniewski SR, et al. Insomnia in patients with depression: a STAR*D report. CNS Spectr. 2010;15(6):394–404.)*

Fear of dying as well as the physical effects of sleep deprivation, oxygen desaturation, and hypercarbia may all play a role. The severity of hypoxia and the degree of excessive daytime sleepiness are independent predictors of reduced quality of life in patients with severe OSA.[65]

The presence of depression affects the presentation of OSA. Depressed OSA patients tend to present with more prominent sleepiness than those without depression.[66] Indeed, one study found that the presence of depression correlated more strongly with sleepiness than did the severity of sleep apnea. OSA severity explained 4.2% of variance in sleepiness while depressive symptoms explained an additional 42.3%. In another cross-sectional evaluation of patients with REM-related OSA (in which the severity of sleep apnea does not correlate well with sleepiness), depressive symptoms were associated with worse quality of life and elevated sleepiness scores.[67]

Patients with RLS also report poorer health-related quality of life in all physical domains as well as in the Mental Health and Vitality domain.[68] In RLS patients with MDD, the frequency of RLS symptoms has been associated with depression severity.[16]

■ COURSE AND NATURAL HISTORY

Given the association between various sleep problems and the severity of depression at presentation, it is not surprising that sleep disturbance also predicts a more prolonged course of the mood disorder with more negative consequences. Suicidal thoughts and behaviors have been the focus of much attention. Sleep disturbances (in particular insomnia and nightmares) consistently predict both suicidal ideation and suicide attempts. This association persists after adjustment for depression severity and other psychiatric comorbidity. One meta-analysis found that the presence of any sleep disturbance increased the risk of suicidal ideation (RR = 1.86), suicide attempts (RR = 2.01), and completed suicide (RR = 1.96).[69] There were insufficient data to draw definitive conclusions about the differential risk associated with specific sleep disorders. Not all participants carried a diagnosis of MDD, but the lack of a modifying effect of depressive symptoms indicates that this association is likely to hold in both depressed and nondepressed patients.

The course of both depression and sleep disorders is often marked by absenteeism from work or school and short- and long-term disability. Thus, both insomnia and OSA are independent predictors of subsequent long-term sick leave.[70] Insomnia is also a risk factor for days out-of-role[71] and delay in returning to work among those on sick leave.[72] Depression is also a major cause of disability.[73,74] Most evidence suggests that insomnia and depression independently increase the risk of absenteeism-related outcomes, with the highest risk occurring in those with both conditions.[71,72] In addition to the lost productivity, the absence of a regular daily schedule is likely to perpetuate sleep problems, and lack of structure and social stimulation may perpetuate depression. Thus, depression, insomnia, and disability status are mutually exacerbating conditions that likely prolong the course of all three.

Sleep problems often persist in patients whose depression has remitted. In a large sample of patients whose depression was in remission, insomnia was found in 19.3% and nightmares in 9.3%.[75] Those with residual sleep disturbance were also more likely to have persistent anxiety (**Box 18-2**) symptoms. Another study found a significantly higher rate of insomnia (53%) among remitters when any positive response on the HAM-D insomnia items was included. Among this group, residual insomnia was associated with persistent social and occupational functional impairment.[76]

Given the association between insomnia and new-onset depression, several investigators have examined the effect of residual insomnia symptoms on the risk of relapse to MDD. In two studies of patients with late-life depression,[77,78] insomnia increased the risk of

relapse, but another study did not replicate this finding in younger patients.[79]

■ ASSESSMENT AND DIFFERENTIAL DIAGNOSIS

The symptoms of depression overlap considerably with those of various primary sleep disorders. Whereas fatigue, nonrestorative sleep, low sex drive, decreased concentration, and irritability are common to many sleep disorders and to depression, other symptoms can be identified that are unique to each condition (**Box 18-3**). Feelings of guilt and worthlessness, tearfulness, and suicidality generally are not attributable solely to the sleep disorder and should prompt serious consideration of a primary mood disorder. Conversely, true sleepiness is highly predictive of a primary sleep disorder. Thus, it is important to distinguish fatigue (a common mood symptom) from sleepiness. This distinction can be made by careful history. One may ask, "if you sit down to read a book, do you begin to nod off" or "do you have difficulty staying awake on a long drive?" Provided the patient is allocating adequate time for sleep, an affirmative answer suggests an underlying sleep disorder. The Epworth Sleepiness Scale is a useful tool to quantify the degree of sleepiness (**Fig. 18-4**). It can be completed in <5 minutes and provides feedback to both clinician and patient regarding the likelihood of a sleep disorder.

BOX 18-2
SLEEP DISORDERS AND ANXIETY

- There is a strong association between sleep disorders and nearly every type of anxiety disorder.
- Causation is likely bidirectional: sleep deprivation potentiates anxiety, and the arousal response due to anxiety impairs sleep.
- Treatment of sleep disorders mitigates sleep disruption and frequently improves anxiety.
- Patients with post-traumatic stress disorder frequently suffer from disturbing nightmares. Both CBT and medications directed at nightmares are effective.
- Obsessive-compulsive disorder is strongly associated with delayed sleep phase disorder.
- Nocturnal panic attacks occur in >50% of patients with panic disorder. These should be distinguished from other causes of disturbing arousals, including obstructive sleep apnea and nightmares.

BOX 18-3
IMPORTANT SYMPTOMS

Common to both:
Fatigue
Nonrestorative sleep
Low sex drive
Decreased concentration
Irritability
More typical of depression:
Feelings of guilt and worthlessness
Tearfulness
Suicidality
More typical of sleep disorders:
Sleepiness (as opposed to fatigue)
Involuntary dozing
Snoring, gasping (OSA)
Cataplexy, HH, SP (narcolepsy)

SITUATION	CHANCE OF DOZING
Sitting and reading	0 1 2 3
Watching TV	0 1 2 3
Sitting inactive in a public place (e.g., theater or meeting)	0 1 2 3
Sitting as a passenger in a car for an hour without a break	0 1 2 3
Lying down to rest in the afternoon when circumstances permit	0 1 2 3
Sitting and talking to someone	0 1 2 3
Sitting quietly after lunch without alcohol	0 1 2 3
In a car when stoped for a few minutes in traffic	0 1 2 3

0 = no chance of dozing
1 = slight chance of dozing
2 = moderate chance of dozing
3 = high chance of dozing

Figure 18-4 *Epworth Sleepiness Scale. Scores are summed to produce overall Epworth Sleepiness Score. A score of <10 is normal; 11 to 17 is moderately sleepy; ≥18 is severely sleepy.*

Distinguishing between sleep disorders and depression may be particularly complex in patients also suffering from other comorbid major medical conditions. As discussed elsewhere in this text, MDD is over-represented in a variety of medical disorders. The prudent clinician evaluating a medical patient for depression should also consider that sleep disorders are frequently over-represented in these conditions. For instance, patients with cardiovascular disease suffer disproportionately from both depression and OSA, both of which may present with fatigue and psychomotor retardation. Similarly, those with end-stage renal disease on hemodialysis are at risk for both depression and RLS, disorders that may be easily confused in those presenting with nocturnal agitation. When evaluating a patient with major medical conditions associated with both depressive disorders and sleep disorders, the distinguishing features discussed above should be carefully borne in mind in order to arrive at an accurate diagnosis, leading to appropriate treatment.

■ TREATMENT

In depressed patients with a sleep disorder, treatment of the sleep disorder is crucial, as this may provide substantial alleviation of depressive symptoms (**Box 18-4**). The choice of therapy for depression may also affect sleep, for better or for worse. When embarking on treatment of a patient with comorbid sleep and mood disorders, it is helpful to consider the impact of each intervention on both conditions.

■ GENERAL ISSUES IN THE TREATMENT OF DEPRESSION IN THE PATIENT WITH A SLEEP DISORDER

Most medications used for treatment of depression also affect sleep. Selective serotonin reuptake inhibitors (SSRIs) and serotonin–norepinephrine reuptake inhibitors (SNRIs) are first-line antidepressants in many patients. In addition to suppressing REM sleep, studies in depressed patients indicate that these agents increase sleep onset latency (SOL—time from bedtime to first onset of sleep), increase arousal index (AI—number of awakenings per hour of sleep), increase wake after sleep onset (WASO), and decrease total sleep time.[80,81] Clinically, serotonergic antidepressants variably produce hypersomnia in some patients with depression and insomnia in others.[82] Few head-to-head studies have compared the various SSRIs and SNRIs with regard to their effects on sleep and alertness. Where the evidence exists, it generally indicates no difference.[83–85] SSRI medications have also been associated with abnormal muscle

activity during REM sleep and dream enactment behavior. The latter may be associated with significant injury to the patient or bedpartner and should prompt consideration of downtitrating or changing antidepressants. Bupropion, an NDRI, avoids this side effect and may be more effective than SSRIs for treating MDD-associated fatigue and sleepiness.[86,87] Although bupropion could theoretically exacerbate insomnia, this has not been consistently demonstrated in clinical trials.[87]

On the other hand, several antidepressants have been shown to improve subjective and objective sleep parameters. Trazodone, an atypical antidepressant commonly used in low doses to treat depressed patients with insomnia,[88] tends to decrease SOL and increase TST. These features have led to its consideration as a single-agent treatment of depression and insomnia. Trazodone been compared to SSRIs in several studies and is generally found to have comparable efficacy for mood symptoms while improving sleep more.[89] Mirtazapine is another antidepressant with sleep-enhancing properties. One meta-analysis examined response rate and side-effect profiles of mirtazapine used for MDD in comparison to SSRIs.[90]

BOX 18-4
TREATMENTS FOR DEPRESSION IN PATIENTS WITH SLEEP DISORDERS

Antidepressants specifically promoting sleep:
Trazodone
Mirtazapine (worsens RLS)

Antidepressants thought to adversely affect sleep:
SSRIs and SNRIs (can suppress REM, increase sleep latency, and decrease overall sleep time. SSRIs may also affect muscle activity during REM, and worsen RLS)
Bupropion (concerns of causing insomnia are likely overstated)

Other agents:
Atypical antipsychotics (promotes sleep)
Stimulants (as augmenting agents can promote wakefulness)
Eszopiclone (may augment antidepressants)
Pramipexole (in addition to effect on RLS, may have antidepressant effects)
Bright light therapy
Cognitive behavioral therapy for insomnia (CBT-i)
Behavioral chronotherapy

Mirtazapine was associated with less insomnia but more daytime sleepiness and fatigue. In contrast, a more recent study using mirtazapine (albeit open-label) demonstrated objective improvement in sleepiness using the MSLT, presumably due to the concomitant improvement in nocturnal sleep.[91] Thus, trazodone or mirtazapine may be appropriate choices for depressed patients with prominent insomnia.

Several other classes of drugs used adjunctively in the treatment of depression also have well-established effects on sleep. Second-generation antipsychotics tend to increase total sleep time and subjective sleep quality.[80] Alerting agents (e.g., modafinil, armodafinil, atomoxetine) and stimulants (e.g., amphetamine) may be helpful to augment antidepressant therapy in the patient with sleepiness related to OSA or another primary sleep disorder.[92]

Psychotherapy and behavioral interventions for depression may also affect sleep. Overall, there does not seem to be any difference between CBT and pharmacotherapy with regard to efficacy to treat accompanying insomnia.[93] In addition to conventional CBT, treatment of depression using manipulation of chronobiology ("behavioral chronotherapy") has been studied. The beneficial effects of bright-light therapy (BLT) in SAD are well-accepted and encompass improvements in sleep, alertness, and mood.[94] In a study of elderly patients with nonseasonal MDD, BLT improved mood, augmented sleep efficiency, and increased the upslope of melatonin rise, a marker of the robustness of circadian rhythm. In addition, BLT was associated with ongoing mood enhancement after discontinuation of treatment.[95] Sleep deprivation therapy (SDT) also produces a rapid antidepressant response, likely through a resetting of abnormal circadian machinery.[96] Although this effect is generally not sustained after recovery sleep, combining SDT with medications and/or other chronotherapeutic interventions (BLT, sleep phase advance) may provide sustained improvement.[97]

■ PHARMACOLOGIC TREATMENT OF INSOMNIA IN THE DEPRESSED PATIENT

In depressed patients with prominent complaints of insomnia, it is often unclear whether the sleep disorder is a cause and/or a symptom of depression. However, it is clear that treatment of insomnia in this group improves both sleep and quality of life, although the effect size may be somewhat smaller than in primary insomnia patients.[98] Although observational studies have suggested an association between the use of hypnotics and increased mortality, these data are severely limited by the lack of adjustment for the presence and severity of insomnia itself as well as comorbid psychiatric conditions.[99,100] Thus, it is difficult to draw any conclusions based on these results. Clinicians are advised to weigh carefully the benefits that have been shown in randomized controlled trials (as outlined below) prior to deciding to withhold these agents based on concerns generated by methodologically suspect observational data.

The most commonly used drugs in the treatment of both primary insomnia and insomnia comorbid with depression are the benzodiazepine receptor agonists (BZRA). Several BZRA have been studied as adjuncts to antidepressants as initial therapy for MDD. In one study, zolpidem extended-release in combination with escitalopram was compared to escitalopram alone. Zolpidem extended-release improved total sleep time, morning energy, concentration, and the impact of insomnia on daily activities. However, zolpidem did not significantly augment the antidepressant response to escitalopram.[101] In contrast, another study compared eszopiclone in combination with fluoxetine to fluoxetine alone. In addition to improvement in sleep, the eszopiclone group also showed a faster onset of antidepressant response and a greater magnitude of the antidepressant effect.[102] At the end of this study, fluoxetine was continued open-label while eszopiclone was discontinued in a 2-week single-blind run-out. Remarkably, both mood and insomnia symptoms remained significantly improved in the combination therapy group during the 2 weeks after discontinuation of eszopiclone.[103] This finding suggests that patients with MDD can be safely treated with an adjunctive hypnotic without concern for rebound/withdrawal and with possible continued benefit after the hypnotic is stopped. Whether a true difference exists between zolpidem and eszopiclone with respect to their effects on mood remains to be seen. In the absence of head-to-head data, eszopiclone, with its somewhat broader activity on GABA(A) receptors, may be the hypnotic of choice in this group.

Benzodiazepine receptor agonists have also been studied for residual insomnia during otherwise successful treatment of MDD. In a placebo-controlled trial of zolpidem in adults with persistent insomnia following successful depression treatment, zolpidem was associated with improved subjective sleep quality, fewer awakenings, less daytime sleepiness, and improved concentration.[104] As with eszopiclone, there was no evidence of dependence or withdrawal during a wash-out placebo substitution.

■ BEHAVIORAL TREATMENT OF INSOMNIA IN THE DEPRESSED PATIENT

Although medications can be helpful, cognitive behavioral therapy for insomnia (CBT-i) improves sleep acutely with a comparable or superior effect size and provides a more durable response.[105] CBT-i is often used adjunctively with medications, and the most effective approach may be a combined treatment.[106] Although CBT-i encompasses a variety of domains, including sleep hygiene, relaxation techniques, and cognitive restructuring, the two components of CBT-i with established efficacy are sleep restriction and stimulus control.

Stimulus control is based on principles of operant and classical conditioning. In this model, the bedroom and the process of attempting to sleep become stimuli that interfere with sleep and perpetuate insomnia due to their association with negative cognitive and physiological states. Accordingly, in CBT-i the patient is instructed to get out of bed when awake and alert in order to preserve the bed as a place for drowsiness/sleep. Other activities, such as watching television and reading, should ideally be moved into another room. Sleep restriction, the other key intervention in CBT-i, involves limiting the total time in bed. The estimated length of the sleep period prior to the intervention should be used to determine the length of the scheduled time in bed, limiting the minimum duration to 6 hours. A regular bedtime and wakeup time should be chosen that vary by no more than an hour on different days (e.g., on weekends, a patient may choose to delay the scheduled time in bed by 1 hour on both ends). Although initially total sleep time will decrease relative to baseline, the increased sleep drive that ensues can help to re-establish a pattern of regular sleep, reduce anxiety, and increase confidence in the sleep setting.

Depressed patients may have difficulty implementing both stimulus control and sleep restriction techniques. Amotivation may impede the implementation of a strict sleep schedule required in sleep restriction. Lack of energy and psychomotor slowing may be obstacles to the physical displacement of stimulus control. Despite these theoretical barriers, however, there is evidence that depressed patients are able to benefit from CBT-i. Several studies have demonstrated that the efficacy of CBT-i for insomnia symptoms is not different between patients with and without depression.[107,108] There is also evidence that a brief behavioral intervention utilizing CBT-i principles may be successfully implemented by those without advanced training in the technique. As such, clinicians should not hesitate to introduce these techniques to depressed patients with insomnia. For those with more severe or refractory symptoms, referral to a therapist trained in CBT-i is appropriate.[109]

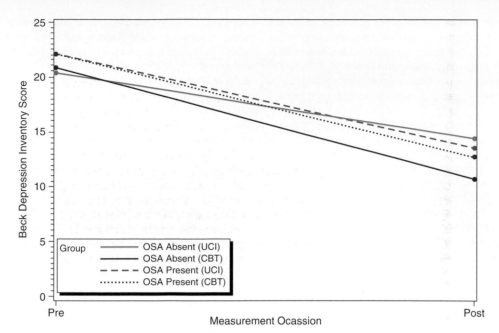

UCI, usual care; CBT, cognitive behavioral therapy for depression. In two groups without OSA, CBT provided substantial benefit compared to UCL in contrast, the change in BDI between the two OSA groups is nearly identical.

Figure 18-5 *Treatment of patients with coronary heart disease and MDD treated with sertraline. (Reproduced with permission from Freedland KE, Carney RM, Hayano J, et al: Effect of obstructive sleep apnea on response to cognitive behavior therapy for depression after an acute myocardial infarction, J Psychosom Res. 2012;72(4):276–281)*

■ TREATMENT OF COMORBID DEPRESSION AND OSA

In patients with comorbid depression and OSA, treatment of each disorder may affect the other. Untreated sleep apnea interferes with the response of MDD to both cognitive behavioral therapy[110] and antidepressants.[111] Roest et al. analyzed data from 105 patients with coronary heart disease who were receiving treatment with sertraline for MDD (**Fig. 18-5**). Moderate to severe OSA was detected in approximately 30% of patients. Patients with OSA had significantly higher scores on the BDI and HAM-D at the end of the 10-week treatment period. This result remained significant after controlling for baseline depression scores, demographic variables, and serum inflammatory markers.

The mechanism by which OSA interferes with antidepressant response is unknown, but it stands to reason that normalization of sleep continuity and oxygenation may mitigate or eliminate this effect. The most effective treatment for OSA is CPAP. CPAP therapy involves use of a mask at night that delivers positive pressure to stent open the upper airway and prevent the repetitive collapse that characterize OSA. Adherence with CPAP is a challenge for many, but there is evidence that depressed patients are just as likely as their euthymic counterparts to use CPAP successfully.[112–114] As in other populations, the ability of depressed patients to successfully implement CPAP is best predicted by measures of self-efficacy and expectation of benefit.[114]

Data have been mixed regarding the effect of CPAP therapy on mood in depressed OSA patients.[115–127] Although most patients with moderate to severe sleep apnea should be offered CPAP regardless of its effect on mood, the value of treatment for those with mild OSA and depression is a subject that requires further study.

Despite the use of CPAP, current or prior depression is a risk factor for residual sleepiness in OSA patients. In one study, over 200 patients with sleep apnea were treated with appropriate CPAP therapy for ≥6 months, with confirmed compliance.[128] Of the 44 patients with a history of depression, none showed resolution of subjective sleepiness, whereas 57% of those with no history of a mood disorder demonstrated such improvement. Although interpretation is limited by lack of information about medication use and current mood state, these data emphasize the complex and bidirectional relationship between OSA symptoms and depression.

■ TREATMENT CONSIDERATIONS IN THE DEPRESSED PATIENT WITH RLS

In addition to the aforementioned effects of antidepressants on sleep continuity and architecture, these agents may also affect sleep quality in susceptible individuals through their effect on RLS symptoms and PLMS. Most antidepressants tend to worsen RLS symptoms and may provoke new-onset symptoms in susceptible individuals. Although one study suggested that SSRIs improve RLS symptoms,[129] most subsequent reports concur that they are more likely to cause or exacerbate both RLS and PLMS.[130,131] Atypical antipsychotics, because of their dopamine blocking effects, would be expected to share this property, although one report suggests that the prevalence of this side effect is low.[132] Mirtazapine exacerbates RLS and has been shown to provoke PLMS even in those without baseline RLS or PLMS.[130,133,134] On the other hand, bupropion may have modest benefit for both RLS symptoms[135] and PLMS.[131,136]

Although informed choice of antidepressant may ameliorate (or at least not exacerbate) RLS, drug therapy directed at RLS symptoms is often indicated. Both dopamine agonists (pramipexole, ropinirole) and drugs active at the $\alpha 2\delta$ calcium channel receptor (gabapentin, pregabalin) are appropriate first-line options. Both classes may confer psychiatric side effects. Dopamine agonists tend to have positive effects on mood and may be used as antidepressants themselves. In one meta-analysis, pramipexole showed a consistent and large effect size ($d = 0.6$–1.1) for improvement in depressive symptoms.[137] This benefit also seems to extend to RLS patients, in whom pramipexole improves RLS-related mood symptoms.[138] One rare side effect of dopamine agonists is the emergence of compulsive behaviors (e.g., gambling, shopping, overeating, hypersexuality), but there is evidence that this is not more common in patients with mood disorders.[137] Therefore, dopamine agonists may be a good choice for treatment of RLS in the depressed patient. Gabapentin and pregabalin, on the other hand, may worsen mood and increase suicidality in some circumstances, although this has not been convincingly demonstrated.[139,140]

■ TREATMENT OF OTHER SLEEP DISORDERS

Narcolepsy usually requires pharmacologic treatment. This generally includes an alerting agent (e.g., modafinil) and/or psychostimulant (e.g., amphetamines), both of which tend to have positive repercussions for mood. In some cases, REM-suppressing antidepressants are added for treatment of cataplexy and might help with mood, though the doses are usually below those used in depression. If cataplexy and/or excessive sleepiness do not respond adequately to these medications, sodium oxybate may be added. However, caution should be exercised when considering sodium oxybate in the patient with depression as it may worsen mood in some cases and can be fatal in overdose.

Treatment for nightmare disorder may include behavioral and/or pharmacologic approaches. During image rehearsal therapy (IRT), the patient is asked to recount the nightmare; create a modified, more positive version of the story; and practice image rehearsal with the new scenario. There is evidence that depressed patients with nightmares benefit from IRT, although this benefit may be less than nightmare sufferers without comorbid depression. In the study by Thunker et al., IRT was associated with decreased nightmare frequency as well as improvements in depression and anxiety.[141] Pharmacologic treatment is also an option in nightmare disorder; prazosin has the most established efficacy. Although data are strongest in patients with comorbid PTSD, prazosin may also be used in others with nightmares.[142,143] In depressed patients with nightmares, prazosin improves mood in parallel to decreased nightmare frequency.[142] Given the benefits of both IRT and prazosin, enquiring about nightmares in the depressed patient may facilitate improved treatment.

■ SUMMARY

Sleep disorders and depression share complex bidirectional relationships. Nearly all primary sleep disorders are associated with increased risk of mood disorders (**Box 18-5**). This is likely due to a combination of shared risk factors, overlapping pathophysiology, and complex causative relationships involving both social and biological elements. Although the observed associations between sleep disorders and depression are strong, the neurologic substrate mediating these relationships remains elusive. Future research is needed to clarify this issue. The ramifications of various treatment approaches for sleep disorders with respect to mood (and vice versa) have also not been fully explored. Given the high prevalence of comorbidity, this remains a compelling area of investigation.

In addition to its implications for the research community, consideration of the relationship between sleep disorders and depression

should prompt clinicians to explore the sleep experience of every depressed patient. While sleep complaints may be a part of the mood disorder itself, a subset of sleep complaints are (alternatively or additionally) attributable to a primary sleep disorder warranting independent treatment. This distinction may be subtle, but it is not trivial. Appropriate treatment of comorbid sleep disorders and consideration of the implications of these disorders in the management of depression is likely to substantially improve both physical and mental health.

REFERENCES

1. Loomis AL, Harvey EN, Hobart GA. Cerebral states during sleep, as studied by human brain potentials. *J Exp Psychol.* 1937; 21(2):127–144.

2. Aserinsky E, Kleitman N. Regularly occurring periods of eye motility, and concomitant phenomena, during sleep. *Science.* 1953;118(3062):273–274.

3. Kupfer DJ. REM latency: a psychobiologic marker for primary depressive disease. *Biol Psychiatry.* 1976;11(2):159–174.

4. Palagini L, Baglioni C, Ciapparelli A, Gemignani A, Riemann D. REM sleep dysregulation in depression: State of the art. *Sleep Med Rev.* 2013;17:377–390.

5. Staner L. Comorbidity of insomnia and depression. *Sleep Med Rev.* 2010;14(1):35–46.

6. Baglioni C, Battagliese G, Feige B, et al. Insomnia as a predictor of depression: a meta-analytic evaluation of longitudinal epidemiological studies. *J Affect Disord.* 2011;135(1–3):10–19.

7. Sivertsen B, Salo P, Mykletun A, et al. The bidirectional association between depression and insomnia: the HUNT study. *Psychosom Med.* 2012;74(7):758–765.

8. Ohayon MM, Roth T. Place of chronic insomnia in the course of depressive and anxiety disorders. *J Psychiatr Res.* 2003;37(1): 9–15.

9. Kaplan KA, Harvey AG. Hypersomnia across mood disorders: a review and synthesis. *Sleep Med Rev.* 2009;13(4):275–285.

10. Jaussent I, Bouyer J, Ancelin M-L, et al. Insomnia and daytime sleepiness are risk factors for depressive symptoms in the elderly. *Sleep.* 2011;34(8):1103–1110.

11. Billiard M, Dolenc L, Aldaz C, Ondze B, Besset A. Hypersomnia associated with mood disorders: a new perspective. *J Psychosom Res.* 1994;38(Suppl 1):41–47.

12. Wheaton AG, Perry GS, Chapman DP, Croft JB. Sleep disordered breathing and depression among U.S. adults: National Health and Nutrition Examination Survey, 2005–2008. *Sleep.* 2012;35(4):461–467.

13. Ohayon MM. The effects of breathing-related sleep disorders on mood disturbances in the general population. *J Clin Psychiatry.* 2003;64(10):1195–1200-quiz-1274–1276.

14. Winkelmann J, Prager M, Lieb R, et al. "Anxietas tibiarum." Depression and anxiety disorders in patients with restless legs syndrome. *J Neurol.* 2005;252(1):67–71.

15. Froese CL, Butt A, Mulgrew A, et al. Depression and sleep-related symptoms in an adult, indigenous, North American population. *J Clin Sleep Med.* 2008;4(4):356–361.

16. Li Y, Mirzaei F, O'Reilly EJ, et al. Prospective study of restless legs syndrome and risk of depression in women. *Am J Epidemiol.* 2012; 176(4):279–288.

17. Szentkiralyi A, Völzke H, Hoffmann W, Baune BT, Berger K. The relationship between depressive symptoms and restless legs

syndrome in two prospective cohort studies. *Psychosom Med*. 2013;75(4):359–365.

18. Hornyak M, Kopasz M, Berger M, Riemann D, Voderholzer U. Impact of sleep-related complaints on depressive symptoms in patients with restless legs syndrome. *J Clin Psychiatry*. 2005;66(9):1139–1145.

19. Szentkiralyi A, Molnar MZ, Czira ME, et al. Association between restless legs syndrome and depression in patients with chronic kidney disease. *J Psychosom Res*. 2009;67(2):173–180.

20. Drake CL, Roehrs T, Richardson G, Walsh JK, Roth T. Shift work sleep disorder: prevalence and consequences beyond that of symptomatic day workers. *Sleep*. 2004;27(8):1453–1462.

21. Besiroglu L, Agargun MY, Inci R. Nightmares and terminal insomnia in depressed patients with and without melancholic features. *Psychiatry Res*. 2005;133(2–3):285–287.

22. Fortuyn HA, Mulders PC, Renier WO, Buitelaar JK, Overeem S. Narcolepsy and psychiatry: an evolving association of increasing interest. *Sleep Med*. 2011;12(7):714–719.

23. Vignatelli L, Plazzi G, Peschechera F, Delaj L, D'Alessandro R. A 5-year prospective cohort study on health-related quality of life in patients with narcolepsy. *Sleep Med*. 2011;12(1):19–23.

24. Fortuyn HA, Lappenschaar MA, Furer JW, et al. Anxiety and mood disorders in narcolepsy: a case-control study. *Gen Hosp Psychiatry*. 2010;32(1):49–56.

25. Riemann D, Spiegelhalder K, Feige B, et al. The hyperarousal model of insomnia: a review of the concept and its evidence. *Sleep Med Rev*. 2010;14(1):19–31.

26. Bonnet MH, Arand DL. Hyperarousal and insomnia: state of the science. *Sleep Med Rev*. 2010;14(1):9–15.

27. Roehrs TA, Randall S, Harris E, Maan R, Roth T. MSLT in primary insomnia: stability and relation to nocturnal sleep. *Sleep*. 2011;34(12):1647–1652.

28. Manconi M, Ferri R, Zucconi M, et al. Dissociation of periodic leg movements from arousals in restless legs syndrome. *Ann Neurol*. 2012;71(6):834–844.

29. Clark LA, Watson D. Tripartite model of anxiety and depression: psychometric evidence and taxonomic implications. *J Abnorm Psychol*. 1991;100(3):316–336.

30. Olbrich S, Sander C, Minkwitz J, et al. EEG vigilance regulation patterns and their discriminative power to separate patients with major depression from healthy controls. *Neuropsychobiology*. 2012;65(4):188–194.

31. Hegerl U, Wilk K, Olbrich S, Schoenknecht P, Sander C. Hyperstable regulation of vigilance in patients with major depressive disorder. *World J Biol Psychiatry*. 2012;13(6):436–446.

32. Kemp AH, Quintana DS, Gray MA, Felmingham KL, Brown K, Gatt JM. Impact of depression and antidepressant treatment on heart rate variability: a review and meta-analysis. *Biol Psychiatry*. 2010;67(11):1067–1074.

33. Veith RC, Lewis N, Linares OA, et al. Sympathetic nervous system activity in major depression. Basal and desipramine-induced alterations in plasma norepinephrine kinetics. *Arch Gen Psychiatry*. 1994;51(5):411–422.

34. Jarcho MR, Slavich GM, Tylova-Stein H, Wolkowitz OM, Burke HM. Dysregulated diurnal cortisol pattern is associated with glucocorticoid resistance in women with major depressive disorder. *Biol Psychol*. 2013;93(1):150–158.

35. Kufoy E, Palma J-A, Lopez J, et al. Changes in the heart rate variability in patients with obstructive sleep apnea and its response to acute CPAP treatment. *PLoS ONE*. 2012;7(3):e33769.

36. Henley DE, Russell GM, Douthwaite JA, et al. Hypothalamic-pituitary-adrenal axis activation in obstructive sleep apnea: the effect of continuous positive airway pressure therapy. *J Clin Endocrinol Metab*. 2009;94(11):4234–4242.

37. Donadio V, Liguori R, Vetrugno R, et al. Daytime sympathetic hyperactivity in OSAS is related to excessive daytime sleepiness. *J Sleep Res*. 2007;16(3):327–332.

38. Waradekar NV, Sinoway LI, Zwillich CW, Leuenberger UA. Influence of treatment on muscle sympathetic nerve activity in sleep apnea. *Am J Respir Crit Care Med*. 1996;153(4 Pt 1):1333–1338.

39. Scalco AZ, Rondon MU, Trombetta IC, et al. Muscle sympathetic nervous activity in depressed patients before and after treatment with sertraline. *J Hypertens*. 2009;27(12):2429–2436.

40. Ryan S, Taylor CT, McNicholas WT. Systemic inflammation: a key factor in the pathogenesis of cardiovascular complications in obstructive sleep apnoea syndrome? *Postgrad Med J*. 2009;85(1010):693–698.

41. Miller AH, Maletic V, Raison CL. Inflammation and its discontents: the role of cytokines in the pathophysiology of major depression. *Biol Psychiatry*. 2009;65(9):732–741.

42. Campbell S, Marriott M, Nahmias C, MacQueen GM. Lower hippocampal volume in patients suffering from depression: a meta-analysis. *Am J Psychiatry*. 2004;161(4):598–607.

43. Joo EY, Kim SH, Kim S-T, Hong SB. Hippocampal volume and memory in narcoleptics with cataplexy. *Sleep Med*. 2012;13(4):396–401.

44. Riemann D, Voderholzer U, Spiegelhalder K, et al. Chronic insomnia and MRI-measured hippocampal volumes: a pilot study. *Sleep*. 2007;30(8):955–958.

45. Noh HJ, Joo EY, Kim ST, et al. The relationship between hippocampal volume and cognition in patients with chronic primary insomnia. *J Clin Neurol*. 2012;8(2):130–138.

46. Plante DT, Jensen JE, Schoerning L, Winkelman JW. Reduced γ-aminobutyric acid in occipital and anterior cingulate cortices in primary insomnia: a link to major depressive disorder? *Neuropsychopharmacology*. 2012;37(6):1548–1557.

47. Morgan PT, Pace-Schott EF, Mason GF, et al. Cortical GABA levels in primary insomnia. *Sleep*. 2012;35(6):807–814.

48. Cross RL, Kumar R, Macey PM, et al. Neural alterations and depressive symptoms in obstructive sleep apnea patients. *Sleep*. 2008;31(8):1103–1109.

49. Morrell MJ, Jackson ML, Twigg GL, et al. Changes in brain morphology in patients with obstructive sleep apnoea. *Thorax*. 2010;65(10):908–914.

50. Macey PM, Henderson LA, Macey KE, et al. Brain morphology associated with obstructive sleep apnea. *Am J Respir Crit Care Med*. 2002;166(10):1382–1387.

51. Feng J, Wu Q, Zhang D, Chen B-Y. Hippocampal impairments are associated with intermittent hypoxia of obstructive sleep apnea. *Chin Med J*. 2012;125(4):696–701.

52. Molendijk ML, Bus BA, Spinhoven P, et al. Serum levels of brain-derived neurotrophic factor in major depressive disorder: state-trait issues, clinical features and pharmacological treatment. *Mol Psychiatry*. 2011;16(11):1088–1095.

53. Frodl T, Schüle C, Schmitt G, et al. Association of the brain-derived neurotrophic factor Val66Met polymorphism with reduced hippocampal volumes in major depression. *Arch Gen Psychiatry*. 2007;64(4):410–416.

54. Verhagen M, van der Meij A, van Deurzen PA, et al. Meta-analysis of the BDNF Val66Met polymorphism in major depressive

disorder: effects of gender and ethnicity. *Mol Psychiatry*. 2010; 15(3):260–271.

55. Bachmann V, Klein C, Bodenmann S, et al. The BDNF Val66Met polymorphism modulates sleep intensity: EEG frequency- and state-specificity. *Sleep*. 2012;35(3):335–344.

56. Faraguna U, Vyazovskiy VV, Nelson AB, Tononi G, Cirelli C. A causal role for brain-derived neurotrophic factor in the homeo-static regulation of sleep. *J Neurosci*. 2008;28(15):4088–4095.

57. Gooneratne NS, Bellamy SL, Pack F, et al. Case-control study of subjective and objective differences in sleep patterns in older adults with insomnia symptoms. *J Sleep Res*. 2011;20(3):434–444.

58. Merica H, Blois R, Gaillard JM. Spectral characteristics of sleep EEG in chronic insomnia. *Eur J Neurosci*. 1998;10(5):1826–1834.

59. Giese M, Unternährer E, Hüttig H, et al. BDNF: an indicator of insomnia? *Mol Psychiatry*. 2014;19(2):151–152.

60. Léger D, Morin CM, Uchiyama M, Hakimi Z, Cure S, Walsh JK. Chronic insomnia, quality-of-life, and utility scores: comparison with good sleepers in a cross-sectional international survey. *Sleep Med*. 2012;13(1):43–51.

61. Espie CA, Kyle SD, Hames P, Cyhlarova E, Benzeval M. The day-time impact of DSM-5 insomnia disorder: comparative analysis of insomnia subtypes from the Great British Sleep Survey. *J Clin Psychiatry*. 2012;73(12):e1478–e1484.

62. O'Brien EM, Chelminski I, Young D, Dalrymple K, Hrabosky J, Zimmerman M. Severe insomnia is associated with more severe presentation and greater functional deficits in depression. *J Psychiatr Res*. 2011;45(8):1101–1105.

63. Sunderajan P, Gaynes BN, Wisniewski SR, et al. Insomnia in patients with depression: a STAR*D report. *CNS Spectr*. 2010; 15(6):394–404.

64. van Mill JG, Hoogendijk WJ, Vogelzangs N, van Dyck R, Penninx BW. Insomnia and sleep duration in a large cohort of patients with major depressive disorder and anxiety disorders. *J Clin Psychiatry*. 2010;71(3):239–246.

65. Akashiba T, Kawahara S, Akahoshi T, et al. Relationship between quality of life and mood or depression in patients with severe obstructive sleep apnea syndrome. *Chest*. 2002;122(3):861–865.

66. Jacobsen JH, Shi L, Mokhlesi B. Factors associated with exces-sive daytime sleepiness in patients with severe obstructive sleep apnea. *Sleep Breath*. 2013;17:629–635.

67. Pamidi S, Knutson KL, Ghods F, Mokhlesi B. Depressive symp-toms and obesity as predictors of sleepiness and quality of life in patients with REM-related obstructive sleep apnea: cross-sectional analysis of a large clinical population. *Sleep Med*. 2011;12(9):827–831.

68. Winkelman JW, Finn L, Young T. Prevalence and correlates of restless legs syndrome symptoms in the Wisconsin Sleep Cohort. *Sleep Med*. 2006;7(7):545–552.

69. Pigeon WR, Pinquart M, Conner K. Meta-analysis of sleep dis-turbance and suicidal thoughts and behaviors. *J Clin Psychiatry*. 2012;73(9):e1160–e1167.

70. Sivertsen B, Björnsdóttir E, Øverland S, Bjorvatn B, Salo P. The joint contribution of insomnia and obstructive sleep apnoea on sickness absence. *J Sleep Res*. 2013;22(2):223–230.

71. Hajak G, Petukhova M, Lakoma MD, et al. Days-out-of-role asso-ciated with insomnia and comorbid conditions in the America Insomnia Survey. *Biol Psychiatry*. 2011;70(11):1063–1073.

72. Øverland S, Glozier N, Sivertsen B, et al. A comparison of insom-nia and depression as predictors of disability pension: the HUNT Study. *Sleep*. 2008;31(6):875–880.

73. Mykletun A, Øverland S, Dahl AA, et al. A population-based cohort study of the effect of common mental disorders on dis-ability pension awards. *Am J Psychiatry*. 2006;163(8):1412–1418.

74. Knudsen AK, Øverland S, Aakvaag HF, Harvey SB, Hotopf M, Mykletun A. Common mental disorders and disability pension award: seven year follow-up of the HUSK study. *J Psychosom Res*. 2010;69(1):59–67.

75. Li SX, Lam SP, Chan JW, Yu MW, Wing Y-K. Residual sleep distur-bances in patients remitted from major depressive disorder: a 4-year naturalistic follow-up study. *Sleep*. 2012;35(8):1153–1161.

76. Romera I, Pérez V, Ciudad A, et al. Residual symptoms and func-tioning in depression, does the type of residual symptom mat-ter? A post-hoc analysis. *BMC Psychiatry*. 2013;13:51.

77. Buysse DJ, Reynolds CF, Hoch CC, et al. Longitudinal effects of nortriptyline on EEG sleep and the likelihood of recurrence in elderly depressed patients. *Neuropsychopharmacology*. 1996; 14(4):243–252.

78. Dombrovski AY, Mulsant BH, Houck PR, et al. Residual symp-toms and recurrence during maintenance treatment of late-life depression. *J Affect Disord*. 2007;103(1–3):77–82.

79. Yang H, Sinicropi-Yao L, Chuzi S, et al. Residual sleep disturbance and risk of relapse during the continuation/maintenance phase treatment of major depressive disorder with the selective sero-tonin reuptake inhibitor fluoxetine. *Ann Gen Psychiatry*. 2010;9:10.

80. DeMartinis NA, Winokur A. Effects of psychiatric medications on sleep and sleep disorders. *CNS Neurol Disord Drug Targets*. 2007;6(1):17–29.

81. Wilson S, Argyropoulos S. Antidepressants and sleep: a qualita-tive review of the literature. *Drugs*. 2005;65(7):927–947.

82. Beasley CM, Sayler ME, Weiss AM, Potvin JH. Fluoxetine: acti-vating and sedating effects at multiple fixed doses. *J Clin Psychopharmacol*. 1992;12(5):328–333.

83. Thaler KJ, Morgan LC, Van Noord M, et al. Comparative effective-ness of second-generation antidepressants for accompanying anxiety, insomnia, and pain in depressed patients: a systematic review. *Depress Anxiety*. 2012;29(6):495–505.

84. Gartlehner G, Hansen RA, Morgan LC, et al. *Second-Generation Antidepressants in the Pharmacologic Treatment of Adult Depression: An Update of the 2007 Comparative Effectiveness Review*. Rockville, MD: Agency for Healthcare Research and Quality (US); 2011.

85. Fava M, Hoog SL, Judge RA, Kopp JB, Nilsson ME, Gonzales JS. Acute efficacy of fluoxetine versus sertraline and paroxetine in major depressive disorder including effects of baseline insom-nia. *J Clin Psychopharmacol*. 2002;22(2):137–147.

86. Papakostas GI, Nutt DJ, Hallett LA, Tucker VL, Krishen A, Fava M. Resolution of sleepiness and fatigue in major depressive disor-der: A comparison of bupropion and the selective serotonin reuptake inhibitors. *Biol Psychiatry*. 2006;60(12):1350–1355.

87. Gaynes BN, Farley JF, Dusetzina SB, et al. Does the presence of accompanying symptom clusters differentiate the comparative effectiveness of second-line medication strategies for treating depression? *Depress Anxiety*. 2011;28(11):989–998.

88. Walsh JK. Drugs used to treat insomnia in 2002: regulatory-based rather than evidence-based medicine. *Sleep*. 2004;27(8): 1441–1442.

89. Fagiolini A, Comandini A, Catena Dell'Osso M, Kasper S. Rediscovering trazodone for the treatment of major depressive disorder. *CNS Drugs*. 2012;26(12):1033–1049.

90. Papakostas GI, Homberger CH, Fava M. A meta-analysis of clinical trials comparing mirtazapine with selective serotonin reuptake

inhibitors for the treatment of major depressive disorder. *J Psychopharmacol (Oxford)*. 2008;22(8):843–848.

91. Shen J, Hossain N, Streiner DL, et al. Excessive daytime sleepiness and fatigue in depressed patients and therapeutic response of a sedating antidepressant. *J Affect Disord*. 2011;134(1–3):421–426.

92. Krystal AD, Harsh JR, Yang R, Yang RR, Rippon GA, Lankford DA. A double-blind, placebo-controlled study of armodafinil for excessive sleepiness in patients with treated obstructive sleep apnea and comorbid depression. *J Clin Psychiatry*. 2010;71(1):32–40.

93. Carney CE, Segal ZV, Edinger JD, Krystal AD. A comparison of rates of residual insomnia symptoms following pharmacotherapy or cognitive-behavioral therapy for major depressive disorder. *J Clin Psychiatry*. 2007;68(2):254–260.

94. Golden RN, Gaynes BN, Ekstrom RD, et al. The efficacy of light therapy in the treatment of mood disorders: a review and meta-analysis of the evidence. *Am J Psychiatry*. 2005;162(4):656–662.

95. Lieverse R, Van Someren EJ, Nielen MM, Uitdehaag BM, Smit JH, Hoogendijk WJ. Bright light treatment in elderly patients with nonseasonal major depressive disorder: a randomized placebo-controlled trial. *Arch Gen Psychiatry*. 2011;68(1):61–70.

96. Bunney BG, Bunney WE. Mechanisms of rapid antidepressant effects of sleep deprivation therapy: clock genes and circadian rhythms. *Biol Psychiatry*. 2012;73(12):1164–1171.

97. Tuunainen A, Kripke DF, Endo T. Light therapy for non-seasonal depression. *Cochrane Database Syst Rev*. 2004;(2):CD004050.

98. Krystal AD, McCall WV, Fava M, et al. Eszopiclone treatment for insomnia: effect size comparisons in patients with primary insomnia and insomnia with medical and psychiatric comorbidity. *Prim Care Companion CNS Disord*. 2012;14(4):pii: PCC.11m01296.

99. Kripke DF, Langer RD, Kline LE. Hypnotics' association with mortality or cancer: a matched cohort study. *BMJ Open*. 2012;2(1): e000850.

100. Kripke DF, Klauber MR, Wingard DL, Fell RL, Assmus JD, Garfinkel L. Mortality hazard associated with prescription hypnotics. *Biol Psychiatry*. 1998;43(9):687–693.

101. Fava M, Asnis GM, Shrivastava RK, et al. Improved insomnia symptoms and sleep-related next-day functioning in patients with comorbid major depressive disorder and insomnia following concomitant zolpidem extended-release 12.5 mg and escitalopram treatment: a randomized controlled trial. *J Clin Psychiatry*. 2011;72(7):914–928.

102. Fava M, McCall WV, Krystal A, et al. Eszopiclone co-administered with fluoxetine in patients with insomnia coexisting with major depressive disorder. *Biol Psychiatry*. 2006;59(11):1052–1060.

103. Krystal A, Fava M, Rubens R, et al. Evaluation of eszopiclone discontinuation after cotherapy with fluoxetine for insomnia with coexisting depression. *J Clin Sleep Med*. 2007;3(1):48–55.

104. Asnis GM, Chakraburtty A, DuBoff EA, et al. Zolpidem for persistent insomnia in SSRI-treated depressed patients. *J Clin Psychiatry*. 1999;60(10):668–676.

105. Mitchell MD, Gehrman P, Perlis M, Umscheid CA. Comparative effectiveness of cognitive behavioral therapy for insomnia: a systematic review. *BMC Fam Pract*. 2012;13:40.

106. Morin CM, Vallières A, Guay B, et al. Cognitive behavioral therapy, singly and combined with medication, for persistent insomnia: a randomized controlled trial. *JAMA*. 2009;301(19):2005–2015.

107. Manber R, Bernert RA, Suh S, Nowakowski S, Siebern AT, Ong JC. CBT for insomnia in patients with high and low depressive symptom severity: adherence and clinical outcomes. *J Clin Sleep Med*. 2011;7(6):645–652.

108. Manber R, Edinger JD, Gress JL, San Pedro-Salcedo MG, Kuo TF, Kalista T. Cognitive behavioral therapy for insomnia enhances depression outcome in patients with comorbid major depressive disorder and insomnia. *Sleep*. 2008;31(4):489–495.

109. Watanabe N, Furukawa TA, Shimodera S, et al. Brief behavioral therapy for refractory insomnia in residual depression: an assessor-blind, randomized controlled trial. *J Clin Psychiatry*. 2011;72(12):1651–1658.

110. Freedland KE, Carney RM, Hayano J, Steinmeyer BC, Reese RL, Roest AM. Effect of obstructive sleep apnea on response to cognitive behavior therapy for depression after an acute myocardial infarction. *J Psychosom Res*. 2012;72(4):276–281.

111. Roest AM, Carney RM, Stein PK, et al. Obstructive sleep apnea/hypopnea syndrome and poor response to sertraline in patients with coronary heart disease. *J Clin Psychiatry*. 2012;73(1):31–36.

112. Wells RD, Freedland KE, Carney RM, Duntley SP, Stepanski EJ. Adherence, reports of benefits, and depression among patients treated with continuous positive airway pressure. *Psychosom Med*. 2007;69(5):449–454.

113. Lewis KE, Seale L, Bartle IE, Watkins AJ, Ebden P. Early predictors of CPAP use for the treatment of obstructive sleep apnea. *Sleep*. 2004;27(1):134–138.

114. Stepnowsky CJ, Bardwell WA, Moore PJ, Ancoli-Israel S, Dimsdale JE. Psychologic correlates of compliance with continuous positive airway pressure. *Sleep*. 2002;25(7):758–762.

115. Engleman HM, Martin SE, Deary IJ, Douglas NJ. Effect of continuous positive airway pressure treatment on daytime function in sleep apnoea/hypopnoea syndrome. *Lancet*. 1994; 343(8897):572–575.

116. Engleman HM, Kingshott RN, Wraith PK, Mackay TW, Deary IJ, Douglas NJ. Randomized placebo-controlled crossover trial of continuous positive airway pressure for mild sleep Apnea/Hypopnea syndrome. *Am J Respir Crit Care Med*. 1999;159(2): 461–467.

117. Means MK, Lichstein KL, Edinger JD, et al. Changes in depressive symptoms after continuous positive airway pressure treatment for obstructive sleep apnea. *Sleep Breath*. 2003;7(1):31–42.

118. Schwartz DJ, Karatinos G. For individuals with obstructive sleep apnea, institution of CPAP therapy is associated with an amelioration of symptoms of depression which is sustained long term. *J Clin Sleep Med*. 2007;3(6):631–635.

119. Schwartz DJ, Kohler WC, Karatinos G. Symptoms of depression in individuals with obstructive sleep apnea may be amenable to treatment with continuous positive airway pressure. *Chest*. 2005;128(3):1304–1309.

120. Habukawa M, Uchimura N, Kakuma T, et al. Effect of CPAP treatment on residual depressive symptoms in patients with major depression and coexisting sleep apnea: contribution of daytime sleepiness to residual depressive symptoms. *Sleep Med*. 2010;11(6):552–557.

121. Millman RP, Fogel BS, McNamara ME, Carlisle CC. Depression as a manifestation of obstructive sleep apnea: reversal with nasal continuous positive airway pressure. *J Clin Psychiatry*. 1989; 50(9):348–351.

122. Derderian SS, Bridenbaugh RH, Rajagopal KR. Neuropsychologic symptoms in obstructive sleep apnea improve after treatment with nasal continuous positive airway pressure. *Chest*. 1988;94(5): 1023–1027.

123. Yu BH, Ancoli-Israel S, Dimsdale JE. Effect of CPAP treatment on mood states in patients with sleep apnea. *J Psychiatr Res.* 1999;33(5):427–432.

124. Borak J, Cieślicki JK, Koziej M, Matuszewski A, Zieliński J. Effects of CPAP treatment on psychological status in patients with severe obstructive sleep apnoea. *J Sleep Res.* 1996;5(2):123–127.

125. Muñoz A, Mayoralas LR, Barbé F, Pericás J, Agusti AG. Long-term effects of CPAP on daytime functioning in patients with sleep apnoea syndrome. *Eur Respir J.* 2000;15(4):676–681.

126. Lee I-S, Bardwell W, Ancoli-Israel S, Loredo JS, Dimsdale JE. Effect of three weeks of continuous positive airway pressure treatment on mood in patients with obstructive sleep apnoea: a randomized placebo-controlled study. *Sleep Med.* 2012;13(2):161–166.

127. Haensel A, Norman D, Natarajan L, Bardwell WA, Ancoli-Israel S, Dimsdale JE. Effect of a 2 week CPAP treatment on mood states in patients with obstructive sleep apnea: a double-blind trial. *Sleep Breath.* 2007;11(4):239–244.

128. Koutsourelakis I, Perraki E, Economou NT, et al. Predictors of residual sleepiness in adequately treated obstructive sleep apnoea patients. *Eur Respir J.* 2009;34(3):687–693.

129. Dimmitt SB, Riley GJ. Selective serotonin receptor uptake inhibitors can reduce restless legs symptoms. *Arch Intern Med.* 2000;160(5):712.

130. Hoque R, Chesson AL. Pharmacologically induced/exacerbated restless legs syndrome, periodic limb movements of sleep, and REM behavior disorder/REM sleep without atonia: literature review, qualitative scoring, and comparative analysis. *J Clin Sleep Med.* 2010;6(1):79–83.

131. Yang C, White DP, Winkelman JW. Antidepressants and periodic leg movements of sleep. *Biol Psychiatry.* 2005;58(6):510–514.

132. Jagota P, Asawavichienjinda T, Bhidayasiri R. Prevalence of neuroleptic-induced restless legs syndrome in patients taking neuroleptic drugs. *J Neurol Sci.* 2012;314(1–2):158–160.

133. Ağargün MY, Kara H, Ozbek H, Tombul T, Ozer OA. Restless legs syndrome induced by mirtazapine. *J Clin Psychiatry.* 2002; 63(12):1179.

134. Fulda S, Kloiber S, Dose T, et al. Mirtazapine Provokes Periodic Leg Movements during Sleep in Young Healthy Men. *Sleep.* 2013;36(5):661–669.

135. Bayard M, Bailey B, Acharya D, et al. Bupropion and restless legs syndrome: a randomized controlled trial. *J Am Board Fam Med.* 2011;24(4):422–428.

136. Nofzinger EA, Fasiczka A, Berman S, Thase ME. Bupropion SR reduces periodic limb movements associated with arousals from sleep in depressed patients with periodic limb movement disorder. *J Clin Psychiatry.* 2000;61(11):858–862.

137. Aiken CB. Pramipexole in psychiatry: a systematic review of the literature. *J Clin Psychiatry.* 2007;68(8):1230–1236.

138. Montagna P, Hornyak M, Ulfberg J, et al. Randomized trial of pramipexole for patients with restless legs syndrome (RLS) and RLS-related impairment of mood. *Sleep Med.* 2011;12(1): 34–40.

139. Schmitz B. Effects of antiepileptic drugs on mood and behavior. *Epilepsia.* 2006;47(Suppl 2):28–33.

140. Ettinger AB. Psychotropic effects of antiepileptic drugs. *Neurology.* 2006;67(11):1916–1925.

141. Thünker J, Pietrowsky R. Effectiveness of a manualized imagery rehearsal therapy for patients suffering from nightmare disorders with and without a comorbidity of depression or PTSD. *Behav Res Ther.* 2012;50(9):558–564.

142. Raskind MA, Peskind ER, Hoff DJ, et al. A parallel group placebo controlled study of prazosin for trauma nightmares and sleep disturbance in combat veterans with post-traumatic stress disorder. *Biol Psychiatry.* 2007;61(8):928–934.

143. Aurora RN, Zak RS, Auerbach SH, et al. Best practice guide for the treatment of nightmare disorder in adults. 2010;6:389–401.

CHAPTER 19

Depression and Substance Use Disorders

Joji Suzuki, MD

INTRODUCTION

The comorbidity of major depression and substance use disorder (SUD), which includes both alcohol and drugs, remains very common in medical and psychiatric settings (**Fig. 19-1**).[1-3] Both major depression and SUD are among of the most common psychiatric disorders, each leading to significant morbidity and mortality and placing a heavy burden on the health care system.[4] In clinical settings, however, SUDs are often underdiagnosed or missed entirely. Even if the SUD is correctly identified, treatment is often inadequate or not offered at all.[5,6] Studies have consistently noted that patients with both depression and SUD present with worse symptoms and have poorer outcomes, including a higher incidence of suicide attempts, than patients with either disorder alone (**Fig. 19-2**).[7,8] Research on the dually diagnosed population is still in its early stages, and significant gaps still remain.[9] Research on the comorbidity between dual diagnosis and medical illness is even less frequently studied. Nevertheless, when approaching a depressed patient with comorbid SUD, clinicians need to be aware of the specific issues unique to this population.

EPIDEMIOLOGY

The comorbidity between SUD and psychiatric disorders has been documented in all major epidemiological studies conducted to date. The Epidemiological Catchment Area (ECA) study reported a lifetime prevalence of 5.9% for major depression and 16.7% for any SUD in the general population.[3] Individuals with a diagnosis of major depression or other affective disorders showed elevated rates for SUD—16.5% for alcohol use disorder and 18% for drug use disorder. Conversely, individuals with any SUD were 1.9 times and 4.7 times more likely to have a diagnosis of depression or other affective disorders, respectively.

The National Epidemiological Survey of Alcohol and Related Conditions study (NESARC)[10] utilized face-to-face surveys with a broad sample of noninstitutionalized US citizens. It provided significant advantages over prior surveys by using the DSM criteria, differentiating primary mood disorders from substance-induced mood disorders, and including both substance abuse and dependence. Overall, 9.4% of the US population met DSM-IV criteria for any SUD within the past year. Among respondents meeting criteria for any SUD in the past year, 19.7% also met criteria for at least one independent mood disorder in the past year, and 17.7% met criteria for at least one anxiety disorder in the past year (**Box 19-1**; Fig. 19-2). For those with drug use disorder, 31.8% of respondents also had an independent mood disorder, compared to 12.3% for those with any alcohol use disorder. Similarly, 25.4% of all respondents with any drug use disorder also met criteria for an independent anxiety disorder, as compared to 17.1% for those with any alcohol use disorder. Overall, the most common comorbid diagnoses for respondents with any SUD were major depressive disorder (MDD) at 14.5% and specific phobia at 10.5%.[10]

Comorbidity with mood disorders was lower in those with substance disorder than in those with substance dependence. For instance, 40.0% of those with drug dependence had any mood disorder in the past year, compared to 15.8% of those with drug abuse. Of those with alcohol dependence, 20.5% also had any mood disorder in the past year, compared to 8.2% of those with alcohol abuse only.[10]

When the index disorder is any mood disorder, study results indicated that 20.0% also met criteria for any SUD in the past year. When

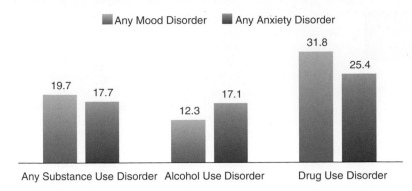

Figure 19-1 *Prevalence of comorbid mood and anxiety disorders in the general population with SUD. (Data from Grant BF, Dawson DA, Stinson FS, et al: The 12-month prevalence and trends in DSM-IV alcohol abuse and dependence: United States, 1991–1992 and 2001–2002, Drug Alcohol Depend 2004;74(3):223–234.)*

the index disorder is any anxiety disorder, 15.0% also met criteria for any SUD in the past year. Respondents endorsing any mania or hypomania had the highest rates of comorbid SUD, reporting 27.9% and 26.6%, respectively. Overall, for those respondents with an alcohol use disorder, the odds ratio of having any mood disorder was 2.6. When separated by race, the odds ratio are as follows: whites 2.4, blacks 3.3, Native Americans 2.8, Asians 3.7, and Hispanics 2.6.[10]

The prevalence of depression is significantly higher in patients seeking treatment for SUD than in the general population. The lifetime prevalence of major depression was 42.2% in treatment-seeking alcohol-dependent patients and 43.7% in patients enrolled in substance disorder treatment programs.[11] In the NESARC study,[9] among individuals with any mood disorder seeking treatment, about 20% also met criteria for any SUD. These findings demonstrate the very high rates of SUD and mood disorder co-occurring, particularly in the treatment-seeking population.

PATHOPHYSIOLOGY

The relationship between depression and SUD has been debated for some time. A frequently cited link is that depression is a risk factor for SUD. In this model, individuals experiencing depression or anxiety attempt to "self-medicate" and control distressing symptoms by using substances (**Box 19-2**).[12] For example, a patient with anxiety might choose to consume alcohol for its anxiolytic effects. Up to a quarter of individuals in the general population with a mood disorder admit to using substances to relieve symptoms,[13] and the majority of them report self-medicating using alcohol only. Research in the use of antidepressants for those with co-occurring alcohol

dependence and depression may support this theory. In a trial of depressed patients with comorbid alcohol dependence, those receiving fluoxetine showed greater improvement in both depression and drinking outcomes than those on placebo.[14] Nevertheless, the self-medication hypothesis has not been empirically tested, and research has failed to identify specific mood changes that are associated with specific drugs.[15]

Another theory proposes that chronic use of substances leads to mood or anxiety symptoms.[16] Acute intoxication as well as withdrawal can both be associated with significant affective, psychotic, or anxiety symptoms.[17] However, such symptoms often remit rapidly after a period of abstinence.[18,19] Indeed, in order to diagnose a substance-induced mood disorder, as opposed to an independent mood disorder, the DSM suggests that the mood or anxiety symptoms remit within approximately 4 weeks after cessation of substance use. Nevertheless, even though substance use clearly plays a role in producing depressive symptoms, the prevalence of substance-induced mood disorders is much lower than that of independent mood disorders in those with SUD.[10]

Another theory posits that mood disorders and SUDs are related through a shared genetic vulnerability, since both disorders have a high heritability.[20,21] Based on twin studies, shared environmental factors likely contribute only about 1% of the variance in the risk for alcohol dependence, while genetic factors contribute over 40% of the variance.[22] However, the evidence remains inconsistent. The risk of depression is three times higher in the offspring of parents with histories of major depression than it is in the offspring of parents without major depression.[23] The same study revealed a nonsignificant trend for greater incidence of substance dependence in the offspring

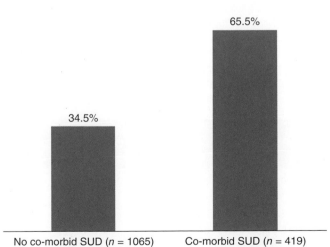

Figure 19-2 *Suicide attempts in depressed patients with and without comorbid SUD. (Data from Davis LL, Rush JA, Wisniewski SR, et al: Substance use disorder comorbidity in major depressive disorder: an exploratory analysis of the Sequenced Treatment Alternatives to Relieve Depression cohort, Compr Psychiatry 2005;46(2):81–89.)*

BOX 19-1
MANAGING ANXIETY IN THE PATIENT WITH SUBSTANCE USE DISORDERS: PEARLS TO CONSIDER

Anxiety is a frequent comorbidity in patients with substance use disorders, notably PTSD, GAD, and social phobia

Patients frequently cite self-medication of anxiety as a major reason for using alcohol, cannabis, sedatives, and opioids

Clinicians should rule out intoxication with cocaine and stimulants, or withdrawal from alcohol, benzodiazepines, cannabis, and opioids

Benzodiazepines should be used with caution in patients with substance use disorders, with preference for using them only for acute management of withdrawal or agitation

Whenever possible, treatment should target the underlying substance use disorder simultaneously as the mood and anxiety disorders, focusing on psychosocial interventions and medications other than benzodiazepines

"Self-medication" hypothesis
Secondary hypothesis (i.e., substance use causes mood disorders)
Shared genetic vulnerabilities

of parents with histories of depression compared to offspring of parents without depression. In another long-term study, the offspring of depressed parents reported more symptoms of depression than the offspring on nondepressed parents,[24] but the incidence of alcohol or tobacco use did not differ in these two groups of offspring.[25]

Research examining the pathophysiology of SUDs has strongly implicated the involvement of the mesolimbic reward pathway.[26] In response to both substances and natural rewards (i.e., food, sex, social interactions), an increase in dopamine in the nucleus accumbens appears to function as a prediction–error signal that helps the organism efficiently obtain rewards.[27] Although this system helps to shape survival behaviors related to procuring food and mates, substances appear to hijack this system. Even though research on the pathophysiology of depression has largely focused on the role of hippocampal and frontal cortical regions, there is now increasing recognition that the mesolimbic reward pathways may also play a significant role in the manifestation of depression.[28] While it remains unclear what role the reward pathway plays in depression, this line of research points to the possibility of a shared therapeutic target for both depression and SUDs.

Thus, the relationship between depression and substance use is a complex interaction between genetics and environment, and no single theory can capture this relationship sufficiently.

CLINICAL PRESENTATIONS

The current DSM 5 diagnostic criteria for SUD are listed in **Table 19-1**. It is important to recognize that tolerance and withdrawal are elements

TABLE 19-1 DSM5 Diagnostic Criteria for Substance Use Disorder

Criteria	Diagnosis and Modifiers
1. Tolerance	**Mild:** 2–3 criteria
2. Withdrawal	**Moderate:** 4–5 criteria
3. Persistent desire or inability to cut down substance use	**Severe:** >5 criteria
4. Substance often taken in larger amounts than intended	**Early remission:** 3–12 months without meeting any SUD criteria except cravings
5. Continued use despite knowledge of harm	
6. Great deal of time obtaining using, and recovering from the substance	**Sustained remission:** >12 months without meeting any SUD criteria except cravings
7. Important social, occupational, and other activities are given up due to substance use	**In controlled environment:** Incarcerated, hospitalized, or otherwise restricted access to substance
8. Craving, or strong desire, to use the substance	
9. Recurrent use of substance in hazardous situations	**On maintenance therapy:** On medication-assisted treatment
10. Failure to meet role obligations	
11. Continued use despite persistent or recurrent social or interpersonal problems	

Data from American Psychiatric Association: Diagnostic and Statistical Manual of Mental Disorders, 5th ed. Arlington, VA: American Psychiatric Association; 2013.

of "physiologic dependence." Although physiologic dependence may be prominent in many patients with SUD, physiologic dependence alone is neither sufficient nor necessary for the diagnosis. Indeed, physiologic dependence can be observed from using medications that have no abuse liability. For example, a patient taking pain medications for chronic pain may report the development of tolerance and withdrawal, but may not manifest any behaviors of SUD. The central feature of the SUD diagnosis is the loss of control over the use of the substance, that is, inability to cut down, using more than intended, using despite knowledge of harm. Therefore, it is the inability to regulate the consumption of the substance that is the core feature of a SUD.

Comorbid SUD is found in about a fifth of those patients seeking treatment for a mood disorder, and depression is found in about half of those patients seeking treatment for SUD.[10] The symptoms of major depression are likely to overlap with the symptoms of SUD. For example, a patient with alcohol dependence may present with chronic sleep problems, loss of appetite, difficulty concentrating, and depressed mood, all driven largely by the effects of alcohol. A patient with opioid dependence may present with anhedonia, weight loss, and psychomotor retardation. A cocaine-dependent patient may present with psychomotor agitation, perceptual disturbances, sleep and appetite disturbances, and poor concentration. Clinicians should routinely screen for substance use in patients seeking treatment for depression, and should assess not just current symptoms but the longitudinal history and the relationship of these symptoms to the use of substances.

In the Sequenced Treatment Alternatives to Relieve Depression (STAR*D) trial, 28% of depressed patients reported symptoms consistent with current SUD.[8] When compared to those without a current SUD, these individuals were more likely to be male, be divorced or never married, have a younger age of onset of depression, and to have had more suicide attempts (**Box 19-3**). Those with comorbid SUD also reported higher levels of hypersomnia, anxious mood, and suicidal ideation.

Patients frequently present in clinical settings with depressed mood in the context of acute intoxication with a variety of substances, notably alcohol. Although the acute mood effects of alcohol include euphoria and anxiolysis, alcohol is a CNS depressant and acts to inhibit executive functions, leading to agitation, irritability, and anger. Paranoia, and suicidal ideation may be present in severe situations.[24] Given that a large proportion of suicides occur in the context of substance use,[29] patients endorsing suicidal thoughts require close observation even when acutely intoxicated. Acute intoxication with alcohol can worsen depression while intoxication from stimulants, hallucinogens, or dissociatives can cause anxiety and paranoia. Acute withdrawal from alcohol, benzodiazepines, cocaine, and opioids may present with depressed, anxious, or irritable mood. Affective symptoms are particularly common and often very prominent in acute withdrawal, and so this constellation of symptoms alone may not aid in differentiating the effects

Sociodemographic

Younger age

Men

Hispanic

Separated, divorced, or never married

Family history of SUD

Clinical

Anxiety

Self-medication of negative affect

BOX 19-4
IMPORTANT SYMPTOMS

Many symptoms of withdrawal and intoxication overlap with depression, including many of the cardinal symptoms of depression: dysphoric/irritable mood, anxiety, anhedonia, low energy, appetite changes, poor concentration, insomnia or hypersomnia, fatigue, poor concentration, and suicidal ideation

of acute withdrawal from a substance-induced mood disorder or an independent mood disorder. Nevertheless, many patients will experience a rapid improvement in mood following detoxification.[19]

In order to diagnose a patient with a substance-induced mood disorder, the DSM 5 requires the remission of mood symptoms within a substantial period of time (e.g., 4 weeks) following cessation of substance use. However, in clinical practice, continuous abstinence for 4 weeks is often difficult to maintain regardless of the presence of mood symptoms. While the mood symptoms are likely to lessen after cessation of substance use, relapse is a common occurrence early in treatment, and the persisting mood symptoms can hinder the patient's ability to remain abstinent. Thus, distinguishing an independent mood disorder from a substance-induced mood disorder at the time of detoxification is difficult and requires careful review of the patient's history (**Box 19-4**).[30]

Several medical illnesses commonly associated with SUD can also present with depression. Depression may be a presenting complaint for nutritional deficiencies in alcohol-dependent patients. Pellagra, caused by niacin deficiency, is a disease characterized by dermatitis, diarrhea, and dementia. However, early in the course of illness, depression may be prominent.[31] Wernicke–Korsakoff syndrome, a potential complication of thiamine deficiency, may be complicated by depression.[32] Depression can also be a prominent complaint in chronic pain patients (see Chapter 17) who are using opioids for nonmedical reasons. Depressed chronic pain patients are less likely to experience analgesia from opioids, and are more likely to misuse their pain medications.[33] Finally, hepatitis C is an extremely common diagnosis in opioid-dependent patients, with reports indicating prevalence rates as high as 66%.[34] Although newer treatments have now become available, depression is a well-described complication of interferon treatment.[35]

Finally, regardless of the history, given the high prevalence of depression in the substance using population, the index of suspicion for an independent mood disorder should remain high, especially in those seeking treatment for SUD.

COURSE AND NATURAL HISTORY

The natural history of major depression with comorbid SUD tends to follow a characteristic course: depression outcomes are worse in those who also use substances even though such patients are more likely to receive more intensive treatment.[36] Depressed patients with comorbid SUD are also more likely to attempt suicide, and experience greater social and personal dysfunction.[37] In a study of fluoxetine treatment for depression, the degree of alcohol consumption at baseline was a strong predictor of worse treatment outcomes.[38] In a study of veterans with depression and SUD, greater frequency of substance use predicted worse depressive symptoms at every time point during the follow-up period.[39] In the STAR*D study, the individuals with major depression and comorbid SUD reported more severe depression, longer duration of depression, more anxiety, and more atypical and melancholic features than those without comorbid SUD.[40,41] Interestingly, the comorbidity with alcohol dependence alone, or drug dependence alone, did not significantly alter the rates of response or time to achieve response.[42] However, those with both alcohol and drug use had significantly lower rates of remission and

an increased time to remission from both depression and substance use. Furthermore, participants with a comorbid SUD experienced more psychiatric adverse events (e.g., suicidal ideation, suicide attempts) and psychiatric hospitalizations.

Studies have consistently shown that patients seeking treatment for their SUD will experience worse SUD outcomes if they are also depressed. Alcohol-dependent patients with depression are more likely to relapse and begin drinking sooner after inpatient treatment than comparable patients without depression. Among individuals with alcohol dependence, the diagnosis of major depression at the time of entry into treatment predicted relapse (hazard ratio 2.12) and a shorter time to relapse (hazard ratio 2.03) within 1 year of the hospitalization.[43] In addition, the more severe the depression, the greater is the likelihood of relapse after inpatient treatment. Thus, male veterans with *mild-to-moderate* depression and alcohol dependence were 2.9 times more likely to relapse to alcohol use within 1 year following treatment than those without any depression; individuals with *severe* depression were 4.9 times more likely to relapse to alcohol use.[44] Among methamphetamine users, the presence of depression at baseline was negatively correlated with abstinence, and predicted more frequent use of methamphetamine at follow-up, as well as a greater likelihood of attempting suicide.[45]

The relationship between major depression that precedes the initiation of substance use and the subsequent risk of relapse to substance use has been examined.[46] SUD patients with a history of depression that pre-dated their substance use were significantly less likely to achieve remission of their substance dependence than those whose depression did not pre-date their substance use.[44] In addition, individuals who experienced depression during periods of abstinence were significantly more vulnerable to SUD relapse than those with a lifetime history of depression but not during periods of abstinence.

ASSESSMENT AND DIFFERENTIAL DIAGNOSIS

As in all clinical evaluations, depressed patients should be assessed for any indication of a SUD. In addition to guiding treatment, a complete history assists in determining whether the depression is an independent mood disorder, is substance-induced, or a combination of the two (**Box 19-5**). Given that moods typically improve after cessation of substance use, making the correct diagnosis during ongoing use of substance may be challenging. Whenever possible, collateral information should also be obtained from family members, other individuals close to the patient, and other treating clinicians.

Patients may be reluctant to share or disclose sensitive information that is shameful or embarrassing, especially if it includes activities that are illegal. Clinicians should be mindful that these patients may have had negative interactions with other clinicians, and therefore a nonjudgmental and empathic approach is especially critical in building a therapeutic alliance. Studies have shown that outcomes are better when patients are able to form strong alliances with their providers.[47]

BOX 19-5
DIFFERENTIAL DIAGNOSIS

Affective symptoms not usually helpful, as they are common to substance use disorders as well as mood disorders

Suggestive of independent mood disorder

- Initiation of substance use after the emergence of mood symptoms as a young adult
- Prominent mood symptoms during extended periods of abstinence
- Persistence of mood symptoms following detoxification for a substantial period of time (e.g., 4 weeks or more)

At the least, enquiring about the use of alcohol, opioids, stimulants, sedative/hypnotics, and cannabinoids should be routine for all depressed patients. The clinician should try to ascertain, for each substance used, the duration of use, frequency and quantity of use, the route, first use, last use, and longest period of sobriety. In addition, clinicians should enquire about prior treatment episodes, including detoxification and AA attendance, history of severe withdrawal (i.e., delirium tremens or withdrawal seizures), family history of SUD, legal problems stemming from substance use, and social and occupational impairment due to substance use.

At the time of the assessment, there is no definitive method for determining whether the depressive symptoms represent a primary, independent mood disorder or a substance-induced mood disorder. To diagnose an independent mood disorder, the DSM 5 requires that the mood symptoms persist for a substantial period of time (e.g., 4 weeks) following cessation of all substance use. However, this can be difficult for many patients, especially if the mood symptoms are persistent or severe. The complete resolution of mood symptoms following cessation of substance use is clearly a strong indicator of a substance-induced mood disorder. Additionally, if the mood symptoms clearly preceded the initiation of substance use or are prominent during extended periods of abstinence, then an independent mood disorder is highly likely.

TREATMENT

■ PHARMACOLOGICAL TREATMENT

The treatment of comorbid SUD and depression has been a controversial topic for some time. Many clinicians have adopted the view that depression cannot be treated unless the patient first achieves complete abstinence from substance use (**Box 19-6**).[48] However, the emerging evidence on the treatment of dually diagnosed patients has begun to challenge this outdated view.[49] While it remains true that achieving abstinence, or at least reducing the substance use, will likely lead to improvements in mood, the current approach would recommend that treatment for both disorders be initiated even if the patient is unable to first achieve complete abstinence.

The role of antidepressants in treating depression in patients with comorbid SUD has not been clear because the results from controlled trials are mixed.[50] Nunes and Levin helped to clarify the role of antidepressants in an important systematic review and meta-analysis. They included patients with MDD and alcohol, opioid, or cocaine dependency who received selective serotonin reuptake inhibitors, tricyclic antidepressants, and other antidepressants. The pooled effect size of the antidepressants on depression outcomes was 0.38 (95% CI 0.18–0.58), and on substance use outcomes was 0.25 (95% CI 0.08–0.42). These results suggest that antidepressants offer a modest benefit for patients in terms of depression and substance use outcomes, similar to the effect size (0.43) found in antidepressant trials for patients with major depression.[51] However, the authors caution interpreting this finding because there was significant heterogeneity in the effect sizes (ranging from near 0 to 0.5) across studies and widely varying placebo response rates. In addition, the study revealed that the use of manual-guided psychosocial interventions led to lower

---

BOX 19-6
TREATMENTS FOR DEPRESSION IN PATIENTS WITH SUBSTANCE USE DISORDERS

Antidepressants (mixed data)

Cognitive behavioral therapy

Specific substance disorder interventions (motivational interviewing, self-help groups) have limited data but may help adherence in depressed substance users

---

antidepressant effect sizes, possibly due to the antidepressant effect of the psychosocial interventions. For example, cognitive behavioral therapy (CBT) itself may improve mood by reducing substance use, or may confer antidepressant effects through CBT modules that specifically address dysphoric symptoms.[50] The authors, therefore, suggest a clinical approach that focuses on providing evidence-based psychosocial interventions first, and then incorporating medications if depression does not improve.[49] If antidepressants are used, however, the overall treatment should still focus on the substance use itself because the impact of antidepressants on substance use remains modest at best.[52]

■ ALCOHOL

In those depressed individuals with alcohol dependence, an important treatment option for the latter is naltrexone, a mu-opioid receptor antagonist. Naltrexone has been studied extensively for the treatment of alcohol dependence, and systematic review of 50 randomized clinical trials disclosed a significant reduction in heavy drinking, drinking days, heavy drinking days, and amount of alcohol consumed.[53] Unfortunately, the impact of naltrexone on depression has not been systematically investigated, but the available evidence does not indicate naltrexone significantly improves mood in depressed alcohol-dependent patients.[54,55] Clinically, naltrexone is well tolerated, with GI effects and somnolence being the most common adverse effects. However, like other pharmacotherapies for SUD, adherence remains a big challenge. Pettinati and colleagues conducted the only trial to date examining the use of naltrexone and an antidepressant for the treatment of co-occurring major depression and alcohol dependence.[56] Depressed alcohol-dependent patients were randomly assigned to treatment with sertraline (200 mg/d), naltrexone (100 mg/d), combined sertraline plus naltrexone, or placebo. Every patient also received weekly CBT. The results showed a significantly higher proportion of patients receiving the combination treatment remained abstinent throughout the 14-week study (**Fig. 19-3**). In addition, the number of patients in the combination group not depressed by the end of the trial approached significance when compared to the other groups (**Fig. 19-4**).

The mean time to relapse was also greater in patients receiving combination treatment. Although there was only a nonsignificant trend in the treatment effect for depression across the groups, a larger proportion of subjects were no longer depressed in the combination group than in the other groups. Taken together, the results suggest that if pharmacotherapy is undertaken in depressed patients who are alcohol dependent, combination treatment of naltrexone and an antidepressant may be superior to using either agent alone.

Disulfiram has also been studied for the treatment of alcohol dependence. A systematic review revealed that just over half the studies reported greater rates of abstinence in patients taking disulfiram.[57] Disulfiram was also associated with longer duration until relapse, and fewer drinking days. In a trial of naltrexone and disulfiram for alcohol-dependent patients, 55% of whom had major depression, the presence of depression did not affect drinking outcomes, psychiatric symptoms, and side effects.[58] Although depression scores improved in those receiving disulfiram, naltrexone, or placebo, medications provided no additional benefit over placebo in improving mood. However, patients receiving naltrexone or disulfiram reported significantly fewer drinking days per week and more consecutive days abstinent compared to patients receiving placebo. Nevertheless, taking both disulfiram and naltrexone did not provide additional improvements in drinking outcomes compared to taking either medication alone.

■ OPIOIDS

Historically, agonist replacement with methadone, a synthetic mu-opioid agonist, has been the treatment of choice.[59] Patients treated

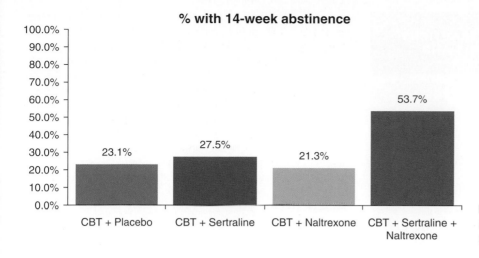

% with 14-week abstinence

Figure 19-3 *Efficacy of combination therapy (proportion of patients remaining abstinent throughout 14-week trial).*

with methadone show improvement in opioid use outcomes, especially at doses greater than 80 mg/d.[60] However, methadone use is associated with dangerous adverse effects, notably respiratory depression and drug–drug interactions (**Box 19-7**),[61] and can only be prescribed federally licensed methadone clinics. Thus, although methadone maintenance is an effective treatment option, acceptability by patients has been limited. More recently, buprenorphine has become available.[62,63] Buprenorphine is a partial mu-opioid agonist that is available as a sublingual tablet that also contains naloxone. Studies have consistently shown that patients treated with buprenorphine report improvement in opioid use outcomes.[64] In addition, unlike methadone, buprenorphine can be prescribed in office practice, though physicians must obtain a special license to prescribe it.

Depression is a common comorbidity in patients with opioid dependence. Studies of patients with both disorders have largely been limited to those enrolled in maintenance with methadone or buprenorphine. A systematic review of the use of antidepressants in this population found no difference from placebo in opioid use outcomes or treatment retention, but did find greater dropouts due to side effects in those receiving an antidepressant.[65] As such, to date, there is no clear role for antidepressants in depressed opioid-dependent patients who are currently maintained on opioid agonist treatment. One exception has been the study by Nunes and colleagues, where depressed opioid-dependent patients were randomly assigned to either imipramine or placebo.[66] Patients receiving imipramine were significantly more likely to report improvement in depression than patients on placebo. There is also evidence to suggest depressed opioid-dependent patients on buprenorphine fare better in terms of opioid use outcomes than those without depression: patients with a comorbid depression were 1.6 times more likely to achieve successful opioid use outcomes than patients without depression.[67] Even when the depressed patients were divided into patients who are and who are not receiving psychiatric treatment, no difference was found in opioid use outcomes. Agonist maintenance may itself ameliorate depressive symptoms sufficiently so that additional treatment provides no incremental benefit. It is also possible that the greater severity of depressive symptoms in opioid-dependent patients may act to motivate the patient more to engage with treatment. Taken together, these data suggest that depressed opioid-dependent patients should first be offered agonist maintenance treatment with clearly established efficacy.

■ COCAINE

For patients with cocaine dependence, there are no evidence-based pharmacotherapy options.[68] Likewise, in depressed cocaine users, there are few evidence-based pharmacotherapy options. A controlled clinical trial of fluoxetine (40 mg/d) for cocaine-dependent patients with comorbid depression found no benefit in cocaine use or depression outcomes.[69] Trials of nefazodone (400 mg/d) and

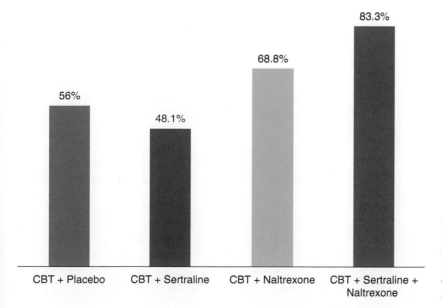

Figure 19-4 *Not depressed by the end of 14-week treatment. (Data from Pettinati HM, Oslin DW, Kampman KM, et al: A double-blind, placebo-controlled trial combining sertraline and naltrexone for treating co-occurring depression and alcohol dependence, Am J Psychiatry 2010;167(6):668–675.)*

venlafaxine (300 mg/d) were also negative.[70,71] In the only positive trial to date, desipramine (300 mg/d) was superior to placebo in treating depression but not cocaine disorder.[72]

On the other hand, psychosocial interventions do show more promise in the treatment of cocaine dependence.[73] Taken together, depressed cocaine-dependent patients should not be routinely offered antidepressants, but treatment should initially focus on psychosocial interventions.

■ CANNABIS

Research is limited on the comorbidity between cannabis dependence and major depression. While studies do point to a possible causal relationship between cannabis use and psychosis, the causal relationships with depression, suicidal thoughts, and anxiety remain uncertain.[74] Nevertheless, epidemiological studies do indicate depressed adults are more likely to be users of cannabis.[75] In a randomized, controlled trial of fluoxetine for depressed cannabis users, the patients receiving fluoxetine had significantly fewer depressive symptoms, and used less cannabis.[76] However, more recently, escitalopram conferred no benefit over placebo in terms of cannabis use, abstinence, depression, or anxiety.[77] Similarly, venlafaxine did not produce any therapeutic benefit in abstinence or depression when given to depressed cannabis-dependent patients.[78] Therefore, the available evidence so far does not support the routine use of antidepressants in this population.

PSYCHOSOCIAL TREATMENTS

■ COGNITIVE BEHAVIORAL THERAPY

CBT is one of the most widely used psychosocial treatments that has been rigorously studied for depression as well as SUD.[79] CBT focuses on providing new strategies and skills for dealing with a wide variety of target behaviors, including substance use, depression, anxiety, insomnia, and PTSD.[80] However, very few studies have examined the use of CBT specifically for depressed substance users. In one such study, when CBT was compared to 12-step facilitation (TSF) for depressed patients with SUD,[81] reduction in drinking and depression was more stable in the CBT group. In another example, Carroll and colleagues found that CBT was superior to a control condition in achieving greater periods of abstinence for depressed cocaine users.[82] Therefore, although few studies have assessed CBT in depressed substance users, it remains an important treatment option to target both depressive and substance use symptoms.

■ MOTIVATIONAL INTERVIEWING

Motivational interviewing (MI) is a psychosocial intervention with extensive empirical support for a wide range of target behaviors, including substance use.[83–85] It has emerged as an important option for treatment of patients with SUD.[85,86] MI focuses on creating a collaborative environment in which particular attention is paid to exploring and eliciting the patient's own arguments and reasons for change, while demonstrating empathy and respect for patient autonomy. MI is best understood as a method of helping patients to engage and adhere to treatment. Unfortunately, like other psychosocial treatments, few studies have focused on using MI specifically for depressed substance users. In one study of depressed cocaine-dependent patients receiving MI or treatment-as-usual, those receiving MI were significantly more likely to adhere to aftercare treatment sessions, and were significantly less likely to be hospitalized within 1 year of discharge.[87] Because of its strong empirical support in patients with SUD, clinicians are strongly encouraged to incorporate MI into the treatment of all patients with SUD.

■ SELF-HELP

Twelve-step programs such as Alcoholics Anonymous (AA) are a key treatment option for dually diagnosed patients. A systematic review demonstrated that 12-step participation provides general benefit for both mental health and substance use.[88] For example, Laudet et al. found that ongoing attendance in a 12-step program was associated with a significantly greater likelihood of abstinence.[89] In order to increase engagement with AA, clinicians can use a manual-guided approach to recommending AA or related services, called 12-step facilitation (TSF).[90] There are also approaches that nonspecialists can use to help increase patients' engagement with 12-step programs.[91] However, research on depressed substance users shows that CBT likely leads to more stable reduction in substance use than TSF.[81,92] Nevertheless, these findings suggest that it is reasonable for clinicians to refer appropriate patients to 12-step programs.

CONCLUSION

The co-occurrence of depression and SUD is frequently encountered in clinical populations. Although effective treatment exists for both disorders, SUD treatments are often underutilized. The research shows, however, that both disorders can be effectively treated simultaneously. In fact, attempting to treat the depression without also addressing the substance use is not optimal therapy (**Box 19-8**). All depressed patients should be routinely screened for substance use, and appropriate treatments provided, and clinicians should gather a comprehensive history in an empathic and nonjudgmental approach. Diagnostically, it is important to tease out independent mood disorders from substance-induced disorders, given that depressive symptoms are common in patients actively using substances. The initial goal is to achieve abstinence, or at least reduction in substance use, while closely monitoring the patient's mood and safety risk. Specific pharmacologic treatment for the substance use should be considered (e.g., buprenorphine, naltrexone, disulfiram). After a short period (1–2 weeks), psychosocial treatments targeting the depression should be initiated if the depression has not improved. Evidence-based approaches include CBT, MI, 12-step facilitation, and contingency management. Antidepressant treatment should not be routinely offered unless patients do not respond to this initial psychosocial intervention.

BOX 19-8
SUMMARY

- Given the high rates of comorbidity, patients with depression should be routinely screened for SUD and vice versa
- Despite proven efficacy, SUD treatments are often underutilized; both disorders can be treated successfully and addressing them separately is not optimal treatment
- Antidepressants should be initiated if depressive symptoms fail to resolve with psychosocial treatments

REFERENCES

1. Hasin D, Kilcoyne B. Comorbidity of psychiatric and substance use disorders in the United States: current issues and findings from the NESARC. *Curr Opin Psychiatry*. 2012;25(3):165–171.

2. Kessler RC, Chiu WT, Demler O, Merikangas KR, Walters EE. Prevalence, severity, and comorbidity of 12-month DSM-IV disorders in the National Comorbidity Survey Replication. *Arch Gen Psychiatry*. 2005;62(6):617–627.

3. Regier DA, Farmer ME, Rae DS, et al. Comorbidity of mental disorders with alcohol and other drug abuse. Results from the Epidemiologic Catchment Area (ECA) Study. *JAMA*. 1990;264(19):2511–2518.

4. Mark TL. The costs of treating persons with depression and alcoholism compared with depression alone. *Psychiatr Serv*. 2003;54(8):1095–1097.

5. Mark TL, Kranzler HR, Song X, Bransberger P, Poole VH, Crosse S. Physicians' opinions about medications to treat alcoholism. *Addict Abingdon Engl*. 2003;98(5):617–626.

6. Substance Abuse and Mental Health Services Administration. Results from the 2011 National Survey on Drug Use and Health: Summary of National Findings, NSDUH Series H-44, HHS Publication No. (SMA) 12–4713. [Internet]. Substance Abuse and Mental Health Services Administration; 2012 [cited 2013 Jul 23]. Available at http://www.samhsa.gov/data/NSDUH/2k11Results/NSDUHresults2011.htm

7. Ritsher JB, McKellar JD, Finney JW, Otilingam PG, Moos RH. Psychiatric comorbidity, continuing care and mutual help as predictors of five-year remission from substance use disorders. *J Stud Alcohol*. 2002;63(6):709–715.

8. Davis LL, Rush JA, Wisniewski SR, et al. Substance use disorder comorbidity in major depressive disorder: an exploratory analysis of the sequenced treatment alternatives to relieve depression cohort. *Compr Psychiatry*. 2005;46(2):81–89.

9. McLellan T. Revisiting the past for a look toward future research: A final editorial. *J Subst Abuse Treat*. 2009;36(4):352–354.

10. Grant BF, Dawson DA, Stinson FS, Chou SP, Dufour MC, Pickering RP. The 12-month prevalence and trends in DSM-IV alcohol abuse and dependence: United States, 1991–1992 and 2001–2002. *Drug Alcohol Depend*. 2004;74(3):223–234.

11. Schuckit MA, Tipp JE, Bucholz KK, et al. The life-time rates of three major mood disorders and four major anxiety disorders in alcoholics and controls. *Addiction* 1997;92(10):1289–1304.

12. Khantzian EJ. Addiction as a self-regulation disorder and the role of self-medication. *Addiction*. 2013;108(4):668–669.

13. Bolton JM, Robinson J, Sareen J. Self-medication of mood disorders with alcohol and drugs in the National Epidemiologic Survey on Alcohol and Related Conditions. *J Affect Disord*. 2009;115(3):367–375.

14. Cornelius JR, Salloum IM, Ehler JG, et al. Fluoxetine in depressed alcoholics. A double-blind, placebo-controlled trial. *Arch Gen Psychiatry*. 1997;54(8):700–705.

15. Weiss RD, Griffin ML, Mirin SM. Drug abuse as self-medication for depression: an empirical study. *Am J Drug Alcohol Abuse*. 1992;18(2):121–129.

16. Boden JM, Fergusson DM. Alcohol and depression. *Addiction*. 2011;106(5):906–914.

17. Schuckit MA. Comorbidity between substance use disorders and psychiatric conditions. *Addiction*. 2006;101(Suppl 1):76–88.

18. Satel SL, Southwick SM, Gawin FH. Clinical features of cocaine-induced paranoia. *Am J Psychiatry*. 1991;148(4):495–498.

19. Brown SA, Schuckit MA. Changes in depression among abstinent alcoholics. *J Stud Alcohol*. 1988;49(5):412–417.

20. Schuckit MA. An overview of genetic influences in alcoholism. *J Subst Abuse Treat*. 2009;36(1):S5–S14.

21. McGuffin P, Cohen S, Knight J. Homing in on depression genes. *Am J Psychiatry*. 2007;164(2):195–197.

22. Rietschel M, Treutlein J. The genetics of alcohol dependence. *Ann N Y Acad Sci*. 2013;1282:39–70.

23. Weissman MM, Wickramaratne P, Nomura Y, Warner V, Pilowsky D, Verdeli H. Offspring of depressed parents: 20 years later. *Am J Psychiatry*. 2006;163(6):1001–1008.

24. Phillips TJ, Shen EH. Neurochemical bases of locomotion and ethanol stimulant effects. *Int Rev Neurobiol*. 1996;39:243–282.

25. Timko C, Cronkite RC, Swindle R, Robinson RL, Turrubiartes P, Moos RH. Functioning status of adult children of depressed parents: a 23-year follow-up. *Psychol Med*. 2008;38(3):343–352.

26. Hyman SE, Malenka RC. Addiction and the brain: the neurobiology of compulsion and its persistence. *Nat Rev Neurosci*. 2001;2(10):695–703.

27. Hyman SE. Addiction: a disease of learning and memory. *Am J Psychiatry*. 2005;162(8):1414–1422.

28. Nestler EJ, Carlezon WA. The mesolimbic dopamine reward circuit in depression. *Biol Psychiatry*. 2006;59(12):1151–1159.

29. Substance Abuse and Mental Health Services Administration. *Drug Abuse Warning Network 2009: Area profiles of drug-related mortality. HHS Publication No (SMA) 11–4639, DAWN series D-24*. Rockville, MD: Substance Abuse and Mental Health Services Administration; 2011.

30. Schuckit MA, Smith TL, Kalmijn J. Relationships among independent major depressions, alcohol use, and other substance use and related problems over 30 years in 397 families. *J Stud Alcohol Drugs*. 2013;74(2):271–279.

31. Badawy AA-B. Pellagra and alcoholism: a biochemical perspective. *Alcohol Alcohol*. 2014;49(3):238–250.

32. Cocksedge KA, Flynn A. Wernicke-Korsakoff syndrome in a patient with self-neglect associated with severe depression. *JRSM Open*. 2014;5(2):2042533313518915.

33. Wasan AD, Michna E, Edwards RR, et al. Psychiatric comorbidity is associated prospectively with diminished opioid analgesia and increased opioid misuse in patients with chronic low back pain. *Anesthesiology*. 2015;123(4):861–872.

34. Hagan H, Pouget ER, Des Jarlais DC, Lelutiu-Weinberger C. Meta-regression of hepatitis C virus infection in relation to time since onset of illicit drug injection: the influence of time and place. *Am J Epidemiol*. 2008;168(10):1099–1109.

35. Lucaciu LA, Dumitrascu DL. Depression and suicide ideation in chronic hepatitis C patients untreated and treated with interferon: prevalence, prevention, and treatment. *Ann Gastroenterol*. 2015;28(4):440–447.

36. Watkins KE, Paddock SM, Zhang L, Wells KB. Improving care for depression in patients with comorbid substance misuse. *Am J Psychiatry*. 2006;163(1):125–132.

37. Davis L, Uezato A, Newell JM, Frazier E. Major depression and comorbid substance use disorders. *Curr Opin Psychiatry*. 2008;21(1):14–18.

38. Worthington J, Fava M, Agustin C, et al. Consumption of alcohol, nicotine, and caffeine among depressed outpatients.

Relationship with response to treatment. *Psychosomatics*. 1996; 37(6):518–522.

39. Worley MJ, Trim RS, Roesch SC, Mrnak-Meyer J, Tate SR, Brown SA. Comorbid depression and substance use disorder: longitudinal associations between symptoms in a controlled trial. *J Subst Abuse Treat*. 2012;43(3):291–302.

40. Rush AJ, Fava M, Wisniewski SR, et al. Sequenced treatment alternatives to relieve depression (STAR*D): rationale and design. *Control Clin Trials*. 2004;25(1):119–142.

41. Howland RH, Rush AJ, Wisniewski SR, et al. Concurrent anxiety and substance use disorders among outpatients with major depression: clinical features and effect on treatment outcome. *Drug Alcohol Depend*. 2009;99(1–3):248–260.

42. Davis LL, Wisniewski SR, Howland RH, et al. Does comorbid substance use disorder impair recovery from major depression with SSRI treatment? An analysis of the STAR*D level one treatment outcomes. *Drug Alcohol Depend*. 2010;107(2–3): 161–170.

43. Greenfield SF, Weiss RD, Muenz LR, et al. The effect of depression on return to drinking: a prospective study. *Arch Gen Psychiatry*. 1998;55(3):259–265.

44. Curran GM, Flynn HA, Kirchner J, Booth BM. Depression after alcohol treatment as a risk factor for relapse among male veterans. *J Subst Abuse Treat*. 2000;19(3):259–265.

45. Glasner-Edwards S, Mooney LJ, Marinelli-Casey P, et al. Risk factors for suicide attempts in methamphetamine-dependent patients. *Am J Addict*. 2008;17(1):24–27.

46. Hasin D, Liu X, Nunes E, McCloud S, Samet S, Endicott J. Effects of major depression on remission and relapse of substance dependence. *Arch Gen Psychiatry*. 2002;59(4):375–380.

47. Meier PS, Barrowclough C, Donmall MC. The role of the therapeutic alliance in the treatment of substance misuse: a critical review of the literature. *Addict Abingdon Engl*. 2005;100(3): 304–316.

48. Pettinati HM, O'Brien CP, Dundon WD. Current status of co-occurring mood and substance use disorders: a new therapeutic target. *Am J Psychiatry*. 2013;170(1):23–30.

49. Kelly TM, Daley DC, Douaihy AB. Treatment of substance abusing patients with comorbid psychiatric disorders. *Addict Behav*. 2012;37(1):11–24.

50. Nunes EV, Levin FR. Treatment of depression in patients with alcohol or other drug dependence: a meta-analysis. *JAMA*. 2004;291(15):1887–1896.

51. Walsh BT, Seidman SN, Sysko R, Gould M. Placebo response in studies of major depression: variable, substantial, and growing. *JAMA*. 2002;287(14):1840–1847.

52. Nunes EV, Levin FR. Treating depression in substance abusers. *Curr Psychiatry Rep*. 2006;8(5):363–370.

53. Rösner S, Hackl-Herrwerth A, Leucht S, Vecchi S, Srisurapanont M, Soyka M. Opioid antagonists for alcohol dependence. *Cochrane Database Syst Rev*. 2010;(12):CD001867.

54. Salloum IM, Cornelius JR, Thase ME, Daley DC, Kirisci L, Spotts C. Naltrexone utility in depressed alcoholics. *Psychopharmacol Bull*. 1998;34(1):111–115.

55. Krystal JH, Gueorguieva R, Cramer J, Collins J, Rosenheck R, VA CSP No. 425 Study Team. Naltrexone is associated with reduced drinking by alcohol dependent patients receiving antidepressants for mood and anxiety symptoms: results from VA Cooperative Study No. 425, "Naltrexone in the treatment of alcoholism." *Alcohol Clin Exp Res*. 2008;32(1):85–91.

56. Pettinati HM, Oslin DW, Kampman KM, et al. A double-blind, placebo-controlled trial combining sertraline and naltrexone for treating co-occurring depression and alcohol dependence. *Am J Psychiatry*. 2010;167(6):668–675.

57. Jørgensen CH, Pedersen B, Tønnesen H. The efficacy of disulfiram for the treatment of alcohol use disorder. *Alcohol Clin Exp Res*. 2011;35(10):1749–1758.

58. Petrakis I, Ralevski E, Nich C, et al. Naltrexone and disulfiram in patients with alcohol dependence and current depression. *J Clin Psychopharmacol*. 2007;27(2):160–165.

59. Fullerton CA, Kim M, Thomas CP, et al. Medication-assisted treatment with methadone: assessing the evidence. *Psychiatr Serv*. 2014;65(2):146–157.

60. Faggiano F, Vigna-Taglianti F, Versino E, Lemma P. Methadone maintenance at different dosages for opioid dependence. *Cochrane Database Syst Rev*. 2003;(3):CD002208.

61. Kapur BM, Hutson JR, Chibber T, Luk A, Selby P. Methadone: a review of drug-drug and pathophysiological interactions. *Crit Rev Clin Lab Sci*. 2011;48(4):171–195.

62. Thomas CP, Fullerton CA, Kim M, et al. Medication-assisted treatment with buprenorphine: assessing the evidence. *Psychiatr Serv*. 2014;65(2):158–170.

63. Clark W. The state of buprenorphine treatment [Internet]. 2010 [cited 2012 Aug 30]; Buprenorphine in the treatment of opioid addiction: Reassessment 2010. Available at http://buprenorphine.samhsa.gov/bwns/2010_presentations_pdf/01_Clark_508.pdf

64. Ling W, Wesson DR, Charuvastra C, Klett CJ. A controlled trial comparing buprenorphine and methadone maintenance in opioid dependence. *Arch Gen Psychiatry*. 1996;53(5):401–407.

65. Pani PP, Vacca R, Trogu E, Amato L, Davoli M. Pharmacological treatment for depression during opioid agonist treatment for opioid dependence. *Cochrane Database Syst Rev*. 2010;(9): CD008373.

66. Nunes EV, Quitkin FM, Donovan SJ, et al. Imipramine treatment of opiate-dependent patients with depressive disorders. A placebo-controlled trial. *Arch Gen Psychiatry*. 1998;55(2):153–160.

67. Griffin ML, Dodd DR, Potter JS, et al. Baseline characteristics and treatment outcomes in prescription opioid dependent patients with and without co-occurring psychiatric disorder. *Am J Drug Alcohol Abuse*. 2014;40(2):157–162.

68. de Lima MS, de Oliveira Soares BG, Reisser AA, Farrell M. Pharmacological treatment of cocaine dependence: a systematic review. *Addiction*. 2002;97(8):931–949.

69. Schmitz JM, Averill P, Stotts AL, Moeller FG, Rhoades HM, Grabowski J. Fluoxetine treatment of cocaine-dependent patients with major depressive disorder. *Drug Alcohol Depend*. 2001;63(3):207–214.

70. Ciraulo DA, Knapp C, Rotrosen J, et al. Nefazodone treatment of cocaine dependence with comorbid depressive symptoms. *Addict Abingdon Engl*. 2005;100(Suppl 1):23–31.

71. Raby WN, Rubin EA, Garawi F, et al. A randomized, double-blind, placebo-controlled trial of venlafaxine for the treatment of depressed cocaine-dependent patients. *Am J Addict*. 2014;23(1):68–75.

72. McDowell D, Nunes EV, Seracini AM, et al. Desipramine treatment of cocaine-dependent patients with depression: a placebo-controlled trial. *Drug Alcohol Depend*. 2005;80(2):209–221.

73. Farronato NS, Dürsteler-Macfarland KM, Wiesbeck GA, Petitjean SA. A systematic review comparing cognitive-behavioral

therapy and contingency management for cocaine dependence. *J Addict Dis*. 2013;32(3):274–287.

74. Moore TH, Zammit S, Lingford-Hughes A, et al. Cannabis use and risk of psychotic or affective mental health outcomes: a systematic review. *Lancet*. 2007;370(9584):319–328.

75. Shi Y. At high risk and want to quit: Marijuana use among adults with depression or serious psychological distress. *Addict Behav*. 2013;39(4):761–767.

76. Cornelius JR, Salloum IM, Haskett RF, et al. Fluoxetine versus placebo for the marijuana use of depressed alcoholics. *Addict Behav*. 1999;24(1):111–114.

77. Weinstein AM, Miller H, Bluvstein I, et al. Treatment of cannabis dependence using escitalopram in combination with cognitive-behavior therapy: a double-blind placebo-controlled study. *Am J Drug Alcohol Abuse*. 2014;40(1):16–22.

78. Levin FR, Mariani J, Brooks DJ, et al. A randomized double-blind, placebo-controlled trial of venlafaxine-extended release for co-occurring cannabis dependence and depressive disorders. *Addict Abingdon Engl*. 2013;108(6):1084–1094.

79. McHugh RK, Hearon BA, Otto MW. Cognitive behavioral therapy for substance use disorders. *Psychiatr Clin North Am*. 2010;33(3):511–525.

80. Carroll KM. Behavioral therapies for co-occurring substance use and mood disorders. *Biol Psychiatry*. 2004;56(10):778–784.

81. Brown SA, Glasner-Edwards SV, Tate SR, McQuaid JR, Chalekian J, Granholm E. Integrated cognitive behavioral therapy versus twelve-step facilitation therapy for substance-dependent adults with depressive disorders. *J Psychoactive Drugs*. 2006;38(4):449–460.

82. Carroll KM, Nich C, Rounsaville BJ. Differential symptom reduction in depressed cocaine abusers treated with psychotherapy and pharmacotherapy. *J Nerv Ment Dis*. 1995;183(4):251–259.

83. Hettema J, Steele J, Miller WR. Motivational interviewing. *Annu Rev Clin Psychol*. 2005;1:91–111.

84. Lundahl B, Burke BL. The effectiveness and applicability of motivational interviewing: a practice-friendly review of four meta-analyses. *J Clin Psychol*. 2009;65(11):1232–1245.

85. Smedslund G, Berg RC, Hammerstrøm KT, et al. Motivational interviewing for substance abuse. *Cochrane Database Syst Rev Online*. 2011;(5):CD008063.

86. Matching alcoholism treatments to client heterogeneity: treatment main effects and matching effects on drinking during treatment. Project MATCH Research Group. *J Stud Alcohol*. 1998;59(6):631–639.

87. Daley DC, Salloum IM, Zuckoff A, Kirisci L, Thase ME. Increasing treatment adherence among outpatients with depression and cocaine dependence: results of a pilot study. *Am J Psychiatry*. 1998;155(11):1611–1613.

88. Aase DM, Jason LA, Robinson WL. 12-step participation among dually-diagnosed individuals: a review of individual and contextual factors. *Clin Psychol Rev*. 2008;28(7):1235–1248.

89. Laudet AB, Magura S, Cleland CM, Vogel HS, Knight EL, Rosenblum A. The effect of 12-step based fellowship participation on abstinence among dually diagnosed persons: a two-year longitudinal study. *J Psychoactive Drugs*. 2004;36(2):207–216.

90. Donovan DM, Floyd AS. Facilitating involvement in twelve-step programs. *Recent Dev Alcohol*. 2008;18:303–320.

91. Kelly JF, McCrady BS. Twelve-step facilitation in non-specialty settings. *Recent Dev Alcohol*. 2008;18:321–346.

92. Lydecker KP, Tate SR, Cummins KM, McQuaid J, Granholm E, Brown SA. Clinical outcomes of an integrated treatment for depression and substance use disorders. *Psychol Addict Behav*. 2010;24(3):453–465.

SECTION IV
Special Populations and Settings

CHAPTER 20

Depression in Medically Ill Children

Eleni Maneta, MD
David DeMaso, MD

Each day children and adolescents[†] face a wide range of medical illnesses including allergies, asthma, epilepsy, cancer, diabetes, and obesity, all of which appear to be increasing in prevalence.[1] According to the 2005 to 2006 National Survey of Children with Special Health Care Needs Chartbook, the two most common are allergies (53%) and asthma (38.8%).[2] The increasing prevalence of these has been partly attributed to medical advances that have reduced mortality rates, so that children with chronic medical conditions now live longer.[3,4] The increased prevalence of childhood illnesses is also related to increased exposure to toxic stress, sedentary lifestyle, and an unhealthy diet leading to increased childhood obesity and subsequently other comorbid medical disorders.[3]

Ten to twenty million children in the United States have a medical condition, and about 10% of them are impacted by it in their daily lives.[5] Illnesses affect the emotional and social wellbeing of children and their parents, and increase the stress-level of the family system as well.[6] For example, illness characteristics (such as pain or fatigue) and required treatments (such as steroid medication) can interfere with school participation, which in turn can lead to academic difficulties and social isolation as well as increased caregiving and financial demands on their parents. Children with chronic illness are also more prone to bullying by peers,[7] which can then further exacerbate their physical symptoms and lead to greater psychological distress.[8] While the majority of children with medical illness are resilient,[5] when compared to their healthy counterparts, they have an increased risk for the development of psychiatric problems.[6,9,10] It is estimated that 20% of children with chronic health conditions will have psychiatric problems.[5]

Children with medical illness can present with both internalizing and externalizing psychiatric problems. Internalizing problems are manifested in symptoms of depression, anxiety and somatic complaints whereas externalizing problems are reflected in hyperactivity, aggression, or "acting-out" (**Table 20-1**). That said, internalizing problems tend to occur more frequently in medically ill children.[11,12] For example, a meta-analysis assessing behavioral outcomes of children with medical illness concluded that internalizing symptoms were more prominent than externalizing symptoms.[13] It is hypothesized that certain characteristics associated with physical illness, such as the sense of losing control, restrictions of positive activities, isolation from peers, and pain, are the driving force for the development of internalizing symptoms.

This chapter focuses specifically on diagnostic considerations and challenges in psychiatric assessment and differential diagnosis of depression in children with medical illness. Asthma, obesity, epilepsy, cancer, and diabetes mellitus are specifically reviewed. Treatment-related issues and the recommendations of the American Academy of Child and Adolescent Psychiatry are considered.

DEPRESSION IN MEDICALLY ILL CHILDREN— WHAT DOES IT LOOK LIKE?

Children with medical illness are more prone to develop depressive disorders.[14,15] The overall prevalence of depressive disorders in the general population is approximately 2% in children and 6% in adolescents,[16] with another estimated 5% to 10% having subsyndromal symptoms of depression.[17] Children with physical illness are approximately twice as likely to develop depression as their healthy

---

[†]Hereafter, "children" refers to both children and adolescents unless specifically noted otherwise.

TABLE 20-1 Internalizing and Externalizing Symptoms in Children

Internalizing Symptoms	Externalizing Symptoms
Anxiety	Anger
Somatic complaints	Oppositionality
Depression	Aggression
Withdrawn	Hyperactivity
Low self-esteem	Low self-esteem

counterparts,[18] and because they often present with subsyndromal symptoms they are not always accurately diagnosed.[19]

Though the evidence suggests that acute medical illness increases the risk of developing depression in childhood, the long-term effects of childhood medical illness on adult psychological adjustment are less clear. One important study found no difference in prevalence of psychiatric disorders among young adults who had experienced childhood medical illness and those who had not;[20] however, the severity of psychiatric symptoms in the adults was greater in those who had experienced more severe illnesses in childhood. A comprehensive literature review reported that the overall prevalence of psychiatric disorders in young adult survivors of childhood medical illness was similar to that of their healthy counterparts, but that social adjustment was significantly more impaired in those who had experienced chronic childhood illnesses.[19] It also appears that subsyndromal symptoms of depression in medically ill children and adolescents may have an effect on social and functional outcomes in adulthood.[19] This underscores the need for early detection and treatment of psychiatric comorbidity in these children.

Depression in children presents with a similar picture to that in adults. According to the *Diagnostic and Statistical Manual, 5th Edition* (DSM-5)[21] children can be diagnosed with major depressive disorder (MDD) if they have persistent depressed or irritable mood for at least 2 weeks accompanied by loss of pleasure and interest in activities, changes in sleep and appetite and feelings of worthlessness and suicidal ideation. While the DSM-5 criteria for MDD are similar for adults and children, there are some important differences when it comes to clinical presentation, which are attributed to the developmental stage of the child.

Children tend to present with fewer melancholic symptoms and are less likely to verbalize feelings of depression. Instead they may present with temper tantrums, irritability, social isolation, and somatic symptoms.[17] The high rates of somatic symptoms present a challenge when trying to diagnose depression in a medically ill child because the symptoms of the illness can either be misperceived as depression, or a diagnosis of depression may be delayed because of attributing such symptoms directly to the medical illness.[22] Children's developmental stage, their understanding of their medical illness and their ability to express their feelings may present an additional challenge when evaluating the presence of a depressive disorder.

Similar to MDD, the diagnostic criteria for persistent depressive disorder are comparable in children and adults, with the exception of the duration of illness which is one year of persistent low or irritable mood along with changes in sleep, appetite, and energy levels instead of 2 years in adults.[21]

Depressive symptoms in medically ill children may range from a transient mood change requiring no treatment to a severe clinical disorder requiring psychiatric hospitalization.[18] Thus, mental health classification systems, with their focus on diagnosable disorder may be of little value to primary care physicians who deal with the whole spectrum of mental health symptoms.[18] In order to address the wide range of symptoms, the American Academy of Pediatrics introduced

The Classification of Child and Adolescent Mental Diagnoses in Primary Care, Child and Adolescent Version which provides a system to classify symptoms ranging from developmental variation to problem to disorder.[23]

Underdiagnosis of depression in the face of medical illness[24] is a missed opportunity to improve quality of life, increase adherence to treatment and shorten hospital stays, all of which are themselves associated with improvement in depressive symptoms.[18] There are many different reasons for underdiagnosis and misdiagnosis of depression in children with illnesses. For example, irritable mood and somatic symptoms may be more prominent than depressed mood. Parents and children are more likely to focus on somatic complaints than mood or cognitive symptoms. Primary care clinicians may be reluctant to raise concerns of psychiatric symptoms to avoid stigmatizing patients.[25] These facts further highlight the importance of early screening and accurate assessment of depression in children who are ill.

Diagnosing depression in children is not infrequently complicated by the presence of co-occurring anxiety. Box 20-1 presents some of the psychological factors that may contribute to clinically significant anxiety in medically ill children (**Box 20-1**).

THE ASSESSMENT OF DEPRESSION—FACTORS TO CONSIDER

The assessment of depression in children who are ill begins with a psychiatric examination for psychological and somatic symptoms consistent with the DSM-5 criteria for a depressive episode. The examination should lead to accurate diagnosis along with a developmentally informed biopsychosocial formulation[26] whereby the child's presentation should be seen in light of a continuum of depressive symptoms.[23] In the examination, the following factors are important to consider when developing an accurate biopsychosocial formulation for medically ill children.

BOX 20-1
POTENTIAL PSYCHOLOGICAL FACTORS THAT MAY CONTRIBUTE TO DISABLING ANXIETY AND/OR DEPRESSION IN MEDICALLY ILL CHILDREN[89]

Factors	Effects
Diagnosis	– Fear, worry, and/or sadness around time of diagnosis, particularly if there is a family history of a specific medical condition. – Fear, worry, and sadness in the context of abnormal lab tests but absence of concrete diagnosis
Physical Integrity	– Worry and/or unhappiness about bodily integrity in pre-school children – Worry and/or unhappiness about cosmetic effects of illness in adolescents
Hospitalization	– Fear, sadness, and/or anger in young children about being separated from caretakers during their hospitalization – Fear, sadness, and/or anger in an adolescent separated from peers
Impact of illness	– Concern about missing school or falling behind – Concern about difference from peers
Prognosis	– Fear, worry, and/or sadness about recurrence or death particularly when there is family history of death from the same medical condition

■ CHILD-RELATED FACTORS

The level of psychological distress experienced will depend on certain personal characteristics. Low IQ and low self-esteem are two risk factors that can predispose medically ill children to develop depressive disorders.[26] The child's coping style (i.e., maladaptive, catastrophizing) can also influence their psychological adjustment.[26]

■ DEVELOPMENTAL FACTORS

While children's approach to their illnesses will in part be shaped by their prior experiences with medical conditions,[27] developmental stage is a critical consideration as children's understanding of their illness directly affects their cognition and emotions.[28] Very young children are limited in their cognitive understanding and ability to remember information about their condition, which may result in adverse behaviors around medical procedures.[29,30]

Although various theories have been proposed to explain children's understanding of illness,[31] Piaget's stages of cognitive development still offer a pragmatic approach to comprehending their view of medical illness (**Fig. 20-1**).[32,33] Young children who are in the *pre-operational* phase classically interpret their illness as a form of punishment and feel that they have caused the illness by doing something wrong or being bad. They may attribute illness to magic or evil[34] and assume that all illnesses are contagious. By school age, children develop *concrete operations*, and become aware of other factors (i.e., "germs") that can cause illness. These older children are prone to feeling a loss of control, anxiety, and significant fear about harm to their bodies,[28] which can put them at higher risk for the development of depression.

Adolescents who are in the process of developing *formal operations*, have a more complex understanding of illness including the interactions of various organ systems.[35] Illness in this age group has the potential to significantly interfere with the adolescent developmental tasks of individuation, identity formation and sexuality, particularly in the presence of medical conditions that can cause loss of function or change in appearance.[28] A young child experiencing hair loss due to chemotherapy may be less affected than an adolescent in a similar situation. The interference with normal developmental tasks can heighten the risk for depression in adolescents.

■ FAMILY FACTORS

Childhood medical illness affects family dynamics, caregiver burden and parental vulnerability to stress.[6] At the same time the family's ability to manage a child's illness in turn impacts the child's ability to cope with his/her illnesses.[25,28] Thus, when assessing medically ill children, it is important to consider the developmental stage of the family.

The life cycle of the family, and the developmental tasks associated with each stage, have been described and characterized as families with young children, families with adolescents, and families with children who are young adults.[36] Families with young children have to focus on children's development while building confidence in their parenting skills. In contrast families with adolescents have to embrace the adolescent's gradual independence while continuing to maintain family boundaries and responsibilities. As adolescents transition into young adulthood families continue to promote the establishment of new relationships outside the family along with medical and financial independence. When childhood illness occurs at any of these phases it can impact the developmental tasks of the entire family. When a young child is ill, the family may have trouble setting appropriate limits, which can lead to "acting-out." When adolescents are ill, they may not be able to work on achieving independence, which may lead to feelings of insecurity and depression as well as frustration for the family. Similarly, young adults who become ill may be prevented from achieving developmental milestones, such as higher level of education, or financial independence and career planning, which can add more burdens to the individual and the family system. Parental divorce, insufficient funds, and poor parental adjustment to the child's condition have been associated with poor adjustment in children with medical illness.[35]

■ SUICIDAL RISK

Unlike adult studies, pediatric studies have not found an association between suicidal thoughts and specific medical conditions (such as cancer).[37] However, studies in children have noted increased rates of suicidal behaviors when the chronic medical illness co-occurs with significant psychiatric disorder.[38,39] Medically ill children who attempt suicide have similar risk factors to physically healthy children.[18] Exposure to childhood sexual abuse, unsupportive parental relationships, and limited parental involvement as well as mood disorders, substance abuse, and antisocial behaviors have all been linked with increased risk for suicide in children.[40] Family history and prior history of suicidality are additional risk factors, as is access to lethal means.

DIFFERENTIAL DIAGNOSIS IN MEDICALLY ILL CHILDREN

In the medical setting, it is important to consider the following three diagnostic categories in the differential diagnosis—primary depressive disorder, depressive disorder as a reaction to medical illness, and secondary depressive disorder due to a general medical condition. All three entities can be involved to some degree in any single patient and as a result can create a significant challenge in determining which is the primary diagnosis underlying the depressive symptoms.

■ PRIMARY DEPRESSIVE DISORDERS

Children with medical illness who meet DSM-5 criteria can be diagnosed with a co-occurring major depressive episode. While there is overlap in neurovegetative symptoms between the direct effects of a general medical condition and a depressive disorder, the preoccupation with worthlessness, hopelessness, inappropriate guilt, and suicidality are more consistent with a primary depressive disorder than either of the other two categories.[18] The Children's Depression Rating Scale Revised,[41] which focuses on nonoverlapping symptoms and excludes somatic symptoms, has demonstrated high sensitivity for the clinical diagnosis of a primary depressive disorder in children with cancer.[42] The Children's Depression Inventory (CDI) accurately identified clinical depression in medically ill children and has been recommended for screening in the medical setting.[21] The anhedonia subscale is the most highly correlated scale with a primary depressive disorder.[21]

As in the general population, prior episodes of depression and significant genetic loading through a family history of mood disorders are two major risk factors for the development of a primary depression in children with medical illness. Depression in the family of origin is the most important risk factor for the development of a depressive disorder.[42,43]

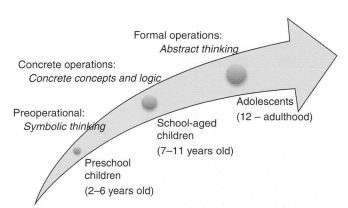

Figure 20-1 *Cognitive stages of development. (Reproduced with permission from Piaget J: The child's conception of the world. New York, NY: Harcourt Brace; 1929.)*

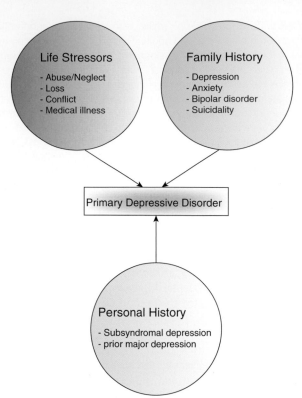

Life Stressors

- Abuse/Neglect
- Loss
- Conflict
- Medical illness

Family History

- Depression
- Anxiety
- Bipolar disorder
- Suicidality

Primary Depressive Disorder

Personal History

- Subsyndromal depression
- prior major depression

Figure 20-2 *Factors contributing to the development of depression.*

Environmental factors such as abuse, neglect, loss, conflicts and stress, including that imposed by the presence of the medical illness, may contribute to the development of a primary mood disorder. There is an interaction effect between life stressors, subsyndromal depressive symptoms and a family history of depression that can lead to the development of a primary depressive disorder (**Fig. 20-2**).[16]

Somatic complaints, neurovegetative symptoms, and mood lability in children with medical illness can also stem from anxiety disorders, which are commonly comorbid with depressive disorders. Anxiety disorders are one of the most common psychiatric diagnoses in children, and frequently co-occur with medical illness with an estimated rate of up to 40%.[44] There is also some evidence that bipolar disorders, which are significantly less frequent in childhood and have an estimated lifetime prevalence of 1% in the general population,[45] may be more prevalent among medically ill individuals.[46] While the treatment of anxiety disorders parallels that of depressive disorders, management of bipolar differs greatly and therefore accurate diagnosis is imperative.

DEPRESSIVE DISORDER AS A REACTION TO MEDICAL ILLNESS

Psychological distress in the context of a medical illness is common[47] and can present with sadness and feelings of helplessness, which may resemble a depressive episode. The distress experienced after a new medical diagnosis may be an understandable reaction in the face of the illness. In such cases, children and families are generally able to work through their feelings of anger and sadness during the initial phase of the illness and eventually discover ways to cope adaptively with the stress.[18]

When children's reactions to illness become maladaptive or interfere persistently with their ability to function, consider the diagnosis of adjustment disorder with depressed mood. The DSM-5 criteria for adjustment disorder require the presence of an identifiable stressor;[21] in this case it is the diagnosis of a medical condition. Children with adjustment disorder present with a milder dysphoric mood (without anhedonia) than that seen in a primary depressive disorder. Adjustment disorder is the most common diagnosis given to children who are medically ill and present with psychological distress,[19] and may represent a risk factor for the development of major depressive disorder under continued stress. Adjustment disorder is most prevalent in the initial phases of disease and frequently remits over time.[48] A "watchful waiting approach"[49] is warranted in order to determine whether the adjustment disorder will remit or convert into a primary depressive disorder.

Depressed mood in children adjusting to medical illness can also manifest itself in the form of behavioral and emotional regression.[18] Regressive behavior can be recognized as excessive clinginess toward caregivers, disproportionate tearfulness and constant demands for attention. Anna Freud has described regression in medically ill children as an adaptive mechanism by which they return to an earlier state in which they can be cared for and protected by their caregivers.[50] Similar to adjustment disorders, regressed behavior is most commonly seen in the initial phases of the illness, particularly during hospitalization, and often remits on its own as the stress of the illness decreases.

Children with medical illnesses and particularly those facing a terminal illness may present with bereavement, which can further complicate the differential diagnosis of depression. Bereavement has been associated with symptoms of helplessness, irritable or sad mood, somatic complaints and fear.[51] In bereavement, however, self-esteem tends to be preserved and the thought content is often associated directly with the loss rather than the generalized hopelessness seen in primary depressive disorders.[21] Bereavement can present with passive thoughts about dying, however, active suicidality is more suggestive of a primary depressive disorder and warrants further evaluation and treatment (**Fig. 20-3**).[52]

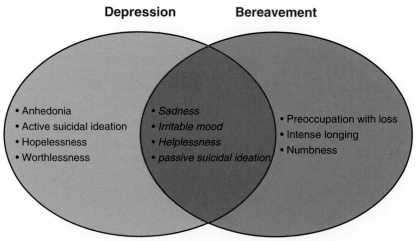

Depression

Bereavement

- Anhedonia
- Active suicidal ideation
- Hopelessness
- Worthlessness

- *Sadness*
- *Irritable mood*
- *Helplessness*
- *passive suicidal ideation*

- Preoccupation with loss
- Intense longing
- Numbness

Figure 20-3 *Overlap between depression and bereavement.*

■ SECONDARY DEPRESSIVE DISORDER DUE TO A GENERAL MEDICAL CONDITION

Children can develop depressive disorders that are the direct result of their general medical condition, referred to as secondary depressive disorders. For example, conditions such as hypothyroidism, systemic lupus erythematosus, and Wilson disease have all been associated with mood disturbances. In secondary depressive disorders, onset of symptoms is temporally related to the development of the medical condition. There is often malaise, mood is typically more flat in quality and other physical changes are often present (e.g., abnormal neurological signs, weight loss, abnormal laboratory studies, etc.).[25]

The relationship between physical illness and depression however is not one-directional. Research in adults has suggested that depression can be not only a consequence but also a cause of certain conditions. For example, depression may have an etiological role in conditions, such as heart disease, cancer, and epilepsy, which further highlights the importance of early diagnosis and treatment, of both the depressive disorder and medical illnesses.[49]

SPECIFIC MEDICAL CONDITIONS

While so far, we have taken a noncategorical approach to depression in children who are ill, a diagnosis specific approach[49] views the illness experience in the context of specific medical disorders. Although the noncategorical approach has helped in understanding the effects of general medical conditions on children,[53] the American Academy of Child and Adolescent Psychiatry recommends incorporating a diagnosis specific approach during assessment of medically ill children,[28] particularly since certain physical conditions, such as neurological disorders, have been associated with greater vulnerability to psychological distress.[35] In that context, we provide overviews of selected specific illnesses in relation to their comorbidity with depression.

■ ASTHMA

Asthma afflicts over 7 million US children with a prevalence of 9.6%.[54] The incidence and prevalence of asthma is increasing over time[1] and now represents a major public health problem, particularly given the morbidity associated with acute asthma attacks.[54] Asthma has been associated with comorbid psychiatric disorders, particularly depression and anxiety[55,56] with which it is thought to have a bi-directional relationship.[57]

There are three theoretical explanations of the link between asthma and psychiatric disorders: (1) the presence of a psychiatric condition affects the management of asthma (i.e., children with psychiatric diagnoses are less treatment adherent); (2) the burden of having asthma is internalized and leads to the development of psychiatric illness; and (3) the development of asthma is associated with the development of psychiatric illness.[55] There are reports of a higher prevalence of mood disorders in mothers and extended families of asthmatic children compared to healthy children, raising the question of a genetic link particularly since both disorders are known to be heritable.[57] Asthma and depression are each independently associated with an inflammatory state, and their co-occurrence has been shown to lead to further increases in inflammatory markers.[58] There is also evidence of underlying cholinergic dysregulation in both depression and asthma.[57] The hypothesis of neurotransmitter dysregulation affecting both asthma and depression is being investigated by using antidepressants to treat asthma-related symptoms.[56] However, only a few small studies have been conducted to date and additional research is needed to further delineate the relationship between asthma and depression.

■ OBESITY

Childhood obesity is a major public health concern due to its rising incidence and prevalence in the last 30 years.[1] Nearly 17% of children were obese in 2009 and another 31.8% were overweight.[59] Obese children are at risk for serious medical comorbidities as well as social and psychological problems throughout their life span. Children with obesity are more likely to have lower self-esteem and depressed mood compared to their healthy counterparts.[56]

Increasingly, obesity and depression are viewed as having a bi-directional relationship. Depression in adolescence has been found to be an independent risk factor for the development of obesity.[57] Research is underway into the common symptoms and underlying pathways that may be contributing to the co-occurrence of obesity and depression. Sleep disturbances, sedentary behavior, changes in appetite, and low self-esteem are common to both depression and obesity, and can have a bi-directional relationship, both resulting from and exacerbating each condition.[60] There is evidence of some common underlying biologic mechanisms involved in the development of obesity and depression: Both conditions have been linked with a pro-inflammatory state through increased levels of the inflammatory marker interleukin-6 and with hypothalamic–pituitary–adrenal axis dysfunction (**Fig. 20-4**).[60]

■ EPILEPSY

Epilepsy affects 4 to 5 of every 1,000 children.[61,62] It has been associated with numerous psychiatric comorbidities, at rates as high as 50%, which is far above that of other chronic medical conditions.[63] Depression is more common in children with epilepsy with a prevalence rate of 23% to 26%[64,65] compared to 2% to 6% in the general pediatric population. Several factors have been identified that play a role in the co-occurrence of epilepsy and depression including central nervous system involvement, social and family factors (e.g., stigma), and the iatrogenic effects of antiepileptic medications.[18]

Comorbid depression may increase the risk for suicidal behavior in children with epilepsy and can complicate the course of the disease itself.[63] It is important to provide appropriate treatment for depression with antidepressant medications that may also help to decrease seizure severity by stabilizing the noradrenergic and serotonergic systems in the central nervous system, both of which have been implicated in seizure predisposition.[65] Selective serotonin reuptake inhibitors (SSRIs) are considered safe for the treatment of children with comorbid epilepsy and depression[66] whereas older generation antidepressants, such as tricyclic antidepressants, have been associated with an increased risk for seizures.[67]

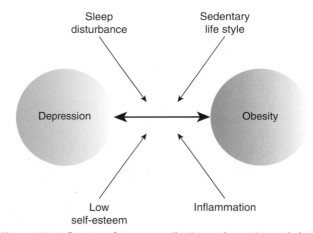

Figure 20-4 *Common factors contributing to depression and obesity.*

■ CANCER

Childhood cancer is a devastating illness that can significantly impact youngsters and their families. Cancer remains the second leading cause of death in children despite significant improvements in survival rates over the past decades.[68] Cancer treatment poses challenges for the family particularly as it is frequently associated with significant side effects that affect quality of life.

Depressive symptoms are common in children with cancer, with prevalence estimates ranging from 7% to 32%.[69] Accurate diagnosis, however, may be difficult because of overlapping symptoms, such as weight loss, anorexia, and fatigue. Depressed mood in the context of cancer can occur secondary to the psychological burden of the diagnosis, as a side effect of antineoplastic treatment, or due to underlying neurological problems, endocrine problems or metastatic disease. It can also represent the recurrence of a pre-existing mood disorder. The co-occurrence of depression and cancer in children can result in greater illness morbidity and prolonged hospitalizations.[70]

Childhood Cancer survivors are at increased risk for depressive symptoms, even after recovery from the acute illness. Adolescent survivors of childhood cancer are 1.5 times more likely to have depressive symptoms compared to siblings of cancer survivors.[66] Disfigurement as a result of the cancer treatment further increases the risk for depression.

■ DIABETES MELLITUS

Diabetes Mellitus is an insidious disease that can start in childhood and have long lasting-effects into adulthood. During 2002 to 2005, 15,600 children were diagnosed annually with type I diabetes and 3,600 youths with type II.[71] The prevalence of type II diabetes is rising among youths and now accounts for 45% of new cases compared to 3% 15 years ago.[72]

Depression frequently co-occurs with diabetes, and is thought to be the most common psychiatric comorbidity with prevalence rates as high as 27.5%.[73] It is most prevalent within the first year after diagnosis, and factors such as maternal psychopathology and pre-existing psychiatric illness further increase the likelihood of developing a depressive disorder.[73] Overall, girls with diabetes have higher rates of depression than boys, but boys with type II diabetes report more depressive symptoms than those with type I.[74] Co-occurring depression and diabetes are associated with increased suicidality.[38]

Accurate diagnosis of depression and prompt treatment are imperative because depression is associated with worse outcomes in youths with diabetes. Children with diabetes and inappropriately treated comorbid depression, for example, are at higher risk for both poorer glycemic control and juvenile retinopathy.[75,76] Depression in youths with diabetes is also been associated with nonadherence to treatment and lower self-esteem.[77,78]

TREATMENT

The high rates of depression in children with medical illness underscore the importance of accurate diagnosis and appropriate treatment on the outcome of the child's physical and mental health. Research shows untreated depression in medically ill patients can worsen prognosis and decrease survival by interfering with treatment adherence and physical and cognitive functioning.[49]

The treatment of depression in medically ill children follows the same guidelines that have been established by the American Academy of Child and Adolescent Psychiatry for the treatment of depression in all children.[17] Mild forms can initially be treated with psychotherapeutic interventions, whereas more severe forms should receive integrated psychotherapy and psychopharmacology (**Table 20-2**). The final treatment choice depends to some extent on the specific medical condition of children (for example hepatic

TABLE 20-2 First-Line Treatment Recommendations for Depression in Children and Adolescents

Level of Depression	Treatment Recommendations
Mild	Supportive therapy/CBT/IPT
Moderate	CBT/IPT
Severe (or moderate not responding to therapy alone)	Antidepressants (SSRIs) + CBT/IPT

CBT, cognitive-behavioral therapy; IPT, interpersonal therapy; SSRIs, selective serotonin re-uptake inhibitors.

illness may prevent the use of certain psychotropic medications) as well as on other factors including the child's age, availability of trained clinicians, and/or family preferences.

Psychoeducation of the child and family regarding depression is the critical first step of all treatment approaches whether psychotherapeutic or psychopharmacologic. Explaining the symptoms of depression, its expected course and the available treatments to the child and family is necessary to ensure their active participation and collaboration in the intervention.

■ PSYCHOTHERAPEUTIC INTERVENTIONS

The psychological distress resulting from a medical condition can lead to feelings of sadness or anger and a transient depression. Supportive psychotherapy in this context can be used to help child and family develop coping mechanisms to better manage the medical condition and its associated life changes. Specific challenges that are present in the face of medical illness and need to be taken into consideration in the course of psychotherapy include loss of independence, loss of control, diminished low self-esteem, as well as significant changes to the child and family's plans for the future. Medical procedures can further impact children and families through experiences of pain, loss of bodily integrity, and resultant cosmetic effects (e.g., scars or amputations).[79] These factors present challenges to the mental health clinician who has to help the child express feelings about the medical condition and accompanying treatments, and enhance the child's understanding of the process while also helping child and family develop new future goals that may need to take into account new physical limitations.

In mild forms of depression, supportive psychotherapy is as efficacious as other therapeutic modalities, such as cognitive behavioral therapy (CBT) or interpersonal therapy (IPT).[17,80] Supportive psychotherapy in the context of medical illness can be used to provide problem-solving, particularly around treatment adherence, restoration of hope and development of coping strategies.

When symptoms do not respond to supportive treatment or when the symptoms are deemed to be more severe, then CBT or IPT should be considered. The effects of psychotherapy in the treatment of adolescent depression are modest,[81] and CBT and IPT appear more effective in the treatment of moderate depression than supportive management.[17,82,83,84] In children with illnesses, CBT techniques for depression often aim to identify maladaptive cognitions about the physical illness and/or its treatment that may lead to the development and maintenance of depressed mood. For example a child with obesity may feel inherently at fault for his or her condition and therefore become hopeless about the proposed weight loss plan. Identifying the distorted thoughts and helping the child generate alternative explanations may promote treatment adherence and lessen the burden of the depressed mood. Severe depression accompanied by intense suicidality and hopelessness generally requires the addition of psychopharmacology. Other indications for the use of psychotropic medication include moderate

TABLE 20-3 Prescribing Considerations in Specific Childhood Medical Illnesses

Illness	Considerations
Hepatic disease	– Drug distribution and clearance changes – Increased serum drug levels
Gastrointestinal disease	– Drug absorption – Drug-induced GI side effects (i.e., anticholinergic-induced gastroparesis)
Renal disease	– Effects of hemodialysis (decreased drug plasma levels followed by rebound after dialysis) – Starting doses at 2/3 the regular dose
Cardiac disease	– Decreased perfusion of absorption sites – Drug-induced cardiac side effects (i.e., hypotension, QTc prolongation)

depression that has not responded to CBT or IPT; lack of trained CBT or IPT clinicians; and/or child and family preference.

■ **PSYCHOPHARMACOLOGIC TREATMENT**

Although psychopharmacologic treatment is an important intervention that can significantly reduce the burden of depression in children,[85] several factors should be taken into account when prescribing medications to children with medical illnesses. First, it is important to remember that "children are not little adults," when it comes to pharmacokinetics (effects of the body on the drug, i.e., absorption and elimination, etc.) and pharmacodynamics (effects of the drug on the body, i.e., receptor binding). Dosing adjustments must be considered. For example, drug metabolism that is primarily dependent on the liver may be different in children who have lower levels of drug-metabolizing enzymes and different metabolizing capacities. This can result in either higher or lower drug plasma levels depending on the drugs pharmacokinetic properties.[86]

The physical illness that afflicts the child has to be taken into account when it comes to psychopharmacologic interventions to avoid adverse interactions (**Table 20-3**). For example, illnesses that affect the liver (i.e., cirrhosis) can affect its ability to metabolize medications and thereby elevate their plasma levels. At the same time treatment of the underlying medical condition has to be taken into consideration when prescribing psychotropic medications to avoid drug–drug interactions. Antidepressants for example inhibit the cytochrome P450 system and can therefore raise levels of other medications by inhibiting their metabolism.

The effectiveness of psychopharmacological treatments for depression in medically ill adults has been well established.[49] The most evidence for the treatment of depression in children has been gathered for selective serotonin receptor inhibitors (SSRIs), and particularly Fluoxetine, which is approved by the U.S. Food and Drug Administration (FDA) for treatment of youths.[17] While dosing of antidepressants is similar to that of adults, the American Academy of Child and Adolescent Psychiatry recommends low initial doses and avoidance of early dose adjustments to minimize side effects.[17]

In general, SSRIs are well tolerated by children and the side effect profile is similar to that of adults. Because of differences in pharmacokinetic properties however, children may metabolize some of the shorter-acting SSRIs faster than adults, which makes them more prone to daily serotonin withdrawal symptoms.[17] This can be avoided by using fluoxetine, which has a long half-life that does not appear to be significantly altered in the pediatric population. Given the FDA black box warning and the small but significant association between antidepressants and suicidality,[87] the early phases of antidepressant treatment should include close monitoring of the patient for the emergence of suicidal thoughts. It is important to note here that the clinical significance of the association between antidepressants and suicidality has yet to be determined.[87] Therefore, given the data indicating that suicide rates have dramatically decreased with the rising use of antidepressants in children,[88] prescribers should not be deterred from using antidepressants when clinically warranted.

CONCLUSION

Children with medical illness are at greater risk for the development of depression. Despite the high rates of co-occurrence, depression is often misdiagnosed and undertreated. A developmentally informed biopsychosocial approach to the psychiatric evaluation of medically ill children is important for the accurate diagnosis and differentiation of their depressed mood, which can stem from a primary depressive disorder, a depressive disorder in reaction to medical illness, or a secondary depressive disorder due to a general medical condition. Depression and medical illness in children has a bi-directional relationship such that the direct effect of each illness can worsen the severity and outcome of the other illness. Strong evidence is emerging that supports the effectiveness of psychotherapies for mood disorders in medically ill children; there is somewhat less evidence about the effectiveness of psychopharmacology in this population.[18] Given that troubling depressive symptoms can significantly complicate medical treatment, they should be identified early and treated aggressively.

REFERENCES

1. Van Cleave J, Gortmaker SL, Perrin JM. Dynamics of obesity and chronic health conditions among children and youth. *JAMA*. 2010;303(7):623–630.

2. The National Survey of Children with Special Health Care Needs Chartbook 2005–2006. In: Services USDoHaH, ed. Rockville, MD: U.S.: Department of Health and Human Services; 2007.

3. Halfon N, Newacheck PW. Evolving notions of childhood chronic illness. *JAMA*. 2010;303(7):665–666.

4. Compas BE, Jaser SS, Dunn MJ, Rodriguez EM. Coping with chronic illness in childhood and adolescence. *Annu Rev Clin Psychol*. 2012;8:455–480.

5. American Academy of Pediatrics Committee on Children With Disabilities and Committee on Psychosocial Aspects of Child and Family Health: Psychosocial risks of chronic health conditions in childhood and adolescence. *Pediatrics*. 1993;92(6): 876–878.

6. Wamboldt MZ, Wamboldt FS. Role of the family in the onset and outcome of childhood disorders: Selected research findings. *J Am Acad Child Adolesc Psychiatry*. 2000;39(10):1212–1219.

7. Shaw SR, McCabe PC. Hospital-to-school transition for children with chronic illness: meeting the new challenges of an evolving health care system. *Psychol Sch*. 2008;45(1):74–87.

8. Fekkes M, Pijpers FI, Fredriks AM, Vogels T, Verloove-Vanhorick SP. Do bullied children get ill, or do ill children get bullied? A prospective cohort study on the relationship between bullying and health-related symptoms. *Pediatrics*. 2006;117(5): 1568–1574.

9. Burke P, Elliott M. Depression in pediatric chronic illness: A diathesis-stress model. *Psychosomatics*. 1999;40(1):5–17.

10. Wallander JL, Thompson RJ, Alriksson-Schmidt A. Psychosocial adjustment of children with chronic physical conditions. In: Roberts MC, ed. *Handbook of Pediatric Psychology*. 3rd ed. New York, NY: Guilford; 2003:141–158.

11. Lavigne JV, Faier-Routman J. Psychological adjustment to pediatric physical disorders: a meta-analytic review. *J Pediatr Psychol*. 1992;17(2):133–157.

12. Stuber ML. Psychiatric sequelae in seriously ill children and their families. *Psychiatr Clin North Am*. 1996;19(3):481–493.

13. Pinquart M, Shen Y. Behavior problems in children and adolescents with chronic physical illness: A meta-analysis. *J Pediatr Psychol*. 2011;36(9):1003–1016.

14. Bennett DS. Depression among children with chronic medical problems: A meta-analysis. *J Pediatr Psychol*. 1994;19(2):149–169.

15. Barlow JH, Ellard DR. The psychosocial well-being of children with chronic disease, their parents and siblings: an overview of the research evidence base. *Child Care Health Dev*. 2006; 32(1):19–31.

16. Birmaher B, Arbelaez C, Brent D. Course and outcome of child and adolescent major depressive disorder. *Child Adolesc Psychiatr Clin N Am*. 2002;11(3):619–637, x.

17. Birmaher B, Brent D, Bernet W, et al. Practice parameter for the assessment and treatment of children and adolescents with depressive disorders. *J Am Acad Child Adolesc Psychiatry*. 2007;46(11):1503–1526.

18. Benton T, DeMaso D. Mood disorders. In: Shaw RJ, DeMaso DR, eds. *Textbook of Pediatric Psychosomatic Medicine*. Washington, DC: American Psychiatric Publishing, Inc.; 2010:77–100.

19. LeBlanc LA, Goldsmith T, Patel DR. Behavioral aspects of chronic illness in children and adolescents. *Pediatr Clin North Am*. 2003;50(4):859–878.

20. Kokkonen J, Kokkonen ER. Prevalence of mental disorders in young adults with chronic physical diseases since childhood as identified by the Present State Examination and the CATEGO program. *Acta Psychiatr Scand*. 1993;87(4):239–243.

21. American Psychiatric Association. *Diagnostic and Statistical Manual of Mental Disorders*. 5th ed. Arlington, VA: American Psychiatric Association; 2013.

22. Shemesh E, Yehuda R, Rockmore L, et al. Assessment of depression in medically ill children presenting to pediatric specialty clinics. *J Am Acad Child Adolesc Psychiatry*. 2005;44(12):1249–1257.

23. Wolraich ML, Felice ME, Drotar D. *Classification of Child and Adolescent Mental Diagnoses in Primary Care, Child and Adolescent Version*. Elk Grove Village, IL: American Academy of Pediatrics; 1996.

24. Wells KB, Kataoka SH, Asarnow JR. Affective disorders in children and adolescents: addressing unmet needs in primary care settings. *Biol Psychiatry*. 2001;49:1111–1120.

25. Shaw RJ, DeMaso DR. *Clinical Manual of Pediatric Psychosomatic Medicine: Mental Health Consultation with Physically Ill Children and Adolescents*. Washington, DC: American Psychiatric Publishing, Inc.; 2006.

26. Goldman S, Shaw RJ, DeMaso DR. The pediatric psychosomatic medicine assessment. In: Shaw RJ, DeMaso DR, eds. *Textbook of Pediatric Psychosomatic Medicine*. Washington, DC: American Psychiatric Publishing, Inc; 2010.

27. Lewis M, Vitulano LA. Biopsychosocial issues and risk factors in the family when the child has a chronic illness. *Child Adolesc Psychiatr Clin N Am*. 2003;12(3):389–399.

28. DeMaso DR, Martini DR, Cahen LA, et al. Practice parameter for the psychiatric assessment and management of physically ill children and adolescents. *J Am Acad Child Adolesc Psychiatry*. 2009;48(2):213–233.

29. Melamed BG, Robbins RL, Fernandez J. Factors to be considered in psychological preparation for surgery. In: Routh D, Wolraich ML, ed. *Advances in Developmental and Behavioral Pediatrics*. New York, NY: JAI; 1982:51–72.

30. Simeonsson RJ, Buckley L, Munson L. Conceptions of illness causality in hospitalized children. *J Pediatr Psychol*. 1979;4: 77–84.

31. Eiser C. Children's concepts of illness: Towards an alternative to the "stage" approach. *Psychology & Health*. 1989;3(2): 93–101.

32. Piaget J. *The Child's Conception of the World*. New York, NY: Harcourt Brace; 1929.

33. Bibace R, Walsh ME. Children's conceptions of illness. In: Bibace R, Walsh ME, eds. *Children's Conceptions of Health Illness and Bodily Functions*. San Francisco, CA: Jossey-Bass; 1981.

34. Perrin EC, Gerrity PS. There's a demon in your belly: Children's understanding of illness. *Pediatrics*. 1981;67:841–849.

35. Perrin JM, Gnanasekaran S, Delahaye J. Psychological aspects of chronic health conditions. *Pediatr Rev*. 2012;33(3):99–109.

36. Carter B, McGoldrick M. Overview: the expanded family life cycle. In: Carter B, McGoldrick M, eds. *The Expanded Family Life Cycle: Individual, Family and Social Perspectives*, 3rd ed. Boston, MA: Allyn and Bacon; 2005:1–26.

37. Hughes D, Kleespies P. Suicide in the Medically Ill. *Suicide Life Threat Behav*. 2001;31:48–59.

38. Goldston DB, Kovacs M, Ho VY, Parrone PL, Stiffler L. Suicidal ideation and suicide attempts among youth with insulin-dependent diabetes mellitus. *J Am Acad Child Adolesc Psychiatry*. 1994; 33(2):240–246.

39. Robins LN. Suicide attempts in teen-aged medical patients. *Report of the Secretary's Task Force on Youth Suicide*. Vol 4: Strategies for the Prevention of Youth Suicide. Washington, DC: US Government Printing Office; 1989.

40. Beautrais AL, Joyce PR, Mulder RT. Risk factors for serious suicide attempts among youths aged 13 through 24 years. *J Am Acad Child Adolesc Psychiatry*. 1996;35(9):1174–1182.

41. Poznanski E, Mokros H. *Children's Depression Rating Scale- Revised (CDRS-R)*. Los Angeles, CA: WPS; 1996.

42. Nomura Y, Wickramaratne PJ, Warner V, Mufson L, Weissman MM. Family discord, parental depression, and psychopathology in offspring: ten-year follow-up. *J Am Acad Child Adolesc Psychiatry*. 2002;41(4):402–409.

43. Weissman MM, Wickramaratne P, Nomura Y, et al. Families at high and low risk for depression: a 3-generation study. *Arch Gen Psychiatry*. 2005;62(1):29–36.

44. Pao M, Bosk A. Anxiety in medically ill children/adolescents. *Depress Anxiety*. 2011;28(1):40–49.

45. McClellan J, Kowatch R, Findling RL Work Group on Quality Issues. Practice parameter for the assessment and treatment of

children and adolescents with bipolar disorder. *J Am Acad Child Adolesc Psychiatry*. 2007;46(1):107–125.

46. Krishnan KR. Psychiatric and medical comorbidities of bipolar disorder. *Psychosom Med*. 2005;67:1–8.

47. Borowsky IW, Mozayeny S, Ireland M. Brief psychosocial screening at health supervision and acute care visits. *Pediatrics*. 2003; 112(1 Pt 1):129–133.

48. Gledhill J, Rangel L, Garralda E. Surviving chronic physical illness: psychosocial outcome in adult life. *Arch Dis Child*. 2000; 83(2):104–110.

49. Evans DL, Charney DS, Lewis L, et al. Mood disorders in the medically ill: scientific review and recommendations. *Biol Psychiatry*. 2005;58(3):175–189.

50. Freud A. The role of bodily illness in the mental life of children. *Psychoanal Study Child*. 1952;7:69–81.

51. Freyer DR, Kuperberg A, Sterken DJ, Pastyrnak SL, Hudson D, Richards T. Multidisciplinary care of the dying adolescent. *Child Adolesc Psychiatr Clin N Am*. 2006;15(3):693–715.

52. Block SD. Assessing and managing depression in the terminally ill patient. ACP-ASIM End-of-Life Care Consensus Panel. American College of Physicians—American Society of Internal Medicine. *Ann Intern Med*. 2000;132(3):209–218.

53. Perrin EC, Newacheck P, Pless IB, et al. Issues Involved in the Definition and Classification of Chronic Health Conditions. *Pediatrics*. 1993;91(4):787–793.

54. Akinbami LJ, Moorman JE, Liu X. *Asthma Prevalence, Health Care Use and Mortality: United States, 2005–2009*. In: NHSR, ed. Vol no. 32. Hyattsville, MD: National Center for Health Statistics; 2011.

55. Ortega AN, Huertas SE, Canino G, Ramirez R, Rubio-Stipec M. Childhood asthma, chronic illness, and psychiatric disorders. *J Nerv Ment Dis*. 2002;190(5):275–281.

56. Zielinski TA, Brown ES, Nejtek VA, Khan DA, Moore JJ, Rush AJ. Depression in asthma: prevalence and clinical implications. *Prim Care Companion J Clin Psychiatry*. 2000;2(5):153–158.

57. Galil N. Depression and asthma in children. *Curr Opin Pediatr*. 2000;12(4):331–335.

58. Shanahan L, Copeland WE, Worthman CM, Angold A, Costello EJ. Children with both asthma and depression are at risk for heightened inflammation. *J Pediatr*. 2013;163(5):1443–1447.

59. Ogden CL, Carroll MD, Kit BK, Flegal KM. Prevalence of obesity and trends in body mass index among US children and adolescents, 1999–2010. *JAMA*. 2012;307(5):483–490.

60. Reeves GM, Postolache TT, Snitker S. Childhood obesity and depression: connection between these growing problems in growing children. *Int J Child Health Hum Dev*. 2008;1(2): 103–114.

61. Waaler PE, Bloom BH, Skeidsvoll H, Mykletun A. Prevalence, classification and severity of epilepsy in children in western Norway. *Epilepsia*. 2000;41:802–810.

62. Eriksson KJ, Koivikko MJ. Prevalence, classification and severity of epilepsy and epileptic syndromes in children. *Epilepsia*. 1997; 38(12):1275–1282.

63. Davies S, Heyman I, Goodman R. A population survey of mental health problems in children with epilepsy. *Dev Med Child Neurol*. 2003;45:292–296.

64. Dunn DW, Austin JK, Huster GA. Symptoms of depression in adolescents with epilepsy. *J Am Acad Child Adolesc Psychiatry*. 1999;38(9):1132–1138.

65. Ekinci O, Titus JB, Rodopman AA, Berkem M, Trevathan E. Depression and anxiety in children and adolescents with epilepsy: Prevalence, risk factors, and treatment. *Epilepsy Behav*. 2009; 14(1):8–18.

66. Thome-Souza MS, Kuczynski E, Valente KD. Sertraline and fluoxetine: safe treatments for children and adolescents with epilepsy and depression. *Epilepsy Behav*. 2007;10(3):417–425.

67. Montgomery SA. Antidepressants and seizures: emphasis on newer agents and clinical implications. *Int J Clin Pract*. 2005; 59(12):1435–1440.

68. Jemal A, Siegel R, Ward E, Hao Y, Xu J, Thun MJ. Cancer statistics, 2009. *CA Cancer J Clin*. 2009;59(4):225–249.

69. Kersun LS, Elia J. Depressive symptoms and SSRI use in pediatric oncology patients. *Pediatr Blood Cancer*. 2007;49(7):881–887.

70. Apter A, Farbstein I, Yaniv I. Psychiatric aspects of pediatric cancer. *Child Adolesc Psychiatr Clin N Am*. 2003;12(3):473–492, vii.

71. Centers for Disease Control and Prevention. *National Diabetes Fact Sheet: national estimates and general information on diabetes and prediabetes in the United States*. Atlanta, GA: U.S. Department of Health and Human Services, Centers for Disease Control and Prevention, 2011.

72. Pinhas-Hamiel O, Zeitler P. The global spread of type 2 diabetes mellitus in children and adolescents. *J Pediatr*. 2005;146(5): 693–700.

73. Kovacs M, Goldston D, Obrosky DS, Bonar LK. Psychiatric disorders in youths with IDDM: rates and risk factors. *Diabetes Care*. 1997;20(1):36–44.

74. Lawrence JM, Standiford DA, Loots B, et al. Prevalence and correlates of depressed mood among youth with diabetes: the SEARCH for Diabetes in Youth study. *Pediatrics*. 2006;117(4):1348–1358.

75. Kovacs M, Mukerji P, Drash A, Iyengar S. Biomedical and psychiatric risk factors for retinopathy among children with IDDM. *Diabetes Care*. 1995;18(12):1592–1599.

76. Kovacs M, Mukerji P, Iyengar S, Drash A. Psychiatric disorder and metabolic control among youths with IDDM. *Diabetes Care*. 1996;19(4):318–323.

77. Jacobson AM, Hauser ST, Willett JB, et al. Psychological adjustment to IDDM: 10-year follow-up of an onset cohort of child and adolescent patients. *Diabetes Care*. 1997;20(5):811–818.

78. Hood KK, Huestis S, Maher A, Butler D, Volkening L, Laffel LM. Depressive symptoms in children and adolescents with type 1 diabetes: association with diabetes-specific characteristics. *Diabetes Care*. 2006;29(6):1389–1391.

79. Szigethy E, Noll RB. Individual psychotherapy. In: Shaw RJ, DeMaso DR, eds. *Textbook of Pediatric Psychosomatic Medicine*. Washington, DC: American Psychiatric Publishing, Inc.; 2010.

80. Renaud J, Brent DA, Baugher M, Birmaher B, Kolko DJ, Bridge J. Rapid response to psychosocial treatment for adolescent depression: a two-year follow-up. *J Am Acad Child Adolesc Psychiatry*. 1998;37(11):1184–1190.

81. Weisz JR, McCarty CA, Valeri SM. Effects of psychotherapy for depression in children and adolescents: a meta-analysis. *Psychol Bull*. 2006;132(1):132–149.

82. Barbe RP, Bridge J, Birmaher B, Kolko D, Brent DA. Suicidality and its relationship to treatment outcome in depressed adolescents. *Suicide Life Threat Behav*. 2004;34(1):44–55.

83. Mufson L, Dorta KP, Wickramaratne P, Nomura Y, Olfson M, Weissman MM. A randomized effectiveness trial of interpersonal psychotherapy for depressed adolescents. *Arch Gen Psychiatry*. 2004;61(6):577–584.

84. Szigethy E, Carpenter J, Baum E, et al. Case study: longitudinal treatment of adolescents with depression and inflammatory bowel disease. *J Am Acad Child Adolesc Psychiatry*. 2006;45(4):396–400.

85. Zito JM, Safer DJ, DosReis S, et al. Psychotropic practice patterns for youth: a 10-year perspective. *Arch Pediatr Adolesc Med*. 2003;157(1):17–25.

86. Fernandez E, Perez R, Hernandez A, Tejeda P, Arteta M, Ramos JT. Factors and mechanisms for pharmacokinetic differences between pediatric population and adults. *Pharmaceutics*. 2011;3:53–72.

87. Hammad TA, Laughren T, Racoosin J. Suicidality in pediatric patients treated with antidepressant drugs. *Arch Gen Psychiatry*. 2006;63(3):332–339.

88. Olfson M, Shaffer D, Marcus SC, Greenberg T. Relationship between antidepressant medication treatment and suicide in adolescents. *Arch Gen Psychiatry*. 2003;60(10):978–982.

89. Guite J, Kazak A. Anxiety symptoms and disorders. In: Shaw RJ, DeMaso DR, eds. *Textbook of Pediatric Psychosomatic Medicine*. Washington, DC: American Psychiatric Publishing; 2010.

CHAPTER 21

Depression in the Medically Ill Older Adult

Mark Eldaief, MD, MMSc
Hongtu Chen, PhD
Michael Gaziano, MD
Olivia Okereke, MD, SM

INTRODUCTION

■ OVERVIEW

Depression is among the most common health conditions affecting older adults. Depression may present in a phenotypically distinct manner in older, as opposed to younger, individuals. For example, in the older adult depression is less likely to present with dysphoria and more likely to be accompanied by irritability and somatic symptoms.[1] In addition, psychosocial stressors predisposing to the development of affective symptoms are different with advancing age (e.g., the stressor of losing a loved one becomes more common).[1] Still, one of the major factors affecting the inception and prognosis of depression in the older adult is the co-occurrence of medical conditions.

In this chapter, we will address common medical conditions with which coexistent depression is likely to occur in the older adult. We also will give attention to biological and psychosocial mechanisms that might give rise to both the depressive symptoms and the medical condition, and emphasize how this co-occurrence predicts poorer health outcomes for both conditions. We will then survey methods for screening older adults with medical illness for depression, and review methods of differentiating it from symptoms that could simulate it, but which are more likely due to the medical condition. Next, we explore pharmacologic and nonpharmacologic treatment approaches for major depressive illness in the setting of a medical condition, and survey the considerations that must be taken into account in older adults. Finally, we review future methods of treating depression in this clinical setting, including novel techniques for preventing depression in the medically ill older adult (**Table 21-1**).

■ EPIDEMIOLOGY OF DEPRESSION IN OLDER ADULTS AND ROLES OF MEDICAL COMORBIDITY

Overall, it is clear that the burden and health impacts of depression among older adults, particularly those with medical illness, are high, and that substantial numbers of cases occur in late-life. Current (12-month) prevalence of major depressive disorder and persistent depressive disorder (dysthymia)—is estimated at 2% to 4%.[2,3] However, when one considers presentations of subsyndromal or minor depressions, the current prevalence is much higher for older adults. In a comprehensive meta-analysis of many studies of community-based older adults, the current prevalence of any depressive disorder—major or minor—was estimated to be 13%.[2] Lifetime prevalence is much higher than current prevalence. As is observed in younger persons, there is a gender difference in the lifetime burden of depression such that the ratio of women to men affected is approximately 2:1. For example, one study estimated the lifetime prevalence of depression among men aged 65+ years at 9.6%; while, the lifetime prevalence among women of the same age was 20.4%.[3]

Another important epidemiological consideration is whether depression in the older adult is new in onset, or whether it represents a recrudescence of a prior mood disorder. In the former case, it is incumbent upon the clinician to search for medical conditions/medications that may be mimicking depression (see below), as well as to evaluate unique psychosocial factors related to aging. The distinction can also be important for prognostic reasons, as new onset depression in the elderly has been associated with greater treatment resistance and a worse overall prognosis.[4] An impactful study by Luijendijk et al.[5] demonstrated incidence rates of seven cases per 1,000 person-years for major depression and 19 cases per 1,000 person-years for combined minor and major depression. These rates

TABLE 21-1 Biological Factors Underlying Reciprocal Relationships Between Depression and Medical Illness in the Older Adult

Medical Condition	Biological Factors Linking Depression to the Medical Condition
Parkinson disease	Hypofunctionality of dopaminergic basal ganglia circuits, Lewy Body deposition in limbic regions, increased elaboration of cytokines, activation of the HPA axis, decreased neurotrophic factors and neurogenesis.[6]
Cerebrovascular disease	Disrupted white matter projections between limbic regions and prefrontal cortex[7]
Coronary artery disease	Altered heart rate variability, increased platelet aggregation, alterations in homocysteine metabolism, increases in catecholamine release, activation of the HPA axis, elevated immune response[8]
Cancer	Hypercalcemia from bone metastases, paraneoplastic syndromes (e.g., limbic encephalitis), endocrine abnormalities such as hypoadrenalism and hypothyroidism, depressogenic effects of chemotherapeutic agents (e.g., corticosteroids, vincristine, vinblastine, procarbazine, interferons), depressogenic effects of whole brain radiation.[9]

are comparable to incidence rates of other major diseases in this age group, such as myocardial infarction, stroke, and breast cancer. Furthermore, older people are affected by high recurrence rates of depression—given that depressive episodes in earlier life are a risk factor for depression later in life. Thus, recurrence outpaces incidence by 3 to 4 to 1; overall recurrence rates were 27 cases per 1,000 person-years for major depression and 66 cases per 1,000 person-years for minor and major depressions combined.[5]

This high prevalence of depression in older adults has substantial implications for healthcare costs. For example, in a study of Medicare beneficiaries,[10] patients with depression had significantly higher total healthcare costs than those without ($20,046 compared to $1,196; p< .01). Importantly, the magnitude of the difference in healthcare costs associated with depression was higher with increasing levels of medical comorbidity, as measured by the Charlson index.[10] The costs associated with depression treatment per se were only a small fraction of the incremental healthcare costs. Therefore, results support that, in addition to their benefits for the quality of life, adequate treatment of depression in medically ill older persons could be an important moderator of health care costs.

■ CO-OCCURRENCE OF MEDICAL ILLNESS AND DEPRESSION AMONG OLDER ADULTS

Major depression commonly coexists with other medical conditions. Depression and medical illness often share common biopsychosocial antecedents, and each can impact the clinical course of the other in a deleterious manner. Katon[8] outlined several of the bidirectional influences of depression and medical illness. First, depression is a risk factor for the development of medical illness. In some cases, this causal influence is readily apparent. For example, depression may give rise to poor health habits (such as smoking, an insalubrious diet and/or a sedentary lifestyle), which can serve as risk factors for the development of cardiovascular and cerebrovascular disease. Second, medical illness may catalyze the onset of depression. Thus, the presence of at least one chronic medical condition significantly increases the risk of having depression.[11] In some cases, depression may be an effective

response to the psychological stress of having a medical condition, particularly chronic, painful, and debilitating or life-threatening conditions.[12] Alternatively, certain medical conditions likely induce depression through neurobiological mechanisms. This is supported by the fact that select medical illnesses appear to produce depressive symptoms significantly more commonly than others causing similar amounts of disability and mortality. Moreover, coexistent neurological illnesses can have direct effects upon corticolimbic brain networks that regulate mood. In addition, the medications used to treat a medical illness may themselves have depressogenic actions. Finally, a given medical condition might induce depression through indirect effects on the central nervous system (CNS). For example, proinflammatory cytokines such as interleukin-6 (IL-6), which may be elaborated in the setting of medical disease, are capable of traversing the blood–brain barrier and of stimulating the hypothalamic–pituitary–adrenal (HPA) axis.[7] Given the high proportion of older adults with medical morbidities, all of the above-mentioned potential paths to depression are noteworthy in this population.

MEDICAL COMORBIDITIES AND DEPRESSION

■ IMPLICATIONS OF COMORBIDITY AMONG OLDER ADULTS

In the older adult, the interplay between depression and medical illness is amplified. Depression is increasingly prevalent with advanced age, especially in hospitalized elders.[13] Greater medical comorbidity is associated with more severe depression in the elderly, and with greater utilization of medical resources.[13,14] Several factors increase the strength of this relationship between depression and medical illness in the older adult: (1) the increased likelihood of having one or more chronic medical conditions in individuals over the age of 65;[8] (2) the increased likelihood of functional impairment resulting from a given medical condition; (3) medication factors such as polypharmacy, changes in pharmacokinetics and increases in drug–drug interactions; (4) a higher risk that a given medical illness will directly and/or indirectly impact affective brain networks; (5) changes in neuroendocrine and neuroinflammatory function[12] as well as changes in neuroplasticity[14] with advanced age; (6) changes in sleep architecture;[15] and (7) changes in the nature and extent of certain psychosocial stressors in later life.

Identifying depression in the older adult with medical illness can be challenging, in part because many medical conditions cause symptoms that mirror depressive somatic symptoms (such as apathy, nonspecific physical complaints, fatigue, and anergia). Nonetheless, increasing awareness of the association between depression and medical illness in the older adult is critical, because depression increases the morbidity and mortality of the comorbid medical illness, and because chronic medical conditions are known to increase the morbidity of co-occurring depression.

■ SPECIFIC MEDICAL CONDITIONS WHICH COEXIST WITH DEPRESSION IN THE OLDER ADULT
Depression in Neurological Illness

Certain neurological conditions can induce depressive symptoms by directly disrupting homeostatic neurobiological mechanisms that regulate mood. Specifically, this could occur through alteration of neurotransmitter levels, disruption of anatomical and/or functional connections among corticolimbic networks, and modulation of neuroplasticity (e.g., by changing the expression of trophic factors). Neurological conditions affecting such neurobiological changes become increasingly common with advanced age.

For example, the association between neurodegenerative disease and depression is well supported. When coexistent with depression, cognitive symptoms and signs can be mistaken for a dementing illness—a condition referred to historically as "pseudodementia."

Cognitive deficits induced by mood symptoms can be distinguished from a true neurodegenerative condition by a patient's neuropsychological profile. Depression is associated with dysfunction of frontal-subcortical circuits, and presents with psychomotor slowing, frontally based memory deficits and executive dysfunction[12] In contrast, Alzheimer disease (AD) is typically also attended by deficits with memory consolidation, language deficits and loss of semantic knowledge. In addition, the extent of cognitive impairment can be helpful to differentiate depression from dementia. Finally, the two conditions can be differentiated through the use of biomarkers, such as structural and functional neuroimaging and CSF analysis.

Depressive symptoms can also co-occur with diagnostically established neurodegenerative conditions. In some cases, this occurs because depression and dementia affect shared neural circuits. For example, apathy is a common symptom in depression, frontotemporolobar degeneration and AD. Full depressive symptomatology can also accompany neurodegenerative illnesses. For instance, approximately 35% of patients with Parkinson disease[16] have clinical depression,[6] and the incidence of this is higher than in other chronic debilitating disorders. One explanation for this association is that changes in monoaminergic neurotransmission, specifically dysfunction of dopaminergic basal ganglia relays, predispose PD patients to depressive symptoms (e.g., anhedonia). Lewy body deposition in limbic regions may also contribute to depressive symptoms.[6] The presence of depression in PD is associated with greater physical disability and increased cognitive decline.[17] Finally, it is now well recognized that major depression can be a prodromal condition of PD, predating its presentation by years or decades.[6] Comorbidity between depression and AD is less well established, with some studies suggesting that premorbid depression is a strong predictor of the development of amnestic dementia, and others finding no such relationship.[18] It does appear, however, that individuals with AD are more likely than matched controls to be depressed. Also, similar to PD, the presence of depression in AD is predictive of greater functional decline and overall disability.

Cerebrovascular disease is another factor that is consistently linked to the onset of late life depression. This has given rise to the "vascular depression hypothesis."[7] Cerebrovascular disease giving rise to depression can either take the form of a clinical stroke or occult subcortical white matter hyperintensities revealed on T2-weighted MRI. Several reports have found that late-life depression is more common in adults with high microvascular ischemic disease burden, as compared to age-matched controls. Also, microvascular ischemic disease burden has been preferentially tied to late-onset (as opposed to early-onset) depression, and the extent of this disease burden has been linked to depression severity.[7] Because leukoaraiosis tends to be highest in concentration in prefrontal subcortical white matter, depression due to microvascular ischemic disease presents with a similar neuropsychological profile of frontal-subcortical dysfunction. With respect to clinical strokes, post-stroke patients are more depressed than controls matched for level of functional disability, suggesting a neurobiological, as opposed to psychological, effect of the stroke on mood. Often, these strokes affect the left hemisphere preferentially and tend to involve the prefrontal cortex, the basal ganglia, or cortical-subcortical relays between these structures.[19] Still, following a clinical stroke it is often difficult to disentangle depressive symptoms, such as fatigue or apathy, from other common sequelae of cerebral infarction.[20] Moreover, the exact incidence of post-stroke depression, and the time course of the development of depressive symptoms after a stroke, vary considerably across studies-though it appears to be more evident in the months following an infarct.[20]

Depression and Cardiovascular Illness

Along similar lines, a rich literature now exists detailing a bidirectional relationship between cardiovascular disease and major depression. A myriad of studies have demonstrated that depression is a risk factor for the development of coronary artery disease (CAD), and that it is associated with increases in both the morbidity and the mortality of CAD. Depression predicts myocardial infarction and death, even when controlling for confounding factors which give rise to both CAD and depression (e.g., smoking and other behavioral patterns).[15] Conversely, up to one-third of adults suffering a myocardial infarction will develop depressive symptoms in the year following their cardiac event.[15]

Several mechanisms have been proposed to explicate this bidirectional association, including psychosocial and biological explanations. With respect to the former, older depressed individuals may have less healthy lifestyles, thus predisposing them to heart disease; and depressed individuals with established heart disease may be less likely to adhere to disease-modifying interventions. From a biological perspective, depression could catalyze the development of heart disease through centrally mediated changes in heart rate variability, increased recruitment of the HPA axis, increased inflammatory activation, increases in platelet aggregation or through increases in catecholamine release and sympathetic tone.[12,15] Finally, heart disease and depression may well share common genetic predeterminants, such as alterations in the methylenetetrahydrofolate reductase (MTHFR) gene, which is involved in homocysteine metabolism.[12]

Depression and Cancer

As is the case with other medical conditions, depression in the older adult can worsen the morbidity of cancer. Depression is more likely when a diagnosis of cancer is accompanied by the recent loss of a spouse, the prospect of poorly controlled pain or significant functional disability. Certain types of cancer are also more likely to be accompanied by depression in the older adult, including cancers of the pancreas, head and neck, and lung.[9] Several medications used to treat cancer in the older adult can induce depression (and cognitive changes). These include vincristine, vinblastine, procarbazine, corticosteroids and interferons. Radiotherapy, particularly whole brain radiation, can promote the development of neuropsychiatric symptoms as well.[9]

Depression and Other Medical Illnesses

An assortment of endocrine, pulmonary, renal, and gastrointestinal diseases tend to coexist with depression,[15] and many of these are exacerbated in the older adult. Although somewhat controversial, some authors have posited that declining testosterone levels in older men play a causative role in the development of late-life depression. Others have ascribed a role to decreases in thyroxine levels. Several studies indicate that diabetes and insulin resistance are risk factors for depression.[21] Depression is also more common in older adults suffering from chronic obstructive pulmonary disease (COPD), especially in the setting of oxygen dependence and during periods of COPD exacerbation.[15] Moreover, depression is quite common in end-stage renal disease (ESRD) with prevalence rates of approximately 21%.[15] There have also been links between depression and irritable bowel disease, osteoporosis, and obstructive sleep apnea.[12] Finally, depression has been linked to hearing and visual impairment in the older adult.[21]

ROLE OF DEPRESSION SCREENING IN MEDICALLY ILL OLDER ADULTS

The discussion below specifically focuses on screening for depression in elderly patients. A discussion of depression screening in general is found in Chapter 3.

■ DEPRESSION SCREENING FOR OLDER ADULTS IN PRIMARY CARE

There are important clinical benefits of screening for depression among older adults in medical settings, such as primary care. First, older adults have the highest risk of suicide of all age groups, which is a major public health concern for communities and the nation,[22] and most of these suicidal patients experience depression episodes prior to suicidal attempt. Nearly 50% to 75% of older adults who commit suicide have seen their primary care doctors for medical care during the preceding month, and about 40% saw their doctors during the week prior to their death.[23] Therefore, screening for depression in primary care practice and treating it is a central component of suicide prevention.[22] Second, screening may help clinicians identify older patients earlier in their course of depression. Third, screening may identify patients who may have been previously diagnosed with depression but were ineffectively treated—suggesting the need for modification of treatment.

Depression in older adults can be difficult to diagnose in primary care for a number of reasons:[24,25]

- Multiple medications: Many medications can cause symptoms of depression, such as fatigue, loss of energy insomnia or hypersomnia, appetite change, weight loss, and difficulty concentrating.
- Multiple comorbidities: Depressive screening for older adults is often complicated by comorbid medical conditions that increase in incidence with longevity
- Cognitive or functional impairment: Communication deficits such as hearing impairments, poor vision, and speech problems, or early onset of dementia can all complicate the screening process.
- Reporting bias: Reluctance of older people or family members to complain about problems because of concerns of being ignored, stigmatized, or generating additional, burdensome medical care costs.

■ CURRENT EVIDENCE AND RECOMMENDATIONS FOR DEPRESSION SCREENING

As many as three-quarters of primary care settings performed mental health screening, including screening for depression for older adults[26] in 2010. However, other studies suggest that up to 30~40% of depression cases are missed by primary care providers.[27]

Depression screening for older adults in clinical practice has been recommended.[26] This recommendation is based on some evidence that screening improves the accurate identification of depressed patients in primary care and that treatment of these patients can decrease clinical morbidity. However, trials evaluating the effect of screening on clinical outcomes have shown mixed results: simply providing screening results to primary care clinicians resulted in small benefits, though the communication of screening results in combination with coordinated follow-up and treatment leads to larger benefits.

■ USE OF SCREENING TOOLS FOR ASSESSING DEPRESSION IN OLDER ADULTS

Given the high caseloads of primary care settings, both clinicians and patients prefer efficient depression screening tools. Below are some screening instruments that have been successfully used for detecting depressive symptoms in older adults during primary care.

PHQ-9

The 9-item Patient Health Questionnaire (PHQ-9) is an effective and efficient depression screening tool for older adults in primary care settings.[28] The PHQ-9 was also successfully used to identify depression in homebound older adults.[29] Medicare integrated the full PHQ-9 into the revised Minimum Data Set assessments (MDS 3.0) for nursing home residents.[30]

CES-D

The 20-item standard Center for Epidemiologic Studies Depression Scale (CES-D) has been extensively used and studied, and is considered a reliable valid instrument and a widely recognized research tool for assessing levels of depressive symptoms in adult populations. Specifically in older adults, the CES-D is excellent a screening instrument for major depression.[31] The CES-D can also be used to screen for both depression and anxiety disorders at the same time in very old populations.[32] The abbreviated 10-item version of the CES-D[33] has excellent properties for use as a screening instrument in older adults, while requiring 5 minutes less than the standard 20-item CES-D. However, it should be noted that the CES-D items do not assess the diagnostic criteria items of appetite, anhedonia, guilt, or suicidality.

GDS-15

The Geriatric Depression Scale is a self-report instrument measuring depressive symptoms in older adults.[34] The original 30-item version[35] has been reduced to a short version (GDS-15) with a yes/no response format to decrease fatigue or lack of focus seen in the elderly.[36] The scale is designed to identify symptoms that distinguish depression in the elderly from dementia. The GDS is comprised of the affective (e.g., sadness, apathy, crying) and cognitive (e.g., thoughts of hopelessness, helplessness, guilt, worthlessness) symptoms of depression in the elderly. It contains none of the somatic items (e.g., disturbances in appetite, sleep, energy level, and sexual interest) that are potentially important confounds in older adults.[24] Compared with younger depressed adults, depressed elderly tend to present more often with somatic symptoms (e.g., general and gastrointestinal somatic symptoms), agitation and hypochondriasis, and less guilt and loss of sexual interest.[37]

BDI (or BDI-II)

The Beck Depression Inventory (BDI) is a valid instrument for the diagnosis of depression in older adults.[38] It is composed of cognitive, affective, somatic, and vegetative symptoms of depression. The 7-item BDI–PC is an abbreviated primary care version of the BDI–II, but it has not been specifically tested in elderly medical patients.[39] This self-report scale is generally regarded as a cost-effective option for screening depression in elderly medical patients, but there are concerns about overlapping symptoms between medical conditions and the depressive somatic symptoms in BDI.[40] Moreover, some elderly individuals may not be able to complete the scale due to reading difficulty, physical debility, or compromised cognitive functioning.[41]

DEPRESSION ASSESSMENT IN MEDICALLY ILL OLDER ADULTS

■ APPROACH TO THE DIAGNOSIS OF DEPRESSION IN THE MEDICALLY ILL ODER ADULT

One of the most challenging tasks in detecting depression in the medically ill older adult is distinguishing the symptoms of true affective illness from those of medical disorder. Fatigue, anergia, anorexia, sleep disturbance and apathy can all be due to medical conditions in the elderly. This can lead to misattribution of the medical symptoms to depression. As such, routine tests to exclude a medical condition causing a patient's symptoms are recommended. Among these are evaluations of anemia, hypothyroidism and B12 deficiency.[1] Of equal concern, a diagnosis of depression can be missed if a provider attributes these symptoms solely to the comorbid medical condition, since depression often presents in the older adult with prominent somatic symptoms.[9] One useful approach is to probe for more specific symptoms, such as anhedonia, hopelessness (e.g., hopelessness for the future), frequent crying, pronounced self-reproach/guilt, psychosis, and passive or active suicidal ideation. Structured clinical interviews and selected diagnostic batteries can be helpful in discriminating depression from the symptoms commonly associated with advanced aging, and those of comorbid medical conditions.

TABLE 21-2 Psychological, Social, and Medical Risk and Predisposing Factors for Depression

Psychological and Social Risk Factors	Medical Conditions and Medications as Risk Factors
• Being female • Social isolation, or lack of a supportive social network • Recent loss of a loved one (especially spouse) or other major adverse life-event • Family history of major depressive disorder	• Cerebrovascular disease, coronary heart disease, endocrine disorders (including diabetes, thyroid disease and adrenal insufficiency), sleep disturbance, Parkinson disease, and cancer • Significant physical/functional impairment or mobility limitation, including loss of body part due to medical operation (e.g., amputation, cancer surgery) • Chronic or severe pain • Certain medicines or combinations of medicines (corticosteroids, alcohol, benzodiazepines, narcotics; other CNS depressants; levodopa; antihypertensives; certain cancer chemotherapeutic agents) • Alcohol and/or substance abuse • Previous history of depression or past suicide attempt(s)

■ CURRENT APPROACHES TO DIAGNOSIS AMONG OLDER ADULTS IN PRIMARY CARE

Screening instruments are not sufficient for diagnosing depression, but do indicate the need for more detailed follow-up by a clinician to determine whether the individual meets diagnostic criteria for a depressive disorder, to explore other possible causes for depression (such as medication or substance use), and assess for co-existing psychiatric disorders.

In some patients, it can be difficult to attain an accurate diagnosis of depression in older adults. There are several things to consider:

(1) Fully use the results from assessment tools: Depression screening instruments inform the clinicians about the likelihood of having depression. Some instruments, such as PHQ-9 or GDS-15, have clear cutoff points that, based on empirical evidence, are highly predictive of the diagnosis of major depression. If the screening score is very far above or below the cutoff point, the chance is high that the screening result can be used to obtain or eliminate a diagnosis, with the understanding that it does not replace a formal diagnosis. If the screening result is close to the cutoff point, further assessment often is needed.

(2) Clinical diagnostic interview: With adequate training, and if time is available, primary care providers can conduct a clinical interview, using either an observer-rated instrument, such as the SCID (Structured Clinical Interview for the Diagnostic and Statistical Manual of Mental Disorders [DSM]),[47] or following a reliable process for assessing DSM diagnostic criteria. Many primary care physicians may not have the time or the requisite skills, and prefer a referral to a mental health or geriatric specialist.

(3) Assessing risk factors for depression: At least half of older adults who present with depression have no previous history of depression, suggesting that different pathological mechanisms may be involved in "late-onset depression." Late-onset depression may be associated with specific comorbid diseases, poor physical health, cognitive impairment and structural changes in the brain. Older people with depression who have experienced an episode earlier in life are more likely to have a family history of mental illness. Factors that have been associated with increased risk of depression in the elderly are presented in **Table 21-2**.

Nonetheless, the diagnosis of depression in older people can be challenging when comorbid cognitive impairments (e.g., delirium and dementia) and comorbid physical illness coexist with depression. Sometimes, the symptoms of depression may be similar to those of a chronic illness, such as cancer, and may both warrant treatment. Depressive symptoms, such as feelings of worthlessness, may lead to not complaining of physical illness or not asking for help, and the result may worsen noncompliance with medication and other treatments, foster self-neglect or nonattendance at clinics, which in turn may worsen depression.[43]

The difficulty of achieving accurate diagnosis and effective management of depression in older adults requires or competes for the primary care physician's attention during a time-limited office visit. Therefore, it is critical to develop a systematic approach for managing these patients. Some even argue that depression screening alone may not improve health outcomes unless there are resources available to ensure accurate diagnosis, treatment, and follow-up for patients screening positive.[44–46]

Tools to Aid Assessment of Depression in Older Adults

Table 21-3 summarizes the characteristics and strengths of several depression screening instruments that are commonly used for assessing older adults in primary care settings. In addition to concerns about the correspondence between a screening tool and the DSM criteria, and whether screening instruments can serve as a proxy for diagnosis of major depression (see section below), there are several things to consider when selecting an instrument for assessing depression in elderly medical patients. One involves the somatic symptoms that should not be eliminated when assessing depression in older adults. Omitting the somatic items may lead to under-diagnosing of depression.[47]

TABLE 21-3 Depression Screening Instruments and Respective Strengths

Screening Instrument	Number of Items	Response Format	Strengths[a]				
			DSM-Criteria Based	Including Somatic Symptoms	Including Suicidal Ideation	Having a Diagnostic Cutoff	Respondent Burden (Time to Complete)
PHQ-9	9	0–3	√	√	√	√	<3 min
GDS-15	15	Yes/No	No	No	No	√	2–5 min
CESD-10	10	Yes/No, or 0–3	No	√	No	No	2–7 min
BDI-II	21	0–3	√	√	√	√	5–10 min
CES-D	20	0–3	No	√	No	No	7–12 min

[a]Note: All scales in this table have shown satisfactory to excellent psychometric properties including sensitivity, specificity, validity and reliability.

Another is the inclusion of the item(s) for assessing suicidal ideation. Given the high prevalence of suicidality among older adults, it is critical to screen for suicidal ideation while screening for depression. However, the information gleaned requires clinicians to respond immediately if the screening result indicates positive on the suicidal item.[23]

The third concern is the respondent burden associated with screening. This can be a concern especially, when busy primary care clinicians often expect the elderly person to complete the screen without assistance. Some scales (e.g., BDI, CES-D) are more wordy and cognitively complex than others, which challenges elderly medical patients often with visual deficit and compromised reading ability due to medical illness and other functional impairments.[48]

TREATMENT CONSIDERATIONS FOR DEPRESSION IN MEDICALLY ILL OLDER ADULTS

■ PHARMACOLOGIC APPROACHES
General Principles

There are important general considerations when prescribing antidepressants in the elderly. First, allowances should be made for age-related changes in the ability or speed of drug processing. Slower rates of metabolism (i.e., by hepatic enzyme action), differences in protein binding (e.g., among protein-depleted, medically ill elderly), or alterations in drug clearance due to even mild renal impairment should be considered in the initiation, titration, and maintenance of pharmacotherapy. For example, adjustments by as much as 50% may be required in the starting doses, the titration speeds or the target doses used for older, medically ill patients; however, some clinical judgment is required to determine the extent to which dose adjustment is warranted based on a given patient's constellation of comorbidities.

Second, there are some adverse effects that can be particularly problematic in older populations. For instance, orthostatic hypotension is the cause of significant morbidity in older adults. Another major cause of morbidity in older individuals is agents with anticholinergic properties. Many older persons are vulnerable to confusion when exposed to anticholinergic burden, even in the absence of clinical dementia.[49–52]

Third, older adults benefit from the same principles of rational pharmacologic practice that serve patients of all ages: namely, doses should be increased to the maximum tolerable level necessary to achieve the target effect and should be maintained for a minimum therapeutic duration. Thus, although it may be necessary to lower the starting dose or to apply a slower speed of dose titration, it is important always to treat the older patient with these principles of rational pharmocotherapy in mind. Although a well-known axiom in geriatric pharmacology is to "start low and go slow," this can unfortunately result in many older patients' being treated for too long with subtherapeutic doses of medications. Although caution is indicated when choosing a low starting dose or a slow titration schedule, dose escalation should not stop short of the dosage strength that would have any reasonable expectation of efficacy—provided that the drug is tolerated.

Third, with few exceptions, antidepressant pharmacotherapy in the elderly will be conducted in the presence of other nonpsychotropic medications. Thus, managing polypharmacy and monitoring for its potential hazards are essential.

Antidepressant Agent Choices and Consideration of Side Effects and Interactions

A list of commonly prescribed antidepressants that have been specifically studied in older adults is provided in **Table 21-4**. Agents are arranged by class, and special considerations among older persons, both within drug class and for individual compounds, are addressed. Although many antidepressants are available for the treatment of the older adult, Table 21-4 focuses on those agents and doses that have been examined specifically in trials with older patients. The dose ranges in Table 21-4 reflect commonly suggested and applied doses for older persons, based on published trials and/or safety data.

Selective serotonin reuptake inhibitors (SSRIs) are the first-line, approved agents for pharmacologic treatment of depression. Among the SSRIs, citalopram, escitalopram, and sertraline are regarded as safe for use in older patients and show low to minimal cytochrome P450 interaction potential; however, the recent advisory regarding dose limitations for citalopram to 20 mg/day among persons aged 60+ years may create a relative ceiling on how high doses can be advanced in this population. Fluoxetine, paroxetine and fluvoxamine are also available for use in older persons, but they carry a higher likelihood of drug–drug interactions. An important consideration for all SSRIs is an increased risk of gastrointestinal bleeding, particularly in persons predisposed due to concurrent administration of anticoagulants or nonsteroidal anti-inflammatory agents, which can be frequent in older adults.[49–52]

Serotonin-norepinephrine reuptake inhibitors (SNRIs) are also efficacious among older adults (see **Table 21-4**). Duloxetine also has an indication for treatment of pain conditions; this feature has potential utility in addressing depression among older, medically ill persons with comorbid pain disorders.[49,51,53]

The earliest widely used antidepressants, TCAS, also have demonstrated efficacy among older people. However, the side effect profile of this class—particularly, their potential proarrhythmic and anticholinergic actions—are important to consider. Nortriptyline and desipramine have both been well studied in the elderly and have relatively less anticholinergic activity.

Other antidepressants that have been studied for use in older patients include mirtazapine, nefazodone, bupropion, and the monoamine oxidase inhibitor (MAOI) tranylcypromine. Among these, nefazodone has been noted for safety concerns regarding increased risk of liver toxicity. Bupropion, as a noradrenergic-dopaminergic agent, may have useful stimulating and cognitive-enhancing properties among older patients. A caution with the administration of the MAOIs is the risk of serotonin-syndrome (with concurrent use of contraindicated drugs, including SSRIs, SNRIs, and TCAs) and of hypertensive crises upon ingestion of tyramine-containing foods; therefore, a "washout" period between switching to/from MAOIs and other agents is necessary.[49,50,54–60]

Finally, there is a literature on antidepressant augmentation strategies that have been employed among older persons. While many of these medications do not have Food and Drug Administration-approved indications in the treatment of depression, either as primary or adjunctive therapies, their note here reflects clinical practice. Two long-standing augmentation strategies that have been studied in older patients are the hormone levothyroxine (25–50 μg/day)[61] and the mood stabilizer lithium (dosed to achieve 0.4–1 mmol/L plasma concentration).[49,62,63] In recent years, several atypical antipsychotics (aripiprazole, risperidone, olanzapine, quetiapine) have been studied with regard to augmentation of antidepressant treatment in older patients.[16,62,64–67] Respective typical daily dose ranges for aripiprazole, risperidone, olanzapine, and quetiapine were: 2 to 15 mg/day, 0.25 to 1 mg/day, 2.5 to 15 mg/day, and 50 to 200 mg/day. Important potential side effects include weight gain, akathisia (particularly for aripiprazole and risperidone), somnolence and orthostatic hypotension, and some notable interaction potential exists for CYP 450 enzyme inhibitors, such as with fluoxetine, fluvoxamine, and paroxetine. Finally, a more augmentation tools have come in the form of nutritional agents that target one-carbon/homocysteine-reducing pathways, such as folate/folic acid or L-5-methyltetrahydrofolate.[68–70]

TABLE 21-4 Commonly Prescribed Antidepressants Among Older Adults

Drug	Type	Typical Dose Range (mg/day)	Key Side Effects	Key Interactions	Age Ranges Under Study	Citations
Selective Serotonin Reuptake Inhibitors						
Fluoxetine	SSRI	10–40	Hyponatremia (fatigue, delirium), GI effects (nausea, dry mouth, diarrhea), insomnia, agitation, headache, sexual dysfunction	SSRI inhibition of hepatic cytochrome P-450 isoenzymes affects medications that are metabolized by these isoenzymes (TCAs, steroids, benzodiazepines). Concurrent use with NSAIDs is associated with increased risk of upper GI bleeding.	≥60 years	49–50
Paroxetine	SSRI	10–40				
Citalopram	SSRI	10–20				
Escitalopram	SSRI	5–20				
Sertraline	SSRI	25–150				
Fluvoxamine	SSRI	25–100				
Tricyclic Antidepressants						
Nortriptyline	TCA	10–150	Postural hypotension, anticholinergic effects, cardiac abnormalities, sedation	MAOIs; SSRIs and other medications that inhibit the inhibit the hepatic cytochrome P-450 isoenzymes; anticholinergic agents	≥60 years	49–50
Amitriptyline	TCA	10–150				
Desipramine	TCA	10–200				
Serotonin-Norepinephrine Reuptake Inhibitors						
Duloxetine	SNRI	10–60	Elevated blood pressure (venlafaxine), nausea, dizziness, dry mouth	MAOIs; SSRIs (increased risk of serotonin syndrome)	≥65 years	49,51,53
Venlafaxine	SNRI	37.5–225				
Desvenlafaxine	SNRI	10–50				
Monoamine Oxidase Inhibitors						
Phenelzine	MAOI	30–90	Hypertensive crisis, drowsiness, dry mouth, headaches, weight gain (phenelzine), postural hypotension	Simultaneous use of MAOIs and SSRIs/TCAs can lead to serotonin syndrome. Hypertensive crisis possible with ingestion of tyramine-rich foods	≥19 years	49,54,56,58,60
Isocarboxazid	MAOI	10–40				
Tranylcypromine	MAOI	10–30				
Selegiline	MAOI	6–12				
Others						
Mirtazapine	NaSSA	15–45	Drowsiness, dry mouth, increased appetite, weight gain	MAOIs; SSRIs (increased risk of serotonin syndrome)	≥55 years	50,59
Bupropion	Atypical (NEDI)	50–300	Headache, dry mouth, nausea, insomnia, seizures	MAOIs, alcohol, medications that lower seizure threshold		55,59
Nefazodone	Atypical	50–600	Dizziness, dry mouth, sedation, GI discomfort, liver damage	Antihypertensive medications, SSRIs, MAOIs, alcohol		57
Agomelatine	MASSA	25–50	Sedation, nausea, GI discomfort	SSRIs (fluvoxamine), any acute liver disease		71,72

■ NONPHARMACOLOGIC APPROACHES

A strong evidence base exists for the use of psychotherapies in the treatment of depression in older adults, including numerous major randomized controlled trials, as well as systematic reviews and meta-analyses examining the effects of psychotherapies for depression in persons over 60 or over 65.[73–83] These therapies have been particularly successful when applied in combination with pharmacotherapy.

In an important study, Reynolds et al.[78] reported that nortriptyline (80–120 ng/mL) and interpersonal therapy (IPT) were equally effective for major depression in patients aged 60+ years; however, the greatest benefit was seen in the patients receiving both nortriptyline and IPT. Recurrence rates were lower in the three treatment groups than the placebo group over the 3-year follow-up period; patients in the combined treatment group had a recurrence rate of 20%—lower than that of the placebo group ($p < .001$), the IPT monotherapy group ($p = .003$) and the nortriptyline monotherapy group ($p = 0.06$). In a later trial with elderly primary care patients, Bruce et al.[73] found that a collaborative care (see section on "The

Role of Collaborative Care in Depression Treatment of Medically Ill Older Adults") intervention group had significantly greater decline in depression symptoms than a usual care group, evident at 4-, 8-, and 12-month follow-up. Similarly, Hunkeler et al.[77] studied the effects of the IMPACT collaborative care intervention (including behavioral activation and problem-solving therapy) in primary care patients over age 60 years with major depression, dysthymia, or both. The IMPACT intervention group had significantly lower depression scores than controls at 12-, 18-, and 24-month follow-up.

Several studies specifically address the effects of nonpharmacologic interventions in older patients with high levels of medical morbidity. An RCT in elderly subjects with both major depression and executive dysfunction demonstrated a significant advantage of problem-solving therapy (PST) compared to supportive (control) therapy.[84] Similarly, significant benefits of CBT were found in older adults with depression and recent myocardial infarction: the intervention group had significantly greater average decreases in depression severity compared to the control group.[85] Overall, this literature demonstrates that not only are psychotherapies beneficial for treating depression in the medically ill elderly, but also that the specificity of intervention (established, manualizable interventions such as PST, CBT, or IPT) is important.

THE ROLE OF COLLABORATIVE CARE IN DEPRESSION TREATMENT OF MEDICALLY ILL OLDER ADULTS

■ INTRODUCTION TO THE COLLABORATIVE CARE APPROACH

Implementing a strategy for detecting depression in primary care settings is undoubtedly an effective first step in addressing the problem of depression burden in the medically ill elderly. The greater challenge is the delivery of care after the case of depression is identified. Many primary care providers who are willing to screen for depression in elders do not have the capacity to follow up with treatment for patients who screened positive.[86]

Over the past two decades, numerous studies, including a number of large multi-site randomized controlled trials, have established a robust evidence base for the collaborative care approach.[87] The approach has now been recommended as a best practice by the Surgeon General's Report on Mental Health,[88] the President's New Freedom Commission on Mental Health,[89] and by several federal agencies.[90]

Collaborative care has emerged from the chronic care model proposed by Wagner and colleagues.[91] They recognized that improving the quality of care for patients with chronic medical illnesses required improved self-management and guideline-based care, and that this was difficult during the usual brief primary care visit. They proposed a chronic care model with two core components: a disease registry for identifying cases of the target chronic disease, and timely measurement of treatment by monitoring primary care visits, dosage of medication, and adherence to treatment.

Consistent with the general principles of the chronic care model, the collaborative care model attempts to improve mental health and behavioral health care by integrating them into primary care practice. It typically entails procedures to identify cases of depression and to enhance its management through coordinated team effort aimed at improving patient self-care and adherence to treatment regimens.[87] Mental health care is delivered by a collaborative team that includes primary care providers (e.g., internist or nurse practitioner), care managers (e.g., nurse or clinical social worker), and mental health specialists (e.g., psychiatrist, or clinical psychologist).

Primary care providers typically perform the routine screening. The care manager, who is based in the primary care setting, provides education, care coordination, and, if needed, brief behavioral interventions, as well as periodic contact with the patient to ensure treatment compliance. And the mental health specialist provides clinical support and back-up to primary care providers. This ranges from consultation around diagnosis, conducting more extensive evaluation for difficult or complex cases, and providing advice on treatment options, to developing the initial treatment plan and delivering it in collaboration with primary care providers.[92]

■ EVIDENCE FOR COLLABORATIVE CARE MODELS

Systematic reviews of collaborative depression care have recently provided robust evidence that it increases adherence to treatment by approximately twofold and improves outcomes such as "depression-free days." The literature also suggests that collaborative care provides "good economic value," based on cost-effectiveness and cost-benefit analyses.[93–99]

■ APPLICATION/IMPLEMENTATION IN PRIMARY CARE SETTINGS INVOLVING OLDER ADULTS

The collaborative depression care model has been implemented in several large-scale dissemination efforts.[100–104] These programs for older adults in primary care have been shown to be effective in reducing mortality. In the PROSPECT (Prevention of Suicide in Primary Care Elderly: Collaborative Trial) RCT, older adults who received additional services for intensive depression management had a lower mortality rate than that observed in usual care.[105] Patients with major depression in the intervention practices had a statistically significant 24% relative reduction in mortality compared to those receiving usual care. The mortality risk in the depressed older adults receiving the intervention was similar to the risk among older adults without depression.

Although collaborative care approaches for depressed elderly are highly promising, barriers to successful implementation often arise. These include: (a) limited financial resources to cover the costs of developing registries, care manager time, and physician caseload supervision time; (b) limited time to address goals due to competing tasks and priorities, (c) frequent turnover of key organizational leaders, (d) limited skills and training among team members, and (e) difficulty coordinating activities across care teams on related goals.

FUTURE DIRECTIONS

■ THE POLICY LANDSCAPE

A changing policy landscape is leaning toward supporting the provision of depression care for older adults through primary care. Medicare now covers annual depression screening conducted in primary care settings. For adult beneficiaries covered under the fee-for-service program Medicare Part B reimburses for an annual depression screen lasting up to 15 minutes conducted within a primary care setting that includes staff-assisted depression care supports. At a minimum level, staff-assisted depression care supports consist of clinical staff (e.g., nurse, physician assistant) who can advise the physician of screening results and who can facilitate and coordinate referrals for necessary mental health treatment.

Medicaid programs have begun to design "health homes" to provide comprehensive care coordination for their beneficiaries with chronic conditions. The health home model of service delivery expands on the traditional medical home models that many states have developed in their Medicaid programs, by building additional linkages and enhancing coordination and integration of medical and behavioral health care. Most of the Medicaid Health Home State Plans that have been approved by the Center for Medicare and Medicaid Services have included older adults with behavioral health conditions among the population to be served in the health home programs, where the key components of collaborative depression care could be supported.[104]

As states continue to move forward, Medicaid beneficiaries are likely to be among the first groups to receive integrated primary and behavioral health care. Despite the remaining challenges to obtaining adequate funding for the implementation of care management and behavioral health consultation, the overall prospect is promising for widespread delivery of collaborative depression care to elders using cost-effective clinical models that have been developed with sound empirical evidence.

■ PREVENTING DEPRESSION IN MEDICALLY ILL OLDER ADULTS

Selective Prevention of Depression in Older Adults

An important literature has emerged recently regarding the opportunities to prevent depression in vulnerable older adults. General strategies for preventing depression in older adults have focused on modifying lifestyle factors, including the institution of such modifications much earlier in life. More specifically, increasing emphasis has been placed on dietary modifications, regular aerobic exercise, psychoeducation, psychotherapy (e.g., CBT), sleep pattern normalization and increasing socialization/social connectedness.[4] Recognition of the elevated risk of late-life depression that is posed by serious medical illness and its attendant physical/functional limitations has led to work on preventing depression in this specific group.[106–108]

Application of Depression Prevention Strategies in Medically Ill Older Adults

In addition to modifying lifestyle factors, several recent successful RCTs illustrate the potential of other preventive interventions among older adults with medical conditions.[109–111] For example, an RCT of depression-free elderly patients recovering from recent stroke, Robinson et al. found that patients randomized to placebo had a significantly greater risk of developing post-stroke depression than those randomized to escitalopram.[110] In another RCT ancillary study of older adults with a recent stroke or transient ischemic attack, Almeida et al.[112] reported that patients given folic acid (2 mg/day), vitamin B6 (25 mg/day) and vitamin B-12 (0.5 mg/day) had a significantly lower risk of developing major depression than patients on placebo. Although similar results for depression prevention with folic acid/B-vitamins has not been observed in a larger RCT among older adults in the general population,[113] this study underscores the potential of targeting selected high risk populations for trials of depression prevention.

■ SUMMARY

Depression commonly co-exists with various medical illnesses, particularly neurological and cardiovascular disease. These comorbidities become more common with advanced age. This is partly attributable to the fact that older adults are more likely to have one or more chronic medical illnesses, but psychosocial experiences which are unique to aging, and biological effects of medical illness that preferentially affect the aging brain are also likely to play critical roles. The importance of recognizing depression in the medically ill older adult is underscored by the fact that depression significantly increases the morbidity and mortality of a coexistent medical disease, and by the fact that having medical disease can markedly increase the morbidity of depression. The recognition of depression can be aided by the use of routine screening by primary care physicians and geriatricians, and by clinical batteries and structured interviews. Emphasis should be placed on screening older patients with medical illnesses that are likely to be comorbid with depression, those with multiple medical comorbidities, those who have a personal or strong family history of affective illness, and those with psychosocial risk factors for depression (e.g., significant disability caused by their medical illness). Moreover, preventative measures can be undertaken successfully in potentially vulnerable older adults. Finally, once identified, treatment of depression in the medically ill older adult should be implemented through a multidisciplinary collaborative care model.

REFERENCES

1. Taylor WD. Clinical practice. Depression in the elderly. *N Engl J Med*. 2014;371(13):1228–1236.

2. Beekman AT, Copeland JR, Prince MJ. Review of community prevalence of depression in later life. *Br J Psychiatry*. 1999;174: 307–311.

3. Steffens DC, Skoog I, Norton MC, et al. Prevalence of depression and its treatment in an elderly population: the Cache County study. *Arch Gen Psychiatry*. 2000;57(6):601–607.

4. Madhusoodanan S, Ibrahim FA, Malik A. Primary prevention in geriatric psychiatry. *Ann Clin Psychiatry*. 2010;22(4):249–261.

5. Luijendijk HJ, van den Berg JF, Dekker MJ, et al.. Incidence and recurrence of late-life depression. *Arch Gen Psychiatry*. 2008;65(12):1394–1401.

6. Aarsland D, Påhlhagen S, Ballard CG, Ehrt U, Svenningsson P Depression in Parkinson disease–epidemiology, mechanisms and management. *Nat Rev Neurol*. 2011;8(1):35–47.

7. Disabato BM, Sheline YI. Biological basis of late life depression. *Curr Psychiatry Rep*. 2012;14(4):273–279.

8. Katon W. Clinical and health services relationships between major depression, depressive symptoms, and general medical illness. *Biol Psychiatry*. 2003;54:216–226.

9. Roth AJ, Modi R. Psychiatric issues in cancer patients. *Crit Rev Oncol Hematol*. 2003;48(2):185–197.

10. Unützer J, Schoenbaum M, Katon WJ, et al. Healthcare costs associated with depression in medically ill fee-for-service medicare participants. *J Am Geriatr Soc*. 2009;57(3):506–510.

11. Patten SB. Long-term medical conditions and major depression in a Canadian population study at waves 1 and 2. *J Affect Disord*. 2001;63:35–41.

12. Naismith SL, Norrie LM, Mowszowski L, Hickie IB. The neurobiology of depression in later-life: clinical, neuropsychological, neuroimaging and pathophysiological features. *Prog Neurobiol*. 2012;98(1):99–143.

13. Charlson M, Peterson JC. Medical comorbidity and late life depression: what is known and what are the unmet needs?. *Biol Psychiatry*. 2002;52:226–235.

14. Pascual-Leone A, Freitas C, Oberman L, et al. Characterizing brain cortical plasticity and network dynamics across the age-span in health and disease with TMS-EEG and TMS-fMRI. *Brain Topogr*. 2011;24(3–4):302–315.

15. Gleason OC, Pierce AM, Walker AE, Warnock JK. The two-way relationship between medical illness and late-life depression. *Psychiatr Clin N Am*. 2013;36(4):533–544.

16. Meyers BS, Flint AJ, Rothschild AJ, et al. A double-blind randomized controlled trial of olanzapine plus sertraline vs olanzapine plus placebo for psychotic depression: the study of pharmacotherapy of psychotic depression (STOP-PD). *Arch Gen Psychiatry*. 2009;66(8):838–847.

17. Dobkin RD, Menza M, Bienfait KL, et al. Depression in Parkinson's disease: symptom improvement and residual symptoms following acute pharmacological management. *Am J Geriatr Psychiatry*. 2011;19(3):222–229.

18. Modrego PJ. Depression in Alzheimer's disease. Pathophysiology, diagnosis, and treatment. *J Alzheimers Dis*. 2010;21(4):1077–1087.

19. Whyte E, Mulsant B. Post stroke depression: epidemiology, pathophysiology, and biological treatment. *Biol Psychiatry*. 2002; 52:253–264.

20. Hackett ML, Köhler S, O'Brien JT, Mead GE. Neuropsychiatric outcomes of stroke. *Lancet Neurol*. 2014;13:525–534.

21. Valkanova V, Ebmeier KP. Vascular risk factors and depression in later life: a systematic review and meta-analysis. *Biol Psychiatry*. 2013;73(5):406–413.

22. Goldsmith SK, Pellmar TC, Kleinman AM, Bunney WE. *Reducing Suicide: A National Imperative*. Washington, DC: National Academies Press; 2002.

23. Luoma JB, Martin CE, Pearson JL. Contact with mental health and primary care providers before suicide: a review of the evidence. *Am J Psychiatry*. 2002;159:909–916.

24. Gallo JJ, Bogner HR, Fulmer T, Paveza J. *Handbook Of Geriatric Assessment*. Sudbury, MA; Jones & Bartlett Publishers; 2005.

25. Unützer J. Diagnosis and treatment of older adults with depression in primary care. *Biol Psychiatry*. 2002;52(3):285–292.

26. O'Connor EA, Whitlock EP, Gaynes B, Beil TL. *Screening for Depression in Adults and Older Adults in Primary Care: An Updated Systematic Review*. Available at http://www.ncbi.nlm.nih.gov/books/NBK36406./ Rockville, MD, Agency for Healthcare Research and Quality.

27. Simon GE, Von Korff M. Recognition, management and outcomes of depression in primary care. *Arch Fam Med*. 1995;4: 99–105.

28. Kroenke K, Spitzer RL, Williams JB. The PHQ-9: validity of a brief depression severity measure. *J Gen Int Med*. 2001;16:606–613.

29. Choi NG, Sirey JA, Bruce ML. Depression in homebound older adults: recent advances in screening and psychosocial interventions. *Curr Transl Geriatr Exp Gerontol Rep*. 2013;2(1): 16–23.

30. Saliba D, DiFilippo S, Edelen MO, et al. Testing the PHQ-9 interview and observational versions (PHQ-9 OV) for MDS 3.0. *J Am Med Dir Assoc*. 2012;13:618–625.

31. Lyness JM, Noel TK, Cox C, King DA, Conwell Y, Caine ED. Screening for depression in elderly primary care patients. A comparison of the Center for Epidemiologic Studies-Depression Scale and the Geriatric Depression Scale. *Arch Intern Med*. 1997;157(4):449–454.

32. Dozeman E, van Schaik DJ, van Marwijk HW, Stek ML, van der Horst HE, Beekman AT. The center for epidemiological studies depression scale (CES-D) is an adequate screening instrument for depressive and anxiety disorders in a very old population living in residential homes. *Int J Geriatr Psychiatry*. 2011;26(3):239–246.

33. Irwin M, Artin KH, Oxman MN. Screening for depression in the older adult: criterion validity of the 10-item Center for Epidemiological Studies Depression Scale (CES-D). *Arch Intern Med*. 1999;159(15):1701–1704.

34. Olin JT, Schneider LS, Eaton EM, Zemansky MF, Pollack VE. The geriatric depression scale and the beck depression inventory as screening instruments in an older adult outpatient population. *Psychol Assess*. 1992;4:190–192.

35. Yesavage JA, Brink TL, Rose TL, et al. Development and validation of a geriatric depression screening scale: a preliminary report. *J Psychiatr Res*. 1983;17:37–49.

36. Sheikh J, Yesavage JA. Geriatric Depression Scale (GDS): recent evidence and development of a shorter version. *Clin Gerontol*. 1986;6:165–173.

37. Hegeman JM, Kok RM, van der Mast RC, Giltay EJ. Phenomenology of depression in older compared with younger adults: meta-analysis. *Br J Psychiatry*. 2012;200(4):275–281.

38. Suija K, Rajala U, Jokelainen J, et al. Validation of the Whooley questions and the Beck Depression Inventory in older adults. *Scand J Prim Health Care*. 2012;30(4):259–264.

39. Beck AT, Guth D, Steer RA, Ball R. Screening for major depression disorders in medical inpatients with the Beck Depression Inventory for Primary Care. *Behav Res Ther*. 1997;35(8):785–791.

40. Norris MP, Arnau RC, Bramson R, Meagher MW. The efficacy of somatic symptoms in assessing depression in older primary care patients. *Clin Gerontol*. 2003;27:43–57.

41. Wang YP, Gorenstein C. Assessment of depression in medical patients: A systematic review of the utility of the Beck Depression Inventory-II." *Clinics (Sao Paulo)*. 2013;68(9):1274–1287.

42. Spitzer RL, Williams JBW, Gibbon M, et al. *Structured Clinical Interview for the DSM-III-R*. Washington, DC: American Psychiatric Press; 1990.

43. Ormel J, Kempen GI, Penninx BW, Brilman EI, Beekman AT, van Soderen E. Chronic medical conditions and mental health in older people: disability and psychosocial resources mediate specific mental health effects. *Psychol Med*. 1997;27:1065–1077.

44. Coyne J, Palmer S, Sullivan P. Screening for Depression in Adults. *Ann Intern Med*. 2003;138:767–768.

45. Hickie IB, Davenport TA, Ricci CS. Screening for depression in general practice and related medical settings. *Med J Aust*. 2002;177(Suppl): S111–S116.

46. Pignone MP, Gaynes BN, Rushton JL, et al. Screening for depression in adults: a summary of the evidence for the U.S. Preventive Services Task Force. *Ann Intern Med*. 2002;136:765–776.

47. Gentry RA. Somatic complaints in older adults: aging processes or symptoms of depression. *PSI CHI J Undergraduate Res*. 2002;7(4):176–184.

48. Shumway M, Sentell T, Unick G, Bamberg W. Cognitive complexity of self-administered depression measures. *J Affect Disord*. 2004; 83:191–198.

49. Kairuz T, Zolezzi M, Fernando A. Clinical considerations of antidepressant prescribing for older patients. *N Z Med J*. 2005; 118(1222):U1656.

50. Montgomery SA. Late-life depression: rationalizing pharmacological treatment options. *Gerontology*. 2002;48(6):392–400.

51. Wiese BS. Geriatric depression: the use of antidepressants in the elderly. *BC Med J*. 2011;53(7):341–347.

52. Wilson K, Mottram P. A comparison of side effects of selective serotonin reuptake inhibitors and tricyclic antidepressants in older depressed patients: a meta-analysis. *Int J Geriatr Psychiatry*. 2004;19(8):754–762.

53. Dolder C, Nelson M, Stump A. Pharmacological and clinical profile of newer antidepressants: implications for the treatment of elderly patients. *Drugs Aging*. 2010;27(8):625–640.

54. Amsterdam JD, Shults J. MAOI efficacy and safety in advanced stage treatment-resistant depression—a retrospective study. *J Affect Disord*. 2005;89(1–3):183–188.

55. Hewett K, Chrzanowski W, Jokinen R, et al. Double-blind, placebo-controlled evaluation of extended-release bupropion in elderly patients with major depressive disorder. *J Psychopharmacol*. 2010;24(4):521–529.

56. Kennedy SH Continuation and maintenance treatments in major depression: the neglected role of monoamine oxidase inhibitors. *J Psychiatry Neurosci*. 1997;22(2):127–131.

57. Saiz-Ruiz J, Ibanez A, Diaz-Marsa M, et al. Nefazodone in the treatment of elderly patients with depressive disorders: a prospective, observational study. *CNS Drugs*. 2002;16(9):635–643.

58. Shulman KI, Fischer HD, Herrmann N, Huo CY, Anderson GM, Rochon PA. Current prescription patterns and safety profile of irreversible monoamine oxidase inhibitors: a population-based cohort study of older adults. *J Clin Psychiatry*. 2009;70(12): 1681–1686.

59. Tedeschini E, Levkovitz Y, Iovieno N, Ameral VE, Nelson JC, Papakostas GI. Efficacy of antidepressants for late-life depression: a meta-analysis and meta-regression of placebo-controlled randomized trials. *J Clin Psychiatry*. 2011;72(12):1660–1668.

60. Volz HP, Gleiter CH. Monoamine oxidase inhibitors. A perspective on their use in the elderly. *Drugs Aging*. 1998;13(5):341–355.

61. Abraham G, Milev R, Stuart Lawson J. T3 augmentation of SSRI resistant depression. *J Affect Disord*. 2006;91(2–3):211–215.

62. Cooper C, Katona C, Lyketsos K, et al. A systematic review of treatments for refractory depression in older people. *Am J Psychiatry*. 2011;168(7):681–688.

63. Kok RM,. Heeren TJ, Nolen WA. Continuing treatment of depression in the elderly: a systematic review and meta-analysis of double-blinded randomized controlled trials with antidepressants. *Am J Geriatr Psychiatry*. 2011;19(3):249–255.

64. Alexopoulos GS. Pharmacotherapy for late-life depression. *J Clin Psychiatry*. 2011;72(1):e04.

65. Goforth HW, Carroll BT. Aripiprazole augmentation of tranylcypromine in treatment-resistant major depression. *J Clin Psychopharmacol*. 2007;27(2):216–217.

66. Sheffrin M, Driscoll HC, Lenze EJ, et al.. Pilot study of augmentation with aripiprazole for incomplete response in late-life depression: getting to remission. *J Clin Psychiatry*. 2009;70(2):208–213.

67. Steffens DC, Nelson JC, Eudicone JM, et al. Efficacy and safety of adjunctive aripiprazole in major depressive disorder in older patients: a pooled subpopulation analysis. *Int J Geriatr Psychiatry*. 2011;26(6):564–572.

68. Fava M, Mischoulon D. Folate in depression: efficacy, safety, differences in formulations, and clinical issues. *J Clin Psychiatry*. 2009;70(Suppl 5):12–17.

69. Papakostas GI, Petersen T, Mischoulon D, et al. Serum folate, vitamin B12, and homocysteine in major depressive disorder, Part 1: predictors of clinical response in fluoxetine-resistant depression. *J Clin Psychiatry*. 2004;65(8):1090–1095.

70. Papakostas GI, Shelton RC, Zajecka JM, et al. l-Methylfolate as adjunctive therapy for SSRI-resistant major depression: results of two randomized, double-blind, parallel-sequential trials. *Am J Psychiatry*. 2012;169(12):1267–1274.

71. Heun R, Ahokas A, Boyer P. The efficacy of agomelatine in elderly patients with recurrent major depressive disorder: a placebo-controlled study. *J Clin Psychiatry*. 2013;74(6):587–94.

72. Luzny J. Agomelatine in elderly–finally a patient friendly antidepressant in psychogeriatry? *Actas Esp Psiquiatr*. 2012;40(6):304–07.

73. Bruce ML, Ten Have TR, Reynolds CF 3rd, et al. Reducing suicidal ideation and depressive symptoms in depressed older primary care patients: a randomized controlled trial. *JAMA*. 2004;291(9):1081–1091.

74. Ciechanowski P, Wagner E, Schmaling K, et al. Community-integrated home-based depression treatment in older adults: a randomized controlled trial. *JAMA*. 2004;291(13):1569–1577.

75. Cuijpers P, van Straten A, Smit F. Psychological treatment of late-life depression: a meta-analysis of randomized controlled trials. *Int J Geriatr Psychiatry*. 2006;21(12):1139–1149.

76. Gitlin LN, Harris LF, McCoy MC, et al. A home-based intervention to reduce depressive symptoms and improve quality of life in older African Americans: a randomized trial. *Ann Intern Med*. 2013;159(4):243–252.

77. Hunkeler E M, Katon W, Tang L, et al. Long term outcomes from the IMPACT randomised trial for depressed elderly patients in primary care. *BMJ*. 2006;332(7536):259–263.

78. Reynolds CF 3rd, Frank E, Perel JM, et al. Nortriptyline and interpersonal psychotherapy as maintenance therapies for recurrent major depression: a randomized controlled trial in patients older than 59 years. *JAMA*. 1999;281(1):39–45.

79. Serfaty MA, Haworth D, Blanchard M, Buszewicz M, Murad S, King M. Clinical effectiveness of individual cognitive behavioral therapy for depressed older people in primary care: a randomized controlled trial. *Arch Gen Psychiatry*. 2009;66(12):1332–1340.

80. Thompson LW, Coon DW, Gallagher-Thompson D, Sommer BR, Koin D. Comparison of desipramine and cognitive/behavioral therapy in the treatment of elderly outpatients with mild-to-moderate depression. *Am J Geriatr Psychiatry*. 2001;9(3):225–240.

81. van Schaik A, van Marwijk H, Ader H, et al. Interpersonal psychotherapy for elderly patients in primary care. *Am J Geriatr Psychiatry*. 2006;14(9):777–786.

82. Wilson KC, Mottram PG, Vassilas CA. Psychotherapeutic treatments for older depressed people. *Cochrane Database Syst Rev*. 2008;23(1):CD004853.

83. Zhou W, He G, Gao J, Yuan Q, Feng H, Zhang CK. The effects of group reminiscence therapy on depression, self-esteem, and affect balance of Chinese community-dwelling elderly. *Arch Gerontol Geriatr*. 2012;54(3):e440–e447.

84. Arean PA, Raue P, Mackin RS, Kanellopoulos D, McCulloch C, Alexopoulos GS. Problem-solving therapy and supportive therapy in older adults with major depression and executive dysfunction. *Am J Psychiatry*. 2010;167(11):1391–1398.

85. Berkman LF, Blumenthal J, Burg M, et al. Effects of treating depression and low perceived social support on clinical events after myocardial infarction: the Enhancing Recovery in Coronary Heart Disease Patients (ENRICHD) Randomized Trial. *JAMA*.2003;289(23):3106–3116.

86. Druss BG, Marcus SC, Campbell J, et al. Medical services for clients in community mental health centers: results from a national survey. *Psychiatr Serv*. 2008;59(8):917–920.

87. Katon W. Collaborative depression care models from development to dissemination. *Am J Prev Med*. 2012;42:550–552.

88. National Institute of Mental Health. *Mental Health: A Report of the Surgeon General, Department of Health and Human Services, US Public Health Service*. 1999; Available at http://www.surgeon-general.gov/library/mentalhealth/home.html.

89. New Freedom Commission on Mental Health. *Achieving the Promise: Transforming Mental Health Care in America. Final Report.* (DHHS Pub. No. SMA-03-3832). Rockville, MD; 2003.

90. Butler M, Kane RL, McAlpine D, et al. *Integration of Mental Health/Substance Abuse and Primary Care. Evidence Reports/Technology Assessments, No. 173. Report No.: 09-E003*. Rockville, MD: Agency for Healthcare Research and Quality; 2008.

91. Wagner EH, Austin BT, Von Korff M. Organizing care for patients with chronic illness. *Milbank Q*. 2006;74(4):511–544.

92. Trangle M, Gursky J, Haight R, Hardwig J. Institute for Clinical Systems Improvement. *Adult Depression in Primary Care*. Updated March 2016.

93. Gilbody S, Bower P, Fletcher J, Richards D, Sutton AJ. Collaborative care for depression: a cumulative meta-analysis and review of longer-term outcomes. *Arch Intern Med*. 2006;166(21):2314–2321.

94. Gilbody S, Bower P, Whitty P. Costs and consequences of enhanced primary care for depression: systematic review of randomised economic evaluations. *Br J Psychiatry*. 2006;189:297–308.

95. Jacob V, Chattopadhyay SK, Sipe TA, et al. Economics of collaborative care for management of depressive disorders: a Community Guide systematic review. *Am J Prev Med*. 2012;42(5):539–549.

96. Katon WJ, Schoenbaum M, Fan MY, et al. Cost-effectiveness of improving primary care treatment of late-life depression. *Arch Gen Psychiatry*. 2005;62(12):1313–1320.

97. Simon G, Katon W, Von Korff M, et al. Cost-effectiveness of a collaborative care program for primary care patients with persistent depression. *Am J Psychiatry*. 2001;158:1638–1644.

98. Thota AB, Sipe TA, Byard GJ, et al. Collaborative care to improve the management of depressive disorders: a Community Guide systematic review and meta-analysis. *Am J Prev Med*. 2012;42(5):525–538.

99. Unutzer J, Katon WJ, Fan MY, et al. Long-term cost effects of collaborative care for late-life depression. *Am J Manag Care*. 2008;14(2):95–100.

100. Agency for Healthcare Research & Quality. Integration of Mental Health/Substance Abuse and Primary Care. 2009; AHRQ Evidence Reports Retrieved April 29, 2014.

101. Alexander L, Druss BG. *Behavioral Health Homes for People with Mental Health & Substance Abuse Conditions: The Core Clinical Features*. Washington, DC: SAMHSA-HRSA Center for Integrated Health Solutions; 2012.

102. Katon W, Unützer J, Wells K, Jones L. Collaborative depression care: history, evolution and ways to enhance dissemination and sustainability. *Gen Hosp Psychiatry*. 2010;32:456–464.

103. Smith JL, Williams JW Jr, Owen RR, Rubenstein LV, Chaney E. Developing a national dissemination plan for collaborative care for depression: QUERI Series. *Implement Sci*. 2008;3:59.

104. Unützer J, Harbin H, Schoenbaum M, Druss B. *The Collaborative Care Model: An Approach for Integrating Physical and Mental Health Care in Medicaid Health Homes. Health Home Information Resource Center. Brief, 1–13*. Centers for Medicare & Medicaid Services; 2013; Available at: https://www.medicaid.gov/State-Resource-Center/Medicaid-State-Technical-Assistance/Health-Homes-Technical-Assistance/Downloads/HH-IRC-Collaborative-5-13.pdf.

105. Gallo JJ, Morales KH, Bogner HR, et al. Long term effect of depression care management on mortality in older adults: follow-up of cluster randomized clinical trial in primary care. *BMJ*. 2013;346:f2570.

106. Lyness JM, Yu Q, Tang W, Tu X, Conwell Y. Risks for depression onset in primary care elderly patients: potential targets for preventive interventions. *Am J Psychiatry*. 2009;166(12):1375–1383.

107. Reynolds CF 3rd, Cuijpers P, Patel V, et al. Early intervention to reduce the global health and economic burden of major depression in older adults. *Annu Rev Public Health*. 2012;33:123–135.

108. Schoevers RA, Smit F, Deeg DJ, et al. Prevention of late-life depression in primary care: do we know where to begin? *Am J Psychiatry*. 2006;163(9):1611–1621.

109. Cuijpers P, van Straten A, Smit F, Mihalopoulos C, Beekman A. Preventing the onset of depressive disorders: a meta-analytic review of psychological interventions. *Am J Psychiatry*. 2008;165(10):1272–1280.

110. Robinson RG, Jorge RE, Moser DJ, et al. Escitalopram and problem-solving therapy for prevention of poststroke depression: a randomized controlled trial. *JAMA*. 2008;299(20):2391–2400.

111. Rovner BW, Casten RJ, Hegel MT, Leiby BE, Tasman WS. Preventing depression in age-related macular degeneration. *Arch Gen Psychiatry*. 2007;64(8):886–892.

112. Almeida OP, Marsh K, Alfonso H, Flicker L, Davis TM, Hankey GJ. B-vitamins reduce the long-term risk of depression after stroke: The VITATOPS-DEP trial. *Ann Neurol*. 2010;68(4):503–510.

113. Walker JG, Mackinnon AJ, Batterham P, et al. Mental health literacy, folic acid and vitamin B12, and physical activity for the prevention of depression in older adults: randomised controlled trial. *Br J Psychiatry*. 2010;197(1):45–54.

CHAPTER **22**

The Surgical Patient

Meghan Kolodziej, MD
David Wolfe, MD, MPH
Fremonta Meyer, MD
Samata Sharma, MD
Stanley Ashley, MD

INTRODUCTION

The literature on psychiatric illness in surgical patients is limited and mostly confined to small patient samples within surgical subspecialties. The findings suggest that depression, anxiety, and alcohol use disorders are more prevalent, both pre and postoperatively, than in the general population.[1] In addition to pre-existing psychiatric illness, surgery may be further complicated postoperatively by delirium, acute stress disorder, posttraumatic stress disorder, new onset mood disorders, or substance withdrawal.

Studies suggest that common mood and stress-related disorders may be overlooked in the immediate postsurgical phase.[2] Rates of depression in the immediate postoperative period range between 10% and 14%, with rates in trauma patients nearing 40% within 1 to 3 months of surgery.[3] Untreated, postsurgical depression impacts subjective quality of life scores that may persist several years following surgery and is commonly associated with poorer surgical outcomes.

Psychiatry plays an important role in the care of the surgical patient. This chapter reviews the role of the psychiatrist in evaluating patients preoperatively, and in managing depression and associated psychiatric conditions during the postoperative period. Many surgical subspecialties carry unique risks for the development of depression and these are reviewed in greater detail.

PRESURGICAL CONSIDERATIONS

The preoperative period is a time when information can be collected about a patient's current and past psychiatric history. For certain types of surgeries such as solid-organ transplantation and bariatric surgery, preoperative psychiatric evaluation is routinely recommended in order to identify psychosocial issues that may affect the postoperative course and outcome. Early identification of depression or other psychiatric conditions allows for adequate treatment. Decisions can also be made about maintaining psychiatric medications prior to surgery, ensuring that psychiatric illnesses are monitored postoperatively, and assessing the adequacy of social support postoperatively.

Antidepressant use is prevalent in patients undergoing elective surgery. As many as 35% of patients undergoing elective surgeries take antidepressant medications.[4] It used to be recommended that patients discontinue antidepressant medications prior to surgery. The selective serotonin reuptake inhibitors (SSRIs) and selective serotonin and norepinephrine reuptake inhibitors (SNRIs) impact platelet function, which could affect risk of bleeding. Tricyclic antidepressants have been associated with electrocardiographic changes and vulnerability to arrhythmias during anesthesia. Monoamine oxidase inhibitors raise concern about the risk for adverse effects if combined with sympathomimetic agents, opioids or serotonergic medications during surgery.

For patients with severe depression, however, discontinuation of antidepressant medications may place them at increased risk for recurrence of their depressive symptoms or for discontinuation syndromes. And recent studies suggest that antidepressants may be safely continued prior to surgery. When the use of SSRIs and SNRIs has been examined in cardiac patients, they have not been shown to increase the risk of bleeding in the perioperative period following CABG surgery.[5] Likewise, patients who continued to receive tricyclic and tetracyclic antidepressants prior to surgery had no increased incidence of arrhythmia or hypotension, and had a decreased risk of depressive symptoms or delirium postoperatively.[6] In addition, a study of monoamine oxidase inhibitor use prior to surgery found no increase in the incidence of tachycardia or hypertension during the operative course. In this study, many patients received sympathomimetic drugs during anesthesia and were treated with opioids postoperatively. Only one patient (receiving meperidine) had an adverse reaction.[7] Whenever there is concern about the advisability of continuing a psychiatric medication, particularly with monoamine oxidase inhibitors, collaboration between psychiatry, anesthesia, and surgery is indicated.

POSTSURGICAL CONSIDERATIONS

The immediate postoperative period presents several challenges for the assessment and treatment of depression. Delirium can mimic many psychiatric illnesses, and the hypoactive form of delirium is often misdiagnosed as a primary depressive disorder. Anesthesia, medication changes, and pain all contribute to the complexity of medical management during this period. Adding to the difficulty, patients may be unable to report their symptoms consistently or take medications by mouth for hours to weeks following surgery. Patients with depression report more pain, and conversely, inadequate pain control increases the risk of developing postoperative depression.

DELIRIUM

Delirium, an acute change in mental status marked by impairment of attention, remains a common and serious complication among hospitalized surgical patients. The syndrome of delirium can involve hallucinations, agitation, sleep disturbance, affective changes, and disruption of cognition, causing risk of injury as well as subjective distress.

The prevalence of delirium in the hospital ranges between 14% and 56%, and at least doubles the likelihood of mortality over the subsequent year.[8,9,10] Delirium has also been found to be an independent risk factor for the subsequent development of dementia.[11] One particularly vulnerable period for developing delirium is in the days following surgery, when rates as high as 70% have been reported.[12] Reviews of delirium in patients following orthopedic or cardiac surgeries have found widely varying incidence rates from 3.6% to 53.3% and 13.5% to 41.7%, respectively.[13,14]

The hyperactive type of delirium, marked by agitation and dyssomnia, receives more clinical attention, often requiring medication and restraints. Yet, the hypoactive type where patients appear withdrawn, less interactive, and "quietly confused" is often undiagnosed or misdiagnosed as depression. Hypoactive delirium lacks the physical agitation often targeted by antipsychotic medication.[15] In the ICU setting following cardiac surgery, hypoactive delirium is more common than hyperactive delirium and is an independent risk factor for prolonged mechanical ventilation.[16] Given its relatively high prevalence and morbidity during this period, postoperative changes in mood should be considered delirium until proven otherwise. While clinical presentations can vary widely, **Table 22-1** contrasts the general features of delirium and depression.

Typically patients with hypoactive delirium deny depressed mood, but may endorse associated symptoms, such as low energy, anxiety, difficulty concentrating, and sleep disturbance. Performing a cognitive exam, with special consideration to attentional tasks (e.g., saying the months of the year backward, or reciting digits backward), as well as direct inquiry into the patient's mood are helpful in distinguishing hypoactive delirium from depression. Delirium is more typically associated with visual hallucinations, worsened symptoms at night ("sun-downing"), and acute changes in cognitive impairment.

Difficulties in cognition seen in severe cases of depression, occasionally (and misleadingly) referred to as "pseudo-dementia," generally reflect lack of effort or apathy, as opposed to true cognitive dysfunction. Auditory hallucinations, which can occur in severe cases of either condition, are still relatively more likely to occur in delirium. In some cases, especially in patients with a significant psychiatric history, or a prolonged and complicated hospital stay, distinguishing the two can be difficult. In relatively rare instances, delirious patients can appear quite tearful and endorse several signs

TABLE 22-1 Distinguishing Features of Postoperative Delirium and Depression

Feature	Delirium	Depression
Onset	Acute—associated with medical or surgical event	Acute or gradual—may predate surgery
Affect	Blunted (hypoactive), anxious, or labile (hyperactive)	Dysphoric, hopeless, guilty
Mood	Often "anxious" or "okay"	"Depressed"
Attention impairment	+++	–
Other cognitive impairment	++	+/– (typically from apathy)
Daily course	Some waxing and waning, typically worse at night ("sundowning")	Constant
Sleep disturbance	+++	+
Visual hallucinations	++	–
Auditory hallucinations	+	+/– (in severe cases)
Electroencephalogram (EEG)	Diffuse slowing	Normal

of depression, including suicidal thoughts. In unclear situations, an electroencephalogram (EEG) can be helpful by revealing the diffuse slowing classically seen in delirium, as well in ruling out seizure activity. In a depressed individual without delirium or other neurologic disease, the EEG would be expected to be normal.

It is worth noting that delirium and depression can coexist, though the immediate objectives following surgery should be to treat the underlying causes of delirium, while managing agitation, sleep disturbance, and subjective distress with antipsychotics. Adding antidepressant therapies during this period may actually worsen confusion and is best considered when the delirium has resolved.

The goals of delirium care have moved toward earlier recognition, identifying individuals who are at risk for delirium and screening high risk patients for it, to allow for improved management. Screening tools, including the Confusion Assessment method (CAM) or Confusion Assessment Method ICU (CAM-ICU), are validated measures designed to help nonpsychiatrically trained clinicians identify and monitor cases of delirium.[17,18] Evidence based treatment guidelines, such as those formed by the UK National Institute for Health and Care Excellence, may be helpful in the prevention, diagnosis and management of delirium.[19]

ANTIDEPRESSANT MANAGEMENT IN THE POSTOPERATIVE PATIENT

Most antidepressants require oral administration and absorption. For many patients taking these agents prior to surgery, they are withheld at the time of the procedure, and restarted within a few hours to days. In some situations, however, oral antidepressants may need to be withheld for longer periods. Many antidepressant pills can be crushed and administered through a nasogastric tube, a common approach for patients in surgical intensive care. However, extended release formulations, such as those found with bupropion, venlafaxine, paroxetine, and duloxetine, generally cannot be administered this way. Absorption may be improved with alternative formulations, such as orally disintegrating tablets (mirtazapine) or liquids (citalopram, sertraline, fluoxetine, lithium).

Unfortunately, there are very few parenteral alternatives. Intravenous citalopram, comparable in efficacy and tolerability to the oral version, has been produced but is not routinely available in most hospitals.[20] Transdermal selegiline is approved for treatment of major depression, but as a monamine oxidase inhibitor its use in the hospital is limited by potential drug interactions and risk of serotonin syndrome.[21]

In the confused postsurgical patient, withholding antidepressants may be prudent in some cases. Agents with significant anticholinergic activity, such as amitriptyline, imipramine, nortripyline, doxepin, and paroxetine may directly contribute to the incidence and duration of delirium.[22] Cases of delirium have been reported with bupropion, presumably due to its relatively unique inhibition of dopamine reuptake.[23]

Drug–drug interactions also deserve special consideration. For example, co-administration of the antibiotic linezolid, itself a monamine oxidase inhibitor, with serotonergic agents is associated with an elevated risk of serotonin syndrome.[24] Serotonin toxicity can also arise from concomitant use of SSRIs and tramadol for pain.[25] Fluoxetine and other psychotropic medications have been associated with increased INR and bleeding risk in patients taking warfarin.[26]

When antidepressants need to be discontinued, it is ideal to reduce them gradually, though this is rarely possible in the immediate postoperative period. Nonetheless, every effort should be made to taper the medication, even if briefly, to avoid discontinuation reactions. This is especially important in instances where the half-life of the agent is short and the baseline dose is relatively high. Notably, paroxetine, venlafaxine, desvenlafaxine, duloxetine, all have relatively short half-lives (while that for fluoxetine is 4–6 days). Abrupt discontinuation of these medications rarely causes dangerous adverse reactions, though headache, gastrointestinal symptoms, dysphoria, irritability, dizziness, agitation, and confusion have all been reported.[27] All patients in this situation will require ongoing monitoring for recurrence or worsening of their depressive symptoms, possibly after discharge.

PAIN AND SLEEP

Suboptimal pain control in the peri- and postoperative periods is an independent risk factor for development of postsurgical depression. Recent orthopedic literature highlights the association between pain and depression. One study revealed that preoperative pain predicts postoperative depressive symptoms, and postoperative depressive symptoms predict pain at discharge. This suggests that perioperative pain therapy may require treatment of both pain and depressive symptoms to achieve sufficient analgesia.[28] Other studies have also shown that preoperative depression and anxiety are associated with worse postoperative pain, and poorer functioning and health-related quality of life.[29,30]

Sleep disorders are frequently co-morbid with depression and anxiety. Postsurgical shoulder pain, for example, is closely correlated with depression, anxiety, and sleep disturbances.[30] Treatment of sleep disorders improves depression scores, and vice-versa.[31] Effective pre- and postoperative screening for mood and sleep disorders may lead to earlier recognition and treatment and therefore to improved outcomes. Consultation liaison psychiatric services may be helpful for evaluation of commonly occurring psychiatric illnesses in the surgical patient, and may also be used to assess the need for, and provide access to, ambulatory psychiatric services following the acute surgical recovery phase.

GASTROINTESTINAL SURGERY

■ BARIATRIC SURGERY

A bi-directional relationship between obesity and depression has been described, though the mediating factors are still being investigated.[32] Population-based studies suggest the odds ratio of obesity leading to depression lies between 1.0 and 2.0.[33] Bariatric surgery—

now encompassing the Roux-en-Y gastric bypass, gastric sleeve, and other procedures—continues to gain popularity as an effective treatment for morbid obesity (currently defined BMI $\geq$ 40 kg/m^2). Psychiatric screening of bariatric surgery candidates is recommended and commonplace. As a consequence, relatively high levels of psychiatric co-morbidity have been detected in this population, including mood, personality, and eating disorders.[34] High rates of suicidal thoughts and attempts have also been reported.[35] Although many factors affect surgical outcomes, greater preoperative depression is associated with less postoperative weight loss.[36] Although many patients experience improvement in their mood and quality of life following the procedure,[37] antidepressant use typically remains the same before and after bariatric surgery.[38] In procedures that affect absorption, such as the Roux-en-Y, medications doses may need to be adjusted, as has been suggested in a pharmacokinetic study of sertraline, which revealed significantly lower plasma concentrations and an approximate halving of the mean concentration–time curve in postbariatric surgery patients compared to controls.[39] Liquid formulations of antidepressants may be a useful option in situations where absorption is otherwise altered, though there have been no studies demonstrating their superiority to tablet or capsule formulations in this population.

■ OSTOMIES

The psychological impact of a stoma is often underestimated. Recovery from ostomy creation has been associated with clinically significant psychological symptoms—such as depression, anxiety, and embarrassment—in approximately one quarter of cases.[40] These distressing emotions generally improve over time. Better mood adjustment is associated with stoma acceptance, better interpersonal relationships, and stoma care self-efficacy.[41] Men may be more likely to report depression and lower quality of life[42] though this is controversial since another study did not find this gender difference.[41]

Physical symptoms, such as pain and nausea, affect quality of life, as do social factors such as limitations on travel and interference with intimacy. Routine psychosocial assessment and support, especially in the early weeks following surgery, appears to be beneficial, though there remains a need for further prospective studies on depression incidence and management in this population (**Box 22-1**). For patients with apparent social isolation or more chronic difficulty accepting their stoma, regular monitoring for depressive symptoms and evaluation for antidepressant therapy are recommended.

TRANSPLANTATION

■ GENERAL PRINCIPLES

The psychiatric care of the patient undergoing organ transplantation takes place in three distinct phases: evaluation (and/or listing), surgery, and post-transplant. In the evaluation phase, some combination of psychiatric, psychological, and/or social assessments are common if not required at many centers. This phase includes a careful screening for psychiatric disorder, as many patients have not had formal assessment previously.[43] At this point, the features of depression typically resemble those of patients with end-stage organ disease, though the testing, treatment planning, uncertainty, and risks associated with the transplantation process can worsen the mood of many candidates. For some patients on a waiting list for transplant, a sense of helplessness and hopelessness becomes more pervasive as the disease progresses. Transplant support groups and close monitoring of mood are especially helpful during this period.

Following surgery, complications or deviations from patient expectations can directly impact mood, especially when the recovery is prolonged. Pain, nausea, and fatigue are common complaints even in the absence of complications. Steroids can precipitate depression and affective lability in a subset of patients, especially at the relatively high doses required following transplant. Delirium, sleep disturbance, other drug side effects (such as tremor from the commonly used immunosuppressive agent tacrolimus), and the stress on social supports can all contribute to acute depression.

In the post-transplant phase, depression may arise from guilt when the graft came from a deceased donor, as well as from excessive worry that the transplant may fail. There are also psychiatric consequences from chronic immunosuppression. Post-transplant lymphoproliferative disorder arises from B-cell proliferation following infection with the Epstein–Barr Virus (EBV) and long-term immunosuppression. Most common in the first year following transplant, rare cases can occur several years later. Heralding symptoms resemble those in primary EBV infection, including lymphadenopathy, fever, and malaise. The latter may resemble depression, a presentation potentially confounded by cognitive deficits. Generally, treatment involves a reduction in immunosuppression, as well as antivirals and chemotherapy, depending on the degree of dissemination.

Progressive multifocal leukoencephalopathy (PML), a demyelinating disease stemming from JC virus can lead to mood as well as cognitive changes. While antiretrovirals are the current treatment of choice, two small case series have found some benefit with mirtazpine in preventing the progression of PML in patients with HIV, raising an interesting question of whether antidepressants confer some neuroprotective effect in this process.[44,45]

SOLID-ORGAN TRANSPLANTATION

In the immediate postoperative period, distinguishing among delirium, reactive depression, and the direct effects of steroids can be difficult. Generally speaking, delirium management and supportive care are the primary goals from a psychiatric perspective during this period, with close monitoring of mood, sleep, and appetite. Antipsychotics can provide acute symptomatic improvement, especially if sleep disturbance, anxiety, or hallucinations are present. An open-label 5-week trial of olanzapine demonstrated efficacy at treating depression and mixed mood (or manic) symptoms arising from corticosteroids.[46]

In spite of improvements in health status following transplant, mental distress remains relatively common, with some level of depressive symptoms present in as many as 80% of solid organ recipients in 2 years following surgery.[47] In this time period, the prevalence of more severe major depression in cardiac and lung transplant recipients has been reported as high as 28% and 32%, respectively.[48] A prospective study of renal transplant recipients found a depression prevalence of 22% immediately following surgery, and depression was significantly associated with mortality over the subsequent 5 years.[49] The association of depression with worse surgical outcomes is far from clear, however. In one study of liver and renal failure patients, a Beck Depression Inventory score in the "mild" or higher range at the time of listing was associated with

a threefold decrease in risk of graft failure and mortality during the 18 months following transplant.[50]

FACE TRANSPLANTATION

There is a small but growing literature on the psychological and ethical complications of face transplantation.[51] To date, more than 20 face transplants have been performed worldwide, including 7 transplantations at Brigham and Women's Hospital, primarily for traumatic injuries. There are few data on psychiatric outcomes. Facial disfigurement is clearly associated with major psychological morbidity, including depression and suicidal thoughts.[52] Transplantation has the potential to improve this distress as well social functioning. One case report demonstrated a decrease in depressive symptoms 3 months after successful transplant.[53]

In addition to the unique and devastating social impact of facial disfigurement, hospitalization for the surgeries and the recovery tend to be longer than for most solid-organ transplants. Blindness and speech difficulties are common and interfere with communication. Consequently, a thorough assessment of depressive symptoms may require considerable time and repeated visits.

BURN/TRAUMA SURGERY

Advances in surgical burn trauma care have led to a sharp rise in the number of severe burn injury survivors. These patients face unique psychological adjustments and challenges from loss of function and disfigurement. Psychiatric consultation services may be utilized in any of the commonly recognized three phases of burn care: emergent, acute (reconstitutive), and long-term adjustment phases.[54]

■ EMERGENT PHASE

The emergent phase of burn injury is broadly defined as the time from initial onset of injury through the first 72 hours of treatment. Care during this period focuses on stabilization. Pre-existing substance abuse (percentages range from 20% to 80%) is a well-documented concern among patients with burn injury. Thus, the emergent phase of burn recovery may be complicated by alcohol withdrawal and multifactorial delirium. Burn related delirium generally occurs within the first 3 days following burn injury[54] and may present with emotional lability, tearfulness, withdrawal, apathy and other symptoms that mimic depression. The diagnosis of depression, anxiety, acute stress disorder or PTSD emerges most frequently in the later phases, and after delirium subsides.[54]

■ ACUTE PHASE

The acute (also referred to as the reconstitutive) phase lasts from the end of acute surgical intervention to hospital discharge; or from the emergent phase to the time when the burned area is completely covered by skin grafts and/or wounds are healed. During this phase, promoting sleep, as well as expedient identification and treatment of any acute stress disorder or mood disorder, promotes faster recovery and minimizes the length of hospital stay.[54] Patients with pre-existing depression have longer hospital stays and poorer wound healing than nondepressed patients.[55] This appears to hold true as well for patients who develop depressive symptoms following burn injury. Early pharmacological interventions for burn-related depressive symptoms and optimal pain control may reduce the chances of post-burn depression, and improve functional outcomes and quality of life.[56]

Allostatic load may be a potential explanation linking pain during the acute phase with development of acute stress disorder, depression and poor wound healing. Allostasis, the process of achieving homeostasis during times of stress, is mediated by the hypothalamic–pituitary–adrenal (HPA) axis. Alterations in levels of norepinephrine, epinephrine, glucocorticoids, and proinflammatory cytokines occur in response to physical stressors (such as burn trauma) as well as psychological stressors. Specifically, glucocorticoids and proinflammatory cytokines are involved in the physiological mechanisms underlying both stress and wound healing.[57] During the acute stress, this neuroendorcrine response is advantageous, for example by triggering flight from danger or improving wound healing. However, the response has negative effects if it persists chronically. Chronic elevations in glucocorticoids and proinflammatory cytokines have been linked to depression and depressed patients may have poorer wound healing even during the acute burn phase. Whether depression precedes burn injury or develops after, it exerts an effect long after the acute phase; depression is a stronger predictor of long-term quality of life in burn patients than the extent of total body surface burn area.

Long-Term Adjustment Phase

Up to two thirds of all burn patients have a history of psychiatric illness during their life time, with major depression being most common.[58] Following a burn injury, 30% to 40% of patients develop a new onset psychiatric diagnosis,[59,60] most often major depression (10% of patients), followed by generalized anxiety disorder and PTSD. When new psychiatric symptoms do occur, 57% of patients develop symptoms within the first 12 months, with an additional 21% of patients developing symptoms within 2 years.[60] Depression decreases perceived quality of life in burn patients and affects long term adjustment. This may be related to increased risk of disability and decreased likelihood of returning to work, both major factors in quality of life. Total body surface burn area has not been found to correlate with patient quality of life, which is instead related to preinjury educational level, likelihood of returning to work, postinjury stress disorder,[61] preinjury mental health and social support.[62] Earlier identification and treatment of depression in the acute phase may lead to better patient reported outcomes.

Body image also plays a role in long term adjustment to burn injuries. Patients with pre-burn body image dissatisfaction report increased depressive symptoms and lower perceived quality of life, even without significant disfigurement or functionality loss. Pre-burn body image dissatisfaction has also been found to lead to poor postburn psychosocial adjustment and lower physical functioning at 2 month follow-up.[63]

■ LIMB AMPUTATION

The rates of depression and anxiety range up to 30% in the 1 to 2 years following traumatic limb loss.[64,65,66] Similar rates have been reported in patients with upper limb amputations.[67] The risk of developing depression following amputation appears to fluctuate with the stage of recovery. One study of patients with lower limb amputations found depression levels rose during the immediate postoperative period, then resolved during inpatient rehabilitation, before rising again following discharge. It is suggested that the levels of depression and anxiety following lower limb loss may initially subside during rehabilitation as progress is made toward regaining functionality and then increase following discharge from rehab as patients begin to confront and come to terms with their functional deficits.[68]

Depression and perceived quality of life are closely associated following amputation. Quality of life in patients with lower limb amputations is correlated with seven factors: depression, mobility, social support, number of medical comorbidities, prosthesis problems, age, and social activity participation. Depression is the most significant of these, accounting for approximately 30% of the variance in quality of life; the full model with all seven factors accounts for 42% of the variance in quality of life.[69]

The impact of mood disorders on prosthetic use following lower limb amputation has also been examined. Although it does not appear that a pre-existing mood disorder influences a patient's ability to learn to use a prosthetic,[70] a history of depression has been linked to poorer prosthetic fitting, lower hours of prosthetic use and greater functional restrictions.[71]

Several studies have also examined the role of coping strategies in quality of life and adjustment following limb amputation. Avoidance (cognitive disengagement) is strongly associated with psychological distress and poor adjustment, while problem solving and seeking social support are negatively associated with depression and positively associated with better adjustment.[67,72] Negative beliefs about one's appearance and being self-conscious in public are also associated with increased distress and psychosocial adjustment difficulties.[66] These findings suggest a role for cognitive behavioral therapies in improving cognitive distortions associated with body image alterations, and subsequently improving psychosocial outcomes.

CARDIOTHORACIC SURGERY

■ CORONARY ARTERY BYPASS GRAFTING

Coronary Artery Bypass Grafting (CABG) is the most common type of open heart surgery in the United States. CABG is performed in order to alleviate symptoms of angina, improve quality of life and increase survival. Depression is common among patients undergoing CABG and depressed patients are at increased risk of morbidity and mortality following CABG. Rates of depression in patients undergoing CABG are reported to be 20% to 25%,[73,74] with rates increasing to 38% if patients with mild depressive symptoms are included.[74] Risk factors for depression in CABG encompass biological, social and behavioral factors (**Table 22-2**).

A number of pathophysiological mechanisms may explain the increased risk of morbidity and mortality in depressed CABG patients, including increased sympathetic nervous system activity, activation of the HPA axis, vulnerability to arrhythmias, systemic inflammation, and increased platelet aggregability. These states may individually or synergistically further the progression of atherosclerosis, lead to thrombosis or result in dangerous arrhythmias following CABG surgery. Depression is associated with physical inactivity, obesity, and poor use of cardiac rehabilitation programs, leading to worsened physical health. Individuals with depression are also known to have higher rates of medication nonadherence and more frequent use of tobacco and alcohol, known risks for cardiovascular disease. Depression may also impact the course of CABG by increasing the risk of delirium. In a recent meta-analysis of delirium risk factors, depression was found to increase the risk of delirium by threefold.[75] When delirium does occur, it may complicate the postoperative course by prolonging the length of hospitalization, impeding physical recovery, and increasing mortality.

Depression may increase the likelihood of referral for CABG surgery by amplifying the subjective experience of symptoms. Prior to CABG, patients with depression experience more symptoms of angina than patients without depression. They many also feel

TABLE 22-2 Risk Factors for Depression in CABG Patients[76,77,78]

Prior depression treatment
Comorbid medical conditions
Female gender
Younger age
Limited social support
Unmarried status
Tobacco use
Low health related quality of life
Poor physical functioning

more functionally limited by their symptoms. Thus, patients with depression are more often referred for CABG due to their symptoms than as a result of objective cardiovascular testing.[76]

Depression predicts hospital readmission within 6 months following CABG,[79] and higher rates of myocardial infarction, cardiac arrest or repeat CABG within 12 months.[73] Depression additionally predicts greater progression of atherosclerosis within grafted veins.[77] Over the longer term, depression is a risk factor for recurrence of angina within 5 years of CABG.[80] Given that relief from angina is one of the primary indications for CABG surgery, individuals with depression may have a less satisfactory outcome from surgery.

It is not clear whether the increased risk of mortality in depressed CABG patients is related to cardiac or noncardiac (e.g., infection, COPD or renal failure) causes. Blumenthal et al. conducted the largest trial to date, and found that patients with moderate to severe levels of depression prior to CABG had a greater than twofold risk of all-cause mortality over the ensuing 5.2 years, even after adjusting for age, gender, and severity of illness.[74] In the longest study to date, Connerney et al. found that patients with major depressive disorder had an almost twofold risk of cardiac mortality 10 years after CABG surgery. This indicates that initial depression may continue to impact survival well into the future.[81]

The timing of depression onset may affect mortality risk. Depression starting prior to surgery or postoperatively increases the risk of mortality above that of a past history of depression.[81] When depression is diagnosed at the time of CABG surgery, it is persistent in the majority of patients, with 58% of individuals continuing to meet criteria for depression at 6 month follow-up.[74]

Depression can be challenging to diagnose in the perioperative period. Patients undergoing CABG may experience a wide range of emotions—anxiety about undergoing major surgery, concern about the severity of their medical condition, frustration with the functional limitations they have been experiencing, and concerns about their mortality. Symptoms that are experienced in response to the stresses of surgery may indicate a transient adjustment process or may herald the onset of a more persistent depression. The presence of anhedonia or suicidal ideation are commonly found in depressed patients, but infrequently seen in other conditions, such as adjustment disorders. It is also important to consider the possible role of delirium. Delirium is extremely common following cardiac surgery, with prevalence rates as high as 53.3% of patients. In its hypoactive form, a flat affect, inattention, low energy, poor appetite and insomnia may mimic the symptoms of depression.

In 2008, the American Heart Association issued a scientific advisory recommending screening for depression in all coronary heart disease patients. Subsequently, debate has arisen about the effectiveness of existing screening tools, and whether early identification and treatment actually reduces depression or alters the course of cardiovascular disease. Some of the difficulty in diagnosis may be related to the overlap in somatic symptoms between cardiovascular diseases and depression, specifically fatigue, poor sleep, decreased appetite, weight gain or weight loss, and impaired concentration. There is some evidence, however, that the cognitive symptoms of depression are more important than the somatic symptoms in predicting outcome from CABG surgery. Thus, in the study by Connerney et al., only the cognitive symptoms of depression (sadness, guilt/worthlessness, and irritability) were associated with increased risk of mortality following CABG.[81]

Trials of antidepressant medication and therapy in cardiovascular patients have demonstrated modest improvement in depression. However, they have not shown a substantial benefit in cardiovascular morbidity or mortality. In CABG patients, there has been a specific concern raised regarding the risk of bleeding with SSRIs. Given the role of serotonin in platelet aggregability, SSRIs have the potential to increase the risk of bleeding. Recent studies of CABG patients

have not supported this possibility. A large study of patients receiving SSRIs or SNRIs prior to surgery did not reveal any increased risk for bleeding or in-hospital mortality following CABG. This held true even when the antidepressants were used in combination with antiplatelet agents and anticoagulation for treatment of acute coronary syndromes.[5] Collaborative care models have used to manage depression in patients following CABG, and are effective in reducing depressive symptoms.[78]

■ VENTRICULAR ASSIST DEVICES

In the United States 2,378 heart transplantations were performed in 2012, but 3,498 patients are currently awaiting heart transplantation. Given the shortage of donor hearts and the increasing numbers of patients with end-stage heart failure, mechanical circulatory supports, such as left ventricular assist devices (LVADs), are being used with increased frequency. LVADs are mechanical pumps implanted inside the chest to support heart function and blood circulation. LVADs may be used as a permanent treatment, termed "destination therapy" or may be used as a temporary "bridge-to-transplantation." The use of LVADs has increased greatly following a trial demonstrating that they improved survival and quality of life in end-stage heart failure patients, in comparison to optimal medical management.[82]

Patients undergoing LVAD implantation must be able to comply with frequent medical follow-up visits, perform sterile dressing changes, replace batteries frequently, respond to alarms from the device and must be able to cope with the stress of major surgery and a prolonged recovery. Psychiatric screening of patients who are to undergo LVAD implantation helps to identify individuals who are at higher risk of complications due to psychosocial issues. As there is still a limited knowledge about psychiatric risk factors associated with poor outcome among LVAD recipients, most screening approaches have been based on experience with heart transplant patients. This literature suggests that history of poor medical adherence, current depression, history of alcohol or drug detoxification, and past suicide attempts are associated with decreased survival.[83] A history of suicide attempts may pose a particular risk for patients with LVAD, as the internal pump is connected to an external power supply and controller via a drive line. If a patient disconnects the drive line to his/her LVAD, the device will stop functioning. In patients who develop depression and suicidal ideation following LVAD implantation, rapid evaluation and initiation of treatment is crucial given the ease with which they can harm themselves.

Not all requests to disconnect LVADs are considered suicidal. Some LVAD patients are dissatisfied with the quality of life that is dependent on a mechanical device for circulatory support, and decide to have the pump turned off. This decision should only be made after establishing the individual's capacity to make the decision, identifying treatable sources of suffering, determining whether active psychiatric illness is present, and understanding the familial, religious or cultural beliefs which may be playing a role in the decision.

There are few studies examining the prevalence of depression in LVAD patients, and they are limited by small sample sizes and short follow-up periods. The reported prevalence of depressive disorders following implantation ranges from 20% to 25% of patients, similar to rates seen in other types of cardiovascular illness.[84,85] Patients receiving LVADs have an improvement in their health status, peaking approximately 3 months after LVAD implantation.[86] Increased blood flow in heart failure patients who have chronically been in a low flow state, may improve energy, sleep and concentration. Patients with LVADs may, however, have significant pain, difficulty sleeping with the device, concern about infection, and worry about it malfunctioning.[87] Quality of life following LVAD implantation has been shown to be lower than the quality of life in patients who receive heart transplantation.

The relationship between LVAD implantation and depression may be moderated by the underlying cardiac condition, in most cases congestive heart failure. Congestive heart failure is associated with elevated rates of depression, with the risk increasing in accordance with New York Heart Association functional classification. In addition, patients are at high risk for postoperative delirium and stroke following LVAD implantation, conditions that also carry a relationship to depression. Some reports suggest that a significant proportion of LVAD patients with depression have experienced stroke as a postoperative complication.[85] Finally, there are significant psychological adjustments necessary for a patient to live with an implantable pump, knowing that they are at chronic risk for complications or failure of the device.

GYNECOLOGICAL SURGERY

■ HYSTERECTOMY

In 2003, over 600,000 hysterectomies were performed in the United States.[88] Although the rate has declined over recent decades, hysterectomy remains the most commonly performed gynecological surgery. Hysterectomies are usually performed for benign gynecological conditions; to relieve pain, discomfort and to improve quality of life. The primary indications in premenopausal women are dysfunctional uterine bleeding, endometriosis and fibroids. In postmenopausal women, hysterectomies are commonly performed for prolapsed uterus. The most common age for hysterectomy is 40 – 49, often prior to naturally occurring menopause. In 53.8% of cases, hysterectomy is accompanied by bilateral oophorectomy. Although this rate increases with age, 37% of women receiving bilateral oophorectomy are between 15 and 44 years old.[89]

Historically, a strong association has been described between hysterectomy and depressive symptoms. In 1974, Richards described a post-hysterectomy syndrome in 70% of patients that was characterized by depression, hot flashes, fatigue, and urinary symptoms.[90] Older studies were limited by retrospective designs, small sample sizes and inadequate outcome measures, and more recent prospective studies indicate that hysterectomy does alleviate symptoms for the majority of patients and has high rates of patient satisfaction.[91] In addition to improving physical symptoms, multiple studies have demonstrated reductions in rates of depression postoperatively. In the Maine Women's Health Study, rates of depression decreased from 21% preoperatively to 6% postoperatively.[92] The Maryland Women's Health Study, the largest trial to date, found that 73% of women with preoperative depression experienced remission of depressive symptoms and improvement in quality of life postoperatively.[93] Despite these favorable results, there does appear to be a subset of patients who do not experience symptomatic improvement or who develop new onset depression following hysterectomy. Risk factors for preoperative and postoperative depression include age, psychiatric history, and severity of pain symptoms (**Table 22-3**).

There are many potential mechanisms linking hysterectomy and oophorectomy with depression. Bilateral oophorectomy results in a sharp decline in the circulating levels of estrogen and progesterone.

TABLE 22-3 Risk Factors for Depression in Hysterectomy Patients

Risk Factors for Preoperative Depression[94]	Risk Factors for Postoperative Depression[93,94,95]
Younger age (<50 years)	Preoperative depression
Anxiety	History of psychotherapy
Pain	Anxiety Pain Lower parity

In natural menopause, the ovary continues to secrete small amounts of testosterone, which is converted in body fat to estradiol; however, this does not occur following surgical menopause. Even when ovaries are conserved, hysterectomy itself is associated with an earlier onset of menopause, particularly if unilateral oophorectomy is performed.[96] This may be related to disruption of ovarian blood supply during surgery. There are inconsistent results regarding the impact of hormones on relief from symptoms and risk of depression. The role of hormonal mechanisms is supported by studies showing that bilateral oophorectomy predicted lack of symptom improvement at 2 year follow-up,[93] increased risk for physician diagnosed depression,[97] and reduction of depressive symptoms with estrogen replacement therapy.[98,99] In contrast, other studies restricted to hysterectomy and bilateral oophorectomy patients have not found an association between bilateral oophorectomy and depression risk,[100] androgen levels and psychological health,[101] or alteration in risk for depression with estrogen replacement therapy.[97]

The loss of childbearing ability and perceived loss of femininity are theorized to be important factors in the development of depression post-hysterectomy. Although there is limited literature examining this issue, lower parity and nulliparity were found to be risks for depression post-hysterectomy in a study of Egyptian women.[95] In another study, women who preoperatively stated that they would have liked to have more children had higher depression scores and were more likely to have been in therapy for treatment of psychological symptoms. Postoperatively, these women continued to have elevated levels of depression, in comparison to women who had not wanted additional children.[102]

The benefits of hysterectomy do not appear to vary with the type of hysterectomy performed. In most studies, improvements in depression and quality of life occurred regardless of whether patients had bilateral oophorectomy or conservation of their ovaries.[94] Depression outcomes do not differ depending upon whether laparoscopic or abdominal hysterectomy was performed,[103] or upon whether the hysterectomy was total or subtotal.[104] One study did note that patients with hysterectomy continued to have lower quality of life than age matched women from the community, although their depressive symptoms, somatic symptoms and quality of life all improved preoperative to postoperative.[104]

Most studies have had fairly short follow-up periods and have not compared hysterectomy patients to women in the community. A 10-year, prospective study found that depressive symptoms declined in all women, regardless of whether they underwent natural menopause, had hysterectomy, or hysterectomy with oophorectomy.[100]

Most studies of treatment are based on women with perimenopausal or postmenopausal depression. In these patient groups, estrogen replacement therapy improves hot flashes and sleep, but is not consistently effective in relieving depressive symptoms. Estrogen replacement therapy may augment the efficacy of SSRIs.[105,106] Given that long-term estrogen replacement therapy is associated with an increased risk for stroke, venous thomboembolism, breast cancer and gallbladder disease, the decision to add hormone replacement should be made in collaboration with the patient's gynecologist or primary care physician, while carefully assessing the risks and benefits and conducting appropriate monitoring.

ENDOCRINE SURGERY

Neuropsychological symptoms are common in endocrine conditions, including Cushing disease, primary hyperparathyroidism, and thyroid disease (see also Chapter 14). Cushing disease is characterized by overproduction of adrenocorticotropic hormone (ACTH), most commonly due to a microadenoma, leading to hypercortisolemia. Neuropsychiatric symptoms have been reported in 54% to 86% of patients with Cushing disease.[107,108] Depressive disorders are most frequent, however, anxiety disorders, irritability, and mania have also been reported.[107,108,109] Surgical resection of the microadenoma is the treatment of choice for Cushing disease. Even following correction of hypercortisolism, psychopathology may persist. In a prospective study looking at patients being treated for Cushing disease, initial rates of psychiatric illness were reported to be 54.6% and 53.6% at 3-month visit, 36% at 6-month visit, and 24.1% at 12-month visit.[110] The persistence of neuropsychiatric symptoms may be related to long cortisol-induced effects on brain structure and functioning.[111]

Primary hyperparathyroidism with resultant elevations in parathyroid hormone and serum calcium levels is caused by glandular adenomas (see also Chapter 14) Hyperparathyroidism is frequently associated with psychiatric illness, with symptoms of depression in 23.4% and symptoms of anxiety in 15.6%.[112] Following parathyroidectomy, symptoms of depression and anxiety at 12 months followup have been found to decrease to 15.7% and 7.8%, respectively (Weber, 2007).

Thyroid disease may cause psychiatric symptoms, including depression, anxiety, and cognitive dysfunction.[113] Thyroidectomy is used as a treatment for thyroid cancers, goiter, and in some cases hyperthyroidism. Depending on how much of the thyroid is removed, patients may become hypothyroid postoperatively. In a study of patients undergoing thyroidectomy for thyroid carcinoma, elevated rates of depression and anxiety were found in comparison to normal controls, and the depression was more severe in the hypothyroid state than in those receiving thyroid hormone replacement.[113]

CANCER SURGERY

Patients often eagerly anticipate cancer surgery, despite its potential complications. They focus on the fact that a complete resection ("getting it all out") will increase the likelihood of cure. Clinical lore suggests that patients who receive neoadjuvant chemotherapy and/or radiation prior to surgery have more anxiety and depression than patients who receive it following surgery. This depressogenic effect is particularly strong in the setting of a poor response to neoadjuvant chemotherapy.[114] At times, patients are given the impression that chemotherapy and/or radiation may shrink their tumor sufficiently enough to allow surgery with curative intent; this hope helps them cope with the rigors of their initial treatment. Depression then ensues if their response to chemoradiation is inadequate, dashing their hopes of cure. Several common scenarios include neoadjuvant chemotherapy prior to possible mastectomy for inflammatory breast cancer, or neoadjuvant chemotherapy for pancreatic cancer in an attempt to prepare the patient for a Whipple procedure.

Cancer surgeries that result in permanent sequelae, such as sterility or loss of a body part (e.g. mastectomy, amputation, gynecological, or urological surgery), are more likely to cause depression. Patients who undergo exploratory surgery and are found to have unresectable disease are also at high risk of grief reactions and depression. In these situations, the postoperative period involves not only the usual physical stressors associated with recovery, but also adaptation to loss and confrontation with possible death. Such patients may develop suicidal ideation, and their suicide risk should be carefully assessed prior to discharge from the hospital.

■ BREAST SURGERY

Many women face the choice of either a mastectomy or lumpectomy for management of early stage breast cancer. Difficulty navigating this choice often leads to high anxiety, but usually not depression. A major incentive for developing breast-conserving surgery was to reduce the presumed emotional impact of radical mastectomy. However, in general, studies have not found lumpectomy to be a psychosocial panacea; women demonstrate similar levels of depression and sexual function in the months after surgery, regardless of the

<table>
<tr><td>

BOX 22-2
COMPONENTS OF THE PSYCHOSOCIAL EVALUATION FOR WOMEN CONSIDERING PROPHYLACTIC MASTECTOMY AND/OR PROPHYLACTIC OOPHORECTOMY

Family cancer history
Personal cancer history
Psychiatric history (with emphasis on anxiety, depression, body dysmorphia, and personality disorders)
History of sexual abuse or assault
Sexual, pregnancy, and breastfeeding history
Perception of cancer risk and associated anxiety
Understanding of actual risk
Satisfaction with prior plastic surgeries, if any
Desire for future childbearing
Partner's stance and caregiving role

</td></tr>
</table>

specific procedure, though women who undergo lumpectomy do tend to have less body image disturbance.[115] For those undergoing mastectomy, psychological distress (including depression and anxiety) is apparent immediately and 1 year after surgery, regardless of reconstruction (yes vs. no) or timing of reconstruction (immediate vs. delayed).[116] BRCA mutation carriers sometimes undergo prophylactic mastectomy due to their high lifetime risk of developing breast cancer; in this situation, mastectomy does not appear to raise the risk for depression.[117] Still, a psychosocial assessment of the risk factors for emotional distress after prophylactic mastectomy may help patients and providers in deciding how to proceed (**Box 22-2**). Phantom breast syndrome after mastectomy, which may affect up to 10% to 20% of patients, may be associated with younger age, DCIS, and increased prevalence of depressive symptoms.[118]

Depression and other psychiatric disorders may be associated with postoperative complications in mastectomy patients. Specifically, a recent study suggested that the presence of any psychiatric diagnosis was associated with an increased rate of complications and prolonged hospitalizations, as well as higher average costs of care.[119] In this study, 4.5% of patients had a mental health condition; however, 86.7% of psychiatric disorders were anxiety disorders, and 6% were major depression.[119]

The biological determinants of postmastectomy depression have not been extensively investigated. However, one study suggests that the BDNF Met/Met genotype may be independently linked to depression both 1 week and 1 year after mastectomy, whereas no associations with 5-HTT and 5-HTR2 a genes were identified.[120]

■ HEAD AND NECK CANCER SURGERY

A diagnosis of head and neck cancer often entails surgery that can impair chewing, swallowing, and speaking, as well as sensory functions, such as taste and smell. Some of these surgeries are also physically disfiguring. For example, total laryngectomies result in a permanent stoma and speech loss; communication alternatives, such as the one-way air valve and electrolarynx, are incompletely effective. The laryngectomy stoma is associated with severe halitosis and other functional limitations, such as permanent inability to swim, inability to blow one's nose, difficulty with managing secretions, and difficulty showering. Many patients, even those who do not require total laryngectomy, receive tracheostomies which may be either temporary or permanent. Again, these usually interrupt communication abilities. Other patients require indefinite enteral nutrition and have episodes of aspiration, resulting in frequent bouts of pneumonia.

Anxiety before head and neck surgery is very high in the setting of anticipated cosmetic and functional alterations. Depression tends to peak in the immediate postoperative period but improves as patients adjust to their functional status.[121] Still, follow-up 6 months postoperatively reveals that a subset (perhaps ~10%) of patients meet criteria for major depression.[122] Because head and neck cancer is highly correlated with tobacco and alcohol use, patients are at high risk of withdrawal states in the postoperative period, and guilt over maladaptive health behaviors may further fuel depression.

■ GENITOURINARY AND OTHER CANCER SURGERIES

Prostatectomy, more so than radiotherapy for prostate cancer, can result in troublesome side effects, such as sexual dysfunction and urinary incontinence. However, somewhat surprisingly, a large longitudinal study showed that men with high anxiety around the diagnosis who received prostatectomy reported less anxiety and depression at 6-month follow-up than high-anxiety men receiving radiotherapy alone.[123] In fact, at all postoperative time points, men who underwent prostatectomy reported lower levels of depression than are observed in the general population (9–18% with clinically significant levels vs. 20% in the general population). Several proposed explanations for these findings exist. It is possible that high-anxiety men were sufficiently afraid of surgery that they chose radiotherapy, thus enriching the prostatectomy group with patients who were at lower risk for developing anxiety and/or depression. Alternatively, surgery may have provided more reassurance since the prostate actually is removed. The study suggests that men with localized prostate cancer are surprisingly psychologically resilient, particularly if they receive surgical management.

Patients undergoing surgery for localized renal cell carcinoma (either radical nephrectomy or nephron-sparing surgery) tend to have relatively normal physical and mental health outcomes. For bladder carcinoma, the treatment of choice is radical cystectomy with urinary tract reconstruction. Ileal conduit procedures involve creation of an ureteroenteric anastomosis ultimately leading to a permanent abdominal wall stoma. More recently, surgeons have developed alternate diversion procedures, some of which may be complicated by diarrhea, B12 malabsorption, and incontinence. Quality of life appears to be similar after conduit and continent diversion.[124] Little is known about the true incidence of depression after these procedures, aside from one small study suggesting higher levels of depression in ileal conduit patients than in a control group of patients who received prostatectomy for benign disease.[125]

Ostomies, hysterectomy, and oophorectomy are discussed elsewhere in this section, and psychosocial complications tend to be similar in patients undergoing these procedures for cancer. One final cancer-specific procedure deserves mention, namely pelvic exenteration, in which all pelvic organs (colon, rectum, anus, bladder, prostate, uterus, ovaries, vagina) are removed in order to manage advanced locally invasive tumors. This results in permanent ostomies and severe impairment in sexual function. Little is known about the incidence of depression in pelvic exenteration patients, although a small case series suggests reasonable psychosocial function postoperatively.[126]

CONCLUSION

Depression is prevalent in both the preoperative and postoperative patient but is frequently overlooked. Psychiatric screening allows for the opportunity to identify newly recognized depression and to adequately manage psychiatric medications or treatments, such as cognitive behavioral therapy, in the perioperative period. Each surgical patient population faces unique risks for depression. Preoperatively, rates of depression are elevated in patients undergoing bariatric surgery and CABG. Postoperatively, depression is common following solid-organ transplantation, in burn patients, those with limb amputation, and in patients losing a body part to cancer

surgery. Depression may impact postoperative care, as it increases the risk of suboptimal pain control and may impair compliance with postoperative treatment recommendations. Surgical outcome may also be affected, with depressed bariatric surgery patients having decreased weight loss after surgery and depressed CABG patients having increased morbidity and mortality. However, in some cases surgery may actually decrease rates of depression, as seen in hysterectomy and some types of cancer surgery. The current understanding of the relationship between surgery and depression is still limited, as research has been restricted to specific patient populations with small sample sizes, making the generalizability of the findings unclear. Further research is needed to better understand the complex relationship between surgery and depression, the impact of depression on surgical outcome, and to learn whether treatment of depression improves surgical outcome.

REFERENCES

1. Vaerøy H, Juell M, Høivik B. Prevalence of depression among general hospital surgical inpatients. *Nord J Psychiatry*. 2003;57(1): 13–16.

2. Ni Mhaolain AM, Butler JS, Magill PF, Wood AE, Sheehan J. The increased need for liaison psychiatry in surgical patients due to the high prevalence of undiagnosed anxiety and depression. *Ir J Med Sci*. 2008;177(3):211–215.

3. Conrad EJ, Hansel TC, Pejic NG, Constans J. Assessment of psychiatric symptoms at a level I trauma center surgery follow-up clinic: a preliminary report. *Am Surg*. 2013;79(5):492–494.

4. Scher CS, Anwar M. The self-reporting of psychiatric medications in patients scheduled for elective surgery. *J Clin Anesth*. 1999;11(8):619–621.

5. Kim DH, Daskalakis C, Whellan DJ, et al. Safety of selective serotonin reuptake inhibitor in adults undergoing coronary artery bypass grafting. *Am J Cardiol*. 2009;103(10):1391–1395.

6. Kudoh A, Katagai H, Takazawa T. Antidepressant treatment for chronic depressed patients should not be discontinued prior to anesthesia. *Can J Anaesth*. 2002;49(2):132–136.

7. van Haelst IM, van Klei WA, Doodeman HJ, Kalkman CJ, Egberts TC, Group MS. Antidepressive treatment with monoamine oxidase inhibitors and the occurrence of intraoperative hemodynamic events: a retrospective observational cohort study. *J Clin Psychiatry*. 2012;73(8):1103–1109.

8. Inouye SK. The dilemma of delirium: clinical and research controversies regarding diagnosis and evaluation of delirium in hospitalized elderly medical patients. *Am J Med*. 1994;97(3): 278–288.

9. McCusker J, Cole M, Abrahamowicz M, Primeau F, Belzile E. Delirium predicts 12-month mortality. *Arch Intern Med*. 2002; 162(4):457–463.

10. Kiely DK, Marcantonio ER, Inouye SK, et al. Persistent delirium predicts greater mortality. *J Am Geriatr Soc*. 2009;57(1):55–61.

11. Davis DHJ, Barnes LE, Blossom SCM, et al. The descriptive epidemiology of delirium symptoms in a large population-based cohort study: results from the Medical Research Council Cognitive Function and Ageing Study (MRC CFAS). *BMC Geriatrics*. 2014;14(87):1–8.

12. Guenther U, Radtke FM. Delirium in the postanaesthesia period. *Curr Opin Anaesthesiol*. 2011;24(6):670–675.

13. Bruce AJ, Ritchie CW, Blizard R, Lai R, Raven P. The incidence of delirium associated with orthopedic surgery: a meta-analytic review. *Int Psychogeriatr*. 2007;19(2):197–214.

14. Koster S, Oosterveld FG, Hensens AG, Wijma A, van der Palen J. Delirium after cardiac surgery and predictive validity of a risk checklist. *Ann Thorac Surg*. 2008;86(6):1883–1887.

15. Meagher DJ, Leonard M, Donnelly S, Conroy M, Adamis D, Trzepacz PT. A longitudinal study of motor subtypes in delirium: frequency and stability during episodes. *J Psychosom Res*. 2012;72(3):236–241.

16. Stransky M, Schmidt C, Ganslmeier P, et al. Hypoactive delirium after cardiac surgery as an independent risk factor for prolonged mechanical ventilation. *J Cardiothorac Vasc Anesth*. 2011;25(6):968–974.

17. Inouye SK, van Dyck CH, Alessi CA, et al. Clarifying confusion: the confusion assessment method. A new method for detection of delirium. *Ann Intern Med*. 1990;113(12):941–948.

18. Ely EW, Margolin R, Francis J, et al. Evaluation of delirium in critially ill patients: validation of the Confusion Assessment Method for the Intensive Care Unit (CAM-ICU). *Crit Care Med*. 2001:29(7):1370–1379.

19. National Institute for Health and Care Excellence. Delirium: diagnosis, prevention and management (clinical guideline 103). Published July 2010. Available at www.nice.org.uk/nicemedia/live/13060/49909/49909.pdf. Accessed on January 4, 2016.

20. Guelfi JD, Strub N, Loft H. Efficacy of intravenous citalopram compared with oral citalopram for severe depression. Safety and efficacy data from a double-blind, double-dummy trial. *J Affect Disord*. 2000;58(3):201–209.

21. Robinson DS, Amsterdam JD. The selegiline transdermal system in major depressive disorder: a systematic review of safety and tolerability. *J Affect Disord*. 2008;105(1–3):15–23.

22. Livingston RL, Zucker DK, Isenberg K, Wetzel RD. Tricyclic antidepressants and delirium. *J Clin Psychiatry*. 1983;44(5):173–176.

23. Mack DR, Barbarello-Andrews L, Liu MT. Agitated delirium associated with therapeutic doses of sustained-release bupropion. *Int J Clin Pharm*. 2012;34(1):9–12.

24. Ramsey TD, Lau TT, Ensom MH. Serotonergic and adrenergic drug interactions associated with linezolid: a critical review and practical management approach. *Ann Pharmacother*. 2013;47(4):543–560.

25. Nelson EM, Philbrick AM. Avoiding serotonin syndrome: the nature of the interaction between tramadol and selective serotonin reuptake inhibitors. *Ann Pharmacother*. 2012;46(12):1712–1716.

26. Nadkarni A, Oldham MA, Howard M, Berenbaum I. Drug-drug interactions between warfarin and psychotropics: updated review of the literature. *Pharmacotherapy*. 2012;32(10):932–942.

27. Schatzberg AF, Haddad P, Kaplan EM, et al. Serotonin reuptake inhibitor discontinuation syndrome: a hypothetical definition. Discontinuation Consensus panel. *J Clin Psychiatry*. 1997; 58(Suppl 7):5–10.

28. Goebel S, Steinert A, Vierheilig C, Faller H. Correlation between depressive symptoms and perioperative pain: a prospective cohort study of patients undergoing orthopedic surgeries. *Clin J Pain*. 2013;29(5):392–399.

29. Brander V, Gondek S, Martin E, Stulberg SD. Pain and depression influence outcome 5 years after knee replacement surgery. *Clin Orthop Relat Res*. 2007;464:21–26.

30. Cho CH, Seo HJ, Bae KC, Lee KJ, Hwang I, Warner JJ. The impact of depression and anxiety on self-assessed pain, disability, and quality of life in patients scheduled for rotator cuff repair. *J Shoulder Elbow Surg*. 2013;22(9):1160–1166.

31. Gupta R, Lahan V. Insomnia associated with depressive disorder: primary, secondary, or mixed? *Indian J Psychol Med*. 2011; 33(2):123–128.

32. Luppino FS, de Wit LM, Bouvy PF, et al. Overweight, obesity, and depression: a systematic review and meta-analysis of longitudinal studies. *Arch Gen Psychiatry*. 2010;67(3):220–229.

33. Faith MS, Butryn M, Wadden TA, Fabricatore A, Nguyen AM, Heymsfield SB. Evidence for prospective associations among depression and obesity in population-based studies. *Obes Rev*. 2011;12(5):e438–e453.

34. Black DW, Goldstein RB, Mason EE. Prevalence of mental disorder in 88 morbidly obese bariatric clinic patients. *Am J Psychiatry*. 1992;149(2):227–234.

35. Chen EY, Fettich KC, McCloskey MS. Correlates of suicidal ideation and/or behavior in bariatric-surgery-seeking individuals with severe obesity. *Crisis*. 2012;33(3):137–143.

36. Brunault P, Jacobi D, Miknius V, et al. High preoperative depression, phobic anxiety, and binge eating scores and low medium-term weight loss in sleeve gastrectomy obese patients: a preliminary cohort study. *Psychosomatics*. 2012;53(4): 363–370.

37. Sysko R, Devlin MJ, Hildebrandt TB, Brewer SK, Zitsman JL, Walsh BT. Psychological outcomes and predictors of initial weight loss outcomes among severely obese adolescents receiving laparoscopic adjustable gastric banding. *J Clin Psychiatry*. 2012; 73(10):1351–1357.

38. Cunningham JL, Merrell CC, Sarr M, et al. Investigation of antidepressant medication usage after bariatric surgery. *Obes Surg*. 2012;22(4):530–535.

39. Roerig JL, Steffen K, Zimmerman C, Mitchell JE, Crosby RD, Cao L. Preliminary comparison of sertraline levels in postbariatric surgery patients versus matched nonsurgical cohort. *Surg Obes Relat Dis*. 2012;8(1):62–66.

40. White CA, Hunt JC. Psychological factors in postoperative adjustment to stoma surgery. *Ann R Coll Surg Engl*. 1997;79(1): 3–7.

41. Simmons KL, Smith JA, Bobb KA, Liles LL. Adjustment to colostomy: stoma acceptance, stoma care self-efficacy and interpersonal relationships. *J Adv Nurs*. 2007;60(6):627–635.

42. Mihalopoulos NG, Trunnell EP, Ball K, Moncur C. The psychologic impact of ostomy surgery on persons 50 years of age and older. *J Wound Ostomy Continence Nurs*. 1994;21(4):149–155.

43. Spencer BW, Chilcot J, Farrington K. Still sad after successful renal transplantation: are we failing to recognise depression? An audit of depression screening in renal graft recipients. *Nephron Clin Pract*. 2011;117(2):c106–c112.

44. Lanzafame M, Ferrari S, Lattuada E, et al. Mirtazapine in an HIV-1 infected patient with progressive multifocal leukoencephalopathy. *Infez Med*. 2009;17(1):35–37.

45. Cettomai D, McArthur JC. Mirtazapine use in human immunodeficiency virus-infected patients with progressive multifocal leukoencephalopathy. *Arch Neurol*. 2009;66(2):255–258.

46. Brown ES, Chamberlain W, Dhanani N, Paranjpe P, Carmody TJ, Sargeant M. An open-label trial of olanzapine for corticosteroid-induced mood symptoms. *J Affect Disord*. 2004;83(2–3): 277–281.

47. Baranyi A, Krauseneck T, Rothenhäusler HB. Overall mental distress and health-related quality of life after solid-organ transplantation: results from a retrospective follow-up study. *Health Qual Life Outcomes*. 2013;11:15.

48. Dew MA, DiMartini AF, DeVito Dabbs AJ, et al. Onset and risk factors for anxiety and depression during the first 2 years after lung transplantation. *Gen Hosp Psychiatry*. 2012;34(2): 127–138.

49. Novak M, Molnar MZ, Szeifert L, et al. Depressive symptoms and mortality in patients after kidney transplantation: a prospective prevalent cohort study. *Psychosom Med*. 2010;72(6):527–534.

50. Corruble E, Barry C, Varescon I, et al. Report of depressive symptoms on waiting list and mortality after liver and kidney transplantation: a prospective cohort study. *BMC Psychiatry*. 2011;11:182.

51. Dubernard JM, Lengelé B, Morelon E, et al. Outcomes 18 months after the first human partial face transplantation. *N Engl J Med*. 2007;357(24):2451–2460.

52. Soni CV, Barker JH, Pushpakumar SB, et al. Psychosocial considerations in facial transplantation. *Burns*. 2010;36(7):959–964.

53. Coffman KL, Siemionow MZ. Face transplantation: psychological outcomes at three-year follow-up. *Psychosomatics*. 2013;54:372–378.

54. Ilechukwu ST. Psychiatry of the medically ill in the burn unit. *Psychiatr Clin North Am*. 2002;25(1):129–147.

55. Wisely JA, Wilson E, Duncan RT, Tarrier N. Pre-existing psychiatric disorders, psychological reactions to stress and the recovery of burn survivors. *Burns*. 2010;36(2):183–191.

56. Dalal PK, Saha R, Agarwal M. Psychiatric aspects of burn. *Indian J Plast Surg*. 2010;43(Suppl):S136–S142.

57. Christian LM, Graham JE, Padgett DA, Glaser R, Kiecolt-Glaser JK. Stress and wound healing. *Neuroimmunomodulation*. 2006;13(5–6):337–346.

58. Dyster-Aas J, Willebrand M, Wikehult B, Gerdin B, Ekselius L. Major depression and posttraumatic stress disorder symptoms following severe burn injury in relation to lifetime psychiatric morbidity. *J Trauma*. 2008;64(5):1349–1356.

59. Yabanoğlu H, Yağmurdur MC, Taşkıntuna N, Karakayalı H. Early period psychiatric disorders following burn trauma and the importance of surgical factors in the etiology. *Ulus Travma Acil Cerrahi Derg*. 2012;18(5):436–440.

60. Ter Smitten MH, de Graaf R, Van Loey NE. Prevalence and co-morbidity of psychiatric disorders 1–4 years after burn. *Burns*. 2011;37(5):753–761.

61. Munster AM, Fauerbach JA, Lawrence J. Development and utilization of a psychometric instrument for measuring quality of life in burn patients, 1976 to 1996. *Acta Chir Plast*. 1996;38(4):128–131.

62. Patterson DR, Ptacek JT, Crones F, Fauerbach JA, Engray L. Describing and predicting distress and satisfaction with life for burn survivors. *J Burn Care Rehabil*. 2000;21(6):490–498.

63. Fauerbach JA, Heinberg LJ, Lawrence JW, et al. Effect of early body image dissatisfaction on subsequent psychological and physical adjustment after disfiguring injury. *Psychosom Med*. 2000;62(4):576–582.

64. Senra H. How depressive levels are related to the adults' experiences of lower-limb amputation: a mixed methods pilot study. *Int J Rehabil Res*. 2013;36(1):13–20.

65. Doukas WC, Hayda RA, Frisch HM, et al. The Military Extremity Trauma Amputation/Limb Salvage (METALS) study: outcomes of amputation versus limb salvage following major lower-extremity trauma. *J Bone Joint Surg Am*. 2013;95(2):138–145.

66. Atherton R, Robertson N. Psychological adjustment to lower limb amputation amongst prosthesis users. *Disabil Rehabil*. 2006;28(19):1201–1209.

67. Desmond DM, MacLachlan M. Coping strategies as predictors of psychosocial adaptation in a sample of elderly veterans with acquired lower limb amputations. *Soc Sci Med*. 2006;62(1): 208–216.

68. Singh R, Ripley D, Pentland B, et al. Depression and anxiety symptoms after lower limb amputation: the rise and fall. *Clin Rehabil*. 2009;23(3):281–286.

69. Asano M, Rushton P, Miller WC, Deathe BA. Predictors of quality of life among individuals who have a lower limb amputation. *Prosthet Orthot Int*. 2008;32(2):231–243.

70. Larner S, van Ross E, Hale C. Do psychological measures predict the ability of lower limb amputees to learn to use a prosthesis? *Clin Rehabil*. 2003;17(5):493–498.

71. Webster JB, Hakimi KN, Williams RM, Turner AP, Norvell DC, Czerniecki JM. Prosthetic fitting, use, and satisfaction following lower-limb amputation: a prospective study. *J Rehabil Res Dev*. 2012;49(10):1493–1504.

72. Livneh H, Antonak RF, Gerhardt J. Psychosocial adaptation to amputation: the role of sociodemographic variables, disability-related factors and coping strategies. *Int J Rehabil Res*. 1999;22(1):21–31.

73. Connerney I, Shapiro PA, McLaughlin JS, Bagiella E, Sloan RP. Relation between depression after coronary artery bypass surgery and 12-month outcome: a prospective study. *Lancet*. 2001;358(9295):1766–1771.

74. Blumenthal JA, Lett HS, Babyak MA, et al. Depression as a risk factor for mortality after coronary artery bypass surgery. *Lancet*. 2003;362(9384):604–609.

75. Lin Y, Chen J, Wang Z. Meta-analysis of factors which influence delirium following cardiac surgery. *J Card Surg*. 2012;27(4):481–492.

76. Mallik S, Krumholz HM, Lin ZQ, et al. Patients with depressive symptoms have lower health status benefits after coronary artery bypass surgery. *Circulation*. 2005;111(3):271–277.

77. Saur CD, Granger BB, Muhlbaier LH, et al. Depressive symptoms and outcome of coronary artery bypass grafting. *Am J Crit Care*. 2001;10(1):4–10.

78. Wellenius GA, Mukamal KJ, Kulshreshtha A, Asonganyi S, Mittleman MA. Depressive symptoms and the risk of atherosclerotic progression among patients with coronary artery bypass grafts. *Circulation*. 2008;117(18):2313–2319.

79. Borowicz L, Royall R, Grega M, Selnes O, Lyketsos C, McKhann G. Depression and cardiac morbidity 5 years after coronary artery bypass surgery. *Psychosomatics*. 2002;43(6):464–471.

80. Connerney I, Sloan RP, Shapiro PA, Bagiella E, Seckman C. Depression is associated with increased mortality 10 years after coronary artery bypass surgery. *Psychosom Med*. 2010;72(9): 874–881.

81. Rollman BL, Belnap BH, LeMenager MS, et al. Telephone-delivered collaborative care for treating post-CABG depression: a randomized controlled trial. *JAMA*. 2009;302(19):2095–2103.

82. Rose EA, Gelijns AC, Moskowitz AJ, et al. Long-term use of a left ventricular assist device for end-stage heart failure. *N Engl J Med*. 2001;345(20):1435–1443.

83. Owen JE, Bonds CL, Wellisch DK. Psychiatric evaluations of heart transplant candidates: predicting post-transplant hospitalizations, rejection episodes, and survival. *Psychosomatics*. 2006;47(3):213–222.

84. Wray J, Hallas CN, Banner NR. Quality of life and psychological well-being during and after left ventricular assist device support. *Clin Transplant*. 2007;21(5):622–627.

85. Shapiro PA, Levin HR, Oz MC. Left ventricular assist devices. Psychosocial burden and implications for heart transplant programs. *Gen Hosp Psychiatry*. 1996;18(6 Suppl):30S–35S.

86. Brouwers C, Denollet J, de Jonge N, Caliskan K, Kealy J, Pedersen SS. Patient-reported outcomes in left ventricular assist device therapy: a systematic review and recommendations for clinical research and practice. *Circ Heart Fail*. 2011;4(6):714–723.

87. Dew MA, Kormos RL, Winowich S, et al. Human factors issues in ventricular assist device recipients and their family caregivers. *ASAIO J*. 2000;46(3):367–373.

88. Wu JM, Wechter ME, Geller EJ, Nguyen TV, Visco AG. Hysterectomy rates in the United States, 2003. *Obstet Gynecol*. 2007;110(5):1091–1095.

89. Whiteman MK, Hillis SD, Jamieson DJ, et al. Inpatient hysterectomy surveillance in the United States, 2000–2004. *Am J Obstet Gynecol*. 2008;198(1):34.e31–37.

90. Richards DH. A post-hysterectomy syndrome. *Lancet*. 1974;2(7887):983–985.

91. Kjerulff KH, Rhodes JC, Langenberg PW, Harvey LA. Patient satisfaction with results of hysterectomy. *Am J Obstet Gynecol*. 2000;183(6):1440–1447.

92. Carlson KJ, Miller BA, Fowler FJ. The Maine Women's Health Study: I. Outcomes of hysterectomy. *Obstet Gynecol*. 1994;83(4):556–565.

93. Kjerulff KH, Langenberg PW, Rhodes JC, Harvey LA, Guzinski GM, Stolley PD. Effectiveness of hysterectomy. *Obstet Gynecol*. 2000;95(3):319–326.

94. Vandyk AD, Brenner I, Tranmer J, Van Den Kerkhof E. Depressive symptoms before and after elective hysterectomy. *J Obstet Gynecol Neonatal Nurs*. 2011;40(5):566–576.

95. Helmy YA, Hassanin IM, Elraheem TA, Bedaiwy AA, Peterson RS, Bedaiwy MA. Psychiatric morbidity following hysterectomy in Egypt. *Int J Gynaecol Obstet*. 2008;102(1):60–64.

96. Farquhar CM, Sadler L, Harvey SA, Stewart AW. The association of hysterectomy and menopause: a prospective cohort study. *BJOG*. 2005;112(7):956–962.

97. Rocca WA, Grossardt BR, Geda YE, et al. Long-term risk of depressive and anxiety symptoms after early bilateral oophorectomy. *Menopause*. 2008;15(6):1050–1059.

98. Schiff R, Bulpitt CJ, Wesnes KA, Rajkumar C. Short-term transdermal estradiol therapy, cognition and depressive symptoms in healthy older women. A randomised placebo controlled pilot cross-over study. *Psychoneuroendocrinology*. 2005;30(4):309–315.

99. Nathorst-Böös J, von Schoultz B, Carlström K. Elective ovarian removal and estrogen replacement therapy–effects on sexual life, psychological well-being and androgen status. *J Psychosom Obstet Gynaecol*. 1993;14(4):283–293.

100. Gibson CJ, Joffe H, Bromberger JT, et al. Mood symptoms after natural menopause and hysterectomy with and without bilateral oophorectomy among women in midlife. *Obstet Gynecol*. 2012;119(5):935–941.

101. Aziz A, Brännström M, Bergquist C, Silfverstolpe G. Perimenopausal androgen decline after oophorectomy does not influence sexuality or psychological well-being. *Fertil Steril*. 2005;83(4):1021–1028.

102. Leppert PC, Legro RS, Kjerulff KH. Hysterectomy and loss of fertility: implications for women's mental health. *J Psychosom Res*. 2007;63(3):269–274.

103. Persson P, Wijma K, Hammar M, Kjølhede P. Psychological wellbeing after laparoscopic and abdominal hysterectomy–a randomised controlled multicentre study. *BJOG*. 2006;113(9):1023–1030.

104. Thakar R, Ayers S, Georgakapolou A, Clarkson P, Stanton S, Manyonda I. Hysterectomy improves quality of life and decreases psychiatric symptoms: a prospective and randomised comparison of total versus subtotal hysterectomy. *BJOG*. 2004;111(10):1115–1120.

105. Westlund Tam L, Parry BL. Does estrogen enhance the antidepressant effects of fluoxetine? *J Affect Disord*. 2003;77(1):87–92.

106. Schneider LS, Small GW, Hamilton SH, Bystritsky A, Nemeroff CB, Meyers BS. Estrogen replacement and response to fluoxetine in a multicenter geriatric depression trial. Fluoxetine Collaborative Study Group. *Am J Geriatr Psychiatry*. 1997;5(2):97–106.

107. Cohen SI. Cushing's syndrome: a psychiatric study of 29 patients. *Br J Psychiatry*. 1980;135:120–124.

108. Sonino N, Fava GA, Raffi AR, et al. Clinical correlates of major depression in Cushing's disease. *Psychopathology*. 1998;31(6):302–306.

109. Kelly WF, Kelly MJ, Faragher B. A prospective study of psychiatric and psychological aspects of Cushing's syndrome. *Clin Endocrinol*.1996;45(6):715–720.

110. Dorn LD, Burgess ES, Friedman TC, et al. The longitudinal course of psychopathology in Cushing's syndrome after correction of hypercortisolism. *J Clin Endocrinol Metab*. 1997;82(3):912–919.

111. Starkman MN, Gebarski SS, Berent S, et al. Hippocampal formation volume, memory dysfunction, and cortisol levels in patients with Cushing's syndrome. *Biol Psychiatry*. 1992;32(9):756–765.

112. Weber T, Keller M, Hense I, et al. Effect of parathyroidectomy on quality of life and neuropsychological symptoms in primary hyperparathyroidism. *World J Surg*. 2007;31(6):1202–1209.

113. Constant EL, Adam S, Seron X, et al. Anxiety and depression, attention, and executive functions in hypothyroidism. *J Int Neuropsychol Soc*. 2005;11(5):535–544.

114. Chintamani Gogne A, Khandelwal R, et al. The correlation of anxiety and depression levels with response to neoadjuvant chemotherapy in patients with breast cancer. *JRSM Short Rep*. 2011;2(3):15.

115. Rosenberg SM, Tamimi RM, Gelber S, et al. Body image in recently diagnosed young women with early breast cancer. *Psychooncology*. 2013;22(8):1849–1855.

116. Metcalfe KA, Semple J, Quan ML, et al. Changes in psychosocial functioning 1 year after mastectomy alone, delayed breast reconstruction, or immediate breast reconstruction. *Ann Surg Oncol*. 2012;19(1):233–241.

117. Brandberg Y, Sandelin K, Erikson S, et al. Psychological reactions, quality of life, and body image after bilateral prophylactic mastectomy in women at high risk for breast cancer: a prospective 1-year follow-up study. *J Clin Oncol*. 2008;26(24):3943–3949.

118. Spyropoulou AC, Papageorgiou C, Markopoulos C, Christodoulou GN, Soldatos KR. Depressive symptomatology correlates with phantom breast syndrome in mastectomized women. *Eur Arch Psychiatry Clin Neurosci*. 2008;258(3):165–170.

119. Fox JP, Philip EJ, Gross CP, Desai RA, Killelea B, Desai MM. Associations between mental health and surgical outcomes among women undergoing mastectomy for cancer. *Breast J*. 2013;19(3):276–284.

120. Kim JM, Kim SW, Stewart R, et al. Serotonergic and BDNF genes associated with depression 1 week and 1 year after mastectomy for breast cancer. *Psychosom Med*. 2012;74(1):8–15.

121. Mochizuki Y, Matsushima E, Omura K. Perioperative assessment of psychological state and quality of life of head and neck cancer patients undergoing surgery. *Int J Oral Maxillofac Surg.* 2009;38(2):151–159.

122. Bronheim H, Strain JJ, Biller HF. Psychiatric aspects of head and neck surgery. Part I: New surgical techniques and psychiatric consequences. *Gen Hosp Psychiatry.* 1991;13(3):165–176.

123. Korfage IJ, Essink-Bot ML, Janssens AC, Schröder FH, de Koning HJ. Anxiety and depression after prostate cancer diagnosis and treatment: 5-year follow-up. *Br J Cancer.* 2006;94(8):1093–1098.

124. Porter MP, Penson DF. Health related quality of life after radical cystectomy and urinary diversion for bladder cancer: a systematic review and critical analysis of the literature. *J Urol.* 2005;173(4):1318–1322.

125. Ficarra V, Righetti R, D'Amico A, et al. General state of health and psychological well-being in patients after surgery for urological malignant neoplasms. *Urol Int.* 2000;65(3):130–134.

126. Dempsey GM, Buchsbaum HJ, Morrison J. Psychosocial adjustment to pelvic exenteration. *Gynecol Oncol.* 1975;3(4):325–334.

CHAPTER 23

Delivering Depression Care: Services and Settings

Jane Erb, MD

Emily Benedetto, MSW, LCSW

James Cartreine, PhD

David Kroll, MD

Eliza Park, MD

Sejal Shah, MD

Stuart Pollack, MD

INTRODUCTION

Screening, comprehensive assessment, and effective treatments are necessary but not sufficient to adequately treat individuals with depression. They must be paired with effective and efficient systems for delivering the care. Implementation strategies designed to identify, evaluate, and treat patients wherever they present while seamlessly coordinating their care with other members of the health care team is the challenge. Teams of experts who can communicate with each other and coordinate their therapeutic efforts are essential. Furthermore, a population-based orientation is necessary in order to design systems that are scalable and affordable. Incorporating disease registries allows for efficient monitoring and maximizing patient adherence and optimizing treatment outcomes.[1] This requires the use of computerized technologies to enable tracking and monitoring of symptoms, functioning, and satisfaction over time. Computerized treatment also provides greater access by removing the physical barrier to care and thereby enhancing patient engagement in their care.

In this chapter we discuss the provision of care to medically ill patients with depression, models of depression care delivery in medical outpatient settings, and the components of successful, efficient, and cost-effective delivery models. We also address the role of computerization in delivering care to large populations.

■ THE MEDICAL OUTPATIENT SETTING

In the late 1970s, the first multi-site mental health epidemiological study in the United States identified the primary care system as the "de facto mental health system" for Americans with more prevalent but less severe mental health disorders, including depression.[2] That trend has continued to the present day.[3]

Research has underscored the benefit of identifying and treating depression within the primary care setting and a number of promising care models have been developed. Despite this, mental health care in many primary care settings remains suboptimal. The recent Institute of Medicine report, "Improving Quality of Health Care for Mental and Substance Use Conditions"[4] documented substantial inadequacies in the provision of mental health care, including poor detection, treatment and follow-up care. These findings have documented the need for a wider dissemination of guideline-driven treatment strategies.

According to a recent review, of the 6% to10% of primary care patients who meet diagnostic criteria for MDD, only 50% are accurately diagnosed by primary care providers (PCPs).[5] Primary care patients who are given antidepressants often receive little education about depression and have infrequent follow-up visits, leading to poor treatment adherence. Poor adherence is common across all classes of prescribed antidepressants: only 25% to 50% of primary care patients continue with antidepressant treatment for the guideline-recommended duration, and 15% never start the medication.[5]

A number of barriers to adherence have been identified, including inadequate monitoring, insufficient patient education about depression and its treatment, and inadequate clinician knowledge and skills.[6] Stigma, and legal and financial difficulties are also obstacles.

Integrated care models and treatment strategies, such as collaborative care, have been implemented to bridge these gaps and are promising vehicles to improved and affordable care.[7] Components of these models that have been considered critical are listed in **Table 23-1**.

Screening is essential for efficiently identifying patients at risk. The ideal tool for screening is sensitive yet specific, self-administered, and

TABLE 23-1 Integrated Depression Care: Critical Components

Screening
Patient engagement strategies, e.g., motivational interviewing and patient self-management
Population-based care (e.g., patient registries)
Measurement-based care
Stepped care
Depression Care Manager
Systematic use of treatment algorithms

easily integrated into the work flow. The Patient Health Questionnaire (PHQ-9)[8] has been widely used as the screening tool of choice, though it has not yet universally accepted. (See Chapter 3 for a more complete discussion of screening tools.) Screening is important, but a positive screen is insufficient for a clinical diagnosis of depression. Screening must always be followed by a comprehensive medical and psychiatric evaluation for patients who screen positive.

Algorithmic treatment guidelines have been shown to improve outcomes and reduce costs in a variety of diseases, including depression.[9] Since a high percentage of patients who do receive treatment for depression are not given adequate antidepressant doses for a sufficient duration,[10] guidelines are invaluable in promoting evidence-based care. These guidelines must be integrated into the PCP's workflow so as to be visible to the clinician and actionable in real time. Guidelines can also be used to prompt the clinician to consider important comorbidities, decide when to hospitalize or refer to a specialist, select and dose treatment, and measure progress.

Patient registries are an increasingly important means of tracking patient populations. They allow clinicians to periodically review the progress of individual patients, detect trends within their patient population, and identify patients who are not improving with treatment. Ideally, registries are integrated into the electronic medical record in order to eliminate redundant data entry. These registries allow clinicians and administrators to evaluate the impact of care on outcomes of both individuals and populations, and then iteratively modify programming to improve the quality and efficiency of care. If linked to claims databases, registries make it possible to determine the effects of care on health care costs.

Mental health consultation is the most common and long-standing dimension of integrated care. The consultant is most often a psychiatrist, but may be a nurse, psychologist, or social worker with mental health expertise. Consultants communicate with the PCP in person, by phone, or via email or clinical messaging. Depending on the patient's complexity and the comfort level and experience of the consultee, the questions may be answered informally through a "curbside" consultation. In other instances, a formal interview of the patient is necessary. Pharmacotherapy is generally provided by the PCP with additional consultation as needed. If the patient or pharmacotherapy is too complex, the patient might be treated by the consultant or otherwise referred to a psychiatric outpatient setting. This approach allows more patients to receive optimal care for their depression in the primary care setting. This reduces the need to refer the patient to a psychiatric outpatient setting, in which case at least half of patients never complete the referral and there is a high rate of drop out among those who do.[11] Patient factors (such as forgetting the appointment, interference by the psychiatric symptoms), complicating psychosocial issues (such as homelessness, poor insight, or negative view of psychiatry), as well as clinician factors (such as poor communication, lengthy wait for appointment, and perception of referring clinician devaluing psychiatry) all contribute to the problem of attrition and insufficient care.[12]

The Depression Care Manager (DCM) is often a nurse or social worker with mental health expertise, though a trained bachelors-level person can also be a highly effective DCM. This individual is key in the collaborative care model as he or she assists the PCP in educating the patient about depression and its treatment, reinforcing basic but important activities such as healthy diet and exercise, and tracking and measuring the progress of the patient. The DCM is often trained in motivational interviewing techniques and delivering behavioral activation or problem solving therapy to the patient. Finally, the DCM assists with referrals to therapists when psychotherapy is indicated.

The co-location of mental health clinicians in the primary care setting is another element of integrated care. This provides more opportunities for real-time consultation, increases the opportunities for educating PCPs, and improves the likelihood of a successful mental health referral, since patients receive their specialized care in the familiar primary care setting. The embedded psychiatrist is not only co-located, but is also integrated into the work flow of the primary care team in a standardized, often protocol-driven fashion.

In a stepped care approach, the severity and complexity of the patient's depression determines the level of care. For example, an individual diagnosed with a mild depression might be provided a list of self-help options available in books or over the Internet. An individual with a more severe, acute, or complicated depression (e.g., one associated with other major psychiatric disorders), might be assigned to a psychiatrist for management. Those in between might be co-managed by both the PCP and DCM. Depending on progress, a patient can be reassigned within this spectrum of care. This model allows for limited resources to be distributed or triaged in the most efficient manner.

Collaborative care is an amalgam of all of the components above and truly embraces the team concept for delivering behavioral health care in the primary care setting. The team is composed of clinicians with behavioral health expertise and is called upon by the PCP when needed. A psychiatrist usually serves as a consultant to the behavioral health team who assesses, educates, suggests additional resources, and often provides skills-based therapies and ongoing monitoring. If a medication is recommended, it is prescribed by the PCP.

A number of clinics and health care systems around the United States have developed or are developing models for integrating mental health care into the primary care setting, incorporating some combination of the elements described above. Here we present two successful and well-established models. We also describe the evolving model at our hospital, which is a hybrid of these two models.

Impact

The Improving Mood–Promoting Access to Collaborative Treatment program, or IMPACT, was the first major collaborative care model to undergo rigorous study and wide dissemination. It is both clinically superior to standard treatment[13,14] and cost-effective.[15] This manualized model relies on a clinical algorithm that is carried out under the direction of a DCM, usually a nurse, social worker or psychologist, in collaboration with the primary care doctor, the consulting psychiatrist, and the patient.

In the IMPACT program, older adult patients identified as depressed or dysthymic by referral from their PCP or by a screening questionnaire, are provided educational materials about depression and a referral to the DCM. The DCM assesses the patient, educates, and serves as a coach, engaging the patient in behavioral activation. The DCM helps the patient navigate the clinical algorithm based on his or her assessment of the patient's needs and preferences. For most patients, the initial treatment choice is either an antidepressant medication or a short course of problem solving treatment (PST) administered by the DCM. The treatment is then adjusted as needed according to the algorithm and the patient's progress, monitored by the DCM. For patients who recover, the treatment then focuses on relapse prevention. The consulting psychiatrist reviews cases in which the patient is not responding to treatment and consults on those who pose diagnostic challenges or have a complicated course.[13]

The IMPACT model lends itself well to adaptation in a range of clinical settings.[13] Comprehensive instructions and tools for implementation of the program are available at the IMPACT website.[16] Thus far, IMPACT's benefits have been demonstrated largely in older adult patients with depression; efforts to study it in other populations are in early stages.[17,18]

Mental Health Integration (Intermountain Health Care)

Intermountain Health Care, a network of hospitals and clinics with a tradition of collaboration between medical teams, has developed another model for depression treatment in primary care, called mental health integration (MHI). MHI does not involve a clinical algorithm but rather stratifies patients based on an initial evaluation and screening (using the PHQ-9). Patients with depression are classified as mild, moderate, or severe and/or complicated, and are then triaged to a corresponding level of care. This may include support staff, care management with or without consultation by a mental health specialist, or referral directly to the mental health specialist, respectively.[19]

MHI differs from other models in its emphasis on recruiting family and community support. So far, MHI has been demonstrated to improve the detection of depression without increasing overall health care costs for its patients, and it has been associated with higher levels of patient and provider satisfaction.[20,21]

Brigham and Women's Hospital
The Patient-Centered Medical Home

Brigham and Women's Hospital (BWH) began developing a collaborative care model in the broader context of creating a Patient-Centered Medical Home (PCMH). Before describing the BWH model, it is necessary to understand the PCMH and its origins. PCMH aims to coordinate health care in a patient-centered, technology-enabled manner. The Joint Principles of the Patient-Centered Medical Home outlines seven key principles that appear in **Box 23-1**.[22]

The National Committee for Quality Assurance (NCQA) developed these general principles into specific measurable standards for designation as a PCMH.[23] Their standards and guidelines are divided into six main areas:

- Access and Continuity—including after hours and electronic access, and provision of culturally and linguistically appropriate services
- Identify and Manage Patient Populations—including using registries to proactively remind patients of overdue care
- Plan and Manage Care—including implementing evidence-based guidelines using point-of-care reminders, identifying high-risk patients, and managing medications
- Provide Self-Care Support—including providing educational resources, referring to community resources, providing self-management tools, and creating self-management plans with the patients and their families
- Track and Coordinate Care—including testing and referral tracking and managing care transitions
- Measure and Improve Performance—including patient experience of care

The PCMH model was originally designed to be supported by a blended payment model, in which fee-for-service is supplemented by a capitated fee (per-patient-per-month) to cover additional services that are not covered by current fee-for-service plans, such as care management, preventive interventions, and between-visit communication. PCMH is also considered to be the foundation for the successful implementation of Accountable Care Organizations (ACO).[24]

Successful management of depression is imperative once a system adopts a bundled care model and becomes financially responsible for total cost of care, as in an ACO. For example, many studies have shown that control of diabetes is poorer and care more costly in patients with comorbid depression compared to nondepressed diabetics.[25] Adoption of the Intermountain Mental Health Integration model produced savings of $667 per patient per year in medical expenses, including a 54% decrease in emergency department use.[20]

Although there is no explicit mention of behavioral health within the Joint Principles, such integration is congruent with its principles of comprehensiveness and coordination of care. The 2011 NCQA standards and guidelines require a practice to implement evidence-based guidelines for patients with three important conditions, including one related to unhealthy behaviors or mental health or substance abuse.

The South Huntington Model

It was clear from the outset that the BWH's PCMH model had to include behavioral health services. Because the population we serve has a high rate of trauma-related disorders, bipolar, and psychotic disorders, we incorporated a comprehensive psychiatric assessment early in the process. We wanted to assure that individuals who eventually receive antidepressant medication were at low risk for bipolar disorder, that treatment took comorbidities such as anxiety disorders and substance use disorders into account, and that patients with complicated psychiatric histories were identified at the outset. Ultimately we created a model that is best described as a hybrid of IMPACT and Intermountain (**Fig. 23-1**).

The Behavioral Health Questionnaire is an important component in our program. It allows us to collect important diagnostic information and to screen for other common comorbid conditions. The components of the questionnaire are reviewed in **Box 23-2**.

The process of gathering this information fosters the patient's active involvement in his/her care, and also improves the efficiency of behavioral health team meetings at which we decide whether the patient should be managed in the primary care setting and if so, to develop the treatment plan. The questionnaire also serves as a training tool for our clinicians. This enables them to better

---

BOX 23-1
JOINT PRINCIPLES OF THE PATIENT-CENTERED MEDICAL HOME

- Each patient has a primary care physician who provides comprehensive and continuous care
- The physician leads a team that collectively takes responsibility for a patient's care
- The personal physician and the team have a whole-person orientation, including attention to all stages of life and to prevention
- Care is coordinated and integrated across the health care system and the patient's community, and this is facilitated with technology
- There is a central emphasis on quality and safety
- There is enhanced access to care including through open scheduling and expanded hours
- Payment structure provides compensation for integrative, preventive activities including coordination of care and use of health information technology

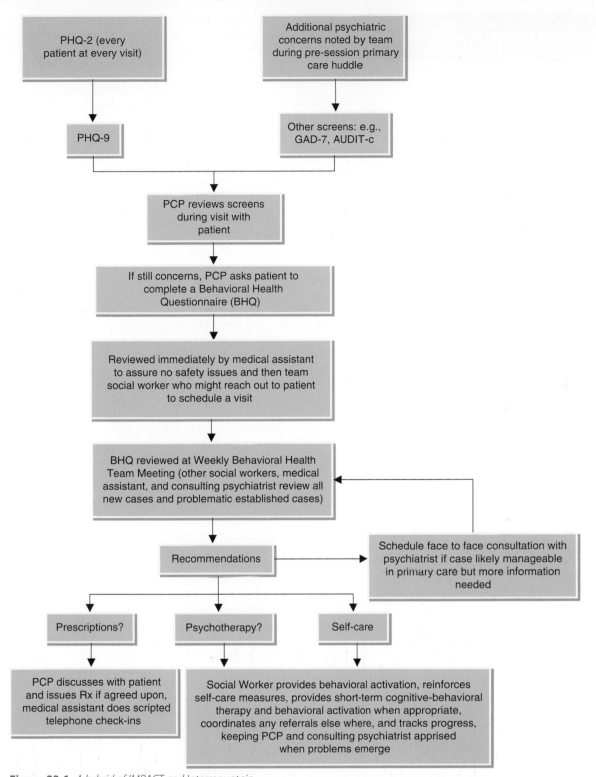

Figure 23-1 *A hybrid of IMPACT and Intermountain.*

implement treatment recommendations. Furthermore, it reduces the need for face-to-face consultations with the psychiatrist, thereby allowing him/her to focus on the most challenging cases (Fig. 23-1).

It can be challenging for some PCPs to shift from the traditional dyadic approach to patient care to team-based care. Fundamental to making this transition is clear role delineation, seamless communication, and trust in the other team members. PCPs learn to slow down and not feel compelled to issue antidepressant prescriptions upon first diagnosing a depression, much as antihypertensives are not routinely prescribed after a single high blood pressure reading. Although the team-based care is not embraced by all patients, most patients report very positive experiences. The feedback about the Behavioral Health Questionnaire from patients has been largely positive. They expressed relief that the team wants to be thorough and is actually interested in the nuances of their mental health.

The Emergency Department
Prevalence of Depression in the Emergency Department

In the United States, more than six million patients with mental health conditions are seen each year in emergency departments (EDs).[26] There has been a 15% increase in psychiatric diagnoses made in EDs between 1992 and 2000,[27] as individuals with psychiatric conditions and no source of primary care increasingly present to EDs.[26] The prevalence of depression among patients in EDs is very high. Patients with depression are almost three times as likely to use emergency department services as those without depression, after adjusting for age, race, gender, and comorbid medical conditions.[28] In a prospective observational study, the prevalence of depression meeting DSM-IV criteria was 22%.[29,30] Another multicenter study estimated the prevalence of depression in EDs at 30%, and it was associated with female gender and lower socioeconomic status.[31]

The rate of suicide is at least eight times higher in people with depression than in the general population.[32] Individuals with mental health problems are more likely to seek care outside the mental health system, from clinicians other than mental health professionals. Seventy-five percent of those completing suicide have had contact with medical care providers within the year of their death, often in emergency departments.[33] Thus, it is imperative that ED personnel become more alert to the possibility of suicide in their patients.

As detailed elsewhere in this book, depression is closely linked to medical illness. This relationship is especially salient in the emergency setting. Thus, for example, a study of inner-city ED patients with diabetes revealed that 60% had some depressive symptoms and 20% screened positive for clinical depression.[34] Many studies have shown that patients with depressive symptoms or diagnosed depression report more health problems, more pain, and more disability.[35,36,37] Not surprisingly, these patients present to EDs with somatic complaints related to their comorbid medical illnesses, but these complaints are in reality often due to depression.[38] It has been widely argued that somatization, or the expression of psychological distress via physical symptoms, is the single most common reason that psychiatric illness goes undetected in medical settings.[39] Some studies suggest that depressed, medically ill patients wait longer to be seen[40] and are assigned a lower-priority triage score in EDs, due to stigma of mental illness.[41]

Depression Assessment in the Emergency Department

The ED is an important site for identifying and referring mentally ill individuals and high utilizing patients, but more work is needed to evaluate screening for depression in this setting.[42] While there are clear recommendations for depression screening in primary care,[43] recommendations for screening in the ED are less clear. However, since so many ED patients have no other source of health care, the ED may represent the only opportunity for identifying depression.

A qualitative analysis of audio-taped ED visits with female patients revealed that depression was rarely addressed. Based on these qualitative analyses, it was suggested that even minimal attention to psychosocial factors could improve the quality of ED care and patient satisfaction.[44] Not surprisingly, the frequency of mental status examinations (MSE) in the ED is low. In one study, an MSE was recorded by the clinician in approximately half of all ED visits for depression, in 44% of visits at which an antidepressant was prescribed, and in 71% of visits involving a self-inflicted injury.[45] More work clearly needs to be done to educate ED physicians regarding the importance of evaluation of at-risk psychiatric patients.

A number of studies examining clinician-administered depression screening tools show promising results. In a study of elderly ED patients, a brief two-question depression screen (inquiring into depressed mood and anhedonia) demonstrated good sensitivity (84%) and fair specificity (64%) in detecting depression.[46] In another study of geriatric patients, a three-item screening instrument (inquiring into depressed mood, helplessness, and feeling "blue") detected depression with a 79% sensitivity and 66% specificity.[47] These self-rated depression screening scales may be a useful alternative to clinician-administered questions,[48,49,50] particularly since the recognition of depression by ED physicians is poor—with a sensitivity of 27% and specificity of 75%.[51] As noted previously, however, a positive depression screen by itself does not make the diagnosis of depression.

The identification of suicidal ideation is one of the most important aspects of psychiatric assessment in the ED. Suicide is now a major public health concern,[52] and approximately 500,000 individuals in the United States receive ED treatment following attempted suicide. The ED is a critical site for suicide screening since so many ED patients lack access to other health care. But in a large multisite study, ED providers reported gaps in their skills and practices for suicide assessment, counseling, and referral.[53] A comprehensive literature review of suicide and the ED identified several key areas for assessment, including previous history of suicide attempts, current lethal plan, recent psychosocial stressor, demographic features (age, race), and psychiatric diagnoses[54] (also see Chapter 3).

Treatment of Depression in the Emergency Department

The indications for initiating depression treatment in the ED are controversial, and the literature on prescribing antidepressants in this setting is sparse.[55] Foremost among the concerns is the potential toxicity and lethality in overdose of antidepressants, particularly tricyclic antidepressant agents. Also of concern is the certainty with which a psychiatric disorder can be reliably diagnosed in a single clinical interview.[56] Other concerns include the delayed therapeutic effects of most antidepressants and obligations for ongoing treatment. Additional considerations include appropriateness of treatment, with attention paid to adherence and accurateness of diagnosis and adequate follow-up. Follow-up in particular may be difficult because so many ED patients have no other source of health care. Follow-up appointments are more often given to those who are provided with a prescription for a psychiatric medication but follow through with aftercare is not more likely in this group.[56] Recent work has focused on agents that may provide more rapid antidepressant effects. One of these agents, ketamine, an N-methyl-D-aspartic (NMDA) glutamate receptor antagonist has shown promise in small open-label study.[57]

An important consideration involves treatment of patients presenting to emergency rooms following overdoses. These overdoses frequently represent intentional suicide attempts, and many involve the medications used to treat depression. Antidepressants accounted for 6% of drug-related illnesses seen in two EDs in one study.[58] Specific medical and toxicity issues arise from overdoses with psychiatric medications, including the serotonin syndrome, changes in cardiac conduction such as QTc prolongation, and neuroleptic malignant syndrome. As more patients treated with psychiatric medications are seen in EDs, clinicians must acquaint themselves with their toxic effects.[59]

The Medical Inpatient Setting

Appropriate recognition and treatment of depression is necessary in medical inpatient settings due to high prevalence of mood disorders in the medically ill, and the unfortunate consequences of untreated depression in this population.[60] Rates of major depressive disorder are higher in medical inpatient settings[61] compared to community samples[62] or outpatients in primary care, affecting as many as 10% to 14% of medical inpatients.[63] The most frequent reason for psychiatric consultation in the inpatient setting is mood disorders.[64,65,66] Proactive psychiatric consultation in medical inpatient settings has been associated with reduced length of stay and cost-savings.[67]

Despite the importance of treating depression in the medically ill, mood disorders tend to be under-recognized and misdiagnosed within medical inpatient settings. In a study of 346 inpatients, the requesting teams' initial diagnosis of depression was accurate in only 53.6% cases.[68]

There are several unique aspects to the evaluation and management of depressive disorders in the medical inpatient setting. The consultant should speak directly with the requesting team when first receiving the request for evaluation given the high likelihood that cognitive disorders, substance use disorders, or personality disorders may be present. After speaking with the medical team, the consultant can then approach the nonphysician staff members who work with the patient on the medical unit. Nurses, patient care observers, and physical or occupational therapists can offer valuable observations about the patient. These staff members often have more contact with the patient than his/her physicians. Indeed, in the inpatient setting, the requesting physician may not know the patient well—a key difference from consultations provided to patients in primary care settings. Review of medication administration records is also important, and unlike the outpatient setting, the inpatient consultant can clearly ascertain the patients' adherence to prescribed medications. Valuable information is also available from the medical record.

After obtaining relevant information, the consultant can then direct his or her assessment of the patient. Understanding the context and trajectory of the patient's symptoms is key to diagnosing depression in the medically ill. Psychiatric consultants must decipher whether the patient is simply experiencing depressed mood or suffering from a depressive disorder. It is imperative to evaluate for potentially reversibly causes of mood deterioration. Medications such as corticosteroids or medical abnormalities such as hypothyroidism, electrolyte or hematologic abnormalities, or vitamin deficiencies (e.g., vitamin B12) may contribute to or even causally explain the depressive symptoms.

The presentations of depression vary widely in the medical inpatient setting. Some patients express frank sadness, tearfulness, or suicidality. In these cases, the referring team may recognize the need for psychiatric consultation early in the course of the patient's illness or hospitalization. For many patients, however, an underlying mood disorder is exhibited in their behavior. Apathy, social withdrawal, or difficulty engaging with the treatment team, are common reasons for psychiatric evaluation of depression. Behaviors that can impede recovery, such as nonadherence or refusal of medical care can suggest an underlying depressive disorder. Other patients may exhibit amplification of somatic symptoms that do not respond to treatment. Many of these behavioral manifestations of depression may create tension between the medical staff and the patient.

Once the patient's symptoms are elicited, the initial differential diagnosis is broad. The consultant's first task is to rule out organic mental syndromes that may either coexist with or mimic depression. Patients with hypoactive delirium, frontal lobe syndrome, dementia, or borderline intellectual functioning may all resemble depression.[69] A thorough cognitive examination is needed to help differentiate these cognitive states. Formal instruments such as the Montreal Cognitive Assessment[70] and the Folstein Mini-Mental Status Examination[71] are useful tools when performing this task. Formal neuropsychological testing is typically unnecessary in the inpatient medical setting though may be useful for particularly difficult cases.

Adjustment disorders merit particular attention because they are frequently diagnosed in the inpatient medical setting.[72] Often, the psychiatric consultant it tasked with differentiating depression due to medical illness from a major depressive episode or an adjustment disorder with depressed mood (see Chapter 3 for further discussion), since these patients have likely just experienced acute medical and/or psychosocial stressors. For patients who have exhibited symptoms for less than 2 weeks, further monitoring may disclose the intensity and chronicity of their depression. In addition, assessment of the patient's hope for the future and motivation for recovery are reflective of underlying mood. Evaluation of the timing of the patient's symptoms and hospital course is also necessary. In the setting of catastrophic news or acute changes in the patient's medical condition, depressive symptoms are exacerbated. When the distinction between these disorders is ambiguous, continued observation is helpful, though not always feasible.

Increasingly, hospital admissions for medical illness are brief, lasting on average 4.6 days.[73] Under these circumstances, the pressing question to the psychiatric consultant is whether pharmacologic treatment for the patient's symptoms is warranted. When deciding on pharmacologic treatment for depression in the medical setting, the consultant should consider the following questions: (1) are there target symptoms that would benefit from symptom-oriented pharmacotherapy? For example, treatment with mirtazapine may serve a dual purpose of promoting appetite and treating depression symptoms[74] while duloxetine may improve chronic pain in addition to its antidepressant effects[75]; (2) are there any deleterious effects of pharmacologic treatment that would compromise the health of the patient? For example, a selective serotonin reuptake inhibitor may increase the risk gastrointestinal hemorrhage in a patient with peptic ulcer disease[76]; (3) is there appropriate follow-up in place to monitor the patient if antidepressant treatment is started?

With careful attention to the presenting symptoms, time course, and precipitating factors, depression in the medically ill can be accurately diagnosed and effectively treated. Attention to the impact of the patient's illness on significant others is also a critical issue to address. Given the frequent rates of hospitalization in the medically ill, psychiatric consultation in the hospital is an effective and appropriate setting for management of depression.

The Role of Computers in Delivering Depression Care

Technology offers new ways to detect, assess, and manage depression; however, it is still in the earliest stages of implementation in clinical practice. Although there are hundreds of mobile health apps and websites to assess and treat depression, few have been evaluated and only one appears to have been cleared by the FDA (ePST; see Berman et al.).[77] Moreover, their quality and security vary widely. And, the technology-delivered assessments and behavioral interventions that have undergone clinical evaluation are rarely commercialized.[78] This leaves only a few computer-delivered tools for depression care that have been evaluated and are available for clinicians to use. Nonetheless, the studies of such tools are increasing and they are likely to become commonplace in the coming years.

Since the first report of a patient interview via computer, in 1966,[79] studies have consistently found that computer programs are acceptable[80,81,82] and valid[83,84,85,86] means of interviewing patients about a wide range of medical and mental health problems. Moreover, computers are often better than live interviewers at eliciting sensitive information, especially when questions are presented via text and audio simultaneously, known as "audio-computer-assisted self-interviewing" (or ACASI). Studies have found that people disclose more high-risk sexual behavior,[81,87,88,89] intimate partner violence,[90] alcohol and drug use,[85,91,92] and suicidal ideation[93,94,95] to a computer than to a live clinician, even when they know that the information will immediately be relayed to a clinician. Several studies have found computer interviews to better predict suicide attempts and self-harm than live clinicians.[94,95] However, data from computerized assessments must be interpreted and combined with clinical observation, rather than relied on as a sole source of information.[96] Comparisons of computer versus paper-and-pencil administration of the same measure reveals that the two formats are equivalent.[97,98] However, two of the most important advantages of assessing patients via computer are the use of branching assessments (to tailor questions to the patient) and the capability of entering the results directly into the electronic medical record.[99]

Among the evidence-based, commercially available, computerized assessments are case-finding screeners, such as *eCHAT*[100,101] which patients access either online or via tablet computers in waiting areas; a computerized version of the *Mini International Neuropsychiatric Interview 6.0*;[102,103] and several web- and mobile-based applications, such as *What's My M3?*.[104,105] Smartphones offer particular promise, as they offer the potential to track patients' symptoms in real time in situ[106] or even to monitor some behaviors, physiology, and environmental variables unobtrusively, sending that data to clinicians in real time.[107]

Another promising use of technology lies in the delivery of behavioral interventions for depression to persons who would otherwise not have access to them. Computer-guided treatment is massively scalable and could help to overcome shortages of clinicians. The use of computers to deliver psychotherapy is not new. The earliest studies of computer-guided therapy appeared in 1966[108] and 1977,[109] and other software to treat depression appeared in the 1990s.[110,111,112] These were predominantly based on cognitive-behavioral therapy[113] and took a psychoeducational approach. More recent programs, such as *MoodManager*[114] and *Mood Gym*[115] have been developed for use via Internet and rely primarily on text and graphics to deliver the intervention. Beyond these, interactive media have also been used, incorporating branching video, audio, animations, and text to provide a more immersive experience and promote user engagement, such as *Electronic Problem-Solving Treatment (ePST)*.[77,116,117,118] These interactive media programs are designed to convey some of the warmth and empathy that clinicians provide. At least one game has been developed to treat depression in teens.[119,120] Many mobile apps for the treatment of depression can also be downloaded and look promising, such as *Mobilyze!*[107]; however, few if any of them have been evaluated in clinical trials. Nonetheless, mobile apps provide great potential to massively disseminate behavioral interventions, and clinical trials of the most promising ones will inevitably be published.

Computer-guided behavioral interventions are remarkably effective. A recent analysis of 75 studies of computer-guided treatment programs for depression, anxiety, drug, alcohol, and nicotine dependence found that computer-guided treatments were more effective than 88% of waitlist comparisons, more effective than 65% of placebo comparisons, and more effective than 48% of active treatment comparisons.[121] A meta-analysis of 31 studies (only some of which used an intent-to-treat analytic strategy) of computerized depression treatment[122] found large effect sizes: $d = 1.35$ in studies where use of the program was overseen by a clinician; $d = 0.95$ in studies where participants had some check-in with an administrative person (not a clinician); and $d = 0.78$ if not supported or followed by anyone. However, dropout from computer-guided depression treatment is high: on average, 74% of participants drop out in studies where there is no support from a live person; however, only 38% drop out if they receive support from an administrative person;

and only 28% drop out if their use of the program is overseen by a clinician who contacts them periodically (typically via telephone or email).[122] By comparison, studies of face-to-face therapy report dropout rates of 30% to 60%.[123,124] Thus, computer-guided treatment can be highly effective, but simply referring patients to a program or website and then leaving them on their own is insufficient. Having some accountability to another person for using the application boosts adherence; a question for the field is how to maximize adherence in settings where live check-in is not feasible.

Although computer-guided interventions for depression have been developed for decades and are generally effective, few have been made available to the public outside of investigational studies. There is a reason for this: although delivery of effective behavioral interventions is extremely appealing from a population management perspective, it has difficulty gaining traction in fee-for-service environments. However, with the rise of accountable care organizations and pay-for-performance health care models, it is likely that computer-guided treatments for depression will become commonplace, as they have in countries with single-payer health care, such as the United Kingdom, the Netherlands, and New Zealand.[78]

There remain a number of important unanswered questions regarding technology-guided assessments and interventions.[125] There are issues around HIPAA compliance, who receives the patient's data (i.e., whether it transmitted to the vendor and other third parties), whether data can be integrated into the patient's electronic health record, and how to respond to patients who are off site and report severe distress or intent to harm themselves or others. In addition, there is little or no regulation of the quality of these tools, although the U.S. Food and Drug Administration has issued guidelines for mobile health technologies,[126] which may steer the field toward tighter regulation and higher quality.

CONCLUSION

Effective care delivery is fundamental to successful treatment of depression and involves much more than simply identifying a case and prescribing an antidepressant. The opportunity to identify and treat depression is not limited to mental health and primary care sites, but is present in all health care settings. The collaborative care models being tested in primary care lead to better outcomes than care delivered in the traditional dyadic doctor–patient model. Involving providers in other settings, such as the emergency department and medical inpatient services, in developing ways to address depression represents the next frontier in depression care delivery. Seamless coordination among all the providers who may cross paths with our patients, along with the use of computerized technologies to track progress, facilitate communication, and provide treatment, will assure that patients with depression receive comprehensive and evidence-based care.

REFERENCES

1. Gawande A. Cowboys and pit crews. *The New Yorker*. May 26, 2011.

2. Regier DA, Goldberg ID, Taube CA. The de facto U.S. mental health services system. *Arch Gen Psychiat*. 1978;35:685–693.

3. Katon W. Collaborative depression care models: From development to dissemination. *Am J Prev Med*. 2012;42(5):550–552.

4. Institute of Medicine Report. *Improving Quality of Health Care for Mental and Substance Use Conditions*. Washington, DC: National Academy Press; 2006.

5. Katon W, Guico-Pabia C. Improving quality of depression care using organized systems of care: A review of the literature. *Prim Care Companion CNS Disord*. 2011;13(1).

6. Meyer F, Peteer J, Joseph R. Models of Care for Co-occurring Mental and Medical Disorders. *Harv Rev Psychiatry*. 2009;17(6): 353–360.

7. Woltmann E, Grogan-Kaylor A, Perron B, Georges H, Kilbourne A, Bauer M. Comparative effectiveness of collaborative chronic care models for mental health conditions across primary, specialty, and behavioral health care settings: systematic review and meta-analysis. *Am J Psychiatry*. 2012;169(8):790–804.

8. Kroenke K, Spitzer RL, Williams JB, Lowe B. The patient health questionnaire somatic, anxiety and depressive symptom scales: a systematic review. *Gen Hosp Psychiatr*. 2010;32:345–359.

9. Farias M, Jenkins K, Lock J, et al. Standardized clinical assessment and management plans (SCAMPs) provide a better alternative to clinical practice guidelines. *Health Affair*. 2013;32(5): 911–920.

10. Kessler R, Berglund P, Demler O, Jin R, Koretz D, Merikangas K. The epidemiology of major depressive disorder: results from the national comorbidity survey replication (NCS-R). *JAMA*. 2003;289(23):3095–3105.

11. Kessler R. Mental health care treatment initiation when mental health services are incorporated into primary care practice. *J Am Board Fam Med*. 2012;25(2):255–259.

12. Mitchell AJ, Selmes T. Why don't patients attend their appointments? Maintaining engagement with psychiatric services. *Advanc Psychiatr Care*. 2007:422–424.

13. Unutzer J, Katon W, Callahan CM, et al. Collaborative care management of late-life depression in the primary care setting: a randomized controlled trial. *JAMA*. 2002;288(22):2836–2845.

14. Hunkeler EM, Katon W, Tang L, et al. Long term outcomes from the IMPACT randomised trial for depressed elderly patients in primary care. *BMJ*. 2006;332(7526):259–263.

15. Katon WJ, Schoenbaum M, Fan M, et al. Cost-effectiveness of improving primary care treatment of late-life depression. *Arch Gen Psychiat*. 2005;62:1313–1320.

16. Impact evidence based depression care. Available at http://impact-uw.org/. Accessed May 13, 2013.

17. Richardson L, McCauley E, Katon M. Collaborative care for adolescent depression: a pilot study. *Gen Hosp Psychiat*. 2009;31(1):36–45.

18. Zatzick D, Rivara F, Jurkovich G, et al. Enhancing the population of collaborative care interventions: mixed method development and implementation of stepped care targeting posttraumatic stress disorder and related comorbidities after acute trauma. *Gen Hosp Psychiat*. 2011;33(2):123–134.

19. Riess-Brennan B, Briot P, Cannon W, James B. Mental health integration: rethinking practitioner roles in the treatment of depression: the specialist, primary care physicians, and the practice nurse. *Ethnic Disparities*. 2006;16(suppl 3):S3-37–S3-43.

20. Reiss-Brennan B, Briot PC, Savitz LA, Cannon W, Staheli R. Cost and quality impact of intermountain's mental health integration program. *J Healthc Manag*. 2010;55(2):97–114.

21. Reiss-Brennan B, Briot P, Daumit G, Ford D. Evaluation of "depression in primary care" innovations. *Adm Policy Ment Health*. 2006; 33(1):86–91.

22. American Academy of Family Physicians, American Academy of Pediatrics, American College of Physicians, American Osteopathic Association. Joint principles of the patient-centered medical home. Available at http://www.aap.org/en-us/professional-resources/practice-support/quality-improvement/Documents/Joint-Principles-Patient-Centered-Medical-Home.pdf. Published March 2007. Accessed May 16, 2013.

23. *Standards and Guidelines for the NCQA's Patient-Centered Medical Home (PCMH)*. Washington, DC: NCQA; 2011.

24. Accountable Care Organizations page. Centers for Medicare and Medicaid Services Web site. Available at http://www.cms.gov/Medicare/Medicare-Fee-for-Service-Payment/ACO/index.html?redirect=/aco/. Accessed May 7, 2013.

25. Lehnert T, Konnopka A, Riedel-Heller S, Konig HH. Diabetes mellitus and comorbid depression: economic findings from a systematic literature review [abstract]. *Psychiatr Prax*. 2011; 38(8):369–375.

26. Larkin GL, Claassen CA, Emond JA, et al. Trends in U.S. emergency department visits for mental health conditions, 1992-2001. *Psychiatr Serv*. 2005;56: 1–7.

27. Hazlett SB, McCarthy ML, Londner MS, Onyike CU. Epidemiology of adult psychiatric visits to U.S. emergency departments. *Acad Emerg Med*. 2004;11:193–195.

28. Himelhoch S, Weller WE, Wu AW, et al. Chronic medical illness, depression, and use of acute medical services among medicare beneficiaries. *Med Care*. 2004; 42: 512–521.

29. Goodwin RD, Jacobi F, Bittner A, Wittchen H. Epidemiology of mood disorders. In: Stein DJ, Kupfer DJ, Schatzberg AF, eds. *Textbook of Mood Disorders*. Washington, DC: American Psychiatric Publishing, Inc.; 2006:43–44.

30. Hoyer D, David E. Screening for depression in emergency department patients. *J Emer Med*. 2012;43:786–789.

31. Kumar A, Clark S, Boudreaux ED, Camargo CA. A multicenter study of depression among emergency department patients. *Acad Emerg Med*. 2004;11:1284–1289.

32. Monk M. Epidemiology of suicide. *Epidemiol Rev*. 1997;9:51–68.

33. Luoma JB, Martin CE, Pearson JL. Contact with mental health and primary care providers before suicide: a review of the evidence. *Am J Psychiatry*. 2002;159:909–916.

34. Hailpern S, Calderon Y, Gosh R, Haughey M. The association between hemoglobin A1c and depression in an inner city diabetic population. *Acad Emerg Med*. 2007;14:S314.

35. Wells KB, Stewart A, Hays RD, et al. The functioning and well-being of depressed patients. Results from the Medical Outcomes Study. *JAMA*. 1989;262:914–919.

36. Yingling KW, Wulsin LR, Arnold LM, Rouan GW. Estimated prevalences of panic disorder and depression among consecutive patients seen in an emergency department with acute chest pain. *J Gen Intern Med*. 1993;8:231–235.

37. Raccio-Robak N, McErlean MA, Fabacher DA, Milano PM, Verdile VP. Socioeconomic and health status differences between depressed and nondepressed ED elders. *Am J Emerg Med*. 2002; 20:71–73.

38. Stephenson DT, Price JR. Medically unexplained physical symptoms in emergency medicine. *Emerg Med J*. 2006;23:595–600.

39. Goldberg DP, Bridges K. Somatic presentations of psychiatric illness in primary care setting. *J Psychosom Res*. 1988;32:137–144.

40. Edmondson D, Newman JD, Chang MJ, Wyer P, Davidson KW. Depression is associated with longer emergency department length of stay in acute coronary syndrome patients. *BMC Emerg Med*. 2012;12:14.

41. Atzema CL, Schull MJ, Tu JV. The effect of a charted history of depression on emergency department triage and outcomes in patients with acute myocardial infarction. *CMAJ*. 2011;183: 663–669.

42. Kowalenko T, Khare RK. Should we screen for depression in the emergency department? *Acad Emerg Med*. 2004;11:177–178.

43. U.S. Preventive Services Task Force. Screening for depression: recommendations and rationale. *Ann Int Med*. 2002;136:760–764.

44. Rhodes KV, Kushner HM, Bisgaier J, Prenoveau E. Characterizing emergency department discussions about depression. *Acad Emerg Med*. 2007;14:908–911.

45. Harman JS, Scholle SH, Edlund MJ. Emergency department visits for depression in the United States. *Psychiatr Serv*. 2004;55:937–939.

46. Hustey FM. The use of a brief depression screen in older emergency department patients. *Acad Emerg Med*. 2005;12:905–908.

47. Fabacher DA, Raccio-Robak N, McErlean MA, Milano PM, Verdile VP. Validation of a brief screening tool to detect depression in elderly ED patients. *Am J Emer Med*. 2002;20:99–102.

48. Meldon SW, Emerman CL, Schubert DS, Moffa DA, Etheart RG. Depression in geriatric ED patients: prevalence and recognition. *Ann Emerg Med*. 1997;30:141–145.

49. Meldon SW, Emerman CL, Schubert DS. Recognition of depression in geriatric ED patients by emergency physicians. *Ann Emerg Med*. 1997;30:442–447.

50. Meldon SW, Emerman CL, Moffa DA, Schubert DS. Utility of clinical characteristics in identifying depression in geriatric ED patients. *Am J Emerg Med*. 1999;17:522–525.

51. Barefoot JC, Schroll M. Symptoms of depression, acute myocardial infarction, and total mortality in a community sample. *Circulation*. 1996;93:1976–1980.

52. Office of the Surgeon General. *The Surgeon General's Call to Action to Prevent Suicide*. Washington, DC: Department of Health and Human Services, U.S. Public Health Service; 1999.

53. Betz ME, Sullivan AF, Manton AP, et al. Knowledge, attitudes, and practices of emergency department providers in the care of suicidal patients. *Depress Anxiety*. 2013;30:1-8.

54. Ronquillo L, Minassian A, Vilke GM, Wilson MP. Literature-based recommendations for suicide assessment in the emergency department: a review. *J Emerg Med*. 2012;43:836–842.

55. Jacobs D. Psychopharmacologic management of the psychiatric emergency patient. *Gen Hosp Psych*. 1984;6:203–210.

56. Ernst CL, Bird SA, Goldberg JF, Ghaemi SN. The prescription of psychotropic medications for patients discharged from a psychiatric emergency service. *J Clin Psychiatry*. 2006;67:720–726.

57. Larkin GL, Beautrais AL. A preliminary naturalistic study of low-dose ketamine for depression and suicide ideation in the emergency department. *Int J Neuropsychopharmacol*. 2011;14:1127–1131.

58. Prince BS, Goetz C, Rihn TL, Olsky M. Drug related emergency department visits and hospital admissions. *Am J Hosp Pharmacy*. 1992;49:1696–1700.

59. Ellison JM, Pfaelzer C. Emergency Pharmacotherapy: the evolving role of medications in the emergency department. *New Dir Ment Health Serv*. 1995Fall;(67):87–98.

60. Frasure-Smith N, Lesperance F, Talajic M. Depression following myocardial infarction. Impact on 6-month survival. *JAMA*. 1993;270:1819–1825.

61. Rapp SR, Parisi SA, Walsh DA. Psychological dysfunction and physical health among elderly medical inpatients. *J Consult Clin Psychol*. 1988;56:851–855.

62. Myers JK, Weissman MM, Tischler GL, et al. Six-month prevalence of psychiatric disorders in three communities 1980 to 1982. *Arch Gen Psychiatry*. 1984;41:959–967.

63. Levenson JL. *The American Psychiatric Publishing Textbook of Psychosomatic Medicine: Psychiatric Care of the Medically Ill*: American Psychiatric Pub; 2011.

64. Arbabi M, Laghayeepoor R, Golestan B, et al. Diagnoses, requests and timing of 503 psychiatric consultations in two general hospitals. *Acta Med Iran*. 2012;50:53–60.

65. Ries RK, Bokan JA, Kleinman A, Schuckit MA. Psychiatric consultation-liaison service: patients, requests, and functions. *Gen Hosp Psychiatry*. 1980;2:204–212.

66. Bourgeois JA, Wegelin JA, Servis ME, Hales RE. Psychiatric diagnoses of 901 inpatients seen by consultation-liaison psychiatrists at an academic medical center in a managed care environment. *Psychosomatics*. 2005;46:47–57.

67. Desan PH, Zimbrean PC, Weinstein AJ, Bozzo JE, Sledge WH. Proactive psychiatric consultation services reduce length of stay for admissions to an inpatient medical team. *Psychosomatics*. 2011;52:513–520.

68. Dilts SL Jr., Mann N, Dilts JG. Accuracy of referring psychiatric diagnosis on a consultation-liaison service. *Psychosomatics*. 2003;44:407–411.

69. Stern TA. *Massachusetts General Hospital Handbook of General Hospital Psychiatry*: Elsevier Health Sciences; 2010.

70. Ismail Z, Rajji TK, Shulman KI. Brief cognitive screening instruments: an update. *Int J Geriatr Psychiatry*. 2010;25:111–120.

71. Folstein MF, Folstein SE, McHugh PR. "Mini-mental state". A practical method for grading the cognitive state of patients for the clinician. *J Psychiatr Res*. 1975;12:189–198.

72. Snyder S, Strain JJ, Wolf D. Differentiating major depression from adjustment disorder with depressed mood in the medical setting. *Gen Hosp Psychiatry*. 1990;12:159–165.

73. Hall MJ, DeFrances CJ, Williams SN, Golosinskiy A, Schwartzman A. National hospital discharge survey: 2007 summary. *Natl Health Stat Report*. 2010;29:1–20.

74. Fava M. Weight gain and antidepressants. *J Clin Psychiatry*. 2000;61(Suppl 11):37–41.

75. Pergolizzi JV Jr, Raffa RB, Taylor R Jr, Rodriguez G, Nalamachu S, Langley P. A review of duloxetine 60 mg once-daily dosing for the management of diabetic peripheral neuropathic pain, fibromyalgia, and chronic musculoskeletal pain due to chronic osteoarthritis pain and low back pain. *Pain Pract*. 2013;13:239–252.

76. Dall M, Schaffalitzky de Muckadell OB, Lassen AT, Hansen JM, Hallas J. An association between selective serotonin reuptake inhibitor use and serious upper gastrointestinal bleeding. *Clin Gastroenterol Hepatol*. 2009;7:1314–1321.

77. Berman MI, Buckey JC Jr, Hull JG, et al. Feasibility study of an interactive multimedia electronic problem solving treatment program for depression: a preliminary uncontrolled trial. *Behav Ther*. 2014;45(3):358–375.

78. Cartreine JA, Ahern DK, Locke SE. A roadmap to computer-based psychotherapy in the United States. *Harvard Review of Psychiatry*. 2010;18(2):80–95.

79. Slack WV, Hicks GP, Reed CE, Van Cura LJ. A computer-based medical history system. *New England Journal of Medicine*. 1966;274:194–198.

80. Slack WV, Kowaloff HB, Davis RB, et al. Evaluation of computer-based medical histories taken by patients at home. *J Am Med Inform Assoc*. 2012;19(4):545–548.

81. Katz LM, Cumming PD, Wallace EL, Abrams PS. Audiovisual touch-screen computer-assisted self-interviewing for donor

health histories: results from two years experience with the system. *Transfusion*. 2005;45(2):171–180.

82. Thornberry J, Bhaskar B, Krulewitch CJ, et al. Audio computerized self-report interview use in prenatal clinics: audio computer-assisted self interview with touch screen to detect alcohol consumption in pregnant women: application of a new technology to an old problem. *Comput Inform Nurs*. 2002;20(2):46–52.

83. Ancill RJ, Rogers D, Carr AC. Comparison of computerised self-rating scales for depression with conventional observer ratings. *Acta Psychiatrica Scandinavica*. 1985;71(3):315–317.

84. Carr AC, Ancill RJ, Ghosh A, Margo A. Direct assessment of depression by microcomputer: A feasibility study. *Acta Psychiatrica Scandinavica*. 1981;64(5):415–422.

85. Kobak KA, Greist JH, Jefferson JW, Katzelnick DJ. Computer-administered clinical rating scales: A review. *Psychopharmacology*. 1996;127(4):291–301.

86. Arunothong W, Ittasakul P. Psychiatric computer interviews: How precise, reliable and accepted are they? *ASEAN Journal of Psychiatry*. 2012;13(1):69–80.

87. Ghanem KG, Hutton HE, Zenilman JM, Zimba R, Erbelding EJ. Audio computer assisted self interview and face to face interview modes in assessing response bias among STD clinic patients. *Sex Transm Infect*. 2005;81(5):421–425.

88. Turner CF, Ku L, Rogers SM, Lindberg LD, Pleck JH, Sonenstein FL. Adolescent sexual behavior, drug use, and violence: increased reporting with computer survey technology. *Science*. 1998;280(5365):867–873.

89. Gates GJ, Sonenstein FL. Heterosexual genital sexual activity among adolescent males: 1988 and 1995. *Fam Plann Perspect*. 2000;32(6):295–297, 304.

90. Mears M, Coonrod DV, Bay RC, Mills TE, Watkins MC. Routine history as compared to audio computer-assisted self-interview for prenatal care history taking. *J Reprod Med*. 2005;50(9):701–706.

91. Simoes AA, Bastos FI, Moreira RI, Lynch KG, Metzger DS. A randomized trial of audio computer and in-person interview to assess HIV risk among drug and alcohol users in Rio De Janeiro, Brazil. *J Subst Abuse Treat*. 2006;30(3):237–243.

92. Metzger DS, Koblin B, Turner C, et al. Randomized controlled trial of audio computer-assisted self-interviewing: utility and acceptability in longitudinal studies. HIVNET Vaccine Preparedness Study Protocol Team. *Am J Epidemiol*. 2000;152(2):99–106.

93. Greist JH, Gustafson DH, Stauss FF, Rowse GL, Laughren TP, Chiles JA. Computer interview for suicide-risk prediction. *Am J Psychiatry*. 1973;130:1327–1332.

94. Levine S, Ancill RJ, Roberts AP. Assessment of suicide risk by computer-delivered self-rating questionnaire: Preliminary findings. *Acta Psychiatrica Scandinavica*. 1989;80(3):216–220.

95. Erdman HP, Greist JH, Gustafson DH, Taves JE, Klein MH. Suicide risk prediction by computer interview: A prospective study. *J Clinl Psychiatry*. 1987;48(12):464–467.

96. Garb HN. Computer-administered interviews and rating scales. *Psychological Assessment*. 2007;19(1):4–13.

97. Coons SJ, Gwaltney CJ, Hays RD, et al. Recommendations on evidence needed to support measurement equivalence between electronic and paper-based patient-reported outcome (PRO) measures: ISPOR ePRO Good Research Practices Task Force report. *Value Health*. 2009;12(4):419–429.

98. Gwaltney CJ, Shields AL, Shiffman S. Equivalence of electronic and paper-and-pencil administration of patient-reported outcome measures: a meta-analytic review. *Value Health*. 2008;11(2):322–333.

99. Office of the National Coordinator for Health Information Technology. Meaningful Use: What is Meaningful Use? 2013; Available at http://www.healthit.gov/policy-researchers-implementers/meaningful-use. Accessed May 10, 2013.

100. Goodyear-Smith F, Arroll B, Coupe N. Asking for help is helpful: Validation of a brief lifestyle and mood assessment tool in primary health care. *Ann Fam Med*. 2009;7(3):239–244.

101. eCHAT (Behavior and Mood Screening). 2013; Available at http://www.myhealthscreenrx.com/tools/behaviour-and-mood-screening. Accessed May 10, 2013.

102. Sheehan DV, Lecrubier Y, Sheehan KH, et al. The Mini-International Neuropsychiatric Interview (M.I.N.I): The development and validation of a structured diagnostic psychiatric interview for DSM-IV and ICD-10. *J Clin Psychiatry*. 1998;59(Suppl 20):22–33.

103. Medical Outcome Systems. Welcome to Medical Outcome Systems. 2013; Available at https://medical-outcomes.com/. Accessed May 10, 2013.

104. Gaynes BN, DeVeaugh-Geiss J, Weir S, et al. Feasibility and diagnostic validity of the M-3 checklist: a brief, self-rated screen for depressive, bipolar, anxiety, and post-traumatic stress disorders in primary care. *Ann Fam Med*. 2010;8(2):160–169.

105. M3 Information. The 3 Minute Test for Depression, Anxiety, Bipolar Disorder and PTSD. 2013; Available at http://www.whatsmym3.com/. Accessed May 10, 2013.

106. Palmier-Claus JE, Myin-Germeys I, Barkus E, et al. Experience sampling research in individuals with mental illness: Reflections and guidance. *Acta Psychiatrica Scandinavica*. 2011;123(1):12–20.

107. Burns MN, Begale M, Duffecy J, et al. Harnessing context sensing to develop a mobile intervention for depression. *J Med Internet Res*. 2011;13(3):158–174.

108. Colby KM, Watt JB, Gilbert JP. A computer method of psychotherapy: Preliminary communication. *J Nerv Ment Dis*. 1966;142(2):148–152.

109. Slack WV, Slack CW. Talking to a computer about emotional problems: A comparative study. *Psychother Theor Res Pract*. 1977;14(2):156–164.

110. Baer L, Greist JH. An interactive computer-administered self-assessment and self-help program for behavior therapy. *J Clin Psychiatry*. 1997;58(Suppl 12):23–28.

111. Selmi PM, Klein MH, Greist JH, Sorrell SP, Erdman HP. Computer-administered cognitive-behavioral therapy for depression. *Am J Psychiatry*. 1990;147(1):51–56.

112. Selmi PM, Klein MH, Greist JH, Sorrell SP, Erdman HP. Computer-administered therapy for depression. *MD Computing*. 1991;8(2):98–102.

113. Cavanagh K, Shapiro DA, Van Den Berg S, Swain S, Barkham M, Proudfoot J. The effectiveness of computerized cognitive behavioural therapy in routine care. *Br J Clin Psychol*. 2006;45(4):499–514.

114. Mohr DC, Duffecy J, Jin L, et al. Multimodal e-mental health treatment for depression: a feasibility trial. *J Med Internet Res*. 2010;12(5):e48.

115. Ellis LA, Campbell AJ, Sethi S, O'Dea BM. Comparative randomized trial of an online cognitive-behavioral therapy program

and an online support group for depression and anxiety. *J CyberTher Rehab*. 2011;4(4):461–467.

116. Cartreine JA, Locke SE, Buckey JC, Sandoval L, Hegel MT. Electronic problem-solving treatment: Description and pilot study of an interactive media treatment for depression. *JMIR Protoc*. 2012;1(2):e11.

117. Carter JA, Buckey JC, Greenhalgh L, Holland AW, Hegel MT. An interactive media program for managing psychosocial problems on long-duration spaceflights. *Aviat Space Environ Med*. 2005;76(Supplement):B213–B223.

118. Cartreine JA, Chang TE, Seville JL, et al. Using self-guided treatment software (ePST) to teach clinicians how to deliver problem-solving treatment for depression. *Depress Res Treat*. 2012;2012:309094, 309011 pgs.

119. Fleming T, Dixon R, Frampton C, Merry S. A pragmatic randomized controlled trial of computerized CBT (SPARX) for symptoms of depression among adolescents excluded from mainstream education. *Behav Cogn Psychother*. 2012;40(5):529–541.

120. Merry SN, Stasiak K, Shepherd M, Frampton C, Fleming T, Lucassen MF. The effectiveness of SPARX, a computerised self

121. Kiluk BD, Sugarman DE, Nich C, et al. A methodological analysis of randomized clinical trials of computer-assisted therapies for psychiatric disorders: Toward improved standards for an emerging field. *Am J Psychiatry*. 2011;168(8):790–799.

122. Richards D, Richardson T. Computer-based psychological treatments for depression: A systematic review and meta-analysis. *Clin Psychol Rev*. 2012;32(4):329–342.

123. Piper WE, Ogrodniczuk JS, Joyce AS, et al. Prediction of dropping out in time-limited, interpretive individual psychotherapy. *Psychother Theor Res Pract Train*. 1999;36(2):114–122.

124. Reis BF, Brown LG. Reducing psychotherapy dropouts: Maximizing perspective convergence in the psychotherapy dyad. *Psychother Theor Res Pract Train*. 1999;36(2):123–136.

125. Freedman J. The diffusion of innovations into psychiatric practice. *Psychiatric Services*. 2002;53(12):1539–1540.

126. Food and Drug Administration. Draft Guidance for Industry and Food and Drug Administration Staff; Mobile Medical Applications; Availability. *Fed Reg*. 2011;76(140):43689–43690.

help intervention for adolescents seeking help for depression: randomised controlled non-inferiority trial. *BMJ*. 2012;344:e2598.

Depression in Medical Illness: Future Directions

David Silbersweig, MD

This book has focused upon the prevalent and important interface of depression and medical illness. The clinical, personal, familial, societal, and financial impacts of this interaction are tremendous. The state of our knowledge and experience concerning this nexus has been detailed, across the spectrum of medical conditions, populations, and settings. Much of this understanding has been facilitated by recent advances in scientific methods, and much has resulted from of careful clinical observation. These converging approaches have been discussed, and resultant principles have been explicated. With this substantial foundation, what are we building toward?

In essence, the goal is a mechanistic understanding that can provide diagnostic and therapeutic tools to improve outcomes, and guide clinical decision making. To accomplish this goal, one must utilize evolving approaches to chart the biopsychosocial intersection of depression and medical illness. This requires a characterization of the heterogeneity of depressive illness, of the range of medical illnesses, and of the types of mechanistic interrelationships among them. It also requires an elucidation of the final common brain pathways mediating depressive symptoms, as well as the pathophysiologic pathways and the etiological factors and interactions affecting those brain pathways in the context of medical illness.

HETEROGENEITY OF DEPRESSIVE ILLNESS

Depression, even Major Depression, is not a unitary phenomenon. It is currently defined descriptively, and a patient can meet clinical criteria with different symptom constellations. Furthermore, there can be considerable overlap with other psychiatric syndromes, including anxiety disorders. With advances in translational research, it will be possible to stratify patients along a dimensional spectrum, within and across DSM categories, through deep phenotyping, multi-modal biomarkers and informatics.[1] This will result in a mechanism-based taxonomy of depressive/mood disorders, with implications for treatment targets that modulate the relevant biological substrate, through pharmacologic, cognitive-behavioral or brain stimulation approaches.[2] For example, there is increasing evidence for an anhedonic syndromic subtype with prominent lack of interest or pleasure in activities, associated with ventral striatum/nucleus accumbens, dopaminergic reward/motivation circuit dysfunction (**Fig. 24-1**).[3,4]

Patterns of distributed brain activity/connectivity may also be able to distinguish patients from healthy subjects, providing a possible foundation for future diagnostic approaches (**Fig. 24-2**).[5]

In addition to systems-level neuroimaging, with both functional and structural elements, other biomarkers can provide cellular and molecular information of relevance. Metabolomics, proteomics, lipidomics, epigenomics, and genomics provide a range of powerful techniques that are starting to provide relevant data.[6] Ultimately, a particular patient may be described in a personalized medicine approach by a profile of abnormalities in these domains, specifying associated therapeutic agents, as happens increasingly with cancer patients.[7]

RANGE OF MEDICAL ILLNESSES

Among the many medical illnesses affecting different organ systems, common underlying biological mechanisms are being identified. These represent pathophysiologies or disruption in signaling pathways that regulate function at the systems or cellular level. Vascular, endocrine, infectious, degenerative, toxic, metabolic, and other etiologies may be implicated.[8] Processes such as inflammation, oxidative stress, and apoptosis can play a critical mediating role, in the context of genetic, developmental, and aging factors.[9,10]

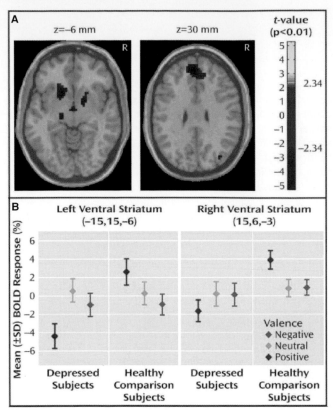

Figure 24-1 *Activation Differences in Ventral Striatal and Dorsomedial Frontal Regions in Response to P Positive Words in Depressed Patients Compared With Healthy Subjects. In part **A**, axial slices reveal significant decreases in activation to positive stimuli in depressed patients compared with healthy subjects; left image: bilateral ventral striatum, with the left contrast maximum falling in the region of the nucleus accumbens (hypothalamic and thalamic decreases are also visible); right image: left dorsomedial frontal gyrus (Brodmann's area 9). In part **B**, within-group, by condition barplots at the statistical maxima of the bilateral ventral striatal findings in the positive between-group condition, revealed these findings to be due to a decrease in activation to positive stimuli in depressed subjects coupled with an increase in healthy comparison subjects.*

■ TYPES OF MECHANISTIC INTERACTIONS AMONG PSYCHIATRIC AND MEDICAL ILLNESSES

Much of this book expounds the importance of understanding the variance and commonalities within and among the psychiatric presentations, as well as the variance and commonalities within and among the medical presentations—and their interactions. In a patient with depression and diabetes, for example, the relationship between these two disease elements may be multidetermined, biologically and psychologically/behaviorally. One condition can play a causal or contributing role in the other (in either direction), they may coincidentally co-occur and interact, and/or they may both result from a common underlying diathesis.[11,12] Stress, inflammation, insulin resistance, eating behavior, and medical adherence may all be involved.[11] There are also intriguing observations, such as demonstration that SSRI medication can improve medical outcome in some cases even in the absence of an improvement in depression.[13,14] Recognizing, addressing, and studying these complex interrelationships can improve clinical care, and can inform impactful translational research strategies. This can also help to extend and transcend the concept of comorbidity.

■ FINAL COMMON BRAIN PATHWAYS MEDIATING DEPRESSIVE SYMPTOMATOLOGY

Ultimately, these effects are mediated via final common pathways of brain dysfunction. The brain regions and circuits that underlie

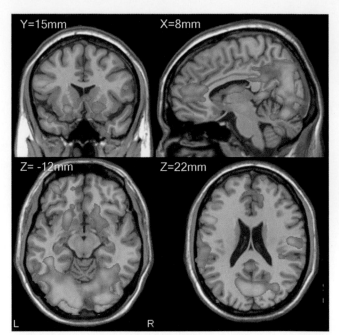

Figure 24-2 *Distributed profile of brain activity identified in a data-driven Principal Component Analysis combining patients with major depression and healthy matched control subjects in a positive emotional word condition, that correlates with group (diagnosis) membership. Note decreased cross-correlated ventral and medial striatal, medial prefrontal and precuneus activity, reflecting reward and default mode processing, in patients. With further developments and testing, such work may suggest patterns of circuit dysfunction distinguishing patients with depression or its subtypes, laying a foundation for future, clinically useful neuroimaging.*

processes such as emotion, motivation, salience, behavior, executive function, and vegetative function are thus critical to distinguish. Excess or diminished activity, abnormal connectivity, aberrant modulation, feedforward/feedback or inhibition, or altered thresholds can produce distinct neuropsychiatric symptoms.[15,16] This is not unlike the localization of neurologic syndromes, due to the hard-wiring of many structure–function relationships in the brain, from those mediating the most basic to the most human behaviors (the biological bases of which are being increasingly understood). Indeed, neuroimaging is identifying key dorsolateral prefrontal, subgenual anterior cingulate, amygdalar, hippocampal, insular, and ventral striatal substrates of depression and its subtypes.[5,17] Neurological lesions or processes that involve such regions and associated circuits can produce depressive phenomenology.[18]

■ RELEVANT NEUROPHYSIOLOGICAL PROCESSES

Critical neurophysiological processes on the local neuronal circuit and cellular level are relevant as well. Neurogenesis in the hippocampus, for instance, is enhanced in all effective treatments of depression, with the involvement of trophic factors, such as brain-derived neurotrophic factor (BDNF).[19] Synaptic plasticity and dendritic arborization (communication and connections among neurons) are implicated.[19] Interneurons and astrocytes have also been implicated due to their important roles regulating the neuronal, neurochemical, and glial micro-environment.[20,21]

■ RELEVANT PATHOPHYSIOLOGICAL PROCESSES

A number of processes have a beneficial or deleterious effect on such local neurophysiology. These processes have been implicated in depression or its treatment, and are of relevance in the medical setting. Excitotoxicity may contribute to stress-mediated hippocampal damage,[22] along with cortisol;[23] and excitatory neurotransmission via glutamatergic NMDA receptor subtypes is a current target for blockade with rapidly acting antidepressants.[20] GABA inhibition-enhancing benzodiazepines can interfere with hippocampal neurogenesis.[24] SSRIs and estrogen may enhance neurogenesis.[25,26] Cytokines play roles in neural signaling and plasticity as well as in inflammation, and proinflammatory cytokines (such as TNF-alpha and IL-6) have been associated with depression (and decrease with treatment, with therapeutic implications being explored).[27] Oxidative stress may also disrupt neurogenesis,[28] and cellular aging (reflected by telemorase activity) has been associated with hippocampal volume in major depression.[29] Abnormal metabolic enzyme and insulin receptor activity have been implicated in pathogenesis.[30] Resting and reactive autonomic (sympathetic/parasympathetic) disruption have been implicated in depression as well.[31] Circadian, menstrual and seasonal biological/hormonal cycles have been shown to have a substantial effect on the relevant basic neurophysiological processes noted above.[32,33] Such observations underlie conditions such as premenstrual dysphoric disorder,[34] and treatments such as bright light therapy.[35]

■ ETIOLOGICAL FACTORS AND INTERACTIONS AFFECTING RELEVANT BRAIN PATHWAYS IN THE CONTEXT OF MEDICAL ILLNESS

As can be imagined, many medical illnesses and treatments involve and affect these biological processes of importance to mood disorders. Vascular, immune, and endocrine disorders and treatments provide numerous examples to be aware of, as described in the chapters of this volume. Psychosis, depression or encephalopathy with lupus and thyroid disease are traditional associations, and even there, new mechanisms are being discovered, such as anti-glutamate/NMDA NR-2 antibodies in such settings.[36,37] Common underlying inflammation and vascular dysfunction may explain elements of both depression and coronary artery disease, and their co-occurrence.[38] For the convergence of depression and diabetes, mechanisms including inflammation, insulin resistance, metabolic, and autonomic dysregulation have been implicated.[39] In this context, the deleterious and beneficial cross-condition effects of antidepressants, steroids, cardiac medications, and diabetes medications need to be considered (beyond drug–drug interactions or side effects).[40,41,42]

Environmental factors can also affect these biological processes via gene–environment, neurodevelopmental and epigenetic mechanisms.[43] Early adversity/trauma, for instance, can affect the mesotemporal and orbitomedial frontal and hypothalamic–pituitary systems, leading to increased stress reactivity and risk for depression in adulthood.[44] Conversely, environmental/social enrichment and support and cognitive-behavioral psychotherapy can promote resilience.[45] There is substantial overlap between these determinants of psychiatric illness and those of medical disease and health behaviors, such as smoking, exercise, and eating habits.[46] Given all these considerations, one can go beyond notions of comorbidity, to develop a more nuanced understanding of the tight interrelationship among depressive and somatic aspects of illness and treatment.

■ MULTIMODAL BIOMARKERS

With all of these factors, processes, and interactions, the challenge and opportunity is to capture the relevant information and analyze it in a manner that can guide clinical decision making and advance care. This requires a multi-modal biomarker approach,[5,47] integrated computationally with clinical psychopathological information, psychosocial measures, and real-time, real-world behavioral, social and physiological data from phones and wearable devices.[48] The resultant individualized profiles can ultimately specify mechanism, suggest therapeutic targets and demonstrate their engagement, identify risk and resilience factors, and predict response to specific interventions as well as outcome (**Fig. 24-3**).

■ TARGETED THERAPEUTICS

Such interventions should evolve beyond the traditional serendipitous, "me-too," monoaminergic drugs, through recent rapidly acting glutamatergic agents, to the targeting of specific receptor subtypes and signaling pathways in affected brain regions. In addition, agents or activities offering neurogenesis-enhancing, plasticity-enhancing, neuroprotection, and anti-inflammatory activity can be developed.[49,50] Ultimately, specific neurorepair with genetic and stem cell approaches may be possible.[51] For circuit neuromodulation, brain stimulation methods should evolve from a relatively nonspecific set of stimulation parameters, to more physiologically sophisticated frequencies, amplitudes and oscillations, guided in a closed-loop fashion by real-time neurophysiological measures.[52] Both less invasive (tDCS, optical) and nano technologies are being developed in this context.[53–55] The optimization and tailored application of cognitive-behavioral, motivational, behavioral activation, and mindfulness interventions will continue.[56,57] Internet-based applications of such modalities are being developed, and would be scalable at relatively low cost.[58]

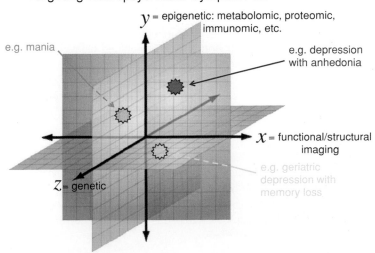

A Multidimensional Biomarker Model for Targeting Neuropsychiatric Symptom Tx

y = epigenetic: metabolomic, proteomic, immunomic, etc.

e.g. mania

e.g. depression with anhedonia

x = functional/structural imaging

e.g. geriatric depression with memory loss

z = genetic

Figure 24-3 *Graphic representation of a future manner of characterizing individual depression patients and sub-syndromes, based upon an informational profile of profiles in a multi-dimensional biomarker space.*

Combination treatments, incorporating more than one synergistic agent or modality, and targeting more than one part of a dysfunctional pathway, should become increasingly utilized. Enhanced knowledge concerning mechanisms of therapeutic action and interaction can guide these developments. Treatment, wellness, and prevention strategies will also increasingly be based on neurodevelopmental and epigenetic knowledge about biopsychosocial and gene–environment interactions.[59,60] From the vantage point of depression and medical illness, this extends to the critical contributions to/of health behaviors and modifiable risk factors.[61]

■ BEHAVIORAL HEALTH CARE REDESIGN

These approaches naturally lead to health care systems redesign. The integration of behavioral healthcare into the primary care medical home bypasses obstacles to care and leverages mental health staffing and expertise to screen and treat more patients, despite resource constraints.[62] Further, the development of wearable devices, smart phone apps, telemedicine, web-based platforms and informatics allow real-world, real-time, data-driven, individualized yet scalable care.[48]

■ EARLY INTERVENTION AND PREVENTION

Ultimately, the aim is to develop personalized, precision medical psychiatry. This will be characterized by evidence-based early detection, early trajectory-altering intervention, and individualized treatment targeting both symptom pathways and pathophysiological mechanisms.[63,64] The focusing of this biomechanistic approach at the interface of depression and medical illness––linking mental and somatic processes, symptoms, and treatments—is particularly impactful and promising.

REFERENCES

1. Scarr E, Millan MJ, Bahn S, et al. Biomarkers for Psychiatry: The Journey from Fantasy to Fact, a Report of the 2013 CINP Think Tank. *Int J Neuropsychopharmacol.* 2015;18(10):pyv042.

2. Phillips ML, Chase HW, Sheline YI, et al. Identifying predictors, moderators, and mediators of antidepressant response in major depressive disorder: neuroimaging approaches. *Am J Psychiatry.* 2015;172(2):124–138.

3. Epstein J, Pan H, Kocsis JH, et al. Lack of ventral striatal response to positive stimuli in depressed versus normal subjects. *Am J Psychiatry.* 2006;163(10):1784–1790.

4. Vrieze E, Demyttenaere K, Bruffaerts R, et al. Dimensions in major depressive disorder and their relevance for treatment outcome. *J Affect Disord.* 2014;155:35–41.

5. Silbersweig D. Default mode subnetworks, connectivity, depression and its treatment: toward brain-based biomarker development. *Biol Psychiatry.* 2013;74(1):5–6.

6. Maes M, Nowak G, Caso JR, et al. Toward Omics-Based, Systems Biomedicine, and Path and Drug Discovery Methodologies for Depression-Inflammation Research. *Mol Neurobiol.* 2016;53(5): 2927–2935.

7. Murck H, Laughren T, Lamers F, et al. Taking Personalized Medicine Seriously: Biomarker Approaches in Phase IIb/III Studies in Major Depression and Schizophrenia. *Innov Clin Neurosci.* 2015;12(3–4):26S–40S.

8. Wang RS, Maron BA, Loscalzo J. Systems medicine: evolution of systems biology from bench to bedside. *Wiley Interdisc Rev Syst Biol Med.* 2015;7(4):141–161.

9. Do KQ, Cabungcal JH, Frank A, Steullet P, Cuenod M. Redox dysregulation, neurodevelopment, and schizophrenia. *Curr Opin Neurobiol.* 2009;19(2):220–230.

10. Nho K, Ramanan VK, Horgusluoglu E, et al. Comprehensive gene- and pathway-based analysis of depressive symptoms in older adults. *J Alzheimers Dis.* 2015;45(4):1197–1206.

11. Holt RI, de Groot M, Golden SH. Diabetes and depression. *Curr Diab Rep.* 2014;14(6):491.

12. Moulton CD, Pickup JC, Ismail K. The link between depression and diabetes: the search for shared mechanisms. *Lancet Diabetes Endocrinol.* 2015;3(6):461–471.

13. Deuschle M. Effects of antidepressants on glucose metabolism and diabetes mellitus type 2 in adults. *Curr Opin Psychiatry.* 2013;26(1):60–65.

14. Goodnick PJ. Use of antidepressants in treatment of comorbid diabetes mellitus and depression as well as in diabetic neuropathy. *Ann Clin Psychiatry* 2001;13(1):31–41.

15. Epstein J, Silbersweig D. The neuropsychiatric spectrum of motivational disorders. *J Neuropsychiatry Clin Neurosci* 2015;27(1):7–18.

16. Perez DL, Pan H, Weisholtz DS, et al. Altered threat and safety neural processing linked to persecutory delusions in schizophrenia: a two-task fMRI study. *Psychiatry Res.* 2015;233(3):352–366.

17. Mayberg HS. Modulating dysfunctional limbic-cortical circuits in depression: towards development of brain-based algorithms for diagnosis and optimised treatment. *Br Med Bull.* 2003;65: 193–207.

18. Benedetti F, Bernasconi A, Pontiggia A. Depression and neurological disorders. *Curr Opin Psychiatry.* 2006;19(1):14–18.

19. Pilar-Cuellar F, Vidal R, Diaz A, et al. Signaling pathways involved in antidepressant-induced cell proliferation and synaptic plasticity. *Curr Pharm Des.* 2014;20(23):3776–3794.

20. Miller OH, Moran JT, Hall BJ. Two Cellular Hypotheses Explaining Ketamine's Antidepressant Actions: Direct Inhibition and Disinhibition. *Neuropharmacology.* 2016;100:17–26.

21. Verkhratsky A, Parpura V. Astrogliopathology in neurological, neurodevelopmental and psychiatric disorders. *Neurobiol Dis.* 2016;85:254–261.

22. Kiss JP, Szasz BK, Fodor L, et al. GluN2B-containing NMDA receptors as possible targets for the neuroprotective and antidepressant effects of fluoxetine. *Neurochem Int.* 2012;60(2):170–176.

23. Moylan S, Maes M, Wray NR, Berk M. The neuroprogressive nature of major depressive disorder: pathways to disease evolution and resistance, and therapeutic implications. *Mol Psychiatry.* 2013;18(5), 595–606.

24. Luscher B, Fuchs T. GABAergic control of depression-related brain states. *Adv Pharmacol.* 2015;73:97–144.

25. McAvoy K, Russo C, Kim S, Rankin G, Sahay A. Fluoxetine induces input-specific hippocampal dendritic spine remodeling along the septotemporal axis in adulthood and middle age. *Hippocampus.* 2015;25(11):1429–1446.

26. McEwen BS, Nasca C, Gray JD. Stress Effects on Neuronal Structure: Hippocampus, Amygdala and Prefrontal Cortex. *Neuropsychopharmacology.* 2015;41(1):3–23.

27. Gadek-Michalska A, Tadeusz J, Rachwalska P, Bugajski J. Cytokines, prostaglandins and nitric oxide in the regulation of stress-response systems. *Pharmacol Rep.* 2013;65(6):1655–1662.

28. Luca M, Luca A, Calandra C. Accelerated aging in major depression: the role of nitro-oxidative stress. *Oxid Med Cell Longev.* 2013;2013:230797.

29. Wolkowitz OM, Mellon SH, Lindqvist D, et al. PBMC telomerase activity, but not leukocyte telomere length, correlates with hippocampal volume in major depression. *Psychiatry Res.* 2015;232(1):58–64.

30. Detka J, Kurek A, Basta-Kaim A, Kubera M, Lason W, Budziszewska B. Neuroendocrine link between stress, depression and diabetes. *Pharmacol Rep.* 2013;65(6):1591–1600.

31. Shinba T. Altered autonomic activity and reactivity in depression revealed by heart-rate variability measurement during rest and task conditions. *Psychiatry Clin Neurosci.* 2014;68(3):225–233.

32. Bunney BG, Li JZ, Walsh DM, et al. Circadian dysregulation of clock genes: clues to rapid treatments in major depressive disorder. *Mol Psychiatry.* 2015;20(1):48–55.

33. Studd J, Nappi RE. Reproductive depression. *Gynecol Endocrinol.* 2012;28(Suppl 1):42–45.

34. Protopopescu X, Tuescher O, Pan H, et al. Toward a functional neuroanatomy of premenstrual dysphoric disorder. *J Affect Disord.* 2008;108(1–2):87–94.

35. Oldham MA, Ciraulo DA. Bright light therapy for depression: a review of its effects on chronobiology and the autonomic nervous system. *Chronobiol Int.* 2014;31(3):305–319.

36. Chiba Y, Katsuse O, Takahashi Y, et al. Anti-glutamate receptor varepsilon2 antibodies in psychiatric patients with anti-thyroid autoantibodies–a prevalence study in Japan. *Neurosci Lett.* 2013; 534:217–222.

37. Lauvsnes MB, Omdal R. Systemic lupus erythematosus, the brain, and anti-NR2 antibodies. *J Neurol.* 2012;259(4):622–629.

38. Mavrides N, Nemeroff CB. Treatment of affective disorders in cardiac disease. *Dialogues Clin Neurosci.* 2015;17(2):127–140.

39. Semenkovich K, Brown ME, Svrakic DM, Lustman PJ. Depression in type 2 diabetes mellitus: prevalence, impact, and treatment. *Drugs.* 2015;75(6):577–587.

40. Hennings JM, Schaaf L, Fulda S. Glucose metabolism and antidepressant medication. *Curr Pharm Des.* 2012;18(36):5900–5919.

41. Ma L, Zhao X, Fu W, et al. Antidepressant medication can improve hypertension in elderly patients with depression. *J Clin Neurosci.* 2015;22(12):1911–1915.

42. Starkman MN. Neuropsychiatric findings in Cushing syndrome and exogenous glucocorticoid administration. *Endocrinol Metab Clin North Am.* 2013;42(3):477–488.

43. Bagot RC, Labonte B, Pena CJ, Nestler EJ. Epigenetic signaling in psychiatric disorders: stress and depression. *Dialogues Clin Neurosci.* 2014;16(3):281–295.

44. Hunter RG, McEwen BS. Stress and anxiety across the lifespan: structural plasticity and epigenetic regulation. *Epigenomics.* 2013;5(2), 177–194.

45. Russo SJ, Murrough JW, Han MH, Charney DS, Nestler EJ. Neurobiology of resilience. *Nat Neurosci.* 2012;15(11):1475–1484.

46. Ward MC, White DT, Druss BG. A meta-review of lifestyle interventions for cardiovascular risk factors in the general medical population: lessons for individuals with serious mental illness. *J Clin Psychiatry.* 2015;76(4), e477–486.

47. Bot M, Chan MK, Jansen R, et al. Serum proteomic profiling of major depressive disorder. *Transl Psychiatry.* 2015;5:e599.

48. Torous J, Staples P, Onnela JP. Realizing the Potential of Mobile Mental Health: New Methods for New Data in Psychiatry. *Curr Psychiatry Rep.* 2015;17(8):602.

49. Bewernick BH, Schlaepfer TE. Chronic depression as a model disease for cerebral aging. *Dialogues Clin Neurosci.* 2013;15(1): 77–85.

50. Hannan AJ. Environmental enrichment and brain repair: harnessing the therapeutic effects of cognitive stimulation and physical activity to enhance experience-dependent plasticity. *Neuropathol Appl Neurobiol.* 2014;40(1):13–25.

51. Liu G, Rustom N, Litteljohn D, et al. Use of induced pluripotent stem cell derived neurons engineered to express BDNF for modulation of stressor related pathology. *Front Cell Neurosci.* 2014;8:316.

52. Ward MP, Irazoqui PP. Evolving refractory major depressive disorder diagnostic and treatment paradigms: toward closed-loop therapeutics. *Front Neuroeng.* 2010;3:7.

53. Chaieb L, Antal A, Masurat F, Paulus W. Neuroplastic effects of transcranial near-infrared stimulation (tNIRS) on the motor cortex. *Front Behav Neurosci.* 2015;9:147.

54. Meron D, Hedger N, Garner M, Baldwin DS. Transcranial direct current stimulation (tDCS) in the treatment of depression: systematic review and meta-analysis of efficacy and tolerability. *Neurosci Biobehav Rev.* 2015;57:46–62.

55. Dominguez A, Suarez-Merino B, Goni-de-Cerio F. Nanoparticles and blood-brain barrier: the key to central nervous system diseases. *J Nanosci Nanotechnol.* 2014;14(1):766–779.

56. Bockting CL, Hollon SD, Jarrett RB, Kuyken W, Dobson K. A lifetime approach to major depressive disorder: The contributions of psychological interventions in preventing relapse and recurrence. *Clin Psychol Rev.* 2015;41:16–26.

57. Strauss C, Cavanagh K, Oliver A, Pettman D. Mindfulness-based interventions for people diagnosed with a current episode of an anxiety or depressive disorder: a meta-analysis of randomised controlled trials. *PLoS One.* 2014;9(4):e96110.

58. Arnberg FK, Linton SJ, Hultcrantz M, Heintz E, Jonsson U. Internet-delivered psychological treatments for mood and anxiety disorders: a systematic review of their efficacy, safety, and cost-effectiveness. *PLoS One.* 2014;9(5):e98118.

59. Chang HS, Won E, Lee HY, Ham BJ, Lee MS. Association analysis for corticotropin releasing hormone polymorphisms with the risk of major depressive disorder and the response to antidepressants. *Behav Brain Res.* 2015;292:116–124.

60. Lopizzo N, Bocchio Chiavetto L, Cattane N, et al. Gene-environment interaction in major depression: focus on experience-dependent biological systems. *Front Psychiatry.* 2015;6:68.

61. Okereke OI, Lyness JM, Lotrich FE, Reynolds CF 3rd. Depression in Late-Life: a Focus on Prevention. *Focus (Am Psychiatr Publ).* 2013;11(1):22–31.

62. Hunkeler EM, Katon W, Tang L, et al. Long term outcomes from the IMPACT randomised trial for depressed elderly patients in primary care. *BMJ.* 2006;332(7536):259–263.

63. Fan HM, Sun XY, Guo W, et al. Differential expression of microRNA in peripheral blood mononuclear cells as specific biomarker for major depressive disorder patients. *J Psychiatr Res.* 2014;59: 45–52.

64. Kaufman J, Gelernter J, Hudziak JJ, Tyrka AR, Coplan JD. The Research Domain Criteria (RDoC) Project and Studies of Risk and Resilience in Maltreated Children. *J Am Acad Child Adolesc Psychiatry.* 2015;54(8):617–625.

INDEX

Note: Page numbers followed by "f" denote figures; "t" denote tables; "b" denote boxes respectively